D1345713

Cancer Neurology in Clinical Practice

David Schiff · Isabel Arrillaga
Patrick Y. Wen
Editors

Cancer Neurology in Clinical Practice

Neurological Complications of Cancer and its Treatment

Third Edition

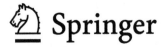 Springer

Editors
David Schiff, MD
Harrison Distinguished Teaching, Professor
    of Neurology, Neurological Surgery, and
    Medicine
University of Virginia
Charlottesville, VA
USA

Patrick Y. Wen, MD
Professor of Neurology, Harvard Medical
    School
Dana-Farber/Brigham and Women's Cancer
    Center, Center for Neuro-Oncology
Boston, MA
USA

Isabel Arrillaga, MD, PhD
Instructor, Harvard Medical School
Massachusetts General Hospital, Department
    of Neurology/Neuro-Oncology
Boston, MA
USA

ISBN 978-3-319-57899-6   ISBN 978-3-319-57901-6   (eBook)
DOI 10.1007/978-3-319-57901-6

Library of Congress Control Number: 2017939916

1st edition: © Springer Science+Business Media New York 2003
2nd edition: © Humana Press, a part of Springer Science+Business Media, LLC 2008
3nd edition: © Springer International Publishing AG 2018

Printed on acid-free paper

This Springer imprint is published by Springer Nature
The registered company is Springer International Publishing AG
The registered company address is: Gewerbestrasse 11, 6330 Cham, Switzerland

Foreword

Cancer Neurology in Clinical Practice comes in its third edition, now edited by David Schiff, Isabel Arrillaga, and Patrick Y. Wen. The overall aim remains to provide a comprehensive overview on neurologic complications of cancer and its treatment. The refined classification of many cancer entities to a molecular level has not only resulted in a better understanding of pathogenesis but also in the development of several rather specific molecularly targeted treatments. Moreover, the last years have seen a wave of new therapeutic approaches in the area of immunotherapy. These were associated not only with striking gains in survival, but also with a changing spectrum of complications from cancer treatment. These developments made a new edition of this textbook timely and necessary.

An overview on the general role of neurologic disease in cancer is followed by parts on diagnostic studies and the overall involvement of the nervous system by systemic cancer. This is then further detailed in a part on the neurologic complications of cancer and of its treatment, and all this with specific consideration of distinct types of cancer. Finally, the last chapter is dedicated to an area of increasing relevance, the neurologic symptoms and signs of long-term cancer survivors.

The editors and their team of distinguished contributors are to be congratulated for having provided an up-to-date and comprehensive source of knowledge of high value for all those involved in the management of patients with cancer.

Prof. Dr. Michael Weller
Department of Neurology
University Hospital Zurich
Zurich, Switzerland

Preface

It is estimated that cancer affects approximately 40% of the population at some time and is responsible for 20% of deaths. Recent years have witnessed substantial advances in the treatment of many malignancies. Targeted molecular therapies have improved outcomes for many cancers including HER2-positive breast cancer, EGFR and ALK-positive non-small cell lung cancer, BRAFV600E-positive melanoma, and a growing number of hematologic malignancies, among others. More recently, checkpoint inhibitor-based immunotherapy has dramatically changed the fortune of some patients with melanoma, non-small cell lung cancer, and a rapidly growing list of other cancers (7 FDA approvals in 2016 alone). However, as therapies for cancer improve and patients live longer, relapse within the nervous system is increasing. Additionally, prolonged survival has exposed more cancer survivors to the long-term neurologic sequelae of radiation therapy and systemic therapies. Finally, newly approved antineoplastic therapies bring new neurologic complications, as seen with immunotherapy. These neurologic complications detract significantly from patients' quality of life.

The diagnosis and treatment of neurologic complications of the nervous system are shared among neuro-oncologists, medical and radiation oncologists, neurologists, and neurosurgeons. While neurologists and neurosurgeons have expertise in the diagnosis and management of neurologic complaints, they are generally less familiar with the biology, behavior, and management of cancer. Conversely, medical and radiation oncologists have expertise in the diagnosis and treatment of cancer but are less familiar with the diagnosis and management of neurologic complaints in cancer patients. The purpose of this Third Edition of *Cancer Neurology in Clinical Practice* is to provide clinicians from various backgrounds and levels of training with information that will allow them to optimally diagnose and manage neurologic complications of the nervous system. This volume begins with an overview of diagnostic studies for neurologic complications involving the nervous system. That is followed by parts on metastatic and non-metastatic complications of cancer involving the nervous system, and the interpretation, diagnosis, and management of common neuro-oncologic symptoms. The next part reviews the neurologic complications of cancer therapy, including corticosteroids, radiation therapy, chemotherapy, targeted molecular therapies, immunotherapies, hematopoietic stem cell transplantation, and infections involving the nervous system. The final part focuses on the most important neurologic complications in cancers arising from specific organs.

We hope that this volume will provide clinicians from varied backgrounds looking after cancer patients with readily accessible, relevant information that will allow them to optimally diagnose and manage neurologic complications in these patients. Prompt diagnosis and effective interventions will ameliorate neurologic outcomes of most of the complications discussed in this volume, translating into improved quality (and in some cases quantity) of life for patients suffering from cancer.

Charlottesville, USA   David Schiff
Boston, USA   Isabel Arrillaga
Boston, USA   Patrick Y. Wen

Acknowledgements

I am very grateful for the addition of Isabel Arrillaga as co-editor; she has provided much-needed new energy, perspective, organization, and talent to this new edition. Patrick Wen, who is responsible for my choosing neuro-oncology as a specialty 25 years ago, remains a mentor, friend, and role model as well as a shining light in the field. My heartfelt appreciation goes to the many excellent chapter authors. Most importantly, I thank my patients and Tanya Nezzer, MD, for teaching me what matters in life.

David Schiff, MD

I am privileged to have worked on this Third Edition of *Cancer Neurology in Clinical Practice* alongside David Schiff and Patrick Wen, both leaders in the field of neuro-oncology and cancer neurology. I am particularly grateful to Patrick for the opportunity to collaborate on this text and for sharing so much of his time and talent over the years as a thoughtful and trusted mentor. I dedicate this book to my husband, Benjamin Rymzo, my greatest supporter and pillar, to my two young daughters, Celina and Camila, whom I hope I can one day inspire to pursue their own passions, and to my parents, Rafael Arrillaga and Celina Romany, who are ever-present sources of encouragement and confidence. Lastly, I humbly acknowledge the patients we treat and the many lessons they have offered about resilience, determination, and grace.

Isabel Arrillaga, MD, Ph.D.

This Third Edition of *Cancer Neurology in Clinical Practice* would not have been possible if not for all the efforts of David Schiff. I am very grateful for his hard work and encyclopedic knowledge of the field, which were both instrumental in making the three editions possible, and, most importantly, for his friendship, support, and always wise counsel over the years. We also were very lucky to have Isabel Arrillaga join us as an editor for this third edition. She is a wonderfully talented neuro-oncologist, and this edition would not have been possible without the hard work and the countless hours she devoted to it. I would also like to thank the expert group of chapter authors for their willingness to contribute to this book despite their very busy schedules. I dedicate this book to my parents, Hsiang-Lai Wen, MD, and Grace Wen, and to my family, May, Katherine, and Jessie.

Patrick Y. Wen, MD

Contents

Contributors

Manmeet S. Ahluwalia MD Cleveland, OH, USA

Dawit Aregawi MD Department of Neurosurgery, Penn State Milton S. Hershey Medical Center, Penn State College of Medicine, Hershey, PA, USA

Isabel Arrillaga MD, Ph.D. Department of Neurology/Neuro-Oncology, Massachusetts General Hospital, Boston, MA, USA

Edward K. Avila DO Department of Neurology, Memorial Sloan Kettering Cancer Center, New York, NY, USA

Joachim M. Baehring MD, DSc Departments of Neurology and Neurosurgery, Yale School of Medicine, New Haven, CT, USA

Tracy Batchelor MD, MPH Department of Neurology, Massachusetts General Hospital, Boston, MA, USA

Christa P. Benit MD Department of Neurology, The Hague Medical Center, The Hague, The Netherlands

Thomas N. Byrne MD Massachusetts General Hospital, Neurology, Boston, MA, USA

Marc C. Chamberlain MD Department of Neurology and Neurological Surgery, Seattle Cancer Care Alliance, University of Washington, Seattle, WA, USA; Cascadian Therapeutics, Inc., Seattle, WA, USA

Amy M. Chan MD Department of Neurology, Yale School of Medicine, New Haven, CT, USA

Ming Chi MD Atlanta Cancer Care, Northside Hospital, Atlanta, GA, USA

Josep Dalmau MD, Ph.D. Hospital Clinic, Institució Catalana de Recerca i Estudis Avançats (ICREA), Institut d' Investigació Biomedica August Pi I Sunyer (IDIBAPS), Barcelona, Catalonia, Spain

Gregory Davis MD Department of Neurological Surgery, George Washington University Hospital, Washington, DC, USA

Lisa M. DeAngelis MD Department of Neurology, Memorial Sloan Kettering Cancer Center, New York, NY, USA

Eli L. Diamond MD Department of Neurology, Memorial Sloan Kettering Cancer Center, New York, NY, USA

Jörg Dietrich MD, Ph.D. Department of Neurology, Harvard Medical School, Massachusetts General Hospital, Boston, MA, USA

Elizabeth S. Duke MD Department of Neurology, Boston Children's Hospital, Boston, MA, USA

Erin M. Dunbar MD Piedmont Hospital, Brain Tumor Center, Atlanta, GA, USA

Alberto Duran-Peña MD Department of Neurology Mazarin, Pitié Salpetrière Hospital, Paris, France

Thomas Durand M.Sc. UMR MD4 8257 Cognition and Action Group, Paris, France

Deborah A. Forst MD Department of Neuro-Oncology, Massachusetts General Hospital, Boston, MA, USA

Federica Franchino MD Department of Neuroscience, University of Turin and City of Health and Science Hospital, Turin, Italy

Christian Grommes MD Department of Neurology, Memorial Sloan Kettering Cancer Center, New York, NY, USA

Amanda C. Guidon MD Department of Neurology, Harvard Medical School, Massachusetts General Hospital, Boston, MA, USA

Raymond Huang MD, Ph.D. Department of Radiology, Brigham and Women's Hospital, Boston, MA, USA

Crystal S. Janani MD Department of Neurology, St. Agnes Hospital, Baltimore, MD, USA

Russell W. Jenkins MD, Ph.D. Department of Medical Oncology, Dana Farber Cancer Institute, Boston, MA, USA

Mark D. Johnson MD, Ph.D. Department of Neurological Surgery, University of Massachusetts Medical School and UMass Memorial Hospital, Worcester, MA, USA

Justin T. Jordan MD Department of Neurology, Massachusetts General Hospital, Boston, MA, USA

Thomas J. Kaley MD Department of Neurology, Memorial Sloan Kettering Cancer Center, New York, NY, USA

Melissa Kerkhof M.Sc., MD Department of Neurology, The Hague Medical Center, The Hague, The Netherlands

Santosh Kesari MD, Ph.D. Department of Translational Neuro-Oncology and Neurotherapeutics, John Wayne Cancer Institute at Providence Saint John's Health Center, Santa Monica, CA, USA

Megan L. Kruse MD Department of Hematology/Oncology, Cleveland Clinic, Cleveland, OH, USA

Emilie Le Rhun MD Department of Neurosurgery and Neuro-oncology, University Hospital, Lille Cedex, France; Breast unit, Department of Medical Oncology, Oscar Lambert Center, Lille Cedex, France; PRISM Inserm U1192, Villeneuve-d'Ascq, France

Delphine Leclercq MD Department of Neuroradiology, Pitié Salpetrière Hospital, Paris, France

Eudocia Q. Lee MD, MPH Center for Neuro-Oncology, Dana-Farber/Brigham and Women's Cancer Center, Boston, MA, USA

Michaela Lee MD Department of Neurosurgery, George Washington University Medical Center, Washington, DC, USA

Andrew L. Lin MD Department of Neurology, Memorial Sloan Kettering Cancer Center, New York, NY, USA

K. Ina Ly MD Stephen E and Catherine Pappas Center for Neuro-Oncology, Massachusetts General Hospital, Boston, MA, USA; Center for Neuro-Oncology, Dana-Farber Cancer Institute, Boston, MA, USA

Rajiv Magge MD Weill Cornell Medicine/New York Presbyterian, Weill Cornell Brain Tumor Center, New York, NY, USA

Hamza Malek MD Department of Neurology, Northwestern University, Chicago, IL, USA

Michelle L. Mauermann MD Department of Neurology, Mayo Clinic, Rochester, MN, USA

Sepideh Mokhtari MD Department of Neurology, H. Lee Moffitt Center, Tampa, FL, USA

Maciej M. Mrugala MD, Ph.D., MPH Department of Neurology, University of Washington Medical School, Fred Hutchinson Cancer Research Center, Seattle, WA, USA; Department of Neurology and Division of Medical Oncology, Mayo Clinic, Phoenix, AZ, USA

Elie Naddaf MD Department of Neurology, Mayo Clinic, Rochester, MN, USA

Lakshmi Nayak MD Department of Neuro-Oncology, Dana-Farber Cancer Institute, Boston, MA, USA

Martha R. Neagu MD, Ph.D. Department of Medical Oncology, Dana Farber Cancer Institute, Boston, MA, USA

Herbert B. Newton MD, FAAN Neuro-Oncology Center, Florida Hospital Cancer Institue & Florida Hospital Orlando, Orlando, FL, USA

Michael W. Parsons Ph.D. Burkhardt Brain Tumor Center and Section of Neuropsychology, Cleveland Clinic, Cleveland, OH, USA

David M. Peereboom MD, FACP Burkhardt Brain Tumor and Neuro-Oncology Center, Cleveland Clinic, Cleveland, OH, USA

Scott L. Pomeroy MD, Ph.D. Department of Neurology, Boston Children's Hospital, Boston, MA, USA

Amy A. Pruitt MD Department of Neurology, Perelman School of Medicine, University of Pennsylvania, Philadelphia, PA, USA

Dimitri Psimaras MD Department of Neurology, Pitié Salpetrière Hospital, Paris, France

Jeffrey Raizer MD Department of Neurology, Northwestern University, Chicago, IL, USA

Surabhi Ranjan MBBS Department of Neurology, University of Virginia, Charlottesville, VA, USA

Leslie A. Ray Pharm.D., BCOP Department of Pharmacy, The James Cancer Hospital, The Ohio State University, Columbus, OH, USA

David Reardon MD Center for Neuro-Oncology, Dana-Farber Cancer Institute, Boston, MA, USA

Damien Ricard MD Department of Neurology, Hôpital d'Instruction des Armées Percy, Clamart, France

Lisa R. Rogers DO Department of Neurology, University Hospitals Cleveland Medical Center, Cleveland, OH, USA

Myrna R. Rosenfeld MD, Ph.D. Institut d'Investigació Biomedica August Pi i Sunyer (IDIBAPS), Barcelona, Catalonia, Spain

Roberta Rudà MD Department of Neuroscience, University of Turin and City of Health and Science Hospital, Turin, Italy

David Schiff MD Neuro-oncology center, University of Virginia, Charlottesville, VA, USA

Mark E. Shaffrey MD Department of Neurological Surgery, University of Virginia Hospital, Charlottesville, VA, USA

Jonathan H. Sherman MD Department of Neurosurgery, The George Washington University Hospital, Washington, DC, USA

Matthew E. Shuman BA Department of Neurosurgery, Brigham and Women's Hospital, Boston, MA, USA

Riccardo Soffietti MD Department of Neuroscience, University of Turin and City of Health and Science Hospital, Turin, Italy

Sophie Taillibert MD Department of Neurology and Department of Radiation Oncology, Pitié-Salpétrière Hospital, UPMC-Paris VI University, Paris, France

Arnault Tauzière-Espariat MD Laboratory of Neuropathology, Sainte-Anne Hospital, Paris, France

Jennie W. Taylor MD, MPH Department of Neurology and Neurosurgery, University of California, San Francisco, CA, USA

Nicole J. Ullrich MD, Ph.D., MMSci Department of Neurology, Boston Children's Hospital, Boston, MA, USA

Craig A. Vargo Pharm.D. Department of Pharmacy, The James Cancer Hospital, The Ohio State University, Columbus, OH, USA

Charles J. Vecht MD, Ph.D. Department of Neurology Mazarin, Pitié Salpetrière Hospital, Paris, France

Yue Wang MD, Ph.D. Department of Neurology, University of Florida, Gainesville, FL, USA

Patrick Y. Wen MD Center for Neuro-Oncology, Dana-Farber/Brigham and Women's Cancer Center, Boston, MA, USA

Annise Wilson MD Department of Neurology, Northwestern University, Chicago, IL, USA

The Prevalence and Impact of Neurological Disease in Cancer

1

Andrew L. Lin and Lisa M. DeAngelis

Abbreviations	
APL	Acute promyelocytic leukemia
CAR T-cell	Chimeric antigen receptor T-cell
CNS	Central nervous system
CSF	Cerebrospinal fluid
CTLA4	Cytotoxic T-lymphocyte-associated protein 4
DIC	Disseminated intravascular coagulation
FDA	Food and Drug Administration
JC virus	John Cunningham virus
HER2	Human epidermal growth factor receptor 2
MEK	Mitogen-activated protein kinase enzyme
MS	Multiple sclerosis
PRES	Posterior reversible encephalopathy syndrome

Introduction

Cancer is a leading cause of disability and death throughout the world. Though regional variations in environmental risk factors and genetic propensities affect the incidence of each type of cancer, as an illness, it afflicts all age and socioeconomic groups worldwide [1]. In the United States, 1 in 4 deaths are due to cancer, making it the second leading cause of death [2]. This sobering statistic is offset by a decline in cancer death rates by as much as 20% over the past 20 years as a result of early treatment and medical advancements which have resulted in some cures, and delays in progression among those with advanced disease.

A large percentage of the cancer population will develop a neurologic complication of their disease. Up to 25% of cancer patients develop a central nervous system

A.L. Lin · L.M. DeAngelis (✉)
Department of Neurology, Memorial Sloan Kettering Cancer Center, 1275 York Ave, New York, NY 10065, USA
e-mail: deangell@mskcc.org

A.L. Lin
e-mail: lina1@mskcc.org

(CNS) metastasis over the course of their illness [3]. Many more develop chemotherapy-associated neuropathy; it occurs commonly in patients receiving both conventional cytotoxic chemotherapy—with an incidence that approaches 100% among patients treated with vincristine—and novel agents, such as the small molecule inhibitor, bortezomib.

For these reasons, in the mid-1980s, almost 50% of patients on a solid tumor service were admitted with a neurologic complaint; Table 1.1 details the most common chief complaints and neurologic diagnoses identified by an inpatient neurology consultant in a population of patients with cancer [4, 5]. During this same time period, a cancer hospital in the Netherlands referred about 15% of their patients for neurologic evaluation [6]. Because patients are living longer after their cancer diagnosis, the number of neurologic complications has increased and more patients suffer the diverse, late effects of treatment and the disease itself.

An estimated 1.7 million Americans will be diagnosed with cancer in 2015, of whom 68% will be alive at 5 years [7]. Many of these 1.2 million cancer survivors will have a neurologic symptom or disability and would benefit from

© Springer International Publishing AG 2018
D. Schiff et al. (eds.), *Cancer Neurology in Clinical Practice*,
DOI 10.1007/978-3-319-57901-6_1

Table 1.1 Categorization of 2137 inpatient neurology consults at a large cancer center by chief complaint and neurologic diagnosis

	Number of patients	Percentage of consults
Chief complaint		
Back pain	385	18
Headache	192	9
Other pain	160	7
Altered mental status	521	24
Weakness	395	18
Sensory deficit	173	8
Ataxia/gait instability	156	7
Seizures	156	7
Vision deficit	54	2
Speech deficit	52	2
Neurologic diagnosis		
Parenchymal brain metastasis	407	19
Epidural metastasis	298	14
Leptomeningeal metastasis	224	10
Other metastasis	407	19
Toxic metabolic encephalopathy	275	12
Cerebrovascular disease	169	8
Headache	67	3
Syncope	45	2
Peripheral neuropathy	40	1
Epilepsy	34	1
Paraneoplastic syndrome	7	0.3
Other	246	12

Patients may have more than one chief complaint or neurologic diagnosis
Used with permission of Oxford University Press from DeAngelis and Posner [5]

neurologic expertise. This book seeks to address the broad scope of these issues and the large unmet clinical needs of these patients.

Management of the Neurologic Complications of Cancer

Neurooncology is the subspecialty of neurology that deals with the neurologic complications of cancer. Neurologic symptoms may arise from primary malignancies of the brain, and for that reason, one focus of neurooncology is the management of gliomas and other primary tumors of the CNS. A second, equally important focus is the diagnosis and management of neurologic complications of systemic cancer and its treatment which is the core of this book. This second focus extends far beyond brain metastases, a problem that is already ten times more common than malignant gliomas [3, 7].

The first step in managing a neurologic complication of cancer is the correct identification of the underlying problem. A cancer patient with a change in gait may have loss of proprioception from prior chemotherapy, disease within the CNS, or severe pain that limits function. Correct diagnosis and treatment of the patient's complaint is contingent upon the same principles of neurology that apply to the non-cancer population. A careful history and detailed exam localizes the deficit in the nervous system to a focal, multifocal, or diffuse process. From that localization, a neurologic differential diagnosis can be developed that is based on specialized knowledge of the characteristic propensities of each cancer, the off-target effects of a wide array of conventional cytotoxic, novel small molecule and biologic therapeutics, and the complications of radiotherapy and surgical treatments. The most common neurologic complications of cancer and their association with different malignancies and treatment are provided in Table 1.2.

Direct Effects of Cancer on the Nervous System

Cancer frequently metastasizes to the nervous system, primarily to the brain, dura, subarachnoid space, spinal cord,

Table 1.2 Neurologic complications of cancer

Location	Complication	Cancer or treatment related causes	
Brain			
Direct complications	Brain metastasis	Lung, melanoma, renal, breast, and colon cancer	
	Primary brain tumor	Meningioma, glioma, pituitary adenoma, and schwannoma	
	Leptomeningeal metastasis	Breast, lung, melanoma, and gastrointestinal cancer	
Complications associated with cancer	Epilepsy/status epilepticus	Brain metastasis, primary brain tumor, paraneoplastic limbic encephalitis, and meningitis/encephalitis	
	Paraneoplastic limbic encephalitis	Anti-VGKC	SCLC and thymoma
		Anti-NMDA	Ovarian teratoma
		Anti-Hu	SCLC and gynecological cancer
		Anti-Ma2	Testicular germ cell
	Paraneoplastic cerebellar degeneration	Anti-Yo	Ovarian and breast cancer
		Anti-Tr	Hodgkin lymphoma
		Anti-Hu	SCLC and gynecological cancer
	Meningitis/encephalitis	Cancer-mediated immunosuppression	Hodgkin lymphoma, CLL, multiple myeloma, and Waldenstrom macroglobulinemia
	Ischemic stroke	Hyperviscosity	Multiple myeloma, Waldenstrom macroglobulinemia, and leukemia
		Cancer-mediated hypercoagulability	Pancreatic cancer, adenocarcinomas
		Tumor emboli	Rhabdomyosarcoma
		DIC	Sepsis from cancer-mediated immunosuppression
		Vasculopathy	Intravascular lymphoma
			Infectious vasculopathy (VZV) from cancer-mediated immunosuppression
	Hemorrhagic stroke	Coagulopathy/DIC	APL
			Sepsis from cancer-mediated immunosuppression
			Liver metastases
		Thrombocytopenia	Leukemia, lymphoma, and multiple myeloma
		Hemorrhage from a metastasis	Renal cell carcinoma, melanoma, choriocarcinoma, and papillary thyroid cancer
Treatment complications	Encephalopathy	Methotrexate, ifosfamide, and 5-FU	
	PRES	Bevacizumab, sorafenib, cyclophosphamide, high-dose corticosteroids, L-asparaginase, cisplatin, gemcitabine, and tacrolimus	
	Ischemic stroke	Bevacizumab, sunitinib, sorafenib, and cisplatin	
		Radiation-induced vasculopathy from treatment of head and neck cancers	
		Infectious vasculopathy and DIC from treatment-induced immunosuppression	
	Hemorrhagic stroke	Chemotherapy-induced thrombocytopia	
		Bevacizumab	
		Hemorrhage due to vascular changes secondary to radiotherapy	
	Venous sinus thrombosis	L-asparaginase	
	Pseudoprogression	Radiation to a primary or metastatic brain tumor	
	Radiation necrosis	Radiation to the head and neck; SRS to brain metastases	
	Bacterial meningitis/abscess/empyema	Neurosurgical procedure	VP shunt, burr hole, craniotomy, transsphenoidal resection, and laminectomy
		Treatment-induced immune suppression	Cytotoxic chemotherapy, hematopoietic stem cell transplant, and immune-modulating biologics

(continued)

Table 1.2 (continued)

Location	Complication	Cancer or treatment related causes	
Spinal cord			
	Leptomeningeal Metastasis	Breast, lung, melanoma, and gastrointestinal cancers	
	Cord compression/cauda equina syndrome	Lung, breast, prostate, renal, colorectal, and hematologic malignancies	
	Paraneoplastic myelopathy	Anti-amphiphysin	Breast cancer
		Anti-CRMP5	SCLC and thymoma
		Anti-Hu	SCLC and gynecological cancer
		Anti-ANNA-3	SCLC
		Anti-NMO	Carcinoma and lymphoma
	Radiation myelopathy	Radiation to the vertebral column, thorax, abdomen, or neck	
	Radiculomyelitis	Cancer-mediated and treatment-induced immunosuppression	
Plexus			
	Neoplastic infiltration	Brachial	Breast and lung cancer
		Lumbosacral	Prostate, colorectal, cervical, bladder cancers, and retroperitoneal sarcoma
	Radiation plexopathy	Radiation near the plexus	
Peripheral nerve			
	Neoplastic infiltration	Leukemia, lymphoma, Waldenstrom macroglobulinemia, prostate cancer, and squamous cell of head and neck (to cranial nerves)	
	Drug-associated neuropathy	Platinum agents, vinca alkaloids, thalidomide, bortezomib, and ipilimumab	
	Immune-mediated neuropathy	POEMS syndrome, MGUS, and multiple myeloma	
	Paraneoplastic neuronopathy	Anti-Hu	SCLC and gynecological cancer
	Peripheral nerve hyper-excitability	Anti-VGKC	SCLC and thymoma
Neuromuscular junction			
	Myasthenia gravis	Anti-acetylcholine receptor	Thymoma
	Lambert–Eaton myasthenic syndrome	Anti-Ca channel	SCLC
Muscle			
	Steroid myopathy	Pituitary adenomas/carcinomas, adrenal adenomas/adrenocortical carcinomas, and exogenous steroids	
	Dermatomyositis/polymyositis	Cervical, lung, ovarian, pancreatic, bladder, and gastric cancer	

Abbreviations APL acute promyelocytic leukemia, *CLL* chronic lymphocytic leukemia; *DIC* disseminated intravascular coagulation, *MGUS* monoclonal gammopathy of unknown significance, *POEMS* polyneuropathy organomegaly endocrinopathy M-protein skin-changes, *PRES* posterior reversible encephalopathy syndrome, *SCLC* small cell lung cancer, *SRS* stereotactic radiosurgery, *VP shunt* ventriculoperitoneal shunt, *VZV* varicella zoster virus, *5-FU* 5-flurouracil

and plexus. Considered together, the direct complications of cancer on the nervous system are responsible for a major burden of disability and death. Ironically, enhanced therapeutics and longer systemic disease control may be responsible for increasing the incidence of these complications, making the need for better therapeutics for CNS disease ever more pressing.

The elucidation of the molecular drivers of cancer has in certain cancer subtypes significantly improved tumor control. For example, trastuzumab, a monoclonal antibody directed against the HER2 receptor which is overexpressed in 25–30% of breast cancers has markedly improved the prognosis of patients with stage IV breast cancer by reducing the hazard rate of relapse by one-half [8, 9]. Unfortunately, the improved systemic control afforded by trastuzumab in appropriately selected patients with HER2 overexpression has not translated into the same degree of control within the CNS. Several retrospective studies have reported an incidence of clinically evident brain metastasis of 25–40% in patients with HER2 positive breast cancer receiving trastuzumab compared with an incidence of only 10–15% in HER2 negative patients with advanced disease [10]. One explanation is that HER2 positive breast cancer has a tropism for seeding the CNS; alternatively, the CNS may function as a sanctuary site because trastuzumab does not penetrate the blood–brain barrier effectively and prolonged systemic control may permit sufficient time for brain metastases to become evident [11]. Both of these and other factors may play a role, and altering this natural history will require unraveling the mechanisms by which it and other malignancies metastasize and circumvent the blood–brain barrier.

Basic and translational research have revealed that the development of metastatic disease is a highly inefficient process; large numbers of circulating tumor cells leave the primary tumor with only a small percentage (<0.01% of metastatic clonal cells in experimental models) surviving and establishing themselves at a distant site, including the brain [12]. The inefficiency of this process is due to the obstacles that these circulating tumor cells must overcome. Some of these obstacles apply to the development of metastases at any organ site, and others appear to be host organ specific.

An emerging concept is that there is a strong and complex interplay between normal brain tissue and tumor cells that develop into brain metastases. For example, it has been recognized that tumor cells thwart the brain's defense against the development of metastases by disrupting the normal function of plasmin. Plasmin is made in the brain to support synaptic plasticity; however, it also protects against the establishment of a metastasis once a tumor cell has extravasated into the brain parenchyma. Plasmin prevents tumor cells from binding to the abluminal surface of brain capillaries and interferes with the required co-option of the cerebral vasculature by the cancer cell to sustain growth [13]. By overexpressing plasminogen activator inhibitory serpins, which inhibit the conversion of plasminogen to plasmin, a subset of tumor cells are able to overcome this obstacle, and they are the cells that successfully develop into a brain metastasis.

Brain and all CNS metastases typically occur late in the cancer course. In autopsy studies, it has been shown consistently that about 30% of individuals with breast cancer have CNS metastases. The rate is even higher for lung cancer and melanoma at 34 and 72%, respectively [14] Cancers with a lower rate of intracranial metastasis include colon and pancreatic cancers; nevertheless, brain metastases develop even in these subtypes (Table 1.3). All told, approximately 25% of all patients with cancer have CNS metastases at death, and in approximately 40% of these patients, the brain is the sole metastatic site [14].

In addition to developing parenchymal brain metastases, patients can develop disease in the subarachnoid space resulting in leptomeningeal metastasis. Leptomeningeal metastasis is another direct complication of cancer that occurs commonly, either in the presence or absence of parenchymal brain metastases. It is found in 4–8% of patients at autopsy and is a particularly challenging diagnosis to establish because the symptoms are highly variable, relatively subtle and nonspecific, and diagnostic tests have a high rate of false negative results [5, 14]. Moreover, outside of cancer, the symptoms of leptomeningeal disease are rarely encountered, except in patients with chronic meningitides, making it more difficult to recognize the clinical syndromes. Leptomeningeal metastasis frequently presents with temporary, postural neurologic symptoms that occur with changes in body position from lying to standing. By history alone, the symptoms seem orthostatic in etiology, but in reality they are due to impaired cerebrospinal fluid (CSF) reabsorption which results in transient, marked elevation in intracranial pressure, typically lasting 5–20 min, known as plateau waves [15]. Alternatively, it may present with symptoms that localize anywhere along the neuraxis such as leg cramping, cranial nerve palsies, radiculopathy, headache, diplopia, and cognitive impairment; the symptoms may occur either alone or in combination.

Metastasis to the CNS contributes significantly to morbidity and mortality in patients with cancer. Unfortunately, the treatment of parenchymal and leptomeningeal metastases has lagged behind the development of treatments for systemic tumors, as trials have historically excluded these patients due to their poor prognosis. Fortunately, this is now beginning to change, particularly for patients with parenchymal brain metastases. There is growing recognition of the need to develop both preventative and therapeutic approaches to metastases in the CNS. Clinical trials are investigating laboratory assays that permit earlier diagnosis, innovative approaches for delivering therapy across the blood–brain barrier, and novel drugs that draw from new insights into the pathogenesis of brain metastases.

Indirect Effects of Cancer on the Nervous System

While neurologic complications of cancer can develop as a consequence of direct metastases to the nervous system, cancer also affects the nervous system indirectly.

Cancer induces an inflammatory state, and certain tumors secrete procoagulant substances. For these reasons, patients with cancer, particularly adenocarcinomas, are at a higher risk for ischemic stroke accounting for the 14.6% incidence of cerebrovascular disease found in an autopsy study [16]. A common mechanism by which individuals with cancer develop ischemic strokes is through the development of nonbacterial thrombotic endocarditis (or marantic endocarditis), but it can be caused by other mechanisms as well

Table 1.3 Prevalence of a primary or secondary brain tumor estimated for 2015

Primary cancer	New cases [7]	Number of deaths [7]	Percentage with intracranial tumor at autopsy [5, 14]	Projected number with intracranial tumor at death
Lung	221,200	158,040	34	53,734
Breast	234,190	40,730	30	12,219
Melanoma	73,870	9940	72	7157
Urinary system	138,710	30,970	23	7123
Leukemia	54,270	24,450	23	5624
Colon	93,090	49,700	7	3479
Non-Hodgkin lymphoma	71,850	19,790	16	3166
Pancreas	48,960	40,560	7	2839
All sites	**1,658,370**	**589,430**	**24**	**141,463**
Brain and spinal cord	**22,850**	**15,320**	**100**	**15,320**

including tumor emboli, infarction secondary to sepsis, and treatment-related hypercoagulability and vasculopathy.

Not only is there a higher incidence of ischemic stroke, population studies also show a higher risk of intracerebral hemorrhage [17, 18]. Primary and secondary brain tumors may hemorrhage; particularly high risk tumors are oligodendrogliomas and brain metastases from choriocarcinoma, melanoma, papillary thyroid cancer, or renal cell carcinoma [19]. Alternatively, cancer can lead to spontaneous intraparenchymal hemorrhage by causing coagulopathy, as in acute promyelocytic leukemia (APL) [20]. Patients with this condition usually have disseminated intravascular coagulation (DIC) at presentation, and until the recent development of effective therapies, death from massive intracranial hemorrhage was common.

A disordered immune response directed against the tumor but cross-reacting with nervous system proteins is another mechanism whereby cancer affects the nervous system. In 1948, Derek Denny-Brown published an early description of a prototypic paraneoplastic neurologic syndrome characterized by a rapidly progressive, debilitating sensory neuronopathy in individuals with small cell lung cancer [21]. The antibody mediating this paraneoplastic syndrome was later identified from the serum of patient H.U. (giving rise to the name anti-Hu); this antibody was found to cause dysfunction at nearly every level of the nervous system. It is associated with limbic encephalitis, cerebellar degeneration, brainstem encephalopathy, autonomic dysfunction, and motor neuron dysfunction [22]. Moreover, anti-Hu co-associates with other paraneoplastic antibodies such as anti-calcium channel antibodies which primarily affect the neuromuscular junction and give rise to the Lambert–Eaton myasthenic syndrome [23].

The true incidence of paraneoplastic syndromes involving the nervous system is unclear, but they are rare. For all cancers, it may be as low as one per 10,000 patients [24]. For

tumors with neuroendocrine proteins, such as small cell lung cancer, the rate is higher, occurring in about 3–5% of patients. In individuals with thymoma and immune dysfunction, myasthenia gravis and other paraneoplastic syndromes are commonplace, occurring in 15–20% of these patients.

Complications of Cancer Treatment

Another category of neurologic dysfunction is the short- and long-term effects of cancer therapies, such as radiotherapy, chemotherapy, and the many procedures that are prescribed. This category of dysfunction may be even more diverse than the others considered.

Peripheral neuropathy is the most common complication of cancer chemotherapy as it affects 30–70% of all patients [25]. Neuropathy can have profound effects on patient function, quality of life, and in one study, was the most troublesome symptom of treatment for one-third of patients with cancer [26]. Importantly, it is also a major dose limiting toxicity of chemotherapy that frequently results in either dose reduction or the premature discontinuation of otherwise effective treatment, and as a consequence, it can adversely affect outcomes.

Conventional cytotoxic chemotherapies are myelosuppressive; hence, treatment may be complicated by hemorrhage from thrombocytopenia or infection due to chronic immunosuppression which may be further compounded by bone marrow suppression and immune dysfunction from the disease itself, as in multiple myeloma. Patients receiving treatment are susceptible to a wide variety of pathogens and often develop more severe disease than is seen in the general population from the same infectious agent. As an example, people who were previously able to clear the West Nile virus with few clinical symptoms may develop a fulminant meningoencephalitis or a poliomyelitis-like syndrome [27]. They can also develop viral, fungal, or atypical bacterial infections such as varicella zoster virus vasculopathy, cytomegalovirus radiculitis, human herpes virus 6 limbic encephalitis, herpes simplex virus meningoencephalitis, aspergillosis, or nocardiosis.

Bacterial meningitis can also occur. Cancer patients who have undergone neurosurgical procedures are susceptible to infections from uncommon bacterial organisms such as gram-negative bacteria; moreover, because their immune response is frequently blunted, clinical manifestations may be subtle and they may not exhibit the classic tetrad of headache, fever, nuchal rigidity and altered mental status, thus delaying recognition and early institution of appropriate antibiotic therapy [28].

Mainstays of cancer treatment, such as methotrexate and ifosfamide, sometimes precipitate encephalopathy syndromes and can be associated with specific neurologic complications, such as venous sinus thrombosis among patients treated with L-asparaginase and posterior reversible leukoencephalopathy syndrome (PRES) among patients receiving cyclophosphamide or cisplatin [5]. With the advent of molecular medicine, a new generation of drugs has emerged that act on cancer by a variety of mechanisms. As these drugs are being tried on an investigational basis and achieve wider use, neurooncologists are being confronted with an unprecedented diversity of unanticipated adverse effects. An illustrative example is the focal neck extensor weakness that can be caused by selumetinib, a MEK inhibitor [29].

Rituximab, a monoclonal antibody against CD20 that revolutionized the treatment of B-cell lymphoma, was Food and Drug Administration (FDA) approved in 1997, but the association between its chronic use and the development of progressive multifocal leukoencephalopathy (PML), a devastating demyelinating condition caused by reactivation of the John Cunningham (JC) virus, was not recognized until 2011 [30]. This association was finally reported by a neurologist with an interest in understanding the development of PML in patients treated with natalizumab, a drug for multiple sclerosis (MS). Research on natalizumab has shown that JC virus serostatus can be used to risk stratify the development of PML [31]. Insights like this from general neurology can form the management of patients with cancer; lymphoma patients on maintenance rituximab and other immunomodulatory drugs may one day benefit from similar serological testing.

Activating the immune system can also have significant neurologic toxicity, as sometimes occurs following the administration of ipilimumab. Ipilimumab is a monoclonal antibody against cytotoxic T-lymphocyte-associated protein 4 (CTLA4); this drug mobilizes the immune system by inhibiting this molecule's ability to downregulate the T-cell response. It extends survival in patients with metastatic melanoma, and has activity against other cancers with high mutational loads and a large number of neoantigens to which the immune system can react [32]. Ipilimumab may cause a number of different autoimmune neurologic syndromes such as hypophysitis (resulting in central hypothyroidism, adrenal insufficiency, and hypogonadism), an axonal motor-predominant polyradiculoneuropathy resembling Guillain–Barre, myasthenia gravis, transverse myelitis, and an inflammatory myopathy [33].

Treatment-related neurotoxicity can also occur following radiotherapy and surgery. These treatments place patients at risk for stroke, radiation necrosis and other forms of direct damage to nearby structures, such as the brachial plexus. Finally, novel treatments are having unanticipated effects on the nervous system by mechanisms that are not completely understood as found in some patients who have received infusions of chimeric antigen receptor T-cells (CAR T-cells) [34]. CAR T-cells are genetically engineered lymphocytes that attack tumor cells and appear highly active against hematologic cancers. Patients treated with this form of cell-based immunotherapy can develop a cytokine storm, which results in striking neurologic symptoms that start with aphasia and progresses to severe encephalopathy, even obtundation, with or without seizures [35]. When the cytokine storm and seizures are appropriately managed, this treatment-related neurologic toxicity is often reversible, but failure to implement treatment rapidly can result in permanent damage, particularly from uncontrolled seizures.

Because neurologic complications of cancer treatments are so common, any team endeavoring to treat these medically complicated patients requires a neurologist to correctly localize the deficit and identify the underlying cause. This is of particular importance in the context of clinical trials because investigational agents commonly have unexpected neurologic consequences which need to be clearly and completely defined so that the safety profile can be assessed adequately and reported.

Conclusion

The nervous system is both a uniquely protected and uniquely vulnerable organ system. Neurologic complications of cancer are common and increasingly prevalent, as patients are surviving longer and are able to experience both the acute and delayed consequences of the disease and its treatment. Compromise of the nervous system by cancer or its therapy is often serious but frequently treatable, particularly if recognized early before serious deficits are fully established, making accurate diagnosis essential. This is where the neurooncologist plays a fundamental role.

Mobility, functional independence, and freedom from pain are of the utmost importance to patients. The neurooncologist works to help patients accomplish these goals, and in this way, neurooncologists strive to improve not only the quantity, but also the quality of life for their patients with cancer. This book was written to provide the neurooncologist, the general neurologist, and the oncologist with a framework for the early recognition and management of the most frequent neurologic complications of cancer, thus minimizing their effect on the increasingly longer life enjoyed by many with this disease.

References

1. Gulland A. Global cancer prevalence is growing at "alarming pace," says WHO. BMJ. 2014;348.
2. Siegel R, Ma J, Zou Z, Jemal A. Cancer statistics, 2014. CA Cancer J Clin. 2014;64(1):9–29.
3. Langer CJ, Mehta MP. Current management of brain metastases, with a focus on systemic options. J Clin Oncol. 2005;23(25):6207–19.
4. Gilbert MR, Grossman SA. Incidence and nature of neurologic problems in patients with solid tumors. Am J Med. 1986;81(6):951–4.
5. DeAngelis LM, Posner JB. Neurologic complications of cancer. 2nd ed. Oxford; New York: Oxford University Press; 2009.
6. Hovestadt A, van Woerkom CM, Vecht J. Frequency of neurological disease in a cancer hospital. Eur J Cancer. 1990;26(6):765–6.
7. Siegel RL, Miller KD, Jemal A. Cancer statistics, 2015. CA Cancer J Clin. 2015;65(1):5–29.
8. Slamon DJ, Godolphin W, Jones LA, Holt JA, Wong SG, Keith DE, et al. Studies of the HER-2/neu proto-oncogene in human breast and ovarian cancer. Science. 1989;244(4905):707–12.
9. Cossetti RJ, Tyldesley SK, Speers CH, Zheng Y, Gelmon KA. Comparison of breast cancer recurrence and outcome patterns between patients treated from 1986 to 1992 and from 2004 to 2008. J Clin Oncol. 2015;33(1):65–73.
10. Lin NU, Winer EP. Brain metastases: the HER2 paradigm. Clin Cancer Res. 2007;13(6):1648–55.
11. Kirsch DG, Ledezma CJ, Mathews CS, Bhan AK, Ancukiewicz M, Hochberg FH, et al. Survival after brain metastases from breast cancer in the trastuzumab era. J Clin Oncol. 2005;23(9):2114–6.
12. Mehlen P, Puisieux A. Metastasis: a question of life or death. Nat Rev Cancer. 2006;6(6):449–58.
13. Valiente M, Obenauf AC, Jin X, Chen Q, Zhang XH, Lee DJ, et al. Serpins promote cancer cell survival and vascular co-option in brain metastasis. Cell. 2014;156(5):1002–16.
14. Posner JB, Chernik NL. Intracranial metastases from systemic cancer. Adv Neurol. 1978;19:579–92.
15. Hayashi M, Kobayashi H, Handa Y, Kawano H, Kabuto M. Brain blood volume and blood flow in patients with plateau waves. J Neurosurg. 1985;63(4):556–61.
16. Graus F, Rogers LR, Posner JB. Cerebrovascular complications in patients with cancer. Medicine (Baltimore). 1985;64(1):16–35.
17. Zoller B, Ji J, Sundquist J, Sundquist K. Risk of haemorrhagic and ischaemic stroke in patients with cancer: a nationwide follow-up study from Sweden. Eur J Cancer. 2012;48(12):1875–83.
18. Navi BB, Reiner AS, Kamel H, Iadecola C, Elkind MS, Panageas KS, et al. Association between incident cancer and subsequent stroke. Ann Neurol. 2014;77(2):291–300.
19. Bernstein M, Berger MS. Neuro-oncology: the essentials. 2nd ed. New York: Thieme; 2008.
20. Chen CY, Tai CH, Tsay W, Chen PY, Tien HF. Prediction of fatal intracranial hemorrhage in patients with acute myeloid leukemia. Ann Oncol. 2009;20(6):1100–4.
21. Denny-Brown D. Primary sensory neuropathy with muscular changes associated with carcinoma. J Neurol Neurosurg Psychiatry. 1948;11(2):73–87.
22. Graus F, Keime-Guibert F, Rene R, Benyahia B, Ribalta T, Ascaso C, et al. Anti-Hu-associated paraneoplastic encephalomyelitis: analysis of 200 patients. Brain. 2001;124(6):1138–48.
23. Lucchinetti CF, Kimmel DW, Lennon VA. Paraneoplastic and oncologic profiles of patients seropositive for type 1 antineuronal nuclear autoantibodies. Neurology. 1998;50(3):652–7.
24. Dalmau J, Rosenfeld MR. Paraneoplastic syndromes of the CNS. Lancet Neurol. 2008;7(4):327–40.
25. Nolan CP, DeAngelis LM. Neurologic complications of chemotherapy and radiation therapy. Continuum (Minneap Minn). 2015;21(2):429–51.
26. Kautio AL, Haanpaa M, Kautiainen H, Kalso E, Saarto T. Burden of chemotherapy-induced neuropathy-a cross-sectional study. Support Care Cancer. 2011;19(12):1991–6.
27. Davis LE, DeBiasi R, Goade DE, Haaland KY, Harrington JA, Harnar JB, et al. West Nile virus neuroinvasive disease. Ann Neurol. 2006;60(3):286–300.
28. Safdieh JE, Mead PA, Sepkowitz KA, Kiehn TE, Abrey LE. Bacterial and fungal meningitis in patients with cancer. Neurology. 2008;70(12):943–7.
29. Chen X, Schwartz GK, DeAngelis LM, Kaley T, Carvajal RD. Dropped head syndrome: report of three cases during treatment with a MEK inhibitor. Neurology. 2012;79(18):1929–31.
30. Clifford DB, Ances B, Costello C, Rosen-Schmidt S, Andersson M, Parks D, et al. Rituximab-associated progressive multifocal leukoencephalopathy in rheumatoid arthritis. Arch Neurol. 2011;68(9):1156–64.
31. Bloomgren G, Richman S, Hotermans C, Subramanyam M, Goelz S, Natarajan A, et al. Risk of natalizumab-associated progressive multifocal leukoencephalopathy. N Engl J Med. 2012;366(20):1870–80.
32. Snyder A, Makarov V, Merghoub T, Yuan J, Zaretsky JM, Desrichard A, et al. Genetic basis for clinical response to CTLA-4 blockade in melanoma. N Engl J Med. 2014;371(23):2189–99.
33. Liao B, Shroff S, Kamiya-Matsuoka C, Tummala S. Atypical neurological complications of ipilimumab therapy in patients with metastatic melanoma. Neuro Oncol. 2014;16(4):589–93.
34. Duong CP, Yong CS, Kershaw MH, Slaney CY, Darcy PK. Cancer immunotherapy utilizing gene-modified T cells: from the bench to the clinic. Mol Immunol. 2015;67(2 Pt A):46–57.
35. Davila ML, Riviere I, Wang X, Bartido S, Park J, Curran K, et al. Efficacy and toxicity management of 19-28z CAR T cell therapy in B cell acute lymphoblastic leukemia. Sci Transl Med. 2014;6 (224):224ra25.

Part II
Diagnostic Studies

Imaging Neurologic Manifestations of Oncologic Disease

Raymond Huang and Patrick Y. Wen

Intracranial Metastasis

Brain metastases are the most common cause of malignant brain tumors in adults. Lung and breast cancers are the most common tumors that metastasize to brain, with melanoma, renal, and colorectal cancers accounting for the majority of the remaining metastases [1]. Among human cancers, melanoma has the highest propensity to metastasize to the brain [2]. The relative anatomical distribution of metastases in brain is associated with regional blood perfusion, with 80% of metastases found in supratentorial compartment, 15% in the cerebellum, and 5% in brainstem [3]. Metastatic tumors can involve either intra-axial or extra-axial compartments, or both.

Radiological Features of Intra-Axial Metastases

When metastases occur in brain parenchyma (intra-axial), the junction of gray and white matters is the most common site of seeding. Intra-axial metastatic lesions can be solid-appearing or demonstrate intratumoral necrosis or cystic changes as rimenhancement on contrast enhancement CT or MRI.

Unless intratumoral hemorrhage is present, metastases are usually isodense on unenhanced CT and often not readily distinguished from adjacent brain tissues. The presence of vasogenic edema characterized by hypodensities outlining

the gray and white matter junction can be an important clue suggesting an underlying metastasis. For larger lesions with cystic or necrotic changes, the lesions appear hypodense compared to normal brain tissues. In a few subtypes of metastatic tumors including germ cell tumors, melanoma, small cell lung cancers, and lymphoma, the tumors cells are highly cellular resulting in increased attenuation on CT. Due to streak and beam hardening artifacts from dense osseous structures in the skullbase, small or isodense posterior fossa lesions can be difficult to detect on CT. Most metastases enhance intensely with iodinated contrast due to absence of blood–brain barrier within tumor vasculature. Contrast-enhanced CT remains a very commonly employed screening test for some tumor types since CT imaging of other body areas can be performed on the same day of brain CT and its cost is lower than that of MRI.

The cellular component of brain metastases on MRI is usually hypointense to isointense relative to gray matter on T1-weighted images and hypointense on T2-weighted images. The necrotic or cystic tumor components generally appear hypointense on T1-weighted images and hyperintense on T2-weighted images. A subset of metastases can exhibit hyperintensity on T1-weighted images due to presence of subacute blood product. The wall of the enhancing rim is usually thick and irregular, and this can be an important sign to differentiate from the usual thin rim of enhancement seen with brain abscesses.

More than half of brain metastases are multifocal, but a significant number will present as a solitary brain mass, making differentiation from primary brain tumors difficult [4]. The enhancing portions of tumor often have distinct sharp margins from adjacent brain parenchyma, in contrast to high-grade primary gliomas that typically exhibit an infiltrative pattern at the tumor–brain interface. In the following sections individual imaging features pertinent to the diagnosis of metastasis will be discussed (Table 2.1).

R. Huang (✉)
Department of Radiology, Brigham and Women's Hospital, 75 Francis Street, Boston, MA 02115, USA
e-mail: ryhuang@partners.org

P.Y. Wen
Center for Neuro-Oncology, Dana-Farber/Brigham and Women's Cancer Center, 450 Brookline Avenue, Boston, MA 02215, USA
e-mail: Patrick_Wen@dfci.harvard.edu

© Springer International Publishing AG 2018
D. Schiff et al. (eds.), *Cancer Neurology in Clinical Practice*,
DOI 10.1007/978-3-319-57901-6_2

Table 2.1 Imaging differential diagnosis for intra-axial mass(es)

		Multifocal enhancing lesions	Solitary enhancing lesion
	Solid	Metastases Multifocal glioma Lymphoma Demyelination Granulomatous disease	High-grade glioma Metastases Lymphoma Medullublastoma Ependymoma
	Cystic	Metastases Infection (bacterial, fungal, parasitic)	High-grade glioma Metastases Hemangioblastoma Pilocytic astrocytoma Ependymoma
	Calcification	Granulomatous disease Metastases (squamous cell carcinoma, mucinous adenocarcinomas, osteosarcoma, chondrosarcoma)	Oligodendrogliomas Gangliogliomas Central neurocytomas
	Hemorrhage	Metastases (melanoma, renal cell carcinoma, and thyroid carcinoma) Fungal septic emboli	High-grade glioma Metastasis Pleomorphic xanthoastrocytoma

Tumor Permeability and Peritumoral Edema

Metastatic tumors to brain resemble the tissue characteristics of the primary tumors and therefore do not possess the blood–brain barrier seen in normal brain tissues. Thus, lesional enhancement is almost always observed for metastases on delayed post-contrast CT or T1-weighted MR images due to extra-vascular leakage of contrast agents. Aggressive primary intra-axial tumors such as higher grade astrocytomas, primitive neuroectodermal tumors, and primary CNS lymphomas also commonly enhance, although the mechanism of enhancement often include disruption of blood brain barrier and secretion of vasoactive substances. Other non-neoplastic intracranial processes can also exhibit contrast enhancement, including infarct, inflammation or infection.

One consequence of increased vascular permeability is accumulation of interstitial water content, resulting in decreased attenuation on CT as well as hyperintense signal on T2-weighted MRI from prolonged T2 relaxation times. A vasogenic pattern is characterized by edema that does not violate the boundary at the gray-white matter junction and can be easily identified by noting the exaggerated difference between gray and white matter attenuation or signal intensities on both CT and MRI. In contrast, cytotoxic edema resulted from direct damage to tissues as seen with ischemic infarction, does not spare the gray matter and there is a reduction in visual contrast at the gray-white matter junction. The extent of edema surrounding intra-axial metastases is often significantly greater than the actual tumor size. Rarely, vasogenic edema can be absent particularly with very small tumors (<1 cm).

When untreated brain metastases in the cortex near cerebral sulci or cerebellar folia are observed without associated edema, involvement of the extra-axial space, i.e. leptomeninges, should be suspected. Extra-axial metastatic tumors, similar to some meningiomas, can produce edema in the adjacent brain due to mass effect causing venous congestion or direct effect on capillary permeability.

Intratumoral Hemorrhage

Among intracranial metastases, hemorrhage more commonly occurs in melanoma, renal cell carcinoma, and thyroid carcinoma. Hemorrhagic metastases demonstrate variable signal intensities depending on the age of hemorrhage, and intratumoral hemorrhages tend to evolve more slowly and often contain blood product of mixed ages as compared to hemorrhages from non-tumor causes. Due to their intrinsic melanin content and frequently intratumoral hemorrhages, hyperintensity on unenhanced T1-weighted images can be observed in melanoma [5–7] (Figs. 2.1a–c and 2.2a–d).

Assessing whether parenchymal hemorrhage in brain is spontaneous or secondary to aneoplastic process is an important task in neuroimaging. Important clues to an underlying tumor include presence of nodular enhancement adjacent or within hematoma, incomplete hemosiderin ring, peritumoral edema more extensive than expected for the age of the hemorrhage, and delay in the expected evolution of signal characteristics in the hematoma. When these imaging signs are not present, short-term follow-up imaging may be required to confirm the nature of hemorrhage.

Venous infarcts can mimic a brain mass with enhancement, vasogenic edema, and hemorrhage. The site of sinus or cortical vein thrombosis can lead to venous infarct in corresponding venous drainage territory. Thus, recognizing

Fig. 2.1 a–c Melanoma hemorrhage. Two melanoma metastases in the *left* temporal and occipital lobes demonstrate hyperintensity on T1-weighted image (**a**). Following contrast administration, subtle enhancement is seen along the margins of hemorrhage. Magnetic susceptibility within the masses confirm presence of hemorrhage (**c**)

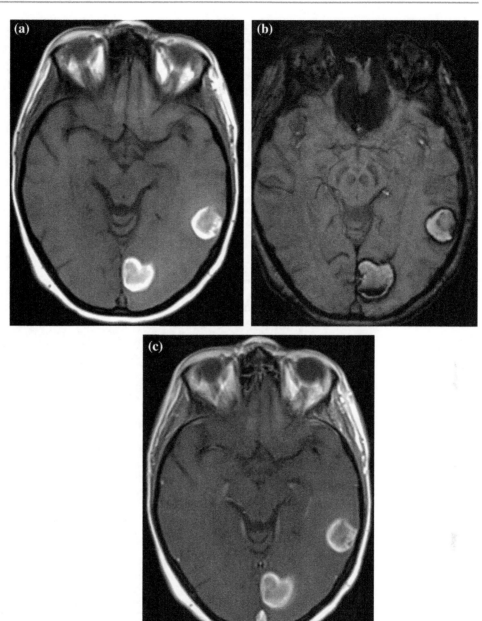

common location of venous infarct corresponding to site of thrombosis can be helpful in making the diagnosis.

Tumor Necrosis and Tumor Associated Cysts

Necrosis is a common imaging feature in brain metastases but also commonly seen with glioblastomas as well as lymphoma in immunocompromised population. Necrosis in metastases can also commonly occur following chemo- or radiation treatment, occasionally accompanied by enlargement of overall tumor size requiring close imaging follow-up to determine durability of treatment response.

Cystic brain metastases are commonly found with tumors of gastrointestinal or genitourinary origins but also occur in lung cancers [8]. In contrast to necrosis, tumor associated cysts tend to have thinner borders. Other primary neoplasms, including hemangioblastoma, pilocytic astrocytoma, and ganglioglioma can contain cysts although these tumors are usually not associated with peritumoral edema. Unlike post-chemotherapy or radiation necrosis often observed during treatment response, enlargement of tumor associated cysts often indicates elevated tumor secretion and can be a sign of tumor growth.

The thin-wall cysts seen in some metastases can appear identical to non-neoplastic cystic brain lesions. It is

Fig. 2.2 a–d Melanoma. 33-year-old female presented with history of melanoma presenting with rapid onset hearing loss. A nodular lesion in the *left* cerebellopontine angle is hyperintense on T1-weighted image (**a**) and hypointense on T2-weighted images (**b**). No magnetic susceptibility is seen associated with this lesion (**c**). Following contrast administration, an enhancing component is difficult to detect in the presence of underlying T1 hyperintensity (**d**)

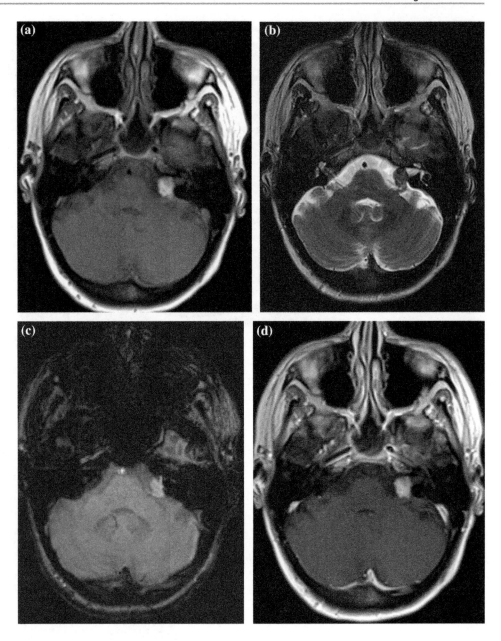

important to consider infectious etiologies such as brain abscesses, which can appear as multifocal rim-enhancing lesions and exhibit surrounding vasogenic edema. Often patients with brain abscess(es) have a distinct clinical history as well as presenting signs and symptoms from those with brain metastases, although it can be challenging to distinguish them clinically on occasions. Diffusion-weighted imaging based on the detection of changes in the random motion of protons in water is particularly helpful in diagnosing brain abscesses since their mucopurulent content tends to have very low diffusivity and exhibits a dark signal on the apparent diffusion coefficient (ADC) maps. In contrast, brain metastases have peripheral low diffusivity due to higher cell density while the necrotic content centrally tends to be of high diffusivity (bright on ADC). However, presence of hemorrhage can affect diffusion characteristics and one should be careful when there is evidence of susceptibility changes within the area of diffusion signal abnormality. Compared to abscesses, metastases are much more likely to be associated with hemorrhage. Furthermore, a small group of metastases, usually from GI or GU origins, may present as mucin-containing cystic lesions that manifest as similarly low diffusivity. On the other hand, atypical infections such as toxoplasmosis may not show low diffusivity within the cyst content.

Calcifications

Intratumoral calcifications rarely observed among untreated brain metastases, although it has been reported in a variety of tumor types, including common tumor metastasizing to brain such as lung and breast cancers as well as more rare tumor types including squamous cell carcinoma, mucinous adenocarcinomas from genitourinary or gastrointestinal origins, osteosarcoma, and chondrosarcoma [9, 10]. On the other hand, calcifications frequently occur in many primary intracranial tumors, most notably oligodendrogliomas, gangliogliomas, neurocytomas, and craniopharyngiomas. Following treatment, calcifications can develop within metastases. CT is both sensitive and specific in detecting macroscopic calcification, and approximately 3% of brain metastases seen on CT exhibited calcification in one series [11]. On MRI, calcifications can result in variable signal intensities depending on the microenvironment of calcium, but most commonly they appear as focal T1 shortening and magnetic susceptibility. These MR imaging findings, however, overlap with iron within blood products although they can be distinguished by differences in phase shifts [12].

Extra-Axial Intracranial Metastases

Within the extra-axial compartment metastases can involve bony structures of calvarium and skull base, dura (pachymeninges), leptomeningeal spaces including cerebral sulci, cerebellar folia, and cranial nerves, or within ventricles. Similar to osseous metastatic tumor elsewhere, metastases to calvarium and skull base can have lytic, sclerotic, or mixed patterns on CT depending on primary tumor subtypes. For example, prostate cancer metastases are generally sclerotic, whereas renal and thyroid metastases tend to present as lytic lesions. Following treatment, lytic metastases frequently produce a sclerotic pattern.

Dural (pachymeningeal) metastases often grow from adjacent calvarium or skull base but can be directly seeded from hematogeneous sources. Breast cancer, lymphoma, leukemia, prostate cancer, and neuroblastoma are tumors most commonly presenting as dural metastases (Fig. 2.3a–c). Meningiomas are the most common benign tumor arising from dura, and it can be difficult to distinguish from dural metastases unless meningiomas contain calcifications or induce hyperostosis of adjacent bone. Intracranial hypotension is a common non-neoplastic cause of dural enhancement but the pattern of enhancement is almost always diffuse and smooth rather than focal or nodular, and is often supported by clinical history of previous cranial or spinal intervention. In severe cases, intracranial hypotension can be associated with subdural hygroma or hematoma, and it is also not uncommon for dural metastases to produce subdural fluid collection or hemorrhage. Contrast-enhanced MRI is best for detecting nodular enhancement along the dural lining of hematomato diagnose dural-based tumor (Fig. 2.3a–c).

Leptomeningeal metastases occur in many types of cancer, particularly breast carcinoma, lung carcinoma, melanoma, lymphoma, and leukemia. Metastatic spread to the meninges can occur hematogenously via meningeal vessels or through direct extension from metastatic lesions at the pial surface. Leptomeningeal metastases are usually not detectable on CT without contrast enhancement, although hydrocephalus can be an indirect sign of leptomeningeal involvement. Contrast-enhanced MRI provides significant better sensitivity in detecting leptomeningeal metastases as planar or nodular enhancement along cerebral sulci, cerebellar folia, or cranial nerves [13] (Fig. 2.4a–c). Other non-tumor processes including ischemic infarction and leptomeningitis can also exhibit enhancement along brain surfaces but often can be distinguished based on clinical history. A nodular pattern of leptomeningeal enhancement is more commonly seen with neoplastic processes but can also be observed in infectious etiologies. CSF analysis should be obtained when leptomeningeal abnormality is identified on imaging but there is uncertainty regarding the diagnosis. On fluid-attenuated inversion recovery (FLAIR) sequence, leptomeningeal tumor can appear as hyperintense signal along sulci as a result of shortened T1 relaxation time but this finding without enhancement is not specific since other CSF pathologies such as hemorrhage or infection can appear identical. Unlike parenchymal metastases, leptomeningeal seeding of tumor commonly does not lead to significant vasogenic edema, although edema and mass effect can be observed when there is florid involvement. Table 2.2 summarizes the main differential diagnoses of extra-axial masses.

General Approach to Imaging of Patients Presenting with Suspected Brain Metastases

When one or more enhancing mass is found on brain imaging of a patient with known progressive or recurrent metastatic cancer, diagnostic certainty for brain metastasis is high. For patients with no or remote history of cancer presenting with newly discovered brain mass(es), the diagnostic possibilities can be broad, including primary brain neoplasms, infection, demyelinating lesions, vascular lesions that can be difficult to distinguish from brain metastasis on both imaging and clinical presentation.

While multiplicity can be helpful in making the diagnosis, solitary metastases are common and can be difficult to distinguish from other intra-axial tumors such as primary glioma or lymphoma, as well as non-neoplastic mass-like

Fig. 2.3 a–c 70-year-old man with metastatic prostate cancer presents with headache. T1-weighted unenhanced image shows a T1 hyperintense collection along right frontal convexity (**a**) consistent with subacute subdural hematoma. Following intravenous contrast administration, extensive dural thickening with multifocal enhancing masses are identified (**b** and **c**), evening along the lining of subdural hematoma (**b**)

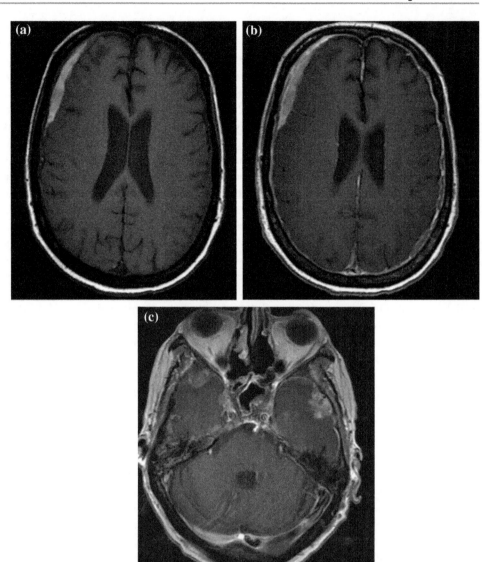

processes such as demyelination, infection, or vascular pathology. When multifocal enhancing brain metastases occur, the extent of T2 signal abnormality surrounding lesions tend to be separated on T2-weighted imaging, whereas multifocal enhancement in high-grade gliomas typically show contiguous areas of infiltrative appearing nonenhancing T2 abnormalities between foci of enhancement. In addition, the areas of T2 abnormality in high-grade glioma often demonstrate infiltration of gray matter.

Demyelination disease can be "tumefactive," mimicking a brain mass clinically and on imaging. These lesions, however, tend to occur in younger patients without history of malignancy. On imaging, an "incomplete ring sign" is an important feature suggesting the presence of a demyelinating lesion. CSF analysis for gamma globulin can help clarify the diagnosis, and follow-up imaging several months later often confirms eventual improvement or resolution.

Vascular lesions including arterial or venous infarction as well as vascular malformations can mimic a brain mass. Ischemic infarcts, particular during subacute phase, can present as enhancing lesions 2–3 days following onset of the ischemic event that persist for several months; diffusion signal changes typically associated with acute infarct usually normalize after 7–10 days [14]. Enhancement associated with ischemic infarct, however, does not exhibit surrounding vasogenic edema. For small enhancing lesions along gray matter that cannot be diagnosed as infarction based on clinical history or lesion location, a short-term follow-up imaging can readily clarify the etiology. It is important to keep in mind that ischemic infarct can coexist with brain metastasis due to a hypercoagulable state associated with malignancy, as well as from embolic events from systemic procedures. In addition, perioperative infarct is not infrequently observed and often located immediately adjacent to

Fig. 2.4 **a–c** Leptomeningeal. 55-year-old man with history of lung cancer presents with acute headache and gait disturbance. Axial T1-weighted post-contrast images demonstrate leptomeningeal carcinomatosis with enhancement along cerebral sulci (**a**), cerebellar folia (**b**), and cranial nerve in the internal acoustic canals (**c**)

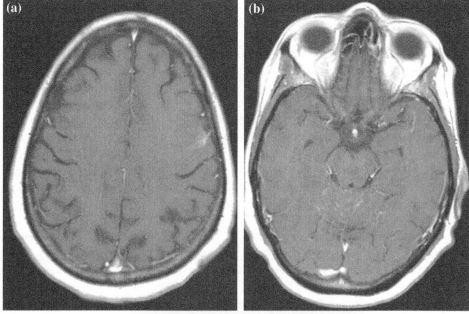

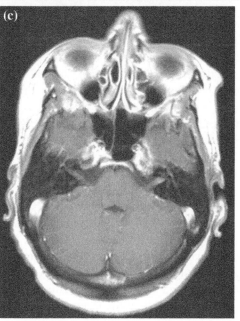

Table 2.2 Differential diagnosis for extra-axial mass(es)

Intraosseous-calvarium	Leptomeningeal	Pachymeningeal
Hemangioma	Metastases	Meningioma
Fibro-osseous lesions	Infectious meningitis	Metastases
Metastasis	Lymphoma	Lymphoma
Langerhans cell histiocytosis	Sarcoidosis	Sarcoidosis
Sarcoma	PNET	Idiopathic pachymeningitis
Meningioma		

the surgical margin. It is important to perform and examine the diffusion- weighted sequence during the immediate postoperative MRI to identify area(s) of peritumoral infarct so the expected subsequent enhancement will not be misinterpreted as tumor recurrence.

When brain imaging reveals findings suggestive of metastatic disease in a patient without history of systemic cancer, imaging for potential primary cancer site or additional extracranial metastases is often necessary to identify an anatomical site that carries a lower risk for diagnostic biopsy. The imaging modalities depend on the patient demographics, but often include CT scan of the chest, abdomen and pelvis. FDG-PET imaging can be highly sensitive in detecting occult primary malignancy and can be used as part of staging in many systematic cancers.

Optimization of Radiological Protocol for Evaluation of Intracranial Metastasis

For staging systemic malignancy in an asymptomatic patient, CT can be the test of choice due to its wider availability and the speed of imaging. While small brain metastases can be difficult to detect by CT unless there is significant surrounding edema, mass effect or intratumoral hemorrhage, CT has the advantage of visualizing lesions that are centered in bone or producing calcifications. CT imaging of the bony margins can help elucidate the underlying pathology. For example, slow-growing lesions are often accompanied by bone remodeling and manifesting as smooth cortical rather than destructive margins. Calcifications are often found in a subset of brain tumors, including meningioma, oligodendroglioma, germ cell neoplasm, and craniopharyngioma, and these are better visualized by CT evaluation. CT may be the only available option for screening if patients have contraindications for MRI such as cardiac pacers, ferromagnetic foreign bodies, implants or surgical devices. While whole-body ^{18}fluoro-D-glucose positron emission tomography (FDG-PET) is commonly used for initial stating of systemic cancers, its sensitivity in detecting brain metastases is generally considered low due to relative high FDG uptake in normal brain tissues. For example, the sensitivity of brain PET/CT for detecting brain metastases in lung cancer was 72% in one series [15].

For most systemic malignancy, MRI is the imaging modality of choice in assessing brain metastases due to its excellent soft tissue contrast and lack of ionizing radiation. Several MRI sequences are generally recommended during evaluation of brain metastases. An isotropic volumetric post-gadolinium T1-weighted sequence allows detection of very small lesions, on the order of 1–2 mm. This high sensitivity can be important since the total number as well as the distribution of metastatic brain lesions contributes to selection of treatment approach. The sensitivity of detecting brain metastasis can be improved by increased time duration following contrast and using contrast agents with longer T1 relaxation time [16–18]. Higher magnet strengths, i.e., 3 versus 1.5 T, can further increase sensitivity [19, 20]. In addition, volumetric acquisition allows multi-planar reformation for better lesion visualization and can be fused with stereotactic equipment for surgical guidance. This type of

acquisition method requires longer acquisition time and is therefore more susceptible to patient motion artifact when performed using lower field strength MR scanners. Finally, it is often helpful to perform a T1-weighted sequence before contrast administration to distinguish true enhancement from other tissue types with short T1 relaxation times such as hemorrhage, fat or proteinaceous cyst.

Mass lesions with a cystic component as well as perilesional edema can be readily delineated by a T2-weighted sequence. Infiltration of tissues with prolonged T2 relaxation time in the cortical gray matter with expansion of gray matter and blurring of the gray-white matter junction is a specific sign of primary glioma and not observed with metastatic tumors. On T2-weighted imaging, the interface of tumor and adjacent brain often appears sharper compared to high-grade gliomas.

Diffusion weighted imaging (DWI) is commonly included during evaluation of brain lesions due to its high sensitivity in detecting a variety of brain pathologies including infarct, abscess, cerebritis, and tumor that manifest as hyperintensity on DWI and hypointensity on apparent diffusion coefficient (ADC) maps that are calculated from DWI. Findings on DWI images are more helpful when they are interpreted alongside conventional imaging sequences and clinical history for improved specificity. For example, subacute infarct can manifest as cortical swelling and enhancement mimicking brain tumor, but a serpiginous pattern of low diffusivity confined to an arterial distribution is characteristic of ischemic infarct rather than neoplasm. When a peripherally enhancing brain lesion is encountered, evidence of low diffusivity within the lesion is suggestive of abscess as discussed previously but the diagnostic specificity can be increased if the enhancing rim is also thin and systemic signs of infection are present.

On MR imaging, DWI has also been correlated with hypercellularity typically manifesting as reduced diffusivity on the ADC map [21]. This imaging marker of cell density can be used to help several tumor types that are characteristically hypercellular, including breast and lung metastases [22]. CNS lymphomas are characteristically cellular [21, 23] and are more commonly located in the periventricular regions of brain. It is important to recognize that intratumoral hemorrhage can appear as hyperdensity on CT, and ADC measurement can also be decreased due to presence of blood product. DWI is also very useful in identifying calvarial and skullbase metastases due to its high lesion to background contrast [24] (Fig. 2.5a, b).

T2*-sensitive techniques such as gradient-echo and susceptibility-weighted imaging are useful for detecting intratumoral hemorrhage, which is common in high-grade gliomas and metastases, but rare in low-grade gliomas and

Fig. 2.5 a–b DWI-Calvarium-Orbit. 46-year-old female with breast cancer developed metastases to calvarium and right orbit. The lesions are seen on both T1-weighted imaging (a) than DWI (b), although more conspicuous on the latter due to greater lesion to background contrast

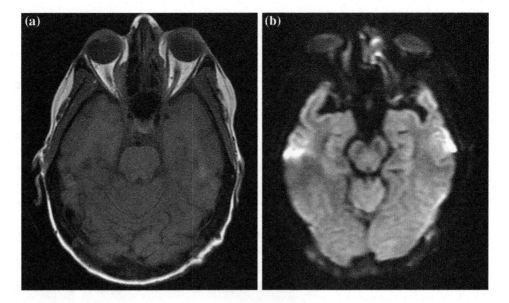

lymphoma. The deoxyhemoglobin causes magnetic suscep-tibility that results in shortened T2* relaxation times and hypointense signal changes on T2*-weighted (T2*W) ima-ges. This phenomenon can improve sensitivity of detecting small metastatic lesions with hemorrhages that do not enhance or elicit peritumoral edema. For example, 7% of melanoma lesions were detected only on this sequence in one series [5]. Susceptibility-weighted imaging (SWI) can amplify the effect of magnetic susceptibility by overlaying magnetic phase changes with high-resolution magnitude images to detect foci of microhemorrhages [25]. These techniques are also helpful in identifying thromboses within dural venous sinuses or cortical veins due to exaggerated magnetic susceptibility from deoxyhemaglobin [26]. The appearance of venous infarction on conventional MRI sequences can mimic brain tumor due to mass effect, edema, and enhancement. If misdiagnosed, this can lead to unnec-essary biopsy or a delay in anticoagulation treatment.

Advanced Techniques in Brain Metastasis Imaging

Several imaging techniques have become increasingly available for evaluation of brain lesions including MR spectroscopy, MR perfusion, and MR diffusion tensor imaging. When combined with conventional imaging sequences, these advanced methods can often provide useful diagnostic information when evaluating brain lesions including metastases. As these advanced imaging methods are being improved and validated, it is important to under-stand their advantages and limitations before incorporating them into clinical imaging protocol.

Magnetic Resonance Spectroscopy (MRS)

MR spectroscopy can provide a noninvasive window to analyze metabolic composition of brain lesions. Similar to most pathological processes observed in brain, metastases show reduced NAA peak on MR spectroscopy [27, 28], and the level of NAA concentration is often absent or much lower than other intrinsic brain pathologies where brain tissues are being infiltrated or damaged as in case of primary brain tumor or inflammation. Choline concentration also typically increases in the enhancing portion of metastases as a result of increased cellular turnover [27, 29]. This meta-bolic marker can be useful in distinguishing peritumoral edema surrounding metastases from infiltrative glioma since reactive or vasogenic edema, unlike tumor infiltration, does not result in greater cellular turnover [30]. Lipids and lactate are also frequently seen in metastases although these are not specific findings and can be found also in high-grade glio-mas [30]. Based on a retrospective analysis of multicenter trial data, automatic brain tumor classification by MRS allows classifications of glioblastoma, meningioma, metas-tasis, and low-grade glial with diagnostic accuracies of near 90% for most diagnostic pairs except for the glioblastoma versus metastasis discrimination [31].

Perfusion-Weighted Imaging (PWI)

Similar to high-grade primary brain neoplasms, metastatic lesions induce neovascularization resulting in greater intravascular blood volume, although the vessels associated with metastases are highly permeable similar to those of the primary systemic tumors [32]. Estimation of intravascular volume in tumors can be performed by dynamic imaging methods such as dynamic contrast-enhanced MRI (DCE-MRI), dynamic susceptibility contrast MRI (DSC-MRI), as well as dynamic contrast-enhanced CT. Due to its short acquisition time of less than 2 min, DSC-MRI can readily be incorporated into standard imaging protocol for evaluation of brain mass. Elevation of regional cerebral blood volume (rCBV) is characteristic of most high-grade gliomas, although metastatic tumors, particularly renal cell carcinoma, choriocarcinoma, and thyroid carcinoma, can also demonstrate high intravascular blood volume making this diagnostic imaging marker less useful [33]. The specificity of DSC-MRI can be improved by using spin-echo (SE) acquisition compared to gradient-echo (GRE) since the former technique appears to correlate with microscopic angiogenesis that is typical with gliomas, while the later technique detects macroscopic intratumoral vessels more commonly

seen in cases of hypervascular metastases [34]. Furthermore, higher rCBV within the peritumoral region is also suggestive of infiltrative tumor rather than vasogenic edema [35, 36].

Diffusion Tensor Imaging (DTI)

The magnitude and directionality of water motion can be quantified by DTI and used as imaging markers to characterize microstructural changes occurring at tissue or cellular levels [37]. This technique can be highly sensitive to pathological changes in brain including both neoplastic and non-neoplastic processes, although its specificity is low without advanced post-processing. For example, fractional anisotropy (FA) values of high-grade gliomas and solitary brain metastases show significant overlap [38, 39]. Similar to

Fig. 2.6 **a–d** Infarct. 48 h postoperative MRI demonstrates no significant enhancement near resection bed on contrast-enhanced T1-weighted image (**a**) but a wedge-shaped DWI abnormality anterior to the resection cavity (**b**). **b** Two weeks following surgery, the regions of previous infarct exhibit enhancement (**c**) (*blue arrow*) with normalization of DWI abnormality (**d**), and the blood product within resection cavity appears hyperintense on T1-weighted image (**c**) (*red arrow*) and bright on DWI (**d**)

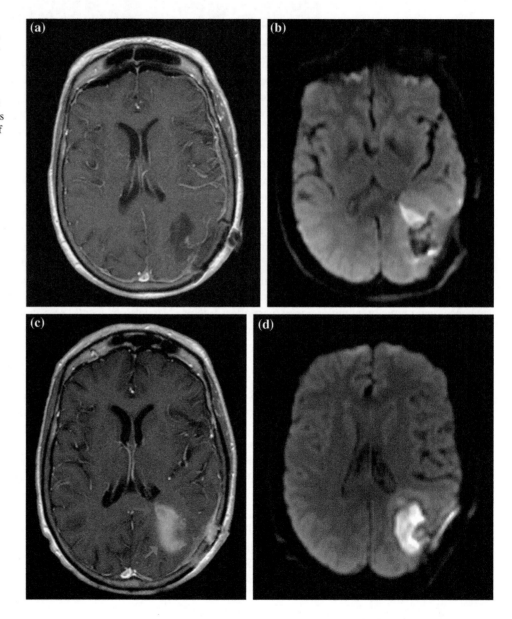

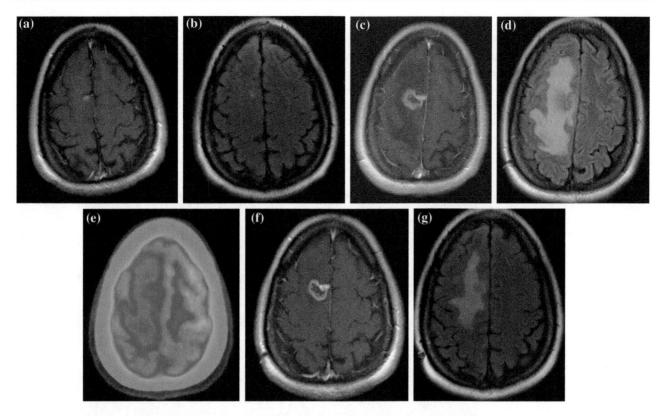

Fig. 2.7 a–g Radiation necrosis. 51-year-old woman with history of breast cancer and brain metastatic received SRS treatment to a superior *right* frontal lesion. Axial enhanced T1W and FLAIR images at one month (**a** and **b**) and 9 month (**c** and **d**) following treatment, demonstrating interval increase in size of enhancement and surrounding edema. FDG-PET shows no significant uptake in the region of enhancement relative to adjacent brain (**e**). At 15 months after treatment, the area of enhancement and surrounding edema decreased in size (**f** and **g**)

Table 2.3 Differential diagnosis for spinal mass(es)

	Multifocal enhancing lesions	Solitary enhancing lesion
Extra-dural	Metastasis Lymphoma Myeloma Granulomatous disease	Metastasis Meningioma Schwannoma Neurofibroma Lymphoma Myeloma/plasmacytoma
Intradural, extramedullary	Metastasis (systemic or CNS origins) Schwannomas Neurofibromas Granulomatous disease	Schwannomas Neurofibromas Metastasis
Intramedullary	Demyelinating disease Hemangioblastomas Metastasis Abscesses Granulomatous disease	Ependymoma Astrocytoma Hemangioblastoma Demyelinating disease Metastasis

PWI and MRS, measuring peritumoral nonenhancing abnormalities result in improved specificity [38, 40]. More recently, using k-means clustering of FA/mean diffusivity (MD) data, metastasis can be differentiated from high-grade glioma and meningioma with high accuracy [41].

Morphological Analysis

While qualitative assessment of tumor morphology based on MR imaging can contribute to diagnosis of brain tumors, the subjective nature of such evaluation methodology introduces significant variability. More recently, quantitative approaches to these imaging features have been developed. Three-dimensional (3D) shape morphology of tumor has been used to build morphometric models of glioblasdtomas and brain metastases pathology [42, 43]. These promising techniques require further validation using larger prospective imaging data. Once validated, software optimization will also be necessary prior routine clinical use.

Post-therapeutic Evaluation of Brain Metastasis

In order to assess presence of residual tumor, postoperative MRIs are usually performed within 48 h following surgical resection prior to onset of enhancement along surgical margins [44, 45]. During this period, enhancement is highly suggestive of residual tumor. In addition, perioperative brain infarction can be detected during early postoperative

Fig. 2.8 **a–c** Spine epidural. 45-year-old male with lung cancer presents with back pain. Sagittal T1 weighted image without contrast enhancement (**a**) shows abnormal marrow signal in the posterior aspect of multiple vertebral bodies in the thoracic spine. Sagittal T1-weighted image without contrast enhancement (**b**) and axial T1W post-contrast image (**c**) show involvement of *left* epidural space and neural foramen with narrowing of thecal sac and flattening of spinal cord

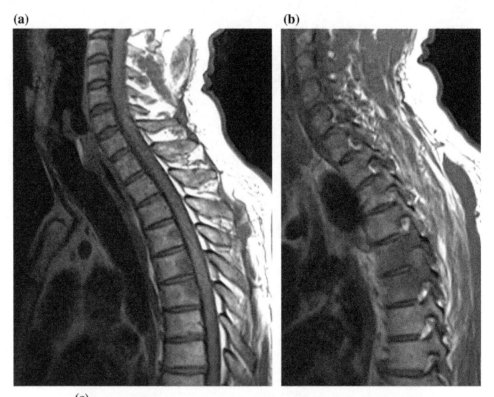

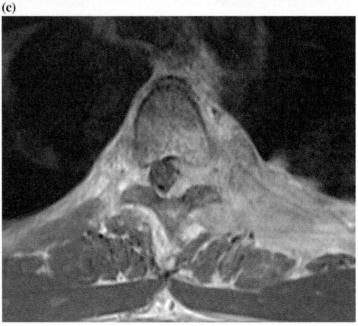

imaging with diffusion weighted imaging. Documenting presence of infarction can be important since enhancement from evolved infarction can mimic tumor residual tumor [14] (Fig. 2.6a–d).

Increased enhancement along surgical margins can also occur during postoperative infection. Enlargement of surgical cavity and increased degree of surrounding edema are suspicious signs for infection. While low diffusivity on diffusion-weighted imaging is a specific imaging sign of an abscess, a small number of brain metastases also exhibit low diffusivity and this finding is also less specific in the postoperative setting in the presence of evolving blood products within resection cavity [46] (Fig. 2.6a–d).

Depending on number, location and types of brain metastases, focal or whole brain radiation therapy is commonly performed alone or following surgical resection. Not infrequently, brain injury following radiation can produce clinical and imaging findings that resemble tumor progression or recurrence. It is important to recognize a number of imaging patterns associated with radiation treatment to avoid unnecessary surgery or cessation of effective chemotherapy.

Radiation-related brain injuries can be categorized by their timing following therapy initiation into acute (within weeks), subacute (within 3–4 months) and late (4 months to years) phases. Acute radiation injuries are transient and can appear normal on imaging or show increased edema and contrast enhancement. Subacute and delayed radiation injuries are often accompanied by increased edema and enhancement at and around original tumor site that can mimic tumor progression (Fig. 2.7a–g). Seventy percent of focal late radiation injuries occur within 2 years after therapy. Demyelination of white matter in periventricular regions is also a common late manifestation of injury following whole brain radiation treatment, characterized by gradually increasing patchy-appearing areas of T2 prolongation without associated mass effect or enhancement. White matter volume loss as a result of radiation injury can be apparent from expansion of ventricular size, although communicating hydrocephalus can be a superimposed clinical imaging finding that may be difficult to distinguish without a shunt trial. Capillary telangiectasias and cavernous malformations are vasculopathies that often develop several years to decades after radiation therapy. These lesions can be readily recognized by multifocal small hemosiderin depositions on T2*-weighted imaging and are not associated with edema or mass effect [47].

While it is usually difficult to distinguish radiation necrosis from tumor recurrence, several imaging features

Fig. 2.9 a–d Pathological Fracture. 88-year-old female with history of breast cancer presents with back pain. Sagittal T1 (**a**) and T2 (**b**) weighted images show compression fracture of L1 vertebral body with abnormal marrow signal involving the entire vertebral body and there is a convex appearance of the posterior cortex. The posterior element also shows abnormal marrow signal (**c**). Trabecular and cortical destructions are readily identified on axial CT imaging (**d**)

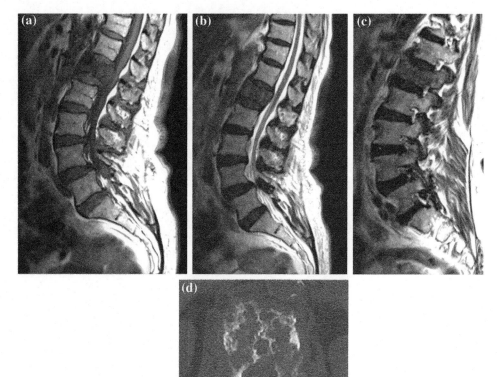

have been observed to help distinguish the two. Following radiosurgery, longer time between radiosurgery and resection and a larger edema/lesion volume ratio are predictive of radionecrosis as opposed to tumor recurrence [48]. Delayed MRI at greater than one hour following contrast injection can differentiate tumor from non-tumor tissues with high sensitivity and positive predictive value to active tumor [49]. Texture features analysis of conventional MRI sequence also provides improved classification accuracy in differentiating brain metastasis and radiation necrosis [50].

Advanced MR imaging techniques including DWI, MRS, and PWI have been used to differentiate radiation necrosis following lesions treated by stereotactic radiosurgery [51]. Radiation necrosis usually shows heterogeneity on DWI images and has significantly higher maximal ADC values compared to recurrent tumors [52]. While the blood volume and blood flow measurements of brain metastases on PWI are highly variable depending on primary tumor histology, a change in PWI parameters between pre-treatment and post-treatment imaging provides greater diagnostic value; a decrease of rCBV values indicates radiation-induced necrosis while elevation of rCBV following treatment is indicative

of tumor recurrence [53]. Based on serial change in the tissue choline/creatine level and lipid–lactate complex, MR spectroscopy can distinguish tumor recurrence from radiation-induced changes [54, 55]. While these advanced MR imaging techniques are undergoing validation for their clinical utility, they also require expertise in imaging quality control and postprocessing to ensure diagnostic consistency.

[18]FDG PET can also distinguish between necrosis and recurrent tumor with modest accuracy raging from 50 to 70% [56, 57]. Residual or recurrent tumor usually demonstrates increased FDG uptake, whereas necrosis from radiation or chemotherapy usually demonstrates isometabolic or decreased FDG uptake, although there is significant overlap in the uptake values. Novel amino acid PET radiotracers with high lesion to background ratio have been evaluated for imaging of metastases. 6-[(18)F]-fluoro-L-3,4-dihydroxyphenylalanine (F-DOPA) PET can differentiate radionecrosis from tumor progression with greater overall accuracy compared to perfusion-MRI [58].

Finally, CNS metastases can respond to systemic treatment differently from tumors at extracranial sites secondary to differences in drug penetration, tumor genetic

Fig. 2.10 a–c Hemangioma. 69-year-old with history of colon adenocarcinoma presented with new lumbar spine mass discovered on abdominal imaging. Axial T1-weighted images before (**a**) and after (**b**) intravenous contrast administration showed an enhancing mass involving the left aspect of vertebral body extending to pedicle and left paravertebral space. Percutaneous needle biopsy did not reveal malignant cells, and mass decreased in size without treatment on subsequent imaging, demonstrating characteristic hyperintensity of hemangioma on unenhanced axial T1-weighted image (**c**)

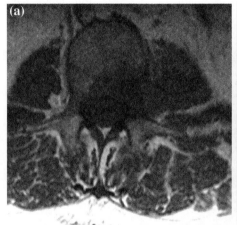
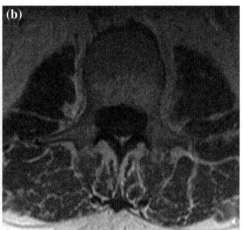
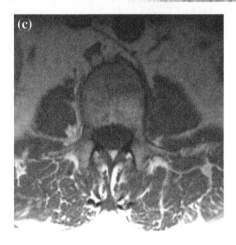

Fig. 2.11 a–d Spine intradural. 54-year-old male with metastatic melanoma presented with progressive right lower extremity weakness. Sagittal and axial T2- (**a** and **c**) and T1-weighted contrast (**b** and **d**) enhanced images show heterogeneously enhancing intradural, extramedullary mass resulting in leftward displacement and flattening of the spinal cord (**d**). There is cord edema on axial T2-weighted image (**c**)

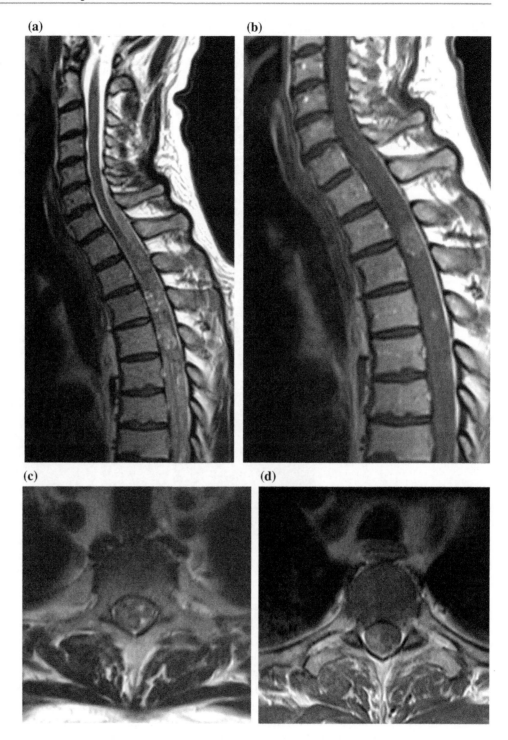

heterogeneity, and tumor microenvironment. On the other hand, localized therapies for CNS lesions including whole brain radiotherapy and stereotactic radiosurgery can produce a local response despite progression of systemic disease. Therefore, two-compartment response assessment criteria has been proposed to account for both CNS and non-CNS tumor burden [59].

Spinal Metastasis

Metastases to the spine can also be classified by their anatomical locations with respect to the dura and involvement of the spinal cord (Table 2.3). Most commonly, metastatic spinal lesions are extra-dural, found predominantly in the vertebral bodies and posterior elements with

Fig. 2.12 a–d Intramedullary metastasis. 63-year-old female with renal cell cancer presents with intramedullary metastasis. Sagittal and axial T2-weighted images (**a** and **c**) show a solitary lesion with central hypointensity and surrounding edema. There is enhancement on post-contrast T1-weighted images (**b** and **d**)

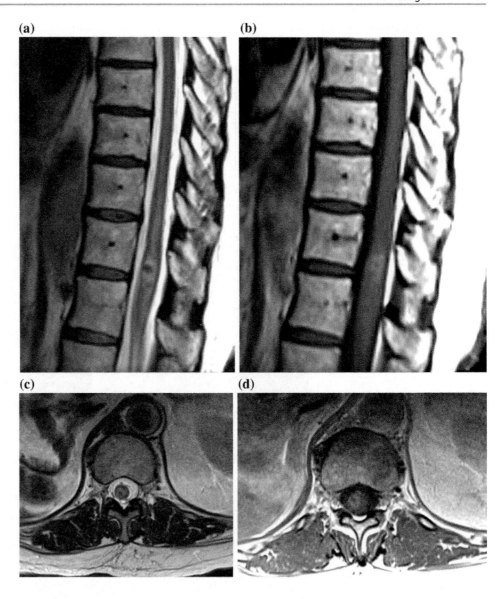

frequent extension to the epidural compartment causing compression of spinal cord or nerve roots. Epidural spinal cord compression occurs in approximately 5% of patients with cancer [60]. MRI, in particular unenhanced T1-weighted imaging, is most sensitive in detecting marrow involvement and diagnosing epidural disease due to replacement of marrow and epidural fat (Fig. 2.8a–c). Flattening of spinal cord contour with or without edema suggests cord compression (Fig. 2.8a–c). While cord compression is usually a clinical diagnosis, imaging is important for confirming locations of tumor to facilitate surgical or radiotherapy planning. Since multiple spinal levels are often simultaneously involved, it is important to obtain imaging of the entire spine.

Occasionally it can be difficult to distinguish pathological vertebral fractures from insufficiency fractures. On MRI, preservation of normal marrow signal in the non-compressed portion of vertebra and linear fluid signal or vacuum favor non-tumor etiologies [61–63]. Retropulsed fracture fragments at the posterior vertebra, usually located at the superior endplate, is highly specific for a benign fracture but has low sensitivity [64]. On the other hand, abnormal marrow signal in the pedicle or posterior element suggests metastatic involvement [65] (Fig. 2.9a–d). A convex posterior border of the vertebral body is also commonly found in metastatic compression fractures [65] (Fig. 2.9a–d). Destruction of cortical bone of the vertebral body or the pedicle provides important clues to underlying malignancy and can be best visualized on CT (Fig. 2.9a–d). DWI methods has been used to differentiate benign from metastatic compression fractures and can improve diagnostic accuracy when added to conventional MR sequences [66–69].

Presence of paraspinal or epidural enhancing soft tissues as well as additional spinal metastatic lesions are signs of tumor involvement [70], although one must also consider fluid or soft tissue findings related to hematoma, infection, or atypical hemangiomas. In particular, findings suggestive of vertebral height loss due to infection have contiguous vertebral, endplate and disk involvement.

Hemangiomas are common benign lesions in spine that are typically diagnosed on the basis of intrinsic short T1 (hyperintense) signal. However, a subset of hemangiomas exhibit atypical imaging appearances including lack of hyperintensity on T1-weighted images and aggressive changes including cortical disruption and epidural/paravertebral extension (Fig. 2.10a–c). Detection of a characteristic "polka dotted" trabellular pattern on both MRI and CT can be helpful in diagnosing hemangiomas.

Intradural, extramedullary metastases are due to tumor seeding within the leptomeninges and can appear as linear or nodular enhancing lesions along the surfaces of cord or cauda equina nerve roots. Large intradural metastases can also compress the spinal cord (Fig. 2.11a–d). While gadolinium contrast is highly valuable in diagnosing leptomeningeal carcinomatosis, subtle nodular thickening of cauda equina nerve roots can be detected by T2-weighted imaging at high resolution (3 mm or less). If MR imaging is contraindicated, CT myelography can also outline the contours of spinal cord and nerve roots.

Intramedullary metastases are rare although they must be considered in the setting of advanced systemic metastatic disease [71, 72]. These lesions usually demonstrate enhancement and adjacent cord edema (Fig. 2.12a–d), although on imaging they are often not distinguishable from other entities affecting spinal cord, including primary cord neoplasms, inflammatory or infectious pathologies.

Conclusion

Imaging plays a critical role in the diagnosis and management of metastatic disease in the central nervous system. Accurate diagnosis of CNS metastases is an important step in staging. While the imaging appearance of metastases can be highly variable depending on histological subtype of primary tumor, there are a number of important imaging features that can help with diagnosis and treatment planning. The imaging approach to CNS metastasis depends on both clinical symptoms and cancer types in order to maximize the sensitivity of lesion detection.

Acknowledgements This work was supported by the ARRS/ASNR Scholar Award.

References

1. Davis FG, Dolecek TA, McCarthy BJ, Villano JL. Toward determining the lifetime occurrence of metastatic brain tumors estimated from 2007 United States cancer incidence data. Neuro Oncol. 2012;14(9):1171–7.

2. Sloan AE, Nock CJ, Einstein DB. Diagnosis and treatment of melanoma brain metastasis: a literature review. Cancer Control. 2009;16(3):248–55.

3. Delattre JY, Krol G, Thaler HT, Posner JB. Distribution of brain metastases. Arch Neurol. 1988;45(7):741–4.

4. Sze G, Milano E, Johnson C, Heier L. Detection of brain metastases: comparison of contrast-enhanced MR with unenhanced MR and enhanced CT. AJNR Am J Neuroradiol. 1990;11 (4):785–91.

5. Gaviani P, Mullins ME, Braga TA, Hedley-Whyte ET, Halpern EF, Schaefer PS, et al. Improved detection of metastatic melanoma by T2*-weighted imaging. AJNR Am J Neuroradiol. 2006;27(3):605–8.

6. Atlas SW, Braffman BH, LoBrutto R, Elder DE, Herlyn D. Human malignant melanomas with varying degrees of melanin content in nude mice: MR imaging, histopathology, and electron paramagnetic resonance. J Comput Assist Tomogr. 1990;14(4):547–54.

7. Enochs WS, Petherick P, Bogdanova A, Mohr U, Weissleder R. Paramagnetic metal scavenging by melanin: MR imaging. Radiology. 1997;204(2):417–23.

8. Hayashi H, Okamoto I, Tanizaki J, Tanaka K, Okuda T, Kato A, et al. Cystic brain metastasis in non–small-cell lung cancer with ALK rearrangement. JCO. 2014;32(36):e122–4.

9. Hwang TL, Valdivieso JG, Yang CH, Wolin MJ. Calcified brain metastasis. Neurosurgery. 1993;32(3):451–454; discussion 454.

10. Tashiro Y, Kondo A, Aoyama I, Nin K, Shimotake K, Tashiro H, et al. Calcified metastatic brain tumor. Neurosurgery. 1990;26 (6):1065–70.

11. Deck MD, Messina AV, Sackett JF. Computed tomography in metastatic disease of the brain. Radiology. 1976;119(1):115–20.

12. Yamada N, Imakita S, Sakuma T, Takamiya M. Intracranial calcification on gradient-echo phase image: depiction of diamagnetic susceptibility. Radiology. 1996;198(1):171–8.

13. Collie DA, Brush JP, Lammie GA, Grant R, Kunkler I, Leonard R, et al. Imaging features of leptomeningeal metastases. Clin Radiol. 1999;54(11):765–71.

14. Pirzkall A, McGue C, Saraswathy S, Cha S, Liu R, Vandenberg S, et al. Tumor regrowth between surgery and initiation of adjuvant therapy in patients with newly diagnosed glioblastoma. Neuro Oncol. 2009;11(6):842–52.

15. Hjorthaug K, Højbjerg JA, Knap MM, Tietze A, Haraldsen A, Zacho HD, et al. Accuracy of 18F-FDG PET-CT in triaging lung cancer patients with suspected brain metastases for MRI. Nucl Med Commun. 2015;36(11):1084–90.

16. Colosimo C, Ruscalleda J, Korves M, La Ferla R, Wool C, Pianezzola P, et al. Detection of intracranial metastases: a multicenter, intrapatient comparison of gadobenate dimeglumine-enhanced MRI with routinely used contrast agents at equal dosage. Invest Radiol. 2001;36(2):72–81.

17. Runge VM, Parker JR, Donovan M. Double-blind, efficacy evaluation of gadobenate dimeglumine, a gadolinium chelate with enhanced relaxivity, in malignant lesions of the brain. Invest Radiol. 2002;37(5):269–80.

18. Yuh WT, Tali ET, Nguyen HD, Simonson TM, Mayr NA, Fisher DJ. The effect of contrast dose, imaging time, and lesion size in the MR detection of intracerebral metastasis. AJNR Am J Neuroradiol. 1995;16(2):373–80.

19. Ba-Ssalamah A, Nöbauer-Huhmann IM, Pinker K, Schibany N, Prokesch R, Mehrain S, et al. Effect of contrast dose and field strength in the magnetic resonance detection of brain metastases. Invest Radiol. 2003;38(7):415–22.

20. Nöbauer-Huhmann I-M, Ba-Ssalamah A, Mlynarik V, Barth M, Schöggl A, Heimberger K, et al. Magnetic resonance imaging contrast enhancement of brain tumors at 3 tesla versus 1.5 tesla. Invest Radiol. 2002;37(3):114–9.

21. Hayashida Y, Hirai T, Morishita S, Kitajima M, Murakami R, Korogi Y, et al. Diffusion-weighted imaging of metastatic brain tumors: comparison with histologic type and tumor cellularity. AJNR Am J Neuroradiol. 2006;27(7):1419–25.

22. Duygulu G, Ovali GY, Calli C, Kitis O, Yünten N, Akalin T, et al. Intracerebral metastasis showing restricted diffusion: correlation with histopathologic findings. Eur J Radiol. 2010;74(1):117–20.

23. Haldorsen IS, Espeland A, Larsson E-M. Central nervous system lymphoma: characteristic findings on traditional and advanced imaging. AJNR Am J Neuroradiol. 2011;32(6):984–92.

24. Nemeth AJ, Henson JW, Mullins ME, Gonzalez RG, Schaefer PW. Improved detection of skull metastasis with diffusion-weighted MR imaging. AJNR Am J Neuroradiol. 2007;28(6):1088–92.

25. Chavhan GB, Babyn PS, Thomas B, Shroff MM, Haacke EM. Principles, techniques, and applications of T2*-based MR imaging and its special applications. Radiographics. 2009;29(5):1433–49.

26. Mittal S, Wu Z, Neelavalli J, Haacke EM. Susceptibility-weighted imaging: technical aspects and clinical applications, part 2. AJNR Am J Neuroradiol. 2009;30(2):232–52.

27. Bruhn H, Frahm J, Gyngell ML, Merboldt KD, Hänicke W, Sauter R, et al. Noninvasive differentiation of tumors with use of localized H-1 MR spectroscopy in vivo: initial experience in patients with cerebral tumors. Radiology. 1989;172(2):541–8.

28. Poptani H, Gupta RK, Roy R, Pandey R, Jain VK, Chhabra DK. Characterization of intracranial mass lesions with in vivo proton MR spectroscopy. AJNR Am J Neuroradiol. 1995;16(8):1593–603.

29. Sijens PE, Knopp MV, Brunetti A, Wicklow K, Alfano B, Bachert P, et al. 1H MR spectroscopy in patients with metastatic brain tumors: a multicenter study. Magn Reson Med. 1995;33(6):818–26.

30. Law M. MR spectroscopy of brain tumors. Top Magn Reson Imaging. 2004;15(5):291–313.

31. García-Gómez JM, Luts J, Julià-Sapé M, Krooshof P, Tortajada S, Robledo JV, et al. Multiproject-multicenter evaluation of automatic brain tumor classification by magnetic resonance spectroscopy. MAGMA. 2009;22(1):5–18.

32. Groothuis DR. The blood-brain and blood-tumor barriers: a review of strategies for increasing drug delivery. Neuro-Oncol. 2000;2(1):45–59.

33. Law M, Cha S, Knopp EA, Johnson G, Arnett J, Litt AW. High-grade gliomas and solitary metastases: differentiation by using perfusion and proton spectroscopic MR imaging. Radiology. 2002;222(3):715–21.

34. Young GS, Setayesh K. Spin-echo echo-planar perfusion MR imaging in the differential diagnosis of solitary enhancing brain lesions: distinguishing solitary metastases from primary glioma. AJNR Am J Neuroradiol. 2009;30(3):575–7.

35. Bertossi M, Virgintino D, Maiorano E, Occhiogrosso M, Roncali L. Ultrastructural and morphometric investigation of human brain capillaries in normal and peritumoral tissues. Ultrastruct Pathol. 1997;21(1):41–9.

36. Cha S. Perfusion MR imaging of brain tumors. Top Magn Reson Imaging. 2004;15(5):279–89.

37. Basser PJ. Inferring microstructural features and the physiological state of tissues from diffusion-weighted images. NMR Biomed. 1995;8(7–8):333–44.

38. Lu S, Ahn D, Johnson G, Cha S. Peritumoral diffusion tensor imaging of high-grade gliomas and metastatic brain tumors. AJNR Am J Neuroradiol. 2003;24(5):937–41.

39. Tsuchiya K, Fujikawa A, Nakajima M, Honya K. Differentiation between solitary brain metastasis and high-grade glioma by diffusion tensor imaging. Br J Radiol. 2005;78(930):533–7.

40. Lu S, Ahn D, Johnson G, Law M, Zagzag D, Grossman RI. Diffusion-tensor MR imaging of intracranial neoplasia and associated peritumoral edema: introduction of the tumor infiltration index. Radiology. 2004;232(1):221–8.

41. Jones TL, Byrnes TJ, Yang G, Howe FA, Bell BA, Barrick TR. Brain tumor classification using the diffusion tensor image segmentation (D-SEG) technique. Neuro-Oncol. 2015;17(3):466–76.

42. Yang G, Jones TL, Howe FA, Barrick TR. Morphometric model for discrimination between glioblastoma multiforme and solitary metastasis using three-dimensional shape analysis. Magn Reson Med. 2016;75(6):2505–16.

43. Blanchet L, Krooshof PWT, Postma GJ, Idema AJ, Goraj B, Heerschap A, et al. Discrimination between metastasis and glioblastoma multiforme based on morphometric analysis of MR images. AJNR Am J Neuroradiol. 2011;32(1):67–73.

44. Albert FK, Forsting M, Sartor K, Adams HP, Kunze S. Early postoperative magnetic resonance imaging after resection of malignant glioma: objective evaluation of residual tumor and its influence on regrowth and prognosis. Neurosurgery. 1994;34(1):45–60–61.

45. Forsting M, Albert FK, Kunze S, Adams HP, Zenner D, Sartor K. Extirpation of glioblastomas: MR and CT follow-up of residual tumor and regrowth patterns. AJNR Am J Neuroradiol. 1993;14(1):77–87.

46. Hartmann M, Jansen O, Heiland S, Sommer C, Münkel K, Sartor K. Restricted diffusion within ring enhancement is not pathognomonic for brain abscess. AJNR Am J Neuroradiol. 2001;22(9):1738–42.

47. Gaensler EH, Dillon WP, Edwards MS, Larson DA, Rosenau W, Wilson CB. Radiation-induced telangiectasia in the brain simulates cryptic vascular malformations at MR imaging. Radiology. 1994;193(3):629–36.

48. Leeman JE, Clump DA, Flickinger JC, Mintz AH, Burton SA, Heron DE. Extent of perilesional edema differentiates radionecrosis from tumor recurrence following stereotactic radiosurgery for brain metastases. Neuro-Oncol. 2013;15(12):1732–8.

49. Zach L, Guez D, Last D, Daniels D, Grober Y, Nissim O, et al. Delayed contrast extravasation MRI: a new paradigm in neuro-oncology. Neuro-Oncol. 2015;17(3):457–65.

50. Larroza A, Moratal D, Paredes-Sánchez A, Soria-Olivas E, Chust ML, Arribas LA, et al. Support vector machine classification of brain metastasis and radiation necrosis based on texture analysis in MRI. J Magn Reson Imaging. 2015;42(5):1362–8.

51. Kang TW, Kim ST, Byun HS, Jeon P, Kim K, Kim H, et al. Morphological and functional MRI, MRS, perfusion and diffusion changes after radiosurgery of brain metastasis. Eur J Radiol. 2009;72(3):370–80.

52. Asao C, Korogi Y, Kitajima M, Hirai T, Baba Y, Makino K, et al. Diffusion-weighted imaging of radiation-induced brain injury for differentiation from tumor recurrence. AJNR Am J Neuroradiol. 2005;26(6):1455–60.

53. Essig M, Waschkies M, Wenz F, Debus J, Hentrich HR, Knopp MV. Assessment of brain metastases with dynamic susceptibility-weighted contrast-enhanced MR imaging: initial results. Radiology. 2003;228(1):193–9.

54. Graves EE, Nelson SJ, Vigneron DB, Verhey L, McDermott M, Larson D, et al. Serial proton MR spectroscopic imaging of recurrent malignant gliomas after gamma knife radiosurgery. AJNR Am J Neuroradiol. 2001;22(4):613–24.

55. Schlemmer HP, Bachert P, Herfarth KK, Zuna I, Debus J, van Kaick G. Proton MR spectroscopic evaluation of suspicious brain lesions after stereotactic radiotherapy. AJNR Am J Neuroradiol. 2001;22(7):1316–24.

56. Griffeth LK, Rich KM, Dehdashti F, Simpson JR, Fusselman MJ, McGuire AH, et al. Brain metastases from non-central nervous system tumors: evaluation with PET. Radiology. 1993;186(1):37–44.

57. Rohren EM, Provenzale JM, Barboriak DP, Coleman RE. Screening for cerebral metastases with FDG PET in patients undergoing whole-body staging of non-central nervous system malignancy. Radiology. 2003;226(1):181–7.

58. Cicone F, Minniti G, Romano A, Papa A, Scaringi C, Tavanti F, et al. Accuracy of F-DOPA PET and perfusion-MRI for differentiating radionecrotic from progressive brain metastases after radiosurgery. Eur J Nucl Med Mol Imaging. 2015;42(1):103–11.

59. Lin NU, Lee EQ, Aoyama H, Barani IJ, Barboriak DP, Baumert BG, et al. Response assessment criteria for brain metastases: proposal from the RANO group. Lancet Oncol. 2015;16(6):e270–8.

60. Schiff D, O'Neill BP, Suman VJ. Spinal epidural metastasis as the initial manifestation of malignancy: clinical features and diagnostic approach. Neurology. 1997;49(2):452–6.

61. Yu C-W, Hsu C-Y, Shih TT-F, Chen B-B, Fu C-J. Vertebral osteonecrosis: MR imaging findings and related changes on adjacent levels. AJNR Am J Neuroradiol. 2007;28(1):42–7.

62. Baur A, Stäbler A, Arbogast S, Duerr HR, Bartl R, Reiser M. Acute osteoporotic and neoplastic vertebral compression fractures: fluid sign at MR imaging. Radiology. 2002;225(3):730–5.

63. Theodorou DJ. The intravertebral vacuum cleft sign. Radiology. 2001;221(3):787–8.

64. Yuh WT, Zachar CK, Barloon TJ, Sato Y, Sickels WJ, Hawes DR. Vertebral compression fractures: distinction between benign and malignant causes with MR imaging. Radiology. 1989;172(1):215–8.

65. Cuénod CA, Laredo JD, Chevret S, Hamze B, Naouri JF, Chapaux X, et al. Acute vertebral collapse due to osteoporosis or malignancy: appearance on unenhanced and gadolinium-enhanced MR images. Radiology. 1996;199(2):541–9.

66. Zhou XJ, Leeds NE, McKinnon GC, Kumar AJ. Characterization of benign and metastatic vertebral compression fractures with quantitative diffusion MR imaging. AJNR Am J Neuroradiol. 2002;23(1):165–70.

67. Chan JHM, Peh WCG, Tsui EYK, Chau LF, Cheung KK, Chan KB, et al. Acute vertebral body compression fractures: discrimination between benign and malignant causes using apparent diffusion coefficients. Br J Radiol. 2002;75(891):207–14.

68. Abanoz R, Hakyemez B, Parlak M. Diffusion-weighted imaging of acute vertebral compression: differential diagnosis of benign versus malignant pathologic fractures. Tani Girisim Radyol. 2003;9(2):176–83.

69. Sung JK, Jee W-H, Jung J-Y, Choi M, Lee S-Y, Kim Y-H, et al. Differentiation of acute osteoporotic and malignant compression fractures of the spine: use of additive qualitative and quantitative axial diffusion-weighted MR imaging to conventional MR imaging at 3.0 T. Radiology. 2014;271(2):488–98.

70. Laredo JD, Lakhdari K, Bellaïche L, Hamze B, Janklewicz P, Tubiana JM. Acute vertebral collapse: CT findings in benign and malignant nontraumatic cases. Radiology. 1995;194(1):41–8.

71. Lee SS, Kim MK, Sym SJ, Kim SW, Kim WK, Kim S-B, et al. Intramedullary spinal cord metastases: a single-institution experience. J Neurooncol. 2007;84(1):85–9.

72. Schiff D, O'Neill BP. Intramedullary spinal cord metastases: clinical features and treatment outcome. Neurology. 1996;47(4):906–12.

Other Diagnostic Tools for Neurological Disease in Cancer: EEG, EMG, and Lumbar Puncture

Crystal S. Janani and Edward K. Avila

Electroencephalography

History

The early works of Galvani and Volta were essential in the discovery of animal and later human electrical circuitry in the nervous system [1]. In 1875, British physician Richard Caton received a grant to explore electrical phenomena in the exposed cerebral hemispheres of monkeys. Caton found that "feeble currents of varying directions pass through the multiplier when the electrodes are placed on two varying points of the external surface." [2] In 1924, Hans Berger performed the first electroencephalogram (EEG) on a human when he performed an EEG on a 17-year-old boy during an open neurosurgical operation. Throughout the 1930s Berger continued to describe different patterns, but it was the work of American pioneers Fredric Gibbs, Erna Gibbs, Herbert Jasper, and William Lenox that defined what we know today about epileptogenic discharges and their role in epilepsy [1, 3]. Recent advances have helped to further the field of epilepsy. While the first EEGs were on paper, the advent of computers has made digitalized EEG easier to read and more accessible to the clinician. Additionally, video monitoring in conjunction with EEG has helped to further correlate semiology types with EEG findings. The discovery of electroencephalography was a milestone in the diagnosis and evaluation of patients with seizures and remains a valuable tool today.

Technical Component

In order to obtain an EEG, an EEG technician places scalp leads, records the EEG for a given amount of time, and transfers the data to a neurologist for interpretation. Most commonly with electroencephalography, scalp electrodes are placed with a gel or putty that makes an electrolyte bridge between the electrode and the skin. An electrical potential is generated between two given positions on the scalp and the signal is amplified via an amplifier and displayed on the computer screen as an upward or downward deflected wave. Ultimately, an EEG recording measures, amplifies, and registers differences between fluctuating electrical field potentials and displays this as a function of time. Frequencies and amplitudes are interpreted by the neurologist. Frequencies include delta (0.5–4 Hz), theta (4–8 Hz), alpha (8–12 Hz), beta (12–30 Hz), and gamma (30–60 Hz) [1]. In adults, the normal wake state consists of alpha, while theta and delta frequencies are considered abnormal. Additionally, sharply contoured epileptiform discharges can be seen and are sometimes pathologic. In the most basic sense, a seizure is a rhythmic build up of epileptogenic discharges with evolution over space and time.

In order to localize pathology of a lesion, one must know where the electrodes are placed on the scalp. In an effort to standardize the recorded data, a committee of the International Federation of Societies for Electroencephalography and Clinical Neurophysiology recommended what is known as the International 10–20 system. This system requires specific measurements to be made from bony structures of the skull to determine the placement of electrodes in order to standardize inter-electrode distance in every patient [4].

An EEG has very good temporal resolution but lacks spatial resolution. Approximately 10 cm^2 of cortical surface must be activated in order to appreciate a response on scalp EEG. EEG has varied sensitivity and specificity. It is sensitive for discharges with a large field as seen in a generalized seizure but lacks sensitivity in small focal seizures.

C.S. Janani
Department of Neurology, St. Agnes Hospital, 900 Caton Avenue, Baltimore, MD 21229, USA
e-mail: crystal.janani@stagnes.org

E.K. Avila (✉)
Department of Neurology, Memorial Sloan Kettering Cancer Center, 1275 York Avenue, New York, NY 10065, USA
e-mail: avilae@mskcc.org

© Springer International Publishing AG 2018
D. Schiff et al. (eds.), *Cancer Neurology in Clinical Practice*,
DOI 10.1007/978-3-319-57901-6_3

EEGs with spike and wave discharges can be relatively specific for certain epilepsy types, but generalized slowing and other patterns are relatively nonspecific in determining the causative source [5]. Thus, interpretation of the EEG should be made with the clinical context of the patient in mind.

Indications and Contraindications

Electroencephalography is a useful tool in the diagnosis of both clinical and subclinical seizures. It is most commonly used in evaluation of patients with suspected seizures but has other utility in the cancer patient. Overall, 20–40% of patients with brain tumors will present with seizures and another 20–45% will develop seizures later in the course of their disease [5–8]. Mental status changes, unresponsiveness, episodic spells, and shaking movements are frequent indications for EEG evaluation. There is mounting evidence that comatose patients, particularly those with structural lesions of the brain, should be monitored with continuous EEG for the evaluation of subclinical seizures. Nearly 10% of all comatose medical intensive care unit patients with no suspicion for seizure have non-convulsive seizures [9]. Up to one-third of patients with central nervous system infections have subclinical seizures [10]. In certain paraneoplastic encephalidities, up to one-half of the patients have seizures and even more have EEG slowing [11]. Supratentorial tumors can have rates exceeding these [8]. Thus, it is imperative that EEG has a low threshold for use as a diagnostic tool in the cancer patient.

There are no true contraindications to EEG. Placing electrodes over skin lesions on the scalp (due to surgical incision or ulcerations from prolonged EEG monitoring) should be avoided, but the electrodes can be placed on a nearby site if needed. EEG can be performed even with the presence of electrical devices such as a cardiac pacemaker, cochlear implant, or deep brain stimulator. Hair weaves or other extensions should be removed in order to allow direct contact between the electrodes and the scalp.

Slow EEG Patterns

Electrocorticography has strengths and weaknesses in evaluating the cancer patient. EEG is reliable at localizing lesions of the superficial cerebral hemisphere but is of limited use in deep lesions, particularly those in the posterior fossa. Tumors are electrically inert and destroy neurons thus augmenting the EEG recording. Studies have shown that direct electrocorticogram (ECog) evaluation of the cortex with the skull removed demonstrates (a) the cortex invaded by tumor has no activity, (b) the cortex abutting the tumor has a burst-suppression pattern, and (c) the most distant cortical zones have continuous slow waves [12].

A common pattern present with primary or metastatic brain tumors is continuous focal polymorphic delta slow activity due to focal lesions of the subcortical white matter. This slow activity is minimally reactive to different physiologic states and persists throughout wake, drowsiness, and even N2, N3 and REM sleep. This is often seen in tumors such as glioblastoma which disrupt subcortical and cortical structures [13].

Another pattern commonly seen is slow rhythmic sinusoidal monomorphic waves occurring in bursts. This intermittent rhythmic delta activity (IRDA) activity can have a frontal predominance (FIRDA) or occipital predominance (OIRDA); the occipital pattern being seen primarily in children. This intermittent monomorphic activity, in contrast to polymorphic delta activity, is much more widespread over bilateral hemispheres and shows reactivity with augmentation with eye closure, hyperventilation, and drowsiness. IRDA ceases during deeper non-REM sleep and reappears in REM sleep. With infratentorial lesions, this IRDA is typically symmetric and bilateral with some shifting asymmetry. With supratentorial lesions, however, this IRDA can show a persistent asymmetry being most prominent over the side of the lesion [13].

Yet another pattern often seen with focal lesions such as primary or metastatic brain tumors is attenuation, or a decrease in amplitude often with drop-out of faster frequencies. It is typically localized to the side of the lesion and can be widespread in distribution over the hemisphere. Attenuation can also be widespread over both hemispheres, and when severe, can become suppressed constituting a burst-suppression pattern [13].

Cancer patients with focal lesions can also have diffuse changes on EEG due to a variety of toxic-metabolic entities. At times, EEG can provide objective criteria for severity of the underlying pathologic process. Table 3.1 lists some common toxic-metabolic derangements that are seen in cancer patients and their EEG findings.

Paroxysmal and Ictal EEG Patterns

According to the International Federation of Societies for Electroencephalography and Clinical Neurophysiology (IFSECN), a transient is an event that clearly stands out against the background EEG and can be a single wave or a sequence of two or more waves. Spikes are transients which are considered epileptiform and are clearly distinguished from the background with a pointed peak and duration between 20 and 70 ms and a sharp wave is a transient clearly distinguished from the background with a pointed peak and duration between 70 and 200 ms [14]. Spikes and sharp

Table 3.1 Common toxic-metabolic derangements in cancer patients and their associated EEG findings

Derangement	EEG findings
Benzodiazepine or barbiturate use	Diffuse beta activity
Hepatic failure	Early—slowed alpha rhythm
	Late—persistent theta or delta activity
	Triphasic wave pattern—2–4 Hz bilaterally synchronous waves with a triphasic morphology
Renal failure	Early—slowed alpha rhythm
	Late—nearly persistent theta or delta activity
	Triphasic waves—also present
Hyponatremia	Early—slowposterior alpha rhythm
	Late—generalized slow activity
	High-voltage IRDA
	Epileptiform discharges are uncommon even with seizures
Hypernatremia	Theta activity
	Often no EEG changes at all
Hypoglycemia	Enhanced response to hyperventilation with FIRDA longer after cessation of hyperventilation
	Glucose 50–80 mg/dl: slowing of alpha rhythm
	Glucose below 40 mg/dl diffuse theta and delta with IRDA activity
	Epileptiform discharges are uncommon even with seizures
Hyperglycemia	Changes typically not seen until glucose greater than 400 mg/dl
	Sporadic epileptiform discharges
Hypothermia	Core temperature 29–30 °C—diffuse theta and delta
	Core temperature 20–22 °C—burst suppression pattern
	Core temperature <18 °C—electrocerebral silence

waves are closely related phenomenon, both of which are associated with an epileptic seizure disorder, although both transients may occur with no prior history of epileptic seizure disorder [1]. These epileptiform and highly epileptogenic potentials are seen in patients with and without structural brain lesions. These discharges are often seen interictally in patients with brain tumors and epilepsy. They are often localized to the region of the brain tumor but in multifocal structural lesions such as brain metastasis, multifocal epileptiform discharges can be seen. It is uncommon for this epileptiform activity to be the only EEG abnormality associated with a tumor. Typically, some degree of focal slowing is present when epileptiform activity is present [13, 15].

While epileptiform activity is commonly seen with indolent or static lesions, periodic lateralized epileptiform discharges are more commonly seen with an acute lesion [13]. Periodic lateralized epileptiform discharges (PLEDs) are sharp waves, spike waves, or more complex wave forms recurring periodically every 1–2 s with a return to background between discharges and occupying a relatively large area of the hemicranium [13, 16]. They can be due to a variety of structural lesions including neoplasms,

hematomas, and infections. While stroke is the most common etiology of PLEDs, 12% of patients with PLEDs have brain tumors, almost all of which are supratentorial brain tumors. PLEDs are considered to be on the ictal-interictal spectrum and are highly associated with conversion to frank seizure activity. Almost 50% of patients with brain tumors and PLEDs have seizures [16].

When a patient has a seizure that persists for a sufficient length of time or repeats frequently enough that recovery between attacks does not occur, it is termed status epilepticus. Mortality with status epilepticus is up to 20%. Convulsive status epilepticus accounts for nearly half of all status epilepticus [17]. Over 4% of patients who present with status epilepticus have brain tumors. In patients who present with status epilepticus with no preexisting history of seizure, almost 9% have brain tumors [18]. Patients with structural brain lesions more often have refractory status epilepticus and over 5% of patients presenting with refractory status epilepticus have this condition secondary to a brain tumor [19].

At times, status epilepticus is partial (as opposed to generalized) in nature. Epilepsia partialis continua is a partial somatomotor status epilepticus that is often seen in the setting of brain tumors. Between 11 and 15% of patients who present with epilepsia partialis continua have brain tumors as the etiology. EEG findings with this can be variable depending on the area of focus and, at times, the EEG can be normal given that it takes a sufficient amount of cortex to elicit a response on EEG [20, 21].

A common cause of altered mental status in the brain tumor population is non-convulsive status epilepticus (NCSE). NCSE can be defined as status epilepticus with reduced or altered consciousness, behavioral and vegetative abnormalities, or subjective symptoms with no major convulsive movements [22]. NCSE is the cause of altered mental status in over 5% of tumor patients [23]. NCSE is more common in patients with gliomas than in those with metastatic tumors [24]. Even in patients with systemic cancer but no brain metastasis, NCSE was the cause of altered mental status in 6% of patients [23]. EEG monitoring can be particularly helpful in the diagnosis of seizures in these patients and should be utilized in any cancer patient with altered mental status [25].

EEG Changes by Tumor Type

EEG changes in patients with brain tumors depend on several factors, including location, size, and growth rate. Although EEG patterns are not specific for the histologic pathology of the tumor, some general correlations can be made.

Extra-axial tumors that are slow growing, like meningiomas, are less likely to produce EEG abnormalities. Meningiomas located in the convexities, especially parasagittally, are more likely to cause changes like focal theta, FIRDA, and diminished or altered frontal beta rhythms. Rolandic meningiomas cause epileptiform discharges in up to 45% of patients with similar incidence of seizure. Meningiomas of other regions are less likely to cause EEG effects; however, approximately 25% of patients with meningiomas present with seizures [26, 27].

Indolent gliomas are more likely to cause EEG changes. Glioneural tumors including gangliogliomas and dysembryoplastic neuroepithelial tumors (DNETs) have the highest rates of epilepsy with 90–100% of patients having seizures, often pharmacoresistant [8, 28]. Diffuse low-grade gliomas cause seizures in 60–88% of patients [8, 29]. Focal polymorphic slow activity is usually a later finding and can occur intermittently. This slowing becomes increasingly persistent as the tumor progresses [30].

Rapidly growing parenchymal tumors, such as glioblastomas, are more likely to cause marked abnormalities on EEG but are less likely to cause seizures. Glioblastomas and other rapidly growing and destructive tumors cause prominent and focal polymorphic delta activity with marked alterations of background rhythms unilaterally and often bilaterally. Areas of necrosis can be electrically silent causing regions of attenuation. FIRDA occurs more frequently in glioblastoma than in other types of supratentorial tumors. With glioblastoma, epileptiform discharges are not present as frequently as they are with more indolent gliomas but PLEDS are more likely to occur [13]. Seizure rates in glioblastoma are approximately 30–50%, which is significantly lower than what is seen with lower grade gliomas [8, 31, 32].

Metastatic tumors to brain occur most commonly with cancers of the lung, breast, kidney, and melanoma. The EEG findings tend to be lateralized to the side of the metastasis. Larger or multiple metastatic lesions cause more EEG abnormalities than do small solitary lesions. The slow activity in metastatic lesions tends to be more theta range, compared to delta slow activity present with glioblastomas. EEG slow activity in metastatic disease also tends to be more episodic rather than persistent as seen with glioblastomas [33]. Metastatic lesions cause epileptogenic discharges in about one-third of patients and seizures in nearly one-half. Overall, metastatic lesions tend to cause more benign EEG changes than do gliomas of any grade [34].

EEG Changes by Tumor Location

EEG findings can vary by location of the tumor. Since the EEG reflects cortical neuron activity, hemispheric tumors affect EEG more markedly and reliably than do deeper tumors and tumors of the posterior fossa.

Frontal lobe tumors often cause local high-voltage delta slow activity. The slow activity can be continuous or episodic and bifrontal with a FIRDA pattern. FIRDA is more common with frontal tumors than in tumors of other locations. The background activity can be relatively preserved in frontal tumors. Epileptiform discharges are seen in almost one-half of frontal tumor patients [26].

Temporal tumors are the easiest to localize with EEG and display moderate to high-voltage focal polymorphic delta slowing lateralized over the tumor in over 80% of cases. In a majority of cases the slow activity is localized to the region of the tumor [33]. The slow activity recorded with temporal tumors tends to be continuous rather than intermittent. Temporal lobe tumors are also likely to cause FIRDA, but less so than frontal lobe tumors [26]. Background rhythms are more likely to be altered in posterior temporal lesions than in anterior temporal lesions.

Parietal tumors are less likely to cause EEG changes than are other supratentorial tumors. Slow activity can be local or more widespread and is more likely to be theta range, only of a moderate voltage, and intermittent or continuous. The background rhythms tend to be disturbed with parietal tumors [33].

Occipital tumors tend to cause focal polymorphic delta activity. Slow activity in surrounding temporal and parietal regions is often seen in conjunction with this. The posterior alpha rhythm is frequently absent ipsilaterally [1].

Tumors of subcortical structures vary in their findings and can be fairly non-localizing. Tumors of deep structures including the hypothalamus, fornix, basal ganglia, internal capsule, and corpus callosum characteristically cause intermittent slow activity. The slow activity is often monorhythmic and bilateral in an IRDA pattern [35]. Up to one-fourth of patients with lesions in these regions will have normal EEG findings [13]. Tumors of the sellar region typically do not cause EEG findings until they expand and obstruct the third ventricle, only then causing IRDA [36]. Thalamic tumors can cause IRDA but have also been shown to cause attenuation, disorganization of background frequencies, and slow activity of the ipsilateral alpha rhythm [37].

Tumors of the third ventricle and posterior fossa tend to be variable and are often normal on EEG. Abnormalities are more frequently found with obstruction of cerebrospinal fluid flow causing obstructive hydrocephalus. If an abnormal EEG is seen, the most common pattern is that of IRDA [1].

EEG Changes with Tumor Treatment

Iatrogenic changes are also seen on EEG in response to treatment therapies. Some are well characterized and others less so. EEG is useful in diagnosing epileptogenic potential with new cancer treatments and chemotherapeutic agents.

Brain irradiation occurs in two forms, whole brain radiation (WBRT) and partial brain radiation. WBRT can cause an acute or delayed reaction with cognitive decline and neurologic deficits. It can also cause generalized slowing of the background rhythms, IRDA, or even focal polymorphic delta slowing due to necrosis. Partial brain radiation can cause necrosis lending to focal slow activity, epileptogenic discharges, and even seizures [38–40].

Numerous medications for cancer treatment have an associated incidence of central nervous system toxicity. Some drugs cause diffuse dysfunction and slow activity on EEG while others are frankly epileptogenic. Table 3.2 lists known electrographic changes associated with common cancer treatments [41, 42].

EEG Changes with Autoimmune and Paraneoplastic Disorders

Paraneoplastic limbic encephalitis is becoming increasingly recognized with the commercial availability of antibody assays. Any paraneoplastic encephalitis involving the cortex or limbic system can cause EEG abnormalities and seizures. There are several autoantibody syndromes that are commonly associated with paraneoplastic epilepsy. These cause marked EEG abnormalities that are sometimes reversible with treatment of the underlying malignancy. Up to 100% of patients with paraneoplastic limbic encephalitis have an abnormal EEG, with seizures occurring in over 50% of these patients. EEG abnormalities include diffuse slowing, focal slowing, multifocal slowing, focal or multifocal epileptiform discharges, periodic lateralized epileptiform discharges (PLEDs), and seizures [43, 44]. Table 3.3 lists autoantibodies and their associated EEG findings [45–50].

Electromyography

History

The groundwork set by Alessandro Volta and Luigi Galvani paved the way for later visionaries in the field of peripheral electrodiagnosis [51, 52]. In 1833, Guillaume-Benjamin Duchenne used cloth-covered electrodes to stimulate nerves from the surface of the skin [53, 54]. Later, in 1850, Helmholtz successfully measured the conduction velocity of a nerve impulse of a frog, and later a human median nerve [54, 55]. In 1882, Wilhelm Erb devised a formula for polar contraction in normal and abnormal nerve states, and is generally cited as the founder of classic electrodiagnostics [54, 56]. On the electromyography front, a sensitive recording apparatus was needed for progress in the study of muscle action potentials. In 1922, Herbert Spencer Gasser and Joseph Erlanger overcame the limitations of a galvanometer with the advent of a cathode ray oscilloscope and laid the ground of the modern electrodiagnostic era [54, 57]. The first electromyogram (EMG) in a patient was performed by R. Proebster in 1928 and, following this, the field continued to expand into common clinical use [54, 58].

The demand for electrical testing of peripheral nerves grew with the two World Wars as physicians treating war casualties needed to know the extent of damaged nerves and the status of regeneration. This sparked a greater interest in the field and the need for peripheral diagnostics was realized. The First International Congress of Electromyography was held in 1961 in Pavia, Italy, and helped standardize values and the understanding of current peripheral electrodiagnostic studies [54]. Today, we continue to use electromyography and nerve conduction measurements to aid in the diagnosis of peripheral nervous system disorders.

Table 3.2 Cancer treatments and their associated EEG findings

Cancer treatment	EEG findings
Busulfan	Diffuse and focal delta
	Resolves within days of treatment discontinuation
	Seizures common and require prophylactic antiepileptic drug administration
Chimeric antigen receptor T-cell therapy	Slow background activity
	Epileptogenic discharges and increased seizure frequency
Cytarabine	Diffuse theta and delta activity
Ifosfamide	Slow alpha rhythm with increased theta and delta
	Triphasic waves
	Epileptogenic discharges and increased seizure frequency
	EEG and encephalopathy improve with benzodiazepine administration
Interferons	Diffuse theta and delta activity
	FIRDA activity
Methotrexate	Both diffuse and localized delta activity
	Seizure incidence increased
Pacitaxel	Diffuse theta activity
Vincristine	Diffuse theta and delta activity
	Epileptogenic discharges
	Increased seizure frequency with focal seizures

FIRDA frontal intermittent rhythmic delta activity

Table 3.3 Autoantibodies and their associated EEG findings

Antibody	Associated cancers	EEG findings
Anti-Hu	Small cell lung cancer	10% EEGs abnormal Temporal, bitemporal, or multifocal epileptiform discharges Seizures, epilepsia partialis continua, status epilepticus
Anti-Ma	Testicular germ cell tumor Breast cancer Non-small cell lung cancer	Epileptiform discharges Seizures and status epilepticus
NMDA	Ovarian teratoma	Irregular or rhythmic delta activity Extreme delta brush pattern Up to 70% with seizures or status epilepticus Tonic, focal, or generalized seizures
AMPA	Thymus Breast Lung	Temporal or bitemporal epileptiform discharges or seizures Diffuse, focal, or multifocal slow activity
GABA-B	Small cell lung cancer	Diffuse slow activity PLEDs Up to 100% with seizures
VGKC	Small cell lung cancer Often no tumor found	Temporal or bitemporal epileptiform discharges Faciobrachial dystonic seizures, tonic seizures, temporal seizures Diffuse slow activity

NMDA N-methyl D-aspartate, *AMPA* α-amino-3-hydroxy-5-methyl-4-isoxazolepropionic acid, *GABA-B* γ-Aminobutyric acid, Type B, *VGKC* voltage-gated potassium channel, *PLEDs* periodic lateralized epileptiform discharges

Technical Component

EMG is a method of recording motor unit potentials with extracellular electrodes. This study is typically performed after a nerve conduction study (NCS) has narrowed the clinical diagnosis and suggested muscles that may be pathologically involved. To perform an EMG, a needle electrode is inserted into the muscle of interest. See Fig. 3.1. The needle may have a reference electrode embedded within it (concentric needle) or a monopolar needle with a surface skin reference electrode can be used. The tip of the needle is the active recording electrode and a triphasic waveform is produced as the muscle action potential approaches, reaches, and leaves the recording electrode. The needle is connected to an EMG machine which records and amplifies the signal and provides a visual and auditory representation of the signal [54, 59].

To perform the test, a needle electrode is placed in the muscle and electrical activity is noted during the insertion. Insertional activity from initial needle insertion should be only a few hundred milliseconds in duration. Insertional activity can be classified as normal, decreased (seen in fibrotic muscle disease) or increased (seen in denervated muscle). Next, the muscle is evaluated while it is at rest for any spontaneous activity. All muscle fibers of a given motor unit will fire at the same time as action potentials are an all-or-none response. Damaged and denervated muscle fibers become unstable and no longer fire with the rest of their motor unit. These damaged fibers can fire spontaneously with no external stimuli, producing spontaneous activity. Fibrillation potentials and positive sharp waves are the most common findings when assessing for spontaneous activity, and typically signify active denervation [54, 59, 60]. The patient is then asked to perform mild voluntary contraction

of the muscle to evaluate motor unit potentials. Motor unit action potentials (MUAP) have typical morphology and characteristics. The duration reflects the number of muscle fibers within the motor unit and is typically 5–15 ms from initial take-off to the return to baseline. The number of phases, or times the waveform crosses baseline, is typically 2–4 in normal MUAPs. Polyphasia can be seen in both neuropathic and myopathic disorders. The amplitude of a MUAP is typically 100 µV–2 mV, and reflects only the few fibers that are nearest to the needle. After the MUAP is assessed with mild voluntary contraction, the patient is asked to perform maximal voluntary contraction of the muscle in order to evaluate recruitment and interference. Normally with muscle contracture, motor units can increase muscle force by increasing the firing rate or by recruiting additional motor units to fire. Decreased recruitment occurs when there is a loss of MUAPs, typically through axonal loss or conduction block, where additional units cannot be recruited easily. In contrast, increased or early recruitment typically occurs with myopathic processes where the individual muscle fibers within a unit cannot produce enough force and require additional motor units to generate a small amount of force. Once all of these factors are evaluated, the needle is moved to another location to repeat the above maneuver. The needle electrode samples muscle motor unit potentials in close proximity to the location of needle insertion; thus, multiple sites must be examined to have a thorough sampling of an area of interest. Typically, sampling is done in at least four directions from any given puncture site and multiple puncture sites are selected in one or several muscles of interest [54, 59, 60].

NCS can be performed to evaluate both nerve compound motor action potentials (CMAP) and sensory nerve action potentials (SNAP). CMAPs are measured in millivolts

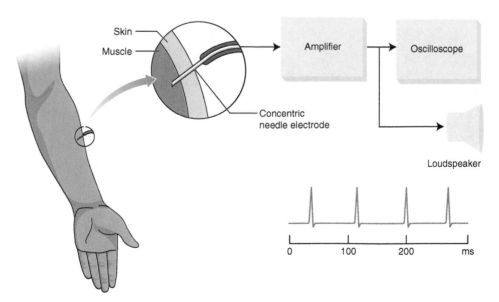

Fig. 3.1 Electromyography showing a needle insertion with EMG tracing

(mV) and are very large compared to SNAPs which are measured in microvolts (μV). While these have some differences in interpretation, much of the technical components remain the same [54, 59].

A stimulating probe is typically used with fixed surface electrodes that consist of a cathode (negative pole) and anode (positive pole) that are two to three centimeters apart. The cathode is positioned closer to the recording site. An electrical current is introduced into the stimulating probe. The current flows from the anode to the cathode, collecting negative charges between the cathode and the underlying nerve surface and depolarizing the underlying nerve. To record the stimulus for a motor nerve, an active recording surface electrode is placed over the belly of a muscle innervated by the nerve of interest, and a second inactive recording surface electrode is placed over the tendon of the muscle. When a stimulating current is given from the stimulating probe, the nerve is depolarized and the propagating muscle action potential is recorded at active recording electrode which is at the motor end point. See Fig. 3.2. Sensory nerves can be stimulated orthodromically (distal-to-proximal or in the direction of sensory flow) or antidromically (proximal-to-distal or opposite of the direction of sensory flow). Orthodromic recording is more commonly used; the active recording surface electrode is placed over the nerve and the second, inactive, recording surface electrode is placed at a remote site. Again, the stimulating probe depolarizes the nerve and propagates an action potential recorded at the given location on the sensory nerve [54, 59].

Several parameters are recorded and analyzed in a NCS. Amplitude (measured from baseline to the negative peak) reflects the number of muscle fibers that are depolarized. Duration (measured from the initial deflection from baseline to the first crossing of baseline) is a measure of synchrony of the muscle fibers. Conduction velocity (the distance traveled divided by the nerve conduction time) measures the speed of the fastest conducting axons. Latency (onset latency the time from the stimulus to the initial deflection from baseline), or peak latency (the time from the stimulus to the midpoint of the first negative peak) reflects the time from stimulation until a response is recorded at recording electrode. With motor studies, the distal motor latency includes the conduction time along the distal nerve, the neuromuscular junction (NMJ) transmission time, and the muscle depolarization time, necessitating two stimulation sites in order to subtract the time across the NMJ and muscle. With sensory studies, only one stimulation is needed to measure the latency and velocity [60].

There are several basic abnormal nerve conduction patterns. With neuropathic lesions one can see axonal loss, with reduced amplitude being the primary finding, or demyelination, with slowed velocity and latency. In myopathic disorders, the sensory NCS remain normal, as do the distal latencies and conduction velocities, with an occasional decrease in CMAP amplitude. These patterns are important in understanding etiologies of disease and correlating this with the clinical picture. See Table 3.4.

Indications and Contraindications

NCS and EMG are used to diagnose disorders of the peripheral nervous system (PNS), including disorders of primary motor neurons (anterior horn cells), sensory neurons (dorsal root ganglia), nerve roots, brachial and lumbosacral plexuses, peripheral nerves, neuromuscular junctions, and muscles. Patients with peripheral pain, paresthesias, sensory loss, atrophy, and weakness are routinely tested via EMG and NCS in order to better delineate an etiology and treatment plan. EMG and NCS have become a staple in our armamentarium and continue to provide useful diagnostic information in cancer patients.

At this time, there are no true contraindications of NCS. They are routinely performed in patients with pacemakers, cochlear implants, vagus nerve stimulators, deep brain stimulators, and other electric hardware as there are insufficient data to suggest significant risk to the patient [54, 59]. Although there is no clearly defined risk, a discussion with the patient's cardiologist may be advised if the NCS is to be performed close to the chest wall, or if dysfunction of the pacemaker may be life threatening [61, 62].

Patients with a bleeding tendency should be screened prior to performing routine EMG examination. The study maybe contraindicated in patients with untreated hemophilia or severe thrombocytopenia (typically considered platelets <20,000/mm [3]). Patients with iatrogenic blood thinning due to oral or intravenous anticoagulation should not

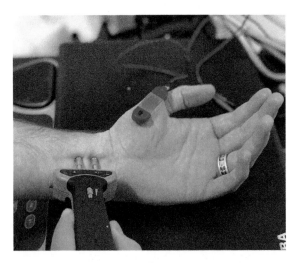

Fig. 3.2 Nerve conduction velocity. Depicting the stimulator with recording electrodes on the thenar eminence

Table 3.4 Comparison of neuropathy versus myopathy

	NCV	CMAP	SNAP	MUAP
Neuropathy—axonal	Normal	Decreased	Decreased	Large
Neuropathy—demyelinating	Decreased	Normal	Normal	Normal
Myopathy	Normal	Decreased	Normal	Small

NCV nerve conduction velocity, *CMAP* compound muscle action potential, *SNAP* sensory nerve action potential, *MUAP* motor unit action potential

undergo EMG until there is some degree of reversal of the prothrombin time or partial thromboplastin time. In addition to bleeding tendency, EMG should not be performed in an area with local skin or soft tissue infection as there is a risk of bacteremia [54].

Local Cancer Invasion

Tumors can enter the peripheral nervous system by direct invasion or hematogenous spread. The tumor can then externally compress the nerve fibers or invade them. Neural compression is more common with many cancers causing local trauma to the nerve with resultant neurologic symptoms and deficits. Neural invasion is less common but has been demonstrated with prostate cancer, breast cancer, lung cancer, pancreatic cancer, and lymphoma [63].

Leptomeningeal metastasis or epidural tumors can cause radiculopathy with irritation or direct compression of the nerve roots. Plexopathies are quite frequent in approximately 1% of cancer patients with some metastatic involvement of their plexi [64]. Invasion of the lumbosacral plexus is more common and is often due to direct extension of abdominal and pelvic tumors including cervical cancer, colorectal cancer, bladder cancer, and retroperitoneal sarcomas. Invasion of the brachial plexus is typically due to breast and lung cancer. The lower trunk of the brachial plexus is most commonly involved due to its proximity to the lateral axillary lymph nodes [64]. Peripheral neuropathies are less frequent, but can be seen with peripheral nervous system infiltration from lymphoma called neurolymphomatosis. This is a well-known disorder and has been described with both B-cell and T-cell lymphomas [65]. It tends to invade multiple nerves or nerve roots and presents clinically as a polyneuropathy or polyradiculopathy [66]. Mononeuropathies are less common with local cancer invasion, but can occur with extension of bony metastasis. Malignant nerve sheath tumors that typically occur in the setting of neurofibromatosis I, or as a result of radiation therapy, can also cause a mononeuropathy [65].

The neurologic symptoms and deficits depend on the topography of the nerve involvement. Electrodiagnostic testing with EMG and NCS can be valuable in localizing nerve involvement to determine if the pathology is in the root, plexus, peripheral nerve, or neuromuscular junction.

Although neurophysiologic testing does not distinguish local cancer invasion from other types of nerve damage, it can help localize the region of pathology so that a specific region can be imaged or biopsied for further investigation and prognostication.

Paraneoplastic and Antibody Mediated

Most paraneoplastic disorders begin acutely or subacutely and progress over time often with some stabilization late in the disease process. The current concept of paraneoplastic syndromes is that the primary tumor ectopically expresses an antigen that is identical in structure to a neural antigen but seen by the host immune system as foreign, thus eliciting an immune attack on both the antigen and the neural structure. The central nervous system or peripheral nervous system can be attacked, leaving the patient with debilitating symptoms. The incidence of paraneoplastic peripheral neuropathy is thought to be 6–8%, with most paraneoplastic neuropathies being sensorimotor and axonal [67]. Paraneoplastic disorders can also occur at the level of the neuromuscular junction or muscle. While antibodies and tissue pathology are more specific, EMG and NCS can be a valuable tool in the diagnosis of peripheral paraneoplastic disorders. Here we describe some common paraneoplastic and antibody-mediated disorders of the peripheral nervous system (motor neuron, nerve, NMJ and muscle) and their associated neurophysiologic findings. See Table 3.5.

Acute Inflammatory Demyelinating Polyneuropathy

An acute inflammatory demyelinating polyneuropathy (AIDP or Guillain–Barre syndrome) with acute to subacute weakness and sensory features has an increased incidence in patients with Hodgkin lymphoma as well as various types of solid cancers [68, 69]. With AIDP, typical findings include prolonged or absent F waves followed by increased distal latencies and conduction block of motor responses. Significant slowing of the motor nerve conduction velocities is not seen until later in the disease course. Sensory NCS can demonstrate absent or slowed conduction velocities. The needle EMG often remains normal or only with decreased recruitment [70].

Table 3.5 Autoantibody, paraneoplastic, and paraproteinemic diseases of the peripheral nervous system and associated EMG/NCV findings

	Associated cancer	NCV	EMG
AIDP	Hodgkin lymphoma, lung cancer, breast cancer	Prolonged F-wave	Normal or decreased recruitment
		Increased distal latencies	
		Conduction block	
CIDP	Lymphoma, leukemia, melanoma, paraproteinemia	Absent or prolonged F-wave	
		Increased distal latencies	
		Abnormal temporal dispersion, conduction block	
Paraproteinemic neuropathy	Amyloid, multiple myeloma, MGUS, Waldenström's macroglobulinemia	Decreased motor and sensory CMAP	Spontaneous activity an acute denervation
Anti-CV2	Small cell lung cancer	Decrease motor sensory CMAP	
Anti-Hu	Small cell lung cancer	Decreased sensory CMAP; Normal motor CMAP	Normal or active denervation
Mononeuritis multiplex	Vasculitic neuropathy, small cell lung cancer, uterine cancer, lymphoma, prostate cancer	Decreased sensory CMAP	
Neuromyotonia	Thymoma, lymphoma, small cell lung cancer		Spontaneous irregular firing of single or MUAP
			Persist during sleep and general anesthesia
Stiff person syndrome	Breast cancer, small cell lung cancer, Hodgkin lymphoma, colon cancer		Sustained continuous MUAP, disappeared during sleep and general anesthesia
Lambert-Eaton myasthenic syndrome	Small cell lung cancer	Decrement with slow rate repetitive nerve stimulation; 3–5 Hz	Single-fiber EMG-increased jitter
		High rate stimulation; 20–50 Hz results in increased CMAP	
Myasthenia gravis	Thymoma, lymphoma	Slow rate repetitive nerve stem; 3–5 Hz decrement in CMAP amplitude	Single-fiber EMG-increased jitter
		High rate stimulation-no increment	

AIDP acute inflammatory demyelinating polyneuropathy; *CIDP* chronic inflammatory demyelinating polyneuropathy; *CMAP* compound muscle action potential; *EMG* electromyography; *MUAP* motor unit action potential

Chronic Inflammatory Demyelinating Polyneuropathy

Chronic inflammatory demyelinating polyneuropathy (CIDP) has been reported in patients with solid and liquid tumors including adenocarcinomas, melanoma, and paraproteinemias [71, 72]. Clinically, these patients have slowly progressive sensory changes with large fiber sensory modalities being most affected. CIDP is distinguished from AIDP on the basis of a prolonged and relapsing course, enlargement of nerves, and responsiveness to corticosteroids. Progression tends to be in a length-dependent manner for the sensory changes. The motor abnormalities are typically not as pronounced but are frequently present. The neuropathy may precede the discovery of the neoplasm. Similar to what is seen with acute inflammatory demyelinating polyneuropathy, the electrophysiologic studies demonstrate prolonged or absent F waves, increased distal latencies, abnormal temporal dispersion, and conduction block of motor responses [73].

Paraproteinemic Neuropathies

The prevalence of peripheral neuropathy is ten times higher in patients with paraproteinemias than it is in the general population. Peripheral neuropathy can occur with primary amyloidosis, multiple myeloma, monoclonal gammopathy of unknown significance, Waldenstrom macroglobulinemia, and other rare conditions. Paraproteinemic neuropathies are a heterogeneous group of disorders but with a great degree of overlap.

Patients with primary amyloidosis of the light chain type can develop a devastating peripheral neuropathy. The neuropathy consists of distal and symmetric progressive sensorimotor and autonomic dysfunction. The sensory symptoms are often small fiber predominant with persistent pain. Nerve conduction studies demonstrate decreased amplitude and, at times, mild slowing of conduction velocity consistent with axonal degeneration due to invasion of the nerves by amyloid. EMG can demonstrate increased spontaneous activity and evidence of acute denervation [67, 74].

Peripheral neuropathy can occur in multiple myeloma (MM) in several settings. With typical osteolytic MM, patients can have a mild sensorimotor axonal neuropathy with decreased motor and sensory amplitudes or a purely sensory axonal neuropathy with only sensory involvement. A demyelinating type of primary motor neuropathy can also be seen and resembles AIDP or CIDP as described above. Patients with MM associated with systemic amyloidosis can have prominent pain and small fiber sensory findings with electrophysiologic findings as seen in primary amyloidosis. Patients with atypical osteosclerotic myeloma tend to be younger and less ill. The neuropathy associated with osteosclerotic myeloma is chronic in nature with distal and symmetric sensorimotor changes. This neuropathy also resembles CIDP with a motor predominance and marked slowing in conduction velocities. These patients can develop a clinical syndrome (POEMS syndrome) with organomegaly, endocrinopathy, and skin changes [67, 74].

Patients with monoclonal gammopathy of unknown significance (MGUS) typically present with distal and symmetric chronic and progressive sensorimotor symptoms. Electrophysiologically, the peripheral neuropathy resembles a chronic inflammatory demyelinating polyneuropathy with slow motor nerve conduction velocities and increased distal latencies on NCS. Some MGUS patients have circulating anti-myelin-associated protein (anti-MAG) antibodies directed against peripheral nerve myelin. The majority of patients with anti-MAG antibodies have IgM-kappa monoclonal proteins in their serum [67, 74, 75].

Patients with Waldenstrom macroglobulinemia (WM) can develop symmetric and distal sensorimotor changes and a primarily demyelinating sensorimotor polyneuropathy on electrophysiologic testing. Similar to MGUS, some WM patients have circulating anti-MAG antibodies damaging the myelin and causing increased distal latency and slowed conduction velocity in motor and sensory nerves. Occasionally, WM is associated with an axonal pattern of neuropathy [67, 74, 75].

Anti-CV2

Anti-CV2 antibodies are seen in association with small cell lung cancer and can cause a variety of nervous system maladies including cerebellar degeneration, peripheral neuropathy, and uveitis. In up to 20% of patients, the anti-Hu antibody is also expressed. Patients with anti-CV2 typically have symmetric distal length-dependent sensory loss in all modalities with concomitant motor weakness. Electrophysiologically, a sensory motor axonal polyneuropathy is seen, but at times there are some demyelinating features. NCS demonstrates decreased amplitude of sensory and motor responses with some decrease in velocity of these responses [76].

Anti-Hu

Anti-Hu antibodies are now recognized as a common cause of paraneoplastic neuronopathy that affects the dorsal root ganglia. It is most commonly associated with small cell lung cancer, but is also present with other malignancies. The onset is typically rapid and painful but, unlike classic peripheral neuropathies, this neuronopathy can be asymmetric or non-length dependent in some patients. All sensory modalities can be affected, but the proprioceptive loss can be so profound that patients can have debilitating sensory ataxia. Anti-Hu was once thought to be only a sensory disorder, but evidence shows that some patients have a mixed sensorimotor picture [77, 78]. Electrophysiologic studies demonstrate axonal degeneration with low amplitude or absent sensory action potentials and preserved or abnormal motor responses on NCS. EMG is typically normal but, at times, can show signs of active denervation including fibrillation potentials and positive sharp waves [77, 79].

Mononeuritis Multiplex

A vasculitic neuropathy can be seen in association with malignancies. Vasculitic neuropathies typically present as mononeuritis multiplex, most commonly with asymmetric and patchy changes in sensory and/or motor nerves. The symptoms can occur acutely or chronically, and are commonly seen with solid tumors, including small cell lung cancer, prostate cancer, uterine cancer, and lymphomas [67, 80]. Anti-Hu antibodies are sometimes associated with this disorder. On NCS, a primarily axonal neuropathy is seen with low amplitude sensory and compound muscle action potentials with minimal reduction of conduction velocities [79, 81].

Neuromyotonia

Neuromyotonia is a disorder characterized by peripheral nerve hyperexcitability due to spontaneous firing of motor unit action potentials. Clinically, patients can present with slow relaxation of muscles, cramps, stiffness, or myokymia. It is thought to be autoimmune mediated and can be associated with voltage-gated potassium channel antibodies or amphiphysin antibodies [67, 82]. Thymoma is the most common cause of paraneoplastic neuromyotonia, which can also be seen with lymphoma and small cell lung cancer [83, 84]. On EMG there is spontaneous irregular firing of single or multiple motor units at a rate of 150–300 Hz that can persist even in sleep and under general anesthesia [67].

Stiff Person Syndrome

Stiff person syndrome is characterized by painful muscle stiffness and rigidity typically involving truncal musculature. It can be autoimmune in nature and most commonly associated with glutamic acid decarboxylase antibodies. The paraneoplastic version of the disorder can have glutamic acid decarboxylase antibodies or more commonly amphiphysin antibodies. Breast cancer, small cell lung cancer, Hodgkin disease, and colon cancer are commonly associated cancers with the paraneoplastic version. On EMG, there are sustained continuous motor unit action potentials that disappear during sleep and with general anesthesia [67, 85].

Lambert–Eaton Myasthenic Syndrome

Lambert–Eaton Myasthenic Syndrome (LEMS) is one of the most common paraneoplastic syndromes although it can also be autoimmune in nature. About one-half of patients with LEMS have an underlying malignancy, with small cell lung cancer being the most likely culprit. Patients with paraneoplastic LEMS have V/Q voltage-gated calcium channel antibodies that bind presynaptically at the cholinergic junction preventing entry of calcium into the terminal axon and inhibiting the release of acetylcholine [86]. Patients present with fatigue and muscle weakness that is typically more proximal and can improve with repeated use. With LEMS, the compound muscle action potential in hand muscles are small at baseline and increase dramatically after exercise. With repetitive nerve stimulation at a slow rate of 3–5 Hz, there is a decrement in the CMAP amplitude due to failure of the neuromuscular junctions. When stimulated at a higher rate of 20–50 Hz, this is overcome with increased release of calcium and there is an increase in the CMAP amplitude. An increase greater than 100% in most muscles tested is suggestive of LEMS. Single-fiber EMG (SFEMG) can also be performed to help establish the diagnosis. With SFEMG, the variability in the timing of discharges of fibers is compared and an increase in this timing, known as jitter, demonstrates the insecurity of the neuromuscular junction [67, 87].

Myasthenia Gravis

In contrast to LEMS, myasthenia gravis (MG) is not considered a classic paraneoplastic syndrome because only a small portion of patients with the disease harbor a malignancy. Thymoma and lymphoma are the most common malignancies associated with the disease. When present, acetylcholine antibodies can aid in the diagnosis of MG but the antibodies do not distinguish paraneoplastic from non-paraneoplastic forms of MG. Clinically, patients have weakness in frequently used muscles and the weakness progresses throughout the day. Similar to LEMS, with repetitive nerve stimulation at a slow rate of 3–5 Hz, there is a decrement in the CMAP amplitude due to failure of the neuromuscular junctions. However, there is no increment with faster stimulation as seen with LEMS. Increased jitter is also seen with MG, again demonstrating the insecurity of the neuromuscular junction [67, 87].

Myopathies

Inflammatory Myopathy

Of the inflammatory myopathies, dermatomyositis (DM) and polymyositis (PM) have a clear relation to malignancy while this relationship is less clear with inclusion body myositis (IBM). DM and PM are associated with a wide range of cancers with lung cancer, ovarian cancer, and non-Hodgkin lymphoma being the most common [88]. With both DM and PM, patients have proximal symmetric weakness that typically evolves over weeks to months; muscle tenderness and pain are associated with this weakness. While muscle biopsy provides the definitive diagnosis, EMG can be a valuable tool in diagnosing inflammatory myopathies. With DM and PM, the EMG demonstrates a myopathic pattern with small amplitude short duration muscle potentials with early recruitment. Later in the disease, fibrillation potentials and positive sharp waves can be seen [67].

Necrotizing Myopathy

Necrotizing myopathy is a rare disorder that has been shown to have an association with gastrointestinal adenocarcinoma, transitional cell carcinoma, prostatic carcinoma, and non-small cell carcinoma. Patients have a rapid and progressive syndrome with symmetric proximal weakness and pain. EMG studies in patients with necrotizing myopathy demonstrate abnormal spontaneous activity and decreased amplitude and duration of the motor unit potentials [89, 90].

Therapy-Induced Pathology

Chemotherapy Induced Pathology

Peripheral neuropathy is a common side effect of multiple chemotherapeutic agents. The taxanes, vinca alkaloids, and platinum compounds are the most notorious classes of agents that produce neuropathic side effects, but other less commonly known agents can be neuropathic as well. There are several patterns of disease caused by these drugs. While many cause diffuse polyneuropathies, some can cause myositis while sparing the peripheral nerves. EMG and NCS findings can be useful in diagnosing and following the recovery of these pathologic changes. Table 3.6 lists electromyographic findings associated with some common cancer treatments [91–97].

Radiation-Induced Pathology

Radiation therapy (RT) is frequently used as adjunctive treatment for malignancy. RT causes damage to both normal and abnormal cells often leaving unwanted side effects. Ionizing radiation causes cellular damage by breaking DNA, damaging RNA, proteins, and lipids, and by stimulating apoptosis [63]. Classically, there are three stages of radiation damage: acute (during the actual course of radiation), early-delayed (within weeks), or late-delayed (within months to years). While the acute and early-delayed stages are often reversible, the late-delayed stage is often chronic and can be progressive with few treatment options. The peripheral nervous system is more resistant than the central nervous system to the adverse side effects of radiation therapy, but despite this, peripheral nerve damage is a frequent complication of RT. The major sites of damage include the brachial plexus (typically after lymphoma, breast, or lung cancer treatment) and the lumbosacral plexus (after pelvic and abdominal treatment for numerous cancers) [63]. Distinguishing local cancer recurrence from radiation-induced plexopathy can be difficult. The clinical picture remains very important as several clinical factors aid in determining the diagnosis. With radiation-induced plexopathy, electromyography and nerve conduction studies can also be useful.

Myokymia on EMG examination may be the single most helpful electrodiagnostic finding in differentiating local cancer recurrence versus radiation-induced plexopathy [59, 98, 99]. Myokymic discharges are caused by the same motor unit and are groups of rhythmic spontaneous repetitive discharges (grouped fasciculations). With myokymia, the firing frequency is typically 5–60 Hz and the firing frequency between bursts is much slower. Myokymic discharges are likely due to spontaneous depolarization along demyelinated nerve segments. Clinically, myokymia looks like continuous involuntary rippling movement of a muscle [59]. Other EMG abnormalities are often seen in patients with radiation-induced injury. Fibrillation potentials, decreased motor unit potential amplitude, and increased motor unit potential duration are frequent findings associated with radiation injury but are nonspecific [99].

NCS abnormalities are also seen in patients with radiation plexopathy. These are not specific and can also be seen with direct neoplastic invasion. One such finding is conduction block due to an acquired demyelinating process. Conduction block is defined as a drop in compound motor action potentials amplitude of at least 20% between proximal and distal stimulation sites. Conduction block is frequently present in early-delayed and late-delayed radiation injury, but at times can also be seen with local neoplastic invasion. Sensory nerve conduction studies can have decreased amplitudes or be absent in patients with radiation injury [59, 98]. While NCS sensory changes are present in local neoplastic invasion, the incidence of abnormal NCS studies is greater in patients with radiation-induced injury [98].

Lumbar Puncture

History

The presence of fluid surrounding the brain was known for centuries. It was described by Hippocrates in the fourth-century B.C., Galen in the second-century A.D., and Valsalva in the 1600s [100]. In 1764, Contungo described fluid within the ventricles and subarachnoid space of 20 adults on whom he did lumbar taps [101]. Later in 1825, Magendie described tapping the cisterna magna in animals and postulated that there was continuity of the subarachnoid space around the brain and spinal cord. However, it was Axel Key and Magnus Retzius in 1875 who discovered what we know about cisternal anatomy today [102]. Soon after, Quincke developed a procedure using a percutaneous needle with a stylet to investigate hydrocephalus and tuberculous meningitis. He recorded the opening pressure with a manometer and was the first to study cell counts, protein, and glucose within the cerebrospinal fluid [103]. Nearly 50 years later, Merritt and Fremont-Smith published nearly 20 years of experience with cerebrospinal fluid studies at Boston City Hospital, providing a valuable reference point [104]. In the past century, the field has further advanced with radioisotopes, polymerase chain reaction (PCR), cytology,

Table 3.6 Cancer treatments and their associated EMG findings

Drug class	Drug names	Common uses	Mechanism of action	Clinical findings	EMG findings	NCS FINDINGS
Vinca alkaloids	Vincristine, vinblastine, vindesine, vinorelbine	Leukemia, lymphoma	Binds intracellular tubulin and inhibits polymerization	Symmetric distal sensory changes ±motor symptoms	EMG: rarely pathologic spontaneous activity in distal muscles	NCS: Axonal neuropathy with reduced amplitude of sensory > motor compound action potentials with late demyelinating features
				Autonomic neuropathy is common. "Coasting" phenomenon—worsening of symptoms despite withdrawal of agent		
Taxanes	Paclitaxel, docetaxel, abraxane, tesetaxel	Breast, ovarian, prostate, bladder, esophageal, head and neck cancers	Microtubule stabilizing agent that interferes with mitotic spindles during mitosis	Symmetric or asymmetric distal sensory changes, mixed small and large fiber	EMG: pathologic spontaneous activity in distal muscles, rarely myopathic changes on EMG	NCS: Axonal neuropathy with reduced amplitude and relative sparing of velocity of sensory > motor compound action potentials
				Motor symptoms are uncommon and mild but can include foot drop		
Platinum compounds	Cisplatin, carboplatin, oxaliplatin	Ovarian, bladder, testicular, lung cancers	DNA is damaged by intrastrand and interstrand crosslinks which induces apoptosis	Symmetric distal sensory changes—primarily large fiber modalities affected. Motor symptoms are extremely rare. "coasting" phenomenon with worsening of symptoms despite withdrawal of agent	EMG: no changes	NCS: Axonal neuropathy with reduced amplitude of sensory compound action potentials with late demyelinating features
Polysulfonated urea	Suramin	Prostate cancer	Inhibits reverse transcriptase	Symmetric distal sensory changes—mixed small and large fiber modalities. Motor symptoms are common but mild	EMG: rarely pathologic spontaneous activity in distal muscles	NCS: Axonal neuropathy with reduced amplitude of sensory and motor compound action potentials
				Guillian-Barre-like syndrome with severe, rapid predominantly motor demyelinating neuropathy can be seen, albeit rare	With the Guillian-Barre-like syndrome there is prolongation of F-wave latencies, decreased sensory and motor compound action potential amplitude and velocities, and temporal dispersion	
Angiogenesis inhibitors	Thalidomide	Myeloma, lymphoma	Inhibits angiogenesis	Symmetric sensory changes—mixed small and large fiber modalities affected. Motor symptoms are uncommon but mild	EMG: rarely pathologic spontaneous activity in distal muscles	NCS: Axonal neuropathy with reduced amplitude of sensory > motor compound action potentials

(continued)

Table 3.6 (continued)

Drug class	Drug names	Common uses	Mechanism of action	Clinical findings	EMG findings	NCS FINDINGS
Proteasome inhibitors	Bortezomib	Myeloma, lymphoma	Breakdown of intracellular molecules	Symmetric sensory changes with small > large fiber modalities affected	EMG: no changes	NCS: Axonal neuropathy with reduced amplitude of sensory compound action potentials
Monoclonal antibody	Ipilimumab	Melanoma	Targets human cytotoxic T-lymphocyte-associated antigen	Symmetric distal sensory changes. Motor symptoms can be seen	EMG: no changes	NCS: Sensorimotor polyneuropathy with demyelinating features with decreased amplitude and conduction velocities with conduction block
Nucleoside analogs	Gemcitabine	Pancreatic cancer	Replaces cytidine in DNA replication causing faulty DNA and apoptosis	Painful, symmetric, mild proximal weakness	EMG: motor unit action potentials with small amplitude, short duration, and early recruitment consistent with myopathic changes	

and other assays leading to widespread use of lumbar puncture as an essential tool for the diagnosis of many neurologic conditions [102].

Technical Component

A lumbar puncture is best performed with the patient in the lateral recumbent position with the craniospinal axis parallel to the floor and the patient in the fetal position with the head, knees, and torso flexed. The most superior part of the iliac crest is palpated and correlates with the L4 vertebral body at midline. Under sterile conditions and after local anesthesia, the spinal needle is advanced at the L3/L4 or L4/L5 vertebral interspace, angling slightly towards the head. Once the subarachnoid space is reached, the patient extends legs and a manometer is placed on the hub of the spinal needle to measure opening pressure. After pressure is measured, cerebrospinal fluid (CSF) is drained into sterile tubes. A total of 5–15 mL of fluid is typically collected during a routine lumbar puncture. However, in the workup of neurologic malignancy, more CSF may increase the yield and at least 10 mL should be collected for cytologic evaluation [102, 105, 106]. Fluoroscopic-guided lumbar puncture may be required if traditional lumbar puncture is failed at the bedside. If lumbar puncture is not possible, then cisternal puncture or cervical puncture may be considered. In modern day, these are done under fluoroscopy.

Indications and Contraindications

Lumbar puncture is useful in the diagnosis of many neurologic conditions including but not limited to: bacterial meningitis, viral meningitis, fungal meningitis, mycobacterial meningitis, vasculitis, subarachnoid hemorrhage, normal pressure hydrocephalus, central demyelinating disease, Guillain–Barre syndrome, central nervous system malignancy, carcinomatous meningitis, autoimmune encephalitis, and paraneoplastic encephalitis. The diagnostic role of lumbar puncture in neurologic malignancies will be discussed below.

There are several relative contraindications to lumbar puncture. Performing a lumbar puncture in a patient with preexisting increased intracranial pressure can precipitate deleterious consequences. Herniation syndromes can arise and can be life threatening. When increased intracranial pressure is suspected, computed tomography (CT) or magnetic resonance imaging (MRI) should be performed first to help assess the risk of herniation associated with lumbar puncture. Lumbar puncture in a patient with a focal mass with midline shift increases the risk of herniation and should be avoided [107].

Local skin infection, spinal epidural abscess, and epidural or vertebral malignancy in the lumbar region near the entry zone of the spinal needle is another relative contraindication. Performing a lumbar puncture through an infection, abscess, or malignancy can seed the CSF, increasing morbidity and mortality [102, 108].

Thrombocytopenia and anticoagulation also pose a risk when performing a lumbar puncture. It is generally advised to withhold lumbar puncture in patients who are actively bleeding, have platelets <50,000/μl, or an international normalized ratio (INR) >1.4. Aspirin and subcutaneous heparin at doses appropriate for deep vein thrombosis prophylaxis are not believed to pose a substantial risk [109–111]. Cisternal puncture is contraindicated in patients with an Arnold–Chiari malformation or posterior fossa tumor.

Composition of Cerebrospinal Fluid

CSF pressure is balanced carefully by the production from the choroid plexus and absorption from arachnoid granulations. Normal CSF opening pressure with a manometer while the patient is lying flat with legs extended is between 60 and 250 mm H_2O [112].

CSF is normal, clear, and colorless. Turbidity is rated from 0 to 4+ by most laboratories. Color is pathologic and can be due to infection, inflammation, or blood product. Three major pigments derived from red blood cells can be detected in CSF: oxyhemoglobin, bilirubin, and methemoglobin. Oxyhemoglobin is derived from lysed red blood cells and present in CSF by 2 h, peaks at 36 h, and typically disappears by 7 days. Bilirubin is first detected in CSF at about 10 h, reaches maximum in 48 h, and can persist up to 2–4 weeks after extensive bleeding. Oxyhemoglobin, and more so bilirubin, are the major pigments responsible for xanthochromia seen with subarachnoid blood. CSF bilirubin can be elevated with liver disease causing xanthochromia that can falsely mimic that found with subarachnoid blood. Methemoglobin, the latest byproduct of blood, is found in encapsulated subdural hematomas and in old loculated intracerebral hemorrhages [102].

Protein is largely excluded from the CSF by the blood–CSF barrier. The protein level in normal CSF is 20–45 mg/dl. A high protein level is nonspecific and can be due to an array of etiologies including but not limited to tumor, infection, trauma, stroke, hemorrhage, vasculitis, and demyelinating disease [105].

CSF glucose level is maintained by facilitated transport and simple diffusion. Glucose in CSF is derived from plasma glucose and is typically two-thirds of the plasma level. Thus, high or low glucose level should be corrected for serum glucose in order to make a proper assessment [105].

Under normal conditions, CSF is acellular. CSF can contain up to 5 white blood cells (WBC) per mm [3] and/or 5 red blood cells (RBC) per mm [3] without being considered pathologic. A cell count greater than this should be investigated. Unfortunately, not all lumbar punctures go as planned and interpreting a traumatic tap is often necessary.

Under normal conditions, there may be an increase of 1 WBC for every 700 RBC introduced into the CSF for a traumatic tap. If there is a significant anemia or leukocytosis, the following formula may be implemented: where WBC_{REAL} is the calculated WBC count of the CSF before the traumatic blood was added, WBC_{CSF} is the WBC count in the bloody spinal fluid, WBC_{SERUM} is the WBC count in the serum, RBC_{CSF} is the RBC count in the bloody spinal fluid, and RBC_{SERUM} is the RBC count in the serum [102].

$$WBC_{REAL} = WBC_{CSF} - (WBC_{SERUM} \times RBC_{CSF})/RBC_{SERUM}$$

Focal Mass and Leptomeningeal Involvement

Brain metastases are a common complication of cancer. The incidence is 9–17% although this number is thought to be low as the incidence of brain metastases is increasing [113]. This increase in incidence may be due, at least in part, to improved imaging techniques. Additionally, the incidence may be increasing as we provide systemic treatments that prolong life, allowing the cancer to disseminate to the brain [114]. Breast cancer, lung cancer, and melanoma are the leading cancers with brain metastasis, and account for over two-thirds of all metastases [113].

Leptomeningeal metastasis is diagnosed in nearly 5% of patients with cancer metastasis. Again, this number is thought to be low as it is found to be much higher at autopsy [115]. The largest risk factor for leptomeningeal metastasis is the presence of parenchymal brain metastasis [116]. Additionally, primary brain tumors including astrocytomas, meduloblastomas, ependymomas, pineoblastomas, and oligodendrogliomas can infiltrate the CSF [117].

With solid tumor invasion of the brain (primary brain tumors and parenchymal metastasis), the CSF typically has a normal cell count, although there can occasionally be a pleocytosis that is most commonly seen with tumors near the ventricular surface or with large infiltrating gliomas. There is often normal glucose but an elevated protein concentration. This is in contrast to leptomeningeal metastasis, which typically demonstrates a more profound pleocytosis (approximately 50%), elevated protein (approximately 75%), and decreased glucose (approximately 30–50%) [102, 118]. The pleocytosis is typically due to lymphocytes, although eosinophilia can be seen with acute lymphoblastic leukemia and Hodgkin lymphoma [119]. Elevated opening pressure is often seen with leptomeningeal metastasis (nearly 50%) and large solid tumors [102, 118]. Although most patients do not have all of these features, completely normal CSF is uncommon [120].

Cytology

Positive cytology remains the gold standard for diagnosis of malignancy in the CSF. Unfortunately, despite having a high specificity, the sensitivity of cytology is between 50 and 90%. With parenchymal involvement alone the sensitivity is even lower [121, 122]. This often necessitates repeat lumbar punctures that can be difficult for both the patient and the physician. Several steps can improve the sensitivity of cytology: (1) A minimum of 10 ml of CSF should be submitted for cytology evaluation, (2) specimens should be fixed in ethanol-based fixative for cytology and should be processed immediately and not left overnight in the laboratory, (3) CSF should be obtained closest to the symptomatic site (lumbar puncture for spinal imaging or clinical findings and cisternal or ventricular puncture for cranial imaging or clinical findings). If these measures continue to provide negative cytology in the setting of clinical suspicion for parenchymal or leptomeningeal involvement, a second tap should be performed, again with the aforementioned measures in place. Although some perform further taps, little additional benefit has been shown for subsequent samplings [122]. Despite these efforts, CSF cytology remains negative in up to 20% of patients with clinical or radiographically unequivocal leptomeningeal carcinomatosis [116, 122]. It is important to note that sensitivity of cytology is reduced in primary CNS lymphoma with recent exposure to corticosteroids, which causes cytolysis [123]. A recent pilot study revealed the utility of rare cell capture technology in the diagnosis of leptomeningeal metastasis from solid tumor with 100% sensitivity and 97% specificity [124].

Flow Cytometry

Flow cytometry is a technique used to measure multiple characteristics of individual cells within a heterogenous population. Immunophenotyping can then be done to determine the composition of a group of cells by detecting cellular protein expression [125]. These methods are particularly useful in determining metastasis from hematologic malignancies. CSF flow cytometry can help identify whether atypical lymphoid cells lines are monoclonal or polyclonal [114, 126]. It can be used as an adjunct to CSF cytology to help increase diagnostic accuracy as almost 50% of patients have a positive flow cytometry in the absence of positive cytology [127]. With cytology and adjunctive flow cytometry, up to 80% of lymphoma cases with CSF involvement can be detected with the first CSF sample. Although rare, peripheral blood of a patient with active systemic lymphoma can contaminate the CSF causing false-positive CSF results. Thus, using CSF from a traumatic tap should be avoided when sending for flow cytometry [127, 128].

After flow cytometry is performed, CSF immunoglobulin heavy chain (IgH) rearrangement testing can be used to analyze the clonality of the antibodies being produced. Using PCR analysis of CSF, regions of the IgH can be amplified. In cases of neoplastic proliferation of lymphocytes, a unique arrangement is produced, resulting in a single sharp band on agarose gel. Conversely, nonneoplastic proliferation of lymphocytes, as seen with inflammatory processes, will reflect a widened band with multiple heavy chain sequences [128]. IgH rearrangement studies in the CSF for the detection of monoclonal antibody production have reported sensitivity of nearly 60% and specificity of nearly 85%. Similar to what is seen with cytology, recent corticosteroid treatment reduces the sensitivity of this study.

Biomarkers

Tumor markers in CSF can be useful when cytology is negative. The most usefulness is found with organ-specific tumor markers such as prostate-specific antigen (PSA-prostate), carcinoembryonic antigen (CEA-colon), carcinoma antigen 15-3 (CA 15-3-breast), carcinoma antigen 125 (CA 125-ovarian), carcinoma antigen 19-9 (CA 19-9-pancreatic), carcinoma antigen 72-4 (CA 72-4-gastric), melanoma antigen recognized by T cells (MART-1-melanoma), alpha fetoprotein (AFP-germ cell), and beta human chorionic gonadotropin (BhCG-germ cell). These can be relatively specific for leptomeningeal involvement when elevated in the CSF with the absence or markedly elevated serum levels [129–139].

Other novel biomarkers have been investigated but need more data in order to be useful clinically. Molecules involved in tumor invasion, angiogenesis, and metastasis (e.g., vascular endothelial growth factor, cathepsins, matrix malloproteinases, and lipid-associated sialic acid) show some promise, but are not sensitive enough at this time to improve cytologic diagnosis [139–145]. With vascular endothelial growth factor (VEGF), the sensitivities were 51.4–100% and specificities 71–100% [126, 140]. Levels of Beta2-microglobulin may be elevated up to 68% in leukemia or lymphoma with CSF involvement, but the false-positive rate was found to be as high as 25% [128]. Additionally, other biomarkers pertaining to brain metabolism have been studied but again with mixed results. In the brain, aerobic isozymes of LDH dominate (LD1 and LD2), reflecting the brain's dependence on aerobic metabolism. With malignant disease states, however, there is increased anaerobic LDH isozymes (LD4 and LD5). Patients with CNS malignancy were found to have higher LD5 anaerobic isozymes, with a 93% sensitivity. Unfortunately, LD5 elevation is also seen in bacterial meningitis and other conditions thus rendering this nonspecific [128, 146]. Proteomic analysis of CSF has revealed several proteins that are differentially expressed in different tumor types. With CNS lymphoma there is some hope that a serine protease inhibitor, antithrombin III, may be useful clinically. Antithrombin III levels above 1.2 g/ml were able to detect CNS lymphoma with 75% sensitivity and 98% specificity [128, 140]. Further investigation of these biomarkers is necessary before they gain wide clinical use.

Paraneoplastic

Paraneoplastic neurologic syndromes are characterized by indolent tumor growth, inflammation of the nervous system, and immune activation against antigens shared by the tumor cell and the nervous system [147]. Paraneoplastic reactions can cause a wide array of neurologic syndromes encompassing the central nervous system and peripheral nervous system, including but not limited to limbic encephalitis, brainstem encephalitis, encephalomyelitis, cerebellar degeneration, and peripheral nerve disorders. Serum should be evaluated for suspected paraneoplastic neurologic syndromes but CSF studies for anti-Hu, anti-Yo, anti-Ma, anti-Ri, anti-CV2, and amphiphysin can be checked as well [148].

Abnormalities in the CSF can be found early on in paraneoplastic neurologic disease and can provide useful adjunctive information. In the vast majority of patients, the CSF is abnormal. Elevated white blood cells (>5 cells/mm [3]) are found in 47% of patients with lumbar punctures performed within one month of clinical symptom onset, but only 28% after the third month. Elevated protein (>50 mg/dl) is found in 71% of patients before the third month and only 61% after the third month. Oligoclonal bands are positive in over 60% of patients and remain stable over time. In up to 10% of patients, oligoclonal bands are the only abnormal finding in the CSF. Completely normal CSF is found in just 3% of patients with paraneoplastic neurologic syndromes with confirmed serum antibody when CSF is measured within the first month of clinical symptom onset [148].

Infections

Neurologic infections pose a serious risk to patients with cancer. Cancer patients are more susceptible to neuroinfectious disease for a number of reasons including cancer infiltrating the bone marrow, immunosuppressive therapies, radiation, neurosurgical procedures, indwelling ventricular catheters, and indwelling vascular catheters [149]. They are at increased risk of infection not only during the time of cancer treatment, but also before and after treatment. A few groups of cancer patients account for a large majority of those afflicted with neuroinfectious disease. Patients with lymphoma or leukemia represent one-fourth of the cancer population with CNS infection, while patients with primary brain tumors represent just over one-sixth of the population [150]. Patients with recent neurosurgery account for over three-fourths of cases of bacterial or fungal infection [151].

The organisms encountered in this population are diverse and differ from those in the general population. Additionally, in this population, two or more independent infectious agents can coexist. This is further complicated by the fact that up to one-third of neutropenic patients with culture positive bacterial or fungal meningitis can have normal CSF [151]. Adding to this complexity is the fact that cancer patients do not present with the classic symptoms of neurologic infection [149]. In fact, in one study only 5% of patients with culture positive meningitis presented with the triad of fever, nuchal rigidity, and mental status change, compared to 44% in the general population. Fever and headache were the most common isolated symptoms associated with meningitis in cancer patients [151]. Meningitis without focal signs is more typical in viruses, Candida, and Cryptococcus, while symptoms and focal deficits are more commonly seen in Toxoplasma gondii and Aspergillus [152]. Thus, lumbar puncture is an essential tool in the workup of infection or headache in patients with cancer even when clinical symptoms are scant.

Infectious patterns are important to recognize when trying to diagnose a suspected neurologic infection with CSF. In a

Table 3.7 CSF findings associated with abscesses, bacterial infections, fungal infections, and viral infections

	Normal	Abscess	Bacterial	Fungal	Viral
Pressure (mmH$_2$O)	60–250	Normal to elevated	Elevated	Normal to elevated	Normal
WBC count (mm^3)	0–5	Normal to elevated	>1000	10–500	10–500
Differential (Predominance)	None	Neutrophil	Neutrophil	Lymphocyte	Lymphocyte
Protein (mg/dl)	20–45	Normal to elevated	Elevated	Elevated	Normal to elevated
Glucose (mg/dl)	45–100 or >50% of serum	Normal	Low	Low	Normal

Table 3.8 Different immunodeficiencies and their associated infectious agents

Reason for infection	Infectious etiologies
Procedures: Craniotomy, Ventricular shunt, Ommaya reservoir, Intracerebral pressure monitoring devices, Central lines, Chemo ports, Feeding tubes	*Staphylococcus aureus, Staphylococcus epidermidis, Escherichia coli*, Enterobacteria, *Candida albicans*
T-lymphocyte deficit or dysfunction (Leukemia, Lymphoma, Hematopoietic stem cell transplantation, T-cell directed immunosuppressive therapies)	Human immunodeficiency virus, Cytomegalovirus, Herpes simplex virus, Epstein–Barr virus, *Cryptococcus neoformans, Candida albicans, Toxoplasma gondii, Listeria monocytogenes*
B-lymphocyte deficit or dysfunction (Paraproteinemias, Splenectomy, B-cell directed immunosuppressive therapies)	*Streptococcus pneumoniae, Haemophilus influenza, Klebsiella pneumonia*, Enteroviruses

clinical situation there are typically limitations to the quantity of CSF that can be obtained and the number of tests that can be sent for. Thus, narrowing the differential diagnosis in order to send the appropriate tests is important. Table 3.7 [102] lists CSF findings associated with abscesses, bacterial infections, fungal infections, and viral infections. Table 3.8 [150, 152] lists different immunodeficiencies and their associated infectious agents.

References

1. Neidermeyer E, De Silva FL. Electroencephalography: basic principles, clinical applications and related fields. Philadelphia: Lippincott, Williams and Wilkins; 2005. p. 1–14.
2. Caton R. The electric currents of the brain. Br Med J. 1875;2:278.
3. Tudor M, Tudor L, Tudor KI. Hans Berger (1873-1941)—the history of electroencephalography. Acta Med Croatica. 2005;59 (4):307–13.
4. Jasper H. Report of committee on methods of clinical exam in EEG. Electroencephalogr Clin Neurophysiol. 1958;10:370–5.
5. Wyllie E. Wyllie's treatment of epilepsy principles and practice. 5th ed. Philadelphia: Lippincot Williams & Wilkins; 2011.
6. Liigant A, Haldre S, Oun A, et al. Seizure disorders in patients with brain tumors. Eur Neurol. 2001;45(1):46–51.
7. Lynam LM, Lyons MK, Drazkowski JF, et al. Frequency of seizures in patients with newly diagnosed brain tumors: a retrospective review. Clin Neurol Neurosurg. 2007;109(7):634–8.
8. Ruda R, Trevisan E, Soffietti R. Epilepsy and brain tumors. Curr Opin Oncol. 2010;22(6):611–20.
9. Towne AR, Waterhouse EJ, Boggs JG, et al. Prevalence of nonconvulsive status epilepticus in comatose patients. Neurology. 2000;54(2):340–5.
10. Carrera E, Claassen J, Oddo M, Emerson RG, Mayer SA, Hirsch LJ. Continuous electroencephalographic monitoring in critically ill patients with central nervous system infections. Arch Neurol. 2008;65(12):1612–8.
11. Kaplan PW, Sutter R. Electroencephalography of autoimmune limbic encephalopathy. J Clin Neurophysiol. 2013;30(5):490–504.
12. Hirsch JF, Buisson-Ferey J, Sachs M, Hirsch JC, Scherrer J. Electrocorticogram and unitary activities with expanding lesions in man. Electroencephalogr Clin Neurophysiol. 1966;21(5):417–28.

13. Daly DD, Pedley TA. Current practice of clinical encephalopathy. 2nd ed. New York: Raven Press; 1990.
14. IFSECN. A glossary of terms commonly used by clinical electroencephalgraphers. Electroencephalogr Clin Neurophysiol. 1974;37:538–48.
15. Blume WT, Girvin JP, Kaufmann JC. Childhood brain tumors presenting as chronic uncontrolled focal seizure disorders. Ann Neurol. 1982;12(6):538–41.
16. Garcia-Morales I, Garcia MT, Galan-Davila L, et al. Periodic lateralized epileptiform discharges: etiology, clinical aspects, seizures, and evolution in 130 patients. J Clin Neurophysiol. 2002;19(2):172–7.
17. Trinka E, Hofler J, Zerbs A. Causes of status epilepticus. Epilepsia. 2012;53(Suppl 4):127–38.
18. Aminoff MJ, Simon RP. Status epilepticus. Causes, clinical features and consequences in 98 patients. Am J Med. 1980;69 (5):657–66.
19. Mayer SA, Claassen J, Lokin J, Mendelsohn F, Dennis LJ, Fitzsimmons BF. Refractory status epilepticus: frequency, risk factors, and impact on outcome. Arch Neurol. 2002;59(2):205–10.
20. Cockerell OC, Rothwell J, Thompson PD, Marsden CD, Shorvon SD. Clinical and physiological features of epilepsia partialis continua. Cases ascertained in the UK. Brain. 1996;119(Pt 2):393–407.
21. Thomas JE, Reagan TJ, Klass DW. Epilepsia partialis continua. A review of 32 cases. Arch Neurol. 1997;34:266–75.
22. Drislane FW. Presentation, evaluation, and treatment of nonconvulsive status epilepticus. Epilepsy Behav. 2000;1(5):301–14.
23. Cocito L, Audenino D, Primavera A. Altered mental state and nonconvulsive status epilepticus in patients with cancer. Arch Neurol. 2001;58(8):1310.
24. Cavaliere R, Farace E, Schiff D. Clinical implications of status epilepticus in patients with neoplasms. Arch Neurol. 2006;63 (12):1746–9.
25. Avila EK, Graber J. Seizures and epilepsy in cancer patients. Curr Neurol Neurosci Rep. 2010;10(1):60–7.
26. Van der Drift JHA. The significance of electroencephalography for the diagnosis and localization of cerebral tumors. Leiden: H. E. Stenfert Kroese; 1957.
27. Lieu AS, Howng SL. Intracranial meningiomas and epilepsy: incidence, prognosis and influencing factors. Epilepsy Res. 2000;38(1):45–52.
28. Prayson RA. Diagnostic challenges in the evaluation of chronic epilepsy-related surgical neuropathology. Am J Surg Pathol. 2010;34(5):e1–13.

29. Danfors T, Ribom D, Berntsson SG, Smits A. Epileptic seizures and survival in early disease of grade 2 gliomas. Eur J Neurol. 2009;16(7):823–31.

30. Daly DD, Thomas JE. Sequential alterations in the electroencephalograms of patients with brain tumors. Electroencephalogr Clin Neurophysiol. 1958;10(3):395–404.

31. Moots PL, Maciunas RJ, Eisert DR, Parker RA, Laporte K, Abou-Khalil B. The course of seizure disorders in patients with malignant gliomas. Arch Neurol. 1995;52(7):717–24.

32. Riva M, Salmaggi A, Marchioni E, et al. Tumour-associated epilepsy: clinical impact and the role of referring centres in a cohort of glioblastoma patients. A multicentre study from the Lombardia Neurooncology Group. Neurol Sci. 2006;27(5):345–51.

33. Fisher-Williams M, Last SL, Lyberi G, Northfield DW. Clinico-EEG study of 128 gliomas and 50 intracranial metastatic tumours. Brain. 1962;85:1–46.

34. Klass DW, Bickford RG. The electroencephalogram in metastatic tumors of the brain. Neurology. 1958;8(5):333–7.

35. Neufield MY, Chistik V, Chapman J, Korczyn AS. Intermittent rhythmic delta activity (IRDA) morphology cannot distinguish between focal and diffuse brain disturbances. J Neurosci. 1999;164(1):56–9.

36. Nau HE, Bock WJ, Clar HE. Electroencephalographic investigations in sellar tumours, with special regard to different methods of operative treatment. Acta Neurochir (Wien). 1978;44(3–4):207–214.

37. Jasper H, Van Buren J. Interrelationship between cortex and subcortical structures. Clinical and electroencephalographic studies. Electroencephalogr Clin Neurophysiol. 1953;4:168–88.

38. Valk PE, Dillon WP. Radiation injury of the brain. AJNR Am J Neuroradiol. 1991;12(1):45–62.

39. Martins AN, Johnston JS, Henry JM, Stoffel TJ, Di Chiro G. Delayed radiation necrosis of the brain. J Neurosurg. 1977;47 (3):336–45.

40. Morris PG, Gutin PH, Avila EK, Rosenblum MK, Lassman AB. Seizures and radionecrosis from non-small-cell lung cancer presenting as increased fluorodeoxyglucose uptake on positron emission tomography. J Clin Oncol. 2011;29(12):e324–6.

41. Tuxen MK, Hansen SW. Neurotoxicity secondary to antineoplastic drugs. Cancer Treat Rev. 1994;20(2):191–214.

42. Salsano E, Rizzo A, Bedini G, et al. An autoinflammatory neurological disease due to interleukin 6 hypersecretion. J Neuroinflammation. 2013;10:29.

43. Lawn ND, Westmoreland BF, Kiely MJ, Lennon VA, Vernino S. Clinical, magnetic resonance imaging, and electroencephalographic findings in paraneoplastic limbic encephalitis. Mayo Clin Proc. 2003;78(11):1363–8.

44. Davis R, Dalmau J. Autoimmunity, seizures, and status epilepticus. Epilepsia. 2015;54:46–9.

45. Dalmau J, Graus F, Rosenblum MK, Posner JB. Anti-Hu–associated paraneoplastic encephalomyelitis/sensory neuronopathy. A clinical study of 71 patients. Medicine (Baltimore). 1992;71(2):59–72.

46. Iizuka T, Sakai F, Ide T, et al. Anti-NMDA receptor encephalitis in Japan: long-term outcome without tumor removal. Neurology. 2008;70(7):504–11.

47. Schmitt SE, Pargeon K, Frechette ES, Hirsch LJ, Dalmau J, Friedman D. Extreme delta brush: a unique EEG pattern in adults with anti-NMDA receptor encephalitis. Neurology. 2012;79 (11):1094–100.

48. Lai M, Hughes EG, Peng X, et al. AMPA receptor antibodies in limbic encephalitis alter synaptic receptor location. Ann Neurol. 2009;65(4):424–34.

49. Lancaster E, Lai M, Peng X, et al. Antibodies to the GABA(B) receptor in limbic encephalitis with seizures: case series and characterisation of the antigen. Lancet Neurol. 2010;9(1):67–76.

50. Pozo-Rosich P, Clover L, Saiz A, Vincent A, Graus F. Voltage-gated potassium channel antibodies in limbic encephalitis. Ann Neurol. 2003;54(4):530–3.

51. Galvani L. De viribus electrocitatis in motu musculari commentaries. Proc Bologna Acad Inst Sci Arts. 1791;7:363.

52. Volta A. Account of some discoveries made by Mr. Galvani of Bologna: with experiments and observations on them. Phil Trans R Soc Lond. 1793;83:10.

53. De Duchenne G. L'ectrisation Localisee et de son application a la Physiologie, a la Pathologie et a la Therapeutique. Paris: JB Bailliere; 1871.

54. Kimura J. Electrodiagnosis in diseases of nerve and muscle: principles and practice. Philadelphia: F.A. Davis; 1985.

55. Helmholtz H. Vorloufiger Bericht uber die Fortpflanzungsgeschwindigkeit der Nervenreinzung. Arch Anat Physiol Wiss Med. 1850;71.

56. Erb W. Handbuch der Electrotherapie. Leipzig: FCW Vogel; 1882.

57. Gasser HS, Erlanger J. A study of the action currents of nerve with the cathode ray oscillography. Am J Physiol. 1922; 62:496.

58. Proebster R. Muskelationsstrome am gesunden und kranken menschen. Zeit fur Orthopadische Chirurgie. 1928;50:1.

59. Preston DC, Shapiro BE. Electromyography and neuromuscular disorders: clinical-electrophysiologic correlations. 2nd ed. Philadelphia: Elsevier; 2005.

60. Daube J. Clinical neurophysiology. 3rd ed. New York: Oxford; 2009.

61. Mallik A, Weir AI. Nerve conduction studies: essentials and pitfalls in practice. J Neurol Neurosurg Psychiatry. 2005;76 Suppl 2:ii23–31.

62. Schoeck AP, Mellion ML, Gilchrist JM, Christian FV. Safety of nerve conduction studies in patients with implanted cardiac devices. Muscle Nerve. 2007;35(4):521–4.

63. DeAngelis LM, Posner JB. Neurologic complications of cancer. New York: Oxford University Press; 2009.

64. Ramchandren S, Dalmau J. Metastases to the peripheral nervous system. J Neurooncol. 2005;75(1):101–10.

65. Antoine JC, Camdessanche JP. Peripheral nervous system involvement in patients with cancer. Lancet Neurol. 2007;6 (1):75–86.

66. Kelly JJ, Karcher DS. Lymphoma and peripheral neuropathy: a clinical review. Muscle Nerve. 2005;31(3):301–13.

67. Darnell RB, Posner JB. Paraneoplastic syndromes affecting the nervous system. Semin Oncol. 2006;33(3):270–98.

68. Vigliani MC, Magistrello M, Polo P, et al. Risk of cancer in patients with Guillain-Barre syndrome (GBS). A population-based study. J Neurol. 2004;251(3):321–6.

69. Lisak RP, Mitchell M, Zweiman B, Orrechio E, Asbury AK. Guillain-Barre Syndrome and Hodgkin's Disease: three cases with immunological studies. Ann Neurol. 1977;1(1):72–8.

70. Gordon PH, Wilbourn AJ. Early electrodiagnostic findings in Guillain-Barre syndrome. Arch Neurol. 2001;58(6):913–7.

71. Antoine JC, Mosnier JF, Lapras J, et al. Chronic inflammatory demyelinating polyneuropathy associated with carcinoma. J Neurol Neurosurg Psychiatry. 1996;60(2):188–90.

72. Bird SJ, Brown MJ, Shy ME, Scherer SS. Chronic inflammatory demyelinating polyneuropathy associated with malignant melanoma. Neurology. 1996;46:822–4.

73. Dalakas MC. Pathogenesis of immune-mediated neuropathies. Biochim Biophys Acta. 2015;1852(4):658–66.

74. Kelly JJ Jr. Peripheral neuropathies associated with monoclonal proteins: a clinical review. Muscle Nerve. 1985;8(2):138–50.

75. Vital A, Vital C, Julien J, Baquey A, Steck AJ. Polyneuropathy associated with IgM monoclonal gammopathy. Immunological

and pathological study in 31 patients. Acta Neuropathol. 1989;79 (2):160–7.

76. Antoine JC, Honnorat J, Camdessanche JP, et al. Paraneoplastic anti-CV2 antibodies react with peripheral nerve and are associated with a mixed axonal and demyelinating peripheral neuropathy. Ann Neurol. 2001;49(2):214–21.

77. Camdessanche JP, Antoine JC, Honnorat J, et al. Paraneoplastic peripheral neuropathy associated with anti-Hu antibodies. A clinical and electrophysiological study of 20 patients. Brain. 2002;125(Pt 1):166–75.

78. Oh SJ, Gurtekin Y, Dropcho EJ, King P, Claussen GC. Anti-Hu antibody neuropathy: a clinical, electrophysiological, and pathological study. Clin Neurophysiol. 2005;116(1):28–34.

79. Abgrall S, Mouthon L, Cohen P, et al. Localized neurological necrotizing vasculitides. Three cases with isolated mononeuritis multiplex. J Rheumatol. 2001;28(3):631–3.

80. Fain O, Hamidou M, Cacoub P, et al. Vasculitides associated with malignancies: analysis of sixty patients. Arthritis Rheum. 2007;57(8):1473–80.

81. Bouche P, Leger JM, Travers MA, Cathala HP, Castaigne P. Peripheral neuropathy in systemic vasculitis: clinical and electrophysiologic study of 22 patients. Neurology. 1986;36 (12):1598–602.

82. Newsom-Davis J, Buckley C, Clover L, et al. Autoimmune disorders of neuronal potassium channels. Ann N Y Acad Sci. 2003;998:202–10.

83. Caress JB, Abend WK, Preston DC, Logigian EL. A case of Hodgkin's lymphoma producing neuromyotonia. Neurology. 1997;49(1):258–9.

84. Walch JC. Neuromyotonia: an unusual presentation of intrathoracic malignancy. J Neurol Neurosurg Psychiatry. 1976;39: 1086–91.

85. Murinson BB. Stiff-person syndrome. Neurologist. 2004;10 (3):131–7.

86. Takamori M. Lambert-Eaton myasthenic syndrome as an autoimmune calcium channelopathy. Biochem Biophys Res Commun. 2004;322(4):1347–51.

87. Mills KR. Specialised electromyography and nerve conduction studies. J Neurol Neurosurg Psychiatry. 2005;76 Suppl 2:ii36–40.

88. Hill CL, Zhang Y, Sigurgeirsson B, et al. Frequency of specific cancer types in dermatomyositis and polymyositis: a population-based study. Lancet. 2001;357(9250):96–100.

89. Levin MI, Mozaffar T, Al-Lozi MT, Pestronk A. Paraneoplastic necrotizing myopathy: clinical and pathological features. Neurology. 1998;50(3):764–7.

90. Zochodne DW, Ramsay DA, Saly V, Shelley S, Moffatt S. Acute necrotizing myopathy of intensive care: electrophysiological studies. Muscle Nerve. 1994;17(3):285–92.

91. Quasthoff S, Hartung HP. Chemotherapy-induced peripheral neuropathy. J Neurol. 2002;249(1):9–17.

92. Chen X, Stubblefield MD, Custodio CM, Hudis CA, Seidman AD, DeAngelis LM. Electrophysiological features of taxane-induced polyneuropathy in patients with breast cancer. J Clin Neurophysiol. 2013;30(2):199–203.

93. Chaudhry V, Eisenberger MA, Sinibaldi VJ, Sheikh K, Griffin JW, Cornblath DR. A prospective study of suramin-induced peripheral neuropathy. Brain. 1996;119(Pt 6):2039–52.

94. Chaudhry V, Cornblath DR, Corse A, Freimer M, Simmons-O'Brien E, Vogelsang G. Thalidomide-induced neuropathy. Neurology. 2002;59(12):1872–5.

95. Richardson PG, Briemberg H, Jagannath S, et al. Frequency, characteristics, and reversibility of peripheral neuropathy during treatment of advanced multiple myeloma with bortezomib. J Clin Oncol. 2006;24(19):3113–20.

96. Thaipisuttikul I, Chapman P, Avila EK. Peripheral neuropathy associated with ipilimumab: a report of 2 cases. J Immunother. 2015;38(2):77–9.

97. Pentsova E, Liu A, Rosenblum M, O'Reilly E, Chen X, Hormigo A. Gemcitabine induced myositis in patients with pancreatic cancer: case reports and topic review. J Neurooncol. 2012;106(1):15–21.

98. Harper CM Jr, Thomas JE, Cascino TL, Litchy WJ. Distinction between neoplastic and radiation-induced brachial plexopathy, with emphasis on the role of EMG. Neurology. 1989;39(4): 502–6.

99. Lederman RJ, Wilbourn AJ. Brachial plexopathy: recurrent cancer or radiation? Neurology. 1984;34(10):1331–5.

100. McHenry LCJ. Garrison's history of neurology. Springfield: Charles C. Thomas; 1969.

101. Viets HR. Domenico Contugno: His description of the cerebrospinal fluid with a translation of part of his "De ischia nervosa commentarius" (1764) and a bibliography of his important works. Bull Hist Med. 1935;3:701–38.

102. Fishman RA. Cerebrospinal fluid in diseases of the nervous system. Philadelphia: W.B. Saunders; 1980.

103. Quincke H. Diseases of the nervous system. New York: Appleton; 1909.

104. Merritt HH, Fremont-Smith F. The cerebrospinal fluid. Philadelphia: W.B. Saunders; 1938.

105. Sternbach G. Lumbar puncture. J Emerg Med. 1985;2(3):199–203.

106. Glantz MJ, Cole BF, Glantz LK, Cobb J, Mills P, Lekos A, et al. Cerebrospinal fluid cytology in patients with cancer: minimizing false-negative results. Cancer. 1998;82(4):733–9.

107. van Crevel H, Hijdra A, de Gans J. Lumbar puncture and the risk of herniation: when should we first perform CT? J Neurol. 2002;249(2):129–37.

108. Reihsaus E, Waldbaur H, Seeling W. Spinal epidural abscess: a meta-analysis of 915 patients. Neurosurg Rev. 2000;23(4):175–204; discussion 205.

109. van Veen JJ, Nokes TJ, Makris M. The risk of spinal haematoma following neuraxial anaesthesia or lumbar puncture in thrombocytopenic individuals. Br J Haematol. 2010;148(1):15–25.

110. Layton KF, Kallmes DF, Horlocker TT. Recommendations for anticoagulated patients undergoing image-guided spinal procedures. AJNR Am J Neuroradiol. 2006;27(3):468–70.

111. Horlocker TT, Wedel DJ, Schroeder DR, et al. Preoperative antiplatelet therapy does not increase the risk of spinal hematoma associated with regional anesthesia. Anesth Analg. 1995;80 (2):303–9.

112. Whiteley W, Al-Shahi R, Warlow CP, Zeidler M, Lueck CJ. CSF opening pressure: reference interval and the effect of body mass index. Neurology. 2006;67(9):1690–1.

113. Nayak L, Lee EQ, Wen PY. Epidemiology of brain metastases. Curr Oncol Rep. 2012;14(1):48–54.

114. Tabouret E, Bauchet L, Carpentier AF. Brain metastases epidemiology and biology. Bull Cancer. 2013;100(1):57–62.

115. Kesari S, Batchelor TT. Leptomeningeal metastases. Neurol Clin. 2003;21(1):25–66.

116. Clarke JL, Perez HR, Jacks LM, Panageas KS, Deangelis LM. Leptomeningeal metastases in the MRI era. Neurology. 2010;74 (18):1449–54.

117. Saito R, Kumabe T, Jokura H, Shirane R, Yoshimoto T. Symptomatic spinal dissemination of malignant astrocytoma. J Neurooncol. 2003;61(3):227–35.

118. Kaplan JG, DeSouza TG, Farkash A, et al. Leptomeningeal metastases: comparison of clinical features and laboratory data of solid tumors, lymphomas and leukemias. J Neurooncol. 1990;9 (3):225–9.

119. Hauke RJ, Tarantolo SR, Bashir RM, Moravec D, Bierman PJ. Central nervous system Hodgkin's disease relapsing with eosinophilic pleocytosis. Leuk Lymphoma. 1996;21 (1–2):173–5.

120. Wasserstrom WR, Glass JP, Posner JB. Diagnosis and treatment of leptomeningeal metastases from solid tumors: experience with 90 patients. Cancer. 1982;49(4):759–72.

121. Glass JP, Melamed M, Chernik NL, Posner JB. Malignant cells in cerebrospinal fluid (CSF): the meaning of a positive CSF cytology. Neurology. 1979;29(10):1369–75.

122. Glantz MJ, Cole BF, Glantz LK, et al. Cerebrospinal fluid cytology in patients with cancer: minimizing false-negative results. Cancer. 1998;82(4):733–9.

123. Balmaceda C, Gaynor JJ, Sun M, Gluck JT, DeAngelis LM. Leptomeningeal tumor in primary central nervous system lymphoma: recognition, significance, and implications. Ann Neurol. 1995;38(2):202–9.

124. Nayak L, Fleisher M, Gonzalez-Espinoza R, Lin O, Panageas K, Reiner A, Liu C-M, DeAngelis LM, Omuro A. Rare cell capture technology for the diagnosis of leptomeningeal metastasis in solid tumors. Neuroology. 2013;80(17):1598–1605.

125. Shapiro HM. Practical flow cytometry. Hoboken: Wiley; 2005.

126. Chamberlain MC, Glantz M, Groves MD, Wilson WH. Diagnostic tools for neoplastic meningitis: detecting disease, identifying patient risk, and determining benefit of treatment. Semin Oncol. 2009;36(4 Suppl 2):S35–45.

127. Bromberg JE, Breems DA, Kraan J, et al. CSF flow cytometry greatly improves diagnostic accuracy in CNS hematologic malignancies. Neurology. 2007;68(20):1674–9.

128. Scott BJ, Douglas VC, Tihan T, Rubenstein JL, Josephson SA. A systematic approach to the diagnosis of suspected central nervous system lymphoma. JAMA Neurol. 2013;70(3):311–9.

129. Hoon DS, Kuo CT, Wascher RA, Fournier P, Wang HJ, O'Day SJ. Molecular detection of metastatic melanoma cells in cerebrospinal fluid in melanoma patients. J Invest Dermatol. 2001;117(2):375–8.

130. Malkin MG, Posner JB. Cerebrospinal fluid tumor markers for the diagnosis and management of leptomeningeal metastases. Eur J Cancer Clin Oncol. 1987;23(1):1–4.

131. Stockhammer G, Poewe W, Burgstaller S, et al. Vascular endothelial growth factor in CSF: a biological marker for carcinomatous meningitis. Neurology. 2000;54(8):1670–6.

132. van Zanten AP, Twijnstra A, Ongerboer de Visser BW, van Heerde P, Hart AA, Nooyen WJ. Cerebrospinal fluid tumour markers in patients treated for meningeal malignancy. J Neurol Neurosurg Psychiatry. 1991;54(2):119–23.

133. Castro MP, McDonald TJ, Qualman SJ, Odorisio TM. Cerebrospinal fluid gastrin releasing peptide in the diagnosis of leptomeningeal metastases from small cell carcinoma. Cancer. 2001;91(11):2122–6.

134. Fujimaki T, Mishima K, Asai A, et al. Levels of beta-human chorionic gonadotropin in cerebrospinal fluid of patients with malignant germ cell tumor can be used to detect early recurrence and monitor the response to treatment. Jpn J Clin Oncol. 2000;30 (7):291–4.

135. Jorda M, Ganjei-Azar P, Nadji M. Cytologic characteristics of meningeal carcinomatosis: increased diagnostic accuracy using carcinoembryonic antigen and epithelial membrane antigen immunocytochemistry. Arch Neurol. 1998;55(2):181–4.

136. Bernstein WB, Kemp JD, Kim GS, Johnson VV. Diagnosing leptomeningeal carcinomatosis with negative CSF cytology in advanced prostate cancer. J Clin Oncol. 2008;26(19):3281–4.

137. Cone LA, Koochek K, Henager HA, et al. Leptomeningeal carcinomatosis in a patient with metastatic prostate cancer: case report and literature review. Surg Neurol. 2006;65(4):372–75, discussion 375–76.

138. Kosmas C, Tsavaris NB, Soukouli G, et al. Changes of cerebrospinal fluid tumor marker levels may predict response to treatment and survival of carcinomatous meningitis in patients with advanced breast cancer. Med Oncol. 2005;22(2):123–8.

139. Walbert T, Groves MD. Known and emerging biomarkers of leptomeningeal metastasis and its response to treatment. Future Oncol. 2010;6(2):287–97.

140. Gomes HR. Cerebrospinal fluid approach on neuro-oncology. Arq Neuropsiquiatr. 2013;71(9B):677–80.

141. van de Langerijt B, Gijtenbeek JM, de Reus HP, et al. CSF levels of growth factors and plasminogen activators in leptomeningeal metastases. Neurology. 2006;67(1):114–9.

142. Reijneveld JC, Brandsma D, Boogerd W, et al. CSF levels of angiogenesis-related proteins in patients with leptomeningeal metastases. Neurology. 2005;65(7):1120–2.

143. Friedberg MH, Glantz MJ, Klempner MS, Cole BF, Perides G. Specific matrix metalloproteinase profiles in the cerebrospinal fluid correlated with the presence of malignant astrocytomas, brain metastases, and carcinomatous meningitis. Cancer. 1998;82 (5):923–30.

144. Katopodis N, Glantz MJ, Kim L, Dafni U, Wu JK, Perides G. Lipid-associated sialoprotein in the cerebrospinal fluid: association with brain malignancies. Cancer. 2001;92(4):856–62.

145. Groves MD, Hess KR, Puduvalli VK, et al. Biomarkers of disease: cerebrospinal fluid vascular endothelial growth factor (VEGF) and stromal cell derived factor (SDF)-1 levels in patients with neoplastic meningitis (NM) due to breast cancer, lung cancer and melanoma. J Neurooncol. 2009;94(2):229–34.

146. Lossos IS, Breuer R, Intrator O, Lossos A. Cerebrospinal fluid lactate dehydrogenase isoenzyme analysis for the diagnosis of central nervous system involvement in hematooncologic patients. Cancer. 2000;88(7):1599–604.

147. Dalmau JO, Posner JB. Paraneoplastic syndromes. Arch Neurol. 1999;56(4):405–8.

148. Psimaras D, Carpentier AF, Rossi C, Euronetwork PNS. Cerebrospinal fluid study in paraneoplastic syndromes. J Neurol Neurosurg Psychiatry. 2010;81(1):42–5.

149. Tan K, Patel S, Gandhi N, Chow F, Rumbaugh J, Nath A. Burden of neuroinfectious diseases on the neurology service in a tertiary care center. Neurology. 2008;71(15):1160–6.

150. Pruitt AA. Central nervous system infections in cancer patients. Semin Neurol. 2010;30(3):296–310.

151. Safdieh JE, Mead PA, Sepkowitz KA, Kiehn TE, Abrey LE. Bacterial and fungal meningitis in patients with cancer. Neurology. 2008;70(12):943–7.

152. Pruitt AA. CNS infections in patients with cancer. Continuum (Minneap Minn). 2012;18(2):384–405.

Part III

Nervous System Involvement of Systemic Cancers

Brain Metastasis as Complication of Systemic Cancers

Riccardo Soffietti, Federica Franchino, and Roberta Rudà

Introduction

Brain metastases represent one of the most common neurological complications of systemic cancer, in many cases resulting in significant morbidity and mortality. The incidence has increased over time as a result of advances in detection and improvements in the treatment of primary tumor and systemic disease, which have led to an increase in survival. They currently represent the most frequent intracranial tumors, outnumbering primary brain tumors.

The majority of patients who develop brain metastases have a relatively short survival, despite the fact that initial treatment is often effective. The short survival may be the result of progressive systemic disease (in more than a half of patients) or uncontrolled neurological disease. The treatment of brain metastases includes corticosteroids, anticonvulsants, surgery, radiosurgery, radiotherapy, chemotherapy, and targeted therapies. Although for many patients effective palliation is transient or not possible, other patients with metastatic brain disease do well for prolonged periods with an aggressive therapeutic approach. Prognostic factors can help to identify subgroups of patients with differing life expectancy, and tailor therapeutic approaches.

This chapter will review the state of the art and advances in the management of patients with brain metastases.

Epidemiology, Natural History and Risk Factors

Few population estimates of brain metastasis are available. The incidence of newly diagnosed brain metastasis is estimated to be 3–10 times the number of newly diagnosed primary malignant brain tumors each year [1, 2]. Brain metastases occur in up to 40% of patients with cancer, being symptomatic during life in 60–75% or discovered incidentally on CT/MRI or autopsy [3–7].

In adults, lung (36–64%), breast (15–25%), and skin (melanoma) (5–20%) are the most frequent sources of brain metastases. Less frequent are cancers from colon rectum, kidney, prostate, testis, ovary, and sarcomas. In general, any malignant tumor is able to metastasize to the brain. The primary site is unknown in up to 10–15% of patients with brain metastases. The propensity of primary tumors to spread to the brain parenchyma ("neurotropism") differs, and is high for melanoma (20–45% of patients), small-cell lung cancer, choriocarcinoma and germ cell tumors; intermediate for breast cancer, nonsmall-cell lung cancers (being more frequent in adenocarcinomas than in squamous tumors) and renal cancer; low for cancers of the prostate, gastrointestinal tract, ovary, thyroid, and sarcomas. Cerebral metastatic disease in children is less frequent than in adults (6–10%) [8]. The childhood solid tumors that more frequently metastasize to the brain are neuroblastomas and a variety of sarcomas, including rhabdomyosarcoma, Wilms' tumor, Ewing's sarcoma, and osteogenic sarcoma. Among children older than 15 years, germ cell tumors have the highest incidence. Brain metastases are more commonly diagnosed in patients with known systemic malignancy (metachronous presentation) and may be the first evidence of the metastatic disease. Less commonly, brain metastases are discovered in patients at the same time as the primary tumor (synchronous presentation, up to 30%) or prior to discovery of primary disease (precocious presentation).

In the CT era around 50% of brain metastases were presumed to be single, while MRI has revealed that multiple

R. Soffietti (✉) · F. Franchino · R. Rudà
Department of Neuroscience, University of Turin and City of Health and Science Hospital, Via Cherasco 15, Turin 10126, Italy
e-mail: riccardo.soffietti@unito.it

F. Franchino
e-mail: fedef8@virgilio.it

R. Rudà
e-mail: rudarob@hotmail.com

© Springer International Publishing AG 2018
D. Schiff et al. (eds.), *Cancer Neurology in Clinical Practice*,
DOI 10.1007/978-3-319-57901-6_4

lesions exist in two-thirds to three-fourths of all cases of brain metastases [9, 10]. Brain metastases from renal and abdominopelvic tumors are often single, whereas malignant melanoma and lung tumors have a greater tendency to produce multiple cerebral lesions.

The overwhelming majority of brain metastases arise from embolization of tumor cells through the arterial circulation (hematogenous spread). The occurrence of metastases in the different locations is roughly proportional to their relative mass and blood flow: lesions are located in the cerebral hemispheres in 80% of patients, in the cerebellum in 15%, in the brainstem in 5%, and are rare in the basal ganglia, pineal gland, and hypophisis [11]. Brain metastases are commonly found at the junction of the gray and white matter, and are overrepresented in "watershed" areas of the brain, consistent with the origin of metastases from tumor cell emboli carried to terminal arterioles. Melanoma is unusual in its predilection to metastasize to the cerebral cortex and basal ganglia rather than to the gray-white matter junction [12]. There are few circumstances in which non-specific hematogenous spread does not explain the observed distribution of brain metastases. Pelvic and abdominal tumors have a predilection to form posterior fossa metastases far in excess of what the proportion of blood flow supply to this region would predict. Dissemination byway of Batson's vertebral venous plexus has long been invoked to explain this phenomenon, but this hypothesis cannot explain why patients with pelvic or abdominal tumors do not a high incidence of spinal and skull metastases as well, as these structures are also drained by Batson's plexus.

Some clinico-pathological and molecular factors are recognized as risk factors for developing brain metastases. In NSCLC an increased risk for brain metastases has been related to an advanced disease stage, large primary tumor size, non-squamous histology (mainly adenocarcinoma) and, more recently, EGFR mutational status [13, 14].

In breast cancer, younger age at first diagnosis, the presence of lung metastases and short disease-free survival are considered as major clinical risk factors for the development of brain metastases. Patients with triple-negative tumors (ER-, PR-, HER2 wild type) are at higher risk of developing brain metastases compared with the luminal or HER2-positive subtypes [15]. HER2-positive patients with metastatic disease receiving the monoclonal antibody against HER2 trastuzumab have a higher incidence of brain metastases (30–55%) than patients with HER2-negative disease [16]. It is still debated whether patients with early breast cancer receiving adjuvant trastuzumab have a significant increase in the risk of CNS relapse as well [17, 18]. CNS disease as the first site of relapse remains relatively rare, but occurs more frequently in HER2-positive compared to HER2-negative patients [19]. There are two hypotheses to explain the higher risk for brain metastases in HER2-positive

patients [20]. The first one is that trastuzumab is not able to cross an intact BBB, thus being active against the systemic disease but not preventing CNS disease. The second hypothesis suggests that there is an increased propensity of the HER-2 lineage to colonize the brain.

Biology and Molecular Pathways

In general, metastasis of cancer cells occurs via the "metastatic cascade," which refers to tumor cell invasion of surrounding tissue, entry into the blood stream (intravasation), attachment to local vasculature (arrest), extravasation, and proliferation at the site of metastasis. The "soil and seed" hypothesis of metastasis formation explains why circulating tumor cells may travel throughout the body, but metastases tend to form in particular organs (as in the brain in absence of lung metastases). The metastasis formation would be the result of an interaction between the organ microenvironment (the "soil") and the adhesive and invasive capabilities of the metastasizing tumor cells (the "seed") [21]. Neoplastic cells with the potential to colonize the brain may express unique molecular determinants and respond to brain-derived growth factors, and thereby be able to invade, proliferate, and induce angiogenesis [22]. Moreover, the brain is a unique target organ because of the presence of the blood–brain barrier (BBB) [23] and the absence of lymphatic drainage.

Several genes that mediate the spread of the different primary tumor types to the brain have been identified. Expression profiling has revealed at least five molecular subtypes of breast cancer that differ in tropism to different organs. The luminal breast cancer subtype tends to affect pleura and bone, while the basal subtype preferentially metastasizes to lung and brain [24]. Recently, a set of specific genes was identified [25] by comparing the expression profiles of murine breast cancer cells preferentially metastasizing to brain with the profiles of breast cancer samples from patients with known cerebral metastases. A distinction was made between genes that are expressed in primary tumors with metastases, and therefore called "metastasis progression-genes," and other genes active in the metastatic tumors but not expressed in the primary tumors. The cyclooxygenase COX2, the EGFR ligand HBEGF and the α26-sialyltransferase ST6GALNAC5 were identified as mediators of cancer cell passage through the BBB. While the EGFR ligand and COX2 are also involved in the development of lung metastases, the sialyltransferase ST6GALNAC5 is more specific to the development of brain metastases. In an invitro model COX2 was found to be crucial in the passage of the tumor cells through the BBB [25], and COX2 knock-down lowered the frequency of brain metastasis. Palmieri and colleagues [26] found hexokinase 2 (HK2) to be upregulated 1.5-fold in tumor cells in the brain and associated with poor survival in patients following craniotomy. Moreover, HER2 overexpression does not appear to affect tumor cell arrival or intravasation into the brain, but it increases brain colonization [27]. STAT3 activation has been implicated as an important driver of brain metastasis in breast cancer and its inhibition has been recently shown to suppress development of brain metastases [28]. Few studies have investigated the genomic drivers of brain metastases from lung cancer. Grinberg-Rashi and colleagues [29] reported 12 candidate genes whose overexpression was associated with brain or systemic metastasis in a large series of NSCLC primary tumors, and three genes (CDH2, KIFC1, FAL2) were able to predict prognosis. Of particular interest is the overexpression of CDH2 (N-cadherin), which is involved in multiple processes, such as invasion, migration, and adhesion. The EGFR pathway and integrins may play a role in helping promote brain metastasis in lung and breast cancers [30]. Cancer cells of neural crest origin such as melanoma and neuroendocrine carcinoma may preferentially migrate to the brain [31]. The TGF-B2 expression by murine melanoma is necessary for the establishment and growth of metastases in the brain [32].

In order to get to the brain, tumor cells must reach the cerebral microvasculature and pass through the BBB [33, 34]. Genes coding for cell surface glycoproteins are involved in the attachment of the cells to local blood vessels, and genes regulating vascular permeability are involved in passing through the vessels. Genes involved in the formation and maintenance of the astrocytic end-feet at the opposite side of the BBB have also been implicated.

In order to proliferate, metastatic tumor cells need to switch on the expression of pro-angiogenic molecules like VEGF, MMP-9, and gelatinase B, as well as molecules degrading the extracellular matrix, allowing the growth of new vessels [35]. Increased expression levels of VEGF are necessary but not sufficient for successful formation of metastases in experimental animals [34, 36]. The absence of neo-angiogenesis in metastatic tumor cell populations keep the tumor dormant, a state of increased apoptosis of tumor cells with normal proliferation [37].

Various genes that suppress the formation of metastases have been identified, including Nm23 and CD44. Overexpression of Nm23 in breast cancer and melanoma negatively affects invasion, colonization, and motility [38], and patients with melanoma with low expression of Nm23 had increased risk of developing brain metastases [39]. The membrane glycoprotein CD44 plays a role in the adherence of circulating tumor cells to endothelium. Downregulation of the gene by DNA hypermethylation prevented the formation of metastases and, conversely, consistent expression was reported in cancers of thyroid, skin, and breast [40]. Interestingly, while the standard CD44 isoform is expressed in

primary brain tumors, the CD44 splicing variant is almost exclusively found in brain metastases [41].

Clinical Presentation

The clinical presentation of brain metastases is similar to the presentation of any intracranial mass lesion. Headache is a presenting symptom in 40–50% of patients, is more common with multiple or posterior fossa metastases, and may be mild. Papilledema is associated with headache in 15–25% of patients only. Up to 40% of patients present with focal neurological deficits, and seizures occur in 15–20% of patients. Another 5–10% of patients present with acute "strokelike" symptoms due to an intratumoral hemorrhage (especially in melanoma, renal carcinoma, and choriocarcinoma). Altered mental status or impaired cognition are frequently seen in patients with multiple metastases and/or increased intracranial pressure, sometimes resembling a metabolic encephalopathy. Conversely, the symptoms and signs at presentation can be subtle. As a general rule, brain metastases should be suspected in any patient with known systemic cancer in whom new neurological findings develop.

Diagnosis by Neuroimaging

MRI is the method of choice for the assessment of brain metastasis. Contrast-enhanced MRI is more sensitive than enhanced CT (including double-dose delayed contrast) or unenhanced MRI in detecting brain metastases, particularly lesions in the posterior fossa or multiple punctate metastases [9, 10]. Although T2-weighted and FLAIR images are sensitive in showing vasogenic edema as areas of increased signal intensity, not all metastatic lesions have sufficient edema to be identified.

There are no specific features on MRI that distinguish brain metastases; however, a peripheral location, spherical shape, ring enhancement with prominent peritumoral edema and multiple lesions all suggest metastatic disease (Fig. 4.1). Differential diagnoses, including primary brain tumors (especially high-grade gliomas and lymphomas) and non-neoplastic conditions (abscesses, infections, hemorrhages) must be considered, even in patients with a history of cancer. Diffusion-weighted (DW) MR imaging may be useful in the diagnosis of ring-enhancing cerebral lesions (restricted diffusion is more typical in abscesses compared to unrestricted diffusion in necrotic glioblastomas or metastases), but the findings are not specific [42–44]. When employing MR perfusion imaging, there is a tendency towards lower cerebral blood volume values within the peritumoral region in brain metastases compared with

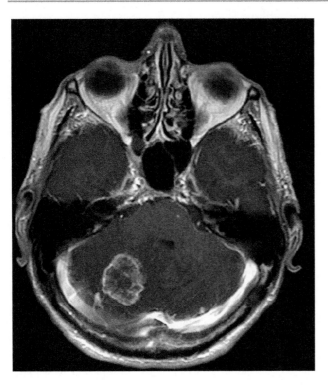

Fig. 4.1 MRI with gadolinium: brain metastasis from colon cancer in the *right* cerebellar hemisphere with edema and mass effect on the 4th ventricle

history or physical exam is suggestive of a specific primary site [53]. Whole-body fluorodeoxyglucose (FDG) PET can be useful [54], but the specificity in differentiating malignant tumors from benign or inflammatory lesions is relatively low. Notably, serial chest CTs may increase the probability of detection of lung cancer in patients with a brain metastasis from an unknown primary tumor, but for these patients early detection provides only limited if any, benefit in survival. [55]. Therefore, a costly extensive evaluation for the undetected primary during the follow-up is not appropriate until more effective cancer therapies are available [53, 55].

A CSF examination is not indicated in the work-up of brain metastases unless there are symptoms, signs or neuroimaging findings that suggest a coexistent leptomeningeal carcinomatosis.

Diagnostic Neuropathology

Routine hematoxylin-eosin stain of biopsy specimens usually reveals the neoplastic nature of the cerebral lesion, and can distinguish between metastases, malignant gliomas, meningiomas, lymphomas, and more rare entities. Immunohistochemical markers may aid in the further characterization of the tumor.

Cerebral Metastasis of Known Primary Tumors

In patients with a known primary tumor, the histology and the marker profile of the primary and the cerebral metastasis will usually show similarities. In general, histologic comparison between the specimen of primary tumor(s) and cerebral metastasis is mandatory, as not infrequently patients may harbor more than one tumor type.

Cerebral Metastasis of Unknown Primary Tumors

For the determination of the lineage of the metastatic tumor, basic morphology provides a first differentiation between carcinomas, lymphomas, or melanomas (Fig. 4.2a–c). In addition, immunohistochemical profiles of metastases may be indicative of the site and lineage of the primary tumor [56]; however, these show variable overlap, and most markers are not specific. In case of a cerebral adenocarcinoma of unknown primary, TTF-1 positivity is strongly associated with lung cancer (Fig. 4.3) and cancer of the thyroid. Negativity for CK7 and positivity for CK20 suggests colorectal cancer. Neuroendocrine differentiation is confirmed by chromogranin, synaptophysin and antibodies directed against specific hormones (insulin, gastrin, glucagon, serotonin and somatostatin). Similarly, there are

glioblastomas [45, 46]. MR spectroscopy more often shows a lower choline to creatinine ratio in brain metastases than in high-grade gliomas [47, 48]. FDG-PET and18F-FET PET do not provide sufficient differentiation between metastases and high-grade glial tumors [49, 50].

Overall, advanced functional imaging techniques cannot reliably identify the histologic origin of an enhancing brain lesion and hence histopathological analysis remains the gold standard. A tissue diagnosis by biopsy should be considered in patients with either unknown primary tumor or well-controlled systemic cancer, especially if a long interval has elapsed since the initial cancer diagnosis, or (less common) in patients with active systemic cancer when the radiographic appearance is atypical. In the modern era there is seldom a justification for irradiating "presumed brain metastases" without a histological diagnosis of cancer.

Staging

A new brain mass suspected to be a metastasis in a patient with no prior history of cancer warrants additional systemic work-up for a primary malignancy. A chest CT is always recommended given the high frequency of brain metastases from lung cancer [51, 52], CT of the abdomen and ultrasound of the testis occasionally reveal the primary tumor. Additional work-up beyond this is low yield, unless the patient's

Fig. 4.2 a–c Hematoxylin-eosin: neoplastic cells from NSCLC with hyperchromatic nuclei, arranged in well demarcated solid foci within brain parenchyma

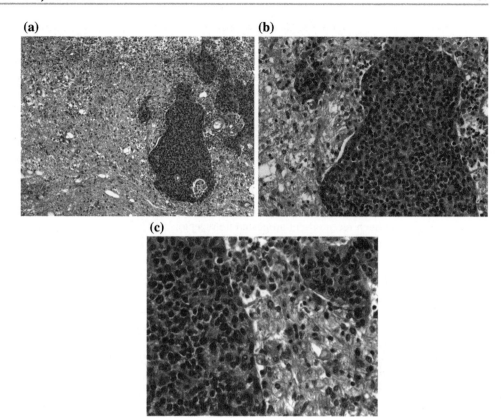

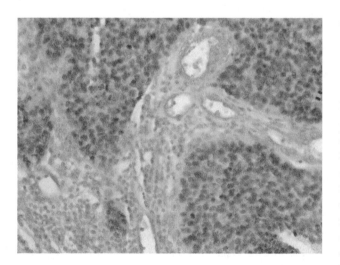

Fig. 4.3 Nuclear immunostaining of neoplastic cells for thyroid transcription factor 1 (TTF 1) in a brain metastasis from lung carcinoma

immunohistochemical panels for mesenchymal tumors (vimentin, desmin, S100).

Attempts to identify unknown primary tumors from their metastases by using RNA expression profiles are ongoing. In general, few studies have focused on the comparison of primary tumors and their cerebral metastases with respect to lineage markers and biomarkers for treatment eligibility [57, 58].

Prognostic Factors

Several factors, including Karnofsky performance status (KPS), age, primary/systemic tumor activity, neurocognitive function, number of brain metastases, primary tumor type and time from primary tumor diagnosis to the brain lesion have individual prognostic significance in patients with brain metastases [59, 60]. Of these, the KPS has consistently been shown to be the major determinant of survival. Based on the most powerful factors, prognostic indices have been developed in order to distinguish subgroups of patients with different prognosis. Utilizing recursive partitioning analysis (RPA) a three-tiered prognostic categorization (RPA Classes I, II and III) was derived from 1200 patients in the Radiation Therapy Oncology Group (RTOG) database who received WBRT [59, 61]. RPA class I represents patients with a KPS greater than 70, age younger than 65 years, controlled primary tumor and no extracranial metastases, with a median survival of 7.7 months; RPA class III represents patients with KPS less than 70, with a median survival of 2.3 months; RPA class II represents the remainder of patients with a median survival of 4.5 months.

A new prognostic index, the Graded Prognostic Assessment (GPA), derived from an analysis of an updated RTOG database of 1960 patients, has been proposed [62]. The GPA uses four factors (age, KPS, status of extra neural disease and number of brain metastases) to subdivide patients into one of four categories with median survival ranging from 2.6 to 11 months. This new index appears equivalent to the RPA in ability to prognosticate, but is less subjective and more quantitative. Additional analysis [63] has shown that the prognostic factors for patients with brain metastases vary according to the histological diagnosis. For both nonsmall-cell and small-cell lung cancer, the significant prognostic factors were KPS, age, presence of extracranial metastases and number of brain metastases, confirming the original GPA. Conversely, for breast cancer, significant prognostic factors were KPS, age and tumor subtype (classified as HER2, estrogen receptor and progesterone receptor status), but not number of brain metastases or status of systemic disease. For melanoma and renal cell carcinoma, the significant prognostic factors were KPS and number of brain metastases. The GPA categorization has now been validated in patients with breast cancer and brain metastases [64, 65], and should be used to stratify future randomized clinical trials, estimate survival and guide the choice of management options. RPA and GPA provide group rather than individual estimates. Recently, a nomogram for the estimation of individual survival probabilities in patients with brain metastases has been proposed with use of data from RTOG database [66].

Additional prognostic scores have been developed for patients with brain metastasis undergoing radiosurgery [67, 68]. Prognosis does not differ between patients with a known and unknown primary tumor [52, 69].

Supportive Care

Corticosteroids are used to control vasogenic cerebral edema and mass effect. Two evidence-based guidelines on the role of steroids in brain metastases have been published in Europe [70] and US [71], and they substantially agree. Dexamethasone is recommended for patients who are symptomatic, with a starting dose of 4–8 mg/day, considering higher doses such as 16 mg/day or more in patients with severe symptoms. Dexamethasone is the steroid of choice because of its minimal mineralocorticoid effect and long half-life, though other corticosteroids can be effective if given in equipotent doses. A neurological improvement within 24–72 h after beginning of treatment is expected in up to 75% of patients. As monotherapy, dexamethasone can relieve symptoms for approximately one month and may slightly increase the 4–6-weeks median survival in comparison to patients who receive no treatment at all. To minimize side effects from chronic dexamethasone administration, including proximal myopathy, tapering of steroid dosing within 1 week of starting therapy and discontinuation within 2 weeks is encouraged. Asymptomatic patients do not need steroids.

The need for anticonvulsant medication is clear in patients who have experienced a seizure. There exists no evidence to support the use of prophylactic anti-epileptic drugs (AEDs) in patients with brain tumors, including metastases. Twelve studies, either randomized trials or cohort studies, investigating the ability of prophylactic AEDs (phenytoin, phenobarbital, valproic acid) to prevent the first seizure, have been examined, and none have demonstrated efficacy [72]. Subtherapeutic levels of anticonvulsants were extremely common and the severity of side effects appeared to be higher (20–40%) in brain tumor patients than in the general population receiving anticonvulsants, probably as a result of drug interactions. Phenytoin, phenobarbital, carbamazepine, and oxcarbazepine stimulate the cytochrome P450 system and accelerate the metabolism of corticosteroids and antineoplastic agents, such as nitroso ureas, paclitaxel, cyclophosphamide, topotecan, irinotecan, thiotepa, adriamycin, methotrexate, imatinib, gefitinib, erlotinib and other tyrosine kinase inhibitors (TKIs), and thus reduce their efficacy. The role of prophylactic anticonvulsants remains to be addressed in subgroups of patients who have a higher risk of developing seizures, such as those with metastatic melanoma, hemorrhagic lesions, or multiple metastases. For patients who undergo a neurosurgical procedure the efficacy of prophylaxis has not been proven. The efficacy of novel AEDs (levetiracetam, topiramate, gabapentin, lamotrigine, lacosamide) has to date not been extensively investigated [73].

Anticoagulant therapy is the standard treatment for acute venous thromboembolism (VTE) in cancer patients. Subcutaneous low-molecular weight heparin(LMWH) is recommended for the initial 5–10 days of treatment for deep vein thrombosis and pulmonary embolism as well as for long-term secondary prophylaxis (for a minimum of 6 months) [74]. Use of novel oral anticoagulants is not currently recommended for patients with malignancy and VTE because of limited data in this patient population [75].

Prophylaxis with LMWH is required for hospitalized patients undergoing major surgery, while in the outpatient setting it is recommended only in selected high-risk patients [76, 77].

Treatment of Newly Diagnosed Brain Metastasis

Surgery

Three randomized trials in single brain metastasis have compared the efficacy of surgical resection followed by WBRT with WBRT alone [78–80]. See Table 4.1.

Table 4.1 Results of phase III trials comparing WBRT alone with surgery plus WBRT in single brain metastasis

Author	Treatment arms	Median survival	Patterns of progression	Median time to progression
Patchell [78]	A1: WBRT ($n = 23$) A2: surgery +WBRT ($n = 25$)	A1: 15 weeks A2: 40 weeks $p < 0.01$	Local A1: 12/23(52%) A2: 5/25(20%) $p < 0.02$ distant A1: 3/23(13%) A2: 5/25(20%) $P = NS$	Local A1: 21 weeks A2: >59 weeks $P < 0.0001$
Vecht [79]	A1: WBRT ($n = 31$) A2: surgery +WBRT ($n = 32$)	A1: 3 months A2: 15 months $p = 0.04$	NR	N
Mintz [80]	A1: WBRT ($n = 43$) A2: surgery +WBRT ($n = 41$)	A1: 6.3 months A2: 5.6 months $P = NS$	NR	NR

NR not reported; *NS* not significant; *A1* Arm 1; *A2* Arm 2

The first two studies showed a survival benefit for patients receiving the combined treatment (median survival 9–10 months vs. 3–6 months). In the Patchell study, patients who received surgery displayed a reduced rate of local relapses (20% versus 52%) and a longer time of functional independence. In the third study, which included more patients with active systemic disease and a low Karnofsky performance status, the addition of surgery to WBRT did not confer a survival benefit, suggesting that this benefit may be limited to a subgroup of patients with controlled systemic disease and good performance status.

In the majority of patients, surgical resection can alleviate symptoms of intracranial hypertension, reduce focal neurological deficits and seizures, and allow for a rapid steroid taper. It should be strongly considered for lesions ≥ 3 cm and/or with significant surrounding edema and/or located in the posterior fossa with mass effect and associated hydrocephalus. Gross total resection of a brain metastasis can be achieved with lower morbidity using contemporary image-guided systems, such as preoperative functional MRI, intraoperative neuronavigation, and cortical mapping [81]. An early postoperative MRI has been recommended to detect residual tumor that is present in up to 20% of patients, and can lead to an increased risk in local recurrence [82]. The same group has suggested that a supramarginal resection (i.e., a resection including a peripheral portion of normal nervous tissue) in eloquent locations could increase the rate of gross total resection [83]. The combined resection of a solitary brain metastasis and a synchronous nonsmall-cell lung carcinoma (stage I and II) yields a median survival of at least 12 months, with 10–30% of patients surviving at 5 years [84].

Leptomeningeal dissemination (LMD) can be a significant complication of the resection of metastasis, especially in case of patients with posterior fossa lesions [85, 86]. A recent retrospective study from MD Anderson Cancer Center [86] in 379 patients with posterior fossa metastases, who underwent either surgery or radiosurgery, revealed a significant increase of LMD in patients whose tumors underwent a "piecemeal" resection (13.8%) compared to *en bloc* resection (5–6%), and the risk of LMD after *en bloc* resection was comparable to that after SRS.

Surgery may be considered for patients with 2–3 surgically accessible brain metastases who are in good neurological condition, have controlled systemic disease and limited comorbidities (Fig. 4.4a–d). Complete surgical resection in this population yields results comparable to those obtained in single lesions [87].

The usefulness of carmustine wafer placement in the resection cavity in newly diagnosed brain metastasis [88] has not been proven in large series of prospective trials.

The GliaSite Radiation Therapy System is an intracavitary high-activity 125-I brachytherapy, performed with a balloon placed in the resection cavity and filled with a radioactive solution. It delivers highly localized doses of radiation to the resection margins (60 Gy to 1 cm depth). A phase II trial in resected single brain metastasis [89] has reported an overall and 1-year local control rate of 83 and 79%, respectively, with a 17% of local failures. Seventeen per cent of patients experienced radiation necrosis. A smaller retrospective study [90] reported the results of 125-I brachytherapy using low-activity permanent seeds placed in the resection cavity. Local tumor control was achieved in 96% of patients, with 4% local failure. The 1-year risk of symptomatic radiation necrosis was lower than that seen in the phase II trial [89] with high-activity seeds (8% vs. 23%).

Stereotactic Radiosurgery

Stereotactic radiosurgery (SRS) is a single, high-dose radiation treatment with precise localization of the target using stereotactic frames or image guidance. Convergence of multiple beams on the target yields a highly therapeutic

Fig. 4.4 a–d 40 year-old woman with node-positive triple-negative breast cancer diagnosed two years earlier presenting with headache and gait ataxia. **a**, **b** Bihemispheric cerebellar metastases on post-contrast T1-weighted MRI at diagnosis. **c**, **d** Same case of **a** and **b** following resection

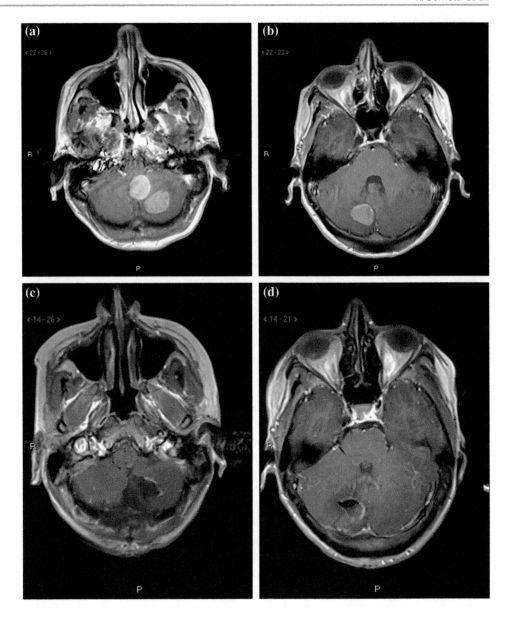

effect, while the steep dose fall-off to surrounding normal structures minimizes the risk of damage. Most brain metastases represent an ideal target for SRS, owing to the small size, spheroid shape, and distinct pathologic margins [91]. The dose is inversely related to tumor diameter and volume. Maximal tolerated doses of SRS were defined in the RTOG 90-05 study [92] in previously irradiated primary brain tumors or brain metastases: 24 Gy for ≤ 20 mm, 18 Gy for 21–30 mm and 15 Gy for 31–40 mm in maximum diameter. As a consequence, the local tumor control decreases as the size of the metastasis increases and the dose that can be given in single fraction decreases. Recently, there has been an increasing interest in hypofractionation for larger metastases (2–5 fractions of smaller doses) with the aim to give radiobiologically higher doses to improve local control and decrease the risk of radionecrosis [93–95].

Comparative studies of hypofractionated SRS versus single dose SRS are awaited.

Several retrospective series have shown single dose SRS to be effective in the treatment of newly diagnosed brain metastases. One-year local control rates of 80-90% with symptom improvement and median survival of 6–12 months have been reported [96–98]. Patients with single lesion, controlled systemic disease and KPS of 70% or greater, have longer survival [99, 100].

Metastases from radio resistant tumors, such as melanoma and renal cell carcinoma, respond to SRS as do metastases from radiosensitive tumors [101]. Radiosurgery allows the treatment of brain metastases in almost any location, including the brainstem [102, 103]. Older patients (≥ 80 years of age) may respond as well as younger patients [104]. The type of radiosurgical procedure, gamma knife or linear accelerator (Linac)-based, does not impact the results. The imaging response to SRS has been reported to correlate with survival only in patients with breast cancer [105].

For patients in RPA classes 1 and 2 with 1–3 brain metastases, SRS has been reported to be more effective than WBRT alone in terms of local tumor control [106].

A randomized phase III study (RTOG95-08) in patients with 1–3 brain metastases, stratified by the RPA system, investigated the value of the addition of a SRS boost to WBRT [107], and reported better local control and performance status at 6 months in the combined therapy group. However, the survival advantage was statistically significant only in a subgroup of patients with single metastasis (6.5 months vs. 4.9 months). Recently, a secondary analysis of RTOG 95-08 that poststratified patients by the GPA classification has reported that the addition of SRS to WBRT conferred a significant survival advantage for patients with a good prognosis (GPA 3.5–4.0) regardless of whether they had 1 or 2 or 3 brain metastases [108]. Conversely, this benefit did not extend to patients with lower GPA and 2 or 3 metastases. It must be stressed that approximately two-third of patient in the trial had lung tumors. A small randomized trial, comparing WBRT alone versus WBRT + SRS in patients with 2–4 metastases, was stopped earlier due to the significant benefit in terms of local failure reduction at 1 year for patients receiving the combined treatment (8% vs. 100%) [109].

The role of SRS alone in patients with up to 3–4 metastases is discussed in the section on WBRT following surgery or radiosurgery.

The role of SRS alone, instead of WBRT, in patients with >4 brain metastases has been investigated in single arm trials. A prospective multicenter Japanese study investigated the use of SRS alone in 1194 patients with one, 2–4 or 5–10 brain metastases, and found similar overall survival (10.8 months) and treatment related toxicity rates between the groups with 2–4 and 5–10 metastases [100]. Salvage SRS was performed in 38% of patients and WBRT in 9%. Cumulative volume of metastases, rather than the number, seems to be a more significant prognostic factor [100, 110]. A consortium in the US is conducting a randomized trial in patients with ≥ 5 metastases to compare SRS to WBRT with neurocognitive outcome as the primary endpoint.

Acute (early) and chronic (late) complications following radiosurgery are reported in 10–40% of patients. Serious complications are rare [111]. Acute reactions (due to edema) occur more often within 2 weeks of treatment, and include headache, nausea and vomiting, worsening of preexistent neurological deficits and seizures. These reactions are generally reversible with steroids. Chronic complications include hemorrhage and radionecrosis (1–17%). Radiographically, a transient increase in the size of the irradiated lesion, with increasing edema and mass effect, with or

without radionecrosis, cannot be distinguished from a tumor progression. FDG-PET, MRI spectroscopy, and MRI perfusion can provide additional information but cannot definitively distinguish between the two diagnoses [112].

Radiation necrosis can be treated with steroids, hyperbaric oxygen, anticoagulants (with risk of bleeding), and more recently with the anti-VEGF agent bevacizumab, which allows a stabilization and normalization of the damaged vascular permeability [113].

A recent review of adverse radiation effects (ARE) following SRS in a large cohort of patients with brain metastases, either radiographic or pathologic, has been published [114]. Although the incidence of ARE after SRS was overall low, the risk increased rapidly with size and volume, leveling off at 1-year cumulative incidence of 13–14%. The authors found a wide range in the time of onset and time to improvement of ARE, and at least 75% probability of improvement over time in conservatively managed AREs. With the exception of capecitabine, neither systemic therapy within 1 month of SRS norarterial hypertension or diabetes [114] appeared to increase the risk of adverse events in the brain.

Surgery Versus SRS

There is no prospective randomized study with sufficient power to compare surgery to SRS. Most comparisons [115–118], including an early terminated small randomized study [119], showed similar outcomes. The one exception is a small series by Bindal and colleagues [120], who reported a superiority of surgery over SRS in terms of OS (16.4 months vs. 7.5 months) and neurologic deaths (19% vs. 50%). However, only 80% of SRS-treated patients were deemed resectable retrospectively, and it is unclear whether this was due to the extent of systemic disease or tumor location.

In general, SRS is less invasive and can be accomplished in an outpatient setting, offering cost-effectiveness advantages over surgery. Patients with larger lesions (2–3 cm), however, may require chronic steroid administration given risk of tumor-related edema and swelling with SRS. Ultimately, the choice between surgery and SRS must be made on a case by case basis, with consideration given to tumor location, size, type of neurological symptoms, patient preference and physician expertise.

Whole Brain Radiotherapy Following Surgery or Radiosurgery

The utility of adjuvant WBRT following surgery or radiosurgery remains controversial. WBRT is believed to eradicate microscopic disease at the original tumor site and at distant intracranial locations. The risk of long-term neurotoxicity and availability of potentially effective salvage treatments [121] are the main arguments against the use of adjuvant WBRT. This needs to be weighted against potential risks of omitting treatment, including CNS progression at distant sites and resultant neurocognitive and neurological sequelae. Moreover, the effectiveness of systemic salvage therapy remains unknown [122].

There are now three phase III trials [123–126], showing that the omission of WBRT in patients with newly diagnosed brain metastases after either surgery or SRS, results in significantly inferior local and distant control, without effect on overall and functionally independent survival. An American-led trial [123] investigating the role of WBRT following surgery, and a Japanese led trial [124] investigating the role of WBRT following SRS, included patients with progressive systemic disease. Conversely, the EORTC 22952-26001 trial focused on patients with stable systemic disease, i.e., on those who could maximally benefit from the addition of early WBRT. This trial randomized 359 patients with 1–3 metastases (81% had one lesion and 19% had two-three lesions), who had previous surgery or SRS, to either WBRT or observation [125]. Adjuvant WBRT significantly reduced the risk of intracranial progression, both locally and at distant sites, by about 50%, but failed to improve functional independence and OS (median 10.9 months vs. 10.7 months). A meta-analysis of the three randomized trials assessing SRS with or without WBRT has challenged our current understanding of the effect of adjuvant WBRT [127]. The investigators reported a survival advantage for SRS alone in those patients presenting with one to four metastases, KPS of 70 or higher and age of 50 years or younger. Moreover, in the subgroup of patients with <50 years, a reduction in the risk of new brain metastases with adjuvant WBRT was not observed. Conversely, in older patients (aged >50 years), WBRT decreases the risk of new brain metastases, but did not affect survival.

A retrospective study [128] has reported that adjuvant WBRT following surgery is of particular value in reducing local and distant recurrence in the brain among patients with metastases >3 cm or with active systemic disease.

The impact of adjuvant WBRT on cognition and quality of life has been examined in several recent studies. Aoyama and coworkers [129] compared the neurocognitive function of patients who underwent either SRS alone or SRS + WBRT. More than 50% of patients experienced significant improvement in the MMSE score shortly after therapy (2–3 months), regardless of treatment, but there was evidence of neurocognitive decline in long-term survivors (up to 36 months) after WBRT. In a randomized controlled trial, Chang and coworkers [130] showed that patients treated

with SRS plus WBRT were at greater risk of a significant decline in learning and memory function by 4 months compared with the group receiving SRS alone.

A recently completed randomized phase III trial (NCCTG N0574) compared SRS alone versus SRS + WBRT in patients with 1–3 brain metastases using a primary neurocognitive endpoint, defined as a decline from baseline in any six cognitive tests at 3 months [131]. Overall, the decline was significantly more frequent after SRS + WBRT versus SRS alone (88% vs. 61.9%, respectively). Specifically, there was more deterioration in the SRS + WBRT arm in immediate recall (31% vs. 8%), delayed recall (51% vs. 20%) and verbal fluency (19% vs. 2%). Intracranial tumor control at 6 and 12 months was higher in the combined arm, but not statistically significant.

Soffietti and coworkers [132] analyzed the quality of life data of the EORTC 22952-26001. They found no significant difference in the global Health-Related Quality of Life over a one-year follow-up period, but patients who underwent adjuvant WBRT had transiently lower physical functioning and lower cognitive functioning scores.

These data suggest that adjuvant WBRT after SRS in patients with a limited number of metastases (up to 3–4) improves intracranial control without improving survival, and carries a high risk of neurocognitive decline, and is therefore not unequivocally recommended. In this regard, the American Society for Radiation Oncology (ASTRO) has recently recommended in their Choose Wisely campaign SRS without adjuvant WBRT for the treatment of limited number of brain metastases [133].

The need for WBRT following surgical resection remains debated, as randomized trials [123, 125] have reported a higher rate of local relapses following surgery alone (about 60% in the EORTC trial) compared with SRS alone.

In general, omission of WBRT, following either SRS or surgery, requires close monitoring with serial imaging (every 3–4 months).

SRS Following Surgery

Postoperative SRS is an approach used to decrease local relapse and avoid the cognitive sequelae of WBRT. Several cohort studies and one phase II trial have reported local control rates of 85–95% [134–136]. The median survival in published studies is around 4 months (range 10–20.5 months). The improved local control and survival rates suggest that postoperative SRS may be as effective as WBRT.

Postoperative SRS is advantageous because it can be delivered within a day or two following surgery and completed in one day. WBRT cannot be initiated for at least

10 days but usually up to two weeks postoperatively to allow for adequate wound healing. For patients receiving systemic therapy, a break from chemotherapy is necessary during WBRT administration, and up to one month following its completion. With postoperative SRS, there is minimal to no interruption of systemic agents, thereby decreasing time off treatment and risk of systemic disease progression.

Despite a growing body of literature [134, 136–139], SRS to the resection cavity does not seem to be superior over WBRT in terms of local control at 1 and 2 years. Moreover, SRS may pose increased risk over WBRT of radionecrosis and other neurological complications, as well as leptomeningeal relapse.

Several questions remain regarding SRS following surgery [135, 140, 141]. The optimal dose and fractionation schedule, especially for large brain metastases (>3 cm) associated with higher risk for local failure, are unknown. The same holds true for the optimal margin around the resection cavity to be included in the treatment field. From a clinical standpoint, there remain little data about the impact of postoperative SRS on HRQOL and neurocognitive function. The timing of SRS after surgery also remains unclear. There is little evidence that SRS administered in the immediate postoperative period is more effective than when administered at the time of tumor progression.

The risk of radionecrosis following postoperative SRS [135, 141–143] is higher (between 9 and 17.5%) than that reported by the EORTC study with WBRT following either surgery or radiosurgery (2.6%), and could increase over time (7% at 1 year and 16% at 2 years) [141]. However, the actual incidence of pathologically proven radionecrosis is unknown, as often the values reported in the different series represent a combination of biopsy proven and MRI suspected cases of radionecrosis. Several advanced neuroimaging techniques (MRS, MRI perfusion, PET with FDG or amino acids) can aid in the diagnosis of radiation necrosis but oftentimes produce conflicting results. Treatment may include the use of bevacizumab [113], but not without significant financial costs. Alternatively, steroids can reduce symptoms and edema related to radiation effects, but their use increases risk of steroid dependency. The average frequency and duration of steroid using following postoperative SRS remains unknown.

The use of SRS to the resection cavity without the addition of WBRT may be associated with increased risk of leptomeningeal disease (LMD). The incidence has been found to range from 8 to 13% [139, 141–146]. Patients with breast histology may be at higher risk (at 1 year 24% vs. 9%) [146]. It is unclear whether the inclusion of WBRT would decrease this risk or whether the increased risk for LMD seen in patients with brain metastases from breast is associated with the biology of this tumor type. To better characterize this risk of LMD, future reports on the use of SRS to the resection cavity should distinguish between compartments of failure: local, distant and leptomeningeal.

In conclusion, the main limitations of available studies on postoperative SRS in single brain metastasis include relatively small sample size, short follow-up, heterogeneous primary histologies, unknown disease stage, and concurrent use of chemotherapy. Given the lack of clear risk/benefit data and increased associated financial costs, additional research in this area is needed before the use of postoperative SRS becomes routine clinical practice [147].

WBRT Alone

WBRT alone is the treatment of choice for patients with any of the following: single or multiple brain metastases not amenable to surgery or radiosurgery, a low KPS (≤ 50) or active systemic disease. Complete and partial responses have been reported in up to 60% of patients, with a neurological improvement that probably is in part attributable to steroids. Tumor volume reduction after WBRT seems to be associated with better neurocognitive function preservation and prolonged survival [148]. Median survival following WBRT alone ranges from 3 to 6 months, with 10–15% of patients alive at 1 year. A meta-analysis of 39 trials involving 10.835 patients concluded that, in comparison to standard fractionation (30 Gy in 10 fractions or 20 Gy in 5 fractions), altered WBRT dose fractionation schemes do not improve overall survival, neurologic function or symptom control [149]. However, a recent randomized trial in patients with NSCLC not candidate for either surgery or radiosurgery, did not show any difference in overall survival and quality of life between WBRT and supportive care alone [150].

Nausea, vomiting, headache, fewer and worsening of neurological symptoms can be observed in the initial phase of therapy, requiring steroid administration for control.

Up to date, radiosensitizers have not provided any clear additional benefit over conventional treatment. Recently, the addition of motexafin gadolinium to early WBRT in patients with brain metastases from NSCLC yielded an improvement in time to neurological progression over WBRT alone (5.5 months vs. 3.7 months) [151]. Likewise, the addition of efaproxiral (RSR 13) to WBRT in patients with brain metastases from breast cancer has reduced the death rate by 46%, while improving quality of life [152].

Cognitive Dysfunctions Following WBRT: Risk Factors, Pathogenesis, and Prevention

A radiation-induced dementia with ataxia and urinary incontinence has been reported in up to 30% of patients by one year from receiving unconventional large size fractions of WBRT (6–8.5 Gy) [153]. The picture on CT/MRI is that of a leukoencephalopathy (diffuse hyperintensity of the periventricular white matter on T2-weighted and FLAIR images) with associated hydrocephalus. Ventriculoperitoneal shunt may be of clinical value in some patients. When using more conventional size fractions (up to 3 or 4 Gy per fraction) the risk is that of milder cognitive dysfunctions, consisting mainly of deficits in learning and memory with associated white matter damage and cortical atrophy on MRI. Patients with arterial hypertension, diabetes or other vascular diseases are at higher risk of developing cognitive dysfunctions. The pathogenesis of this radiation-damage is thought to include injury to the endothelium of small vessels, resulting in accelerated atherosclerosis and ultimately in a chronic ischemia similar to small vessel disease of vascular dementia. For this reason, there is interest in investigating vascular dementia treatments to prevent or reduce radiation-induced cognitive decline. One of these approaches is using memantine in combination with WBRT. Memantine is a non-competitive, low affinity antagonist of the N-methyl-D-aspartate (NMDA) receptor, a receptor activated by the principal excitatory neurotransmitter glutamate. Memantine has the potential to block the excessive NMDA stimulation following ischemia that may lead to excitotoxic damage of the normal brain. In two placebo-controlled phase III trials memantine was well tolerated and effective in treating patients with small vessel disease [154, 155]. In a recently published randomized, double-blind, placebo-controlled phase II trial of RTOG (RTOG 0614) the use of memantine during and after WBRT resulted in better cognitive function over time, specifically delaying time to cognitive decline, and reducing the rates of decline in memory, executive function and processing speed [156].

Radiation-induced cognitive deficits may also result, at least in part, from injury to neuronal stem cells in the subgranular zone of the hippocampus [157, 158]. Stem cell neurogenesis critical in memory function, especially for encoding new episodic memories. Low-dose irradiation in rodents results in a blockade of hippocampal neurogenesis and damage of the neurogenic microenvironment, leading to significant short-term memory impairment. Sparing the hippocampus during WBRT could prevent damage to neuronal progenitor cells and improve memory function [159]. Hippocampal avoidance WBRT (HAWBRT) uses intensity modulated radiotherapy (IMRT) to conformally reduce the radiation dose to the hippocampus, while applying the usual higher dose to the whole brain. A potential concern is whether hippocampal avoidance could lead to loss of control of metastases in or around this region. However, recent studies analyzing the distribution of recurrent brain metastases have shown that the metastatic involvement of the limbic circuit is uncommon [160, 161]. The recent single arm phase II RTOG 0933 suggested that the conformal avoidance of the hippocampus during WBRT spares memory and QoL. Performance at 4 months on standardized memory tests declined 7% from baseline in patients treated with HAWBRT compared with 30% in a historical control group [162]. Importantly, the trial reported that of the patients who developed intracranial progression only 4.5% experienced progression in the hippocampal avoidance area.

Building on results of RTOG 0933 and RTOG 0614, NRGCC001 is a US National Cancer Institute approved phase III trial that will evaluate the potential combined neuroprotective effects of hippocampal avoidance in addition to memantine during WBRT for brain metastases [163]. Given the increased cost of hippocampal avoidance, the trial will also perform a comparative cost-effectiveness analysis.

Treatment of Recurrent Brain Metastasis

Re-resection can afford neurological improvement and prolongation of survival in patients with local accessible brain relapse, high performance status, stable extracranial disease, and relatively long time to recurrence (>6 months) [81, 164–166]. Salvage WBRT following previous WBRT or SRS is now rarely employed. Salvage SRS after WBRT has been widely used during the initial development of SRS, and RTOG 9005 [92] has established the standard doses according to diameter. Several retrospective studies have reported reasonable local control and survival rates with SRS for salvage after WBRT [167–170]. A population-based study has suggested similar survival outcomes following either salvage SRS or boost SRS [171].

Reirradiation with SRS after local recurrence at a site treated with SRS has been employed in a limited number of patients, and the long-term risk of radionecrosis should be considered against the benefit [172].

Multiple courses of SRS for new brain metastases after an initial course of SRS, with continued deferral of WBRT, may yield high rates of local control, low risk of toxicity, and favorable duration of overall and neurologic progression-free survival [100, 173, 174]. A recent large retrospective series [175] has reported that in patients undergoing multiple courses of SRS the aggregate volume, but not the cumulative number of brain metastases, and the GPA score, as recalculated at the second course of SRS, correlate with duration of survival and help guide management.

Chemotherapy and Targeted Therapies

For many years chemotherapy has not been considered to play a major role in the treatment of patients with brain metastases, due to the presence of the blood–brain barrier (BBB) which limits the access of hydrophilic and/or large drugs into the CNS. However, the BBB is partially disrupted in many brain metastases (>1 mm in size) allowing for many chemotherapeutic agents to reach the tumor cells. Intrinsic chemosensitivity of tumor cells is a more critical factor for the response to chemotherapy [176]. Response rates of brain metastases often reflect the sensitivity of the primary tumor: relatively high response rates in SCLC (30–80%), intermediate rates in breast cancer (30–50%) and NSCLC (10–30%), and low rates in melanoma (10–15%).Importantly even in the most chemosensitive tumors response to chemotherapy is typically equivalent to that observed with radiotherapy.

The combination of radiotherapy and chemotherapy may improve response rates compared to radiotherapy alone, but does not improve survival [177], as in the case of radiotherapy combined with temozolomide (TMZ) for brain metastases [178, 179].

At least two theories may help to explain the disappointing results with chemotherapy. First, metastatic tumor cells in the brain may be resistant to chemotherapy. Brain metastases often develop later in the course of disease after multiple rounds of prior chemotherapies, allowing for the development of resistance through the accumulation of different mutations. Second, permeability of BBB in brain metastases is likely heterogeneous, thereby preventing sufficient drug accumulation and distribution. It has been hypothesized [180] that brain metastases from primary tumors with an intrinsic low expression of P-glycoprotein (an ATP-dependent efflux pump linked to chemoresistance) may be more permeable to antineoplastic drugs.

Recent advances in the understanding of the molecular pathways of tumor growth in many solid tumors have allowed the development of agents targeting specific molecular pathways both in extracranial and intracranial disease [181, 182]. Overall, the response rates to targeted agents seem higher than those observed after conventional chemotherapy. However, for some of these agents passage across the BBB remains an issue. Most of these new compounds, similarly to the old chemotherapeutics, have been shown to be substrates of one or more active efflux transporters.

The promising activity of several TKIs in brain metastases from different primaries has led to two main avenues of clinical investigation [183]. The first is the use of targeted agents as radiosensitizers, which has led to the combination of targeted agents with radiotherapy (WBRT, SRS).The second is the upfront use of targeted agents to control micrometastases, which would allow WBRT to be withheld. Clinical and translation work is ongoing to fully characterize the potential utility of TKIs in the management of brain metastases.

The antiangiogenic drug bevacizumab, a monoclonal antibody targeting VEGF with activity in high-grade, is now being investigated in brain metastases from miscellaneous solid tumor types. Its associated risk of bleeding has been shown to be quite low [184].

Two important factors can limit the impact of targeted agents on brain metastases: a lack of molecular concordance between the primary tumor and brain metastasis and the emergence of secondary resistance.

Brain Metastases from NSCLC

Platinum compounds (cisplatin, carboplatin), alone or in combination (etoposide, vinorelbine), are the most commonly used chemotherapeutics against brain metastases from NSCLC, either upfront or after radiation at the time of recurrence [176]. Pemetrexed and temozolomide also have some activity. The role of EGFR tyrosine kinase inhibitors (gefitinib, erlotinib) in the management of brain metastases from NSCLC is emerging. A pooled analysis of published data to evaluate the efficacy of EGFR TKIs in NSCLC patients with brain metastases has been recently published [185]. Sixteen studies were included in the analysis, with a total of 464 enrolled patients. The EGFR mutational status was unknown for 362 (unselected group) and 102 had activating EGFR mutations. A higher response rate (85% vs. 45.1%), and a longer PFS (12.3 months vs. 5.9 months) and OS (16.2 months vs. 10.3 months) were observed in the EGFR mutation group compared with the unselected group. These data strongly suggest that the EGFRTKIs are an effective treatment for NSCLC patients with brain metastases, particularly for those patients harboring activating EGFR mutations. However, even in EGFR wild-type patients EGFR-TKIs represent a valuable second-line therapy with a response rate of around 10% [14].

Based on the high intracranial response rates, TKIs monotherapy may be used in lieu of WBRT in patients harboring activating EGFR mutations and asymptomatic brain metastases (i.e., not needing the palliation from WBRT) [186–188]. However, it is important to note that the discordance rate of EGFR mutations between the primary tumor and brain metastases can be as high as 32%, and the CSF penetration rate of gefitinib (1–10%) and erlotinib (2.5–13%) is limited. A systematic review and metanalysis of the literature has suggested that upfront cranial radiotherapy (SRS or WBRT), alone or with TKIs, may improve survival outcome relative to TKIs alone. On the other hand, the combination of erlotinib with radiation therapy (SRS or WBRT) in patient cohorts not specifically selected for target expression has failed to demonstrate superiority over radiotherapy alone [189–191]. To date, there are no published data on the efficacy for brain metastases of the newer EGFR TKI inhibitors (afatinib, doconitib, and icotinib).

Other "druggable" alterations seen in up to 5% of NSCLC patients include rearrangements of the "anaplastic lymphoma kinase" (ALK) gene. In particular, ALK translocations have been found in 3% of brain metastases from NSCLC, and appear to be concordant between brain metastasis and primary tumor [192]. NSCLC with ALK activating translocations has been shown to be sensitive to treatment with the ALK inhibitor crizotinib. A recent study on brain metastases from ALK-rearranged NSCLC [193] has reported that crizotinib was associated with a 55% rate of disease control within CNS at 3 months of therapy in both RT-naïve and RT-pretreated patients. Moreover, crizotinib was associated with a moderate (18–33%) RECIST-confirmed response rate.

Other multitarget ALK-TKIs, such as ceritinib and alectinib, which are active in patients with ALK-rearranged NSCLC who are either naïve or resistant to crizotinib, are now being investigated in patients with brain metastases. Veliparib, a PARP 1, 2 inhibitor, is another interesting compound currently under investigation in combination with WBRT for the treatment of brain metastases from NSCLC.

Brain Metastases from SCLC

Various combinations of etoposide, teniposide, cisplatinum or carboplatinum are active against brain metastases [176]. So far, there are no effective targeted agents available.

Brain Metastases from Breast Cancer

Chemotherapy regimens, variably combining cyclophosphamide, 5-FU, methotrexate, vincristine, cisplatin, and etoposide are active in patients with brain metastases from breast cancer [176]. Capecitabine monotherapy has activity against breast cancer brain metastases. In a retrospective review conducted at MSKCC [194], three out of four patients showed complete response, and three had stable disease, with a median overall and progression-free survival after treatment of 13 and 8 months respectively. Capecitabine, combined with TMZ, has some efficacy as well [195]. Likewise, high-dose methotrexate has activity in recurrent brain metastases [196]; however, the risk of leukoencephalopathy, especially when administered after WBRT, is a limiting factor.

The dual EGFR and HER2 tyrosine kinase inhibitor lapatinib has shown modest activity in a phase II study in HER2-positive breast cancer patients with brain metastases, following trastuzumab-based systemic chemotherapy and WBRT [197]. CNS objective responses to lapatinib were observed in 6% of patients, and 21% experienced ≥ 20% volumetric reduction in the CNS lesions. A recent phase II single arm study (LANDSCAPE) has shown that the combination of lapatinib and capecitabine in patients with previously untreated brain metastases from HER2-positive metastatic breast cancer yields durable responses in up to 65% of patients [198]. Based on the strength of these data, a randomized trial comparing lapatinib and capecitabine versus WBRT has been launched. In addition, trials of other HER2 directed TKIs, including neratinib and afatinib, are currently in progress.

It is not clear whether trastuzumab, with limited blood–brain barrier penetration, may be active as well [20].

Brain Metastases from Melanoma

Fotemustine (response rate of 5–25%) and temozolomide (response rate 6–10%), either as single agent or in combination with WBRT, are the most active chemotherapeutics against brain metastases from melanoma [176, 199].

BRAF V600E inhibitors are emerging as treatment options for patients with BRAF-mutant melanoma metastatic to the CNS. The activity of vemurafenib is meaningful. Both retrospective [200] and phase II trials [201] have reported an intracranial response rate of 16–50%, despite disappointing results on OS. A phase II study of dabrafenib in patients with BRAF-mutated melanoma and brain metastasis reported an overall intracranial objective response rate of 31%, with little difference between patients who progressed after prior CNS therapy and patients who were treatment naïve [202].

The activity of BRAF inhibitors on brain metastases appears to be superior to that of ipilimumab [203–205], a monoclonal antibody with immunomodulatory activity that has been approved for the treatment of metastatic melanoma. An open-label phase 2 multicenter trial in the US [204] showed that ipilimumab has activity in patients with asymptomatic melanoma brain metastases off steroids. Disease control (CR + PR + SD) after 12 weeks of treatment was 16% in the cohort of asymptomatic patients without steroids compared with 5% in the cohort of symptomatic patients receiving steroids. Steroid use may suppress the immune response thereby limiting the effect of immunotherapy, though this remains to be clearly established. Importantly, the investigators did not report any neurological deterioration as an effect of an inflammatory response to treatment in the CNS, even in patients who had received prior radiation therapy. There is some interest in combining ipilimumab with radiation therapy [206], and new molecular agents, such as trametinib, are being investigated.

Prophylaxis

The brain can be a sanctuary for micrometastases that can become radiologically and/or clinically evident after the primary tumor has been controlled by effective therapies. Thus, treating the subclinical disease could prevent the development of overt brain metastases. This strategy is particularly relevant for SCLC where prophylactic cranial irradiation (PCI) reduces the risk of brain metastases at 2 years and increases overall survival in patients with SCLC who achieve complete remission after upfront therapy [207, 208]. Cognitive decline in SCLC patients after PCI is relatively uncommon up to 2 years after PCI [209, 210]. There is currently insufficient evidence to support PCI in high-risk NSCLC patients [211].

In patients with metastatic HER2-positive breast cancer, PCI or newer drugs with improved penetration of an intact BBB (i.e., TMZ, lapatinib) might be useful. The combination of these agents with radiation could allow a lowering of the PCI dose.

Effective agents are needed to prophylactically treat micrometastatic disease in patients at high risk for brain metastases. Well-designed clinical trials that include detailed neuropsychological assessments are needed to both identify effective agents and establish the role for CNS prophylaxis in different systemic malignancies.

Prevention Strategies: Molecular and Clinical Data

Numerous molecular compounds have been tested in preclinical models in a prevention setting and overall the studies have shown that prevention of brain metastases is feasible [212, 213]. Experimental models have shown that bevacizumab may prevent early angiogenesis and induce prolonged dormancy of micrometastases [214]. Lapatinib, vorinostat, and pazopanib are able to prevent the formation of metastases by brain-topic breast cancer cells [215–217]. The selective PLK1 inhibitor GSK 46I1364A, inhibits the development of large brain metastases and prolongs the survival in a xenograft model of breast cancer brain metastases [218]. Limited clinical data have shown that prevention of brain metastases can also be achieved in clinical settings. In a metastatic breast cancer trial of lapatinib plus capecitabine versus capecitabine alone there was a significant reduction in the incidence of metastases in the brain as first site of relapse after combined treatment [219]. A retrospective review of a sub-cohort of patients with advanced EGFR-mutated NSCLC treated with gefinitib or erlotinib reported 1-year and 2-year CNS relapse rates of 6 and 13%, respectively, an improvement from historical data [220]. A retrospective analysis of the clinical trial data from sorafenib in patients with renal cell cancer(RCC) and brain metastases demonstrated a 75% prevention of brain metastases development, compared with 4% response rate for established metastases [221]. A recent review of patients enrolled in a phase III trial on RCC (TARGET trial) revealed a significantly lower incidence of brain metastases in patients who received sorafenib (3%) than in those who received placebo (12%) [222]. The protective effect of TKIs (sorafenib, sunitinib, pazopanib) on the development of brain metastases from RCC has been recently outlined [223].

A major challenge in the field has been the identification of patients at highest risk of developing brain metastases because of tumor and host factors. Up to date, only HER2-positive breast cancer patients have entered prevention trials to better define the role of lapatinib.

Challenges in Developing Trials in Brain Metastases

The design of clinical trials in brain metastases can be challenging [224–226]. The choice of endpoints is influenced by several factors including the patient population, primary tumor type, phase of trial and the setting (treatment of established brain metastases or prevention). The ideal measure of drug activity in the brain is the assay of target modulation within the tumor obtained after resection in patients treated preoperatively. Moreover, advanced neuroimaging techniques may provide valuable surrogate pharmacodynamic information. Objective response has been commonly used as primary endpoint for phase II trials in patients with brain metastases, being a possible surrogate for other markers of clinical benefit, such as neurological status, neurocognitive decline or neurological deterioration free survival. Unfortunately, none of the standard response criteria (RECIST, WHO, MacDonald, RANO) were designed specifically for brain metastases. There is a need to standardize MRI criteria for lesion measurement (tumor area versus volume) and the definition of response to treatment, including use of both steroids and neurological symptoms in the response criteria. Use of unique therapies such as antiangiogenic agents and immunomodulators will require specific adaptations. A clear distinction between intracranial, extracranial and overall progression-free survival is important. When the concurrent systemic disease is controlled by a standard systemic regimen, the safety (not only the efficacy) of concurrent use of an investigational agent for brain metastasis must be carefully evaluated.

As the number of experimental agents increases and available resources become limited, new trial designs should be considered. Adaptive randomization can make clinical trials more efficient in reaching endpoints with fewer patients than with conventional randomization [227].

The RANO Brain Metastasis Group has recently proposed new response criteria for clinical trials in patients with brain metastases [228]; these need validation in the next generation of studies.

Other Cranial Metastases

The topics of skull and dural metastases are covered in Chap. 23 (Neurological Complications of Breast Cancer and Its Treatment).

References

1. Central Brain Tumor Registry of the US. CBTRUS Statistical Report: Primary Brain and Central Nervous System Tumors Diagnosed in the in 2004.2008. 2012. Available at www.cbtrus. org. Accessed 5 Mar 2012.
2. Davis FG, Dolecek TA, McCarthy BJ, Villano JL. Toward determining the lifetime occurrence of metastatic brain tumors estimated from 2007 United States cancer incidence data. Neuro Oncol. 2012;14(9):1171–7.
3. Schouten LJ, Rutten J, Huveneers HA, Twijnstra A. Incidence of brain metastases in a cohort of patients with carcinoma of the breast, colon, kidney, and lung and melanoma. Cancer. 2002;94 (10):2698–705.
4. Barnholtz-Sloan JS, Sloan AE, Davis FG, Vigneau FD, Lai P, Sawaya RE. Incidence proportions of brain metastases in patients diagnosed (1973–2001) in the metropolitan detroit cancer surveillance system. J Clin Oncol. 2004;22(14):2865–72.
5. Gavrilovic IT, Posner JB. Brain metastases: epidemiology and pathophysiology. J Neurooncol. 2005;75(1):5–14.
6. Fabi A, Felici A, Metro G, Mirri A, Bria E, Telera S, Moscetti L, Russillo M, Lanzetta G, Mansueto G, Pace A, Maschio M, Vidiri A, Sperduti I, Cognetti F, Carapella CM. Brain metastases from solid tumors: disease outcome according to type of treatment and therapeutic resources of the treating center. J Exp Clin Cancer Res. 2011;18(30):10.
7. Nayak L, Lee EQ, Wen PY. Epidemiology of brain metastases. Curr Oncol Rep. 2012;14(1):48–54.
8. Bouffet E, Doumi N, Thiesse P, Mottolese C, Jouvet A, Lacroze M, Carrie C, Frappaz D, Brunat-Mentigny M. Brain metastases in children with solid tumors. Cancer. 1997;79 (2):403–10.
9. Sze G, Milano E, Johnson C, Heier L. Detection of brain metastases: comparison of contrast-enhanced MR with unenhanced MR and enhanced CT. AJNR Am J Neuroradiol. 1990;11 (4):785–91.
10. Schellinger PD, Meinck HM, Thron A. Diagnostic accuracy of MRI compared to CCT in patients with brain metastases. J Neurooncol. 1999;44(3):275–81.
11. Delattre JY, Krol G, Thaler HT, Posner JB. Distribution of brain metastases. Arch Neurol. 1988;45(7):741–4.
12. Byrne TN, Cascino TL, Posner JB. Brain metastasis from melanoma. J Neurooncol. 1983;1(4):313–7.
13. Preusser M, Capper D, Ilhan-Mutlu A, Berghoff AS, Birner P, Bartsch R, Marosi C, Zielinski C, Mehta MP, Winkler F, Wick W, von Deimling A. Brain metastases: pathobiology and emerging targeted therapies. Acta Neuropathol. 2012;123 (2):205–22.
14. Berger LA, Riesenberg H, Bokemeyer C, Atanackovic D. CNS metastases in non-small-cell lung cancer: current role of EGFR-TKI therapy and future perspectives. Lung Cancer. 2013;80(3):242–8.
15. Heitz F, Harter P, Lueck HJ, Fissler-Eckhoff A, Lorenz-Salehi F, Scheil-Bertram S, Traut A, du Bois A. Triple-negative and HER2-overexpressing breast cancers exhibit an elevated risk and

an earlier occurrence of cerebral metastases. Eur J Cancer. 2009;45(16):2792–8.
16. Berghoff AS, Preusser M. Biology in prevention and treatment of brain metastases. Expert Rev Anticancer Ther. 2013;13 (11):1339–48.
17. Yin W, Jiang Y, Shen Z, Shao Z, Lu J. Trastuzumab in the adjuvant treatment of HER2-positive early breast cancer patients: a meta-analysis of published randomized controlled trials. PLoS ONE. 2011;6(6):e21030.
18. Pestalozzi BC, Holmes E, de Azambuja E, Metzger-Filho O, Hogge L, Scullion M, Láng I, Wardley A, Lichinitser M, Sanchez RI, Müller V, Dodwell D, Gelber RD, Piccart-Gebhart MJ, Cameron D. CNS relapses in patients with HER2-positive early breast cancer who have and have not received adjuvant trastuzumab: a retrospective substudy of the HERA trial (BIG 1-01). Lancet Oncol. 2013;14(3):244–8.
19. Olson EM, Najita JS, Sohl J, Arnaout A, Burstein HJ, Winer EP, Lin NU. Clinical outcomes and treatment practice patterns of patients with HER2-positive metastatic breast cancer in the post-trastuzumab era. Breast. 2013;22(4):525–31.
20. Larsen PB, Kümler I, Nielsen DL. A systematic review of trastuzumab and lapatinib in the treatment of women with brain metastases from HER2-positive breast cancer. Cancer Treat Rev. 2013;39(7):720–7.
21. Fidler IJ. The role of the organ microenvironment in brain metastasis. Semin Cancer Biol. 2011;21(2):107–12.
22. Eichler AF, Chung E, Kodack DP, Loeffler JS, Fukumura D, Jain RK. The biology of brain metastases-translation to new therapies. Nat Rev Clin Oncol. 2011;8(6):344–56.
23. Arshad F, Wang L, Sy C, Avraham S, Avraham HK. Blood-brain barrier integrity and breast cancer metastasis to the brain. Patholog Res Int. 2010;29(2011):920509.
24. Smid M, Wang Y, Zhang Y, Sieuwerts AM, Yu J, Klijn JG, Foekens JA, Martens JW. Subtypes of breast cancer show preferential site of relapse. Cancer Res. 2008;68(9):3108–14.
25. Bos PD, Zhang XH, Nadal C, Shu W, Gomis RR, Nguyen DX, Minn AJ, van de Vijver MJ, Gerald WL, Foekens JA, Massagué J. Genes that mediate breast cancer metastasis to the brain. Nature. 2009;459(7249):1005–9.
26. Palmieri D, Fitzgerald D, Shreeve SM, Hua E, Bronder JL, Weil RJ, Davis S, Stark AM, Merino MJ, Kurek R, Mehdorn HM, Davis G, Steinberg SM, Meltzer PS, Aldape K, Steeg PS. Analyses of resected human brain metastases of breast cancer reveal the association between up-regulation of hexokinase 2 and poor prognosis. Mol Cancer Res. 2009;7(9):1438–45.
27. Palmieri D, Bronder JL, Herring JM, Yoneda T, Weil RJ, Stark AM, Kurek R, Vega-Valle E, Feigenbaum L, Halverson D, Vortmeyer AO, Steinberg SM, Aldape K, Steeg PS. Her-2 overexpression increases the metastatic outgrowth of breast cancer cells in the brain. Cancer Res. 2007;67(9):4190–8.
28. Lee H-Te, Xue J, Chou P-C, Zhou A, Yang P, Conrad CA, Aldape KD, Priebe W, Patterson C, Sawaya R, Xie K, Huang S. Stat3 orchestrate interaction between endothelial and tumor cells and inhibition of Stat3 suppresses brain metastasis of breast cancer cells. Oncotarget. 2015;6(12):10016–29.
29. Grinberg-Rashi H, Ofek E, Perelman M, Skarda J, Yaron P, Hajdúch M, Jacob-Hirsch J, Amariglio N, Krupsky M, Simansky DA, Ram Z, Pfeffer R, Galernter I, Steinberg DM, Ben-Dov I, Rechavi G, Izraeli S. The expression of three genes in primary non-small cell lung cancer is associated with metastatic spread to the brain. Clin Cancer Res. 2009;15(5):1755–61.
30. Gril B, Evans L, Palmieri D, Steeg PS. Translational research in brain metastasis is identifying molecular pathways that may lead to the development of new therapeutic strategies. Eur J Cancer. 2010;46(7):1204–10.

31. Marchetti D, Denkins Y, Reiland J, Greiter-Wilke A, Galjour J, Murry B, Blust J, Roy M. Brain-metastatic melanoma: a neurotrophic perspective. Pathol Oncol Res. 2003;9(3):147–58.

32. Zhang C, Zhang F, Tsan R, Fidler IJ. Transforming growth factor-beta2 is a molecular determinant for site-specific melanoma metastasis in the brain. Cancer Res. 2009;69(3):828–35.

33. Nicolson GL, Menter DG, Herrmann JL, Yun Z, Cavanaugh P, Marchetti D. Brain metastasis: role of trophic, autocrine, and paracrine factors in tumor invasion and colonization of the central nervous system. Curr Top Microbiol Immunol. 1996;213(Pt 2):89–115.

34. Yano S, Shinohara H, Herbst RS, Kuniyasu H, Bucana CD, Ellis LM, Davis DW, McConkey DJ, Fidler IJ. Expression of vascular endothelial growth factor is necessary but not sufficient for production and growth of brain metastasis. Cancer Res. 2000;60(17):4959–67.

35. Bergers G, Brekken R, McMahon G, Vu TH, Itoh T, Tamaki K, Tanzawa K, Thorpe P, Itohara S, Werb Z, Hanahan D. Matrix metalloproteinase-9 triggers the angiogenic switch during carcinogenesis. Nat Cell Biol. 2000;2(10):737–44.

36. Kim LS, Huang S, Lu W, Lev DC, Price JE. Vascular endothelial growth factor expression promotes the growth of breast cancer brain metastases in nude mice. Clin Exp Metastasis. 2004;21 (2):107–18.

37. Kirsch M, Schackert G, Black PM. Angiogenesis, metastasis, and endogenous inhibition. J Neurooncol. 2000;50(1–2):173–80.

38. Leone A, Flatow U, King CR, Sandeen MA, Margulies IM, Liotta LA, Steeg PS. Reduced tumor incidence, metastatic potential, and cytokine responsiveness of nm23-transfected melanoma cells. Cell. 1991;65(1):25–35.

39. Sarris M, Scolyer RA, Konopka M, Thompson JF, Harper CG, Lee CS. Cytoplasmic expression of nm23 predicts the potential for cerebral metastasis in patients with primary cutaneous melanoma. Melanoma Res. 2004;14(1):23–7. Erratum in: Melanoma Res. 2004;14(3):239. Lee, Soon C [corrected to Lee, C Soon].

40. Harabin-Słowińska M, Słowiński J, Konecki J, Mrówka R. Expression of adhesion molecule CD44 in metastatic brain tumors. Folia Neuropathol. 1998;36(3):179–84.

41. Li H, Liu J, Hofmann M, Hamou MF, de Tribolet N. Differential CD44 expression patterns in primary brain tumors and brain metastases. Br J Cancer. 1995;72(1):160–3.

42. Desprechins B, Stadnik T, Koerts G, Shabana W, Breucq C, Osteaux M. Use of diffusion-weighted MR imaging in differential diagnosis between intracerebral necrotic tumors and cerebral abscesses. AJNR Am J Neuroradiol. 1999;20(7):1252–7.

43. Hartmann M, Jansen O, Heiland S, Sommer C, Münkel K, Sartor K. Restricted diffusion within ring enhancement is not pathognomonic for brain abscess. AJNR Am J Neuroradiol. 2001;22(9):1738–42.

44. Duygulu G, Ovali GY, Calli C, Kitis O, Yünten N, Akalin T, Islekel S. Intracerebral metastasis showing restricted diffusion: correlation with histopathologic findings. Eur J Radiol. 2010;74 (1):117–20.

45. Law M, Cha S, Knopp EA, Johnson G, Arnett J, Litt AW. High-grade gliomas and solitary metastases: differentiation by using perfusion and proton spectroscopic MR imaging. Radiology. 2002;222(3):715–21.

46. Bulakbasi N, Kocaoglu M, Farzaliyev A, Tayfun C, Ucoz T, Somuncu I. Assessment of diagnostic accuracy of perfusion MR imaging in primary and metastatic solitary malignant brain tumors. AJNR Am J Neuroradiol. 2005;26(9):2187–99.

47. Chiang IC, Kuo YT, Lu CY, Yeung KW, Lin WC, Sheu FO, Liu GC. Distinction between high-grade gliomas and solitary metastases using peritumoral 3-T magnetic resonance

48. spectroscopy, diffusion, and perfusion imagings. Neuroradiology. 2004;46(8):619–27.

48. Server A, Josefsen R, Kulle B, Maehlen J, Schellhorn T, Gadmar Ø, Kumar T, Haakonsen M, Langberg CW, Nakstad PH. Proton magnetic resonance spectroscopy in the distinction of high-grade cerebral gliomas from single metastatic brain tumors. Acta Radiol. 2010;51(3):316–25.

49. Kosaka N, Tsuchida T, Uematsu H, Kimura H, Okazawa H, Itoh H. 18F-FDG PET of common enhancing malignant brain tumors. AJR Am J Roentgenol. 2008;190(6):365–9.

50. Hutterer M, Nowosielski M, Putzer D, Jansen NL, Seiz M, Schocke M, McCoy M, Göbel G, la Fougère C, Virgolini IJ, Trinka E, Jacobs AH, Stockhammer G. [18F]-fluoro-ethyl-L-tyrosine PET: a valuable diagnostic tool in neuro-oncology, but not all that glitters is glioma. Neuro Oncol. 2013;15(3):341–51.

51. Le Chevalier T, Smith FP, Caille P, Constans JP, Rouesse JG. Sites of primary malignancies in patients presenting with cerebral metastases. A review of 120 cases. Cancer. 1985;56(4):880–2.

52. Merchut MP. Brain metastases from undiagnosed systemic neoplasms. Arch Intern Med. 1989;149(5):1076–80.

53. Van de Pol M, van Aalst VC, Wilmink JT, Twijnstra A. Brain metastases from an unknown primary tumor: which diagnostic procedures are indicated? J Neurol Neurosurg Psychiatry. 1996;61(3):321–3.

54. Klee B, Law I, Højgaard L, Kosteljanetz M. Detection of unknown primary tumors in patients with cerebral metastases using whole-body 18F-flouorodeoxyglucose positron emission tomography. Eur J Neurol. 2002;9(6):657–62.

55. Rudà R, Borgognone M, Benech F, Vasario E, Soffietti R. Brain metastases from unknown primary tumor: a prospective study. J Neurol. 2001;248(5):394–8.

56. Monzon FA, Koen TJ. Diagnosis of metastatic neoplasms: molecular approaches for identification of tissue of origin. Arch Pathol Lab Med. 2010;134(2):216–24.

57. Berghoff AS, Bartsch R, Wöhrer A, Streubel B, Birner P, Kros JM, Brastianos PK, von Deimling A, Preusser M. Predictive molecular markers in metastases to the central nervous system: recent advances and future avenues. Acta Neuropatol. 2014;128 (6):879–91.

58. Shen Q, Sahin AA, Hess KR, Suki D, Aldape KD, Sawaya R, Ibrahim NK. Breast cancer with brain metastases: clinicopathologic features, survival, and paired biomarker analysis. Oncologist. 2015;20(5):466–73.

59. Gaspar L, Scott C, Rotman M, Asbell S, Phillips T, Wasserman T, McKenna WG, Byhardt R. Recursive partitioning analysis (RPA) of prognostic factors in three Radiation Therapy Oncology Group (RTOG) brain metastases trials. Int J Radiat Oncol Biol Phys. 1997;37(4):745–51.

60. Lagerwaard FJ, Levendag PC, Nowak PJ, Eijkenboom WM, Hanssens PE, Schmitz PI. Identification of prognostic factors in patients with brain metastases: a review of 1292 patients. Int J Radiat Oncol Biol Phys. 1999;43(4):795–803.

61. Gaspar LE, Scott C, Murray K, Curran W. Validation of the RTOG recursive partitioning analysis (RPA) classification for brain metastases. Int J Radiat Oncol Biol Phys. 2000;47(4):1001–6.

62. Sperduto PW, Berkey B, Gaspar LE, Mehta M, Curran W. A new prognostic index and comparison to three other indices for patients with brain metastases: an analysis of 1960 patients in the RTOG database. Int J Radiat Oncol Biol Phys. 2008;70(2):510–4.

63. Sperduto PW, Chao ST, Sneed PK, Luo X, Suh J, Roberge D, Bhatt A, Jensen AW, Brown PD, Shih H, Kirkpatrick J, Schwer A, Gaspar LE, Fiveash JB, Chiang V, Knisely J, Sperduto CM, Mehta M. Diagnosis-specific prognostic factors,

indexes, and treatment outcomes for patients with newly diagnosed brain metastases: a multi-institutional analysis of 4259 patients. Int J Radiat Oncol Biol Phys. 2010;77(3):655–61.

64. Sperduto PW, Kased N, Roberge D, Xu Z, Shanley R, Luo X, Sneed PK, Chao ST, Weil RJ, Suh J, Bhatt A, Jensen AW, Brown PD, Shih HA, Kirkpatrick J, Gaspar LE, Fiveash JB, Chiang V, Knisely JP, Sperduto CM, Lin N, Mehta M. Effect of tumor subtype on survival and the graded prognostic assessment for patients with breast cancer and brain metastases. Int J Radiat Oncol Biol Phys. 2012;82(5):2111–7.

65. Subbiah IM, Lei X, Weinberg JS, Sulman EP, Chavez-MacGregor M, Tripathy D, Gupta R, Varma A, Chouhan J, Guevarra RP, Valero V, Gilbert MR, Gonzalez-Angulo AM. Validation and development of a modified breast graded prognostic assessment as a tool for survival in patients with breast cancer and brain metastases. J Clin Oncol. 2015;33(20):2239–45.

66. Barnholtz-Sloan JS, Yu C, Sloan AE, Vengoechea J, Wang M, Dignam JJ, Vogelbaum MA, Sperduto PW, Mehta MP, Machtay M, Kattan MW. A nomogram for individualized estimation of survival among patients with brain metastasis. Neuro Oncol. 2012;14(7):910–8.

67. Weltman E, Salvajoli JV, Brandt RA, de Morais Hanriot R, Prisco FE, Cruz JC, de Oliveira Borges SR, Wajsbrot DB. Radiosurgery for brain metastases: a score index for predicting prognosis. Int J Radiat Oncol Biol Phys. 2000;46(5):1155–61.

68. Lorenzoni J, Devriendt D, Massager N, David P, Ruíz S, Vanderlinden B, Van Houtte P, Brotchi J, Levivier M. Radiosurgery for treatment of brain metastases: estimation of patient eligibility using three stratification systems. Int J Radiat Oncol Biol Phys. 2004;60(1):218–24.

69. Nguyen LN, Maor MH, Oswald MJ. Brain metastases as the only manifestation of an undetected primary tumor. Cancer. 1998;83 (10):2181–4.

70. Soffietti R, Cornu P, Delattre JY, Grant R, Graus F, Grisold W, Heimans J, Hildebrand J, Hoskin P, Kalljo M, Krauseneck P, Marosi C, Siegal T, Vecht C. EFNS Guidelines on diagnosis and treatment of brain metastases: report of an EFNS Task Force. Eur J Neurol. 2006;13(7):674–81.

71. Ryken TC, McDermott M, Robinson PD, Ammirati M, Andrews DW, Asher AL, Burri SH, Cobbs CS, Gaspar LE, Kondziolka D, Linskey ME, Loeffler JS, Mehta MP, Mikkelsen T, Olson JJ, Paleologos NA, Patchell RA, Kalkanis SN. The role of steroids in the management of brain metastases: a systematic review and evidence-based clinical practice guideline. J Neurooncol. 2010;96(1):103–14.

72. Glantz MJ, Cole BF, Forsyth PA, Recht LD, Wen PY, Chamberlain MC, Grossman SA, Cairncross JG. Practice parameter: anticonvulsant prophylaxis in patients with newly diagnosed brain tumors. Report of the Quality Standards Subcommittee of the American Academy of Neurology. Neurology. 2000;54 (10):1886–93.

73. Rudà R, Soffietti R. What is New in the management of epilepsy in gliomas? Curr Treat Options Neurol. 2015;17(6):351.

74. Lyman GH, Bohlke K, Khorana AA, Kuderer NM, Lee AY, Arcelus JI, Balaban EP, Clarke JM, Flowers CR, Francis CW, Gates LE, Kakkar AK, Key NS, Levine MN, Liebman HA, Tempero MA, Wong SL, Somerfield MR, Falanga A. American society of clinical oncology. Venous thromboembolism prophylaxis and treatment in patients with cancer: American society of clinical oncology clinical practice guideline update 2014. J Clin Oncol. 2015;33(6):654–6.

75. Sardar P, Chatterjee S, Herzog E, Pekler G, Mushiyev S, Pastori LJ, Visco F, Aronow WS. New oral anticoagulants in patients with cancer: current state of evidence. Am J Ther. 2015;22(6):460–8.

76. Akl EA, Kahale L, Sperati F, Neumann I, Labedi N, Terrenato I, Barba M, Sempos EV, Muti P, Cook D, Schünemann H. Low molecular weight heparin versus unfractionated heparin for perioperative thromboprophylaxis in patients with cancer. Cochrane Database Syst Rev. 2014;6:CD009447.

77. Connors JM. Prophylaxis against venous thromboembolism in patients with cancer. N Engl J Med. 2014;371(13):1263–4.

78. Patchell RA, Tibbs PA, Walsh JW, Dempsey RJ, Maruyama Y, Kryscio RJ, Markesbery WR, Macdonald JS, Young B. A randomized trial of surgery in the treatment of single metastases to the brain. N Engl J Med. 1990;322(8):494–500.

79. Vecht CJ, Haaxma-Reiche H, Noordijk EM, Padberg GW, Voormolen JH, Hoekstra FH, Tans JT, Lambooij N, Metsaars JA, Wattendorff AR, et al. Treatment of single brain metastasis: radiotherapy alone or combined with neurosurgery? Ann Neurol. 1993;33(6):583–90.

80. Mintz AH, Kestle J, Rathbone MP, Gaspar L, Hugenholtz H, Fisher B, Duncan G, Skingley P, Foster G, Levine M. A randomized trial to assess the efficacy of surgery in addition to radiotherapy in patients with a single cerebral metastasis. Cancer. 1996;78(7):1470–6.

81. Vogelbaum MA, Suh JH. Resectable brain metastases. J Clin Oncol. 2006;24(8):1289–94.

82. Kamp MA, Rapp M, Bünher J, Slotty OJ, Reichelt D, Sadat H, Dibué-Adjei M, Steiger H-J, Turowski B, Sabel M. Early postoperative magnet resonance tomography after resection of cerebral metastases. Acta Neuroch. 2015;157(9):1573–80.

83. Kamp MA, Rapp M, Slotty PJ, Turowski B, Sadat H, Smuga M, Dibué-Adjei M, Steiger H-J, Szelényi A, Sabel M. Incidence of local in-brain progression after supramarginal resection of cerebral metastases. Acta Neuroch. 2015;157(6):905–10.

84. Kelly K, Bunn PA Jr. Is it time to reevaluate our approach to the treatment of brain metastases in patients with non-small cell lung cancer? Lung Cancer. 1998;20(2):85–91.

85. Norris LK, Grossman SA, Olivi A. Neoplastic meningitis following surgical resection of isolated cerebellar metastasis: a potentially preventable complication. J Neurooncol. 1997;32 (3):215–23.

86. Suki D, Abouassi H, Patel AJ, Sawaya R, Weinberg JS, Groves MD. Comparative risk of leptomeningeal disease after resection or stereotactic radiosurgery for solid tumor metastasis to the posterior fossa. J Neurosurg. 2008;108(2):248–57.

87. Pollock BE, Brown PD, Foote RL, Stafford SL, Schomberg PJ. Properly selected patients with multiple brain metastases may benefit from aggressive treatment of their intracranial disease. J Neurooncol. 2003;61(1):73–80.

88. Ewend MG, Brem S, Gilbert M, Goodkin R, Penar PL, Varia M, Cush S, Carey LA. Treatment of single brain metastasis with resection, intracavity carmustine polymer wafers, and radiation therapy is safe and provides excellent local control. Clin Cancer Res. 2007;13(12):3637–41.

89. Rogers LR, Rock JP, Sills AK, Vogelbaum MA, Suh JH, Ellis TL, Stieber VW, Asher AL, Fraser RW, Billingsley JS, Lewis P, Schellingerhout D. Shaw EG; Brain Metastasis Study Group. Results of a phase II trial of the GliaSite Radiation Therapy System for treatment of newly diagnosed, resected single brain metastases. J Neurosurg. 2006;105(3):375–8.

90. Dagnew E, Kanski J, McDermott MW, Sneed PK, McPherson C, Breneman JC, Warnick RE. Management of newly diagnosed single brain metastasis using resection and permanent iodine-125 seeds without initial whole-brain radiotherapy: a two institution experience. Neurosurg Focus. 2007;22(3):E3.

91. Baumert BG, Rutten I, Dehing-Oberije C, Twijnstra A, Dirx MJ, Debougnoux-Huppertz RM, Lambin P, Kubat B. A pathology-based substrate for target definition in radiosurgery of brain metastases. Int J Radiat Oncol Biol Phys. 2006;66(1):187–94.

92. Shaw E, Scott C, Souhami L, Dinapoli R, Kline R, Loeffler J, Farnan N. Single dose radiosurgical treatment of recurrent previously irradiated primary brain tumors and brain metastases: final report of RTOG protocol 90-05. Int J Radiat Oncol Biol Phys. 2000;47(2):291–8.

93. Aoyama H, Shirato H, Onimaru R, Kagei K, Ikeda J, Ishii N, Sawamura Y, Miyasaka K. Hypofractionated stereotactic radiotherapy alone without whole-brain irradiation for patients with solitary and oligo brain metastasis using noninvasive fixation of the skull. Int J Radiat Oncol Biol Phys. 2003;56(3):793–800.

94. Minniti G, D'Angelillo RM, Scaringi C, Trodella LE, Clarke E, Matteucci P, Osti MF, Ramella S, Enrici RM, Trodella L. Fractionated stereotactic radiosurgery for patients with brain metastases. J Neurooncol. 2014;117(2):295–301.

95. Eaton BR, LaRiviere MJ, Kim S, Prabhu RS, Patel K, Kandula S, Oyesiku N, Olson J, Curran W, Shu HK, Crocker I. Hypofractionated radiosurgery has a better safety profile than single fraction radiosurgery for large resected brain metastases. J Neurooncol. 2015;123(1):103–11.

96. Mehta MP, Tsao MN, Whelan TJ, Morris DE, Hayman JA, Flickinger JC, Mills M, Rogers CL, Souhami L. The American society for therapeutic radiology and oncology (ASTRO) evidence-based review of the role of radiosurgery for brain metastases. Int J Radiat Oncol Biol Phys. 2005;63(1):37–46.7/s11060-015-1767-4. Epub 2015 Apr 11. Erratum in: J Neurooncol. 2015;123(1):113.

97. Suh JH. Stereotactic radiosurgery for the management of brain metastases. N Engl J Med. 2010;362(12):1119–27.

98. Lippitz B, Lindquist C, Paddick I, Peterson D, O'Neill K, Beaney R. Stereotactic radiosurgery in the treatment of brain metastases: the current evidence. Cancer Treat Rev. 2014;40 (1):48–59.

99. Karlsson B, Hanssens P, Wolff R, Söderman M, Lindquist C, Beute G. Thirty years' experience with Gamma Knife surgery for metastases to the brain. J Neurosurg. 2009;111(3):449–57.

100. Yamamoto M, Serizawa T, Shuto T, Akabane A, Higuchi Y, Kawagishi J, Yamanaka K, Sato Y, Jokura H, Yomo S, Nagano O, Kenai H, Moriki A, Suzuki S, Kida Y, Iwai Y, Hayashi M, Onishi H, Gondo M, Sato M, Akimitsu T, Kubo K, Kikuchi Y, Shibasaki T, Goto T, Takanashi M, Mori Y, Takakura K, Saeki N, Kunieda E, Aoyama H, Momoshima S, Tsuchiya K. Stereotactic radiosurgery for patients with multiple brain metastases (JLGK0901): a multi-institutional prospective observational study. Lancet Oncol. 2014;15(4):387–95.

101. Manon R, O'Neill A, Knisely J, Werner-Wasik M, Lazarus HM, Wagner H, Gilbert M, Mehta M. Eastern cooperative oncology group. Phase II trial of radiosurgery for one to three newly diagnosed brain metastases from renal cell carcinoma, melanoma, and sarcoma: an Eastern cooperative oncology group study (E 6397). J Clin Oncol. 2005;23(34):8870–6.

102. Huang CF, Kondziolka D, Flickinger JC, Lunsford LD. Stereotactic radiosurgery for brainstem metastases. J Neurosurg. 1999;91(4):563–8.

103. Fuentes S, Delsanti C, Metellus P, Peragut JC, Grisoli F, Regis J. Brainstem metastases: management using gamma knife radiosurgery. Neurosurgery. 2006;58(1):37–42.

104. Watanabe S, Yamamoto M, Sato Y, Kawabe T, Higuchi Y, Kasuya H, Yamamoto T, Matsumura A, Barfod BE. Stereotactic radiosurgery for brain metastases: a case-matched study comparing treatment results for patients 80 years of age or older versus patients 65–79 years of age. J Neurosurg. 2014;121(5):1148–57.

105. Iyer A, Harrison G, Kano H, Weiner GM, Luther N, Niranjan A, Flickinger JC, Lunsford LD, Kondziolka D. Volumetric response to radiosurgery for brain metastasis varies by cell of origin. J Neurosurg. 2014;121(3):564–9.

106. Rades D, Pluemer A, Veninga T, Hanssens P, Dunst J, Schild SE. Whole-brain radiotherapy versus stereotactic radiosurgery for patients in recursive partitioning analysis classes 1 and 2 with 1–3 brain metastases. Cancer. 2007;110(10):2285–92.

107. Andrews DW, Scott CB, Sperduto PW, Flanders AE, Gaspar LE, Schell MC, Werner-Wasik M, Demas W, Ryu J, Bahary JP, Souhami L, Rotman M, Mehta MP, Curran WJ Jr. Whole brain radiation therapy with or without stereotactic radiosurgery boost for patients with one to three brain metastases: phase III results of the RTOG 9508 randomised trial. Lancet. 2004;363(9422):1665–72.

108. Sperduto PW, Shanley R, Luo X, Andrews D, Werner-Wasik M, Valicenti R, Bahary J-P, Souhami L, Won M, Mehta M. Secondary analysis of RTOG 9508, a phase 3 randomized trial of whole-brain radiation therapy versus WBRT plus stereotactic radiosurgery in patients with 1–3 metastases; poststratified by the grade prognostic assessment (GPA). Int J Radiat Oncol Biol Phys. 2014;90(3):526–31.

109. Kondziolka D, Patel A, Lunsford LD, Kassam A, Flickinger JC. Stereotactic radiosurgery plus whole brain radiotherapy versus radiotherapy alone for patients with multiple brain metastases. Int J Radiat Oncol Biol Phys. 1999;45(2):427–34.

110. Bhatnagar AK, Flickinger JC, Kondziolka D. Lunsford LD Stereotactic radiosurgery for four or more intracranial metastases. Int J Radiat Oncol Biol Phys. 2006;64(3):898–903.

111. Maldaun MV, Aguiar PH, Lang F, Suki D, Wildrick D, Sawaya R. Radiosurgery in the treatment of brain metastases: critical review regarding complications. Neurosurg Rev. 2008;31 (1):1–8.

112. Chao ST, Ahluwalia MS, Barnett GH, Stevens GH, Murphy ES, Stockham AL, Shiue K, Suh JH. Challenges with the diagnosis and treatment of cerebral radiation necrosis. Int J Radiat Oncol Biol Phys. 2013;87(3):449–57.

113. Boothe D, Young R, Yamada Y, Prager A, Chan T, Beal K. Bevacizumab as treatment for radiation necrosis of brain metastases post stereotactic radiosurgery. Neuro Oncol. 2013;15 (9):1257–63.

114. Sneed P, Mendez J, Vemer-van den Hoek JGM, Seymour ZA, Ma L, Molinaro AM, Fogh SE, Nakamura JL, McDermott MW. Adverse radiation effect after stereotactic radiosurgery for brain metastases: incidence, time course, and risk factor. J Neurosurg. 2015; 123(2):373–86.

115. Auchter RM, Lamond JP, Alexander E, Buatti JM, Chappell R, Friedman WA, Kinsella TJ, Levin AB, Noyes WR, Schultz CJ, Loeffler JS, Mehta MP. A multiinstitutional outcome and prognostic factor analysis of radiosurgery for resectable single brain metastasis. Int J Radiat Oncol Biol Phys. 1996;35(1):27–35.

116. Muacevic A, Kreth FW, Horstmann GA, Schmid-Elsaesser R, Wowra B, Steiger HJ, Reulen HJ. Surgery and radiotherapy compared with gamma knife radiosurgery in the treatment of solitary cerebral metastases of small diameter. J Neurosurg. 1999;91(1):35–43.

117. O'Neill BP, Iturria NJ, Link MJ, Pollock BE, Ballman KV, O'Fallon JR. A comparison of surgical resection and stereotactic radiosurgery in the treatment of solitary brain metastases. Int J Radiat Oncol Biol Phys. 2003;55(5):1169–76.

118. Rades D, Kueter JD, Veninga T, Gliemroth J, Schild SE. Whole brain radiotherapy plus stereotactic radiosurgery (WBRT + SRS) versus surgery plus whole brain radiotherapy (OP + WBRT) for 1–3 brain metastases: results of a matched pair analysis. Eur J Cancer. 2009;45(3):400–4.

119. Muacevic A, Wowra B, Siefert A, Tonn JC, Steiger HJ, Kreth FW. Microsurgery plus whole brain irradiation versus Gamma Knife surgery alone for treatment of single metastases to the brain: a randomized controlled multicentre phase III trial. J Neurooncol. 2008;87(3):299–307.

120. Bindal AK, Bindal RK, Hess KR, Shiu A, Hassenbusch SJ, Shi WM, Sawaya R. Surgery versus radiosurgery in the treatment of brain metastasis. J Neurosurg. 1996;84(5):748–54.

121. Sneed PK, Suh JH, Goetsch SJ, Sanghavi SN, Chappel R, Buatti JM, Regine WF, Weltman E, King VJ, Breneman JC, Sperduto PW, Mehta MP. A multi-institutional review of radiosurgery alone vs. radiosurgery with whole brain radiotherapy as the initial management of brain metastases. Int J Radiat Oncol Biol Phys. 2002; 53(3):519–526.

122. Regine WF, Huhn JL, Patchell RA, St Clair WH, Strottman J, Meigooni A, Sanders M, Young AB. Risk of symptomatic brain tumor recurrence and neurologic deficit after radiosurgery alone in patients with newly diagnosed brain metastases: results and implications. Int J Radiat Oncol Biol Phys. 2002;52(2):333–8.

123. Patchell RA, Tibbs PA, Regine WF, Dempsey RJ, Mohiuddin M, Kryscio RJ, Merkesbery WR, Foon KA, Young B. Postoperative radiotherapy in the treatment of single metastases to the brain: a randomized trial. JAMA. 1998;280(17):1485–9.

124. Aoyama H, Shirato H, Tago M, Nakagawa K, Toyoda T, Hatano K, Keniyo M, Oya N, Hirota S, Shioura H, Kunieda E, Inomata T, Hayakawa K, Katoh N, Kobashi G. Stereotactic radiosurgery plus whole-brain radiation therapy vs stereotactic radiosurgery alone for treatment of brain metastases: a randomized controlled trial. JAMA. 2006;295(21):2483–91.

125. Kocher M, Soffietti R, Abacioglu U, Villà S, Fauchon F, Baumert BG, Fariselli L, Tzuk-Shina T, Kortmann RD, Carrie C, Ben Hassel M, Kouri M, Valeinis E, van den Berge D, Collette S, Collette L, Mueller RP. Adjuvant whole-brain radiotherapy versus observation after radiosurgery or surgical resection of one to three cerebral metastases: results of the EORTC 22952-26001 study. J Clin Oncol. 2011;29(2):134–41.

126. Tsao M, Xu W, Sahgal A. A meta-analysis evaluating stereotactic radiosurgery, whole-brain radiotherapy, or both for patients presenting with a limited number of brain metastases. Cancer. 2012;118(9):2486–93.

127. Sahgal A, Aoyama H, Kocher M, Neupane B, Collette S, Tago M, Shaw P, Beyene J, Chang EL. Phase 3 trials of stereotactic radiosurgery with or without whole-brain radiation therapy for 1–4 brain metastases: individual patient data meta-analysis. Int J Radiat Oncol Biol Phys. 2015;91(4):710–7.

128. McPherson CM, Suki D, Feiz-Erfan I, Mahaian A, Chang E, Sawaya R, Lang FF. Adjuvant whole-brain radiation therapy after surgical resection of single brain metastases. Neuro Oncol. 2010;12(7):711–9.

129. Aoyama H, Tago M, Kato N, Toyoda T, Keniyo M, Hirota S, Shioura H, Inomata T, Kunieda E, Hayakawa K, Nakagawa K, Kobashi G, Shirato H. Neurocognitive function of patients with brain metastasis who received either whole brain radiotherapy plus stereotactic radiosurgery or radiosurgery alone. Iny J Radiat Oncol Biol Phys. 2007;68(5):1388–95.

130. Chang EL, Wefel JS, Hess KR, Allen PK, Lang FF, Kornguth DG, Arbuckle RB, Swint JM, Shiu AS, Maor MH, Meyers CA. Neurocognition in patients with brain metastases treated with radiosurgery or radiosurgery plus whole-brain irradiation: a randomised controlled trial. Lancet Oncol. 2009;10(11):1037–44.

131. Brown PD. NCCTG N0574 (Alliance): a phase III randomized trial of whole brain radiation therapy (WBRT) in addition to radiosurgery (SRS) in patients with 1–3 brain metastases. Paper presented at: 2015 ASCO 51st Annual Meeting 2015; Chicago, IL.

132. Soffietti R, Kocher M, Abacioglu U, Villa S, Fauchon F, Baumert BG, Fariselli L, Tzuk-Shina T, Kortmann RD, Carrie C, Ben Hassel M, Kouri M, Valeinis E, van der Berge D, Mueller RP, Tridello G, Collette L, Bottomley A. A European organisation for research and treatment of cancer phase III trial of adjuvant whole-brain radiotherapy versus observation in patients with one to three brain metastases from solid tumors after surgical resection or radiosurgery: quality-of-life results. J Clin Oncol. 2013; 31(1):65–72.

133. Hahn C, Kavanagh B, Bhatnagar A, Jacobson G, Lutz S, Patton C, Potters L, Steinberg M. Choosing wisely: the American Society for Radiation Oncology's top 5 list. Pract Radiat Oncol. 2014;4(6):349–55.

134. Soltys SG, Adler JR, Lipani JD, Jackson PS, Choi CY, Puataweepong P, White S, Gibbs IC, Chang SD. Stereotactic radiosurgery of the postoperative resection cavity for brain metastases. Int J Radiat Oncol Biol Phys. 2008;70(1):187–93.

135. Brennan C, Yang TJ, Hilden P, Zhang Z, Chan K, Yamada Y, Chan TA, Lymberis SC, Narayana A, Tabar V, Gutin PH, Ballangrud Å. Lis E9, Beal K. A phase 2 trial of stereotactic radiosurgery boost after surgical resection for brain metastases. Int J Radiat Oncol Biol Phys. 2014;88(1):130–6.

136. Amsbaugh MJ, Boling W et al Woo S. Tumor bed radiosurgery: an emerging treatment for brain metastases. J Neurooncol. 2015; 123(2):197–203.

137. Kelly PJ, Lin YB, Yu AY, Alexander BM, Hacker F, Marcus KJ, Weiss SE. Stereotactic irradiation of the postoperative resection cavity for brain metastasis: a frameless linear accelerator-based case series and review of the technique. Int J Radiat Oncol Biol Phys. 2012;82(1):95–101.

138. Hartford AC, Paravati AJ, Spire WJ, Li Z, Jarvis LA, Fadul CE, Rhodes CH, Erkmen K, Friedman J, Gladstone DJ, Hug EB, Roberts DW, Simmons NE. Postoperative stereotactic radiosurgery without whole-brain radiation therapy for brain metastases: potential role of preoperative tumor size. Int J Radiat Oncol Biol Phys. 2013;85(3):650–5.

139. Hsieh J, Elson P, Otvos B, Rose J, Loftus C, Rahmathulla G, Angelov L, Barnett GH, Weil RJ, Vogelbaum MA. Tumor progression in patients receiving adjuvant whole-brain radiotherapy vs localized radiotherapy after surgical resection of brain metastases. Neurosugery. 2015;76(4):411–20.

140. Choi CY, Chang SD, Gibbs IC, Adler JR, Harsh GR 4th, Lieberson RE, Soltys SG. Stereotactic radiosurgery of the postoperative resection cavity for brain metastases: prospective evaluation of target margin on tumor control. Int J Radiat Oncol Biol Phys. 2012;84(2):336–42.

141. Minniti G, Esposito V, Clarke E, Scaringi C, Lanzetta G, Salvati M, Raco A, Bozzao A, Maurizi Enrici R. Multidose stereotactic radiosurgery (9 Gy x 3) of the postoperative resection cavity for treatment of large brain metastases. Int J Radiat Oncol Biol Phys. 2013;86(4):623–9.

142. Ling DC, Vargo JA, Wegner RE, Flickinger JC, Burton SA, Engh J, Amankulor N, Quinn AE, Ozhasoglu C, Heron DE. Postoperative stereotactic radiosurgery to the resection cavity for large brain metastases: clinical outcomes, predictors of intracranial failure, and implications for optimal patient selection. Neurosurgery. 2015;76(2):150–6.

143. Mathieu D, Kondziolka D, Flickinger JC, Fortin D, Kenny B, Michaud K, Mongia S, Niranjan A, Lunsford LD. Tumor bed radiosurgery after resection of cerebral metastases. Neurosurgery. 2008;62(4):817–23.

144. Jensen CA, Chan MD, McCoy TP, Bourland JD, deGuzman AF, Ellis TL, Ekstrand KE, McMullen KP, Munley MT, Shaw EG, Urbanic JJ, Tatter SB. Cavity-directed radiosurgery as adjuvant

therapy after resection of a brain metastasis. J Neurosurg. 2011;114(6):1585–91.

145. Robbins JR, Ryu S, Kalkanis S, Cogan C, Rock J, Movsas B, Kim JH, Rosenblum M. Radiosurgery to the surgical cavity as adjuvant therapy for resected brain metastasis. Neurosurgery. 2012;71(5):937–43.

146. Atalar B, Modlin LA, Choi CY, Adler JR, Gibbs IC, Chang SD, Harsh GR 4th, Li G, Nagpal S, Hanlon A, Soltys SG. Risk of leptomeningeal disease in patients treated with stereotactic radiosurgery targeting the postoperative resection cavity for brain metastases. Int J Radiat Oncol Biol Phys. 2013;87(4):713–8.

147. Roberge D, Parney I, Brown PD. Radiosurgery to the postoperative surgical cavity: who needs evidence? Int J Radiat Oncol Biol Phys. 2012;83(2):486–93.

148. Li J, Bentzen SM, Renschler M, Mehta MP. Regression after whole-brain radiation therapy for brain metastases correlates with survival and improved neurocognitive function. J Clin Oncol. 2007;25(10):1260–6.

149. Tsao MN, Lloyd N, Wong RK, Chow E, Rakovitch E, Laperriere N, Xu W, Sahgal A. Whole brain radiotherapy for the treatment of newly diagnosed multiple brain metastases. Cochrane Database Syst Rev. 2012;4(6):349–55.

150. Mulvenna PM. The management of brain metastases in patients with non-small cell lung cancer-is it time to go back to the drawing board? Clin Oncol (R Coll Radiol). 2010;22(5):365–73.

151. Mehta MP, Shapiro WR, Phan SC, Gervais R, Carrie C, Chabot P, Patchell RA, Glantz MJ, Recht L, Langer C, Sur RK, Roa WH, Mahe MA, Fortin A, Meyers CA, Smith JA, Miller RA, Renschler MF. Motexafin gadolinium combined with prompt whole brain radiotherapy prolongs time to neurologic progression in non-small-cell lung cancer patients with brain metastases: results of a phase III trial. Int J Radiat Oncol Biol Phys. 2009;73(4):1069–76.

152. Scott C, Suh J, Stea B, Nabid A, Hackman J. Improved survival, quality of life, and quality-adjusted survival in breast cancer patients treated with efaproxiral (Efaproxyn) plus whole-brain radiation therapy for brain metastases. Am J Clin Oncol. 2007;30 (6):580–7.

153. DeAngelis LM, Delattre JY, Posner JB. Radiation-induced dementia in patients cured of brain metastases. Neurology. 1989;39(6):789–96.

154. Orgogozo JM, Rigaud AS, Stöffler A, Möbius HJ, Forette F. Efficacy and safety of memantine in patients with mild to moderate vascular dementia: a randomized, placebo-controlled trial (MMM 300). Stroke. 2002;33(7):1834–9.

155. Wilcock GK. Memantine for the treatment of dementia. Lancet Neurol. 2003;2(8):503–5.

156. Brown PD, Pugh S, Laack NN, Wefel JS, Khuntia D, Meyers C, Choucair A, Fox S, Suh JH, Roberge D, Kavadi V, Bentzen SM, Mehta MP, Watkins-Bruner D. Radiation Therapy Oncology Group (RTOG). Memantine for the prevention of cognitive dysfunction in patients receiving whole-brain radiotherapy: a randomized, double-blind, placebo-controlled trial. Neuro Oncol. 2013;15(10):1429–37.

157. Monje ML, Palmer T. Radiation injury and neurogenesis. Curr Opin Neurol. 2003;16(2):12–34.

158. Gibson E, Monje M. Effect of cancer therapy on neural stem cells: implications for cognitive function. Curr Opin Oncol. 2012;24(6):672–8.

159. Gondi V, Tomé WA, Mehta MP. Why avoid the hippocampus? A comprehensive review. Radiother Oncol. 2010;97(3):370–6.

160. Ghia A, Tomé WA, Thomas S, Cannon G, Khuntia D, Kuo JS, Mehta MP. Distribution of brain metastases in relation to the hippocampus: implications for neurocognitive functional preservation. Int J Radiat Oncol Biol Phys. 2007;68(4):971–7.

161. Marsh JC, Herskovic AM, Gielda BT, Hughes FF, Hoeppner T, Turian J, Abrams RA. Intracranial metastatic disease spares the limbic circuit: a review of 697 metastatic lesions in 107 patients. Int J Radiat Oncol Biol Phys. 2010;76(2):504–12.

162. Gondi V, Pugh SL, Tome WA, Caine C, Corn B, Kanner A, Rowley H, Kundapur V, DeNittis A, Greenspoon JN, Konski AA, Bauman GS, Shah S, Shi W, Wendland M, Kachnic L, Mehta MP. Preservation of memory with conformal avoidance of the hippocampal neural stem-cell compartment during whole-brain radiotherapy for brain metastases (RTOG 0933): a phase II multi-institutional trial. J Clin Oncol. 2014;32(34):3810–6.

163. Suh JH. Hippocampal-avoidance whole-brain radiation therapy: a new standard for patients with brain metastases? J Clin Oncol. 2014;32(34):3789–91.

164. Sundaresan N, Sachdev VP, DiGiacinto GV, Hughes JE. Reoperation for brain metastases. J Clin Oncol. 1988;6(10):1625–9.

165. Arbit E, Wroński M, Burt M, Galicich JH. The treatment of patients with recurrent brain metastases. A retrospective analysis of 109 patients with nonsmall cell lung cancer. Cancer. 1995;76 (5):765–73.

166. Bindal RK, Sawaya R, Leavens ME, Hess KR, Taylor SH. Reoperation for recurrent metastatic brain tumors. J Neurosurg. 1995;83(4):600–4.

167. Chao ST, Barnett GH, Vogelbaum MA, Angelov L, Weil RJ, Neyman G, Reuther AM, Suh JH. Salvage stereotactic radiosurgery effectively treats recurrences from whole-brain radiation therapy. Cancer. 2008;113(8):2198–204.

168. Caballero JA, Sneed PK, Lamborn KR, Ma L, Denduluri S, Nakamura JL, Barani IJ, McDermott MW. Prognostic factors for survival in patients treated with stereotactic radiosurgery for recurrent brain metastases after prior whole brain radiotherapy. Int J Radiat Oncol Biol Phys. 2012;83(1):303–9.

169. Kurtz G, Zadeh G, Gingras-Hill G, Millar BA, Laperriere NJ, Bernstein M, Jiang H, Ménard C, Chung C. Salvage radiosurgery for brain metastases: prognostic factors to consider in patient selection. Int J Radiat Oncol Biol Phys. 2014;88(1):137–42.

170. Lucas JT Jr, Colmer HG 4th, White L, Fitzgerald N, Isom S, Bourland JD, Laxton AW, Tatter SB, Chan MD. Competing risk analysis of neurologic versus nonneurologic death in patients undergoing radiosurgical salvage after whole-brain radiation therapy failure: who actually dies of their brain metastases? Int J Radiat Oncol Biol Phys. 2015;92(5):1008–15.

171. Hsu F, Kouhestani P, Nguyen S, Cheung A, McKenzie M, Ma R, Toyota B, Nichol A. Population-based outcomes of boost versus salvage radiosurgery for brain metastases after whole brain radiotherapy. Radiother Oncol. 2013;108(1):128–31.

172. Kim DH, Schultheiss TE, Radany EH, Badie B, Pezner RD. Clinical outcomes of patients treated with a second course of stereotactic radiosurgery for locally or regionally recurrent brain metastases after prior stereotactic radiosurgery. J Neurooncol. 2013;115(1):37–43.

173. Chen JC, Petrovich Z, Giannotta SL, Yu C, Apuzzo ML. Radiosurgical salvage therapy for patients presenting with recurrence of metastatic disease to the brain. Neurosurgery. 2000;46(4):860–6; discussion 866–7.

174. Kondziolka D, Kano H, Harrison GL, Yang HC, Liew DN, Niranjan A, Brufsky AM, Flickinger JC, Lunsford LD. Stereotactic radiosurgery as primary and salvage treatment for brain metastases from breast cancer. Clinical article. J Neurosurg. 2011;114(3):792–800.

175. Shultz DB, Modlin LA, Jayachandran P, Von Eyben R, Gibbs IC, Choi CY, Chang SD, Harsh GR 4th, Li G, Adler JR, Hancock SL, Soltys SG. Repeat courses of stereotactic radiosurgery (SRS), deferring whole-brain irradiation, for new brain metastases after initial SRS. Int J Radiat Oncol Biol Phys. 2015;92(5):993–9.

176. Soffietti R, Rudà R, Trevisan E. Brain metastases: current management and new developments. Curr Opin Oncol. 2008;20 (6):676–84.

177. Mehta MP, Paleologos NA, Mikkelsen T, Robinson PD, Ammirati M, Andrews DW, Asher AL, Burri SH, Cobbs CS, Gaspar LE, Kondziolka D, Linskey ME, Loeffler JS, McDermott M, Olson JJ, Patchell RA, Ryken TC, Kalkanis SN. The role of chemotherapy in the management of newly diagnosed brain metastases: a systematic review and evidence-based clinical practice guideline. J Neurooncol. 2010;96(1):71–83.

178. Liu R, Wang X, Ma B, Yang K, Zhang Q, Tian J. Concomitant or adjuvant temozolomide with whole-brain irradiation for brain metastases: a meta-analysis. Anticancer Drugs. 2010;21(1):120–8.

179. Cao KI, Lebas N, Gerber S, Levy C, Le Scodan R, Bourgier C, Pierga JY, Gobillion A, Savignoni A, Kirova YM. Phase II randomized study of whole-brain radiation therapy with or without concurrent temozolomide for brain metastases from breast cancer. Ann Oncol. 2015;26(1):89–94.

180. Gerstner ER, Fine RL. Increased permeability of the blood-brain barrier to chemotherapy in metastatic brain tumors: establishing a treatment paradigm. J Clin Oncol. 2007;25(16):2306–12.

181. Soffietti R, Trevisan E, Rudà R. Targeted therapy in brain metastasis. Curr Opin Oncol. 2012;24(6):679–86.

182. Lin NU. Targeted therapies in brain metastases. Curr Treat Options Neurol. 2014;16(1):276.

183. Mehta MP. Brain metastases: the changing landscape. Oncology (Williston Park). 2015;29(4):257–60.

184. Besse B, Lasserre SF, Compton P, Huang J, Augustus S, Rohr UP. Bevacizumab safety in patients with central nervous system metastases. Clin Cancer Res. 2010;16(1):269–78.

185. Fan Y, Xu X, Xie C. EGFR-TKI therapy for patients with brain metastases from non-small-cell lung cancer: a pooled analysis of published data. Onco Targets Ther. 2014;10(7):2075–84.

186. Jamal-Hanjani M, Spicer J. Epidermal growth factor receptor tyrosine kinase inhibitors in the treatment of epidermal growth factor receptor-mutant non-small cell lung cancer metastatic to the brain. Clin Cancer Res. 2012;18(4):938–44.

187. Burel-Vandenbos F, Ambrosetti D, Coutts M, Pedeutour F. EGFR mutation status in brain metastases of non-small cell lung carcinoma. J Neurooncol. 2013;111(1):1–10.

188. Zimmermann S, Dziadziuszko R, Peters S. Indications and limitations of chemotherapy and targeted agents in non-small cell lung cancer brain metastases. Cancer Treat Rev. 2014;40(6):716–22.

189. Welsh JW, Komaki R, Amini A, Munsell MF, Unger W, Allen PK, Chang JY, Wefel JS, McGovern SL, Garland LL, Chen SS, Holt J, Liao Z, Brown P, Sulman E, Heymach JV, Kim ES, Stea B. Phase II trial of erlotinib plus concurrent whole-brain radiation therapy for patients with brain metastases from non-small-cell lung cancer. J Clin Oncol. 2013;31(7):895–902.

190. Lee SM, Lewanski CR, Counsell N, Ottensmeier C, Bates A, Patel N, Wadsworth C, Ngai Y, Hackshaw A, Faivre-Finn C. Randomized trial of erlotinib plus whole-brain radiotherapy for NSCLC patients with multiple brain metastases. J Natl Cancer Inst. 2014;106(7).

191. Sperduto PW, Wang M, Robins HI, Schell MC, Werner-Wasik M, Komaki R, Souhami L, Buyyounouski MK, Khuntia D, Demas W, Shah SA, Nedzi LA, Perry G, Suh JH, Mehta MP. A phase 3 trial of whole brain radiation therapy and stereotactic radiosurgery alone versus WBRT and SRS with temozolomide or erlotinib for non-small cell lung cancer and 1–3 brain metastases: radiation therapy oncology group 0320. Int J Radiat Oncol Biol Phys. 2013;85(5):1312–8.

192. Preusser M, Berghoff AS, Ilhan-Mutlu A, Magerle M, Dinhof C, Widhalm G, Dieckmann K, Marosi C, Wöhrer A, Hackl M, Zöchbauer-Müller S, von Deimling A, Schoppmann SF, Zielinski CC, Streubel B, Birner P. ALK gene translocations and amplifications in brain metastases of non-small cell lung cancer. Lung Cancer. 2013;80(3):278–83.

193. Costa DB, Shaw AT, Ou SH, Solomon BJ, Riely GJ, Ahn MJ, Zhou C, Shreeve SM, Selaru P, Polli A, Schnell P, Wilner KD, Wiltshire R, Camidge DR, Crinò L. Clinical experience with crizotinib in patients with advanced ALK-rearranged non-small-cell lung cancer and brain metastases. J Clin Oncol. 2015;33(17):1881–8.

194. Ekenel M, Hormigo AM, Peak S, Deangelis LM, Abrey LE. Capecitabine therapy of central nervous system metastases from breast cancer. J Neurooncol. 2007;85(2):223–7.

195. Rivera E, Meyers C, Groves M, Valero V, Francis D, Arun B, Broglio K, Yin G, Hortobagyi GN, Buchholz T. Phase I study of capecitabine in combination with temozolomide in the treatment of patients with brain metastases from breast carcinoma. Cancer. 2006;107(6):1348–54.

196. Lassman AB, Abrey LE, Shah GD, Panageas KS, Begemann M, Malkin MG, Raizer JJ. Systemic high-dose intravenous methotrexate for central nervous system metastases. J Neurooncol. 2006;78(3):255–60. Erratum in: J Neurooncol. 2006;78(3):261. Shah, Gaurav G [corrected to Shah, Gaurav D].

197. Lin NU, Carey LA, Liu MC, Younger J, Come SE, Ewend M, Harris GJ, Bullitt E, Van den Abbeele AD, Henson JW, Li X, Gelman R, Burstein HJ, Kasparian E, Kirsch DG, Crawford A, Hochberg F, Winer EP. Phase II trial of lapatinib for brain metastases in patients with human epidermal growth factor receptor 2-positive breast cancer. J Clin Oncol. 2008;26(12):1993–9.

198. Bachelot T, Romieu G, Campone M, Diéras V, Cropet C, Dalenc F, Jimenez M, Le Rhun E, Pierga JY, Gonçalves A, Leheurteur M, Domont J, Gutierrez M, Curé H, Ferrero JM, Labbe-Devilliers C. Lapatinib plus capecitabine in patients with previously untreated brain metastases from HER2-positive metastatic breast cancer(LANDSCAPE): a single-group phase 2 study. Lancet Oncol. 2013;14(1):64–71.

199. Agarwala SS, Kirkwood JM, Gore M, Dreno B, Thatcher N, Czarnetski B, Atkins M, Buzaid A, Skarlos D, Rankin EM. Temozolomide for the treatment of brain metastases associated with metastatic melanoma: a phase II study. J Clin Oncol. 2004;22(11):2101–7.

200. Harding JJ, Catalanotti F, Munhoz RR, Cheng DT, Yaqubie A, Kelly N, McDermott GC, Kersellius R, Merghoub T, Lacouture ME, Carvajal RD, Panageas KS, Berger MF, Rosen N, Solit DB, Chapman PB. A retrospective evaluation of vemurafenib as treatment for BRAF-mutant melanoma brain metastases. Oncologist. 2015;20(7):789–97.

201. Dummer R, Goldinger SM, Turtschi CP, Eggmann NB, Michielin O, Mitchell L, Veronese L, Hilfiker PR, Felderer L, Rinderknecht JD. Vemurafenib in patients with BRAF(V600) mutation-positive melanoma with symptomatic brain metastases: final results of an open-label pilot study. Eur J Cancer. 2014;50 (3):611–21.

202. Long GV, Trefzer U, Davies MA, Kefford RF, Ascierto PA, Chapman PB, Puzanov I, Hauschild A, Robert C, Algazi A, Mortier L, Tawbi H, Wilhelm T, Zimmer L, Switzky J, Swann S, Martin AM, Guckert M, Goodman V, Streit M, Kirkwood JM, Schadendorf D. Dabrafenib in patients with Val600Glu or Val600Lys BRAF-mutant melanoma metastatic to the brain (BREAK-MB): a multicentre, open-label, phase 2 trial. Lancet Oncol. 2012;13(11):1087–95.

203. Weber JS, Amin A, Minor D, Siegel J, Berman D, O'Day SJ. Safety and clinical activity of ipilimumab in melanoma patients with brain metastases: retrospective analysis of data from a phase 2 trial. Melanoma Res. 2011;21(6):530–4.

204. Margolin K, Ernstoff MS, Hamid O, Lawrence D, McDermott D, Puzanov I, Wolchok JD, Clark JI, Sznol M, Logan TF, Richards J, Michener T, Balogh A, Heller KN, Hodi FS. Ipilimumab in patients with melanoma and brain metastases: an open-label, phase 2 trial. Lancet Oncol. 2012;13(5):459–65.
205. Queirolo P, Spagnolo F, Ascierto PA, Simeone E, Marchetti P, Scoppola A, Del Vecchio M, Di Guardo L, Maio M, Di Giacomo AM, Antonuzzo A, Cognetti F, Ferraresi V, Ridolfi L, Guidoboni M, Guida M, Pigozzo J, Chiarion Sileni V. Efficacy and safety of ipilimumab in patients with advanced melanoma and brain metastases. J Neurooncol. 2014;118(1):109–16.
206. Patel KR, Shoukat S, Oliver DE, Chowdhary M, Rizzo M, Lawson DH, Khosa F, Liu Y, Khan MK. Ipilimumab and Stereotactic Radiosurgery Versus Stereotactic Radiosurgery Alone for Newly Diagnosed Melanoma Brain Metastases. Am J Clin Oncol. 2015. [Epub ahead of print].
207. Aupérin A, Arriagada R, Pignon JP, Le Péchoux C, Gregor A, Stephens RJ, Kristjansen PE, Johnson BE, Ueoka H, Wagner H, Aisner J. Prophylactic cranial irradiation for patients with small-cell lung cancer in complete remission. Prophylactic cranial irradiation overview collaborative group. N Engl J Med. 1999;341(7):476–84.
208. Meert AP, Paesmans M, Berghmans T, Martin B, Mascaux C, Vallot F, Verdebout JM, Lafitte JJ, Sculier JP. Prophylactic cranial irradiation in small cell lung cancer: a systematic review of the literature with meta-analysis. BMC Cancer. 2001;1:5.
209. Arriagada R, Le Chevalier T, Borie F, Rivière A, Chomy P, Monnet I, Tardivon A, Viader F, Tarayre M, Benhamou S. Prophylactic cranial irradiation for patients with small-cell lung cancer in complete remission. J Natl Cancer Inst. 1995;87 (3):183–90.
210. Gregor A, Cull A, Stephens RJ, Kirkpatrick JA, Yarnold JR, Girling DJ, Macbeth FR, Stout R, Machin D. Prophylactic cranial irradiation is indicated following complete response to induction therapy in small cell lung cancer: results of a multicentre randomised trial. United Kingdom Coordinating Committee for Cancer Research (UKCCCR) and the European Organization for Research and Treatment of Cancer (EORTC). Eur J Cancer. 1997;33(11):1752–8.
211. Lester JF, MacBeth FR, Coles B. Prophylactic cranial irradiation for preventing brain metastases in patients undergoing radical treatment for non-small-cell lung cancer: a Cochrane Review. Int J Radiat Oncol Biol Phys. 2005;63(3):690–4.
212. Steeg PS, Camphausen KA, Smith QR. Brain metastases as preventive and therapeutic targets. Nat Rev Cancer. 2011;11 (5):352–63.
213. Trinh VA, Hwu WJ. Chemoprevention for brain metastases. Curr Oncol Rep. 2012;14(1):63–9.
214. Kienast Y, von Baumgarten L, Fuhrmann M, Klinkert WE, Goldbrunner R, Herms J, Winkler F. Real-time imaging reveals the single steps of brain metastasis formation. Nat Med. 2010;16 (1):116–22.
215. Gril B, Palmieri D, Bronder JL, Herring JM, Vega-Valle E, Feigenbaum L, Liewehr DJ, Steinberg SM, Merino MJ, Rubin SD, Steeg PS. Effect of lapatinib on the outgrowth of metastatic breast cancer cells to the brain. J Natl Cancer Inst. 2008;100(15):1092–103.
216. Palmieri D, Lockman PR, Thomas FC, et al. Vorinostat inhibits brain metastatic colonization in a model of triple-negative breast cancer and induces DNA double-strand breaks. Clin Cancer Res. 2009;15:6148–57.

217. Gril B, Palmieri D, Qian Y, Smart D, Ileva L, Liewehr DJ, Steinberg SM, Steeg PS. Pazopanib reveals a role for tumor cell B-Raf in the prevention of HER2 + breast cancer brain metastasis. Clin Cancer Res. 2011;17(1):142–53.
218. Qian Y, Hua E, Bisht K, Woditschka S, Skordos KW, Liewehr DJ, Steinberg SM, Brogi E, Akram MM, Killian JK, Edelman DC, Pineda M, Scurci S, Degenhardt YY, Laquerre S, Lampkin TA, Meltzer PS, Camphausen K, Steeg PS, Palmieri D. Inhibition of Polo-like kinase 1 prevents the growth of metastatic breast cancer cells in the brain. Clin Exp Metastasis. 2011;28 (8):899–908.
219. Cameron D, Casey M, Press M, et al. A phase III randomized comparison of lapatinib plus capecitabine versus capecitabine alone in women with advanced breast cancer that has progressed on trastuzumab: updated efficacy and biomarker analyses. Breast Cancer Res Treat. 2008;112:533–43.
220. Heon S, Yeap BY, Britt GJ, et al. Development of central nervous system metastases in patients with advanced non-small cell lung cancer and somatic EGFR mutations treated with gefitinib or erlotinib. Clin Cancer Res. 2010;16:5873–82.
221. Stadler WM, Figlin RA, McDermott DF, et al. Safety and efficacy results of the advanced renal cell carcinoma sorafenib expanded access program in North America. Cancer. 2010;116:1272–80.
222. Massard C, Zonierek J, Gross-Goupil M, et al. Incidence of brain metastases in renal cell carcinoma treated with sorafenib. Ann Oncol. 2010;21:1027–31.
223. Verma J, Jonasch E, Allen P, Tannir N, Mahajan A. Impact of tyrosine kinase inhibitors on the incidence of brain metastasis in metastatic renal cell carcinoma. Cancer. 2011;117(21):4958–65.
224. Peereboom DM. Clinical trial design in brain metastasis: approaches for a unique patient population. Curr Oncol Rep. 2012;14:91–6.
225. Lin NU, Lee EQ, Aoyama H, Barani IJ, Baumert BG, Brown PD, Camidge DR, Chang SM, Dancey J, Gaspar LE, Harris GJ, Hodi FS, Kalkanis SN, Lamborn KR, Linskey ME, Macdonald DR, Margolin K, Mehta MP, Schiff D, Soffietti R, Suh JH, van den Bent MJ, Vogelbaum MA, Wefel JS, Wen PY; Response Assessment in Neuro-Oncology (RANO) group. Challenges relating to solid tumour brain metastases in clinical trials, part 1: patient population, response, and progression. A report from the RANO group. Lancet Oncol. 2013;14(10):e396–406.
226. Lin NU, Wefel JS, Lee EQ, Schiff D, van den Bent MJ, Soffietti R, Suh JH, Vogelbaum MA, Mehta MP, Dancey J, Linskey ME, Camidge DR, Aoyama H, Brown PD, Chang SM, Kalkanis SN, Barani IJ, Baumert BG, Gaspar LE, Hodi FS, Macdonald DR, Wen PY; Response Assessment in Neuro-Oncology (RANO) group. Challenges relating to solid tumour brain metastases in clinical trials, part 2: neurocognitive, neurological, and quality-of-life outcomes. A report from the RANO group. Lancet Oncol. 2013;14(10):e407–16.
227. Berry DA. Adaptive clinical trials: the promise and the caution. J Clin Oncol. 2011;29:606–9.
228. Lin NU, Lee EQ, Aoyama H, Barani IJ, Barboriak DP, Baumert BG, Bendszus M, Brown PD, Camidge DR, Chang SM, Dancey J, de Vries EG, Gaspar LE, Harris GJ, Hodi FS, Kalkanis SN, Linskey ME, Macdonald DR, Margolin K, Mehta MP, Schiff D, Soffietti R, Suh JH, van den Bent MJ, Vogelbaum MA, Wen PY; Response Assessment in Neuro-Oncology (RANO) group. Response assessment criteria for brain metastases: proposal from the RANO group. Lancet Oncol. 2015;16(6):e270–8.

Leptomeningeal Metastasis as Complication of Systemic Cancers

5

Sophie Taillibert, Emilie Le Rhun, and Marc C. Chamberlain

Abbreviations

AEDs	Anti epileptic drugs
BBB	Blood brain barrier
BC	Breast cancer
BM	Brain metastases
CSF	Cerebrospinal fluid
CSI	Craniospinal axis irradiation
CT	Computed tomography
CTLA	Cytotoxic T-lymphocyte antigen
CTCs	Circulating tumor cells
EGFR	Epidermal growth factor receptor
EpCAM	Epithelial-cell adhesion molecule
ER	Estrogen receptor
FCI	Flow cytometry immunophenotyping
FLAIR	Fluid attenuation inversion recovery
HD	High dose
IT	Intrathecal
IV	Intravenous
IVent	Intraventricular
LM	Leptomeningeal metastases
LR	Lumbar route
MAPK	Mitogen-activated protein kinase
MR-Gd	Magnetic resonance with gadolinium
MRI	Magnetic resonance imaging

S. Taillibert
Department of Neurology, Pitié-Salpétrière Hospital, UPMC-Paris VI University, 47 bd de l'hôpital, 75013 Paris, France
e-mail: sophie.taillibert@pal.aphp.fr; sophie.taillibert@gmail.com

S. Taillibert
Department of Radiation Oncology, Pitié-Salpétrière Hospital, UPMC-Paris VI University, 47 bd de l'hôpital, 75013 Paris, France

E. Le Rhun
Department of Neurosurgery and Neuro-oncology, University Hospital, 59037 Lille Cedex, France
e-mail: emilie.lerhun@chru-lille.fr

E. Le Rhun
Department of Medical Oncology, Breast Unit, Oscar Lambert Center, 59020 Lille Cedex, France

E. Le Rhun
PRISm Inserm U1191, Villeneuve d'Ascq, France

M.C. Chamberlain (✉)
Cascadian Therapeutics, Inc., 2601 Fourth Ave, Suite 500, Seattle, WA 98121, USA
e-mail: chambemc@uw.edu

© Springer International Publishing AG 2018
D. Schiff et al. (eds.), *Cancer Neurology in Clinical Practice*,
DOI 10.1007/978-3-319-57901-6_5

MTX	Methotrexate
NCCN	National comprehensive cancer network
NSCLC	Non small cell lung cancer
OS	Overall survival
PFS	Progression free survival
PR	Progesterone receptor
PS	Performance status
QoL	Quality of life
RANO	Response assessment in neuro-oncology
RCCT	Rare cell capture technology
RCTs	Randomized clinical trials
RECIST	Response evaluation criteria in solid tumors
RT	Radiation therapy
TKI	Tyrosine kinase inhibitors
TTP	Time to tumor progression
VEGF	Vascular endothelial growth factor
VPS	Ventriculo-peritoneal shunting
WBC	White blood cells
WBRT	Whole brain radiation therapy

Introduction

Leptomeningeal metastases (LM) result from the spread of cancer cells to the leptomeninges. LM is a relevant clinical issue in neuro-oncology due to its increasing incidence and poor prognosis and functional consequences directly impacting patients' quality of life. In recent years, not withstanding advances in earlier diagnosis of LM, the increased recognition has not been accompanied by therapeutic improvements in patient outcomes. This chapter focuses on LM secondary to "solid" primary cancers and excludes those originating from the central nervous system (CNS) or from hematologic malignancies.

Epidemiology and Risk Factors

LM is identified in 4–15% of cancer patients [1–8]. LM is confirmed postmortem in 19% of cancer patients who were neurologically symptomatic antemortem [9]. Brain metastases (BM) are diagnosed in 50–80% of LM patients [10–14]. The cancers that most commonly lead to LM are lymphoma, leukemia, breast and lung cancer, head and neck cancer, melanoma and gastric cancer; however, any histologic type can result in LM (Table 5.1). In most cases (70%), LM occurs in the setting of an advanced systemic disease. Nevertheless, 5–10% of cases are the initial manifestation of the cancer (including occasional cases where no extra-leptomeningeal cancer is identified), or after a prolonged disease-free interval (20%) [1, 5, 15–17]. The three

most common causes of solid tumor-related LM are breast cancer, lung cancer, and melanoma, illustrating the prelection for adenocarcinomas to metastasize to the leptomeninges (Table 5.2) [2, 5, 6].

Although non-small cell cancer lung (NSCLC) and melanoma show a tropism for the leptomeninges (11% and

Table 5.1 Distribution of LM by type of cancer

Type of cancer	%
Breast cancer	12–34
Lung carcinoma	10–26
Melanoma	17–25
Gastrointestinal tract cancer	4–14
Adenocarcinoma of unknown primary	1–7

Data from References [1–6]
Used from Le Rhun E, Taillibert S, Chamberlain MC. Carcinomatous meningitis: Leptomeningeal metastases in solid tumors. Surg Neurol Int. 2013; 4(Suppl 4): S265–S288. Open Access Journal

Table 5.2 Frequency of leptomeningeal metastatic involvement by type of cancer

Type of cancer	Frequency of secondary LM (%)
Melanoma	22–46
Small cell lung cancer	10–25
Breast carcinoma	5
Non-small cell lung cancer	1
Head and Neck	1

Data from References [2, 5, 6]
Used from Le Rhun E, Taillibert S, Chamberlain MC. Carcinomatous meningitis: Leptomeningeal metastases in solid tumors. Surg Neurol Int. 2013; 4(Suppl 4): S265–S288. Open Access Journal

up to 23% respectively) [18, 19], the incidence of LM secondary to breast cancer (BC) is higher, notwithstanding an overall 5% rate of spread to the CSF and leptomeninges [1, 5, 20]. Negative estrogen receptor (ER) , negative progesterone receptor (PR), triple-negative status, and an infiltrating lobular component are all risk factors for LM in BC patients [21–27]. In HER2 positive patients, opposite to the well-established increased incidence of intraparenchymal brain metastases, LM is relatively infrequent with an incidence of 3–5% [28]. According to a recent retrospective study, the occurrence of pulmonary metastases is associated with development of LM in breast cancer [29]. Another retrospective series concluded that breast cancer patients undergoing resection of a brain metastasis had a high risk of leptomeningeal disease [30]. Progressive systemic disease and age younger than 40 years at the time of brain metastasis treatment have also been associated with a higher risk of developing LM in BC patients [31].

Risk factors predisposing metastatic spread to leptomeninges include piecemeal surgical resection of parenchymal cerebellar lesions, and resection of supratentorial BM resulting in a breach of the ventricular system [31–37]. In both situations, direct spillage of tumor cells into the CSF and subsequent dissemination of malignant cells is the presumed mechanism. Improvement in systemic therapy resulting in prolonged survival of patients is another factor that contributes to the increased incidence of LM. By example, the incidence of LM in melanboma has increased since the introduction of recently approved drugs such as anti-cytotoxic T-lymphocyte antigen (CTLA)-4 and PD-1 antibodies and BRAF inhibitors that have improved overall survival (OS) and control of extracranial disease [16]. The poor central nervous system (CNS) penetration of targeted therapies such as antibodies (e.g., trastuzumab in BC) is another factor contributing to the increased incidence of LM [38–41]. The meninges and cerebrospinal fluid (CSF) compartment is a pharmacological sanctuary for many cytotoxic agents that have limited ability to cross an intact blood–CSF barrier.

Pathogenesis

There are many ways by which malignant cells can spread to the leptomeninges: (1) hematogenous spread, mostly by arterial contamination or via the venous plexus of Batson in pelvic cancers; (2) direct dissemination from adjacent BM or primary brain tumors; (3) through centripetal migration, along perineural or perivascular spaces. The latter mechanism is mostly observed in head and neck cancers, and in breast and lung cancers, when there are known vertebral and paravertebral metastases [42–44].

Once circulating tumor cells (CTC) have breached the subarachnoid space (SA), CTC spread through CSF, resulting in diffuse and multifocal seeding of the leptomeninges. The base of brain (especially the basilar cisterns) and dorsal surface of the spinal cord (especially the cauda equina) are predominantly affected [45, 46]. The CSF outflow may be obstructed by ependymal nodules or tumor deposits leading to a communicating hydrocephalus. Obstruction of CSF corridors affects predominantly the IVth ventricle, basal cisterns, cerebral convexity, and spinal SA.

Diagnosis

It is important to diagnose LM in its initial stage, when neurological impairment is minimal, the patient performance status (PS) is maintained, and the tumor burden is low as these factors are correlated with response to treatment and OS.

Clinical Features

LM typically presents with pleomorphic neurological signs and symptoms. The clinical manifestations of LM typically reflect the simultaneous involvement of three distinct neurologic compartments: (1) the cerebral hemispheres; (2) the cranial nerves; and (3) the spinal cord and exiting roots (Table 5.3).

Headache and mental status changes are the most frequent symptoms linked to cerebral hemispheres involvement, followed by confusion, dementia, seizures, and hemiparesis. Diplopia is the most frequent symptom, caused by cranial nerves impairment with a predominant involvement of the VIth cranial nerve followed by cranial nerve III and IV. Trigeminal sensory or motor dysfunction, cochlear impairment, and optic neuropathy are less common. Weakness (mostly of the lower limbs), dermatomal, segmental, or radicular sensory impairment, and pain reflect spinal involvement. In contrast to infectious meningitis, the occurrence of nuchal rigidity is unusual (15% of patients) [2, 5, 6, 16]. Symptoms of increased intracranial pressure such as syncope, headache, nausea, and vomiting may occur when the CSF flow obstruction occurs and results in hydrocephalus. The incidence of seizures is low (<10%) in LM.

Diencephalic storm or paroxysmal sympathetic outflow has been reported in LM. This may manifest as episodic hyperhidrosis, hypertension, tachypnea, tachycardia, and abnormal posturing. The occurrence of diencephalic storm has been reported in many other neurologic conditions, including hydrocephalus. The differential diagnosis includes

Table 5.3 Most frequent symptoms and signs in patients with LM from solid tumors

	Symptom	Initially (%)	At any time (%)	Sign	Initially (%)	At any time (%)
Cerebral	Gait difficulty	46	68	Extensor plantar	50	66
	Headache	38	40	Impaired mental state	50	50
	Mental change	25	30	Seizures	14	15
	Nausea and vomiting	12	20	Papilledema	12	12
Cranial nerve	Diplopia	8	20	Occular muscle palsy	30	38
	Visual Loss	8	12	Facial weakness	25	26
	Hearing Loss	6	9	Hearing Loss	20	20
	Dysphagia	2	4	Trigeminal Neuropathy	12	14
Spinal	Pain	25	40	Lower motor neuron	78	78
	Back pain	18	50	weakness	60	76
	Radicular pain	12	25	Reflex absence/decrease	50	50
	Paresthesia	10	42	Dermatomal sensory loss	16	17
	Weakness	22	50	Nuchal rigidity		

Data from References 1 and 5

seizures, pheochromocytoma, drug withdrawal, thyroid storm, hypertensive crises, and sepsis or anxiety attacks [47].

The clinician should maintain a high index of suspicion in order to diagnose as early as possible the presence of LM. The presence in a cancer patient of neurological signs and symptoms reflecting multifocal neuraxis involvement is highly suggestive of LM. Nevertheless, isolated neurological syndromes may also be seen in patients with LM. The differential diagnosis at initial presentation of LM consists of any underlying cause of chronic meningitis such as tuberculosis, fungal infection, or sarcoidosis. Metabolic and toxic encephalopathies must also be excluded [5, 48].

In known LM, the appearance of new neurological manifestations may reflect progression of LM but other causes must be considered including BM, which can coexist with LM in 30–40% of cases, chemotherapy or radiation related neurological complications, and less commonly paraneoplastic syndromes.

CSF Examination

Cytology

Most cases of LM (90+%) manifest abnormal CSF [49]. Raised opening pressure (>200 mm of H_2O), increased leukocytes rate (>4 mm^3), elevated CSF protein (>50 mg/dl), and hypoglycorrachia (<60 mg/dl) have been reported in respectively 46, 57, 76, and 54% of LM. Nevertheless, these abnormalities are nonspecific. The presence of malignant cells in the CSF shown by cytological analysis is the mainstay of the diagnosis [49, 50]. The sensitivity of a first lumbar puncture is only 45–55%.

There are a few comparatively simple ways to improve the sensitivity of CSF cytological analysis such as providing a nonhemorrhagic CSF sample and by performing a second CSF assessment; the latter will increase the sensitivity to 80%. The benefit of a third CSF assessment is marginal [9]. To decrease the rate of false negative CSF analysis, samples should be obtained from a site compatible with clinical manifestations or based upon radiologic findings [51]. It has been reported that in the absence of CSF flow obstruction, the rate of discrepancy between lumbar and ventricular simultaneous assessments can reach 30% [51]. The minimal recommended volume of CSF sent for cytology should be of 10.5 ml so as to achieve a sensitivity of 97% (vs. 68% for a volume of 3.5 ml) [52]. The processing of the CSF samples should be urgent since the viability of malignant cells depends on time between sampling and laboratory assessment. Only 50% of the CTC remain viable after 30 min, and only 10% after 90 min [53]. The use of CSF fixation in dedicated tubes permits longer intervals between sampling of CSF and laboratory analysis. Nonetheless, approximately 25–30% of patients with clinical LM and normal neuraxis imaging have persistently negative CSF cytology [22, 49, 54–58].

Tumor Biomarkers

A variety of biomarkers of LM have been suggested to assist in achieving an earlier diagnosis of LM as well as to evaluate effectiveness of treatment [22, 57–66]. These markers include nonspecific biomarkers, such as alpha-glucuronidase, lactate dehydrogenase, beta 2-microglobulin, carcinoembryonic antigen, and others that are organ-specific such as CA 15-3, CA 125, CA 19-9, CA724, AFP, NSE, Cyfra 21-1, and EGFR. Two recent studies have reported that increased CSF levels of CA 15-3 in BC-related LM, and the combination of CEA and Cyfra 21.1 in NSCLC patients with LM may assist in the diagnosis of LM [57, 58]. Proangiogenic molecules (vascular endothelial growth factor [VEGF], uPA, and tPA) have been assessed as potential biomarkers for LM. Most series report elevated levels of CSF VEGF in patients with LM, with very variable sensitivity (51.4–100%) and specificity (71–100%) [60, 62, 67–70]. Combinations of different CSF tumor markers may improve the sensitivity though this requires validation [67]. Profiling CSF proteins (using mass spectrometry and multiplex immunoassays), especially those involved in the metastatic process, may be useful for diagnosis and prognosis assessment [62, 71–73]. At present there is no agreement regarding CSF biomarker cutoff levels nor has there been standardization of these various assays. Due to inconsistencies in laboratory methodology, there is considerable variation in sensitivity and specificity of these assays that produces serious challenges for utilizing biomarkers in the management of LM.

Flow Cytometry

Unlike in hematologic LM, flow cytometry is generally not used for the evaluation of suspected solid tumor-related leptomeningeal disease. A recent study explored the contribution of flow cytometry immunophenotyping (FCI) in the diagnosis of LM in solid tumors [74]. Epithelial cells were identified by expression of the epithelial cell adhesion molecule (EpCAM). Compared with cytology, FCI improved the sensitivity and negative predictive value (79% vs. 50%; 68% vs. 52%, respectively), but had a lower specificity and positive predictive value (84% vs. 100%; 90% vs. 100%).

Circulating Tumor Cells

Techniques used for the detection of circulating tumor cells (CTC) in peripheral blood have been applied to CSF with encouraging preliminary results [75–78]. The rare cell capture technology (RCCT) has also been recently utilized in the diagnosis of LM from solid tumors [76]. The sensitivity of this method was reported as superior to conventional CSF cytology (100% vs. 66.7%), demonstrated excellent specificity (97%), and provided an earlier diagnosis that was subsequently confirmed by delayed CSF cytology.

The Cell Search technology (identification of cell surface tumor associated proteins) has been used in BC and melanoma-related LM [75, 78]. It provides a semi-automated molecular analysis that in the future may improve the sensitivity, reliability, objectivity, and accuracy of detecting CSF tumor cells compared to CSF cytology [75]. These techniques are not yet available in daily practice and further evaluation of these novel technologies is ongoing. At present, the pathologic gold standard in diagnosing LM is still based on the detection of malignant cells in the CSF by cytology [50, 79, 80].

Neuroradiographic Studies

Because LM involves the entire neuraxis, imaging of the entire CNS is required. MRI with gadolinium enhancement is the radiologic technique of choice [81–84]. The standard examination should include axial T1-weighted images without contrast, fluid attenuation inversion recovery (FLAIR) sequences and 3D axial T1-weighted sequences with contrast of the brain. The spine is best evaluated with sagittal T1-weighted sequences with and without contrast and sagittal fat suppression T2-weighted sequences, combined with post-contrast axial T1-weighted images through regions of interest. Contrast enhanced T1-weighted and FLAIR sequences are the most sensitive to detect LM [85, 86].

Any leptomeningeal irritation—whether from hemorrhage, infection, or inflammation—of the SA can result in enhancement on MRI. Lumbar puncture may elicit a meningeal reaction resulting in leptomeningeal enhancement; consequently MRI should be obtained before the lumbar puncture [87]. At LM diagnosis, brain involvement may be present in 40–75%. MRI in LM may demonstrate subarachnoid, ventricular or parenchymal enhancing nodules, focal or diffuse pial enhancement, folia (Fig. 5.1a, b), ependymal (Fig. 5.2a, b), sulcal, or cranial nerve and nerve roots enhancement [88]. SA and parenchymal enhancing nodules (10–35%), diffuse or focal pial enhancement (10–20%) are the most common MRI findings. LM should be considered in the differential diagnosis of hydrocephalus in the cancer patient (Fig. 5.3a, b). Spine involvement is present in 15–25% of patients with LM (Fig. 5.4a, b). BM may be associated with LM in 21–82% [13, 56, 89]. The sensitivity of MRI in LM varies by report from 20 to 91% [10, 13, 22, 54, 56, 88–90]. A normal MRI does not exclude the diagnosis of LM. Nonetheless, in cases with a typical clinical presentation, abnormal MRI alone is adequate to establish the diagnosis of LM [49, 50, 88]. Computed tomography (CT) scan is of limited value in the diagnosis of LM [85]. The sensitivity of CT scan is estimated at 23–38%, and CT scan should be performed only in patients for whom MRI is contraindicated [22, 84].

CSF Flow Studies

CSF flow and circulation is best assessed by radionuclide cisternography using either [111]Indium-diethylenetriamine-pentaacetic acid or ^{99}Tc macro-aggregated albumin [44, 91]. Thirty to seventy percent of LM patients have CSF flow abnormalities, mostly located at the skull base, the spinal canal, and over the cerebral convexities [92–94]. Several series have

Fig. 5.1 Gadolinium-enhanced
T1 axial (**a**) and corresponding
FLAIR T2 axial (**b**) brain MRI
demonstrating cerebellar folia
contrast enhancement and FLAIR
hyperintensity in a patient with
breast cancer and leptomeningeal
carcinomatosis

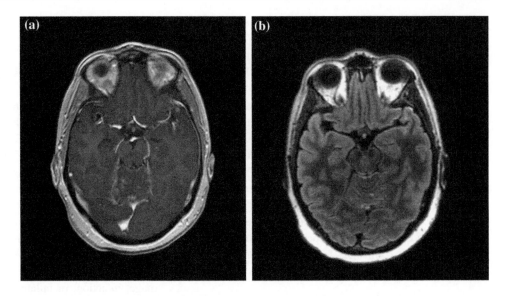

Fig. 5.2 Ependymal contrast
enhancement on
gadolinium-enhanced T1 axial
MRI (**a**) and corresponding
periventricular hyperintensity on
FLAIR MRI (**b**) in breast cancer
with CSF seeding

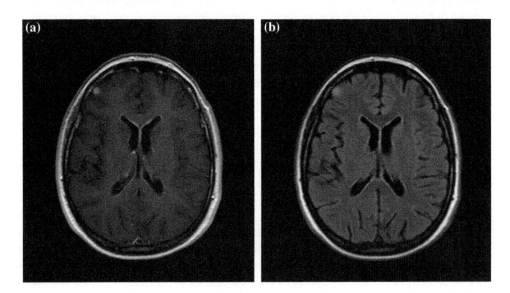

observed a correlation between the presence of CSF flow abnormalities and a shorter survival when compared to LM patients with normal CSF flow [92–95]. CSF flow can be restored to normal in 30% of patients with spinal blockage and 50% of patients with intracranial blockage by targeting the site of CSF flow obstruction with local radiation therapy (RT) [7].

Increased overall survival, less therapeutic morbidity, and decreased mortality from progressive LM have been reported in patients in whom normal CSF flow has been restored following involved-field RT, when compared to the patients with persistent CSF flow obstruction [91, 94]. Indeed, it is likely that altered CSF flow leads to heterogenous distribution of intra-CSF chemotherapy. This may result in an imbalance in drug exposure in the CSF compartments leading to under-treated areas that favor tumor progression and other regions exposed to excess chemotherapy with consequent neurological and systemic side effects.

Fig. 5.3 Gadolinium-enhanced T1 axial MRI (**a**) and corresponding FLAIR T2 axial MRI (**b**) demonstrating hydrocephalus and periventricular FLAIR signal hyperintensity in a breast cancer patient with leptomeningeal carcinomatosis

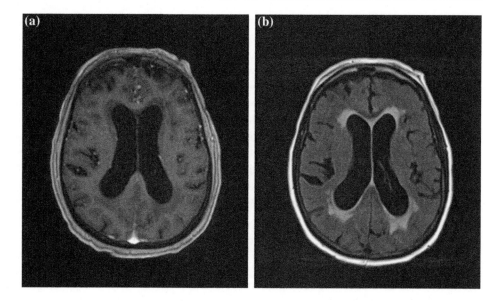

Fig. 5.4 **a**, **b** Spinal MRI. Gadolinium-enhanced T1 sagittal MRI. Perimedullary contrast enhancement in breast cancer

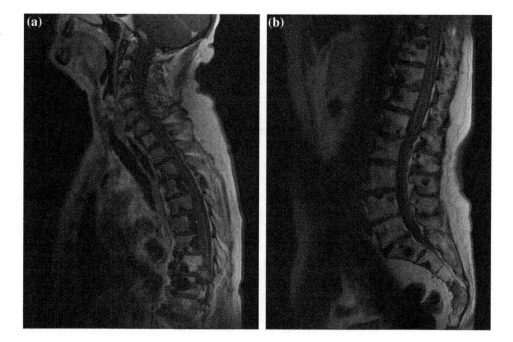

Based on these findings, many authors recommend that intra-CSF treatment be preceded by a CSF flow study, and that focal RT be administered on the sites of blockage prior to any treatment [43, 96]. This systematic approach is recommended by the Response Assessment in Neuro-Oncology (RANO) working group on LM in any clinical trial assessing an intra-CSF therapy in LM [97].

Meningeal Biopsy

Whenever the diagnosis of LM cannot be established and other etiologies of chronic meningitis have been excluded, a meningeal biopsy targeting a symptomatic and/or contrast enhancing area on MRI can be performed [98]. This procedure most often is directed the skull base or the cauda equina [8].

Staging

In summary, patients with suspected LM should undergo, prior to any anticancer treatment, one or two lumbar punctures to establish the presence of CTC, cranial MR-Gd, spinal MR-Gd and a radioisotope CSF flow study (the later only in instances where intra-CSF chemotherapy is to be administered). If cytology and MR are not contributive, a ventricular or lateral cervical CSF analysis may be required. If CSF cytology remains persistently negative despite compelling clinical and radiological manifestations consistent with LM, it is appropriate to commence LM-based therapy.

Differential Diagnosis

In patients with cancer, the diagnosis of LM is often straightforward. The situation is more challenging in patients without any known cancer, or if causality is uncertain (for example, the primary cancer is either in remission or presumed cured) and with a negative CF cytology. Other causes of subacute and chronic meningitis must then be excluded as discussed above [99]. Eventually, if a systemic evaluation does not identify an extraneural cancer, a primary brain tumor should be considered [100–104].

Evaluation of the Response to Treatment

New neurological manifestations must be distinguished from those secondary to parenchymal disease, from complications of intra-CSF treatment, systemic therapies or RT, from concomitant medications, from neurological or extraneurological concurrent disease, and more rarely from paraneoplastic syndromes [82]. Transient manifestations should not be assumed to be LM-related neurological progression. As mentioned earlier, CSF cytological analysis remains the gold standard for the diagnosis of cancer cells in the CSF despite a low sensitivity of a first CSF examination (45–55%), and the usual need of successive CSF samples to adequately assess cytology. The one-dimensional response evaluation criteria in solid tumors (RECIST) criteria are not adapted for the assessment of LM as the imaging characteristics of LM in general are not measurable at least as defined by current brain tumor response criteria [105].

In order to improve the methodology of future clinical trials, a RANO working group critically reviewed published the literature regarding randomized clinical trials (RCT) and trial design in patients with LM [106]. Six RCT have been published regarding the treatment of LM secondary to solid

tumors. As seen in Table 5.4, there were significant differences in the response assessment, such that interpretation of the trial results is challenging. Among these RCT, only a single trial attempted to determine whether intra-CSF chemotherapy was superior to systemic therapy only. Otherwise, this fundamental question has not been prospectively answered in patients with solid cancers and LM. The methodology of the 6 RCT varied considerably regarding pretreatment evaluation, type of treatment, and response to treatment. The RCT all share several common initial assessment features including evaluation of CSF cytology. Positive CSF cytology has been required for participation in all published RCT. Additionally, a neurologic clinical assessment and a predefined performance status were required as inclusion criteria in all RCT. Nevertheless, currently in neuro-oncology there is no standard instrument to assess the neurologic examination and consequently RCT in LM have lacked a rigorous method to determine clinical disease progression [106]. Also poorly defined in the published RCT is the utility of neuroimaging assessment (e.g., how radiographic findings alter treatment and how neuroimaging is used in the response assessment independent of CSF cytology and clinical examination) [106]. The RANO LM working group has developed a series of instruments to address these deficiencies [97] that includes a standardized neurological examination, definitions of CSF cytology and a new radiographic evaluative instrument. The working group recommends that "all patients enrolling in clinical trials undergo CSF analysis (cytology in all cancers; flow cytometry in hematologic cancers), complete contrast-enhanced neuraxis MRI and radioisotope CSF flow studies (in patients treated with intra-CSF therapy only)" [97]. "Response based on CSF cytology is considered when CSF converts from positive to negative and with a second confirmatory determination. CSF cytology is not to be considered in isolation in evaluation of response of patients with solid tumors as patients with persistence of positive cytology may continue on treatment if clinically and radiographically stable or improved" [97]. The committee created a composite score to quantify MRI abnormalities recognizing that most LM lesions are non-measurable. They concluded that "radiographic assessment of LM is subjective, qualitative and graded as stable, progressive or improved. Similar to CSF cytology, radiographic disease progression in isolation, i.e., stable CSF cytology and neurological assessment, would be defined as LM disease progression" [97]. It is hoped that ultimately this work will provide a standardized approach for LM assessment with validated criteria for response to treatment, and defined endpoints for clinical trials.

Table 5.4 Randomized clinical studies in Leptomeningeal metastases

Study	Design	Response	Toxicity
Hitchins [166]	N = 44 Solid tumors and lymphomas IT MTX versus MTX + Ara-C	IT MTX versus IT MTX + Ara-C: RR[a]: 61% versus 45% Median survival:[a] 12 versus 7 wk	IT MTX versus IT MTX + Ara-C: N/V: 36% versus 50% Septicemia, neutropenia: 9% versus 15% Mucositis: 14% versus 10% Pancytopenia: 9% versus 10%. Blocked Ommaya: 17% Intracranial hemorrhage (Ommaya placement): 11%
Grossman [188]	N = 59 Solid tumors and lymphoma (in 90%) IT MTX versus thiotepa	IT MTX versus IT thiotepa: Neurological improvements: none Median survival: 15.9 versus 14.1 wk	IT MTX versus thiotepa: Serious toxicity (47%) Similar between groups Mucositis and neurological AEDs more common in IT MTX group
Glantz [182]	N = 28 Solid tumors L-Ara-C[a] versus MTX	IVent L-Ara-C[a] versus IVent MTX: RR[a]: 26% versus 20% OS[a]: 105 versus 78 d TTP[a]: 58 versus 30 d	L-Ara-C[a] versus MTX: Sensory/motor: 4% versus 10% Altered mental status: 5% versus 2% Headache: 4% versus 2% Bacterial meningitis: 10% versus 3%
Boogerd [193]	N = 35 Breast cancer Systematic therapy and involved-field radiotherapy with versus no IT MTX	Systemic therapy and involved radiotherapy with IT MTX versus no IT MTX: Improved stabilization: 59% versus 67% TTP[a]: 23 versus 24 wk	Systemic therapy and involved radiotherapy with IT MTX versus no IT MTX: Drug-related AEs: 47% versus 6%
Shapiro [310]	Solid Tumors: n = 103 L-Ara-C[a] versus MTX Lymphoma: n = 24 L-Ara-C versus Ara-C	IVent L-Ara-C[a] versus IVent MTX/Ara-C: PFS[a]: 35 versus 43 d IVent L-Ara-C[a] versus IVent MTX: PFS[a]: 35 versus 37.5 d IVent L-Ara-C[a] versus IVent Ara-C: CytR[a]: 33.3% versus 16.7%	IVent L-Ara-C[a] versus IVent MTX/Ara-C: Drug-related AEs: 48% versus 60% Serious AEs: 86% versus 77%

[a]No significant differences between groups; *AE* Adverse event; *Ara-C* Cytarabine; *Cyt R* Cytological response; *d* Days; *L Ara-C* Liposomal Cytarabine; *MTX* Methotrexate; *N/V* Nausea/vomiting; *OS* Overall survival; *PFS* Progression-free survival; *RR* Response rate; *TTP* Time to progression; *wk* Weeks; *IVent* Intraventricular chemotherapy; *IT* Intralumbar chemotherapy
Adapted from Le Rhun E, Taillibert S, Chamberlain MC. Carcinomatous meningitis: Leptomeningeal metastases in solid tumors. Surg Neurol Int. 2013; 4(Suppl 4): S265–S288. Open Access Journal

Survival and Prognostic Factors

The median OS of untreated patients with LM is 4–6 weeks [3, 14, 48, 94, 107–113]. Despite aggressive treatment, LM has a poor prognosis. The survival of patients with combined treatment is usually less than 6 months with a median OS of 2–3 months [3, 10, 13, 14, 22, 48, 54, 56, 89, 90, 109–113]. Table 5.5 illustrates reported survival in patients with LM from the recent literature.

The goal of LM-directed treatment is to improve or stabilize neurologic status, maintain neurological quality of life, and prolong survival. Nevertheless, deciding which patients to treat remains a challenge. The NCCN CNS guidelines (version 1.2012) have attempted to distinguish between patients reasonably considered for treatment versus those patients in whom supportive care is most appropriate [49, 50, 94, 107, 114, 115] (Table 5.6).

Based on the literature, the histology of the primary cancer is known to be the prominent prognostic factor with regard to OS in LM [50, 116]. Multivariate analysis has confirmed the association between survival and primary tumor type and the better prognosis of BC compared with lung cancer or melanoma-related LM [10, 68, 117]. Breast cancer LM has a relatively good prognosis among all solid tumor-related LM, with a median OS of 3.3–5 months [22, 54–56, 109]. Modest improvement in lung cancer-related LM may in part reflect increasing use of targeted agents such as tyrosine kinase inhibitors (TKI) based on recent reports of patients with lung cancer and LM with reported median survival of 3–6 months [13, 89, 118–120]. LM secondary to melanoma continues to demonstrate the worst prognosis of all solid tumor-related LM with a median OS estimated between 10 weeks and 4 months before the era of the immunotherapy and targeted therapies [107–110].

Table 5.5 Median OS in the main cohorts of LM according to the primary type of tumor

Type of the primitive tumor	References	N patients	Median overall survival (Min–Max)
Breast cancer	Grossman [188]	52	14.1–15.9 weeks
	Clamon [311]	22	21–150 days
	Boogerd [196]	58	12 weeks
	Jayson [312]	35	77 days
	Chamberlain [48]	32	7.5 months
	Jaeckle [184]	43	7 weeks
	Boogerd [193]	35	18.3–30.3 weeks
	Regierer [313]	27	9 weeks
	Rudnicka [56]	67	16 weeks
	De Azevedo [54]	60	3.3 months
	Clatot [109]	24	150 days
	Gauthier [22]	91	4.5 months
	Lee [55]	68	4.5 months
	Kim [314]	30	8 months
	Lara-Medina [11]	49	7 weeks
	Le Rhun [185]	103	3.8 months
	Niwinska [125]	149	4.2 months
Melanoma	Chamberlain [94]	16	4 months
	Harstad [110]	110	10 weeks
	Raizer [14]	40	4 months
Lung cancer	Rosen [18]	60	7 weeks
	Chamberlain [190]	32	5 months
	Hammerer [315]	26	57 weeks
	Sudo [316]	37	106 days
	Chuang [317]	34	5.1 weeks
	Morris [13]	50	3 months
	Park [89]	125	4.3 months
	Lee [118]	149	14 weeks
	Riess [120]	30	6 months
	Xu [119]	108	5.3 months

Adapted from Le Rhun E, Taillibert S, Chamberlain MC. Carcinomatous meningitis: Leptomeningeal metastases in solid tumors. Surg Neurol Int. 2013; 4(Suppl 4): S265–S288. Open Access Journal

Table 5.6 Risk categories in patients with in leptomeningeal metastases

High-risk group	Low-risk group
KPS < 60%	KPS ≥ 60%
Major neurological deficits	No major neurological deficits
Extensive systemic disease without any efficient treatment available	Minimal systemic disease
Bulky CNS disease	Manageable with an effective treatment
LM-related encephalopathy	No CSF blockade

Adapted from Le Rhun E, Taillibert S, Chamberlain MC. Carcinomatous meningitis: Leptomeningeal metastases in solid tumors. Surg Neurol Int. 2013; 4(Suppl 4): S265–S288. Open Access Journal
Data from CNS National Comprehensive Cancer Network guidelines
CNS Central Nervous System; *CSF* Cerebrospinal Fluid; *KPS* Karnofsky Performance Status

In addition to tumor histology, multivariate analysis in series including all types of solid tumors confirms the associations between OS and the performance status (PS), the age at LM diagnosis, the presence of a LM-related encephalopathy, time from diagnosis of primary tumor to diagnosis of LC (>67 weeks), the CSF protein level, the treatment modality (administration of systemic therapy), and the presence of a short-term response to treatment [10, 68, 117, 121–124]. In one report, gender was significant in multivariate analysis likely due to an interaction between gender and tumor type [10]. Recently, the quantification of CSF EpCAM+ cells obtained with flow cytometry immunophenotyping (FCI) before any treatment has been reported to be an independent prognostic factor for OS in LM patients with a cutoff value of 8% [74].

In patients with BC and LM, multivariate analysis demonstrates an association between OS and PS as well as PS and treatment (number of prior chemotherapy regimens, receipt of combined treatment modality, coadministration of systemic chemotherapy or intra-CSF chemotherapy) [11, 22,

54, 55, 109, 122, 125]. Histological characteristics (histological grade, hormone receptor status, triple-negative status), the initial CSF protein level, the number of prior chemotherapy regimens, status of systemic disease (i.e., isolated CNS metastases or bone metastases), the presence of an early and/or combined cytological and neurological response to treatment and the initial CSF cyfra 21-1 and protein levels were also identified as significantly associated with prognosis in BC-related LM [11, 22, 54–56, 109, 122–125].

In recent retrospective series of patients with NSCLC and LM, multivariate analysis confirmed that PS, low initial CSF protein level, low initial CSF (white blood cells) WBC count were all significantly associated with a better OS [13, 89, 118]. The treatment modality (systemic therapy and intrathecal chemotherapy) and clinical improvement after intra-CSF chemotherapy were all significant predictors of increased OS [13, 89, 118, 120]. The impact of whole brain radiotherapy (WBRT) in the treatment of LM is unclear [13, 89, 118–120]. In EGFR-mutated NSCLC, EGFR inhibitors have produced durable responses in patients with LM [13, 89, 113, 118, 119, 126–130]. In patients with melanoma, multivariate analysis suggests that a history of a primary melanoma lesion originating on the trunk predicted shorter OS and that intra-CSF chemotherapy predicted longer OS [110]. Nevertheless, unlike prognostic factors present at LM diagnosis and before any treatment, the interpretation of prognostic factors related to treatment and mostly derived from retrospective series remains uncertain. All such series are single-institution retrospective studies in which treated patients are heterogeneous with respect to recognized LM-prognostic features. Because of the retrospective nature of these studies, there were no a priori determinants of treatment such that treatment was defined individually, without apparent standardization making cross-comparisons between treatment groups difficult [131]. Moreover, two series, one in NSCLC and the other in all types of solid tumor LM, report that the placement of a VPS was significantly predictive of improved OS in LM [118, 132]. These observations seem counter-intuitive and are difficult to reconcile.

Treatment

The goals of treatment include palliating neurologic symptoms and whenever possible stabilizing or improving patient neurologic function as well as prolonging survival. Since the prognosis of LM varies noticeably depending upon the primary tumor type and extent of both neurologic and systemic disease, parameters separating poor-risk from good-risk patients are helpful to determine the appropriate therapeutic approach for an individual patient. The poor-risk and good-risk patients categories are illustrated in Table 5.6. LM ideally should be diagnosed early in the disease course before the appearance of fixed and disabling neurological deficits. Early LM-directed treatment may allow maintenance of quality of life and potentially improve survival. A combined treatment approach (i.e., systemic and intra-CSF chemotherapy and site specific radiotherapy) may provide better palliation in patients with LM [133].

Symptomatic Treatment and Supportive Care

Patients with low PS, neurologic deficits interfering with quality of life, encephalopathy due to extensive LM-brain infiltration, or uncontrolled systemic disease with limited therapeutic options have a poor prognosis even with aggressive LM-directed treatment. A palliative approach should be considered in such poor prognosis patients. Regardless, however, supportive care is needed in every patient with LM independent of treatment in order to palliate neurological symptoms and signs associated with LM.

Pain relief is required for headache, back, and radicular pain, and is based on the use of analgesics of increasing efficacy from acetaminophen to opioids. In addition, neuropathic pain often requires use of tricyclic antidepressants (such as amitriptyline or nortriptyline) or antiepileptic drugs (such as gabapentin, pregabalin, carbamazepine, and lamotrigine). Corticosteroids may also improve radicular pain. Focal irradiation of symptomatic sites provides often a good analgesic effect. Seizures are addressed with anticonvulsant drugs (AED) but prophylactic administration of AED is not recommended. Headaches related to edema or increased intracranial pressure can sometimes be managed with steroids, even if the contribution of steroids in the treatment of LM is modest as compared with their efficacy in brain parenchymal metastases. In instances of hydrocephalus secondary to CSF obstruction, steroids in conjunction with whole brain or skull-base radiotherapy may be effective but CSF shunting is often needed [91, 134]. Iterative lumbar punctures when there is no threatening BM may be an alternative method to relieve temporarily headache in patients declining CSF diversion. Depression or fatigue may be managed with serotonin reuptake inhibitors or stimulant medication (modafinil, methylphenidate) as clinically appropriate [45]. Finally a discussion regarding of end of life before institution of LM-directed therapy is recommended in all patients so as to realistically outline the course of disease and palliative treatment goals.

Surgery

The main surgical interventions in LM are ventriculoperitoneal shunting (VPS) for symptomatic hydrocephalus, placement of a ventricular (rarely lumbar) access device (e.g., an Ommaya or Rickham reservoir) to facilitate administration of intra-CSF chemotherapy, and meningeal biopsy. When both a VPS and Ommaya ventricular access device are needed, an on–off valve may be an option but the patient should be able to tolerate having the VPS placed in the off position so as to permit drug installation into the ventricles and time for ventricular transit and distribution into the nonventricular CSF compartments [134–136]. Complications of VPS rarely exceed 10% in recent series [135, 136] but include the potential for peritoneal tumor dissemination, device failure, device malpositioning, device exposure, infection, hemorrhage, and leukoencephalopathy [45, 135, 136].

When a ventricular access device is placed, confirmation post-implantation of correct intraventricular (IVent) placement requires a brain CT or alternatively a radioisotope CSF flow study before intra-CSF drug administration [137–139]. Hemorrhage at the time of device placement occurs in less than 1% of patients. Device infection (4–10% incidence) is due mainly to *Staphylococcus epidermidis* and is either a complication that occurs in relationship to surgery or results from contamination at the time of device access [133, 134, 138–140]. In instances where the ventricular device becomes infected occasionally, the device may be left in situ and treated with both intravenous and IVent antibiotics [93, 140–144]. Most often, however, device infections requires removal and if indicated, replacement of the reservoir [93, 135, 142]. A rare complication in patients with increased intracranial pressure is retrograde tracking of instilled chemotherapy along the catheter, resulting in subgaleal or intraparenchymal collections of CSF that may become symptomatic and require revision or replacement with a ventriculoperitoneal shunt [5].

Radiation Therapy

Craniospinal axis irradiation (CSI) is the only method of radiotherapy that treats the entire neuraxis and that may be reasonably considered as a single modality of treatment for LM. However, in the majority of adults CSI is rarely considered as most patients have previously had some region of the neuraxis irradiated, and as well have poor bone marrow reserve as a consequence of prior exposure to cytotoxic chemotherapy. Consequently, CSI and treatment-associated toxicities of myelosuppression and enteritis is deemed too toxic for routine use in adults with solid tumor-related LM. The role of alternative methods of CSI such as tomotherapy

and proton radiotherapy, which could permit improved precision in radiation dosing and targeted volumes and consequently less hematological toxicity, has not been formally evaluated and may be an option in the future.

The majority of patients with LM receive involved-field radiotherapy to sites of symptomatic disease, bulky disease observed on MRI and to sites of CSF flow block defined by radioisotope ventriculography. Irradiation permits tumor masses not treated by intra-CSF chemotherapy (due to limited diffusion of intra-CSF chemotherapy) to receive palliative radiotherapy [145]. WBRT is most commonly administered at a dose of 30 Gy delivered in 10 fractions over 10 days. While pain relief and stabilization of neurological manifestations are regularly observed, unfortunately significant neurological improvement is exceptional. The failure of neurological improvement is due to demyelination, axonal and neuronal injury, and injury by infiltrating cancer cells, aspects that underscore the need for early treatment of LM [146]. Regardless of MRI findings (e.g., the absence of visible radiographic disease), lumbosacral irradiation is indicated in instances of cauda equine syndrome (low back pain, legs weakness, bladder or bowel dysfunction). Similarly, skull-base RT may be used for cranial neuropathies [8]. RT is also indicated to reestablish normal CSF circulation to improve therapeutic efficacy and reduce side effects of intra-CSF chemotherapy [1–6, 8, 94]. Communicating hydrocephalus is not infrequent in LM and is caused by malignant cells in the subarachnoid space that obstruct normal CSF resorption pathways. In these instances, WBRT or placement of a VPS is often required [147]. Shunting of CSF should be provided in patients with symptomatic or communicating hydrocephalus that does not rapidly respond to WBRT.

Unlike brain metastases, the impact of WBRT on OS is not clearly established in LM, even in radiosensitive cancers such as BC and NSCLC. Contradictory results have been reported that in part reflect the limited survival of patients with LM (<15% survive 1 year) [13, 89, 118–120]. In small case reports WBRT has been reported (as part of a combined modality treatment) to result in prolonged survival (from 13 to 19 months) in patients with melanoma and LM [148–152]. In these case reports, WBRT was either delivered concomitantly or prior to other treatment (intra-CSF or systemic). However, the retrospective nature of the data makes it challenging to determine the role of WBRT in the treatment of LM.

Some authors have posited that WBRT may enhance the efficacy of targeted drug therapy by either by radio sensitization or improving drug penetration into brain/CSF [148, 149]. Improved brain penetration following WBRT has been demonstrated with systemically administered trastuzumab, a monoclonal antibody a low rate of CNS penetration rate [153–155]. In addition to mechanically disrupting the BBB, radiation may hinder the efflux function of multidrug resistance proteins [149]. Indeed, the low CSF concentration of vemurafenib has been related at least partially to the active efflux by P-glycoprotein and breast cancer resistance protein [156].

Side effects of involved-field RT alone are uncommon and manifest mainly as radiation-associated fatigue. However, myelosuppression, mucositis, esophagitis, and leukoencephalopathy have been reported with more extensive radiation fields. Leukoencephalopathy (asymptomatic more often than symptomatic) may be a delayed consequence of WBRT and may be enhanced with coadministered methotrexate (MTX) (either systemic or intra-CSF). Ongoing clinical trials evaluating the safety of concomitant WBRT and intra-CSF liposomal cytarabine will determine if this is a common problem with chemoradiation or unique to MTX when combined with radiotherapy.

Chemotherapy

Chemotherapy is the only treatment aside from CSI to treat simultaneously the entire neuraxis. Chemotherapy may be administered systemically or instilled directly into the CSF. Intra-CSF administration is either intrathecal (IT) by the lumbar route or intraventricular by way of a ventricular access device (IVent).

Intra-CSF Chemotherapy

The benefit of intra-CSF IT or IVent chemotherapy in LM over systemic treatment alone has never been proven in RCT (Table 5.4) [106]. Nonetheless, recent retrospective studies suggest that intra-CSF chemotherapy may be useful in NSCLC patients. This population is rarely treated with intra-CSF chemotherapy treatment because of historic poor prognosis [13, 89]. Park reported on 48 patients with NSCLC-related LM who received intra-CSF chemotherapy with a cytological response rate of 52% [89]. The median survival was 5.5 months in cytological responders and 1.4 months in nonresponders [89].

In a series of 149 patients with NSCLC (mainly adenocarcinoma) and LM, Lee reported a significantly favorable impact of intra-CSF chemotherapy in multivariate analysis [118]. Similarly, the favorable impact of intra-CSF chemotherapy when combined with systemic therapy has been retrospectively reported in BC patients with LM [122]. In melanoma patients, intra-CSF treatment has been reported as a predictive factor of longer survival with occasional long-duration survivors in a retrospective study [110, 150, 151, 157]. However, due to the limited number of patients, heterogeneous intra-CSF treatment and retrospective nature, these results should be interpreted cautiously.

Most anticancer drugs, when given by a systemic route in patients with intact blood–brain and blood–CSF barriers, display poor penetration into the CNS that translates into a CSF exposure less than 5% of the plasma concentration. The blood–CSF barrier in LM undergoes a partial disruption only that varies from one area to another such that with few exceptions (e.g., high-dose methotrexate (MTX) discussed later for breast cancer-associated LM) systemic chemotherapy is rarely a primary treatment of LM.

The goal of intra-CSF chemotherapy is to bypass the blood–CSF barrier, and maximize CSF exposure while decreasing systemic toxicity. Thus, since the distribution volume of CSF is less than that of the plasma (140 vs. 3500 ml), a higher concentration of the active agent can be reached using a lower dose [158]. Moreover, most cytotoxic agents' half-life is longer in the CSF than in plasma, allowing a prolonged CSF exposure that is particularly useful for cell-cycle-specific drugs such as MTX and ara-C. The majority of affected regions in LM is only a few cells in thickness and since intra-CSF chemotherapy can diffuse a relatively short distance (1–2 mm), small volume disease and cells suspended in CSF can be appropriately treated [159, 160]. However, intra-CSF chemotherapy cannot reliably treat radiographically bulky leptomeningeal disease because of limited diffusion into tumor lesions >2 mm in diameter, into the Virchow–Robin spaces, and along nerve root sleeves.

Lumbar Intrathecal or IntraVentricular Route of Administration

Since patient position has an impact on ventricular drug levels after intralumbar administration, patients should remain flat for at least 1 h following injection [161]. On only rare occasion is IT drug administration delivered through a lumbar catheter connected to a subcutaneous reservoir, as such devices frequently fail with repeated use due to the high protein content found in the lumbar cistern.

IVent administration of intra-CSF drug via an Ommaya or Rickham reservoir offers some advantages compared with IT therapy [52]. The procedure is painless for the patient and more time-efficient for the clinician. The drug is also safely administered at the correct place without the 10% risk of epidural or sudural injection observed with IT injections. It is also safe to administer IVent injection in instances of thrombopenia, thus avoiding the risk of epidural or subdural hematoma after lumbar puncture [162]. A better pharmacokinetic profile is also achieved with IVent administration, with improved and more uniform drug distribution in the entire CSF compartment [163–165]. IVent CSF drug concentration following IT injection is only 10% of that achieved after an equivalent IVent dose. Another advantage is that more frequent administrations of smaller doses of drug are an option to achieve lower peak drug concentrations and therefore limit total cumulative dose and neurological side effects. A survival benefit was suggested for IVent compared with IT chemotherapy in one randomized clinical trial [166]. IVent and IT administrations were compared in a subset analysis of a RCT comparing liposomal ara-C with MTX in 100 patients with LM [167]. Overall, intra-CSF chemotherapy was given by IVent and IT route in 72 and 28% of cases, respectively. For patients given liposomal ara-C, there was no statistically significant difference in progression-free survival (PFS) according to the route of administration. For those given MTX, the IVent route appeared superior (PFS 19 vs. 43 days) suggesting that the site of administration affects survival and is dependent upon the CSF half-life of the chemotherapy.

Techniques of Intra-CSF Administration

It is critical to avoid any variation in CSF volume in LM patients, who often are on the edge of the CSF ventricular "pressure-volume" compliance curve. If the total CSF volume is increased, severe intracranial hypertension can occur. Thus equivalent volume of CSF should be removed (so-called isovolumetric withdrawal) prior to chemotherapy administration. During the withdrawal of a large volume of CSF from the ventricles, a transient retro-orbital or frontal headache may result. The headache is often improved with administration of intra-CSF chemotherapy if given in 5–10 ml volume. No prospective trials in adults with LM have proven any benefit to concomitant use of intra-CSF glucocorticoids (hydrocortisone) in combination with intra-CSF chemotherapy.

Drugs Available for Intra-CSF Treatment

Currently, MTX, liposomal ara-C, and less often thiotepa are used in daily practice (Table 5.7). Unfortunately, these agents are not generally considered active systemically against most common solid cancers associated with LM, particularly melanoma and lung cancer. New agents including monoclonal antibodies are currently being investigated in clinical trials and are discussed below.

Methotrexate

Therapeutic CSF concentrations of 1 μM/mL or more are seen 48–72 h after a 12 mg IT dose of MTX in adults and in children aged older than 2 years [3, 165, 168–170]. Usually, MTX is administered on a twice-weekly schedule for 1 month; then the frequency of injections is reduced over a total period of 3–6 months. The optimal duration of treatment is not known, and a prolonged treatment may benefit some patients. Alternative schedules have been reported such as 2 mg of IVent MTX for 5 consecutive days every 2 weeks [169, 171, 172]. A dose-intense regimen of MTX (15 mg/day, 5/7 days, 1 week on 1 week off) has been reported in a retrospective study of BC patients with a median survival of 4.5–5 months [22, 109, 173]. Conversion from positive to negative CSF cytology with intra-CSF MTX occurs in 20–61% of patients with LM [174–176]. The clinical efficacy of different schedules of MTX in retrospective BC LM studies is illustrated in Table 5.8. This table as well reflects coadministered CNS-directed RT given as part of the LM treatment regimen, which makes the interpretation of the impact of one intra-CSF MTX regimen versus another challenging [174–177]. Achievement of a

Table 5.7 Intrathecal chemotherapy regimens in LM

Drugs	Induction regimens		Consolidation regimen		Maintenance regimen	
	Bolus regimen	C × T regimen	Bolus regimen	C × T regimen	Bolus regimen	C × T regimen
Methotrexate	10–15 mg twice weekly (Total 4 weeks)	2 mg/day for 5 days every other week (Total 8 weeks)	10–15 mg once weekly (total 4 weeks)	2 mg/day for 5 days every other week (total 4 weeks)	10–15 mg once a month	2 mg/day for 5 days once a month
Ara-C	25–100 mg 2 or 3 times weekly (Total 4 weeks)	25 mg/day for 3 days weekly (Total 4 weeks)	25–100 mg once weekly (Total 4 weeks)	25 mg/day for 3 days every other week (Total 4 weeks)	25–100 mg once a month	25 mg/day for 3 days once a month
Liposomal cytarabine	50 mg every 2 weeks (Total 8 weeks)		50 mg every 4 weeks (Total 24 weeks)			
Thiotepa	10 mg 2 or 3 times weekly (Total 4 weeks)	10 mg/day for 3 days weekly (total 4 weeks)	10 mg once weekly (Total 4 weeks)	10 mg/day for 3 days every other week (Total 4 weeks)	10 mg once a month	10 mg/day for 3 days once a month

Table 5.8 Intra-CSF treatments in breast cancer

Agent/Reference	N	Other treatments	Response	Median OS (months)
Standard MTX Rudnicka [56]	67	Systemic: 61% RT: 64%	Clinical: NS Cyt: NS MRI: NS Overall: 76%	4
Standard MTX De Azevedo [54]	60	Systemic: 43% RT: 36.7%	Clinical: NS Cyt: NS MRI: NS	3.3
Intensified-MTX Clatot [109]	24	Systemic: 46% RT: 46%	Clinical: 96% Cyt: 46% MRI: NS	5
Intensified-MTX Gauthier [22]	80	Systemic: 78% RT: 29%	Clinical: 73% Cyt: 20% MRI: NS	4.5
L-AraC Le Rhun [185]	103	Systemic: 58.2% RT: 13.5%	Clinical: 56.8% Cyt: 30.6% MRI: 62.5%	3.8

Cyt Cytological; L-*Ara C* Liposomal Aracytine; *MRI* Magnetic Resonance Imaging
NS Not stated; *RT* Radiation Therapy
Adapted from Le Rhun E, Taillibert S, Chamberlain MC. Carcinomatous meningitis: Leptomeningeal metastases in solid tumors. Surg Neurol Int. 2013; 4(Suppl 4): S265–S288. Open Access Journal

cytological response in the first month of IT MTX treatment may be predictive of increase survival (6 vs. 2 months) [177]. Regardless, OS is within a similar range irrespective of the intra-CSF MTX schedule. Considering the short survival of patients with LM and the difficulty differentiating with certainty the respective impact of radiation and intra-CSF chemotherapy, quality of life should be the priority when considering treatment of LM.

MTX is eliminated from the CSF by CSF/venous resorption and subsequent delivery into the systemic circulation. Consequently, conditions that impact CSF resorption increase intra-CSF MTX-related neurotoxicity. Similarly, renal impairment decreases the excretion of MTX and may aggravated systemic MTX toxicity. The presence of pleural or peritoneal effusions (creating a "third space effect") accentuates accumulation of MTX, which may increase systemic MTX side effects such as myelosuppression or mucositis. The concomitant use of drugs that displaces MTX from albumin, such as aspirin, phenytoin, sulfonamides, and tetracycline, may also amplify MTX toxicity. Neurologic complications of intra-CSF MTX include aseptic meningitis, acute encephalopathy, transverse myelopathy, and delayed leukoencephalopathy. Folinic acid (leucovorin) has been suggested to mitigate systemic MTX toxicity and is often prescribed orally 10 mg every 6 h for 1–2 days after each intra-CSF MTX administration. Leucovorin does not cross the blood–brain barrier in sufficient amounts to interfere with the efficacy of intra-CSF MTX. Significant or even lethal complications may occur after an involuntary overdose of intra-CSF MTX. Recommendations have been issued for

such clinical situations including drainage of CSF via lumbar puncture, ventriculostomy with ventriculo-lumbar perfusion, systemic steroids, and systemic leucovorin, and the use of carboxypeptidase-G2 (CPDG2) as an antidote are proposed. CSF MTX concentrations have been reduced by a 400-fold within 5 min of this antidote use according to some pharmacokinetic studies [178].

Cytosine Arabinoside (Cytarabine)

Cytarabine (ara-C) is initially administered at a dosage of 25–100 mg twice weekly. The 4-week induction period is followed by 4 weeks of consolidation and subsequent maintenance. The CSF half-life of ara-C is much longer than in serum because cytidine deaminase, the main catabolic enzyme of ara-C, is present at very low level in the CSF. The rapid deamination that occurs in the systemic circulation leads to a good systemic tolerance profile. A concentration time regimen (i.e., low dose intra-CSF chemotherapy given for consecutive days) has also been reported [179]. Liposomal ara-C, a depot encapsulated formulation (DepoCyt) is a useful intra-CSF agent in patients with LM secondary to solid tumors as conventional ara-C is relatively ineffective due primarily to the short half-life of ara-C (approximately 3.4 h). Intra-CSF administration of the conventional formulation of ara-C results in complete clearance of the drug from the CSF within 1 or 2 days [180, 181]. In contrast, liposomal ara-C with a half-life of 140 h provides a therapeutic ara-C concentration in the CSF for up to 10–12 days. Due to the long half-life of liposomal ara-C, intra-CSF drug administration may be once every 2 weeks. At present, liposomal ara-C is approved only for lymphomatous meningitis but is often used off-label for solid tumor-related LM.

In a RCT with solid tumor patients with LM, assessing intra-CSF liposomal ara-C versus MTX, the median time to neurologic progression was improved (58 vs. 30 days) with a small increase in toxicity but fewer visits to the hospital (75% reduction) with liposomal ara-C [182, 183]. There was no significant difference between arms for median survival (105 vs. 78 days) [182].

The liposomal ara-C regimen showed a better quality-adjusted survival regardless of the quality of life assessment based on time with toxicity and time following disease progression (range, 44–79 days). In BC patients, liposomal ara-C has shown similar cytological response rates (26–30%) and median survival (3–4.6 months) compared with other intra-CSF drugs in nonrandomized series [90, 124, 125, 184, 185] (Table 5.8). Nevertheless, the acceptable tolerance profile of liposomal ara-C and its convenient schedule of administration present some advantages compared to other intra-CSF regimens.

Liposomal ara-C has been used in melanoma-associated LM, in which occasional sustained responses (14–24 months) have been observed [148, 150, 157]. The role of intra-CSF liposomal ara-C in durable response achievement and survival in these case reports is difficult to determine as the majority of patients received systemic therapy, involved-field radiotherapy as well as liposomal ara-C. Liposomal ara-C is mainly complicated by arachnoiditis (i.e., a transient sterile chemical meningitis), but the use of oral dexamethasone (4 mg twice daily during 5 days, onset on the day of liposomal ara-C injection) decreases the occurrence of this side effect [186, 187].

In a retrospective series of 120 patients with LM and treated with liposomal ara-C, neurotoxicity included bacterial meningitis (IVent:IT treatment; 3.75%:0%); chemical meningitis (17.5%:15%); communicating hydrocephalus (3.75%:5%); conus medullaris/cauda equina syndrome (5%:5%); decreased visual acuity (5%:2.5%); encephalopathy (5%:5%); leukoencephalopathy (7.5%:2.5%); myelopathy (2.5%:2.5%); radiculopathy (1.25%:5%); and seizures (1.25%:2.5%) [187]. The toxicity profile was similar in ventricular and lumbar routes. Most side effects were reversible (57% vs. 43%). Hospitalization was needed in 32.2%. The tolerance profile of liposomal ara-C was generally good; however, 12.5% of patients developed serious and permanent neurological side effects that negatively impacted quality of life [187].

Clinicians are advised to inform pathologists when patients are under liposomal ara-C since liposomal particles may be confused microscopically with white blood cells.

A randomized Phase III trial is currently ongoing in France to evaluate intra-CSF liposomal ara-C (vs. no intra-CSF therapy) in BC-related LM.

Thiotepa

Thiotepa, an alkylating agent and therefore cell-cycle-nonspecific, has the shortest half-life (approximately 20 min) of all drugs directly administered in the CSF. CSF clearance is achieved within 4 h. It is usually used as a second-line agent for BC patients, when MTX is ineffective or not tolerated. Thiotepa, unlike other intra-CSF administered drugs, rapidly crosses brain capillaries and consequently may result in meaningful systemic serum levels and associated myelosuppression. Because the half-life is short and the transcapillary movement is rapid, it has been argued that there is no pharmacological advantage to intra-CSF thiotepa. Nonetheless, a RCT has compared intra-CSF thiotepa with intra-CSF MTX in LM patients. Similar median survivals were observed: 14 weeks with intra-CSF thiotepa versus 16 weeks with intra-CSF MTX. The CSF cytological rate was 30%. Less neurotoxicity was reported with thiotepa [188]. Twenty-four BC patients with LM were treated with second-line intra-CSF thiotepa following failure of intra-CSF liposomal ara-C in a retrospective study [189]. Systemic chemotherapy was also coadministered to nine patients. The median PFS and OS with thiotepa was 3.1 months (range 3 days-2 years) and 4.0 months (range 6 days–2.5 years), respectively. The median OS from LM diagnosis was 9.5 months (range 1.3 months–2.7 years). Minimal treatment-related toxicity was observed.

Combination (Multi-agent) Intra-CSF Chemotherapy with Systemic Treatment

Multidrug intra-CSF regimens in LM patients with solid tumor are no more effective than single-drug regimens; moreover, combination therapy is more toxic and associated with a worse tolerance profile [166, 190]. A single RCT compared intra-CSF MTX with intra-CSF MTX plus ara-C plus hydrocortisone in 55 patients [166]. There was a higher rate of cytological response (38% vs. 14%) and a longer median survival (19 vs. 10 weeks) with the multidrug regimen, but these differences did not reach statistical significance and a selection bias (lower risk patients receiving multidrug therapy) cannot be ruled out [191]. In a recent retrospective cohort, the combination of IT MTX and liposomal cytarabine was assessed in 30 LM patients with different types of cancers [192]. Cytologic clearance was achieved in 33% and median OS was 7.5 months in patients with solid tumor-related LM. Considering the retrospective nature of the study, the small number of patients and the heterogeneity of tumor types, interpretation of this study is challenging. Another small randomized study addressed the question of the potential superiority of a combination of systemic and intra-CSF chemotherapy versus systemic treatment alone in LM from BC and failed to show a survival advantage for the intra-CSF chemotherapy treated cohort [193].

Systemic Chemotherapy

Intra-CSF chemotherapy in LM from solid cancers is of modest benefit when compared to results in hematologic cancers. Several factors are responsible such as intrinsic chemoresistance, limited choice of intra-CSF chemotherapeutic agents and the limited accessibility of bulky nodules to intra-CSF chemotherapy [194]. Furthermore, the main cause of death in LM patients is uncontrolled systemic disease [175]. As a consequence, only systemic chemotherapy can simultaneously address the systemic and leptomeningeal disease [173, 175, 195]. Systemic treatment offers several other advantages such as avoiding the risks of the surgical placement of a ventricular access device, being able to treat patients with a CSF flow block or bulky LM disease, as well as having access to a wider range of therapeutic agents that have tumor type specificity [174]. Some authors have suggested that systemic therapy may replace intra-CSF therapy, a hypothesis that has never been adequately evaluated in a prospective trial of LM [13, 120, 122, 125, 148–152, 173, 175, 187, 195–202].

Some have concluded that the addition of intra-CSF chemotherapy to systemic chemotherapy for treatment of BC-related LM does not change the overall response rate, median survival or the long-term survival rate, but does significantly raise the rate of acute, subacute, and delayed neurologic complications [197–199]. Conversely, systemic treatment may not add any benefit for some patients. Another prospective study in LM patients with NSCLC did not show any survival benefit of adding systemic chemotherapy to the combination of radiotherapy and intra-CSF chemotherapy, which could be related to the poor chemosensitivity of NSCLC [190].

An agent selected for use in systemic therapy should be active against the primary cancer. The choice of a systemic agent should be based on its activity profile against potential secondary (acquired) resistance, and upon its capacity to achieve effective intra-CSF concentrations. The later property is related to its chemical properties, e.g., lipophilicity, low protein-binding, low molecular weight, and ionization.

Temozolomide, an alkylating chemotherapy that crosses the BBB, has been evaluated in a phase II trial in first-line therapy of LM secondary to BC and NSCLC [203]. Temozolomide was given according to a 1 week on/1 week off schedule in 19 patients. Only three patients had clinical benefit, median survival was 43 days, and median time to progression was 28 days. These disappointing results likely reflect the absence of clinical efficacy of temozolomide in breast and lung cancer.

High-Dose Methotrexate

High-dose IV methotrexate (HD-MTX) with leucovorin rescue is an alternative to intra-CSF treatment [174]. It has been prescribed up to 8 g/m^2, and its efficacy in this indication has been evaluated in small retrospective studies [174, 176]. Cytotoxic CSF MTX levels were achieved, even with lower doses (700 mg/m^2 initially, followed by a 2800 mg/m^2 23-h continuous infusion), but cytological clearing of malignant cells was variable according to the differing MTX schedules (80% vs. 0% in the "8 g/m^2" vs. "lower dose" regimens, respectively).

High-Dose Cytarabine

Therapeutic CSF levels can be achieved by administering ara-C 3 g/m^2 every 12 h or by continuous infusion >4 g/m^2/72 h [204–207]. However, these schedules are associated with significant systemic toxicity and have not proven beneficial in the treatment of LM from solid tumors.

New Therapeutic Approaches

Investigational Intra-CSF Therapies

Many agents have been assessed in the intra-CSF setting, such as diaziquone (AZQ), mafosfamide, nimustine hydrochloride (ACNU), 4-hydroperoxycyclophosphamide (4-HC), 6-mercaptopurine (6-MP), dacarbazine, and gemcitabine [178, 208–216]. No clear signal of activity was observed with these agents and further development of these drugs in LM has ceased.

Intra-CSF administration of a microcrystalline preparation of busulfan (Spartaject) has been assessed in clinical trials though again with limited clinical efficacy aside from chronic myelogenous leukemia-related LM [217, 218]. A microcrystalline formulation of temozolomide has also been evaluated for intra-CSF use in preclinical studies.

Intra-CSF Etoposide

Intra-CSF etoposide has been assessed in two feasibility studies and one phase II trial [219–221]. In the Phase II study, induction treatment consisted in 0.5 mg etoposide per day for 5 consecutive days per week every other week for 8 weeks. Among the 27 adult patients included, 26% were cytological responders with a stable or improved neurologic status at the end of induction. In responders, time to neurologic progression ranged from 8 to 40 weeks (median, 20 weeks). The 6-month neurologic disease PFS was 11%. The interpretation of these results is not straightforward, since they were obtained in different types of cancers with differing prognoses.

In a recent study, the pharmacokinetic properties of intra-CSF etoposide were determined in 42 patients. An intra-CSF dose of 0.75 mg was administered (over 1–2 min by IVent or IT administration) for 5 consecutive days for 1–3 weeks. Excellent distribution throughout the CSF compartment was achieved, irrespective of delivery route and clearance of etoposide was near complete at 24 h. The dosing regimen was shown to be relatively free of toxicity and considered safe as previously reported [222].

Intra-CSF Topotecan

Topotecan is a topoisomerase I inhibitor that displays a wide spectrum of activity. IVent administration of 1/100th of the systemic dose of topotecan can lead to a 450-fold greater CSF concentration, according to pharmacokinetic studies. A Phase I trial of IT topotecan in a pediatric population of LM patients with primary brain tumors showed 3 out of 13 responders with dose-limiting toxicity aseptic chemical meningitis [223]. A Phase II nonrandomized trial of intra-CSF topotecan in 62 adult patients used 0.4 mg of topotecan administered IVent twice weekly during 6 weeks [224]. The rate of cytological responders was 21% with a 15 week OS in the 65% of patients who completed the 6-week induction period. Arachnoiditis was again the most frequent complication (32% of patients, 5% grade 3). Topotecan displayed a good tolerance profile but its added benefit over other intra-CSF drugs remains unclear since it was evaluated in a heterogeneous population.

Biological Agents

Transduction inhibitors, antiangiogenic agents (angiostatin) or drugs targeting vascular cell adhesion molecules are currently being evaluated [225–229]. Intra-CSF IL-2 has been assessed in melanoma patients with LM [230–232]. As previously reported with systemic treatment, some patients maintain a long duration of response but side effects of treatment are not negligible.

In a phase II study of 22 patients with LM from various solid tumor cancers, intra-CSF alpha interferon showed modest activity (median duration of response: 16 weeks, range 8–40), with transient chemical arachnoiditis and chronic fatigue in the majority of patients [233].

A phase I trial assessed the safety profile of either subcutaneous or IT administered CpG-28, a TRL-9 agonist, in LM patients LM with solid tumors including primary CNS tumors [234]. TLR-9 agonists are immunostimulating agents that have displayed antitumoral activity in preclinical studies. CpG-28 treatment was administered weekly for 5 weeks

in 29 patients, with safety the primary endpoint. The tolerance profile was good at doses up to 0.3 mg/kg subcutaneously and 18 mg intrathecally. Treatment-related adverse events were low-grade lymphopenia, anemia and neutropenia, local erythema at injection sites, fever, and seizures. Serious adverse events consisted of confusion episodes, infections of ventricular devices, grade 4 thrombocytopenia, and neutropenia. The median PFS was 7 weeks and median OS was 15 weeks.

Monoclonal Antibodies

When administered systemically in LM patients, biological response modifiers such as trastuzumab (humanized monoclonal antibody targeting HER2/neu) and SU5416 (inhibitor of the tyrosine kinase activity of the VEGF receptor) penetrate poorly into the CSF [235–237].

A few long-term clinical responses (7–26 months) have been achieved in clinical trials that enrolled LM patients with primary solid tumors (melanoma, ovarian, and breast primaries) to assess the efficacy of intra-CSF injection of I [131] combined to monoclonal antibodies against tumor antigens [227, 238–242]. The creation of specific monoclonal antibodies directed against an individual tumor, the difficulty to reach distant cancer cells from the tumor cell/monoclonal antibody complex, and the potential systemic complications of the released radiolabeled compound exemplify the potential pitfalls of this approach.

Intra-CSF immunotoxins, coupled to monoclonal antibodies or biological ligands, such as epidermal growth factor or transferrin, have been evaluated in preclinical studies and in a pilot study of eight patients [243–247]. In four patients, the CSF cancer cells were reduced by 50%, but progression was observed in seven of eight patients. Toxicity was transient and manageable with steroids and CSF drainage.

LM is relatively infrequent (3–5% incidence) in the HER2/neu positive BC patients as compared with parenchymal BM (approximately 30% incidence) [27, 38, 248]. There is concordance regarding the tumor HER 2/neu status between the primary cancer and CSF CTC, unlike what has been demonstrated in parenchymal brain metastasis [249]. Trastuzumab CSF/serum ratios have been reported prior to and after WBRT completion and vary from 0.0023 to 0.013 mg/dL and up to 0.02 mg/dL in patients with LM [155, 250, 251]. These pharmacological studies suggest very limited entrance of trastuzumab into the CNS regardless of the presence or absence of CNS metastasis or application of WBRT.

In a toxicology study, intra-CSF trastuzumab was administered to monkeys, and CSF concentrations exceeded those reported after systemic administration [252]. Intra-CSF trastuzumab has been administered at varying doses

(5–100 mg) with clinical and cytological success reported in case studies of patients with LM and HER-2/neu positive breast cancer [236, 251–262]. Additionally, occasional prolonged survival has been reported (>72 months). Intra-CSF trastuzumab has also been given in combination with intra-CSF MTX with encouraging preliminary results [259, 263, 264]. Intra-CSF trastuzumab has also been administered with intra-CSF thiotepa after progression following single agent intra-CSF trastuzumab [265]. This drug combination was chosen based on previous preclinical studies that showed a significant synergism between these two agents [266]. A clinical benefit was seen in this case report. A systematic literature review (17 patients in 13 articles) concluded that IT trastuzumab appears unassociated with severe adverse event (SAE) in most cases [267]. Clinical improvement was observed in 68.8% of patients as reflected by a cytological response rate of 66.7%. The median OS was 13.5 months and the median CNS-PFS was 7.5 months.

A longer CNS-PFS was observed in clinical and CSF responders. These data are promising but the intra-CSF use of trastuzumab cannot be considered standard yet, as confirmatory studies are needed in order to determine dose, interval, maintenance duration, and combination drugs. Efforts to develop intra-CSF use of trastuzumab in HER-2 positive BC and LM are ongoing with two Phase I/II studies, one in France and the other in US (NCT01325207 (US) Phase I/II Dose Escalation Trial to Assess Safety of Intrathecal Trastuzumab for the Treatment of Leptomeningeal Metastases in HER2 Positive Breast Cancer and NCT01373710 (France) Phase 1–2 Study (HIT) of Safety and Efficacy of Intrathecal Trastuzumab Administration in Metastatic HER2 Positive Breast Cancer Patients Developing Carcinomatous Meningitis). The final results of the phase I component of the French phase I/II study have been reported recently [268]. IT trastuzumab was administered once weekly for 8 consecutive weeks in a dose escalation study (dose range 30–150 mg) in 19 patients [268]. The primary endpoint was to determine the maximum tolerated dose and to achieve a trastuzumab target concentration in CSF similar to that known to be effective in plasma (30 µg/mL). The maximum tolerated dose was not reached and the safety profile was excellent without high-grade toxicity. The CSF trastuzumab target concentration was reached at dose level 4 (150 mg) and was recommended as the Phase II dose to be administered weekly. The primary endpoint of the study will be neurological progression-free survival at 2 months [12–40].

Bevacizumab is a monoclonal antibody targeting the VEGF ligand. Bevacizumab can be used safely without an increase of bleeding in parenchymal CNS metastases that are otherwise small in volume and asymptomatic, according to

retrospective analyses [269]. LM patients have shown significantly elevated CSF levels and CSF/serum indices of VEGF in several studies, suggesting a contributory role of angiogenesis in LM. Survival was also inversely correlated to the level of VEGF [70, 270, 271]. Prospective trials in LM are ongoing to assess efficacy of intra-CSF bevacizumab. In a pilot study of 15 patients with LM, CSF VEGF levels were significantly decreased over time with bevacizumab treatment. Clinical, radiological, and cytological responses or stable disease were obtained in 54–73% of patients [272].

Investigational Systemic Treatment

Breast Cancer
Capecitabine

A small number of BC patients with LM benefited from capecitabine, an oral prodrug of 5-fluorouracil, with long-lasting responses and stabilizations; however, the role of capecitabine in BC-related LM is uncertain given the paucity of patients reported to date [273–277].

Hormonal Treatment

Tamoxifen, letrozole, anastrozole, and megestrol have occasionally benefited BC patients with LM, but these reports are usually comprised of very small numbers of patients and consequently the interpretation of the data remains speculative [278–280].

Non-Small Cell Lung Cancer
Chemotherapy

Previous reports suggesting systemic chemotherapy improves survival in patients with LM have primarily been in patients with chemoresponsive cancers such as BC or hematologic malignancies. There are recent reports of a similar benefit with administration of systemic chemotherapy in patients with NSCLC and LM [89, 120]. In a series of 22 patients (44%) with NSCLC and LM, systemic chemotherapy (cytotoxic chemotherapy or EGFR inhibitor) combined with intra-CSF chemotherapy showed improved survival relative to patients treated without systemic therapy (11.5 vs. 1.4 months) [89]. Similarly, Riess reported improved survival in a series of 30 patients with LM secondary to lung adenocarcinoma treated with combined systemic and CNS-directed therapy [120].

Targeted Therapies/Epidermal Growth Factor Inhibitors

The epidermal growth factor receptor (EGFR) tyrosine kinase inhibitors (TKI) erlotinib and gefitinib are particularly effective in NSCLC patients with adenocarcinoma and

Table 5.9 Neurological toxicities of intra-CSF treatments and systemic treatments using high-dose systemic methotrexate and ara-C in patients with leptomeningeal metastases

Nature	Timing	Drugs	Clinical, biological and MR findings	Pathological findings	Treatment and course
Myelopathy	48 h to months after treatment	MTX, AraC, L-AraC Thiotepa	Myelopathy CSF: ↑protein MR: spinal cord swelling, ↑T2WI signal	demyelination	Poor prognosis with persistent paraparesis (60%)
Aseptic meningitis	Hours after treatment	Any IT agent	Mimics bacterial meningitis CSF: pleocytosis, ↑protein		Oral antipyretics, Antiemetics and steroids Reversible within 1–3 days Further treatment possible Usually totally reversible
Acute cerebellar syndrome	2–5 days after treatment	HD IV AraC (>3 g/m^2)	Encephalopathy immediately followed by cerebellar syndrome MR: cerebellar atrophy, reversible and diffuse leukoencephalopathy	Diffuse loss of Purkinje cells ± WM demyelination	Further treatment possible Recovery after treatment discontinuation, But may be permanent
Acute encephalopathy	24–48 h after treatment	IT MTX IT AraC, IV HD MTX	Seizures, confusion, disorientation and lethargy		
Acute/subacute encephalopathy	48–72 h/5–6 days after treatment	IT MTX HD IV MTX	Stroke-like syndrome Normal CSF and Restricted diffusion on MR		Folinic acid/steroids, Reversible within 48–72 h, MR normalization may take up to 4 weeks
Posterior reversible encephalopathy syndrome	Within 48–72 h	IT MTX	Headache, change in mental status and seizures. MR: reversible cortical and subcortical changes consisting of high-intensity lesions on T2-WI and FLAIR sequences with postGd↑, ↓signal intensity on diffusion-WI and ↑apparent diffusion coefficient	Not fully understood, vasogenic edema in areas of the brain supplied by the posterior circulation	Total resolution within days following causal agent withdrawal
Delayed leucoencephalopathy	Months to years after treatment	High risk if cumulative dose IT MTX > 140 mg Typically combined RT + HD IV/IT CT	Subcortical-frontal syndrome Mutism-akinetism CSF: ↑protein MR: cortical atrophy, diffuse WM ↑T2WI and FLAIR signal, ventricular dilatation	Disseminated foci of demyelination, axonal loss Necrotizing lesions	No treatment Not reversible

(continued)

Table 5.9 (continued)

Nature	Timing	Drugs	Clinical, biological and MR findings	Pathological findings	Treatment and course
Other: seizures, radiculopathy, visual loss, communicating hydrocephalus, pseudo-tumor cerebri like syndrome, conus medullaris/cauda equine syndrome, ↓VA		Typically combined RT + HD IV/and IT MTX, or LAra-C			May recover partially or remain permanent

Data from References [187, 298–309]

CSF Cerebrospinal fluid; *CT* Chemotherapy; ↓ Decreased; ↑ Elevated; *FLAIR* Fluid attenuation inversion recovery; *Gd* Gadolinium; *H* Hours; *HD* High doses; *IT* Intrathecal

IV Intravenous; *L* Liposomal; *MR* Magnetic resonance; *MTX* Methotrexate; *RT* Radiotherapy; *T2WI* T2 weighted images; *VA* Visual acuity; *WM* White matter

Adapted from Le Rhun E, Taillibert S, Chamberlain MC. Carcinomatous meningitis: Leptomeningeal metastases in solid tumors. Surg Neurol Int. 2013; 4(Suppl 4): S265–S288. Open Access Journal

specific EGFR-activating mutations. Among all NSCLC patients, women, nonsmokers, and patients of Asian ethnicity are the most responsive. Published data have shown that patients with NSCLC-related LM and activating EGFR mutations may benefit from treatment with an EGFR-TKI at normal or higher doses [13, 39, 119, 126, 130, 281–297]. Promising results have been observed in patients with EGFR-activating mutations in NSCLC and LM, according to four recent and one large retrospective series [13, 89, 118, 119]. Xu reported a median survival of 5.5 months in a series of 108 NSCLC patients with LM [118]. Forty-two patients were treated with a EGFR-TKI, and had better survival when compared to patients who did not receive the targeted treatment (11.1 vs. 4.4 months). Lee reported a median survival of 3.5 months in a series of 149 patients with LM from NSCLC (95% adenocarcinoma) [127]. EGFR-TKIs were used in 24 patients. Compared to patients not treated with EGFRI, these patients had overall longer survival (38 weeks vs. 13 weeks). In multivariate analysis, EGFR-TKI therapy was a statistically significant factor associated with a favorable survival [118].

Whether erlotinib should be prescribed in LM at standard dose or at intermittent pulsatile high-dose is not clear [39, 281, 288–293, 297]. Some authors report a pharmacokinetic and therapeutic advantage of a high-dose intermittent pulsatile schedule with EGFR-TKIs (1000–1500 mg/week) in patients with LM [39, 281, 289, 294]. A Phase 1 study of high-dose gefitinib for patients with LM and NSCLC has recently been reported [291]. Eligible patients had known EGFR mutations and/or prior response to EGFR-TKI. Two weeks of high-dose daily gefitinib (dose levels: 750, 1000, 1250 mg) were given alternating with 2 weeks of standard dose maintenance therapy (500 mg daily). Primary endpoints were safety and toxicity. Seven patients were treated: three at the 750 mg dose level and four at the 1000 mg dose level. Toxic epidermal necrolysis was the dose-limiting toxicity at the 1000 mg dose level. The study was stopped due to slow accrual. Median neurologic progression-free survival was 2.3 months (range 1.6–4.0 months); median overall survival was 3.5 months (range 1.6–5.1 months). Despite the absence of documented radiologic response, four patients were clinically improved (not defined as to what constituted improvement) and one patient converted from positive to negative CSF cytology [291]. Long-lasting LM responses have been reported with erlotinib after prior progression on gefitinib and vice versa [89, 127, 128, 130, 291–296]. The authors conclude that in NSCLC and LM with activating mutations in EGFR, EGFR TKI may be systemic therapy option not necessitating intra-CSF chemotherapy.

Melanoma

Patients with LM from melanoma have the worst prognosis among all patients with solid tumor-related LM with a median survival of only 2.5–4 months before the era of immunotherapy and targeted therapies [14, 110]. Intra-CSF chemotherapy may postpone clinical neurologic progression, but systemic chemotherapy (for example temozolomide, DTIC, fotemustine) is usually of modest efficacy. Currently, the impact of new drugs such as anti-cytotoxic T-lymphocyte antigen (CTLA)-4 antibody, anti-PD-1 antibodies and selective BRAF inhibitors in the clinical evolution of patients with melanoma and LM is not established [148]. Nevertheless, several recently published case studies have reported prolonged survival with clinical, cytological, and radiological responses using an intensive schedule of temozolomide, ipilimumab, vemurafenib, or the combination of dabrafenib and trametinib [148, 149, 152, 157, 202, 297]. It remains difficult to evaluate the role of targeted agents, since most patients undergo multi-modality therapy [148, 149, 152, 157]. However, as in NSCLC, selected melanoma patients with LM and druggable targets may be candidates for these novel targeted therapies.

Toxicity and Complications of LM-Directed Treatment

Most published data of patients under evaluation during a treatment for LM report a iatrogenic morbidity rate of 70% (all grades of toxicity) with 15–20% severe side effects, and iatrogenic mortality rate less than 5% [174, 182, 187, 192, 198]. Neurologic side effects are classified according to their time of occurrence (acute, subacute, and delayed) and ascribed to the type of treatment (intra-CSF or systemic chemotherapy) as illustrated in Table 5.9 [187, 298–309]. It remains challenging to differentiate neurologic side effects secondary to LM-directed treatment from underlying disease progression and from other associated comorbidities. Previous or concomitant treatments (whole brain radiotherapy, intra-CSF chemotherapy, HD-MTX, or HD ara-C) appear to increase intra-CSF drug (MTX and liposomal ara-C) toxicities, independently of the route (lumbar or ventricular) of administration [187].

Conclusion

- The incidence of LM is increasing mostly due to increased overall survival in patients with cancer—a reflection of improved control of systemic disease with newly approved systemic targeted therapies that are characterized by their poor CNS penetration rate.
- The prognosis of LM remains poor as a consequence of late diagnosis and current suboptimal therapies.
- To address the challenge in diagnosis, new techniques such as flow cytometry immunophenotyping and techniques used for the detection of circulating tumor cells are currently in development and remain investigational.
- Improvement in the treatment of breast cancer, NSCLC, and melanoma in part reflects the introduction of new targeted therapies which may prove beneficial in the treatment of LM as well. Of urgent need are new clinical trials in LM driven in part by tumor specific therapies as well as molecular biomarkers that define druggable targets.
- There is an additional need for improved standardization of response assessment in LM both within and outside of clinical trials. It is hoped that the development of such guidelines will lead to standardization of clinical trials in LM.

References

1. Olson ME, Chernik NL, Posner JB. Infiltration of the leptomeninges by systemic cancer. A clinical and pathologic study. Arch Neurol. 1974;30:122–37.

2. Little JR, Dale AJ, Okazaki H. Meningeal carcinomatosis. Clinical manifestations. Arch Neurol. 1974;30:138–43.

3. Shapiro WR, Posner JB, Ushio Y, Chemik NL, Young DF. Treatment of meningeal neoplasms. Cancer Treat Rep. 1977;61:733–43.

4. Theodore WH, Gendelman S. Meningeal carcinomatosis. Arch Neurol. 1981;38:696–9.

5. Wasserstrom WR, Glass JP, Posner JB. Diagnosis and treatment of leptomeningeal metastases from solid tumors: experience with 90 patients. Cancer. 1982;49:759–72.

6. Kaplan JG, DeSouza TG, Farkash A, Shafran B, Pack D, Rehman F, Fuks J, Portenoy R. Leptomeningeal metastases: comparison of clinical features and laboratory data of solid tumors, lymphomas and leukemias. J Neurooncol. 1990;9:225–9.

7. Chamberlain MC, Corey-Bloom J. Leptomeningeal metastases: 111indium-DTPA CSF flow studies. Neurology. 1991;41(11):1765–9.

8. Posner JB, Chernik NL. Intracranial metastases from systemic cancer. Adv Neurol. 1978;19:579–92.

9. Glass JP, Melamed M, Chernik NL, et al. Malignant cells in cerebrospinal fluid (CSF): the meaning of a positive CSF cytology. Neurology. 1979;29(10):1369–75.

10. Clarke JL, Perez HR, Jacks LM, et al. Leptomeningeal metastases in the MRI era. Neurology. 2010;74:1449.

11. Lara-Medina F, Crismatt A, Villarreal-Garza C, et al. Clinical features and prognostic factors in patients with carcinomatous meningitis secondary to breast cancer. Breast J. 2012;18(3):233–41.

12. Umemura S, Tsubouchi K, Yoshioka H, et al. Clinical outcome in patients with leptomeningeal metastasis from non-small cell lung cancer: Okayama Lung Cancer Study Group. Lung Cancer. 2012;77:134.

13. Morris PG, Reiner AS, Szenberg OR, et al. Leptomeningeal metastasis from non-small cell lung cancer: survival and the impact of whole brain radiotherapy. J Thorac Oncol. 2012;7:382.

14. Raizer JJ, Hwu WJ, Panageas KS, et al. Brain and leptomeningeal metastases from cutaneous melanoma: survival outcomes based on clinical features. Neuro Oncol. 2008;10:199–207.

15. van Oostenbrugge RJ, Twijnstra A. Presenting features and value of diagnostic procedures in leptomeningeal metastases. Neurology. 1999;53(2):382–5.

16. Balm M, Hammack J. Leptomeningeal carcinomatosis. Presenting features and rognostic factors. Arch Neurol. 1996;53(7):626–32.

17. Sorensen SC, Eagan RT, Scott M. Meningeal carcinomatosis in patients with primary breast or lung cancer. Mayo Clin Proc. 1984;59(2):91–4.

18. Rosen ST, Aisner J, Makuch RW, et al. Carcinomatous leptomeningitis in small cell lung cancer: a clinicopathologic review of the National Cancer Institute experience. Medicine (Baltimore). 1982;61(1):45–53.

19. Amer MH, Al Sarraf M, Baker LH, et al. Malignant melanoma and central nervous system metastases: incidence, diagnosis, treatment and survival. Cancer. 1978;42(2):660–8.

20. Yap HY, Yap BS, Tashima CK, et al. Meningeal carcinomatosis in breast cancer. Cancer. 1978;42(1):283–6.

21. Altundag K, Bondy ML, Mirza NQ, et al. Clinicopathologic characteristics and prognostic factors in 420 metastatic breast cancer patients with central nervous system metastasis. Cancer. 2007;110:2640.

22. Gauthier H, Guilhaume MN, Bidard FC, Pierga JY, Girre V, Cottu PH, et al. Survival of breast cancer patients with meningeal carcinomatosis. Ann Oncol. 2010;21(11):2183–7.

23. Lamovec J, Zidar A. Association of leptomeningeal carcinomatosis in carcinoma of the breast with infiltrating lobular

carcinoma. An autopsy study. Arch Pathol Lab Med. 1991;115:507.

24. Lamovec J, Bracko M. Metastatic pattern of infiltrating lobular carcinoma of the breast: an autopsy study. J Surg Oncol. 1991;48:28.

25. Lin NU, Claus E, Sohl J, Razzak AR, Arnaout A, Winer EP. Sites of distant recurrence and clinical outcomes in patients with metastatic triple-negative breast cancer: high incidence of central nervous system metastases. Cancer. 2008;113(10):2638–45.

26. Le Rhun E, Taillibert S, Zairi F, Devos P, Pierret MF, Dubois F, et al. Clinicopathological features of breast cancers predict the development of leptomeningeal metastases: a case-control study. J Neurooncol. 2011;105(2):309–15.

27. Lin M, Chen ZQ, Bao Y, Li Q, Du ZG, Xu ZD, Tang F. Relationship between breast cancer molecular subtypes with clinicopathological characteristics and prognosis. Zhonghua Bing Li Xue Za Zhi. 2010;39(6):372–6.

28. Rakha EA, El-Sayed ME, Green AR, Lee AH, Robertson JF, Ellis IO. Prognostic markers in triple-negative breast cancer. Cancer. 2007;109:25–32.

29. Trifiletti DM, Romano KD, Xu Z, Reardon KA, Sheehan J. Leptomeningeal disease following stereotactic radiosurgery for brain metastases from breast cancer. J Neurooncol. 2015;124(3):421–7.

30. Atalar B, Modlin LA, Choi CY, Adler JR, Gibbs IC, Chang SD, et al. Risk of leptomeningeal disease in patients treated with stereotactic radiosurgery targeting the postoperative resection cavity for brain metastases. Int J Radiat Oncol Biol Phys. 2013; 87(4):713–8.

31. Jong-myung J, Sohee K, Jungnam J, Kyung HS, Ho-Shin G, Seung Hoon L. Incidence and risk factors for leptomeningeal carcinomatosis in breast cancer patients with parenchymal brain metastases. J Korean Neurosurg Soc. 2012;52(3):193–9.

32. DeAngelis LM, Mandell LR, Thaler HT, et al. The role of postoperative radiotherapy after resection of single brain metastases. Neurosurgery. 1989;24:798.

33. Norris LK, Grossman SA, Olivi A. Neoplastic meningitis following surgical resection of isolated cerebellar metastasis: a potentially preventable complication. J Neurooncol. 1997;32:215.

34. Sawaya R, Hammoud M, Schoppa D, Hess KR, Sz Wu, Shi WM, et al. Neurosurgical outcomes in a modern series of craniotomies for treatment of parenchymal tumors. Neurosurgery. 1998;42:1044–56.

35. Ahn JH, Lee SH, Kim S, Joo J, Yoo H, Lee SH, et al. Risk for leptomeningeal seeding after resection for brain metastases: Implication of tumor location with mode of resection. J Neurosurg. 2012;116:984–93.

36. Elliott JP, Keles GE, Waite M, et al. Ventricular entry during resection of malignant gliomas: effect on intracranial cerebrospinal fluid tumor dissemination. J Neurosurg. 1994;80:834.

37. van der Ree TC, Dippel DW, Avezaat CJ, Sillevis Smitt PA, Vecht CJ, van den Bent MJ. Leptomeningeal metastasis after surgical resection of brain metastases. J Neurol Neurosurg Psychiatry. 1990;66:225–7.

38. Bendell JC, Domchek SM, Burstein HJ, et al. Central nervous system metastases in women who receive trastuzumab-based therapy for metastatic breast carcinoma. Cancer. 2003;97:2972–7.

39. Omuro AM, Kris MG, Miller VA, et al. High incidence of disease recurrence in the brain and leptomeninges in patients with nonsmall cell lung carcinoma after response to gefitinib. Cancer. 2005;103:2344–8.

40. Groves MD. Leptomeningeal disease. Neurosurg Clin N Am. 2011;22(1):67–78, vii.

41. Lai R, Dang CT, Malkin MG, Abrey LE. The risk of central nervous system metastases after trastuzumab therapy in patients with breast carcinoma. Cancer. 2004;101:810.

42. Gonzalez-Vitale JC, Garcia-Bunuel R. Meningeal carcinomatosis. Cancer. 1976;37(6):2906–11.

43. Grossman SA, Krabak MJ. Leptomeningeal carcinomatosis. Cancer Treat Rev. 1999;25(2):103–19.

44. Chamberlain MC. Radioisotope CSF flow studies in leptomeningeal metastases. J Neuro Oncol. 1998;38(2–3):135–40.

45. Chamberlain MC. Carcinomatous meningitis. Arch Neurol. 1997;54(1):16–7.

46. Boyle R, Thomas M, Adams JH. Diffuse involvement of the leptomeninges by tumour—a clinical and pathological study of 63 cases. Postgrad Med J. 1980;56(653):149–58.

47. Soriano A, Gutgsell TL, Davis MP. Diencephalic storms from leptomeningeal metastasis and leukoencephalopathy: a rare and clinically important complication. Am J Hosp Palliat Care. 2014;31(1):98–100.

48. Chamberlain MC, Kormanik PR. Carcinomatous meningitis secondary to breast cancer: predictors of response to combined modality therapy. J Neuro Oncol. 1997;35(1):55–64.

49. Chamberlain MC. Leptomeningeal metastasis. Curr Opin Oncol. 2010;22:627–35.

50. Chamberlain MC, Glantz M, Groves MD, Wilson WH. Diagnostic tools for neoplastic meningitis: detecting disease, identifying patient risk, and determining benefit of treatment. Semin Oncol. 2009;36:S35–45.

51. Chamberlain MC, Kormanik PA, Glantz MJ. A comparison between ventricular and lumbar cerebrospinal fluid cytology in adult patients with leptomeningeal metastases. Neuro-Oncology. 2001;3:42–5.

52. Glantz MJ, Cole BF, Glantz LK, Cobb J, Mills P, Lekos A, et al. Cerebrospinal fluid cytology in patients with cancer: minimizing false-negative results. Cancer. 1998;82:733–9.

53. Dux R, Kindler-Röhrborn A, Annas M, Faustmann P, Lennartz K, Zimmerman CW. A standardized protocol for flow cytometric analysis of cells isolated from cerebrospinal fluid. J Neurol Sci. 1994;121:74–8.

54. de Azevedo CR, Cruz MR, Chinen LT, Peres SV, Peterlevitz MA, de Azevedo Pereira AE, et al. Meningeal carcinomatosis in breast cancer: prognostic factors and outcome. J Neurooncol. 2011;104:565–72.

55. Lee S, Ahn HK, Park YH, Nam do H, Lee JI, Park W, et al. Leptomeningeal metastases from breast cancer: intrinsic subtypes may affect unique clinical manifestations. Breast Cancer Res Treat. 2011;129:809–17.

56. Rudnicka H, Niwinska A, Murawska M. Breast cancer leptomeningeal metastasis: the role of multimodality treatment. J Neurooncol. 2007;84:57–62.

57. Wang P, Piao Y, Zhang X, Li W, Hao X. The concentration of CYFRA 21-1, NSE and CEA in cerebro-spinal fluid can be useful indicators for diagnosis of meningeal carcinomatosis of lung cancer. Cancer Biomark. 2013;13(2):123–30.

58. Le Rhun E, Kramar A, Salingue S, Girot M, Rodrigues I, Mailliez A, et al. CSF CA 15-3 in breast cancer-related leptomeningeal metastases. J Neurooncol. 2014;117(1):117–24.

59. Chamberlain MC. Cytologically negative carcinomatous meningitis: usefulness of CSF biochemical markers. Neurology. 1998;50:1173–5.

60. Corsini E, Bernardi G, Gaviani P, Silvani A, de Grazia U, Ciusani E, et al. Intrathecal synthesis of tumor markers is a highly sensitive test in the diagnosis of leptomeningeal metastasis from solid cancers. Clin Chem Lab Med. 2009;47:874–9.

61. Gaucher AS, Pez E, Boutonnat J, Bourre JC, Pelleter L, Payan R, et al. Early detection of leptomeningeal metastasis in patients with metastatic breast carcinoma: validation of CA 15-3 measurement in cerebrospinal fluid. Ann Biol Clin. 2007;65:653–8.

62. Grewal J, Saria MG, Kesari S. Novel approaches to treating leptomeningeal metastases. J Neurooncol. 2012;106(2):225–34.

63. Kang SJ, Kim KS, Ha YS, Huh SY, Lee JH, Kim JK, et al. Diagnostic value of cerebrospinal fluid level of carcinoembryonic antigen in patients with leptomeningeal carcinomatous metastasis. J Clin Neurol. 2010;6:33–7.

64. Shi Q, Pu CQ, Huang XS, Tian CL, Cao XT. Optimal cut-off values for tumor markers in cerebrospinal fluid with ROC curve analysis. Front Biosci (Elite Ed). 2011;3:1259–64.

65. Shingyoji M, Kageyama H, Sakaida T, Nakajima T, Matsui Y, Itakura M, et al. Detection of epithelial growth factor receptor mutations in cerebrospinal fluid from patients with lung adenocarcinoma suspected of neoplastic meningitis. J Thorac Oncol. 2011;6:1215–20.

66. van Zanten AP, Twijnstra A, Ongerboer de Visser BW, van Heerde P, Hart AA, Nooyen WJ. Cerebrospinal fluid tumour markers in patients treated for meningeal malignancy. J Neurol Neurosurg Psychiatry. 1991;54:119–23.

67. Groves MD, Hess KR, Puduvalli VK, Colman H, Conrad CA, Gilbert MR, et al. Biomarkers of disease: cerebrospinal fluid vascular endothelial growth factor (VEGF) and stromal cell derived factor (SDF)-1 levels in patients with neoplastic meningitis (NM) due to breast cancer, lung cancer and melanoma. J Neurooncol. 2009;94:229–34.

68. Herrlinger U, Fösrschier H, Küker W, Meyermann R, Bamberg M, Dichgans J, et al. Leptomeningeal metastasis: survival and prognosis in 155 patients. J Neurol Sci. 2004;223:167–78.

69. Stockhammer G, Poewe W, Burgstaller S, Deisenhammer F, Mulgg A, Kiechl S, et al. Vascular endothelial growth factor in CSF: a biological marker for carcinomatous meningitis. Neurology. 2000;54:1670–6.

70. van de Lagerijt B, Gijtenbeek JM, de Reus HP, Sweep FC, Geurts-Moespot A, Hendricks JC, et al. CSF levels of growth factors and plasminogen activators in leptomeningeal metastases. Neurology. 2006;67:114–9.

71. Brandsma D, Voest EE, de Jager W, Bonfrer H, Algra A, Boogerd W, et al. CSF protein profiling using multiplex immuno-assay: a potential new diagnostic tool for leptomeningeal metastases. J Neurol. 2006;253:1177–84.

72. Dekker LJ, Boogerd W, Stockhammer G, Dalebout JC, Siccama I, Zheng P, et al. MALDI-TOF mass spectrometry analysis of cerebrospinal fluid tryptic peptide profiles to diagnose leptomeningeal metastases in patients with breast cancer. Mol Cell Proteomics. 2005;4:1341–9.

73. Römpp A, Dekker L, Taban I, Jenster G, Boogerd W, Bonfrer H, et al. Identification of leptomeningeal metastasis-related proteins in cerebrospinal fluid of patients with breast cancer by a combination of MALDI-TOF, MALDI-FTICR and nano LC-FTICR MS. Proteomics. 2007;7:474–81.

74. Subirá D, Simó M, Illán J, Serrano C, Castañón S, Gonzalo R, et al. Diagnostic and prognostic significance of flow cytometry immunophenotyping in patients with leptomeningeal carcinomatosis. Clin Exp Metastasis. 2015;32(4):383–91.

75. Patel AS, Allen JE, Dicker DT, Peters KL, Sheehan JM, Glantz MJ, et al. Identification and enumeration of circulating tumor cells in the cerebrospinal fluid of breast cancer patients with central nervous system metastases. Oncotarget. 2011;2(10):752–60.

76. Nayak L1, Fleisher M, Gonzalez-Espinoza R, Lin O, Panageas K, Reiner A, et al. Rare cell capture technology for the diagnosis of leptomeningeal metastasis in solid tumors. Neurology. 2013;80(17):1598–605.

77. Le Rhun E, Tu Q, De Carvalho Bittencourt M, Farre I, Mortier L, Cai H, et al. Detection and quantification of CSF malignant cells by the cellsearch technology in patients with melanoma leptomeningeal metastasis. Med Oncol. 2013;30(2):538.

78. Le Rhun E, Massin F, Tu Q, Bonneterre J, Bittencourt Mde C, Faure GC. Development of a new method for identification and quantification in cerebrospinal fluid of malignant cells from breast carcinoma leptomeningeal metastasis. BMC Clin Pathol. 2012;12:21.

79. Groves MD. New strategies in the management of leptomeningeal metastases. Arch Neurol. 2010;67:305–12.

80. Weston CL, Glantz MJ, Connor JR. Detection of cancer cells in the cerebrospinal fluid: current methods and future directions. Fluids Barriers CNS. 2011;8:14.

81. Chamberlain MC, Sandy AD, Press GA. Leptomeningeal metastasis: a comparison of gadolinium-enhanced MR and contrast-enhanced CT of the brain. Neurology. 1990;40:435–8.

82. Chamberlain MC. Neoplastic meningitis. Oncologist. 2008;13:967–77.

83. Schumacher M, Orszagh M. Imaging techniques in neoplastic meningiosis. J Neurooncol. 1998;38:111–20.

84. Sze G, Soletsky S, Bronen R, Krol G. MR Imaging of the cranial meninges with emphasis on contrast enhancement and meningeal carcinomatosis. Am J Roentgenol. 1989;153:1039–49.

85. Dietemann JL, Correia Bernardo R, Bogorin A, Abu Eid M, Koob M, Nogueira T, et al. Normal and abnormal meningeal enhancement: MRI features. J Radiol. 2005;86:1659–83.

86. Singh SK, Leeds NE, Ginsberg LE. Imaging of leptomeningeal metastases: comparison of three sequences. Am J Neuroradiol. 2002;23:817–21.

87. Mittl RL Jr, Yousem DM. Frequency of unexplained meningeal enhancement in the brain after lumbar puncture. Am J Neuroradiol. 1994;15:633–8.

88. Chamberlain MC. Neuraxis imaging in leptomeningeal metastasis: a retrospective case series. CNS tumors 2046. J Clin Oncol. 2012;30 (Abstract 2046).

89. Park JH, Kim YJ, Lee JO, Lee KW, Kim JH, Bang SM, et al. Clinical outcomes of leptomeningeal metastasis in patients with non-small cell lung cancer in the modern chemotherapy era. Lung Cancer. 2012;76:387–92.

90. Zairi F, Kotecki N, Rodrigues I, Baranzelli MC, Andre C, Dubois F, et al. Prospective follow-up of a cohort of 112 patients with leptomeningeal metastases of breast cancer recruited from 2007 to 2011: prognostics factors. J Clin Oncol. 2012;30 (General poster session, Central nervous system, abstract 2070, American Society of Clinical Oncology, Annual meeting, 2012; June, Chicago, IL).

91. Glantz MJ, Hall WA, Cole BF, et al. Diagnosis, management, and survival of patients with leptomeningeal cancer based on cerebrospinal fluid-flow status. Cancer. 1995;75(12):2919–31.

92. Chamberlain MC. Comparative spine imaging in leptomeningeal metastases. J Neuro Oncol. 1995;23(3):233–8.

93. Trump DL, Grossman SA, Thompson G, et al. CSF infections complicating the management of neoplastic meningitis. Clinical features and results of therapy. Arch Intern Med. 1982;142 (3):583–6.

94. Chamberlain MC, Kormanik PA. Prognostic significance of 111indium-DTPA CSF flow studies in leptomeningeal metastases. Neurology. 1996;46(6):1674–7.

95. Mason WP, Yeh SD, DeAngelis LM. 111Indium-diethylenetriamine pentaacetic acid cerebrospinal fluid flow studies predict distribution of intrathecally administered chemotherapy and outcome in patients with leptomeningeal metastases. Neurology. 1998;50(2):438–44.

96. Chamberlain MC, Kormanik P, Jaeckle KA, et al. 111Indium-diethylenetriamine pentaacetic acid CSF flow studies predict distribution of intrathecally administered chemotherapy and outcome in patients with leptomeningeal metastases. Neurology. 1999;52(1):216–7.

97. Chamberlain MC, Raizer J, Soffietti R, Ruda R, Brandsma D, Boogerd W, et al. Leptomeningeal Assessment in Neuro-Oncology (Lano): a rano proposed model of evaluation in leptomeningeal metastasis. Neuro-Oncology. 2013;15:105–105.

98. Cheng TM, O'Neill BP, Scheithauer BW, Piepgras DG. Chronic meningitis: the role of meningeal or cortical biopsy. Neurosurgery. 1994;34:590–595; discussion 596.

99. Pradat PF, Delattre J-Y. MeÅLningites chroniques. Encycl Med Chir (Elsevier, Paris), Neurologie. 1995;17–160-C-130, 113.

100. Siegal T, Mildworf B, Stein D, Melamed E. Leptomeningeal metastases: reduction in regional cerebral blood flow and cognitive impairment. Ann Neurol. 1985;17:100–2.

101. Aichner F, Schuler G. Primary leptomeningeal melanoma. Diagnosis by ultrastructural cytology of cerebrospinal fluid and cranial computed tomography. Cancer. 1982;50:1751–6.

102. Savitz MH, Anderson PJ. Primary melanoma of the leptomeninges: a review. Mt Sinai J Med. 1974;41:774–91.

103. Silbert SW, Smith KR Jr, Horenstein S. Primary leptomeningeal melanoma: an ultrastructural study. Cancer. 1978;41:519–27.

104. Smith MT, Armbrustmacher VW, Violett TW. Diffuse meningeal rhabdomyosarcoma. Cancer. 1981;47:2081–6.

105. Wen PY, Macdonald DR, Reardon DA, Cloughesy A, Sorensen AG, Galanis E, et al. Updated response assessment criteria for high grade gliomas: response assessment in neuro-oncology working group. J Clin Oncol. 2010;28:1963–72.

106. Chamberlain MC, Soffietti R, Raizer J, Rudà R, Brandsma D, Boogerd W, et al. Leptomeningeal metastasis: a response assessment in neuro-oncology critical review of endpoints and response criteria of published randomized clinical trials. Neuro Oncol. 2014;16(9):1176–85.

107. Brem SS, Bierman PJ, Black P, Blumenthal DT, Brem H, Chamberlain MC, et al. Central nervous system cancers: clinical practice guidelines in oncology. J Nat Compr Cancer Netw. 2005;3:644–90.

108. Chamberlain MC, Kormanik PA. Prognostic significance of coexistent bulky metastatic central nervous system disease in patients with leptomeningeal metastases. Arch Neurol. 1997;54:1364–8.

109. Clatot F, Philippin-Lauridant G, Ouvrier MJ, Nakry T, Laberge-Le-Couteulx S, Guillemet C, et al. Clinical improvement and survival in breast cancer leptomeningeal metastasis correlate with the cytologic response to intrathecal chemotherapy. J Neurooncol. 2009;95:421–6.

110. Harstad L, Hess KR, Groves MD. Prognostic factors and outcomes in patients with leptomeningeal melanomatosis. J Neurooncol. 2008;10:1010–8.

111. Jaeckle KA. Neoplastic meningitis from systemic malignancies: diagnosis, prognosis, and treatment. Semin Oncol. 2006;33:312–23.

112. Siddiqui F, Marr L, Weissman DE. Neoplastic meningitis# 135. J Palliat Med. 2009;12:88–9.

113. Waki F, Masashi A, Takashima A, Yonemori K, Nokihara H, Miyake M, et al. Prognostic factors and clinical outcomes in patients with leptomeningeal metastasis from solid tumors. J Neurooncol. 2009;93:205–12.

114. Chamberlain MC. Neoplastic meningitis: deciding who to treat. Expert Rev Neurother. 2004;4:89–96.

115. Chamberlain MC, Tsao-Wei D, Groshen S. Neoplastic meningitis-related encephalopathy: prognostic significance. Neurology. 2004;63:2159–61.

116. Taillibert S, Laigle-Donadey F, Chodkiewicz C, Sanson M, Hoang-Xuan K, Delattre JY. Leptomeningeal metastases from solid malignancy: a review. J Neurooncol. 2005;75:85–99.

117. Oechsle K, Lange-Brock V, Kruell A, Bokemeyer C, de Wit M. Prognostic factors and treatment options in patients with leptomeningeal metastases of different primary tumors: a retrospective analysis. J Cancer Res Clin Oncol. 2010;136:1729–35.

118. Lee SJ, Lee JI, Nam DH, Ahn YC, Han JH, Sun JM, et al. Leptomeningeal carcinomatosis in non-small-cell lung cancer patients: impact on survival and correlated prognostic factors. J Thorac Oncol. 2013;8(2):185–91.

119. Xu Q, Chen X, Qian D, Wang Y, Meng S, Liu H, et al. Treatment and prognostic analysis of patients with leptomeningeal metastases from non-small cell lung cancer. Thoracic Cancer. 2015;6:407–12.

120. Riess JW, Nagpal S, Iv M, Zeineh M, Gubens MA, Ramchandran K, et al. Prolonged survival of patients with non-small-cell lung cancer with leptomeningeal carcinomatosis in the modern treatment era. Clin Lung Cancer. 2014;15(3):202–6.

121. Chamberlain MC, Johnston SK, Glantz MJ. Neoplastic meningitis-related prognostic significance of the Karnofsky performance status. Arch Neurol. 2009;66:74–8.

122. Li N, Yang BY, Li JL, Zhu JQ, Zou BH, Wang YF, et al. Clinical features and prognostic factors in patients with leptomeningeal metastases. Zhonghua Zhong liu za zhi [Chin J Oncol]. 2013;35(11):867–70.

123. Palma JA, Fernandez-Torron R, Esteve-Belloch P, Fontes-Villalba A, Hernandez A, Fernandez-Hidalgo O, et al. Leptomeningeal carcinomatosis: prognostic value of clinical, cerebrospinal fluid, and neuroimaging features. Clin Neurol Neurosurg. 2013;115(1):19–25.

124. Fusco JP, Castañón E, Carranza OE, Zubiri L, Martín P, Espinós J, et al. Neurological and cytological response as potential early predictors of time-to-progression and overall survival in patients with leptomeningeal carcinomatosis treated with intrathecal liposomal cytarabine: a retrospective cohort study. J Neurooncol. 2013;115(3):429–35.

125. Niwińska A, Rudnicka H, Murawska M. Breast cancer leptomeningeal metastasis: the results of combined treatment and the comparison of methotrexate and liposomal cytarabine as intra-cerebrospinal fluid chemotherapy. Clin Breast Cancer. 2015;15(1):66–72.

126. Clarke JL, Pao W, Wu N, Miller VA, Lassman AB. High dose weekly erlotinib achieves therapeutic concentrations in CSF and is effective in leptomeningeal metastases from epidermal growth factor receptor mutant lung cancer. J Neurooncol. 2010;99:283–6.

127. Katayama T, Shimizu J, Suda K, Onozato R, Fukui T, Ito S, et al. Efficacy of erlotinib for brain and leptomeningeal metastases in patients with lung adenocarcinoma who showed initial good response to gefitinib. J Thorac Oncol. 2009;4:1415–9.

128. Masuda T, Hattori N, Hamada A, Iwamoto H, Ohshimo S, Kanehara M, et al. Erlotinib efficacy and cerebrospinal fluid concentration in patients with lung adenocarcinoma developing leptomeningeal metastases during gefitinib therapy. Cancer Chemother Pharmacol. 2011;67:1465–9.

129. Wagner M, Besse B, Balleyguier C, Soria JC. Leptomeningeal and medullary response to second-line erlotinib in lung adenocarcinoma. J Thorac Oncol. 2008;3:677–9.

130. Yi HG, Kim HJ, Kim YJ, Han SW, Oh DY, Lee SH, et al. Epidermal growth factor receptor (EGFR) tyrosine kinase inhibitors (TKIs) are effective for leptomeningeal metastasis from non-small cell lung cancer patients with sensitive EGFR mutation or other predictive factors of good response for EGFR TKI. Lung Cancer. 2009;65:80–4.

131. Chamberlain MC. Are prognostic factors for leptomeningeal metastases defined sufficiently to permit tailored treatment? J Thorac Oncol. 2013;8:e66–7.

132. Tae-Young J, Woong-Ki C, In-Jae O. The prognostic significance of surgically treated hydrocephalus in leptomeningeal metastases. Clin Neurol Neurosurg. 2014;119:80–3.

133. Chamberlain MC. Combined-modality treatment of leptomeningeal gliomatosis. Neurosurgery. 2003;52:324–9.

134. DeAngelis LM. Current diagnosis and treatment of leptomeningeal metastasis. J Neurooncol. 1998;38:245–52.

135. Zairi F, Le Rhun E, Bertrand N, Boulanger T, Taillibert S, Aboukais R, et al. Complications related to the use of an intraventricular access device for the treatment of leptomeningeal metastases from solid tumor: a single centre experience in 112 patients. J Neurooncol. 2015;124(2):317–23.

136. Lin N, Dunn IF, Glantz M, Allison DL, Jensen R, Johnson MD, et al. Benefit of ventriculoperitoneal cerebrospinal fluid shunting and intrathecal chemotherapy in neoplastic meningitis: a retrospective, case-controlled study. J Neurosurg. 2011;115:730–6.

137. Machado M, Salcman M, Kaplan RS, Montgomery E. Expanded role of the cerebrospinal fluid reservoir in neurooncology: indications, causes of revision, and complications. Neurosurgery. 1985;17:600–3.

138. Obbens EA, Leavens ME, Beal JW, Lee YY. Ommaya reservoirs in 387 cancer patients: a 15-year experience. Neurology. 1985; 35:1274–8.

139. Sundaresan N, Suite ND. Optimal use of the Ommaya reservoir in clinical oncology. Oncology (Huntingt). 1989;3:15–22.

140. Siegal T. Toxicity of treatment for neoplastic meningitis. Curr Oncol Rep. 2003;5:41–9.

141. Siegal T, Pfeffer MR, Steiner I. Antibiotic therapy for infected Ommaya reservoir systems. Neurosurgery. 1988;22:97–100.

142. Chamberlain M. Leptomeningeal metastases: a review of evaluation and treatment. J Neurooncol. 1998;37:271–84.

143. Dinndorf PA, Bleyer WA. Management of infectious complications of intraventricular reservoirs in cancer patients: low incidence and successful treatment without reservoir removal. Cancer Drug Deliv. 1987;4:105–17.

144. Chamberlain MC, Kormanik PA, Barba D. Complications associated with intraventricular chemotherapy in patients with leptomeningeal metastases. J Neurosurg. 1997;87:694–9.

145. Blasberg RG, Patlak C, Fenstermacher JD. Intrathecal chemotherapy: brain tissue profiles after ventriculocisternal perfusion. J Pharmacol Exp Ther. 1975;195:73–83.

146. Novak LJ. Radiotherapy of the central nervous system in acute leukemia. Am J Pediatr Hematol Oncol. 1989;11:87–92.

147. Chang EL, Maor MH. Standard and novel radiotherapeutic approaches to neoplastic meningitis. Curr Oncol Rep. 2003;5: 24–8.

148. Kim DW, Barcena E, Mehta UN, Rohlfs ML, Kumar AJ, Penas-Prado M, et al. Prolonged survival of a patient with metastatic leptomeningeal melanoma treated with BRAF inhibition-based therapy: a case report. BMC Cancer. 2015;15:400.

149. Lee JM, Mehta UN, Dsouza LH, Guadagnolo BA, Sanders DL, Kim KB. Long-term stabilization of leptomeningeal disease with whole-brain radiation therapy in a patient with metastatic melanoma treated with vemurafenib: a case report. Melanoma Res. 2013;23(2):175–8.

150. Schaefer N, Rasch K, Moehlenbruch M, Urbach H, Stuplich M, Blasius E, et al. Leptomeningeal melanomatosis: stabilization of disease due to radiation, temozolomide and intrathecal liposomal cytarabine. Acta Oncol. 2011;50(8):1260–2.

151. Pan Z, Yang G, Wang Y, Yuan T, Gao Y, Dong L. Leptomeningeal metastases from a primary central nervous system melanoma: a case report and literature review. World J Surg Oncol. 2014;20(12):265.

152. Bot I, Blank CU, Brandsma D. Clinical and radiological response of leptomeningeal melanoma after whole brain radiotherapy and ipilimumab. J Neurol. 2012;259(9):1976–8.

153. d'Avella D, Cicciarello R, Albiero F, Mesiti M, Gagliardi ME, Russi E, et al. Quantitative study of blood-brain barrier permeability changes after experimental whole-brain radiation. Neurosurgery. 1992;30(1):30–4.

154. Qin DX, Zheng R, Tang J, Li JX, Hu YH. Influence of radiation on the blood-brain barrier and optimum time of chemotherapy. Int J Radiat Oncol Biol Phys. 1990;19(6):1507–10.

155. Stemmler HJ, Schmitt M, Willems A, Bernhard H, Harbeck N, Heinemann V. Ratio of trastuzumab levels in serum and cerebrospinal fluid is altered in HER2-positive breast cancer patients with brain metastases and impairment of blood-brain barrier. Anticancer Drugs. 2007;18(1):23–8.

156. Mittapalli RK, Vaidhyanathan S, Sane R, Elmquist WF. Impact of P-glycoprotein (ABCB1) and breast cancer resistance protein (ABCG2) on the brain distribution of a novel BRAF inhibitor: vemurafenib (PLX4032). J Pharmacol Exp Ther. 2012;342: 33–40.

157. Pape E, Desmedt E, Zairi F, Baranzelli MC, Dziwniel V, Dubois F, et al. Leptomeningeal metastasis in melanoma: a prospective clinical study of nine patients. In Vivo. 2012; 26(6):1079–86.

158. Oplack D, Bleyer WA, Horowitz M. Pharmacology of antineoplastic agents in cerebrospinal fluid. New York: Plenum Press; 1980.

159. Benjamin JC, Moss T, Moseley RP, Maxwell HB. Cerebral distribution of immunoconjugate after treatment for neoplastic meningitis using an intrathecal radiolabeled monoclonal antibody. Neurosurgery. 1989;25:253–8.

160. Burch PA, Grossman SA, Reinhard CS. Spinal cord penetration of intrathecally administered cytarabine and methotrexate: a quantitative autoradiographic study. J Natl Cancer Inst. 1988;80:1211–6.

161. Blaney S, Poplack D, Godwin K, McCully C, Murphy RF, Balis F. The effect of body position on ventricular cerebrospinal fluid methotrexate following intralumbar administration. J Clin Oncol. 1995;13:177–9.

162. Larson SM, Schall GL, Di Chiro G. The influence of previous lumbar puncture and pneumoencephalography on the incidence of unsuccessful radioisotope cisternography. J Nucl Med. 1971;12:555–7.

163. Chamberlain MC, Khatibi S, Kim JC, Howell SB, Chatelut E, Kim S. Treatment of leptomeningeal metastasis with intraventricular administration of depot cytarabine (DTC 101). A phase I study. Arch Neurol. 1993;50:261–4.

164. Kim S, Chatelut E, Kim JC, Howell SB, Cates C, Kormanik PA, et al. Extended CSF cytarabine exposure following intrathecal administration of DTC 101. J Clin Oncol. 1993;11:2186–93.

165. Shapiro WR, Young DF, Mehta BM. Methotrexate: distribution in cerebrospinal fluid after intravenous, ventricular and lumbar injections. N Engl J Med. 1975;293:161–6.

166. Hitchins RN, Bell DR, Woods RL, Levi JA. A prospective randomized trial of single-agent versus combination chemotherapy in meningeal carcinomatosis. J Clin Oncol. 1987;5:1655–62.

167. Glantz MJ, Van Horn A, Fisher R, Chamberlain MC. Route of intracerebrospinal fluid chemotherapy administration and efficacy of therapy in neoplastic meningitis. Cancer. 2010;116:1947–52.

168. Bleyer WA, Drake J, Chabner B. Neurotoxicity and elevated cerebrospinal fluid methotrexate concentration in meningeal leukemia. N Engl J Med. 1973;289:770–3.

169. Bleyer WA, Poplack DG, Simon RM. "Concentration-time" methotrexate via a subcutaneous reservoir: a less toxic regimen

for intraventricular chemotherapy of central nervous system neoplasms. Blood. 1978;51:835–42.

170. Kramer K, Cheung NK, Humm JL, Dantis E, Finn R, Yeh SJ, et al. Targeted radioimmunotherapy for leptomeningeal cancer using (131) I-3F8. Med Pediatr Oncol. 2000;35:716–8.

171. Chamberlain MC, Dirr L. Involved-field radiotherapy and intra-Ommaya methotrexate/cytarabine in patients with AIDS-related lymphomatous meningitis. J Clin Oncol. 1993;11:1978–84.

172. Petit T, Dufour P, Korganov AS, Maloisel F, Oberling F. Continuous intrathecal perfusion of methotrexate for carcinomatous meningitis with pharmacokinetic studies: two case studies. Clin Oncol. 1977;9:189–90.

173. Fizazi K, Asselain B, Vincent-Salomon A, Jouve M, Dieras V, Palangie T, et al. Meningeal carcinomatosis in patients with breast carcinoma. Clinical features, prognostic factors, and results of a high-dose intrathecal methotrexate regimen. Cancer. 1996;77:1315–23.

174. Glantz MJ, Cole BF, Recht L, Akerley W, Mills P, Saris S, et al. High-dose intravenous methotrexate for patients with non-leukemic leptomeningeal cancer: is intrathecal chemotherapy necessary? J Clin Oncol. 1998;16:1561–7.

175. Siegal T, Lossos A, Pfeffer MR. Leptomeningeal metastases: analysis of 31 patients with sustained off-therapy response following combined-modality therapy. Neurology. 1994;44:1463–9.

176. Pfeffer MR, Wygoda M, Siegal T. Leptomeningeal metastases-treatment results in 98 consecutive patients. Israel J Med Sci. 1988;24:611–8.

177. Sause WT, Crowley J, Eyre HJ, Rivkin SE, Pugh RP, Quagliana JM, et al. Whole brain irradiation and intrathecal methotrexate in the treatment of solid tumor leptomeningeal metastases: a Southwest Oncology Group study. J Neurooncol. 1988;6:107–12.

178. Adamson PC, Balis FM, Arndt CA, Holcenberg JS, Narang PK, Murphy RF, et al. Intrathecal 6-mercaptopurine: preclinical pharmacology, phase I/II trial, and pharmacokinetic study. Cancer Res. 1991;51:6079–83.

179. Zimm S, Collins JM, Miser J, Chatterji D, Poplack D. Cytosine arabinoside cerebrospinal fluid kinetics. Clin Pharmacol Ther. 1984;35:826–30.

180. Fulton DS, Levin VA, Gutin PH, Edwards MS, Seager ML, Stewart J, et al. Intrathecal cytosine arabinoside for the treatment of meningeal metastases from malignant brain tumors and systemic tumors. Cancer Chemother Pharmacol. 1982;8:285–91.

181. Esteva FJ, Soh LT, Holmes FA, Plunket W, Meyers CA, Forman AD, et al. Phase II trial and pharmacokinetic evaluation of cytosine arabinoside for leptomeningeal metastases from breast cancer. Cancer Chemother Pharmacol. 2000;46:382–6.

182. Glantz MJ, Jaeckle KA, Chamberlain MC, Phuphanich S, Recht L, Swinnen LJ, et al. A randomized controlled trial comparing intrathecal sustained-release cytarabine (DepoCyt) to intrathecal methotrexate in patients with neoplastic meningitis from solid tumors. Clin Cancer Res. 1999;5:3394–402.

183. Cole BF, Glantz MJ, Jaeckle KA, Chamberlain MC, Mackowiak JI. Quality-of-life-adjusted survival comparison of sustained-release cytosine arabinoside versus intrathecal methotrexate for treatment of solid tumor neoplastic meningitis. Cancer. 2003;97:3053–60.

184. Jaeckle KA, Phuphanich S, Bent MJ, Aiken R, Batchelor T, Campbell T, et al. Intrathecal treatment of neoplastic meningitis due to breast cancer with a slow-release formulation of cytarabine. Br J Cancer. 2001;84:157–63.

185. Le Rhun E, Taillibert S, Zairi F, Kotecki N, Devos P, Mailliez A, et al. A retrospective case series of 103 consecutive patients with leptomeningeal metastasis and breast cancer. J Neurooncol. 2013;113(1):83–92.

186. Jahn F, Jordan K, Behlendorf T, Globig C, Schmoll HJ, Müller-Tidow C, et al. Safety and efficacy of liposomal cytarabine in the treatment of neoplastic meningitis. Oncology. 2015;89(3):137–42.

187. Chamberlain MC. Neurotoxicity of intra-CSF liposomal cytarabine (DepoCyt) administered for the treatment of leptomeningeal metastases: a retrospective case series. J Neuro-Oncol. 2012;109:143–8.

188. Grossman SA, Finkelstein DM, Ruckdeschel JC, Trump DL, Moynihan T, Ettinger DS. Randomized prospective comparison of intraventricular methotrexate and thiotepa in patients with previously untreated neoplastic meningitis, Eastern Cooperative Oncology Group. J Clin Oncol. 1993;11:561–9.

189. Le Rhun E, Taillibert S, Devos P, Zairi F, Turpin A, Rodrigues I, et al. Salvage intracerebrospinal fluid thiotepa in breast cancer-related leptomeningeal metastases: a retrospective case series. Anticancer Drugs. 2013;24(10):1093–7.

190. Chamberlain MC, Kormanik P. Carcinomatous meningitis secondary to nonsmall cell lung cancer: combined modality therapy. Arch Neurol. 1998;55:506–12.

191. Kim DY, Lee KW, Yun T, Park SR, Jung JY, Kim DW, et al. Comparison of intrathecal chemotherapy for leptomeningeal carcinomatosis of a solid tumor: methotrexate alone versus methotrexate in combination with cytosine arabinoside and hydrocortisone. Jpn J Clin Oncol. 2003;33:608–12.

192. Scott BJ, van Vugt VA, Rush T, Brown T, Chen CC, Carter BS, et al. Concurrent intrathecal methotrexate and liposomal cytarabine for leptomeningeal metastasis from solid tumors: a retrospective cohort study. J Neurooncol. 2014;119(2):361–8.

193. Boogerd W, van den Bent MJ, Koehler PJ, Heimans JJ, van der Sande JJ, Aaronson NK, et al. The relevance of intraventricular chemotherapy for leptomeningeal metastasis in breast cancer: a randomised study. Eur J Cancer. 2004;40:2726–33.

194. Mellett LB. Physicochemical considerations and pharmacokinetic behavior in delivery of drugs to the central nervous system. Cancer Treat Rep. 1977;61:527–31.

195. Grant R, Naylor B, Greenberg HS, Junck L. Clinical outcome in aggressively treated meningeal carcinomatosis. Arch Neurol. 1994;51:457–61.

196. Boogerd W, Hart AA, van der Sande JJ, Engelsman E. Meningeal carcinomatosis in breast cancer. Prognostic factors and influence of treatment. Cancer. 1991;67:1685–95.

197. Bokstein F, Lossos A, Siegal T. Leptomeningeal metastases in solid tumors: exclusion of intra-CSF chemotherapy does not affect treatment outcome. Comparison of two prospective series. Neurology. 1997;48:A35.

198. Bokstein F, Lossos A, Siegal T. Leptomeningeal metastases from solid tumors: a comparison of two prospective series treated with and without intra-cerebrospinal fluid chemotherapy. Cancer. 1998;82:1756–63.

199. Siegal T. Leptomeningeal metastases: rationale for systemic chemotherapy or what is the role of intra-CSF-chemotherapy? J Neurooncol. 1998;38:151–7.

200. Le Rhun E, Taillibert S, Zairi F, Boulanger 2, Farre I, Deligny N, et al. Prolonged response with bevacizumab + Navelbine as third line of treatment of breast cancer leptomeningeal metastases: a case report. Case Rep Oncol. 2015;8(1):72–7.

201. Vincent A, Lesser G, Brown D, Vern-Gross T, Metheny-Barlow L, Lawrence J, et al. Prolonged regression of metastatic leptomeningeal breast cancer that has failed conventional therapy: a case report and review of the literature. J Breast Cancer. 2013;16(1):122–6.

202. Hottinger AF, Favet L, Pache JC, Martin JB, Dietrich PY. Delayed but complete response following oral temozolomide treatment in melanoma leptomeningeal carcinomatosis. Case Rep Oncol. 2011;4(1):211–5.

203. Segura PP, Gil M, Balana C, Chacon I, Langa JM, Martin M, et al. Phase II trial of temozolomide for leptomeningeal metastases in patients with solid tumors. J Neurooncol. 2012;109:137–42.

204. Morra E, Lazzarino M, Brusamolino E, Pagnucco G, Castagnola C, Bernasconi P, et al. The role of systemic high-dose cytarabine in the treatment of central nervous system leukemia. Clinical results in 46 patients. Cancer. 1993;72:439–45.

205. Slevin ML, Piall EM, Aherne GW, Harvey VJ, Johnston A, Lister TA. Effect of dose and schedule on pharmacokinetics of high-dose cytosine arabinoside in plasma and cerebrospinal fluid. J Clin Oncol. 1983;1:546–51.

206. Donehower R, Karp J, Burke P. Pharmacology and toxicity of high-dose cytarabine by 72-hour continuous infusion. Cancer Treat Rep. 1986;70:1059–65.

207. Frick J, Ritch PS, Hansen RM, Anderson T. Successful treatment of meningeal leukemia using systemic high-dose cytosine arabinoside. J Clin Oncol. 1984;2:365–8.

208. Berg SL, Balis FM, Zimm S, Murphy RF, Holcenberg J, Sato J, et al. Phase I/II trial and pharmacokinetics of intrathecal diaziquone in refractory meningeal malignancies. J Clin Oncol. 1992;10:143–8.

209. Blaney S, Balis F, Murphy RF, Arndt CA, Gillepsie A, Poplack DG. A phase I study of intrathecal mafosfamide (MF) in patients with refractory meningeal malignancies, Abstract 274. Am Soc Clin Oncol. 1992;11:113.

210. Levin VA, Chamberlain M, Silver P, Rodriguez L, Prados M. Phase I/II study of intraventricular and intrathecal ACNU for leptomeningeal neoplasia. Cancer Chemother Pharmacol. 1989;23:301–7.

211. Champagne MA, Silver HK. Intrathecal dacarbazine treatment of leptomeningeal malignant melanoma. J Natl Cancer Inst. 1992;84:1203–4.

212. Chen YM, Chen MC, Tsai CM, Perng RP. Intrathecal gemcitabine chemotherapy for non-small cell lung cancer patients with meningeal carcinomatosis: a case report. Lung Cancer. 2003;40:99–101.

213. Balis FM, Poplack DG. Central nervous system pharmacology of antileukemic drugs. Am J Pediatr Hematol Oncol. 1989;11:74–86.

214. List J, Moser RP, Steuer M, Loudon WG, Blacklock JB, Grimm EA. Cytokine responses to intraventricular injection of interleu-kin 2 into patients with leptomeningeal carcinomatosis: rapid induction of tumor necrosis factor alpha, interleukin 1 beta, interleukin 6, gamma-interferon, and soluble interleukin 2 receptor (Mr 55,000 protein). Cancer Res. 1992;52:1123–8.

215. Strong JM, Collins JM, Lester C, Poplack DG. Pharmacokinetics of intraventricular and intravenous N, N', N'-triethylenethi-ophosphoramide (thiotepa) in rhesus monkeys and humans. Cancer Res. 1986;46:6101–4.

216. Witham TF, Fukui MB, Meltzer CC, Burns R, Kondziolka D, Bozik ME. Survival of patients with high grade glioma treated with intrathecal thiotriethylenephosphoramide for ependymal or leptomeningeal gliomatosis. Cancer. 1999;86:1347–53.

217. Cokgor I, Friedman AH, Friedman HS. Current options for the treatment of neoplastic meningitis. J Neurooncol. 2002;60:79–88.

218. Gururangan S, Petros WP, Poussaint TY, Hancock ML, Philips PC, Friedman HS, et al. Phase I trial of intrathecal spartaject busulfan in children with neoplastic meningitis: a Pediatric Brain Tumor Consortium Study (PBTC-004). Clin Cancer Res. 2006;12:1540–6.

219. Chamberlain MC, Tsao-Wei DD, Groshen S. Phase II trial of intracerebrospinal fluid etoposide in the treatment of neoplastic meningitis. Cancer. 2006;106:2021–7.

220. Fleischhack G, Reif S, Hasan C, Jaehde U, Hettmer S, Bode U. Feasibility of intraventricular administration of etoposide in patients with metastatic brain tumours. Br J Cancer. 2001;84:1453–9.

221. Slavc I, Schuller E, Falger J, Günes M, Pillwein K, Czech T, et al. Feasibility of long-term intraventricular therapy with mafosfamide ($n = 26$) and etoposide ($n = 11$): experience in 26 children with disseminated malignant brain tumors. J Neurooncol. 2003;64:239–47.

222. Meijer L, Veal G, Walker D, Grundy R. Etoposide pharmacokinetics following intra-cerebrospinal fluid administration in patients with leptomeningeal metastases Neuro Oncol. 2014;16 (Suppl 6):vi20–1.

223. Blaney SM, Heideman R, Berg S, Adamson P, Gillespie A, Geyer JR, et al. Phase I clinical trial of intrathecal topotecan in patients with neoplastic meningitis. J Clin Oncol. 2003;21:143–7.

224. Groves MD, Glantz MJ, Chamberlain MC. A multicenter phase II trial of intrathecal topotecan in patients with meningeal malignancies. Neuro Oncol. 2008;10:1010–8.

225. Archer GE, Sampson JH, Lorimer IA, McLendon RE, Kuan CT, Friedman AH, et al. Regional treatment of epidermal growth factor receptor VIII—expressing neoplastic meningitis with a single-chain immunotoxin, MR-I. Clin Cancer Res. 1999;5:2646–52.

226. Bigner DD, Archer GE, McLendon RE, Friedman HS, Fuchs HE, Pai LH, et al. Efficacy of compartmental administration of immunotoxin LMB-1 (B3-LysPE38) in a rat model of carcinomatous meningitis. Clin Cancer Res. 1995;1:1545–55.

227. Brown MT, Coleman RE, Friedman AH, Friedman HS, McLendon Reiman R, et al. Intrathecal 131 I-labeled antitenascin monoclonal antibody 81C6 treatment of patients with leptomeningeal neoplasms or primary brain tumor resection cavities with subarachnoid communication: phase I trial results. Clin Cancer Res. 1996;2:963–72.

228. Cokgor I, Akabani G, Friedman HS, Friedman AH, Zatusky MR, Zehngebot LM, et al. Long term response in a patient with neoplastic meningitis secondary to melnoma treated with (131) I-radiolabeled ant chondroitin proteoglycan sulfate Mel-14 F(ab′) (2): a case study. Cancer. 2001;91:1809–13.

229. Reijneveld JC, Taphoorn MJ, Kerckhaert OA, Drixler TA, Boogerd W, Voest EE. Angiostatin prolongs the survival of mice with leptomeningeal metastases. Eur J Clin Invest. 2003;33: 76–81.

230. Herrlinger U, Weller M, Schabet M. New aspects of immunotherapy of leptomeningeal metastasis. J Neurooncol. 1998;38:233–9.

231. Mitchell MS. Relapse in the central nervous system in melanoma patients successfully treated with biomodulators. J Clin Oncol. 1989;7:1701–9.

232. Samlowski WE, Park KJ, Galinsky RE, Ward JH, Schumann GB. Intrathecal administration of interleukin-2 for meningeal carcinomatosis due to malignant melanoma: sequential evaluation of intracranial pressure, cerebrospinal fluid cytology, and cytokine induction. J Immunother Emphasis Tumor Immunol. 1993;13:49–54.

233. Chamberlain MC. A phase II trial of intra-cerebrospinal fluid alpha interferon in the treatment of neoplastic meningitis. Cancer. 2002;94:2675–80.

234. Ursu R, Taillibert S, Banissi C, Vicaut E, Bailon O, Le Rhun E, et al. Immunotherapy with CpG-ODN in neoplastic meningitis: a phase I trial. Cancer Sci. 2015;106(9):1212–8.

235. Laufman LR, Forsthoefel KF. Use of intrathecal trastuzumab in a patient with carcinomatous meningitis. Clin Breast Cancer. 2001;2:235.
236. Renbarger J, Aleksic A, McGuffey L, Dauser R, Berg S, Blaney S. Plasma and cerebrospinal fluid pharmacokinetics of SU5416 after intravenous administration in nonhuman primates. Cancer Chemother Pharmacol. 2004;53:39–42.
237. Robins HI, Liu G, Hayes L, Mehta M. Trastuzumab for breast cancer-related carcinomatous meningitis. Clin Breast Cancer. 2002;2:316.
238. Coakham HB, Kemshead JT. Treatment of neoplastic meningitis by targeted radiation using (131) I-radiolabelled monoclonal antibodies, results of responses and long term follow-up in 40 patients. J Neurooncol. 1998;38:225–32.
239. Hisanaga M, Kawai S, Maekawa M, Hattori Y, Kotoh K. Neoplastic aneurysms due to cerebral metastasis of choriocarcinoma. Report of two cases. Neurol Med Chir (Tokyo). 1988;28:398–403.
240. Kemshead JT, Papanastassiou V, Coakham HB, Pizer BL. Monoclonal antibodies in the treatment of central nervous system malignancies. Eur J Cancer. 1992;28:511–3.
241. Lashfford LS, Davies AG, Richardson RB, Bourne SP, Bullimore JA, Eckert H, et al. A pilot study of 131I monoclonal antibodies in the therapy of leptomeningeal tumors. Cancer. 1988;61:857–68.
242. Moseley RP, Benjamin JC, Ashpole RD, Sullivan NM, Bullimore JA, Coakham HB, et al. Carcinomatous meningitis: antibody-guided therapy with I-131 HMFG1. J Neurol Neurosurg Psychiatry. 1991;54:260–5.
243. Hall WA, Fodstad O. Immunotoxins and central nervous system neoplasia. J Neurosurg. 1992;76:1–12.
244. Johnson VG, Wrobel C, Wilson D, Zovickian J, Greenfield L, Oldfield EH, et al. Improved tumor-specific immunotoxins in the treatment of CNS and leptomeningeal neoplasia. J Neurosurg. 1989;70:240–8.
245. Myklebust AT, Godal A, Fodstad O. Targeted therapy with immunotoxins in a nude rat model for leptomeningeal growth of human small cell lung cancer. Cancer Res. 1994;54:2146–50.
246. Youle RJ. Immunotoxins for central nervous system malignancy. Semin Cancer Biol. 1996;7:65–70.
247. Zovickian J, Youle RJ. Efficacy of intrathecal immunotoxin therapy in an animal model of leptomeningeal neoplasia. J Neurosurg. 1988;68:767–74.
248. Nam BH, Kim SY, Han HS, Kwon Y, Lee KS, Kim TH, et al. Breast cancer subtypes and survival in patients with brain metastases. Breast Cancer Res. 2008;10:R20.
249. Park IH, Kwon Y, Ro JY, Lee KS, Ro J. Concordant HER2 status between metastatic breast cancer cells in CSF and primary breast cancer tissue. Breast Cancer Res Treat. 2010;123:125–8.
250. Pestalozzi BC, Brignoli S. Trastuzumab in CSF. J Clin Oncol. 2000;18:2349–51.
251. Stemmler HJ, Schmitt M, Harbeck N, Willems A, Bernhard H, Lässig D, et al. Application of intrathecal trastuzumab (Herceptin) for treatment of meningeal carcinomatosis in HER2-overexpressing metastatic breast cancer. Oncol Rep. 2006;15:1373–7.
252. Braen AP, Perron J, Tellier P, Catala AR, Kolaitis G, Geng W. A 4-week intrathecal toxicity and pharmacokinetic study with trastuzumab in cynomolgus monkeys. Int J Toxicol. 2010;29: 259–67.
253. Hofer S, Mengele K, Stemmler HJ, Schmitt M, Pestalozzi B. Intrathecal trastuzumab: dose matters. Acta Oncol. 2012;51: 955–6.
254. Mir O, Ropert S, Alexandre J, Lemare F, Goldwasser F. High-dose intrathecal trastuzumab for leptomeningeal metastases

255. Oliveira M, Braga S, Passos-Coelho JL, Fonseca R, Oliveira J. Complete response in HER2 + leptomeningeal carcinomatosis from breast cancer with intrathecal trastuzumab. Breast Cancer Res Treat. 2011;127:841–4.
256. Platini C, Long J, Walter S. Meningeal carcinomatosis from breast cancer treated with intrathecal trastuzumab. Lancet Oncol. 2006;7:778–80.
257. Stemmler HJ, Mengele K, Schmitt M, Harbeck N, Laessig D, Hermann KA, et al. Intrathecal trastuzumab (Herceptin) and methotrexate for meningeal carcinomatosis in HER-2 overexpressing metastatic breast cancer: a case report. Anticancer Drugs. 2008;19:832–6.
258. Dumitrescu C, Lossignol D. Intrathecal trastuzumab treatment of the neoplastic meningitis due to breast cancer: a case report and review of the literature. Case Rep Oncol Med. 2013;154:674.
259. Park WY, Kim HJ, Kim K, Bae SB, Lee N, Lee KT, et al. Intrathecal trastuzumab treatment in patients with breast cancer and leptomeningeal carcinomatosis. Cancer Res Treat. 2016; 48(2):843–7.
260. Colozza M, Minenza E, Gori S, Fenocchio D, Paolucci C, Aristei C, et al. Extended survival of a HER-2-positive metastatic breast cancer patient with brain metastases also treated with intrathecal trastuzumab. Cancer Chemother Pharmacol. 2009;63 (6):1157–9.
261. Bousquet G, Darrouzain F, de Bazelaire C, Ternant D, Barranger E, Winterman S, et al. Intrathecal trastuzumab halts progression of CNS metastases in breast cancer. J Clin Oncol. 2016;34(16):e151–5.
262. Brandt DS. Intrathecal trastuzumab: 46 months and no progression. Commun Oncol. 2012;9:232–4.
263. Martens J, Venuturumilli P, Corbets L, Bestul D. Rapid clinical and radiographic improvement after intrathecal trastuzumab and methotrexate in a patient with HER-2 positive leptomeningeal metastases. Acta Oncol. 2013;52(1):175–8.
264. Mego M, Sycova-Mila Z, Obertova J, Rajec J, Liskova S, Palacka P, et al. Intrathecal administration of trastuzumab with cytarabine and methotrexate in breast cancer patients with leptomeningeal carcinomatosis. Breast. 2011;20:478–80.
265. Ferrario C, Davidson A, Bouganim N, Aloyz R, Panasci LC. Intrathecal trastuzumab and thiotepa for leptomeningeal spread of breast cancer. Ann Oncol. 2009;20:792–5.
266. Pegram M, Hsu S, Lewis G, Pietras R, Beryt M, Sliwkowski M, et al. Inhibitory effects of combinations of HER-2/neu antibody and chemotherapeutic agents used for treatment of human breast cancers. Oncogene. 1999;18:2241–51.
267. Zagouri F, Sergentanis TN, Bartsch R, Berghoff AS, Chrysikos D, de Azambuja E, et al. Intrathecal administration of trastuzumab for the treatment of meningeal carcinomatosis in HER2-positive metastatic breast cancer: a systematic review and pooled analysis. Breast Cancer Res Treat. 2013;139(1):13–22.
268. Gutierrez M, Mouret-Foutme E, Le Rhun E, tredan O, Dieras V, Tresca P, et al. Final results of the phase I "HIT" study: a multicenter phase I-II study evaluating trastuzumab administered by intrathecal injection for leptomeningeal meningitis of HER2 + metastatic breast cancer (MBC). SABCS. 2014;P5-19-17.
269. Besse B, Lasserre SF, Compton P, Huang J, Augustus S, Rohr UP. Bevacizumab safety in patients with central nervous system metastases. Clin Cancer Res. 2010;16:269–78.
270. Groves MD. CSF levels of angiogenesis-related proteins in patients with leptomeningeal metastases. Neurology. 2006;66:1609–10.
271. Reijneveld JC, Brandsma D, Boogerd W, Bonfrer JG, Kalmijn S, Voest EE, et al. CSF levels of angiogenesis-related proteins in

secondary to HER-2 overexpressing breast cancer. Ann Oncol. 2008;19:1978–80.

patients with leptomeningeal metastases. Neurology. 2005;65: 1120–2.

272. Groves MD, DeGroot J, Tremont I, Forman A, Kang S, Pei BL, et al. A pilot study of systemically administered bevacizumab with neoplastic meningitis NM: imaging, clinical, CSF and biomarker outcomes. Neuro Oncol (OT-02). 2011;13:iii85–91.

273. Ekenel M, Hormigo AM, Peak S, Deangelis LM, Abrey LE. Capecitabine therapy of central nervous system metastases from breast cancer. J Neurooncol. 2007;85:223–7.

274. Giglio P, Tremont-Lukats IW, Groves MD. Response of neoplastic meningitis from solid tumors to oral capecitabine. J Neurooncol. 2003;65:167–72.

275. Rogers LR, Remer SE, Tejwani S. Durable response of breast cancer leptomeningeal metastasis to capecitabine monotherapy. Neuro Oncol. 2004;6:63–4.

276. Shigekawa T, Takeuchi H, Misumi M, Matsuura K, Sano H, Fujiuchi N, et al. Successful treatment of leptomeningeal metastases from breast cancer using the combination of trastuzumab and capecitabine: a case report. Breast Cancer. 2009;16:88–92.

277. Tham YL, Hinckley L, Teh BS, Elledge R. Long-term clinical response in leptomeningeal metastases from breast cancer treated with capecitabine monotherapy: a case report. Clin Breast Cancer. 2006;7:164–6.

278. Boogerd W, Dorresteijn LD, van Der Sande JJ, de Gast GC, Bruning PF. Response of leptomeningeal metastases from breast cancer to hormonal therapy. Neurology. 2000;55:117–9.

279. Chamberlain MC. Response of leptomeningeal metastases from breast cancer to hormonal therapy. Neurology. 2001;56:425–6.

280. Ozdogan M, Samur M, Bozcuk HS, Sagtas E, Yildiz M, Artac M, et al. Durable remission of leptomeningeal metastasis of breast cancer with letrozole: a case report and implications of biomarkers on treatment selection. Jpn J Clin Oncol. 2003;33:229–31.

281. Hashimoto N, Imaizumi K, Honda T, Kawabe T, Nagasaka T, Shimokata K, et al. Successful re-treatment with gefitinib for carcinomatous meningitis as disease recurrence of non-small-cell lung cancer. Lung Cancer. 2006;53:387–90.

282. Jackman DM, Holmes AJ, Lindeman N, Wen PY, Kesari S, Borras AM, et al. Response and resistance in a non-small cell lung cancer patient with an epidermal growth factor receptor mutation and leptomeningeal metastases treated with high-dose gefitinib. J Clin Oncol. 2006;24:4517–20.

283. Kanaji N, Bandoh S, Nagamura N, Kushida Y, Haba R, Ishida T. Significance of an epidermal growth factor receptor mutation in cerebrospinal fluid for carcinomatous meningitis. Internal Med. 2007;46:1651–5.

284. Sakai M, Ishikawa S, Ito H, Ozawa Y, Yamamoto T, Onizuka M, et al. Carcinomatous meningitis from non-small-cell lung cancer responding to gefitinib. Int J Clin Oncol. 2006;11:243–5.

285. So T, Inoue M, Chikaishi Y, Nose N, Sugio K, Yasumoto K. Gefitinib and a ventriculo-peritoneal shunt to manage carcinomatous meningitis from non-small-cell lung cancer: report of two cases. Surg Today. 2009;39:598–602.

286. Tetsumoto S, Osa A, Kijima T, Minami T, Hirata H, Takahashi R, et al. Two cases of leptomeningeal metastases from lung adenocarcinoma which progressed during gefitinib therapy but responded to erlotinib. Int J Clin Oncol. 2012;17:155–9.

287. Dhruva N, Socinski MA. Carcinomatous meningitis in non-small-cell lung cancer: response to high-dose erlotinib. J Clin Oncol. 2009;27:e31–2.

288. Grommes C, Oxnard GR, Kris MG, Miller VA, Pao W, Holodony AI, et al. "Pulsatile" high-dose weekly erlotinib for CNS metastases from EGFR mutant non-small cell lung cancer. Neuro Oncol. 2011;13:1364–9.

289. Kuiper JL, Smit EF. High-dose, pulsatile erlotinib in two NSCLC patients with leptomeningeal metastases–one with a remarkable thoracic response as well. Lung Cancer. 2013;80(1):102–5.

290. Jackman DM, Cioffredi LA, Jacobs L, Sharmeen F, Morse LK, Lucca J, et al. A phase I trial of high dose gefitinib for patients with leptomeningeal metastases from non-small cell lung cancer. Oncotarget. 2015;6(6):4527–36.

291. Choong NW, Dietrich S, Seiwert TY, Tretiakova MS, Nallasura V, Davies GC, et al. Gefitinib response of erlotinib-refractory lung cancer involving meninges-role of EGFR mutation. Nat Clin Pract Oncol. 2006;3:50–7.

292. Hata A, Katakami N, Kaji R, Fujita S, Imai Y. Erlotinib for whole-brain-radiotherapy-refractory leptomeningeal metastases after gefitinib failure in a lung adenocarcinoma patient. J Thorac Oncol. 2012;7:770–1.

293. Togashi Y, Masago K, Hamatani Y, Sakamori Y, Nagai H, Kim YH, et al. Successful erlotinib rechallenge for leptomeningeal metastases of lung adenocarcinoma after erlotinib-induced interstitial lung disease: a case report and review of the literature. Lung Cancer. 2012;77:464–8.

294. Xing P, Li J, Shi Y, Zhang X. Recurrent response to advanced lung adenocarcinoma with erlotinib developing leptomeningeal metastases during gefitinib therapy and two case reports. Thoracic Cancer. 2014;5:38–42.

295. Nakamichi S, Kubota K, Horinouchi H, Kanda S, Fujiwara Y, Nokihara H, et al. Successful EGFR-TKI rechallenge of leptomeningeal carcinomatosis after gefitinib-induced interstitial lung disease. Jpn J Clin Oncol. 2013;43(4):422–5.

296. Kawamura T, Hata A, Takeshita J, Fujita S, Hayashi M, Tomii K, et al. High-dose erlotinib for refractory leptomeningeal metastases after failure of standard-dose EGFR-TKIs. Cancer Chemother Pharmacol. 2015;75(6):1261–6.

297. Schafer N, Scheffler B, Stuplich M, Schaub C, Kebir S, Rehkamper C, et al. Vemurafenib for leptomeningeal melanomatosis. J Clin Oncol. 2013;31(11):e173–4.

298. Waters KD. Leucoencephalopathy in patients on methotrexate. Lancet. 1978;2:46.

299. Tufekci O, Yilmaz S, Karapinar TH, Gozmen S, Cakmakci H, Hiz S, et al. A rare complication of intrathecal methotrexate in a child with acute lymphoblastic leukemia. Pediatr Hematol Oncol. 2011;28:517–22.

300. Teh HS, Fadilah SAW, Leong CF. Transverse myelopathy following intrathecal administration of chemotherapy. Singap Med J. 2007;48:e46–9.

301. Rollins N, Winick N, Bash R, Booth T. Acute methotrexate neurotoxicity: findings on diffusion-weighted imaging and correlation with clinical outcome. Am J Neuroradiol. 2004;25:1688–95.

302. Agarwal A, Vijay K, Thamburaj K, Ouyang T. Transient leukoencephalopathy after intrathecal methotrexate mimicking stroke. Emerg Radiol. 2011;18:345–7.

303. Aradillas E, Arora R, Gasperino J. Methotrexate-induced posterior reversible encephalopathy syndrome. J Clin Pharm Ther. 2011;36:529–36.

304. Ostermann K, Pels H, Kowoll A, Kuhnhenn J, Schlegel U. Neurological complications after intrathecal liposomal cytarabine in combination with systemic polychemotherapy in primary CNS lymphoma. J Neurooncol. 2010;103:635–40.

305. Dicuonzo F, Salvati A, Palma M, Lefons V, Lasalandra G, De Leonardis F, et al. Posterior reversible encephalopathy syndrome associated with methotrexate neurotoxicity: conventional magnetic resonance and diffusion-weighted imaging findings. J Child Neurol. 2009;24:1013–8.

306. Gallego Perez-Larraya J, Palma JA, Carmona-Iragui M, Fernandez-Torron R, Irimia P, Rodrıguez-Otero P, et al. Neurologic complications of intrathecal liposomal cytarabine administered prophylactic ally to patients with non-Hodgkin's lymphoma. J Neurooncol. 2010;103:603–9.

307. Gütling E, Landis T, Kleihues P. Akinetic mutism in bilateral necrotizing leucoencephalopathy after radiation and chemotherapy: electrophysiological and autopsy findings. J Neurol. 1992;239:125–8.

308. Hilgendorf I, Wolff D, Junghanss C, Kahl C, Leithaeuser M, Steiner B, et al. Neurological complications after intrathecal liposomal cytarabine application in patients after allogenic hematopoietic stem cell transplantation. Ann Hematol. 2008;87:1009–12.

309. Jabbour E, O'Brien S, Kantarjian H, Garcia-Manero G, Ferrajoli A, Ravandi F, et al. Neurological complications associated with intrathecal liposomal cytarabine given prophylactically in combination with high dose methotrexate and cytarabine to patients with acute lymphocytic leukemia. Blood. 2007;109:3214–8.

310. Shapiro WR, Schmid M, Glantz M, et al. A randomized phase III/IV study to determine benefit and safety of cytarabine liposome injection for treatment of neoplastic meningitis. J Clin Oncol. 2006;24:(June 6 suppl):1528 s.

311. Clamon G, Doebbeling B. Meningeal carcinomatosis from breast cancer: spinal cord versus brain involvement. Breast Cancer Res Treat. 1987;9(3):213–7.

312. Jayson GC, Howell A, Harris M, Morgenstern G, Chang J, Ryder WD. Carcinomatous meningitis in patients with breast cancer. An aggressive disease variant. Cancer. 1994;74(12):3135–41.

313. Regierer AC, Stroux A, Kühnhardt D, Dieing A, Lehenbauer-Dehm S, Flath B, Possinger K, Eucker J. Contrast-enhancing meningeal lesions are associated with longer survival in breast cancer-related leptomeningeal metastasis. Breast Care. 2008;3:118–23.

314. Kim KH, Im SA, Keam B. Clinical outcomes of central nervous system metastases from breast cancer: differences in survival depending on systemic treatment. J Neurooncol. 2012;106:303–13.

315. Hammerer V, Pauli G, Quoix E. Retrospective study of a series of 26 carcinomatous meningitis secondary to lung cancer. Bull Cancer. 2005;92(11):989–94.

316. Sudo J, Honmura Y, Kurimoto F, Komagata H, Sakai H, Yoneda S. Meningeal carcinomatosis in patients with lung cancer. Nihon Kokyuki Gakkai Zasshi. 2006;44(11):795–9.

317. Chuang TY, Yu CJ, Shih JY, Yang PC, Kuo SH. Cytologically proven meningeal carcinomatosis in patients with lung cancer: clinical observation of 34 cases. J Formos Med Assoc. 2008;107(11):851–6.

Spinal Metastasis as Complication of Systemic Cancers

6

Gregory Davis, Michaela Lee, Dawit Aregawi, Mark E. Shaffrey, David Schiff, and Jonathan H. Sherman

Introduction

Metastatic spinal cord disease represents a common complication of systemic cancer and is a major cause of morbidity in cancer patients [1, 2]. Since the first report of spine metastasis by Dr. William Spiller in 1925 [3], this disease entity has proven to be a challenge to physicians both with regard to diagnosis and management. Symptomatic spine metastasis is seen in 5–10% of patients with cancer and such lesions must be caught early and treated in an effective manner in order to preserve residual neurologic function and to prevent new neurologic deficits [4, 5]. These patients present with signs and symptoms such as pain, weakness, autonomic dysfunction, sensory loss, and ataxia [6]. A variety of prognostic factors have been evaluated in order to adequately assess the appropriate treatment options for these patients. Such factors include extent of metastatic disease, aggressiveness of the cancer, and preoperative function. By assessing the patient's prognosis, the appropriate treatment options that minimize additional morbidity and maximize the patient's quality of life can be selected. These treatment options range from palliative measures, such as radiation therapy, to curative resection; the type of treatment must be individualized for each patient [7, 8].

Epidemiology

1.7 million new cases of cancer are expected to be diagnosed in the U.S. in 2015 [9]. Systemic neoplasia is seen in 60–70% of these patients at the time of their death with bone as the most common site for metastatic disease [10]. Post-mortem studies report the prevalence of skeletal metastasis in cancer patients to range from 7 to 27%. The prevalence is similar for both men and women [11]. Of those with skeletal metastasis, 36–70% have lesions to the spine [12–14]. Metastatic disease to the spine can present in a variety of ways and causes significant morbidity in these patients.

Metastatic lesions can be intradural intramedullary, intradural extramedullary, or extradural in location. Extradural disease can be isolated to the bony spine, or an epidural component can be present with or without compression of the spinal cord or thecal sac. Approximately 94–98% of patients with metastasis to the spine have either vertebral or epidural involvement [11]. On the other hand, intradural extramedullary and intradural intramedullary seeding are only seen in 5–6% and 0.9–2.1% of patients, respectively [15]. Intradural extramedullary lesions of metastatic origin typically arise via seeding of the spinal subarachnoid space (e.g., lymphoma). This topic will

G. Davis
Department of Neurological Surgery, George Washington University Hospital, 2150 Pennsylvania Ave. NW, Suite 7-408, Washington, DC 20037, USA
e-mail: gdavis7@gwu.edu

M. Lee
Department of Neurosurgery, George Washington University Medical Center, 2150 Pennsylvania Avenue, NW, Suite 7-420, Washington, DC 20037, USA
e-mail: mlee@gwmail.gwu.edu

D. Aregawi
Department of Neurosurgery, Penn State Milton S. Hershey Medical Center, Penn State College of Medicine, 30 Hope Drive, P.O. Box 859 Hershey, PA 17033, USA
e-mail: daregawi@hmc.psu.edu

M.E. Shaffrey
Department of Neurological Surgery, University of Virginia Hospital, P.O. Box 800212 Charlottesville, VA 22908, USA
e-mail: mes8c@virginia.edumbt2a@virginia.edu

D. Schiff
Neuro-oncology center, University of Virginia, Hospital West, Room 6225, Jefferson Park Avenue, Charlottesville, VA 22908, USA
e-mail: ds4jd@virginia.edu

J.H. Sherman (✉)
Department of Neurosurgery, The George Washington University Hospital, 2150 Pennsylvania Avenue, NW, Suite 7-408, Washington, DC 20037, USA
e-mail: jsherman@mfa.gwu.edu

© Springer International Publishing AG 2018
D. Schiff et al. (eds.), *Cancer Neurology in Clinical Practice*, DOI 10.1007/978-3-319-57901-6_6

Table 6.1 Site of primary tumor with epidural spinal metastasis

Primary	Incidence (%)
Breast	13–22
Lung	15–19
Prostate	10–18
Lymphoma	8–10
Sarcoma	7.5–9
Kidney	6–7
Gastrointestinal	4–5
Melanoma	2–4
Myeloma	4.5–5
Unknown	4–11

primarily be discussed in another chapter. Epidural spinal metastases (ESM) are most commonly seen in the thoracic spine (70% of cases). Disease is also seen in the lumbar spine (20% of cases) and less commonly the cervical spine (10% of cases) [12, 16]. Despite the incidence of metastasis, ESM are symptomatic in only 5–10% of patients with cancer [17–19].

The incidence of metastatic spine disease varies among different tumor types. A higher index of suspicion must be maintained with particular cancer patients in an attempt to retain and possibly restore neurologic function. The most common malignancies to result in symptomatic ESM include breast cancer, lung cancer, and prostate cancer. Lymphoma, sarcoma, and renal cancers display a high prevalence as the primary source for ESM, and less frequently melanoma, myeloma, and gastrointestinal tract tumors will metastasize to the epidural spine. However, it is not infrequent that the primary site for ESM remains unknown [19–21]. Table 6.1 displays the incidence of each of these primary sites as a source of metastasis. Loblaw and colleagues analyzed the cumulative incidence of ESM in the 5 years preceding death among different cancer types and found an overall incidence of 2.5% for all cancer types with a range of 0.2% in pancreatic carcinoma to 7.9% in myeloma [22].

Pathogenesis and Pathophysiology

Batson, through his cadaveric experiments, identified the low-pressure valveless vertebral-venous plexus, which extends from epidural and perivertebral veins to veins of the thoraco-abdominal wall and veins of the head and neck. Venous blood can bypass the portal, caval, and pulmonary veins via Valsalva, venous obstruction, or increased intra-thoracic and intra-abdominal pressure resulting in flow inversion to the vertebral-venous plexus. This provides a pathway for distant organs to spread disease to the spine [23, 24].

An alternative route for metastasis to the bony spine and epidural space is via arterial emboli through the rich vascular network that supplies the bony spine. The vertebral body has a large blood supply, while the posterior elements are less highly vascular. Spinal lesions arise more often from the vertebral body; [5] however, isolated involvement of the vertebral body is rarely observed—only in 3.8% of cases—while 75% of ESM involve the vertebral body, pedicle and posterior elements [25]. These tumors can grow within the anterior or posterior bony elements or spread to the epidural space via venous drainage [26]. In addition, invasion into the spine can occur via direct extension from the paraspinal region to the nerve roots through the neural foramina [1].

The pathophysiology by which spine metastasis causes neurologic injury is a matter of some debate. Spinal cord compression is associated with endogenous neurochemical changes that lead to neuronal injury. This compression was initially thought to result in arterial ischemia. Subsequent animal and human studies have demonstrated that compression and obstruction of the vertebral-venous plexus result in vasogenic spinal cord edema, venous hemorrhage, and ischemia [20, 27]. In addition to venous obstruction, spinal auto-regulatory mechanisms induce arteriolar dilatation and increased edema via induction of such enzymes as nitric oxide synthase. Cytokine production, e.g., PGF_2, IL-1, IL-6, locally promotes an inflammatory response with vasodilatation and increased edema formation. In addition, animal studies display myelin loss secondary to ischemia and compression [28–31].

Presentation

Patients harboring spinal metastases can present in a variety of ways. Symptoms secondary to metastasis are the same symptoms by which a primary spinal malignancy is discovered. Also, 20% of patients with metastatic cancer have signs and symptoms of ESM as the initial manifestation of their disease [32]. Patients with bony spine metastasis with or without an epidural component commonly present with a prolonged period of persistent back pain with a median time course of 8 weeks. Unfortunately, although back pain is a frequent complaint among the general populace, the physician must consider spine metastasis in the differential diagnosis. This is especially true in older patients and patients with pain at the level of the thoracic spine, as pain at this level is uncommon in degenerative disc disease. Even with the diagnostic modalities available to the modern physician, patients are diagnosed very late in the course of their disease. Levack and colleagues performed a prospective observational study of 319 patients and found that 82% of patients at diagnosis of ESM were either unable to walk or only able to do so with help. 94% of these patients reported approximately a 3-month history of axial spine pain [33]. It is important to note that patients with compression secondary to epidural disease can still present with isolated axial spine pain without neurologic deficit or radicular symptoms. Epidural spinal compression cannot be excluded because a patient with back pain does not manifest myelopathy or radiculopathy.

Pain may occur for a variety of reasons including pathologic fracture, local compression resulting in axial spine pain, or via nerve root impingement resulting in radicular pain. Radicular pain affecting the upper or lower extremities is seen in cervical and lumbar disease, whereas thoracic cord lesions present with bilateral pain radiating around the chest or upper abdomen [34].

The location of pain can help guide the physician; however, pain can be a false localizing sign and may not always correlate directly with the level of the metastasis. The differential diagnosis must also include more common entities such as herniated disc disease, which can be distinguished by a history of trauma or other inciting event as a well an acute onset of pain, rather than the more common insidious onset of pain symptoms seen in spine metastasis [35, 36].

Weakness is the second or third most common complaint of patients with spine metastasis and is both a symptom and sign of disease. Subjective weakness may be a manifestation of axial or radicular pain without true weakness evident on examination and is present in a high percentage of patients with ESM. Objective weakness is seen in 84% of patients with compressive ESM. At the time of diagnosis, approximately 50% are ambulatory, 35% are paraparetic, and 15% are paraplegic. Rapid diagnosis and treatment are critical in these patients as 30% of those individuals presenting with weakness become paraplegic within one week [21].

Patients with spinal metastasis commonly present with numbness and paresthesias such that 51% have subjective sensory symptoms on presentation, and 78% of patients have sensory deficits found on examination [21]. These deficits can assist in localizing the metastatic lesion. Dermatomal sensory loss or reflex loss is more predictive than a sensory level, as the sensory level may be apparent between one and four levels below the level of disease. Patients with cervical and thoracic disease can also present with Lhermitte's sign [37].

Bowel or bladder dysfunction is seen in as many as 57% of patients. Urinary retention is the most common form of dysfunction, more common than both urinary and fecal incontinence. The degree of autonomic abnormality often correlates with the severity of motor and sensory deficits and is considered a late finding. In addition to the aforementioned presenting signs and symptoms, patients may also present with other forms of autonomic dysfunction such as the absence of sweating below the lesion level and Horner's syndrome as well as ataxia, spasticity, and syringomyelia [20, 21].

In assessing patients with ESM, it is important to differentiate between lesions causing myelopathy from spinal cord compression and those causing deficits from cauda equina syndrome (CES) . Patients with either lesion can present with back pain, weakness, sensory deficits, or bowel and bladder dysfunction. However, the former results in upper motor neuron signs such as clonus, Babinski sign, and hyperactive reflexes. On the other hand, the latter displays unique sensory deficits such as saddle anesthesia as well as lower motor neuron signs such as hypoactive reflexes and muscle wasting [38, 39].

Diagnostic Work-up

The diagnosis of spine metastasis is continually evolving as the diagnostic tools available to the physician continue to improve. Plain X-rays are a valuable tool in analyzing the bony spine. Plain radiographs detect bony erosion better in cortical bone than in cancellous bone. The pedicle is primarily composed of cortical bone as compared to the vertebral body, so metastasis to the pedicle is identified first on plain radiographs despite the higher degree of involvement in the vertebral body [16]. Metastatic tumors are commonly lytic lesions that present with vertebral body compression. Plain radiographs also show paraspinal soft-tissue shadows and pathological fracture-dislocation [40, 41]. Despite these advantages, false-negative plain radiographs occur in 10–17% of patients with ESM [18]. The osteoblastic tumors seen in prostate and breast metastases as well as paraspinal tumors that invade the neural foramen are difficult to identify on plain radiographs.

Bone scans are more sensitive in assessing metastatic disease than plain radiographs. Bone scans use technetium diphosphonate to identify diseased bone which present as "hot spots." This diagnostic method has the advantage of providing a survey of the entire skeleton. Degenerative changes seen in elderly patients can show up as "hot spots" and complicate the diagnosis [42, 43]. As an alternative to a conventional bone scan, whole body positron emission tomography (PET) can be used to assess bony metastases. This imaging modality has been shown to have equal sensitivity and improved accuracy in detecting metastatic bone lesions when compared to a bone scan [44]. The improved accuracy is related to the mechanism by which the modalities detect tumor involvement—technetium scanning relies upon osteoblastic bone response to tumor, while PET measures glucose uptake in the tumor itself by the use of a radiotracer [45–48]. Consequently, PET scans are more likely to detect tumors that are at an earlier stage of growth, while bone scans are less likely to detect osteolytic and slow growing metastases [48, 49].

Myelography, as first brought forward by Jean Athanase Sicard, has been an important diagnostic technique in the evaluation of spinal metastasis [50]. Prior to the advent of MRI, myelography was the gold standard for evaluation of these tumors [51]. Myelography can still be used to identify the site and extent of metastasis when MRI is not readily available, a patient is unable to tolerate MRI, or MRI is contraindicated as in patients with ferromagnetic implants [41, 52]. The relationship of the metastasis to the spinal cord, dura, and nerve roots can also be discerned. Myelography is primarily performed via lumbar injection of radio-opaque dye. However, some metastases can present in multiple locations; a tumor causing complete obliteration of the spinal canal results in failure to identify additional rostral metastases, in which case a cisternal injection is required to complete the evaluation [41].

Computed tomography (CT) can be used either as a separate modality or in combination with myelography. CT imaging is primarily useful in assessing the bony elements surrounding the spinal cord. CT in combination with myelography can greatly improve the data available from each study alone and can provide better anatomical detail of the spinal axis and extent of the tumor both inside and outside the spinal canal [41, 53].

While the aforementioned modalities can be of value in assessing spinal metastasis, magnetic resonance imaging (MRI) is considered the modality of choice. MRI provides multi-planar imaging of the spine that is noninvasive. In addition, paravertebral soft-tissue masses and bone marrow involvement can also be detected [51]. MRI has been shown to be equivalent if not superior to CT myelography in detecting cord compression in ESM as well as cord atrophy [54]. MRI has been shown to be the most accurate and noninvasive method to assess the entire spinal axis so that the appropriate treatment modality can be initiated [55].

Laboratory and radiographic assessment are important in assessing systemic disease. Metabolic panels, blood counts, and prealbumin should be obtained to assess the nutritional status and immunological status of the patient. Renal dysfunction and liver dysfunction via metastasis or primary disease can be assessed via blood urea nitrogen and creatinine and liver function tests [41]. Tumor markers such as prostate specific antigen, serum and urine protein electrophoresis for myeloma, CA-125 for ovarian cancer, and CEA for colorectal cancer can assist with diagnosis [56]. Urinalysis, chest radiography, abdominal ultrasound, and CT imaging of the chest, abdomen, and pelvis are useful screening methods for systemic malignancy [41].

Prognosis

In discussing the various treatment options of spinal metastasis, multiple factors must be considered in order to determine the patient's prognosis. Prognosis can be a key item in patient assessment that can influence how aggressive the treatment is for a particular patient. Tokuhashi generated such a system for assessing prognosis that is useful in based on length of survival (Table 6.2). This system includes such items as general condition, number of extraspinal metastasis, the number of spinal metastasis, the extent of metastasis to internal organs, the primary site of the tumor, and the degree of spinal cord injury. This scoring system has been correlated with prognosis such that patients with a score between 9 and 12 are predicted to survive greater than 12 months, while patients with a score from 0 to 5 are predicted to survive less than 3 months [57].

In general, the median time of survival after diagnosis of ESM is approximately 6 months. Patients who are ambulatory at the time of diagnosis display a median survival of 8–10 months as compared to 2–4 months for non-ambulatory patients. In addition, patients with slow growing cancers such as breast and prostate cancer tend to liver longer than faster growing cancers such as lung cancer. The former has a

Table 6.2 Tokuhashi's evaluation for prognosis

	Score		
Symptoms	0	1	2
Karnofsky score	10–40	50–70	80–100
Extraspinal metastasis	>3	1–2	0
Internal organ metastasis	Unresectable	Resectable	No metastasis
Primary site of tumor	Lung, stomach	Kidney, liver, uterus	Thyroid, prostate, breast, rectum
Spinal metastasis	>3	2	1
Spinal cord injury	Complete	Incomplete	None

median survival of 9–10 months, while the latter has a median survival of 3 months [58, 59].

Pharmacotherapy

The treatment options for spinal metastasis are divided into three categories. These options include pharmacologic therapy, radiation therapy, and surgical resection with or without fusion. Treatment of the patient's symptoms and adjuvant therapy, e.g., corticosteroids or chemotherapy, are two roles of pharmacologic therapy. The physician combines medications for analgesia as well as for the control of neuropathic pain with radiation therapy and/or surgical intervention. Opiates are the primary treatment for analgesia, while amytriptiline and gabapentin or pregabalin are effective treatment options for neuropathic pain. These medications are a key component to palliative therapy [34].

Pain develops not only from bony infiltration but also from pathologic fractures. In addition to pain, fractures can lead to spinal instability requiring surgical intervention. Pharmacotherapy directed at bone turnover can provide a method in preventing pathologic compression fractures. Bisphosphonates inhibit osteoclast activity and bony resorption, decreasing the risk of pathologic fracture. Such therapy has shown a benefit in patients with bony metastasis from multiple myeloma and breast cancer [60, 61].

Corticosteroids have been shown in experimental models to reduce peritmoral vasogenic spinal cord edema and transiently improve neurologic function. After initiation of steroid therapy, patients have significant improvement in pain symptoms [34, 41, 62]. A randomized trial by Sorensen and colleagues compared outcome in patients receiving high-dose radiation therapy with or without dexamethasone. In the former group, 81% of patients were ambulatory after treatment and 59% of patients remained ambulatory after 6 months. In contrast, only 63% of patients in the latter group were ambulatory after treatment and 33% of patients remained ambulatory after 6 months. These differences displayed statistical significance identifying the importance of corticosteroids as adjuvant treatment in patients with ESM [63].

Studies have also focused on the effect of high-dose bolus dexamethasone (100 mg) versus moderate-dose bolus dexamethasone (10 mg) versus no corticosteroid treatment. These studies displayed equivalent efficacy between doses with regard to improvement in pain, ambulatory status, and bladder function. The physician must consider the side effect profile of corticosteroids, especially at higher dosages. Significant adverse side effects include severe psychoses, gastric ulcers, rectal bleeding, and gastrointestinal perforations [63–66]. Heimdal and colleagues performed a retrospective study of patients who received radiation therapy in combination with corticosteroids. All patients received pretreatment with antacids or H2 blockers prior to high-dose corticosteroid therapy. Despite preventive measures, two patients developed gastric perforations and two patients developed gastrointestinal bleeding, one of which proved fatal. A subsequent cohort of patients received a lower dose corticosteroid regimen of 16 mg tapered over 2 weeks. These patients did not experience serious side effects and the ambulatory outcome was similar to those patients receiving the high-dose corticosteroid regimen [66]. In addition, the use of corticosteroids has been analyzed in patients with less severe metastatic disease. Maranzano and colleagues analyzed 20 consecutive patients with ESM causing less than 50% narrowing of the spinal canal and no neurologic deficit in a phase II trial. Patients treated with corticosteroids and radiation therapy showed no additional survival benefit and equivalent return of neurologic function in comparison to patients treated with radiation therapy alone [67].

Chemotherapeutic agents can be a valuable treatment option in ESM. The primary use of these agents is dependent on the chemosensitivity or chemoresistance of the particular tumor. Treatment must be designed to maintain neurologic function and maximize quality of life. Consequently, chemotherapy is typically used as adjuvant therapy along with radiation therapy and/or surgical resection in tumors with uncertain or limited chemosensitivity. On the other hand, the role of chemotherapy in chemosensitive tumors has been a matter of debate. Patients with symptomatic chemosensitive metastases have most often been given chemotherapy in combination with other therapeutic modalities. However, patients with chemosensitive tumors have shown good neurologic improvement with chemotherapy alone. Especially early in the course of the disease, chemosensitive tumors are likely to respond to chemotherapy. These tumors include germ cell tumors and hematological malignancies, such as lymphoma [68, 69]. In addition, chemotherapy can be considered as a single mode of treatment for patients who have previously received radiation or surgery and are not candidates for further treatment [34].

Radiation Therapy

Historically, decompression via laminectomy was considered the primary treatment for spinal metastasis. Studies were conducted in the 1970s and 1980s comparing radiation therapy alone to laminectomy followed by adjuvant radiation therapy. These studies displayed similar rates of neurologic improvement. Consequently, radiation therapy became the standard as primary treatment, while surgery was reserved for patients who deteriorated during or failed to improve after radiation therapy [70–72]. As more advanced surgical techniques for resection and stabilization have been developed, the role of radiotherapy has also been modified.

Prognosis for patients with spinal metastasis receiving radiotherapy is highly dependent upon the radiosensitivity of the primary tumor. The most radiosensitive tumors that commonly metastasize to the spine include breast cancer, small cell lung cancer, prostate cancer, myeloma, and lymphoma. Patients with these tumors tend to show improved functional recovery and better tumor control rates as compared to patients with radioresistant tumors such as melanoma and renal cell carcinoma. Patients with radioresistant tumors can, however, still obtain significant pain control and quality of life improvement from radiotherapy [73–75].

A variety of techniques are available for the effective delivery of radiotherapy. Such techniques include but are not limited to conventional radiotherapy and stereotactic ablative radiation therapy. In general, the use of radiotherapy is limited by the level of radiation tolerance of the spinal cord. Hypertension, advanced age, prior spinal cord pathology, combination chemotherapy, and immunosuppression are factors which lower the spinal cord's tolerance to radiation [76]. This tolerance level is not fully understood, which makes it necessary to limit the radiation dose provided to the spinal cord in order to prevent such serious complications as radiation myelitis or myelopathy. When radiation myelopathy occurs, patients have progressive rostral spread of sensorimotor symptoms within months of radiation therapy. Within 1 year of symptomatic onset, MRI displays cord swelling as high T2 signal within the cord with gadolinium enhancement. The combination of clinical and imaging characteristics is used to differentiate between radiation toxicity and tumor recurrence [77–80].

Although utilized with decreasing frequency now, conventional external beam radiation therapy (EBRT) has been historically considered an excellent treatment option for pain associated with bony spinal metastases commonly seen in lung, breast, and prostate cancer. This pain can be treated with various dose schedules with equal efficacy [81–83]. Notably, a retrospective analysis of 1300 patients compared five different treatment regimens between 8 Gy in 1 fraction and 40 Gy in 20 fractions. Functional outcome was similar between all groups; however, the more protracted regimens were associated with a lower rate of local recurrence [84]. A protracted regimen is subsequently advantageous in patients with a longer life expectancy, versus a short course of radiation for palliation for short life expectances [85].

Stereotactic ablative body radiation therapy (SABR) provides an alternate modality for focused high-dose radiation to the tumor while minimizing radiation to the adjacent spinal cord, and has become the dominant modality of radiation delivery to spinal metastases. Accurate targeting requires localization of multiple radiation beams to converge on the lesion of interest at a high dose. The typical dose ranges from 8 to 18 Gy. This treatment can be administered over multiple sessions, which makes outpatient treatment convenient. Gerstzen and colleagues presented 500 consecutive lesions treated with high-dose (15–22.5 Gy) single-fraction SABR with a median follow-up of 21 months. They reported long-term tumor control of 88% overall with 100% for breast, lung, and renal metastases [86]. A series by Bate and colleagues followed 57 patients treated with SABR with or without surgery, the SABR-only group achieved local tumor control of 96% overall [87]. In another study, the tumor control rate was 100% in lesions without previous irradiation [88]. SABR following surgery should be considered when mechanical stability and local tumor control both are required. Laufer and colleagues reported 186 patients with ESM treated with local debulking and spinal stabilization plus SABR, and compared radiotherapy groups. Both groups of high-dose therapy following decompression surgery achieved local recurrence rates below 10% [89]. Radiosurgery is considered safer for recurrent tumors than traditional methods as repeat traditional radiotherapy poses a significant risk at surpassing the radiation tolerance of the spinal cord. Moreover, recent review of the literature advocates SABR as the first-line treatment for palliative symptom control for those with symptomatic radioresistant tumors with no neurologic deficit (Fig. 6.1a–c) [90]. Overall, SABR is becoming a common method for delivering safe doses of radiation to spinal tumors. Radiosurgery, like other forms of radiotherapy, does not address the issue of spinal instability.

Surgical Management

The role of surgery in the treatment of spine metastasis has changed as the techniques available for spinal reconstruction have improved. Despite the variety of options in a surgeon's armamentarium, the ability to maintain a patient's quality of life remains of utmost importance and extensive spinal instrumentation correlates with a longer and more painful recovery period, in addition to the recovery required for treatment of the primary disease. Consequently, prognosis is a key factor in deciding the aggressiveness of treatment for a particular patient.

Various scoring systems have been proposed to help guide treatment strategies and the role of surgical intervention. Tomita and colleagues clarified the correlation between length of survival and surgical treatment goals. In this study, they analyzed the growth rate of primary tumor, the presence of visceral metastasis, and the presence and number of bone metastasis. Slow growth tumors such as breast and thyroid cancer equated to 1 point; moderate growth tumors such as

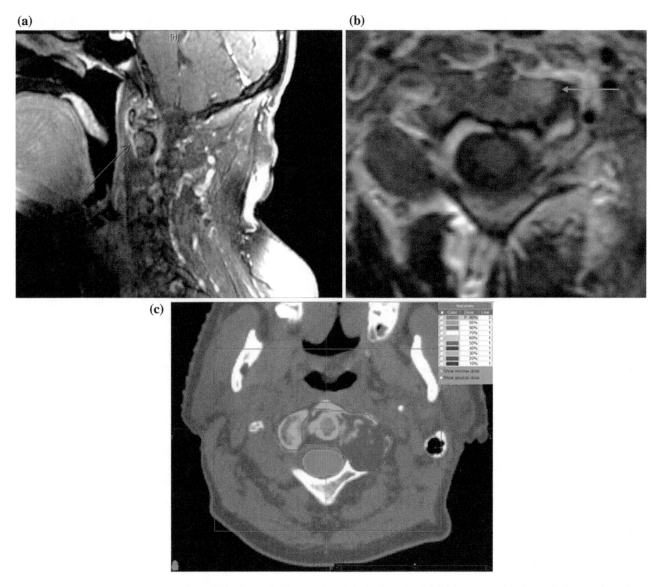

Fig. 6.1 **a–c** 61-year-old male presenting with a 2-month history of progressively worsening neck pain. The patient was neurologically intact on examination. He was recently diagnosed with metastatic thyroid carcinoma; a relatively radioresistant tumor. Pretreatment sagittal (**a**) and axial (**b**) T1 post-gadolinium MR image displaying a tumor in the left C2 vertebral body (*green arrow*). **c** CTV (*red circle*) and PTV (*purple circle*) for SABR treatment planning

renal cell carcinoma equated to 2 points; rapid growth tumors such as lung and gastrointestinal cancer equated to 4 points. Visceral metastases equated to 2 points if they were treatable, while untreatable lesions equated to 4 points. Finally, solitary or isolated bony metastasis equated to 1 point, while multiple metastases equated to 2 points. The group then separated patients into prognostic scores from 2 to 10. Patients with a prognostic score of 2–3 had a treatment goal of long-term local control via wide or marginal excision, e.g., en bloc spondylectomy, with a mean survival time of 38.2 months. Patients with a prognostic score of 4–5 had a treatment goal of middle term local control via intralesional excision with a mean survival time of 21.5 months. Patients

with a prognostic score of 6–7 had a treatment goal of short-term palliation via simple decompression and stabilization with a mean survival time of 10.1 months. Finally, patients with a prognostic score of 8–10 had supportive care only with a mean survival time of 5.3 months [7].

Bilsky and coworkers developed a scoring system that integrates neurologic assessment, oncologic assessment, assessment of mechanical instability, and an assessment of systemic disease burden and medical co-morbidity (NOMS). The neurologic component addresses myelopathy, radiculopathy, and degree of epidural compression. Oncologic assessment evaluates the radiosensitivity of the tumor. Radiosensitive tumors include multiple myeloma and lymphoma while highly radioresistant tumors include renal cell carcinoma, thyroid carcinoma, melanoma, and sarcoma [91].

On the other hand, the Spinal Instability Score Neoplastic Score (aka, SINS) can help the surgeon predict spinal stability with respect to neoplastic lesions. A composite score of six different factors will help determine if a spine is stable (score 0–6), intermediate (score 7–12), or unstable (score 13–18). Those factors are: location of lesion in the spine, mechanical or postural pain, bone lesion quality, spinal alignment, vertebral body involvement (i.e., collapse), and the posterolateral involvement of spinal elements [92].

The simplest therapeutic option—percutaneous vertebroplasty or kyphoplasty—is a valuable option for treating pain from lesions either isolated to the vertebral body or lesions with a mild epidural component. In this treatment, the surgeon injects polymethylmethacrylate (PMMA) either directly into the vertebral body in vertebroplasty or after expansion of the collapsed vertebral body with a balloon in kyphoplasty. The surgeon usually injects bone cement via a transpedicular route; however, anterolateral, intercostovertebral, and posterolateral routes are used in the cervical, thoracic, and lumbar regions, respectively. Patients can experience pain relief within 24–48 h following therapy and have shown to maintain improved pain control upon 2-year follow-up examination [93, 94].

Compressive lesions in the vertebral body not amenable to percutaneous vertebroplasty or kyphoplasty require alternate avenues by which the spinal cord can be accessed. The surgeon typically performs decompression with a corpectomy via an anterior or anterolateral approach. Anterior approaches require access through the neck, thorax, or abdomen or retroperitoneal space, which can present a surgical challenge. For lumbar lesions, the lateral approach is also used to obtain a retroperitoneal plane to the spinal column. Following a corpectomy/vertebrectomy, the space filled by the vertebral body must be reconstructed to the appropriate height. The typical material in degenerative spine disease is autologous bone or bone allograft. Patients with metastatic lesions will or have already received radiation therapy that decreases the rate of bony fusion. PMMA is used for reconstruction in the cervical or thoracic spine or a titanium expandable cage in the thoracic or lumbar spine. The former requires the addition of a plate and screw construct to aid in stability [95]. Sawaya and coworkers studied 72 patients with thoracic spine anterior column disease that underwent a vertebrectomy and fusion procedure. 76% of these patients displayed improvement in neurologic function. In addition, 77% of patients non-ambulatory prior to surgery regained ambulatory capacity postoperatively [12].

While the anterior approach to metastatic disease can be effective in treating the majority of patients, the extent of a patient's primary disease may not warrant such an extensive tumor resection. Simple decompressive laminectomy and fusion with pedicle screw instrumentation provides a palliative surgical option. In a retrospective study by Oda e al., 32 patients with extensive metastatic disease in the cervico-thoracic spine underwent posterior decompression and fusion. 94% of these patients maintained pain relief, neurologic function, and spinal stability throughout the survival period [96–98].

Patchell's seminal paper compared 50 patients treated by the surgical procedure appropriate to the site of the metastasis followed by radiation therapy with 51 patients treated with radiation alone. In this randomized, multi-institutional, non-blinded trial, the treatment group randomly assigned patients with metastatic spinal cord compression to two different treatment arms. In comparing the two groups after treatment, 84% of patients were ambulatory in the surgery/radiation group while only 57% were ambulatory in the radiation-only group. 32 patients were non-ambulatory prior to treatment, 50% in each group. Of these patients, 62% of the combined group were ambulatory after treatment, while only 19% of the latter group were ambulatory after treatment. Finally, patients in the former group were able to retain the ability to walk for a mean of 122 days, while patients in the latter group were only able to retain the ability to walk for a mean of 13 days. This study showed that direct surgical decompression, and fusion where appropriate, followed by radiation therapy was superior to radiation therapy alone. Only patients with single levels of metastatic epidural spinal cord compression were included in this study [99].

Out of Patchell's study was born the idea of separation surgery. Separation surgery is a simple concept, but one that incorporates all the surgical techniques discussed above, as well as the efficacy of SABR. Separation surgery starts with the goal of resecting the tumor off the thecal sac and spinal cord and reconstituting the CSF space. As the majority of tumors present in the vertebral body, these tumors can commonly infiltrate the posterior longitudinal ligament (PLL). Consequently, to adequately decompress the spinal cord, a bilateral pediculectomy must be performed and the PLL must be dissected off of the overlying dura. This approach requires stabilization through the placement of pedicle screws. A gross total resection of tumor is not required as at approximately 2 weeks after surgery, SABR can be delivered to the residual tumor and resection cavity up to the dural edge. The surgical resection allows the CSF to provide an appropriate distance between the desired radiation dose and the spinal cord to minimize risk of radiation myelopathy. A CT myelogram is utilized to best identify the dural margin used for radiation planning with minimal artifact generated by the instrumentation (Fig. 6.2a–f). Studies using this technique demonstrate local progression rates less than 5% at 1 year [87, 89].

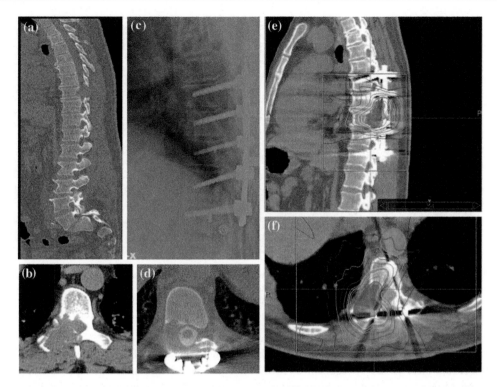

Fig. 6.2 **a–f** 53-year-old male presenting with progressive back pain and lower extremity weakness. The patient displayed 4+/5 weakness in the right lower extremities. He was recently diagnosed with renal cell carcinoma status-post a nephrectomy. **a** Preoperative sagittal CT displaying a tumor at T9. **b** Preoperative axial CT displaying a tumor at the right T9 pedicle and transverse process encroaching on the spinal cord. **c** Postoperative sagittal CT displaying instrumentation placed for stabilization following a T9/10 laminectomy and right T9 pediculectomy and tumor resection. **d** Postoperative axial CT myelogram image displaying reconstitution of the thecal sac. **e, f** GTV (*red circle*) for SABR treatment planning

Intradural Intramedullary Spinal Cord Metastasis

Intradural intramedullary spinal cord metastasis (ISCM) is an uncommon event, diagnosed in only 0.9–2.1% of cancer patients [100–102]. Approximately 50% of ISCM arise from lung carcinoma and the majority of these cases are small cell carcinoma. Breast cancer, lymphoma, kidney cancer, melanoma, gastrointestinal cancer, ovarian cancer, and tumors of unknown primary are other causes of ISCM [102–107]. Table 6.3 displays the incidence of each of these primary sites as a source of metastasis with regard to ISCM. Most ISCM are thought to spread via emboli through a secondary capillary network to penetrating arteries of the spinal cord [23, 105, 107]. Alternatively, ISCM may originate via direct extension from leptomeningeal disease and subsequently spread to the cord parenchyma [102, 107].

Pain is a common presenting sign in ISCM. In addition, patients may present with weakness and display a similar clinical course to ESM, including rapid progression to paraplegia [108]. However, true motor weakness typically follows sensory disturbances in ISCM as they are most commonly located in the posterior cord [109]. The presence of a Brown-Sequard syndrome can also be a common initial

Table 6.3 Site of primary tumor with intradural intramedullary spinal metastasis

Primary	Incidence (%)
Lung	47–54
Breast	11–14.5
Lymphoma	4–12
Kidney	4–9
Melanoma	3.6–9
Gastrointestinal	3–7.3
Ovarian	0.8–1.1
Unknown	1.8–6

finding and help differentiate between ISCM and ESM [109]. MRI (Fig. 6.3a, b) is the primary imaging modality for detecting cord enlargement, contrast enhancement, and surrounding edema in ISCM. As in ESM, opiates for analgesia and gabapentin for neuropathic pain are commonly used. Patients have shown significant relief of pain symptoms as well as transient improvement in neurologic function with the use of corticosteroids [102].

Treatment of ISCM has primarily been based on anecdotal experience and case series, as no prospective trials on

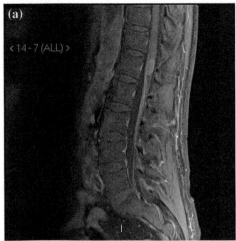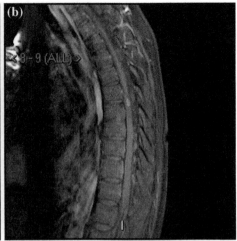

Fig. 6.3 **a**, **b** 57-year-old male with a history of a parasagittal oligodendroglioma for 10 years who presented with new bilateral numbness from the belt line down, Lhermitte's phenomenon, and radicular leg pain worsened with cough. He also noted urinary and fecal retention. Sagittal lumbar (**a**) and thoracic (**b**) post-contrast T1-weighted sequences showed ovoid ring-enhancing masses in the conus and mid-thoracic cord. Chest CT demonstrated a large left upper lobe lung mass, and bronchoscopic biopsy confirmed small cell lung cancer

treatment have been performed. EBRT with or without corticosteroids has been the most effective treatment of ISCM [107]. Clinical response primarily depends on the duration of symptoms, the degree of neurologic deficit, and the radiosensitivity of the tumor. As pathologic evidence indicates that ISCM are multifocal in as many as 30% of patients, radiation therapy to the entire spinal cord could be a treatment option [110, 111]. However, the consequences of bone marrow suppression associated with total spinal irradiation has limited this extensive treatment modality [106, 110]. Stereotactic radiosurgery has a potential role in treating these lesions; however, this modality has only been shown in the literature to be effective in primary vascular tumors [112]. The true issue is discerning the proximity of tumor to functioning spinal cord and limiting radiation exposure to this tissue.

The role of surgery in ISCM remains a matter of debate. 75% of patients with ISCM develop paraplegia within one month from the first symptom of disease. However, patients with rapidly progressive neurologic deficit have shown improved neurologic outcome with early surgical management [102]. In such patients, the objective of surgery is maximal removal of the lesion via microsurgical resection with preservation of existing neurologic function [108]. Focal radiation can then be applied to the involved area, especially in patents with evidence of residual disease [104].

Conclusions

Spinal cord metastases are a common complication of systemic malignancy. ESM most commonly stem from lung, breast, and prostate cancer, while greater than 50% of ISCM stem from lung cancer alone. Patients may present with a variety of symptoms, most notably pain and weakness. The ultimate goals in managing these patients include maximizing both length of survival and quality of life. These goals can best be reached via early, accurate diagnosis followed by the appropriate treatment for a particular patient. As imaging modalities have improved, delineating the exact location and extent of disease has become significantly more accurate. Despite the advantages of MR imaging, other imaging modalities such as CT and plain radiographs still play a valuable role in diagnosis.

Pharmacotherapy plays an important role in treatment for these patients not only for analgesia but also for treatment of edema with corticosteroids and adjuvant treatment with chemotherapy. The patient's prognosis defines the appropriate treatment for spinal metastasis, with the goal of maintaining that patient's quality of life. Radiation therapy continues to be a primary treatment option and a variety of new techniques are now available to maximize the radiation dose to the tumor while minimizing the dose to the spinal cord. Surgical resection and spinal stabilization also have critical roles in the treatment armamentarium. The combination of these different modalities will certainly continue to be a vital component in the treatment of metastatic spinal cord disease as the treatment algorithm continues to evolve with advancements from all fields.

References

1. Schiff D. Spinal cord compression. Neurol Clin N Am. 2003;21:67–87.

2. Mut M, Schiff D, Shaffrey ME. Metastasis to nervous system: spinal epidural and intramedullary metastases. J Neurooncol. 2005;75(1):43–56.
3. Spiller WG. Rapidly developing paraplegia associated with carcinoma. Arch Neurol Psychiatry. 1925;13:471.
4. Bilsky MH, Shannon FJ, Sheppard SS, Prabhu V, Boland PJ. Diagnosis and management of a metastatic tumor in the atlantoaxial spine. Spine. 2002;27(10):1062–9.
5. Barron KD, Hirano A, Araki S. Experiences with metastatic neoplasms involving the spinal cord. Neurology. 1959;9:91–106.
6. Townsend CM. Intraspinal tumors. In: Sabiston textbook of surgery, 17th ed. Philadelphia: Saunders; 2004. p. 2150–2.
7. Tomita K, Kawahara N, Kobayashi T, Yoshida A, Murakami H, Akamaru T. Surgical strategy for spinal metastasis. Spine. 2001;26(3):298–306.
8. Weigel B, Maghsudi M, Neumann C, Kretschmer R, Muller FJ, Nerlich M. Surgical management of symptomatic spinal metastasis. Spine. 1999;24(21):2240–6.
9. American Cancer Society. Cancer facts and figures 2015. Atlanta: American Cancer Society; 2015.
10. Wise JJ, Fischgrund JS, Herkowitz HN, Montgomery D, Kurz LT. Complication, survival rates, and risk factors of surgery for metastatic disease of the spine. Spine. 1999;24(18):1943–51.
11. Tubiana-Hulin M. Incidence, prevalence and distribution of bone metastasis. Bone. 1991;12(Suppl 1):9–10.
12. Perrin RG McBroom RJ. Anterior versus posterior decompression for symptomatic spinal metastasis. Can J Neurol Sci. 1987;14:75–80.
13. Raj PP. Cancer pain syndromes. In: Textbook of regional anesthesia, 1st ed. UK: Churchill Livingstone; 2002. p. 565–6.
14. Browner B. Metastatic disease of the spine. In: Skeletal trauma: basic science, management, and reconstruction, 3rd ed. Philadelphia: Saunders; 2003. p. 405–19.
15. Goetz CG. Direct metastatic disease. In: Textbook of clinical neurology, 2nd ed. Philadelphia: Saunders; 2003. p. 1042–51.
16. Gokaslan ZL, York JE, Walsh GL, McCutcheon IE, Lang FE, Putnam JB, Wildrick DM, Swisher SG, Abi-said D, Sawaya R. Transthoracic vertebrectomy for metastatic spinal tumors. J Neurosurg. 1998;89:599–609.
17. Kim RY. Extradural spinal cord compression from metastatic tumor. Ala Med. 1990;60:10–5.
18. Bach F, Larsen BH, Rohde K, Borgersen SE, Gjerris F, Boge-Rasmussen T, Agerlin N, Rasmussen B, Stjernholm P, Sorensen PS. Metastatic spinal cord compression. Occurrence, symptoms, clinical presentations and prognosis in 398 patients with spinal cord compression. Acta Neurochir (Wien) 1990; 107:37–43.
19. Sorenson PS, Borgeson SE, Rasmussen B, Bach F, Boge-Rasumssen T, Stjernholm P, Larsen BH, Agerlin N, Gjerris F. Metastatic epidural spinal cord compression: results of treatment and survival. Cancer. 1990;65(7):1502–8.
20. Gabriel K, Schiff D. Metastatic spinal cord compression by solid tumors. Semin Neurol. 2004;24(4):375–83.
21. Grant R, Papadopoulos SM, Greenberg HS. Metastatic epidural spinal cord compression. Neurol Clin. 1991;9:825–41.
22. Loblaw DA, Laperriere NJ, Mackillop WJ. A population-based study of malignant spinal cord compression in Ontario. Clin Oncol. 2003;15:211217.
23. Batson OV. The role of the vertebral veins in metastatic process. Ann Intern Med. 1942;16:38.
24. Abeloff MD. Bone metastasis. In: Clinical oncology, 3rd ed. UK: Churchill Livingstone; 2004. p. 1091–123.
25. Khaw FM, Worthy SA, Gibson MJ, Gholkar A. The appearance on MRI of vertebrae in acute compression of the spinal cord due to metastases. J Bone Joint Surg Br. 1999;81-B(5):830–4.
26. Arguello F, Baggs LB, Duerst RE, et al. Pathogenesis of vertebral metastasis and epidural spinal cord compression. Cancer. 1990;65:98–106.
27. Byrne TN. Spinal cord compression from epidural metastasis. N Engl J Med. 1992;327(9):614–9.
28. Siegal T. Spinal cord compression: from laboratory to clinic. Eur J Cancer. 1995;31A(11):1748–53.
29. Siegal T, Siegal TZ, Sandback U, et al. Experimental neoplastic spinal cord compression: evoked potentials, edema, prostaglandins, and light and electron microscopy. Spine. 1987;12(5): 440–8.
30. Ishikawa M, Sekizuka E, Krischek B, et al. Role if nitric oxide in the regulation of spinal arteriolar tone. Neurosurgery. 2002;50 (2):371–7.
31. Kato A, Ushio Y, Hayakawa T, et al. Circulatory disturbance of the spinal cord with epidural neoplasm in rats. J Neurosurg. 1985;63(2):260–5.
32. Schiff D, O'Neil BP, Suman VJ. Spinal epidural metastasis as the initial manifestation of malignancy: clinical features and diagnostic approach. Neurology. 1997;49:452–6.
33. Levack P, Graham J, Collie D, et al. Don't wait for a sensory level—listen to the symptoms: a prospective audit of the delays in diagnosis of malignant cord compression. Clin Oncol (R Coll Radiol). 2002;14(6):474–80.
34. Spinazzé S, Caraceni A, Schrijvers D. Epidural spinal cord compression. Crit Rev Oncol Hematol. 2005;56(3):397–506.
35. Gilbert RW, Kim JH, Posner JB. Epidural spinal cord compression from metastatic tumor: diagnosis and treatment. Ann Neurol. 1978;3:40–51.
36. Love JG. The differential diagnosis of intraspinal tumors and protruded intervertebral disks and their surgical treatment. J Neurosurg. 1944;1:275–90.
37. Prasad D, Schiff D. Malignant spinal-cord compression. Lancet Oncol. 2005;6:15–24.
38. Maxwell M, Chir MB, Borges LF, Zervas NT. Renal cell carcinoma: a rare source of cauda equina metastasis. J Neurosurg (Spine 1). 1999;90:129–32.
39. Shapiro S. Medical realities of cauda equina syndrome secondary to lumbar disk herniation. Spine. 2000;25(3):348–51.
40. Brice J, McKissock WS. Surgical treatment of malignant extradural spinal tumors. BMJ. 1965;i:1341–4.
41. Jacobs WD, Perrin RG. Evaluation and treatment of spinal metastasis: an overview. Neurosurg Focus. 2001;11(6):1–11.
42. Buckwalter JA, Brandser EA. Metastatic disease of the spine. Am Fam Physician. 1997;55:1761–8.
43. Ayyathurai R, Mahaptra R, Rajasudaram R, Srinivasan V, Archard NP, Toussi H. A study on staging bone scans in newly diagnosed prostate cancer. Urol Int. 2006;76:209–12.
44. Hsia TC, Shen YY, Yen RF, Kao CH, Changlai SP. Neoplasma. 2002;49(4):267–71.
45. Thrupkaew AK, Henkin RE, Quinn IL. False negative bone scans in disseminated metastatic disease. Radiology. 1974;113:383–6.
46. Gulenchyn KY, Papoff W. Technetium-99 m MDP scintigraphy; an insensitive tool for the detection of bone marrow metastasis. Clin Nucl Med. 1987;12:45–6.
47. Moog F, Bangerter M, Kotzerke J, Guhlmann A, Frickhofen N, Reske SN. 18-F-fluorodeoxyglucose-positron emission tomography as a new approach to detect lymphomatous bone marrow. J Clin Oncol. 1998;16:603–9.
48. Wu HC, Yen RF, Shen YY, Kao CH, Lin CC, Lee CC. Comparing whole body 18F-2-deoxyglucose positron emission tomography and technetium-99 m methylene diphosphate bone scan to detect bone metastasis in patients with renal cell carcinomas—a preliminary report. J Cancer Res Clin Ocol. 2002;128:503–6.

49. Jacobson AF. Bone scanning in metastatic disease. In: Collier BD Jr, Fogelman I, Rosenthall L, editors. Skeletal nuclear medicine. St. Louis: Mosby; 1996. p. 87–123.

50. Sicard JA, Forestier J. Méthode radiographique d'expolration de la cavité épidurale par le lipiodol. Rev Neurol. 1921;37:1264–6.

51. Husband DJ, Grant KA, Romaniuk CS. MRI and the diagnosis and treatment of suspected malignant spinal cord compression. Br J Radiol. 2001;74:15–23.

52. Stark RJ, Henson RA, Evans SJ. Spinal metastasis: a retrospective survey from a general hospital. Brain. 1982 Mar;105(Pt 1):189–213.

53. Resjó M, Harwood-Nash DC, Fitz CR, Chuang S. CT metrizamide myelography for intraspinal and paraspinal neoplasms in infants and children. AJR. 1979;132:367–72.

54. Karnaze MG, Gado MH, Sartor KJ, Hodges FJ 3rd. Comparison of MR and CT myelography in imaging the cervical and thoracic spine. AJR Am J Roentgenol. 1988;150(2):397–403.

55. Cook AM, Lau TN, Tomlinson MJ, Vaidya M, Wakeley CJ, Goddard P. Magnetic resonance imaging of the whole spine in suspected malignant spinal cord compression: impact on management. Clin Oncol (R Coll Radiol). 1998;10(1):39–43.

56. Perkins GL, Slater ED, Sanders GK. Serum tumor markers. Am Fam Physician. 2003;68(6):1075–82.

57. Tokuhashi Y, Mastsuzaki H, Toriyama S, et al. Scoring system for the perioperative evaluation of metastatic spine tumor prognosis. Spine. 1990;15:1110–3.

58. Marazano E, Latini P, Beneventi S, et al. Comparison of two different radiotherapy schedules for spinal cord compression in prostate cancer. Tumori. 1998;84:472–7.

59. Maranzano E, Latini P. Effectiveness of radiation therapy without surgery in metastatic spinal cord compression: final results from a prospective trial. Int J Radiation Oncol Biol Phys. 1995;32:959–67.

60. Berenson JR, Lichtenstein A, Porter L, et al. Long-term pamidronate treatment for advanced multiple myeloma patients reduces skeletal events. Myeloma Aredia Study Group. J Clin Oncol. 1998;16:593–602.

61. Hortobagyi GN, Theriault RL, Lipton A, et al. Long-term prevention of skeletal complications of metastatic breast cancer with pamidronate. Protocol 19 Aredia Breast Cancer Study Group. J Clin Oncol. 1998;16:2038–44.

62. Ushio Y, Posner R, Kim JH, et al. Experimental spinal cord compression by epidural neoplasm. Neurology. 1977;27:422–9.

63. Sorensen S, Helweg-Larsen S, Mouridsen H, et al. Effect of high-dose dexamethasone in carcinomatous metastatic spinal cord compression treated with radiotherapy: a randomized trial. Eur J Cancer. 1994;30A:22–7.

64. Loblaw DA, Perry J, Chambers A, Laperriere NJ. Systematic review of diagnosis and management of malignant extradural spinal cord compression: the cancer care Ontario practice guidelines initiative's neuro-oncology disease site group. J Neurooncol. 2005;23(9):2028–37.

65. Vecht CJ, Haaxma-Reiche H, van Putten WL, et al. Initial bolus of conventional versus high-dose dexamethasone in metastatic spinal compression. Neurology. 1989;39:1255–7.

66. Heimdal K, Hirschberg H, Slettebo H, Watne K, Nome O. High incidence of serious side effects of high-dose dexamethasone treatment in patients with epidural spinal cord compression. J Neurooncol. 1992;12:141–4.

67. Maranzano E, Latini P, Beneventi S, et al. Radiotherapy without steroids in selected metastatic spinal cord compression patients: a phase II trial. Am J Clin Oncol. 1996;19:179–83.

68. Siegal T. Spinal epidural involvement in haematological tumors: clinical features and therapeutic options. Leuk Lymphoma. 1991;5:101–10.

69. Cooper K, Bajorin D, Shapiro W, et al. Decompression of epidural metastasis from germ cell tumors with chemotherapy. J Neurooncol. 1990;8(3):275–80.

70. Barcena A, Lobato RD, Rivas JJ, Cordobes F, de Castro S, Cabrera A, et al. Spinal metastatic disease: analysis of factors determining functional prognosis and the choice of treatment. Neurosurgery. 1984;15:820–7.

71. Klimo P Jr, Kestle JR, Schmidt MH. Clinical trials and evidence-based medicine for metastatic spinal disease. Neurosurg Clin N Am. 2004;15:549–64.

72. Wu AS, Fourney DR. Evolution of treatment for metastatic spine disease. Neurosurg Clin N Am. 2004;15:401–11.

73. Helweg-Larsen S, Sorensen PS, Kreiner S. Prognostic factors in metastatic spinal cord compression: a prospective study using multivariate analysis of variables influencing survival and gait function in 153 patients. Int J Radiat Oncol Biol Phys. 2000;46:1163–9.

74. Helwig-Larsen S, Rasmussen B, Sorensen PS. Recovery of gait after radiotherapy in paralytic patients with metastatic epidural spinal cord compression. Neurology. 1990;40:1234–6.

75. Gagnon GJ, Nasr NM, Liao JJ, et al. Treatment of spinal tumors using CyberKnife fractionated stereotactic radiosurgery: pain and quality-of-life assessment after treatment in 200 patients. Neurosurgery. 2009;64:297–307.

76. Schultheiss TE. Spinal cord radiation tolerance. Int J Radiat Oncol Biol Phys. 1994;30:735–6.

77. Murakami H, Kawahara N, Yahata T, Yokoyama K, Komai K, Tomita K. Radiation myelopathy after radioactive iodine therapy for spine metastasis. Br J Radiol. 2006;79:e45–9.

78. Maddison P, Southern P, Johnson M. Clinical and MRI discordance in a case of delayed radiation myelopathy. J Neurol Neurosurg Psychiatry. 2000;69:563–4.

79. Wang PY, Shen WC, Jan JS. MR imaging in radiation myelopathy. Am J Neuroradiol. 1992;13:1049–55.

80. Michikawa M, Wada Y, Sano M, et al. Radiation myelopathy: significance of gadolinium-DTPA enhancement in the diagnosis. Neuroradiology. 1991;33:286–9.

81. Chow E, Danjoux C, Wong R, Szumacher E, Franssen E, Fung K, Finkelstein J, Andersson L, Connolly R. Palliation of bone metastasis: a survey of patterns of practice among Canadian oncologists. Radiother Oncol. 2000;56:305–14.

82. Wu JS, Wong RK, Lloyd NS, Johnston M, Bezjak A, Whelan T. Radiotherapy fractionation for the palliation of uncomplicated painful bone metastasis—an evidence-based practice guideline. BMC Cancer. 2004;4:71.

83. Rades D, Stalpers LJ, Schulte R, Veninga T, Basic H, Engenhart-Cabilic R, Schild SE, Hoskin PJ. Defining the appropriate radiotherapy regimen for metastatic spinal cord compression in non-small cell lung cancer patients. Eur J Cancer. 2006;42(8):1052–6.

84. Rades D, Stalpers LJ, Veninga T, et al. Evaluation of five radiation schedules and prognostic factors for metastatic spinal cord compression. J Clin Oncol. 2005;23:3366.

85. Marazano E, Bellavita R, Rossi R, et al. Short-course versus split-course radiotherapy in metastatic spinal cord compression: results of a phase III, randomized, multicenter trial. J Clin Oncol. 2005;23:3358.

86. Gersten PC, Burton SA, Ozhasoglu C, Welch WC. Radiosurgery for spinal metastases: clinical experience from 500 cases from a single institution. Spine. 2007;32:193–9.

87. Bate BG, Khan NR, Kimball BY, et al. Stereotactic radiosurgery for spinal metastases with or without separation surgery. J Neurosurg Spine. 2015;22:209–15.

88. Witham TF, Khavkin YA, Gallia GL, Wolinsky JP, Gokaslan ZL. Surgery Insight: current management of epidural spinal cord

compression from metastatic spine disease. Nat Clin Pract Neurol. 2006;2(2):87–94.

89. Laufer I, Iorgulescu JB, Chapman T, et al. Local disease control for spinal metastases following "separation surgery" and adjuvant hypofractionated or high-dose single-fraction stereotactic radiosurgery: outcome analysis in 186 patients. J Neurosurg Spine. 2013;18:207–14.

90. Kaloostian PE, Yurter A, Etame AB, et al. Palliative strategies for the management of primary and metastatic spinal tumors. Cancer Control. 2014;21:140–3.

91. Laufer I, Rubin DG, Lis E, et al. The NOMS framework: approach to the treatment of spinal metastatic tumors. Oncologist. 2013;18:744–51.

92. Fourney DR, Frangou EM, Ryken TC, et al. Spinal instability neoplastic score: an analysis of reliability and validity from the spine oncology study group. J Clin Oncol. 2011;29:3072–7.

93. Purkayastha S, Gupta AK, Kapilamoorthy TR, Kesavadas C, Thomas B, Krishnamoorth T, Bodhey NK. Percutaneous vertebroplasty in the management of vertebral lesions. Neurol India. 2005;53(2):167–73.

94. Huang TJ, Hsu RWW, Li YY, Cheng CC. Minimal access spinal surgery (MASS) in treating thoracic spine metastasis. Spine. 2006;31(16):1860–3.

95. Miller DJ, Lang FF, Walsh, GL, Abi-Said D, Wildrick DM, Gokaslan ZL. Coaxial double-lumen methylmethacrylate reconstruction in the anterior cervical and upper thoracic spine after tumor resection. J Neurosurg (Spine 2). 2000;92:181–90.

96. Fourney DR, Abi-Said D, Lang FF, McCutcheon I, Gokaslan ZL. Use of pedicle screw fixation in the management of malignant spinal disease: experience in 100 consecutive patients. J Neurosurg (Spine 1). 2001;94:25–37.

97. Oda I, Abumi K, Ito M, Kotani Y, Oya T, Hasegawa K, Minami A. Palliative spinal reconstruction using pedicle screws for metastatic lesions of the spine: a retrospective analysis of 32 cases. Spine. 2006;31(13):1439–44.

98. Mazel C, Hoffmann E, Antonietti P, Grunenwald D, Henry M, Williams J. Posterior cervicothoracic instrumentation in spine tumors. Spine. 2004;29(11):1246–53.

99. Patchell DA, Tibbs PA, Regine WF, Payne RP, Saris S, Kryscio RJ. Direct decompressive surgical resection in the treatment of spinal cord compression caused by metastatic cancer: a randomized trial. Lancet. 2005;366(9486):643–8.

100. Chason JL, Walker FB, Landers JW. Metastatic carcinoma in the central nervous system and dorsal root ganglia. Cancer. 1963;16:781–7.

101. Costigan DA, Winkelman MD. Intramedullary spinal cord metastasis. A clinicopathological study of 13 cases. J Neurosurg. 1985;62:227–33.

102. Kalaycı M, Çağavi F, Güi S, Yenidünya S, Açıkgöz B. Intramedullary spinal cord metastasis: diagnosis and treatment—and illustrated review. Acta Neurochir (Wien). 2004;146:1347–54.

103. Connolly S, Winfree C, McCormick P, et al. Intramedullary spinal cord metastasis: report of three cases and review of the literature. Surg Neurol. 1996;46:329–39.

104. Schiff D, O'Neil BP. Intramedullary spinal cord metastasis: clinical features and treatment outcomes. Neurology. 1996;47:906–12.

105. Edelson RN, Deck MDF, Posner JB. Intramedullary spinal cord metastasis. Neurology. 1972;22:1222–31.

106. Grem JL, Burgess J, Trump D. Clinical features and natural history of intramedullary spinal cord metastasis. Cancer. 1985;56:2305–14.

107. Villegas AE, Guthrie TH. Intramedullary spinal cord metastasis in breast cancer: clinical features, diagnosis, and therapeutic consideration. Breast J. 2004;10(6):532–5.

108. Conill C, Sanchez M, Puig S, Planas I, Castel T. Intramedullary spinal cord metastasis and melanoma. Melanoma Res. 2004;14:431–3.

109. Aryan HE, Azadeh F, Nakaji P, Imbesi SG, Abshire BB. Intramedullary spinal cord metastasis of lung adenocarcinoma presenting as Brown-Sequard syndrome. Surg Neurol. 2004; 61(1):72–6.

110. Winkelman MD, Adelstein DJ, Karling NL. Intramedullary spinal cord metastasis: diagnosis and therapeutic considerations. Arch Neurol. 1987;44:526–31.

111. Siegal T, Siegal T. Spinal metastasis. In: Principles of neuro-oncology, 1st ed. USA: McGraw-Hill; 2005. p. 581–606.

112. Jawahar A, Kondziolka D, Graces YI. Stereotactic radiosurgery for hemangioblastomas of the brain. Acta Neurochir. 2000;142:641–4.

Peripheral Nervous System Metastases as Complications of Systemic Cancer

Amanda C. Guidon

Introduction

Clinically apparent involvement of the peripheral nervous system (PNS) is common in cancer and occurs in approximately 10% of cases. The interaction between cancer and the PNS is multifaceted and complex [1]. First, cancer affects the PNS by different mechanisms. These mechanisms include: (1) compression or infiltration by the tumor; (2) treatment effect (radiation or chemotherapy), which may be delayed; (3) nutritional and metabolic factors; (4) infectious complications related to immunosuppression; and (5) paraneoplastic disorders. Second, precise anatomic localization is important. Cancer can affect any portion of the PNS and can be multifocal. Motor neuron, sensory or autonomic ganglia, nerve roots, plexus, cranial and peripheral nerve, neuromuscular junction and muscle can all be affected. Third, different cellular structures can be damaged including neuronal cell body, axon, or myelin. Finally, different cancers have different mechanisms for producing PNS lesions. For example, hematologic malignancies infiltrate peripheral nerve more frequently than solid tumors [1]. With this framework in mind, this chapter will review metastases to the peripheral nervous system.

Metastases to Nerve Roots

Leptomeningeal metastasis occurs when malignant cells seed the leptomeninges (the pia, arachnoid and cerebrospinal fluid (CSF) within the subarachnoid space). Patients with involvement of plexus or nerve from lymphoma, leukemia and rarely small cell lung cancer may develop leptomeningeal disease and sometimes even cord compression when neoplastic cells track into the epidural space or meninges. In general, leptomeningeal disease is diagnosed in 1–5% of patients with solid tumors (carcinomatous meningitis), 5–15% of patients with leukemia (leukemic meningitis) and lymphoma (lymphomatous meningitis), and 1–2% of patients with primary brain tumors. Melanoma, breast, and lung cancer are the most common primary sites to metastasize to the leptomeninges. Adenocarcinoma is the most common histological subtype. Leptomeningeal disease can rarely be the first manifestation of cancer (5–10%) or present after a period of remission (20%). However, more typically, it presents in patients with widespread and progressive systemic cancer (>70%) [2].

Cancer cells can spread to the meninges by several paths: hematogenous spread, either through Batson's plexus or arterial dissemination, direct extension from adjacent tumor deposits and through centripetal migration from systemic tumors along perineural or perivascular spaces. Once cancer cells arrive in the subarachnoid space, CSF flow disseminates them. This process results in potentially multifocal seeding of the leptomeninges. Conversely, impairment of CSF flow may also occur due to tumor-related adhesions [2].

See Figs. 7.1a–d and 7.2.

Presentation

Spinal nerve roots and cranial nerves can be affected by leptomeningeal disease. The finding of disease at several points along the neuraxis in a patient with known malignancy suggests leptomeningeal disease. However, patients may also present with isolated findings such as a cranial mononeuropathy or cauda equina syndrome. Patients may appear clinically to have a polyradiculopathy or lower motor neuron disease. Differential diagnosis at presentation includes other forms of chronic meningitis such as fungal infection, sarcoid, and tuberculosis [2]. Inflammatory processes, which can be related to immunotherapy for the patient's cancer, can also present with nerve root or leptomeningeal enhancement [3].

A.C. Guidon (✉)
Department of Neurology—Harvard Medical School,
Massachusetts General Hospital, Neuromuscular Diagnostic
Center, 165 Cambridge Street Ste 820, Boston, MA 02114, USA
e-mail: aguidon@partners.org

© Springer International Publishing AG 2018
D. Schiff et al. (eds.), *Cancer Neurology in Clinical Practice*,
DOI 10.1007/978-3-319-57901-6_7

(a)   (b)

(c)   (d)

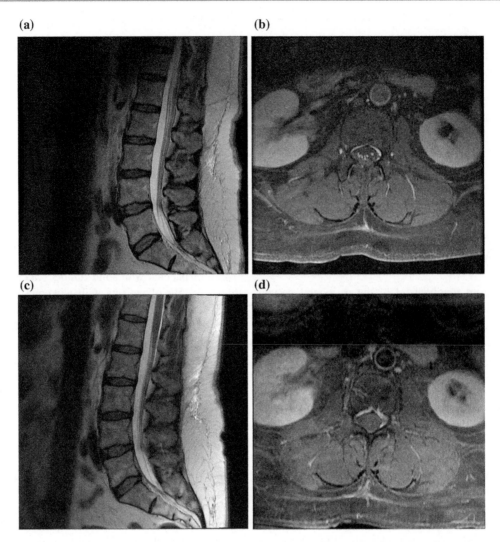

Fig. 7.1 A 56 year old patient with a T1bN0M0 melanoma, not on immunotherapy, presented with bilateral, asymmetric lower extremity and left upper extremity weakness with associated back pain and without significant sensory symptoms. EDX demonstrated polyradiculopathy. Three separate lumbar punctures showed normal cell count, elevated protein and negative cytology. Extensive infectious work-up was negative. MRI lumbar spine showed smooth linear enhancement of the cauda equine (**a, b**). Deficits and MRI abnormalities improved over 1 year with IVIG therapy (**c, d**). Diagnosis was an immune-mediated polyradiculopathy (Copyright by Amanda C. Guidon, MD)

Imaging and Evaluation

Magnetic resonance imaging with gadolinium enhancement is the preferred imaging modality to evaluate patients with suspected leptomeningeal disease. When diffuse leptomeningeal disease is suspected, imaging of the brain and entire spine is required. A normal MRI does not exclude the diagnosis, as a 30% false negative rate exists [2]. Additionally, the diagnostic value of MRI may be less in patients with hematologic malignancies than with solid tumors [4]. This is likely attributable to the propensity of solid tumors to adhere to neural structures and form nodules [5]. In a patient with known malignancy and a typical presentation for leptomeningeal disease, however, an abnormal MRI alone can establish the diagnosis [2].

CSF examination with intracranial pressure measurement is the most useful laboratory test in the diagnosis of leptomeningeal metastasis. Cytology is considered the gold standard for diagnosis. The presence of malignant cells in CSF is diagnostic of leptomeningeal disease. However, cytologic analysis frequently cannot attribute the cells to a specific primary tumor. Abnormal CSF may be merely suggestive of but not diagnostic for leptomeningeal disease. The sensitivity for detecting malignancy when present is 65% on initial LP, which then increases to 80% after a second LP. Even after three lumbar punctures, false negative

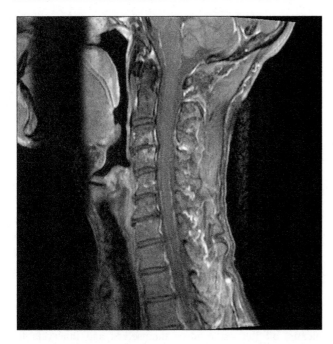

Fig. 7.2 A 54 year old patient with metastatic melanoma treated with nivolumab followed by ipilimumab, presented with diplopia, back pain, progressive sensory symptoms, weakness and gastroparesis. Lumbar puncture showed elevated protein, normal glucose, normal cell count and no evidence of malignancy. MRI brain showed abnormal enhancement along multiple cranial nerves and coating the dorsal and ventral brainstem. Leptomeningeal enhancement also involved the cervical and thoracic spinal cord, conus medularis and cauda equina. He subsequently developed a CIDP-like peripheral neuropathy. Symptoms and enhancement improved after stopping immunotherapy and treatment with high dose corticosteroids and intravenous immunoglobulin (*IVIG*) (Copyright by Amanda C. Guidon, MD)

rate can be approximately 10% [2, 5]. Dissociation between cell count and cytology results may also exist [6]. Further complicating CSF analysis is the potential variability of CSF protein, glucose, and malignant cell at different levels of the neuraxis, even in the absence of CSF obstruction. Obtaining CSF from a site that is not symptomatically or radiographically affected, withdrawing small amounts of CSF (<10 ml), delayed processing, and analyzing only one sample are all associated with false negative results. Low sensitivity poses a challenge to diagnosis of leptomeningeal disease as well as assessing response to therapies [2]. CSF flow cytometry is useful in evaluating hematologic tumors and may be superior to cytology when evaluating for leptomeningeal disease [6]. MR imaging looking for enhancement should preferentially be obtained prior to LP; lumbar puncture itself can rarely cause a meningeal reaction leading to dural-arachnoid enhancement. In situations where there is no systemic manifestation of malignancy, CSF is inconclusive and the suspicion for leptomeningeal disease remains high, meningeal or nerve root biopsy from an enhancing region may be diagnostic [2].

Treatment

Early diagnosis of neoplastic leptomeningeal disease can afford a better prognosis. Treatment is intended primarily to stabilize neurologic function and prolong survival. Median survival with treatment still remains poor and for solid tumors is 2.3 months and for hematopoietic tumors is 4.7 months [5]. Response to treatment is difficult to assess, as there is a lack of standardized treatments and most studies treat all subtypes equivalently. Treatment may include a combination of surgery, radiation, systemic, and intrathecal chemotherapy, and supportive care. Radiation is often used for bulky disease or if CSF flow is obstructed [2].

Metastases to Plexus

Approximately one in a hundred patients with cancer will experience neoplastic plexopathy. Two large retrospective reviews from cancer hospitals showed a frequency of neoplastic brachial plexopathy at 0.43% and lumbosacral plexopathy 0.71%. However, the incidence is higher in certain cancer subtypes. For example, up to 5% of patients with breast cancer may experience neoplastic plexopathy within 5 years following treatment [7, 8]. Knowledge of plexus anatomy helps the clinician localize the area of abnormality. Differential diagnosis of plexopathy in cancer patients includes: radiation plexopathy (most common alternate consideration), epidural cord compression, neoplastic meningitis, primary plexus tumor, chemotoxicity (intraarterial therapy), (paraneoplastic) immune-mediated plexopathy, and postinfectious plexopathy [9].

Cervical Plexus

Cervical Plexus Anatomy

The cervical plexus is formed by the ventral rami of the first four spinal nerves (C1–C4), in a series of irregular loops. The plexus is situated close to the upper four vertebrae, between the deep anterior and lateral muscles of the neck, anterior to the middle scalene and deep to the sternocleidomastoid. Braches form cutaneous, muscular, and communicating nerves. The cutaneous branches (lesser occipital, great auricular, supraclavicular, and transverse cutaneous nerves of the neck) contain sensory information from the skin and soft tissues of the scalp and neck. The cervical plexus also provides motor innervation to several muscles including the diaphragm (via the phrenic nerve), sternocleidomastoid and trapezius (via the accessory nerve) and other deep cervical and hyoid muscles [9, 10]. There are also communicating branches to the accessory, hypoglossal, vagus, and sympathetic nerves [11].

Presentation of Cervical Plexopathy

Metastatic spread to cervical plexus typically occurs from neighboring tissue. Cancer may invade the plexus directly or indirectly via regional lymph nodes or bone (clavicle, first rib, or cervical vertebral bodies). Squamous cell carcinoma of the head and neck, lymphoma and adenocarcinoma of the lung and breast are the most commonly associated tumors [9].

Patients who develop metastatic disease in this area most commonly describe pain and stiffness in the neck, shoulder or throat. The pain is typically unrelenting and may worsen with coughing, swallowing and neck movement. General examination may be surprisingly normal or may demonstrate tender neck musculature unilaterally, palpable tumors or firm anterior or posterior cervical or supraclavicular lymph nodes. Patients often describe vague numbness, paresthesias, pressure, or burning; however, objective sensory loss may be difficult to identify. Additionally prior surgery in the area which can produce numbness in the skin of the anterior neck and submandibular area may complicate assessment of new sensory deficits. Clarifying the temporal relationship of symptom onset and surgery can help distinguish between these two etiologies [9].

Additional clinical manifestations depend on the area of the cervical plexus involved. Abnormality of the spinal accessory nerve or C3/4 roots may produce weakness of the trapezius. This typically manifests as shoulder weakness and scapular depression and winging, most notable with shoulder abduction. Phrenic involvement can present with an elevated and/or paralyzed hemi-diaphragm. Patients describe dyspnea, which is worse when supine. Unilateral weakness of the sternocleidomastoid, deep cervical, and hyoid muscles is typically asymptomatic. A history or exam suggestive of myelopathy raises the suspicion for epidural spread. Given the close proximity, manifestations of skull base, or brachial plexus involvement may also be present [9, 12].

Electrodiagnostic Findings in Cervical Plexopathy

EMG (Electromyography) and NCS (nerve conduction studies) are more limited in the assessment of involvement of the cervical plexus than the brachial or lumbosacral plexus but can add important information. In phrenic neuropathy, the phrenic CMAP (compound muscle action potential) may be abnormal and neurogenic changes may be seen on needle EMG of the diaphragm. In spinal accessory neuropathy, the CMAP of the spinal accessory nerve may be abnormal when recording from the trapezius and needle EMG of the trapezius and/or sternocleidomastoid may reveal neurogenic changes. These abnormalities in the phrenic nerve/diaphragm and spinal accessory nerve/trapezius can

also be seen in a radiculopathy or segmental myelopathy affecting the C3/4/5 and C3/4 myotomes, respectively. Needle EMG of the upper and mid-cervical paraspinals can also reveal abnormal spontaneous activity suggestive of neurogenic abnormality. If metastatic disease is confined to the cervical plexus, routine median, ulnar and radial sensory, and motor responses should be normal [11].

Brachial Plexus

Brachial Plexus Anatomy

The brachial plexus supplies the motor and sensory innervation of most of the upper limb. It is an arrangement of nerve fibers that runs from the spine (C5-T1 roots) through the neck, axilla, and into the arm. As the nerve fibers run proximally to distally, they are arranged into trunks, divisions, cords and individual nerve branches. The phrenic, dorsal scapular, and long thoracic nerve exit proximal to the plexus, off the nerve roots themselves and innervate the diaphragm, rhomboids and serratus anterior respectively. The ventral rami of the C5-T1 nerve roots then form three trunks: upper (C5/6), middle (C7) and lower (C8/T1). They are named with respect to their orientation to one another. They occupy a superficial position as they traverse the posterior cervical triangle. The lower trunk is adjacent to the lung apex and near the subclavian artery. Each trunk then divides into two divisions, anterior, and posterior. These divisions are retroclavicular and run between the middle third of the clavicle and the first rib. The three posterior divisions then form the posterior cord. The anterior divisions of the upper and middle trunk form the lateral cord and the anterior division of the lower trunk continues as the medial cord. The cords are named for their orientation to the axillary artery and are situated proximally in the axilla, next to the axillary lymph node chain. The posterior cord gives rise to the thoracodorsal nerve (latissimus dorsi), subscapular nerve (subscapularis), axillary nerve (deltoid), and radial nerve (triceps, brachioradialis, wrist, and finger extensors) and provides sensory supply to the posterior arm and forearm. The lateral cord divides into two branches: the musculocutaneous nerve and a branch, which joins a portion of the medial cord to form the median nerve. The rest of the medial cord forms the median and ulnar nerves and gives off the medial brachial cutaneous nerves of the arm and forearm, which supply sensation to the medial portion of the arm and forearm. The five terminal nerves of the upper extremity (musculocutaneous, axillary, median, ulnar, and radial) are distally situated in the axilla [11, 13].

Neoplastic Syndromes of the Brachial Plexus

Approximately 70% of tumors involving the brachial plexus come from either lung or breast. The remaining 30% percent arise from a combination of lymphoma, sarcoma, or others [8]. Most metastases to the brachial plexus involve the lower trunk or medial cord. Rarely, primary head or neck neoplasms grow inferiorly and invade the upper portions of the plexus. Sometimes plexus involvement is patchy. Neoplastic invasion of the plexus is rarely the earliest manifestation of cancer, except in Pancoast syndrome, which is typically caused by carcinoma at the apex of the lung invading the lower trunk/medical cord of the brachial plexus [11].

Pain is the most common presenting symptom of neoplastic brachial plexopathy. Typically, the pain originates in the shoulder or axilla and radiates along the medial arm and forearm and into the fourth and fifth digits and can be severe. In a large series, pain upon initial presentation was present in 75% of cases [8]. Sensory loss can follow the same distribution. Motor deficits most commonly (75%) affect the lower plexus. As such, patients will typically have weakness in intrinsic hand muscles, finger and wrist flexion and extension. Approximately one in five patients have an associated Horner's syndrome due to involvement of the sympathetic trunk or ganglia near the first thoracic vertebrae. Given the proximity of this lesion to the spinal cord, a Horner's syndrome should prompt a thorough evaluation for intraspinal disease [8].

Differential diagnosis of neoplastic brachial plexopathy depends on whether the patient has received radiation therapy (RT). In patients who have received RT, the principal alternate diagnosis is radiation-induced brachial plexopathy. In patients who have received prior radiation and have a delayed brachial plexopathy, a radiation-induced nerve sheath tumor of the brachial plexus is also a consideration. This is much less common than radiation-induced brachial plexopathy and may develop 4–40 years after RT. Often presenting as a painful enlarging mass, these tumors are usually malignant. Radiation-induced arteritis may also be seen in patients with radiation-induced plexopathies. Chronic ischemic symptoms and signs can present in the arm and hand or they may have episodic discoloration in the fingers from emboli. This may appear similar to atherosclerotic disease on arteriography. In a patient with known malignancy who has not undergone radiation to the upper chest, the main alternate diagnoses are perioperative brachial plexus trauma or an unrelated episode of acute brachial plexus neuropathy. Primary tumors of the brachial plexus are rare. Most are benign peripheral nerve sheath tumors, including neurofibromas and benign schwannomas [11].

Lumbrosacral Plexus

Lumbosacral Plexus Anatomy

The lumbosacral plexus is derived from the ventral rami of the L1-S4 nerve roots and is made up of two sections. The upper portion is the lumbar plexus, which arises from the L1–L4 nerves roots with variable contribution from T12. The lower portion is the lumbosacral plexus, which arises from the L4-S4 nerve roots. The lumbosacral plexus lies within the psoas major muscle and exits from the lateral edge of the muscle. In general, the lumbosacral plexus supplies motor and sensory functions to the ipsilateral leg and pelvic girdle. The upper portion of the plexus gives rise to several major nerves: the iliohypogastric nerve (T12-L1), the ilioinguinal nerve (L1), the genitofemoral nerve (L1–2), the lateral femoral cutaneous nerve (L2–4), and the obturator nerve (L2–4). Major motor functions include hip flexion and adduction, and knee extension. The upper plexus supplies sensation to the groin, thigh (anterior, lateral, medial), and the medial portion of the leg. The lower portion of the plexus also gives rise to several major nerves: superior gluteal nerve (L4-S1), the inferior gluteal nerve (L5-S2), the sciatic nerve (L4-S3, consisting of the tibial and peroneal components), the posterior femoral cutaneous nerve (S1–S3), and the pudendal nerve. Major motor functions include hip abduction, hip extension, knee flexion, ankle movements, and control of the urinary and anal sphincters. It provides sensory function from the lower extremity distal to the knee (except the medial lower leg), posterior thigh, buttocks, and perineal region [14].

Neoplastic Syndromes of the Lumbrosacral Plexus

Metastatic lumbosacral plexopathy occurs most commonly from direct extension of abdominal and pelvic tumors. Occasionally, however, the plexus is affected by growth from metastases to regional lymph nodes or bony structures. Colorectal cancer is the most common primary tumor. Colorectal cancer along with retroperitoneal sarcoma and breast cancer account for almost half the cases. Lymphoma, cervical cancer, and other malignancies account for the remaining cases. In approximately 15% of patients, plexopathy is part of the initial presentation of cancer. Tumor can either directly invade the plexus or can track along connective tissue or epineurium. When tumor cells track, the presence of cancer can be difficult to demonstrate on imaging. Metastatic plexopathy is typically unilateral, but is bilateral in 25% of patients [9].

Metastatic lumbosacral plexopathy begins with leg pain in nearly all patients, which is followed by numbness and weakness. In a series of 85 patients, pain was so common during the course (98%) and at presentation (91%), that the authors indicated its absence should prompt consideration of alternate diagnoses [7]. Like with brachial plexopathy, the pain is typically constant, dull and aching. Sharp, radicular pain often coexists. Valsalva may exacerbate pain. Patients describe difficulty finding a comfortable position but lying supine may be particularly uncomfortable. Lying with hips flexed can relieve the pain if there is involvement of the iliopsoas [7].

Weakness and sensory disturbance develops in the majority of patients. Leg weakness (86%), sensory loss (73%), reflex loss (64%), and leg edema (47%) are the most common presenting features. A rectal mass may also be present. The distribution of numbness or weakness depends on which part of the plexus is affected. In this same series of 85 patients, the upper plexus (L1–4) was involved in 31% of patients, and the lower plexus (L5-S3) in 51%, while 18% had a pan-plexopathy [7]. In colorectal neoplasms and cervical carcinoma, the sacral plexus is most commonly involved. Accordingly, these patients typically have pain in the posterior thigh, leg or calf and weakness of ankle plantar flexion and knee flexion. Sensory disturbance may involve the posterior leg and sole of the foot [7]. Approximately 20–30% of patients describe a unilateral "hot dry foot." The foot is objectively warm and has hypohydrosis. This is a manifestation of interruption of sympathetic ganglia or postganglionic fibers along the lumbosacral plexus or the peripheral nerves below the L3 segment. This can be an important localizing feature. Autonomic disturbances are not present with lesions of the nerve roots or cauda equina. These autonomic symptoms may precede the onset of weakness or numbness by several months or occur simultaneously [15]. When the upper plexus is involved, patients typically experience pain and sensory changes in the anterior thigh, groin and into the dorsum of the foot. Sarcoma is the most common neoplasm to present in this fashion. Loss of strength affects thigh muscles producing difficulty arising from a low-seated position or walking down stairs. Involvement of the lumbosacral trunk can produce foot drop, which is distinguished from a peroneal neuropathy by weakness of ankle inversion. Incontinence and impotence may be present, typically with bilateral plexus involvement. Pan-plexopathies, most commonly caused by genitourinary malignancies, can cause a combination of these findings [7, 9].

Imaging Evaluation of Brachial and Lumbosacral Plexus

CT, MR, and FDG-PET imaging are primary imaging modalities used to distinguish between malignant plexopathy, radiation-induced plexopathy, and radiation-induced tumor. MRI with and without contrast is generally the preferred method to confirm the diagnosis of suspected malignant plexopathy. The sensitivity of MRI for detecting malignant plexopathy is approximately 80% [9, 16]. Additionally, the presence of tumor recurrence either on imaging or clinical exam in the region of the plexus further supports the diagnosis of plexopathy. Therefore, for example, MRI of the lumbar spine and the pelvis complement plexus imaging in the case of suspected malignant lumbosacral plexopathy.

Typically, a mass is seen in direct contact with the plexus or the expected course of a nerve that is clinically affected. Less commonly, thickening of the components of the plexus or abnormal signal in a nerve may be seen [17]. MR evidence of epidural lesions strongly suggests metastatic disease. However, malignant tissue may also infiltrate the plexus without distorting tissue planes and CT/MRI may not detect it. If MRI is normal or inconclusive, FDG-PET/CT is a reasonable next step. It may show increased uptake in the region of the plexus involved by the metastasis [18]. Additionally, combining diffusion weighted MR neurography with conventional MRI may improve detection of brachial plexopathy in symptomatic patients with known malignancy [19]. Plain radiographs or bone scan may support the diagnosis of malignant plexopathy if there is tumor in adjacent bones or lung. Finally, if there is a high suspicion for malignant plexopathy and the initial imaging is negative, repeating the MRI 4–6 weeks later may reveal a tumor that was not apparent on initial scans.

Radiation-induced plexopathy also produces variable appearance on MRI. Radiation fibrosis may appear as (1) diffuse thickening and enhancement of the brachial plexus without a focal mass or (2) soft tissue changes with low signal intensity (similar to muscle) on both T1- and T2-weighted images. T2-weighted images sometimes help distinguish radiation-induced fibrosis from tumor infiltration, as the former more frequently demonstrates low signal intensity and the later more frequently demonstrates a higher signal intensity. Routine administration of gadolinium is less helpful as both radiation-induced fibrosis and metastatic disease can show some degree of post-contrast enhancement [20]. Surgical exploration to obtain a biopsy should be considered in the event of persistent diagnostic uncertainty, however, even biopsy can be inconclusive [11].

Electrodiagnosis of Plexopathy

Electrodiagnostic studies (EDX) serve as an extension of the physical examination to help localize the lesion to plexus and exclude disorders of the nerve roots or peripheral nerve. In general, the sensory responses are spared in root lesions and affected in plexus lesions. EDX can also further delineate which root(s) and/or which part(s) of the plexus are affected. EDX also help delineate severity and chronicity of the process and exclude alternate peripheral neuropathic etiologies for symptoms.

The hallmark EDX abnormality which supports lower trunk/medial cord plexopathy is the combination of an abnormal or absent ulnar SNAP (sensory nerve action potential), ulnar CMAP, and median CMAP, with a normal median SNAP. Additionally, the radial SNAP and lateral antebrachial cutaneous responses are normal and the medial antebrachial cutaneous response is abnormal. EMG shows neurogenic changes in muscles with a C8/T1, medial cord, and lower trunk distribution.

In a lumbar plexopathy, nerve conduction study abnormalities may be limited to an abnormal femoral motor and saphenous sensory response. Needle EMG reveals abnormalities in the quadriceps, hip flexors, and adductors. In a low lumbosacral plexopathy, additional sensory and motor responses are abnormal and needle EMG of muscles with an L5/S1 innervation are abnormal [21]. In both cases, lumbar paraspinal muscles are expected to be spared; however, in reality, this can be variable. EDX for assessment of metastatic lumbosacral plexopathy can be limited or inconclusive for several reasons. First routine studies do not assess the inferior portion of the sacral plexus with contribution from the S2–S4 roots. Additionally, in this patient population, prior treatment with chemotherapy or age alone can affect the sensory responses in the lower extremities. Structural lumbar spine disease may coexist with cancer. All these factors can complicate interpretation of EDX for plexopathy. As such, EDX are used as one piece of the evaluation in combination with imaging [22].

Radiation-Induced Plexopathy

In patients previously treated with radiation, clinicians often must distinguish between radiation-induced brachial or lumbosacral plexopathy and recurrent tumor. At times, these conditions coexist. Radiation-induced plexopathy sometimes occurs as a mild reversible syndrome. Much more commonly it presents after a latent period ranging from several months to many years, with onset of neurologic symptoms most commonly 2–4 years after radiation. The precise pathophysiology of delayed radiation-induced plexopathy remains unclear. RT can injure the plexus both by direct toxic effects on axons and the vasa nervorum and also secondary microinfarction. Widespread fibrosis within and surrounding nerve, with demyelination and axonal loss, are consistently found at surgery and/or autopsy [23].

Presentation

Radiation plexopathy is more common than neoplastic plexopathy. However, reliably estimating the incidence is challenging for several reasons. (1) Reviews may have limited follow-up periods. Studies with longer follow-up report a higher incidence due to delayed onset, (2) The possible connection of presenting symptoms with prior RT may be overlooked and (3) Many different RT protocols have been used. As an example, in breast cancer, the incidence of radiation-induced brachial plexopathy varies in accordance to radiation technique. Incidence ranges from approximately 66% with 60 Gy in 5 Gy fractions as was

used in the 1960s to approximately 1% with the regimen of 50 Gy in 2 Gy fractions used in contemporary treatment [24]. The risk of radiation-induced brachial plexopathy may be increased with the use of large RT fields, two separate courses of "subthreshold" RT and possibly when patients receive concurrent chemotherapy with RT [9, 23]. The majority of patients with radiation-induced brachial plexopathy will worsen gradually over the course of several years to severe neurologic disability whereas others will stabilize after 1–3 years. Recovery of function is unusual.

Radiation-induced injury of the lumbosacral plexus most frequently occurs after treatment of pelvic or testicular tumors and tumors involving para-aortic lymph nodes. Patients may present after external bean photon therapy, interstitial or intracavitary radiation implants, or combined photon and proton beam RT. Bowel or bladder symptoms are unusual and more often attributed to RT induced proctitis or bladder fibrosis. RT lumbosacral plexopathy also tends to progress slowly over months to years, though a few patients may progress more rapidly or demonstrate spontaneous stabilization or improvement [23].

Electrodiagnostic Evaluation

Electrodiagnostic studies can lend support for a diagnosis of radiation-induced brachial plexopathy or lumbosacral plexopathy. Most characteristics of radiation-induced brachial plexopathy look identical to neoplastic plexopathy. Nerve conduction studies are abnormal in the vast majority (90%) of both neoplastic brachial plexopathy and radiation-induced brachial plexopathy. On needle EMG, abnormal spontaneous activity (fibrillations/positive sharp waves and fasciculations) are seen in both entities, as are reinnervation changes in motor unit potential morphology. Myokymic discharges are the only electrodiagnostic feature, which can be useful in distinguishing radiation-induced brachial or lumbosacral plexopathy. In one series, this finding was present in approximately 60% of patients, compared to <5% of patients with neoplastic brachial plexopathy [25]. Myokymic discharges are spontaneous, grouped repetitive discharges of the same motor unit seen on needle EMG. Clinically, these discharges can sometimes be seen as involuntary rippling or quivering of muscle on physical examination. Additionally, these myokymic discharges are present in a larger percentage of muscles (approximately 25%) in the radiation plexopathy group, most commonly in the pronator teres and abductor pollicis brevis. Interestingly, in this cohort, the patients with neoplastic plexopathy who had myokymic discharges had received prior radiation therapy. Fibrillation potentials can also be seen in paraspinal muscles in a larger percentage of patients (approximately 20%) in the radiation plexopathy group, possibly due to inclusion of the posterior rami, nerve roots or the paraspinal muscles themselves in the field of radiation. Conduction block with proximal stimulation for CMAPs may sometimes be observed; however, these proximal responses can be technically challenging [25].

Treatment for Malignant and Radiation-Induced Plexopathies

Treatment for malignant plexopathy due to metastatic cancer is mainly symptom-based and aimed at eliminating or shrinking the tumor, if possible, with chemotherapy and/or radiation. Typically, pain remains prominent and pharmacologic and interventional strategies for pain management are required. Patients may benefit from being seen in a pain clinic. Treatment for radiation-induced brachial and lumbosacral plexopathy has generally been studied only in case reports or case series. Treatments have included surgical intervention and hyperbaric oxygen therapy, both of which showed no improvement and patients may actually worsen with surgery [23]. Anticoagulation has provided anecdotal improvement in symptoms and conduction block on EDX but is not standard of care [26]. Physical therapy can be important to help prevent secondary musculoskeletal complications in brachial plexopathy and aide in mobility with lumbosacral plexopathy. Primary prevention using the lowest dose and most targeted radiotherapy is paramount [9].

Metastases to Peripheral Nerve

As secondary malignant tumors, metastases must be distinguished from other mass lesions arising from peripheral nerve, including primary malignant peripheral nerve tumors. In general, these lesions fall into several categories: benign non-neoplastic nerve tumors (e.g., neuroma, lipoma), benign neoplasms of non-neural sheath origin (e.g., hemangioma), benign nerve sheath neoplasms (e.g., neurofibroma, schwannoma), and malignant peripheral nerve sheath tumors (e.g., MPNSTs).

Presentation

In general, benign lesions tend to be slowly progressive whereas malignant tumors tend to grow rapidly with progressive pain and/or neurologic deficit. Taking a careful family history to assess for the possibility of an underlying neurogenic disorder such as neurofibromatosis or schwannomatosis is important, particularly in patients without a known primary malignancy [27].

Cancer infrequently affects peripheral nerve; however, it can do so in several ways. The first is through direct compression of the nerve from nearby metastasis. Metastases to the skull base, which occur most commonly in prostate, breast, and lung cancer as well as lymphoma, can cause compression of surrounding nerves [28]. This is most commonly a late stage of cancer where patients already have widespread bone metastases. Craniofacial pain with accompanying cranial nerve palsies alerts the clinician to this complication. The symptoms correlate with the location of the metastasis and which adjacent nerve is compressed. Syndromes include orbital syndrome (frontal headache, proptosis, ophthamoplegia, decreased vision), cavernous sinus syndrome (ophthalmoplegia, facial numbness, and periorbital swelling), middle fossa syndrome/gasserian ganglion syndrome (atypical facial pain and paresthesias), jugular foramen syndrome (occipital pain, hoarseness, dysphagia), and occipital condyle syndrome (occipital pain, dysarthria due to CN XII palsy). Metastases to the mandible or skull base can cause compression of the inferior alveolar nerve. This causes "numb chin" syndrome characterized by oral and facial numbness in the distribution of the mental nerve over the chin and lower lip [28].

In addition to compression of nearby nerves, metastases can also spread via local extension to cranial or peripheral nerves with resulting neurologic dysfunction. One example of this is a vocal cord paralysis from lung cancer through invasion of the recurrent laryngeal nerve from invasion of mediastinal lymph nodes [29]. Other intraneural metastases are rare, presumably due to a protective blood-nerve barrier; however, case reports exist [30–32].

Presentation of Neurolymphomatosis

Neurolymphomatosis (NL) is infiltration of the peripheral nervous system by lymphoma. Malignant lymphocytic infiltrates can occur in root, plexus, or peripheral nerve. NL is distinct from other disorders affecting peripheral nerve associated with lymphoma such as irradiation, chemotherapy or paraneoplastic phenomenon [33]. The vast majority of cases are diffuse large B cell lymphoma. T cell lymphomas and acute leukemias have been reported rarely [34]. NL is rare but precise incidence is unknown. One series estimated an annual incidence of 3 cases per 100 new cases of intermediate/high-grade B cell NHL [35]. Clinical presentation is variable but generally follows 4 typical patterns: (1) Painful involvement of multiple peripheral nerves or nerve roots; (2) cranial neuropathy with or without pain; (3) painless involvement of multiple peripheral nerves; (4) painful or painless involvement of a single peripheral nerve [33]. Additionally, NL affects more than one anatomic structure in approximately 60% of patients and involvement of plexus may also occur. In approximately 25% of patients, NL is the initial manifestation of malignancy. Alternatively, NL can present as a relapse or progression of previously treated disease. When neuropathy is present, a mixed sensory and motor neuropathy is most common. Pure motor neuropathies have been reported and a pure sensory neuropathy has been described in one patient [34]. Some patients may have demyelinating features on EDX, which, at times, can fulfill criteria for diagnosis of chronic inflammatory demyelinating polyradiculoneuropathy (CIDP). As such, diagnosis can be challenging. Some patients even respond temporarily to treatment for CIDP [steroids and/or intravenous immunoglobulin (IVIG)], further clouding diagnosis [36]. In older series, diagnosis was established only at autopsy in almost half of patients [33]. This rate of postmortem diagnosis has reduced substantially to less than 10% in more recent series likely due to increased awareness of NL and advances in imaging. Despite these advances, diagnosis is often delayed and remains challenging [34].

Diagnosis of Neurolymphomatosis

Diagnostic evaluation includes electrodiagnostic studies for localization and characterization, imaging (MRI and sometimes FDG-PET-CT scan), CSF analysis typically including cytology and flow cytometry and nerve biopsy if the rest of the evaluation is inconclusive. Diagnostic yield of MRI and PET-CT is high, with abnormal findings observed in 77 and 84%, respectively, in one series [34]. MRI abnormalities include abnormal enhancement of the affected neural structure. Nerve thickening is observed in approximately 50% of patients and can be diffuse (17%) or nodular (30%). These MRI findings, however, are non-specific and can sometimes be seen in acute or chronic polyradiculoneuropathies, neurofibromatosis, and malignant peripheral nerve sheath tumors [34].

CSF findings in NL have also been reported in detail. In one series, protein was elevated in 61%, glucose low in 11%, elevated cell count (>5 cells/mm^3) in 44%. Cytology was malignant in 40% or suspicious in 13%. Some patients have abnormal or suspicious cytology in the face of a normal cell count. Additionally, CSF cell count may be elevated in patients who have no abnormality on imaging studies [34]. In this series, nerve biopsy was performed in just over 50% of patients and was abnormal, demonstrating NL, in 88% of patients. Nerve biopsy must be performed of a clinically affected structure, which can be challenging based on which areas are commonly affected; common and less invasive biopsy sites, including the sural nerve, may be unaffected [34]. These insights highlight the importance of multi-modal evaluation to arrive at the correct diagnosis of NL, particularly in patients who do not have an established diagnosis of hematologic malignancy.

See Figs. 7.3a–c, 7.4a, b, and 7.5a, b [37].

Treatment of Neurolymphomatosis

Treatment of NL consists of chemotherapy or chemotherapy combined with radiation. Defined standards are lacking and optimal management is unknown. Intra-CSF chemotherapy and standard craniospinal radiation fields will not treat all involved areas as NL often involves nerve roots within and beyond the subarachnoid space, and multiple sites are often involved. Chemotherapy protocols are often based on those to treat CNS involvement by lymphoma. Limited field radiotherapy can be effective in treating refractory pain from a particular area of nerve, plexus, or root involvement. Clinical improvement (reduction of pain and/or functional recovery) and radiographic resolution (improvement of nerve root enlargement/enhancement or normalization of FDG-PET uptake) has been observed in 50–70% of treated patients. Limited data exist about overall survival in this group and this may depend on whether the NL was part of the primary presentation or secondary. In general, in one series, median survival from diagnosis of NL was 10 months with 24% surviving at least 36 months [34]. Some patients may relapse solely with NL despite ongoing complete remission in sites outside the nervous system [35].

Metastases to Muscle

Overall, the prevalence of skeletal muscle metastasis is low and depending on the series of patients and modality used to detect them, ranges from 0.03 to 17.5%. Because they are rare, trauma, hematoma and abscess should be considered on the differential. Several benign and malignant entities including muscle hemangioma, intramuscular ganglion, myxoma and ischiogluteal bursitis, and sarcoma can mimic intramuscular metastases [38].

Several mechanisms for intramuscular metastatic spread have been proposed. Arterial hematologic spread, including through arterial emboli of tumor cells, is the most likely primary method. Malignant tumors can also metastasize through venous circulation, especially through paravertebral venous plexus. Spread from intramuscular lymph nodes and perineural spread are also possible though less likely. Although muscle can accounts for approximately 50% of total body mass and has an abundant blood supply, skeletal muscle metastases are rare, occurring in less than 5% of patients with any malignancy subtype. As such, muscle may be resistant both to primary and to metastatic cancer. Several mechanisms of resistance have been hypothesized. These mechanisms include secretion of factors, which inhibit proliferation of tumor cells, variable blood flow, and involvement in lactic acid metabolism [38, 39].

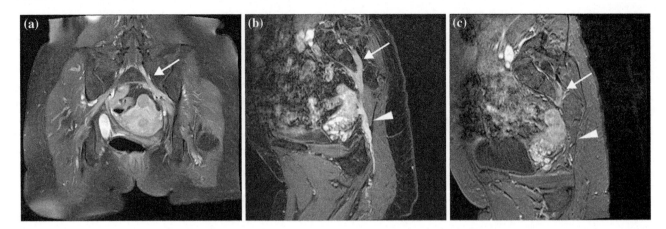

Fig. 7.3 A previously healthy 57 year old patient with progressive left leg weakness, numbness and pain over 3 months. The pelvis MRI showed abnormal thickening and enhancement at left lumbosacral nerve roots, plexus and sciatic nerve (**a**, **b**) with resolution after treatment (**c**) (images reprinted with permission of BMJ Publishing Group from Tsai et al. [37], August 2015)

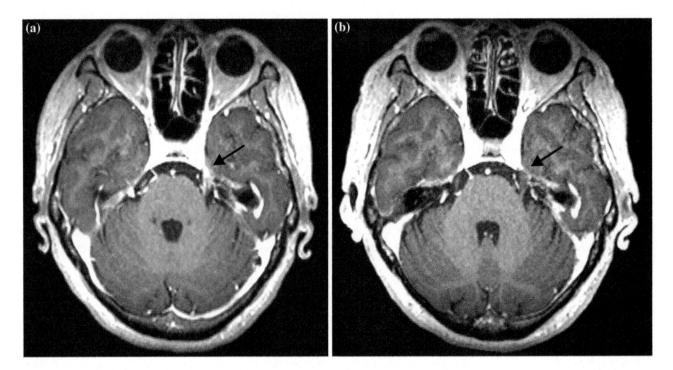

Fig. 7.4 The brain MRI study revealed abnormal enhancement at left trigeminal nerve (**a**) which resolved after chemotherapy (**b**) (images reprinted with permission of BMJ Publishing Group from Tsai et al. [37], August 2015)

Presentation

Metastatic disease to muscle should be considered in patients with cancer who develop a soft tissue mass within muscle. These masses are frequently asymptomatic and discovered incidentally on staging imaging. Conversely, they can be painful and associated with swelling, erythema of the over-lying skin, and restricted movement. Those that are painful typically may be larger and associated with massive muscle infiltration or destruction. Skeletal muscle metastases can occur in upper extremity, lower extremity, abdominal or thoracic wall and paravertebral muscles. Certain locations are more common. In one large series, the most common location was the iliopsoas, followed by paravertebral and then gluteal muscles, together accounting for over 60% of the metastases. The most common tumor types were genital, gastrointestinal, urological, and melanoma. Most commonly, skeletal muscle metastasis exist in the context of other metastatic lesions; however, rarely they can be the only manifestation of metastatic disease. Muscle metastases tend

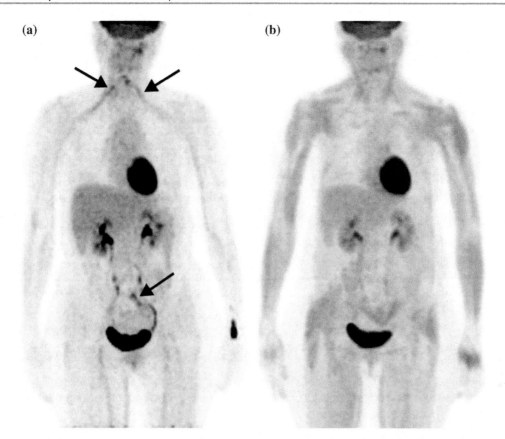

Fig. 7.5 The whole body positron emission tomography (*PET*) showed increased metabolism at bilateral brachial plexuses, left lumbosacral nerve roots and left sciatic nerve (**a**) which resolved after chemotherapy (**b**). The cytology of repeated cerebrospinal fluid studies proved large B cell lymphoma. The bone marrow study did not show evidence of hematologic malignancy (images reprinted with permission of BMJ Publishing Group from Tsai et al. [37], August 2015)

to present in five different patterns: solitary or multiple round/oval masses, multiple intramuscular calcifications, abscess-like lesions, diffuse infiltration with muscle swelling and intramuscular hemorrhage. The first two types tend to be painless and found incidentally on imaging and the later three clinically symptomatic and painful. Secondary abscesses can develop [38].

Diagnosis

MRI is thought to be superior to CT in detection of muscle metastases. Imaging findings, however, are non-specific and most often a complete histological examination is needed. CT guidance can be useful in obtaining biopsy tissue for analysis [40].

Treatment

Therapy includes surgical resection if metastases are isolated. Extensive disease or residual tumor after incomplete resection warrants radiation or chemotherapy. Prognosis in patients with clinically evident metastases to muscle is poor despite treatment, with a median survival of less than 12 months [40].

Radiation-Induced Myopathy

Radiation itself can also adversely affect muscle. Radiation exposure can cause a delayed onset radiation-induced myopathy manifesting 2 to over 40 years after therapy. This typically occurs after neck and/or upper torso radiation and presents with head drop and periscapular muscle weakness. Neuromuscular respiratory failure rarely occurs. CKs are typically normal to only mildly elevated. The presentation is quite distinct from metastatic disease to muscle [41].

Conclusion

Peripheral nervous system metastatic disease is diverse and complex. Two major challenges face the clinician [1]. The first is suspecting an underlying malignancy in a patient with a PNS disorder without an established diagnosis of cancer. The patient's presentation depends on the anatomic location of involvement. However, in general, severe pain and/or relentless progression of deficits typically are hallmarks of underlying PNS metastatic disease. The second is identifying a PNS disorder in patients with malignancy and determining whether symptoms are due to the malignancy itself or to treatment associated factors. This diagnostic process can be challenging since investigations for tumor involvement can be initially negative, even with tumor is present. Clinicians must implement a multi-modal evaluation including several complementary imaging exams, lab studies and repeated evaluation as needed. Early diagnosis and treatment of the cancer hold the most promise for alleviating pain, eliminating the cancer, when possible, improving symptoms and preventing further neurologic deficit.

References

1. Antoine J-C, Camdessanché J-P. Peripheral nervous system involvement in patients with cancer. Lancet Neurol. 2007;6 (1):75–86.
2. Chamberlain MC. The role of chemotherapy and targeted therapy in the treatment of intracranial meningioma. Curr Opin Oncol. 2012;24(6):666–71.
3. Ali S, Lee S-K. Ipilimumab therapy for melanoma: a mimic of leptomeningeal metastases. AJNR Am J Neuroradiol. 2015;36(12): E69–70.
4. Pauls S, Fischer A-C, Brambs H-J, Fetscher S, Höche W, Bommer M. Use of magnetic resonance imaging to detect neoplastic meningitis: Limited use in leukemia and lymphoma but convincing results in solid tumors. Eur J Radiol. 2012 May 1;81(5):974–8.
5. Clarke JL, Perez HR, Jacks LM, Panageas KS, Deangelis LM. Leptomeningeal metastases in the MRI era. Neurology. 2010;74 (18):1449–54.
6. Ahluwalia MS, Wallace PK, Peereboom DM. Flow cytometry as a diagnostic tool in lymphomatous or leukemic meningitis. Cancer. 2011;118(7):1747–53.
7. Jaeckle KA, Young DF, Foley KM. The natural history of lumbosacral plexopathy in cancer. Neurology. 1985;35(1):8–15.
8. Kori SH, Foley KM, Posner JB. Brachial plexus lesions in patients with cancer: 100 cases. Neurology. 1981;31(1):45–50.
9. Jaeckle KA. Neurological manifestations of neoplastic and radiation-induced plexopathies. Semin Neurol. 2004;24(4):385–93.
10. Ramchandren S, Dalmau J. Metastases to the peripheral nervous system. J Neurooncol. 2005;75(1):101–10.
11. Stewart JD. Focal peripheral neuropathies. 4th ed. West Vancouver: JBJ Publishing; 2010. p. 1.
12. Stewart JD. Focal peripheral neuropathies. 4th ed. West Vancouver: JBJ Publishing; 2010. p. 225–333.
13. Ferrante MA. Brachial plexopathies. Continuum (Minneap Minn). 2014 Oct;20(5 Peripheral Nervous System Disorders):1323–42.
14. Dyck PJB, Thaisetthawatkul P. Lumbosacral plexopathy. Continuum (Minneap Minn). 2014 Oct;20(5 Peripheral Nervous System Disorders):1343–58.
15. Dalmau J, Graus F, Marco M. "Hot and dry foot" as initial manifestation of neoplastic lumbosacral plexopathy. Neurology. 1989;39(6):871–2.
16. Thyagarajan D, Cascino T, Harms G. Magnetic resonance imaging in brachial plexopathy of cancer. Neurology. 1995;45(3 Pt 1): 421–7.
17. Brejt N, Berry J, Nisbet A, Bloomfield D, Burkill G. Pelvic radiculopathies, lumbosacral plexopathies, and neuropathies in oncologic disease: a multidisciplinary approach to a diagnostic challenge. Cancer Imaging. 2013;13(4):591–601.
18. Ahmad A, Barrington S, Maisey M, Rubens RD. Use of positron emission tomography in evaluation of brachial plexopathy in breast cancer patients. Br J Cancer. 1999;79(3–4):478–82.
19. Andreou A, Sohaib A, Collins DJ, Takahara T, Kwee TC, Leach MO, et al. Diffusion-weighted MR neurography for the assessment of brachial plexopathy in oncological practice. Cancer Imaging. 2015;15(1):1023.
20. Wittenberg KH, Adkins MC. MR imaging of nontraumatic brachial plexopathies: frequency and spectrum of findings. Radiographics. 2000;20(4):1023–32.
21. Krarup C, Crone C. Neurophysiological studies in malignant disease with particular reference to involvement of peripheral nerves. J Neurol. 2002;249(6):651–61.
22. Tavee J, Mays M, Wilbourn AJ. Pitfalls in the electrodiagnostic studies of sacral plexopathies. Muscle Nerve. 2007;35(6):725–9.
23. Dropcho EJ. Neurotoxicity of radiation therapy. Neurol Clin NA. 2010 Feb 1;28(1):217–34.
24. Delanian S, Lefaix J-L, Pradat P-F. Radiation-induced neuropathy in cancer survivors. Radiother Oncol. 2012 Dec 1;105(3):273–82.
25. Harper CM, Thomas JE, Cascino TL, Litchy WJ. Distinction between neoplastic and radiation-induced brachial plexopathy, with emphasis on the role of EMG. Neurology. 1989;39(4):502–6.
26. Soto O. Radiation-induced conduction block: resolution following anticoagulant therapy. Muscle Nerve. 2005;31(5):642–5.
27. Bhattacharyya AK, Perrin R, Guha A. Peripheral nerve tumors: management strategies and molecular insights. J Neurooncol. 2004;69(1–3):335–49.
28. Laigle-Donadey F, Taillibert S, Martin-Duverneuil N, Hildebrand J, Delattre J-Y. Skull-base metastases. J Neurooncol. 2005;75(1):63–9.
29. Paquette CM, Manos DC, Psooy BJ. Unilateral vocal cord paralysis: a review of CT findings, mediastinal causes, and the course of the recurrent laryngeal nerves. Radiographics. 2012;32 (3):721–40.
30. Hansen JM, Rasti Z, Smith T, Lassen LH. Sciatic neuropathy as first sign of metastasising prostate cancer. Case Rep. 2010 Oct 11;2010 (Oct 08 2):bcr1220092529–9.
31. Matsumine A, Kusuzaki K, Hirata H. Intraneural metastasis of a synovial sarcoma to a peripheral nerve. Bone Joint J. 2005;87 (11):1553–5.
32. Cantone G, Rath SA, Richter HP. Intraneural metastasis in a peripheral nerve. Acta Neurochir (Wien). 2000;142(6):719–20.
33. Baehring JM, Damek D, Martin EC, Betensky RA, Hochberg FH. Neurolymphomatosis. Neuro-Oncol. 2003;5(2):104–15.
34. Grisariu S, Avni B, Batchelor TT, van den Bent MJ, Bokstein F, Schiff D, et al. Neurolymphomatosis: an International Primary CNS Lymphoma Collaborative Group report. Blood. 2010 Jun 17;115 (24):5005–11.
35. Gan HK, Azad A, Cher L, Mitchell PLR. Neurolymphomatosis: diagnosis, management, and outcomes in patients treated with rituximab. Neuro-Oncol. 2010;12(2):212–5.
36. Tomita M, Koike H, Kawagashira Y, Iijima M, Adachi H, Taguchi J, et al. Clinicopathological features of neuropathy associated with lymphoma. Brain. 2013;136(8):2563–78.

37. Tsai H-H, Chen Y-F, Hsieh S-T, Chao C-C. Neurolymphomatosis as the primary presentation of non-Hodgkin's Lymphoma. J Neurol Neurosurg Psychiatry. 2015;86(8):929–30.

38. Surov A, Hainz M, Holzhausen H-J, Arnold D, Katzer M, Schmidt J, et al. Skeletal muscle metastases: primary tumours, prevalence, and radiological features. Eur Radiol. 2009;20(3):649–58.

39. Seely S. Possible reasons for the high resistance of muscle to cancer. Med Hypotheses. 1980;6(2):133–7.

40. Tuoheti Y, Okada K, Osanai T, Nishida J, Ehara S, Hashimoto M, et al. Skeletal muscle metastases of carcinoma: a clinicopathological study of 12 cases. Jpn J Clin Oncol. 2004;34(4):210–4.

41. Ghosh PS, Milone M. Clinical and laboratory findings of 21 patients with radiation-induced myopathy. J Neurol Neurosurg Psychiatry. 2015;1(86):152–8.

Headache as Complication of Cancer

Surabhi Ranjan and David Schiff

List of Abbreviations	
MRI	Magnetic resonance imaging
ICHD	International classification of headache disorders
CSF	Cerebrospinal fluid
ICP	Intracranial pressure
CNS	Central nervous system
ATAC trial	Arimidex, Tamoxifen, Alone or in combination trial
SMART syndrome	Stroke-like migraine attacks after radiation therapy syndrome
PRES	Posterior reversible encephalopathy syndrome
AZT	Azidothymidine
DDI	Didanosine
PCNU	1-(2-chloroethyl)-3-(2,6-dioxo-1-piperidyl)-1-nitrosourea
OKT3	Murine monoclonal anti-CD3 antibody
GM-CSF	Granulocyte-macrophage colony-stimulating factor

Introduction

Patients with headaches constitute a sizeable fraction of the patient population encountered by neurologists, who are well versed in the red flags associated with headaches. For a physician, the implications of missing a brain tumor headache can be profound. The physician has the challenging task of reassuring the patient with primary headache and adequately investigating the patient with a suspected brain tumor headache.

While only a small subset of patients presenting with headaches are found to have an underlying brain tumor, headaches are a frequent accompaniment of both primary and metastatic brain tumors. Knowledge of the epidemiology, pathophysiology, and characteristics of brain tumor headaches helps the clinician to decide how to approach and investigate the patient presenting with an undiagnosed headache. In the management of patients with central nervous system tumors, a key issue is preservation of quality of life. As headaches are a significant symptom in patients with brain tumors, their management can help improve the quality of life. The understanding of the pathophysiology of the brain tumor headache and identification of the specific etiology of headache may allow for more precise interventions.

Epidemiology and Clinical Presentation of Brain Tumor Headaches (Table 8.1)

Headaches are frequently assumed to be the first sign of an underlying brain tumor. Yet in reality, only a small subset of patients with brain tumor present with headaches as the only complaint. In patients presenting with headache as an

S. Ranjan (✉)
Department of Neurology, University of Virginia, PO Box 800394, Charlottesville, VA 22908, USA
e-mail: surabhiranjan18@gmail.com

D. Schiff
Neuro-oncology center, University of Virginia, Hospital West, Room 6225, Jefferson Park Avenue, Charlottesville, VA 22908, USA
e-mail: ds4jd@virginia.edu

© Springer International Publishing AG 2018
D. Schiff et al. (eds.), *Cancer Neurology in Clinical Practice*,
DOI 10.1007/978-3-319-57901-6_8

Table 8.1 Clinical characteristics of brain tumor headaches

Clinical history suggesting a brain tumor headache	Cancer patient with a new headache or a change in headache pattern Unrelenting crescendo headache Headache resistant to all medical interventions Pain location invariant
Characteristics of brain tumor headaches	
Frequent symptoms	Intermittent headaches Headache building up and resolving in hours Pain of pressure-like/ tightening/ dull aching quality Moderate to severe intensity Bilateral pain Ipsilateral headaches in hemispheric tumors, with laterality usually being predictive for ipsilateral tumor location
Less frequent symptoms	Morning headaches Daily headaches Progressive headaches Constant pain Headaches worsening with bending over or with Valsalva's maneuver Headaches waking patients from sleep or interfering with falling asleep Association with nausea and vomiting
Accompanying sign and symptoms	Diffuse weakness Anorexia Malaise Hyperreflexia Positive Babinski Papilledema Cognitive changes Depression Fatigue Personality changes Seizures

initial symptom, posterior fossa tumor and hydrocephalus are frequently present. The prevalence of headaches is similar in primary and metastatic brain tumors [1]. Three studies have demonstrated the prevalence of headaches in patients with brain tumors as 71, 48, and 58% [2–4]. Various studies have suggested that the "classic" brain tumor headache, which is usually progressive, worse in the morning and aggravated by Valsalva-like maneuvers, was an uncommon occurrence in clinical practice. This unfortunately implies that there is no exclusive signature of the brain tumor headache.

Although brain tumor headaches are usually nonspecific in character, they are usually accompanied by other symptoms suggesting either a focal lesion or increased intracranial pressure. Typically, either tension-type or migraine-like headaches are predominant, though a smaller subset of patient will have a mix of headache types. In a prospective study of 111 patients with brain tumors, the "classic" brain tumor type headache occurred in a meager 17% of patients. 67% patients of this subtype of "classic" brain tumor headaches had evidence of increased intracranial pressure. Headaches were worse in the morning in 36%, worse with bending over in 32%, worse with Valsalva in 23% and woke patients from sleep or interfered

with falling sleep in 32% of the patients with headache. Nausea and vomiting associated with headaches were present in 48% patients. The headache was the worst symptom in only 45% patients [3]. In patients with a known history of brain tumor, the development of a headache late in the clinical course may signify the possibility of a change in the tumor structure or tumor recurrence.

Headache location may have a localizing value. Patients with unilateral headache without increased intracranial pressure is likely to have an ipsilateral location of the brain tumor. A frontal headache is the least valuable in localizing a brain tumor. Occipital headaches are associated with posterior fossa and infratentorial tumors. Patients with supratentorial tumors have headaches that more often correspond to the side of tumor than patients with infratentorial tumors. It has also been reported that headaches are more common with infratentorial tumors than supratentorial ones [1–3, 5].

The third edition of the International Classification of Headache Disorders (ICHD-3) has extensively described the diagnostic criteria of classification of headaches due to intracranial neoplasms [6]. While it is useful to have a description and classification of the brain tumor headache, a strict use of this guideline is not recommended as it places emphasis on the "classic" brain tumor headache. According to ICHD-3, the characteristic headache attributed to intracranial neoplasm is a headache that is usually progressive, worse in the morning and aggravated by Valsalva maneuvers, caused by one or more space-occupying intracranial tumors. Evidence of causation should be demonstrated by at least two of the following three criteria: headache has developed in a temporal relationship to the tumor or had led to its discovery; headache has significantly worsened in parallel with the worsening of tumor or headache has improved in parallel with the successful treatment of the tumor; and headache has at least one of the following characteristics-progressive, worse in the morning or after daytime napping, aggravated by Valsalva maneuver. When a patient develops headache for the first time or has a new headache type, and develops a brain tumor in unison, the headache should be attributed to the intracranial tumor, even when the headache character is a migraine, tension-type headache, or a cluster headache. On the other hand, when the patient has a history of a primary headache, which becomes worse in a close temporal relationship to the occurrence of an intracranial neoplasm, it is challenging to say if the intracranial neoplasm is the etiology of the worsened headache. There may be three possible explanations: the finding is coincidental, this is an aggravation of primary headache, or it represents a new headache, causally related to the intracranial neoplasm.

Pathophysiology of the Brain Tumor Headaches (Table 8.2)

In people with a predisposition to headaches, brain tumor headaches may present similarly to primary headaches. This can lead to delay in tumor diagnosis, particularly when headache is the presenting or an isolated symptom. It also suggests that the primary and tumor-associated headaches may have a mutually shared biology. Progressive headache is more common in high grade tumor and secreting pituitary adenomas. Slow growing tumors are less likely to cause headaches [5, 7].

It is important to understand that increased intracranial pressure is not essential to the development of the brain tumor headache. Headaches in brain tumors may be caused by traction or compression of the pain-sensitive structures, release of potential signal substances, or neuroendocrine abnormalities. A direct mass effect or inflammation of intracranial and extracranial structures such as cranial nerves, vasculature, dura, periosteum, etc., can contribute to the headache. The pain-sensitive extracranial tissues include the galea, fascia, arteries, and the scalp muscles and the periosteum along the inferior, frontal, temporal, and occipital skull base. Intracranially, the pain-sensitive structures are the dura

at the skull base and near the major venous sinuses, the tentorium cerebelli, cranial nerves V, IX, X, XI, and the proximal trunks of the main dural arteries. Pain-insensitive structures include the cranial bones, extracranial diploic and emissary veins, cerebral and cerebellar parenchyma, choroid plexus, the ependymal lining of the ventricles, pia-arachnoid, arachnoid granulation, and most of the dura covering the cerebral convexities [8]. Experimental observations suggest that stimulation of pain-sensitive structures on or above the superior surface of the tentorium resulted in pain transmitted by CN V located in the anterior half of the head. Stimulation of the pain-sensitive intracranial structures on or below the inferior surface of the tentorium resulted in pain over the posterior half of the head via CN IX and X and the upper three cervical nerves. Since lesions of remotely separated structures can cause headache in identical areas, the use of tumor location as a localizing tool can be challenging [9].

Cerebrospinal fluid (CSF) obstruction due to a mass lesion may cause increased intracranial pressure (ICP) and can stretch the pain-sensitive structures. Rapid distention or drainage of the ventricular system can produce diffuse headache due to traction on the cortical veins entering the dural sinuses. Third ventricular distention can cause a headache due to stretch of the arteries of the circle of Willis. Tumors may also produce signal substances like nitric oxide synthase, calcitonin gene-related peptide, tumor necrosis factor alpha, vasoactive intestinal peptide, tachykinin (substance P), and prostaglandin endoperoxide synthase, which may cause headaches [1]; however, this finding has not been well substantiated. Neuroendocrine abnormalities have been postulated as a cause of headache in patients with pituitary tumors. Patients with prolactinomas have a higher incidence of headache than those with growth hormone-related pituitary tumor, implicating a potentially greater role for the dopamine-prolactin axis in pain.

Brain Tumor Headache Associated with Increased Intracranial Pressure (Table 8.2)

Approximately 86–95% of patients with increased intracranial pressure have headaches [5]. These headaches can be distinguished from other types of brain tumor headaches due to their severity, association with nausea or vomiting and resistance to common analgesics, rather than their quality or location. Etiologies for the development of increased intracranial pressure include intracranial mass effect due to tumor, cerebral edema, intratumoral hemorrhage, obstructive hydrocephalus, communicating hydrocephalus, and leptomeningeal spread of the tumor. The presence of increased intracranial pressure may slightly decrease the localizing

Table 8.2 Causes of headache in cancer patients

Tumor-related causes

Acute	Intratumoral hemorrhage Acute venous sinus thrombosis CSF obstruction with resulting increase in intracranial pressure Pressure wave headache
Chronic	Persistent or new tumor growth New metastatic lesion involving skull, meninges, brain, skull base, sinuses, orbits, etc. Invasion of tumor into calvarium, skull base, meninges, leptomeninges. Increased intracranial pressure with midline shift causing traction on veins, arteries, nerves, etc.

Nontumor-related causes

Treatment-related causes	Hormones (e.g., tamoxifen) Differentiation agents (retinoic acids) Antibiotics Reverse transcriptase inhibitors (e.g., AZT, DDI) Conventional agents (e.g., L-asparaginase, procarbazine, nitrosoureas, fludarabine, fazarabine, gallium nitrate) Cytokines (e.g., tumor necrosis factor, OKT3, interferons, interleukins, levamisole, GM-CSF) Intrathecal therapy (e.g., methotrexate, Ara-C)
Radiotherapy	Acute radiation encephalopathy Subacute demyelinating encephalopathy Cerebral radiation necrosis SMART syndrome
Supportive therapies	Corticosteroids, cimetidine, ondansetron, narcotics (withdrawal), metoclopramide, anticoagulants (intratumoral hemorrhage), dipyridamole, ibuprofen (aseptic meningitis)
Surgery	Hemorrhage, vascular injury, perioperative stroke, cerebrospinal fluid leak

Other causes of headache

Acute	Cerebral infarcts Fever Infection (abscess, meningitis) Metabolic (hypoxemia, hypercarbia, and hypoglycemia)
Chronic	Referred pain from extracranial structures (cervical metastases, lung tumors, etc.) Post lumbar-puncture headache

Courtesy of Robert Cavaliere, MD, author of a chapter on this subject in the previous edition of this book, in which this table appeared [49]

value of ipsilateral headaches. Traction and displacement of periventricular pain-sensitive structures in obstructive hydrocephalus may be the mechanism of the headache pain. The common signs and symptoms associated with increased intracranial pressure are headache, nausea, vomiting, lethargy, papilledema, visual obscuration, diplopia, tinnitus, and somnolence.

The description of headaches associated with plateau waves is worth mentioning. Plateau waves, first described by Lundberg in 1960, are episodic increase in ICP that arise from rapid cerebrovascular vasodilatation that can cause stereotypical paroxysmal neurological symptoms like headache, blurred vision, diplopia, imbalance, and fainting spells. Impaired intracranial compliance is a prerequisite in the development of plateau waves. In the patient with a brain tumor, the intracranial compliance may be decreased due to the mass effect of the tumor or development of hydrocephalus [10, 11].

Plateau wave headache is also known as pressure wave headache or paroxysmal headache. This headache is usually severe in intensity and builds to peak intensity in seconds.

The duration of the symptoms may be minutes or a few hours and the episode terminates quickly. Headache is frequently associated with plateau waves, but this phenomenon may be challenging to diagnose due to the patient's impaired mental status and inability to describe their symptoms during this paroxysmal spell. These episodes may frequently be misdiagnosed as seizures. Awareness of this phenomenon of plateau waves is important as it may herald impending herniation [8].

Headaches in Pituitary Tumors

With the recent widespread use of sensitive imaging for head trauma, chronic sinusitis and headache, it is quite common for the clinician to find an unexpected sellar lesion. If the patient has a headache, then the question becomes whether the headache is related to the sellar lesion. Intrasellar tumors commonly manifest with headaches, which are often disabling. The reported incidence of headache associated with pituitary adenomas varies from 33 to 72% [2, 12].

A prospective study on 84 patients presenting with pituitary tumors classified patients' headaches using the International Headache Society diagnostic criteria [13]. Headaches were found to be chronic migraines (46%), episodic migraines (30%), primary stabbing headache (27%), short-lasting unilateral neuralgiform headache attacks with conjunctival injection and tearing (SUNCT; 5%), cluster headache (4%), hemicrania continua (1%), and non-specific in 7% of patients. Half of the patients had a family history of headaches. It was posited that migraine patients have an increased sensitivity to changes in the internal or external milieu and that the development of pituitary tumors may have lowered the threshold for migraine attacks in this pre-disposed population. Migraines were found in a higher frequency in prolactinomas and growth hormone-secreting tumors, suggesting that functional activity may be an important trigger. Cluster headaches and SUNCT were overrepresented in pituitary disease.

Of the patients who underwent surgical treatment, 49% reported an improvement in headaches. Treatment with radiotherapy had a poor response in terms of headache alleviation. 64% of acromegalics who were treated with somatostatin analogues had improvement in their headaches. This suggests a shared biology between tumor activity and headache. Somatostatin analogues are known to interfere with the opioidergic system, which may explain an improvement in headache [14, 15]. Octretotide may be useful in the acute treatment of cluster headache [16]. Patients responded unpredictably to treatment with dopamine agonists; some had an improvement in their headaches while others had an exacerbation. It was hypothesized that an improvement in headache could be due to reduction in tumor size in large prolactinomas. The dopamine-prolactin axis plays an important role in several primary headaches like migraines and cluster headaches. Conversely, dopamine agonists may act on the trigeminovascular system, causing headache exacerbation [13, 17–19].

It has been suggested that the headache in pituitary tumors is related to dural traction on pain-sensitive structures, tumor size and cavernous sinus invasion. The expansion of pituitary tumor within the sella turcica stimulates the afferent fibers innervating the dura, causing pain. Invasion of the cavernous sinus by the pituitary tumor causes pain as the cavernous sinus contains the ophthalmic branch of the trigeminal nerve and the internal carotid artery, both of which are pain-sensitive structures. Another cause of headache in pituitary tumor may be the presence of tumor activity and neuroendocrinological signaling alteration. This is supported by the fact that headache can be present in small tumors and can be improved or worsened by endocrine treatment. Regarding the role of cavernous sinus invasion and tumor size in the causation of headaches, studies have reported conflicting results. While two studies found no association between cavernous sinus invasion, pituitary volume and headache, another prospective study in pituitary adenoma showed a positive association between the presence of headache with tumor size and cavernous sinus invasion [20–22]. Given the contradictory findings, further studies are needed to explain the mechanism of headache in pituitary tumors.

Headache in Systemic Cancer (Table 8.2)

In the patient with a systemic cancer, headache is a common complaint. It is usually not a harbinger of an ominous intracranial pathology but nonetheless warrants careful clinical assessment. Patients with systemic cancer, like the general population, commonly suffer from migraine, tension headaches, and other primary headaches. Any change in the patient's preexisting headache, crescendo headaches, headaches unresponsive to treatment, vomiting, lethargy, or abnormal neurological exam should raise suspicion of a secondary cause of headache due to intracranial pathology. A study examining 97 patients with an undiagnosed headache in the setting of systemic cancer found that 61% did not have a structural cause of headache. The majority of these patients with a non-structural cause of headache had migraine, tension headache, or headache due to systemic illness like fever or sepsis. 39% of patients had a structural cause of headache. The common structural causes of headache were cerebral metastases, skull base metastasis, or intracranial hemorrhage. Rare structural causes of headaches included leptomeningeal metastases, upper cervical spine metastasis, and primary brain tumor [23].

Patients with systemic cancers, especially breast cancer, lung cancer, and melanoma, may develop leptomeningeal spread of the tumor. Leptomeningeal disease frequently presents with headache. Usually, other multifocal neurological signs like cranial nerve palsy, evidence of spinal dysfunction, radiculopathies, or acute mental status change accompany the headache. The spread of tumor to the base of brain, arachnoid villi and reactive fibrosis may impede or block the CSF flow pathways leading to the development of hydrocephalus and increased intracranial pressure. The etiology of headache in leptomeningeal carcinomatosis may include hydrocephalus, increased ICP or cranial nerve infiltration.

A rare cause of headache in cancer patients is headache associated with dural venous sinus thrombosis. Venous thrombosis is a well-known complication of cancer. Though thrombotic events usually present as deep venous thrombosis or pulmonary embolism, cerebral venous thrombosis and dural sinus thrombosis may be an uncommon manifestation. A prospective study on 624 patients with cerebral venous thrombosis reported that 7.4% patients with cerebral vein

Table 8.3 Headache accompanying metastasis to the base of the skull

Base of the skull metastasis syndrome	Clinical features
1. Orbital syndrome	Continuous and progressive pain around the supraorbital area of the affected eye Occasionally dull aching frontal headache Periorbital swelling, exophthalmos, ptosis, ophthalmoplegia, diplopia and rarely blurred vision
2. Parasellar syndrome	Metastasis to parasellar region or cavernous sinus Unilateral dull aching frontal headache associated with diplopia, ophthalmoparesis, usually without proptosis
3. Middle cranial fossa syndrome	Metastasis to gasserian ganglion Usually dull aching pain to cheek or jaw Rarely pain typical of trigeminal neuralgia Pain and numbness in the maxillary and mandibular division of trigeminal nerve
4. Jugular foramen syndrome	Chronic unilateral pain, often located behind the ear, occasionally glossopharyngeal neuralgia Dysphagia, hoarseness, unilateral palate weakness, ipsilateral weakness of sternocleidomastoid and upper trapezius
5. Occipital condyle syndrome	Severe pain in the unilateral occipital region, worse with neck flexion Neck stiffness, ipsilateral tongue weakness

and dural sinus thrombosis had malignancy as a risk factor. Of these, 2.2% patients had central nervous system (CNS) tumors, 3.2% patients had solid tumors outside the CNS and 2.9% had hematological malignancies. The presence of malignancy was noted to be an important prognostic factor for death or dependence [24, 25]. Cerebral venous thrombosis may present as headache, projectile vomiting, focal onset seizures, focal neurological deficits, and papilledema. Headache is the most common symptom. The superior sagittal sinus is quite frequently involved [26, 27], representing a neurological emergency that requires expeditious diagnosis and treatment. Unfortunately, most patients present to the emergency room after focal deficits have already occurred. Therefore, for a favorable outcome, it is necessary to identify this cohort of patients early with the use of vessel imaging like MRA, MRV or CTA, in addition to standard MRI or CT and promptly treat them with anticoagulation.

Headaches secondary to metastatic cancer may occur in relation to metastasis to the base of the skull (Table 8.3), particularly in breast and prostate cancer. Five different syndromes have been described according to the site of metastasis. These are the orbital, parasellar, middle-fossa, jugular foramen. and occipital condyle syndromes [28, 29].

Headache Related to Cancer Treatment (Table 8.2)

Headache may be a side effect of drugs used in cancer treatment. Commonly used drugs like ondansetron, steroids, and metoclopramide may cause headaches. Headache can also be a symptom of opioid withdrawal. Tamoxifen is a selective estrogen-receptor modifier used in the treatment of breast cancer. Headache is an infrequent side effect of tamoxifen. In the ATAC trial in postmenopausal women with operable breast cancer who received adjuvant tamoxifen therapy, headache occurred in 8% [30]. Retinoids used in the treatment of leukemia and cutaneous T cell lymphoma may cause headache, with or without the development of pseudotumor cerebri [31–34].

Craniotomy for surgical resection of tumor may cause postsurgical headache. Craniofacial pain may occasionally last for many months after the surgery. Radiation therapy, which is commonly used for the treatment of primary and metastatic brain tumor, can cause headache as an immediate or a delayed side effect. Acute radiation encephalopathy may be seen at initiation of radiotherapy and may present with headaches and other neurological symptoms. Headache can also be a manifestation of a subacute demyelinating encephalopathy, presenting 1–6 months after radiation. Late complications of radiation therapy, occurring months to years after treatment, include cerebral radiation necrosis, which may present with headache and focal neurologic symptoms. Another rare late complication of radiation therapy is stroke-like migraine attacks after radiation therapy (SMART) syndrome, described below [35].

SMART Syndrome

The syndrome of stroke-like migraine attacks after radiation therapy (SMART) is a rare late complication of cerebral radiation. This syndrome, a constellation of reversible episodic neurological dysfunction, headaches and seizures, was first described in a retrospective series of 4 children with brain

Table 8.4 Childhood headache epidemiology

Study	Number of Patients	Headaches prevalence (%)	Headache as initial symptom
Gilles [40]	3291	62	–
Wilne et al. [43]	200	56	41%
Reulecke et al. [42]	245	59.6	–
Hayashi et al. [47]	60	26.7	16.6%
Molineus et al. [48]	79	66.7	–

tumors who had undergone craniospinal irradiation [36]. SMART syndrome has a phenotypic similarity to posterior reversible encephalopathy syndrome (PRES), though seizures are more common in PRES. The attacks are usually subacute and involve stroke-like neurological deficits like hemiparesis, aphasia, homonymous hemianopsia, hemisensory deficits, and transient visual loss, with or without seizures. Most patients have headaches, which are typically described as migraines and may be accompanied by aura. Recovery is usually complete in most cases, although some cases with incomplete clinical recovery have been reported [37].

The pathophysiology of SMART syndrome is poorly understood. The typical MRI findings are focal gyral thickening of the affected cortex and gyriform contrast enhancement. Reported cases have frequently shown a predilection for the involvement of parietooccipital cortex. It has been hypothesized that the parietooccipital cortex is more vulnerable to the effects of radiation or chemotherapy. The underlying mechanism may be postradiation neuronal dysfunction that may cause impairment of the trigemino-vascular system or a lowered threshold for cortical spreading depression. Another hypothesis is a reversible radiation vasculopathy, similar to the mechanism of the development of PRES [38, 39].

Headache in Childhood Brain Tumors

Brain tumors have a long symptom interval to diagnosis in comparison with other childhood malignancies. The presentation of headaches associated with childhood brain tumors is unique due to the small brain size, an open fontanel, open cranial sutures, and the age-dependent capability of the patients to express their symptoms. The data on the epidemiology of headache in childhood brain tumor are largely derived from the Childhood Brain Tumor Consortium databank, which has a registry of 3291 patients. 62% of the children with brain tumor experienced significant headaches prior to their first hospitalization. Headache was present in 58% of children with supratentorial tumors and 70% of children with infratentorial tumors. Less than 1% of children with headache and brain

tumor had no other symptom. Less than 3% of children with headache and a brain tumor had no abnormality on neurological examination. Children with headaches were found to have a greater number of neurological signs and symptoms than children without headaches. Infants and very young children had a lower rate of headache. This may be due the capacity of the infant skull to expand or due to the inability to express the headache pain. There were more neurological signs when the headache was associated with infratentorial tumors as compared to the supratentorial tumors. Headache was found more frequently in supratentorial craniopharyngioma, ependymomas and protoplasmic astrocytomas than astrocytomas and pilocytic astrocytomas. Headaches occurred more frequently with infratentorial pilocytic astrocytomas as compared to infratentorial anaplastic astrocytomas, astrocytomas, ependymomas, and other unclassifiable tumors [40]. See Table 8.4.

The key challenge is to determine when the child with a headache should undergo neuroimaging. Often headache is perceived as a symptom too common and non-specific to warrant imaging of the brain, leading to a delayed diagnosis of childhood brain tumors. Serious intracranial pathology is rarely the cause of chronic headaches in children [41, 42]. On examination, a significant fraction of children may have cranial nerve signs or papilledema without other accompanying signs. A study documented that a third of children had an abnormality of visual field or acuity, and in the majority this was the only cranial nerve abnormality [43]. This emphasizes the importance of cranial nerve examination, fundoscopy, and assessment of vision in a child with suspected brain tumor.

Treatment of the Brain Tumor Headache

It can be gathered from the preceding discussion that brain tumor headache is a clinically and biologically heterogeneous entity. Therefore, the treatment should be tailored according to the etiology of headache, the type of brain tumor, the stage of the disease and the functional status of the patient.

When the headache is secondary to edema, corticosteroids are the standard treatment. Steroids control the peritumoral edema, which also helps mitigate the associated signs and symptoms. Dexamethasone is usually the preferred treatment due to its lack of mineralocorticoid activity. Dexamethasone has a long half-life of 36–54 h. While it is common to see dexamethasone dosed every 6 h, due to the long half-life, it can be given more conveniently twice daily. Although the conventional starting dose of dexamethasone is 16 mg/day, a systemic review and evidence-based clinical practice guideline suggested that in patients with mild symptoms related to mass effect, a starting dose of 4–8 mg/day should be considered. A higher dose of dexamethasone such as 16 mg/day or more is appropriate when patients have severe symptoms consistent with increased intracranial pressure [44, 45].

The treatment of headaches in brain tumor has not been formally studied. Despite the shared biology of the primary headaches with the brain tumor headaches, there are no formal studies investigating the use of non-steroidal anti-inflammatory medications, ergots, or triptans in the patient population with brain tumors. Opioid medications are typically the standard treatment for symptomatic relief of headache. Headaches associated with brain tumor progression should be managed as per the general principles of pain management. Initial treatment may be started with acetaminophen. If the headache is unresponsive to acetaminophen, then codeine or oxycodone should be added. The starting dose of opioid should be done in consideration of safety rather than the patient's expression of pain.

After establishing a safety profile, the dose of opioid medication can be adjusted as appropriate. Patients who have a chronic headache may need to have regularly dosed opioids, with an extended release formulation. For breakthrough pain, they should be given immediate release opioids (10% of the daily regular opioid dose). Constipation and nausea are common side effects of treatment with opioids, which should be treated with the use of laxatives and anti-emetics. The nausea associated with opioids usually improves after a few days [8, 46].

When headache is due to brain metastasis, treatment is usually palliative due to the patient's limited life expectancy. Such patients frequently require multidisciplinary care that includes surgical resection, radiosurgery, radiation therapy, and chemotherapy. Surgical resection of a brain metastatic lesion can decrease the risk of immediate life-threatening mass effect and the source of peritumoral edema. Whole brain radiation can be used either alone or in conjunction with surgery. For oligometastatic disease, stereotactic radiosurgery may be used. For the treatment of headaches due to hydrocephalus, intracranial pressure monitoring and ventriculoperitoneal shunting may be required. Patients with leptomeningeal metastasis usually have a poor prognosis and the headache treatment should be aimed at palliation.

Conclusion

Review of the clinical presentations of the brain tumor headache suggests that the classic brain tumor headache, which is severe, progressive, worse in the morning and associated with nausea or vomiting, is in fact an uncommon clinical entity. Therefore, it is very important to realize that the brain tumor headache does not have an exclusive signature. It is best to maintain a high index of suspicion and not rely on a classic presentation to decide to pursue imaging. Patients with a history of headaches should undergo neuroimaging if the headache is accompanied by new symptoms, abnormal neurological exam, or different features from their usual headache. New onset headache patients should be imaged if the headache is progressive, severe, associated with nausea or vomiting or an abnormal neurological exam [3]. Imaging should invariably be obtained in patient with a known history of brain tumors who develop a headache as this may suggest a structural change in the underlying tumor due to bleed, expansion or a tumor recurrence. Treatment of the brain tumor headache should be individualized tailored, according to the etiology and pathophysiology of the headache. Headache can compromise the quality of life in patients with brain tumor; therefore, aggressive management of this symptom may have a positive impact.

References

1. Kahn K, Finkel A. It is a tumor—current review of headache and brain tumor. Curr Pain Headache Rep. 2014;18(6):421.
2. Suwanwela N, Phanthumchinda K, Kaoropthum S. Headache in brain tumor: a cross-sectional study. Headache. 1994;34(7):435–8.
3. Forsyth PA, Posner JB. Headaches in patients with brain tumors: a study of 111 patients. Neurology. 1993;43(9):1678–83.
4. Pfund Z, Szapary L, Jaszberenyi O, Nagy F, Czopf J. Headache in intracranial tumors. Cephalalgia. 1999;19(9):787–90; discussion 65.
5. Nelson S, Taylor LP. Headaches in brain tumor patients: primary or secondary? Headache. 2014;54(4):776–85.
6. The International Classification of Headache Disorders, 3rd edition (beta version). Cephalalgia. 2013;33(9):629–808.
7. Taylor LP. Mechanism of brain tumor headache. Headache. 2014;54(4):772–5.
8. Jaeckle KA. Causes and management of headaches in cancer patients. Oncology (Williston Park). 1993;7(4):27–31; discussion-2, 4.
9. Kunkle EC, Ray BS, Wolff HG. Studies on headache: the mechanisms and significance of the headache associated with brain tumor. Bull N Y Acad Med. 1942;18(6):400–22.

10. Lundberg N. Continuous recording and control of ventricular fluid pressure in neurosurgical practice. Acta Psychiatr Scand Suppl. 1960;36(149):1–193.

11. Rosner MJ, Becker DP. Origin and evolution of plateau waves. Experimental observations and a theoretical model. J Neurosurg. 1984;60(2):312–24.

12. Yokoyama S, Mamitsuka K, Tokimura H, Asakura T. Headache in pituitary adenoma cases. J Jpn Soc study Chron Pain. 1994;13:79–82.

13. Levy MJ, Matharu MS, Meeran K, Powell M, Goadsby PJ. The clinical characteristics of headache in patients with pituitary tumours. Brain. 2005;128(Pt 8):1921–30.

14. Connor M, Bagley EE, Mitchell VA, Ingram SL, Christie MJ, Humphrey PP, et al. Cellular actions of somatostatin on rat periaqueductal grey neurons in vitro. Br J Pharmacol. 2004;142 (8):1273–80.

15. Otsuka F, Kageyama J, Ogura T, Makino H. Cluster headache dependent upon octreotide injection. Headache. 1998;38(8):629.

16. Matharu MS, Levy MJ, Meeran K, Goadsby PJ. Subcutaneous octreotide in cluster headache: randomized placebo-controlled double-blind crossover study. Ann Neurol. 2004;56(4):488–94.

17. Goadsby PJ. Pathophysiology of cluster headache: a trigeminal autonomic cephalgia. Lancet Neurol. 2002;1(4):251–7.

18. Peres MF, Sanchez del Rio M, Seabra ML, Tufik S, Abucham J, Cipolla-Neto J, et al. Hypothalamic involvement in chronic migraine. J Neurol Neurosurg Psychiatry. 2001;71(6):747–51.

19. Peroutka SJ. Dopamine and migraine. Neurology. 1997;49(3):650–6.

20. Levy MJ, Jager HR, Powell M, Matharu MS, Meeran K, Goadsby PJ. Pituitary volume and headache: size is not everything. Arch Neurol. 2004;61(5):721–5.

21. Gondim JA, de Almeida JP, de Albuquerque LA, Schops M, Gomes E, Ferraz T. Headache associated with pituitary tumors. J Headache Pain. 2009;10(1):15–20.

22. Abe T, Matsumoto K, Kuwazawa J, Toyoda I, Sasaki K. Headache associated with pituitary adenomas. Headache: J Head Face Pain. 1998;38(10):782–6.

23. Clouston PD, DeAngelis LM, Posner JB. The spectrum of neurological disease in patients with systemic cancer. Ann Neurol. 1992;31(3):268–73.

24. Jena SS, Nayak S, Behera IC, Mohapatra D, Tripathy SK. Cerebral venous sinus thrombosis: an unusual initial presentation of mucinous adenocarcinoma of stomach. Neurol India. 2014;62(6):695–7.

25. Ferro JM, Canhão P, Stam J, Bousser M-G, Barinagarrementeria F. Prognosis of cerebral vein and dural sinus thrombosis results of the international study on cerebral vein and dural sinus thrombosis (ISCVT). Stroke. 2004;35(3):664–70.

26. Raizer JJ, DeAngelis LM. Cerebral sinus thrombosis diagnosed by MRI and MR venography in cancer patients. Neurology. 2000;54(6):1222–6.

27. Iurlaro S, Silvani A, Mauri M, Truci G, Beretta S, Zilioli A, et al. Headache in cerebral venous thrombosis associated with extracranial tumors: a clinical series. Neurol Sci. 2015;36(Suppl 1):149–51.

28. Greenberg HS, Deck MD, Vikram B, Chu FC, Posner JB. Metastasis to the base of the skull: clinical findings in 43 patients. Neurology. 1981;31(5):530–7.

29. Laigle-Donadey F, Taillibert S, Martin-Duverneuil N, Hildebrand J, Delattre J-Y. Skull-base metastases. J Neurooncol. 2005; 75(1):63–9.

30. Tamoxifen tablets [package insert]. Morgantown, WV: Mylan Pharmaceuticals Inc.; 2013.

31. Sul JK, DeAngelis LM. Neurologic complications of cancer chemotherapy. Semin Oncol. 2006;33(3):324–32.

32. Ganguly S. All-trans retinoic acid related headache in patients with acute promyelocytic leukemia: prophylaxis and treatment with acetazolamide. Leuk Res. 2005;29(6):721.

33. Thielen AM, Saurat JH. Retinoids. In: Bolognia JL, Jorizzo JL, Schaffer JV, editors. Dermatology. 3rd ed. China: Elsevier; 2012. p. 2089–103.

34. Colucciello M. Pseudotumor cerebri induced by all-trans retinoic acid treatment of acute promyelocytic leukemia. Arch Ophthalmol. 2003;121(7):1064–5.

35. Kirby S, Purdy RA. Headaches and brain tumors. Neurol Clin. 2014;32(2):423–32.

36. Shuper A, Packer R, Vezina L, Nicholson H, Lafond D. Complicated migraine-like episodes' in children following cranial irradiation and chemotherapy. Neurology. 1995;45(10):1837–40.

37. Black DF, Morris JM, Lindell EP, Krecke KN, Worrell GA, Bartleson JD, et al. Stroke-like migraine attacks after radiation therapy (SMART) syndrome is not always completely reversible: a case series. AJNR Am J Neuroradiol. 2013;34(12):2298–303.

38. Kerklaan JP, Lycklama á Nijeholt GJ, Wiggenraad RGJ, Berghuis B, Postma TJ, Taphoorn MJB. SMART syndrome: a late reversible complication after radiation therapy for brain tumours. J Neurol. 2011;258(6):1098–104.

39. Farid K, Meissner WG, Samier-Foubert A, Barret O, Menegon P, Rouanet F, et al. Normal cerebrovascular reactivity in stroke-like migraine attacks after radiation therapy syndrome. Clin Nucl Med. 2010;35(8):583–5.

40. Gilles F. The epidemiology of headache among children with brain tumor. J Neurooncol. 1991;10(1):31–46.

41. Abu-Arafeh I, Macleod S. Serious neurological disorders in children with chronic headache. Arch Dis Child. 2005;90(9):937–40.

42. Reulecke BC, Erker CG, Fiedler BJ, Niederstadt T-U, Kurlemann G. Brain tumors in children: initial symptoms and their influence on the time span between symptom onset and diagnosis. J Child Neurol. 2008;23(2):178–83.

43. Wilne SH, Ferris RC, Nathwani A, Kennedy CR. The presenting features of brain tumours: a review of 200 cases. Arch Dis Child. 2006;91(6):502–6.

44. Ryken TC, McDermott M, Robinson PD, Ammirati M, Andrews DW, Asher AL, et al. The role of steroids in the management of brain metastases: a systematic review and evidence-based clinical practice guideline. J Neurooncol. 2010; 96(1):103–14.

45. Schiff D, Lee EQ, Nayak L, Norden AD, Reardon DA, Wen PY. Medical management of brain tumors and the sequelae of treatment. Neuro Oncol. 2015;17(4):488–504.

46. Bruera E, Paice JA. Cancer pain management: safe and effective use of opioids. Am Soc Clin Oncol Educ Book. 2015;35:e593–9.

47. Hayashi N, Kidokoro H, Miyajima Y, Fukazawa T, Natsume J, Kubota T, et al. How do the clinical features of brain tumours in childhood progress before diagnosis? Brain Dev. 2010;32(8):636–41.

48. Molineus A, Boxberger N, Redlich A, Vorwerk P. Time to diagnosis of brain tumors in children: a single-centre experience. Pediatr Int. 2013;55(3):305–9.

Seizures as Complications in Cancer

9

9

Christa P. Benit, Melissa Kerkhof, Alberto Duran-Peña, and Charles J. Vecht

Introduction

Epilepsy is common in cancer. In fact, epilepsy can be the consequence of any structural or functional brain lesion. As such, seizures represent a large number of cancer complications, resulting directly or indirectly from disease or its treatment. Primary brain tumors are associated with a higher incidence of epilepsy compared to metastatic disease of the brain. The main focus of this chapter is seizures in gliomas, including epidemiology and underlying mechanism, but we will also discuss seizures related to brain metastases and cancer therapies. Both antitumor therapy and symptomatic management with antiepileptic drugs (AEDs) contribute to seizure control. Management of brain tumor-related epilepsy (BTE) is often complicated by adverse effects of AEDs, drug resistance, and drug–drug interactions with chemotherapy. For practical use, a guideline on the medical management of seizure control including dosing regimens is provided.

Seizures as Complication of Cancer

Seizures can be the manifestation of primary brain tumors, metastatic disease, vascular complications, opportunistic infections, surgical complications, or secondary to a host of medical treatments, including surgery, chemotherapy, and rarely radiation [1]. During the course of disease, many circumstances may cause seizures. Most commonly, these are due to metabolic or toxic encephalopathies secondary to organ dysfunction. Additionally, drugs used to treat cancer or its complications, including chemotherapeutic drugs, antibiotic therapy and opioids, can precipitate seizure activity. Chemotherapeutic drugs associated with seizures are listed in Table 9.1 [2, 3]. For semiology and causes of seizures in cancer, see Table 9.2 [2].

Brain Tumors

Epilepsy occurs in 13% of all cancer patients and accounts for 5% of neurological manifestations. Half of all seizures in systemic cancer are associated with brain or leptomeningeal metastasis [1, 2]. Epilepsy may be the first sign of cancer either as manifestation of a primary brain tumor or from systemic cancer that presents with brain metastasis. Seizures are also an early sign of paraneoplastic encephalomyelitis, an intriguing albeit rare manifestation of cancer.

Brain Metastasis

Seizures occur as the presenting symptom in 18% of patients with brain metastases; another 15% develop seizures later in the course of the disease [1, 4, 5]. The incidence varies from 16% with breast cancer, 21% with gastrointestinal metastases, 29% in lung cancer patients and up to 70% with melanoma, possibly due to its predisposition for intratumoral hemorrhage. In a retrospective study of 470 patients with brain metastases of any type, 24% of patients had one or more seizures at any point in their disease course [6]. The incidence can be higher for patients with metastases involving or adjacent to brain regions of high epileptogenicity, such as motor cortex, and in patients with multiple brain metastases.

C.P. Benit (✉) · M. Kerkhof
Department of Neurology, The Hague Medical Center, Lijnbaan 32, 2512 VA The Hague, The Netherlands
e-mail: chrben@mchaaglanden.nl

M. Kerkhof
e-mail: m.kerkhof@mchaaglanden.nl

A. Duran-Peña · C.J. Vecht
Department of Neurology Mazarin, Pitié Salpetrière Hospital, 47 Boulevard de l'hôpital, 75013 Paris, France
e-mail: betitodu@gmail.com

C.J. Vecht
e-mail: charlesvecht@icloud.com

© Springer International Publishing AG 2018
D. Schiff et al. (eds.), *Cancer Neurology in Clinical Practice*,
DOI 10.1007/978-3-319-57901-6_9

Table 9.1 Chemotherapeutic drugs associated with seizures

l-Asparaginase	Chlorambucil	Interferon-a
Bevacuzimab	Cyclosporin A	Lomustine
Carmustine	Etoposide	Methotrexate
Cisplatin	5-Fluorouracil	Procarbazine
Busulphan	Ifosfamide	Vincristine

Table 9.2 Semiology and aetiology of new-onset seizures in cancer

Semiology	Aetiological condition
Isolated generalized tonic–clonic seizures/seizure clusters	Most drug-induced seizures Metabolic encephalopathy Endocrine tumors Intracranial metastasis CNS infections Viral encephalitis Parenchymal space-occupying infections Cerebral venous sinus thrombosis
Myoclonic seizures	Busulfan
Photosensitive seizures	Interferon-alpha
Multiple focal seizures/varying semiology	Intracranial metastasis Multifocal parenchymal infections Paraneoplastic encephalomyelitis
Status epilepticus	Cyclosporine Toxic drug overdose Drug-induced seizures in the setting of impaired clearance
Non-convulsive status epilepticus (a) Generalized (b) Complex partial	Ifosfamide Paraneoplastic limbic encephalitis Limbic encephalitis due to herpes virus Cyclosporine
Epilepsia partialis continua	Paraneoplastic encephalomyelitis Venous sinus thrombosis with venous infarct
Unprovoked recurrent seizures, easily controlled with epilepsy drugs Unprovoked seizures	Methotrexate-radiation Leukoencephalopathy Following cerebral ischemia or hemorrhage CNS infections
Intractable complex partial seizures/epilepsy	Paraneoplastic limbic encephalitis Delayed radiation necrosis Herpes virus-induced encephalitis

Used with permission of BMJ Publishing Group from Singh et al. [2]

Meningiomas

About one-third of patients with meningioma present with epilepsy, of whom 70% have secondary generalized and 30% partial seizures. Seizures are more frequently seen with convexity-based lesions than with tumors in other regions, and are more common in the presence of manifest peritumoral edema [7–9]. Epileptic seizures occur in 30% of patients before surgery and in 26.6% patients after surgery. Of patients with preoperative epilepsy, 59.0% become seizure-free after surgery, and 20% of those without preoperative seizures will develop epilepsy after surgery. Risk factors for postoperative epilepsy are preoperative epilepsy, surgical complications including CNS infections, repeat craniotomy, intracranial hemorrhage, and tumor progression. Postoperative improvement or recovery from preoperative neurologic deficits is associated with improved seizure control [8, 9].

Neuroepithelial Tumors

DNETs

In dysembryoblastic neuroepithelial tumors (DNETs), seizures affect essentially 100% of patients with an average age of 15 years at presentation, and 50% of patients have complex partial seizures with or without secondary generalization. On MRI, 80% of the tumors are located in the temporal lobe, 16% in the frontal lobe, and the remainder in other cortical regions [10, 11].

Gangliogliomas

Among patients with gangliogliomas, 80–90% have seizures, usually as the first and only clinical symptom, at an average age of onset of 17–21 years. Of these, 74% are complex partial, 43% generalized tonic-clonic/mixed, 12% simple partial, and 6% absence seizures. The majority of gangliogliomas are located in the temporal lobe and display staining for the CD34 glycoprotein, in contrast to gangliogliomas located elsewhere [11–13].

Gliomas

Astrocytomas are frequently located in temporal or insular locations, while oligodendrogliomas have a predilection for the frontal lobe [14, 15]. Oligodendroglial tumors more often involve the cortex and result in a higher risk of seizures as compared to astrocytomas, which tend to occur in the white matter. Frontal, temporal, insular, and parietal lobe tumors are more commonly associated with seizures as opposed to occipital and midline tumors. Localization to functional cortex renders tumors particularly epileptogenic.

Anaplastic astrocytomas and high-grade gliomas with temporal lobe or cortical involvement can be associated with preoperative seizures. In contrast, older age and larger tumor size are less commonly associated with preoperative seizures. Seizure-free outcome at 12 months following surgery is 77% [16]. A lower incidence of seizures is seen in de novo GBMs compared to secondary GBMs (e.g., those that developed from prior low-grade gliomas) [17, 18].

Tumor Location

In addition to tumor type and grade, tumor location influences the incidence of epilepsy. Tumors located in superficial cortical areas are more likely to be associated with seizures as are as lesions centered in the temporal lobe, frontal lobe, or insula [5, 19–21]. Inherent epileptogenicity of structures in the mesial temporal lobe contributes to seizure generation in this region [22, 23]. Additionally, localization of tumor to eloquent or near-eloquent brain increases risk for seizures [24–26].

Molecular Biological Factors of Seizure Development

Low-grade brain tumors have a stronger predilection for epileptogenesis than more malignant brain cancers. In comparison to higher grade tumors such as glioblastoma, low-grade brain malignancies including gliomas more frequently present with seizures despite being larger in size at the time of discovery [21, 27]. This may be explained by the slow growth rate associated with low-grade lesions which favors development of seizure-prone changes like de-afferentation and disconnection of cortical areas leading to denervation hypersensitivity [28]. This slower rate of growth may also permit adaptive changes of the surrounding brain tissue to occur, thereby diminishing the development of focal neurological deficits.

Brain tumors can also affect the brain network distant to the original site, leading to disruptions in functional connectivity in remote areas [29]. Alterations in microenvironment including hypoxia and acidosis induce swelling and cell damage together with deregulation of sodium and calcium influx with generation of electrical impulses. Overexpression of voltage-gated sodium channels as well as changes in the SV2A synaptic vesicle protein associated with calcium accumulation may facilitate recurring generation of action potentials around tumor cells [30].

Molecular genotypes also contribute to seizures. Solitary 19q loss associated with anaplastic tumors and temporal lobe location [14] has been associated with secondary generalized seizures [31]. The presence of mutations in the mTOR pathway and BRAF V600E mutations as seen in 50% of gangliogliomas increases the risk for seizures [32]. Likewise mutations of codon 132 isocitrate-dehydrogenase 1 (IDH1), which are present in 71–88% of grade II astrocytomas and oligodendrogliomas are associated with seizures [33–36]. The IDH1 enzyme belongs to the Krebs citric acid cycle, catalyzing the conversion of isocitrate into alpha-ketoglutarate. Instead, the enzymatic product of the mutated gene produces 2-hydroxyglutarate. The latter structurally resembles glutamate, which may activate NMDA receptors with ensuing seizure activity. Altered expression of glutamate transporters, including the cysteine-glutamate transporter (xCT) system, increases the concentration of extracellular glutamate, which contributes to epileptic discharge, tumor proliferation, and peripheral excitotoxicity [37, 38]. Furthermore, dysregulation of intracellular chloride promotes glioma cell mitosis and migration, and γ-aminobutyric acid (GABA) signaling suppresses proliferation. In neurons, however, chloride accumulation leads to aberrant depolarization on GABA receptor activation, thereby promoting epileptic activity [26, 38]. Disturbances of chloride balance in gliomas are secondary to changes in chloride cotransporters by reduced KCC2 and increased NKCC1 expression with accompanying changes in GABA metabolism [39]. Glutamergic stimulation of NMDA- and AMPA-receptors activates intracellular mTOR, AKT, and MAPK signaling pathways leading both to cell growth and to epileptogenesis [40, 41].

Seizure Semiology

In about half of cases, the first epileptic event presents as a generalized seizure, while partial seizures predominate thereafter [42]. In low-grade gliomas, seizures most frequently present as secondarily generalized seizures (70%), followed by simple partial seizures (24%), and complex partial (7%) [24]. In glioblastoma, the most frequent presenting seizure semiology is that of secondary generalization in 40% of cases, followed by partial seizures in 37% and both partial and generalized seizures in 14.4% [16, 43]. Status epilepticus is observed in 12% of cases [43].

Factors in Seizure Control

In patients presenting with epilepsy, the number of seizures and their duration prior to surgery are predictive of postoperative seizure behavior [24, 44]. Furthermore, *the underlying tumor histology can* influence *seizure control*. DNETs show a postoperative seizure control of 83% compared to 78% in patients with gangliogliomas (Table 9.3) [13, 45].

Surgery plays an important role in seizure control. Rates of complete seizure freedom postoperatively range from 45 to 100%. In a systematic review on DNETs and gangliogliomas, 80% of patients with tumor-related epilepsy preoperatively became seizure free after surgery [13, 45–47]. The presence of preoperative partial seizures was associated with 87% seizure freedom after resection, as compared to 73% for generalized seizures. Duration of seizures shorter than one year and extensive tumor resection are both favorable prognostic factors for postoperative seizure control. This suggests that earlier intervention may lead to better control and that residual tumor increases the risk of postoperative seizures [45].

In low-grade gliomas, prognostic factors for good postoperative seizure control include generalized seizures, preoperative seizure control, extra-temporal location, and a gross tumor resection within <1 year after presentation [24, 48, 49]. Overall, seizure freedom is achieved in 74% of patients with generalized or mixed type epilepsy, in 63% with complex partial, and 53% with simple partial epilepsy (Table 9.3) [24]. In oligodendrogliomas, seizure control is linked to tumor control, independent of the presence of seizures as the first clinical sign [50]. AED-resistant seizures are not rare, occurring in 40% of patients.

In GBM, preoperative uncontrolled seizures and parietal lobe involvement are negative prognostic factors. Prolonged seizure control is associated with a better Karnofsky performance score [16].

Table 9.3 Seizure characteristics in patients with neuroepithelial tumors

	Glioneuronal		LGG[c]	GBM[d]
	DNET[a]	Ganglioglioma[b]		
Age at presentation (median)	15 years	17–21 years	38 years	60 years
Seizures				
At presentation (%)	100	60–95	65–85	42.1
Incidence (%)		80–90	70–90	30–60
Type of epilepsy				
Partial (%)	50.7	86		
Simple partial	*na*	12%	23.7%	20.3–27%
Complex partial (%)	52	74	6.6	3.1–10
Generalized or mixed (%)	49.3	43	69.7	35
Location of tumor				
Temporal (%)	79.4	35–76	37	24–27
Extra-temporal (%)	20.6	24	63	73–76
Frontal (%)	13.8	7–13	71	28–43
Parietal (%)	3.4	6–10	9	19–27
Insular (%)	*na*	*na*	21	*na*
Occipital (%)	3.4	2.0–3.2	0	5–9

Used with permission of John Wiley and Sons from Kerkhof and Vecht [188]
LGG low-grade glioma, *HGG* high-grade glioma, *na* not available
[a]Grewal et al. [1], Lynam et al. [5]
[b]Singh et al. [2], Verstappen et al. [3], Zaatreh et al. [20]
[c]Lieu and Howng [189], Oberndorfer et al. [6]
[d]Kerkhof et al. [43]

Seizures in Relation to Survival

Seizure as the presenting symptom of brain tumors is a favorable prognostic factor for survival, as are the number of seizures and duration of preoperative seizures [24, 44].

In low-grade gliomas, seizures without other neurological symptoms at presentation are associated with longer overall survival time (HR: 0.27) [50, 51]. Conversely, neurological deficits or a poor performance status at presentation are associated with worse longevity [49]. Overall, the presence of seizures, smaller tumor volume and extent of surgical resection are all associated with longer survival in low-grade gliomas [11].

In oligodendroglial tumors, uni- and multivariate analysis reveal that the presence of IDH1 mutation, co-deletion of 1p and 19q and frontal tumor location are positive prognostic factors regardless of presence of seizures [14, 52, 53]. Nonetheless, the relation between seizures and survival is remarkable. Patients with a single seizure prior to surgery (14% of all patients) do extraordinarily well, showing a 90% 10 year survival. In contrast, one-third of the small subgroup presenting with other neurological deficits (10% of all patients) die within 1 or 2 years. The remaining patients have either occasional or clearly relapsing seizures, and both groups show a steadily decreasing survival slope with a median survival of 10 years. However, patients with refractory seizures tend to do worse than those with controlled seizures [50].

Nevertheless, seizures as a good prognostic feature seem mainly a secondary phenomenon [38]. In low-grade gliomas, initial epilepsy as favorable prognostic factor could be explained by the association of the IDH1 mutation with formation of D-2HG, which may generate epileptic activity [36, 54]. In glioblastomas, new-onset epilepsy is associated with presentation at younger age, better overall health status and substantially smaller tumor size, which are all independent favorable factors for survival [55, 56].

Seizure Recurrence

Reappearance or worsening of seizures following a relatively long period of seizure control may signal progression or recurrence of glioma. In low-grade gliomas, relapse of seizures after a period of 6 months or more of seizure freedom is an indicator of tumor progression in about 50% of patients [24, 57]. Approximately 15% of glioblastoma patients have ongoing seizure activity despite multiple antitumor regimens [43]. Recurrence or worsening of seizures following a stable period in GBM heralds progression in approximately two-third of patients following first-line antitumor therapy [16, 24, 58]. This necessitates adjustment of seizure treatment and reevaluation of the tumor status of the patient. Thus, while early seizures in gliomas represent a favorable prognostic indicator with respect to survival, late recurring seizures are more likely to indicate progressive disease, often accompanied by adverse effects on cognition and quality of life.

Effects of Antitumor Therapy on Seizure Control

Surgery

Surgical resection is a crucial part of tumor therapy as well as being effective for seizure control. Large series of low-grade gliomas indicate an overall seizure-free rate of 67–87% following surgery [10, 20, 24, 49]. Refractory seizures benefit most from gross tumor surgery. In high-grade gliomas, tumor resection renders 77% of patients seizure-free [16]. For temporal lobe tumors, higher rates of seizure freedom (90–95%) are achieved by using electrocorticography (ECoG) for performing additional hippocampectomy, corticectomy or both as compared to the lower rates (79%) with gross total lesionectomy alone [59]. The most consistent finding in surgical studies of brain tumor-related epilepsy is that gross total resection is associated with greatly improved seizure outcome compared to subtotal resection.

Radiotherapy

Radiation therapy contributes to improved seizure control in low- and high-grade gliomas. A randomized EORTC trial of early versus delayed radiation in low-grade glioma found that 75% of patients became seizure-free following early radiation compared to 59% in the control arm [60]. Retrospective studies in low-grade glioma reveal that 56–77% of patients experience a 50% reduction in seizure frequency with 38–80% becoming seizure-free [61–64]. In a series of combined low- and high-grade gliomas, 77% of patients showed 50% seizure reduction and 38% seizure freedom at 12 months following radiation therapy, although patients were unable to discontinue AEDs [60].

Chemotherapy

The efficacy of chemotherapeutic drugs for treating low-grade gliomas, either as initial treatment or following surgery and radiotherapy, is well established. These agents also contribute to seizure control [44, 65, 66]. Upfront temozolomide chemotherapy in low-grade gliomas is associated with 50% seizure reduction in 50–60% of patients, with 13–55% becoming seizure-free [65, 67, 68]. In recurrent low-grade gliomas, 78% of patients achieve 50% seizure reduction with either temozolomide, PCV chemotherapy or bevacuzimab (in some cases in conjunction with preceding surgery) [65–70].

Symptomatic Treatment with Anticonvulsant Drugs

Symptomatic management of seizures in cancer patient is in principle not different from other causes for focal epilepsy. Antiepileptic drugs can be initiated after the occurrence of a single seizure attributable to a brain tumor [71, 72]. In general, the choice of a specific AED is primarily based on the type of the epilepsy. Epilepsy in patients with brain tumors belongs to the type of partial epilepsy in adults, either with or without secondary generalized seizures, and is essentially based on focal lesion or brain damage. For this type of seizures, the International League against Epilepsy (ILAE) has updated the most appropriate AEDs based on a meta-analysis of large number of randomized controlled trials [73]. As such, levetiracetam (LEV), carbamazepine, phenytoin, and zonisamide are considered class A anticonvulsants, based on trial quality for efficacy. Valproic acid (VPA) represents the only class B anticonvulsant. Gabapentin, lamotrigine, oxcarbazepine, phenobarbital, topiramate, and vigabatrin are class C agents [73]. Subsequently, the choice of the most fitting AED among the approved agents depends on individual patient factors, most importantly age, sex, weight, comorbidities, and concomitant therapy including drug interactions [74]. Regarding concurrent treatment, in neuro-oncology a consensus exists to avoid enzyme-inducing anti-epileptic drugs (EIAEDs)—phenobarbital, carbamazepine and phenytoin—as these accelerate the metabolism of many chemotherapeutic agents [71, 75]. For zonisamide, there is still limited experience with brain tumors [76]. Table 9.4 provides pharmacological details on anticonvulsant drugs.

Monotherapy

Levetiracetam as monotherapy demonstrates a high seizure control rate of 70–100% in low- and high-grade gliomas, although preceding surgery and associated antitumor treatment contribute to these excellent results [43, 77]. Levetiracetam may also be effective with brain metastasis [78].

There are several advantages of levetiracetam over other AEDs, including good tolerability and lack of drug–drug interactions. A comparative trial in the early postoperative period showed a better efficacy and tolerability than phenytoin [79]. However, approximately 5% of patients develop irritability, aggression or psychosis, for which dose adjustment or withdrawal of levetiracetam is usually indicated [80]. Intriguingly, cognition improves in around 25% of patients taking levetiracetam in both general epilepsy and BTE [81–83].

Valproic acid monotherapy in BTE is extensively utilized for low- and high-grade gliomas and provides improved or complete seizure control in 55–78% [16, 43, 58]. Valproic acid is a broad-spectrum, well-tolerated AED although it may cause increased appetite, hand tremor, and thrombocytopenia as side effects. It is contraindicated in pregnant women.

With regard to class C agents, there is little information on gabapentin and lamotrigine in BTE, although both AEDs are generally well-tolerated. Topiramate is a broad-spectrum AED that often causes substantial cognitive side effects. Oxcarbazepine monotherapy in BTE produces complete seizure control in 40–63%, though with a relatively high rate of cognitive adverse effects [84, 85]. Lacosamide is a well-tolerated AED that has recently been approved as monotherapy in the US. With add-on lacosamide in BTE, 43% of patients became seizure-free, and 40–50% of patients showed a 50+% seizure reduction [86, 87]. Adjunctive perampanel in drug-resistant partial seizures produces about a 40% response rate and sustained seizure frequency improvement with a generally favorable safety profile [88, 89].

Polytherapy

When the initial anticonvulsant provides insufficient seizure control, one can switch to a second agent as monotherapy, though there is a trend to rather apply polytherapy as the next step by adding a second AED to the first one [90, 91]. Meta-analysis in drug-resistant epilepsy has indicated that add-on levetiracetam is remarkably effective both in general epilepsy as in BTE, producing 50+% seizure reduction in 65% of patients [43, 77]. This might suggest synergistic qualities of levetiracetam, particularly in combination with AEDs that have GABAergic or antiglutaminergic activity [92]. In neuro-oncology, a crucial advantage of synergistic therapy is that effective lower doses of AEDs carry smaller risks of toxicity, although this requires confirmation in prospective studies.

In BTE, we favor levetiracetam as the anticonvulsant of choice, if necessary to be combined with valproic acid, as both agents are well tolerated in the partial epilepsies [93, 94]. A good alternative anticonvulsant is lacosamide based on efficacy, good tolerability, and absence of drug interactions [87, 95, 96]. In glioblastoma, VPA may be given as first line AED in based on the evidence as class B agent for focal epilepsy together with emerging activity of antitumor

Table 9.4 Main characteristics of AEDs (in alphabetical order) including dose range

AED	Usual dosage (mg/day)	Therapeutic range (mg/l)	Common/ important side effects	Main mechanism of action	Oral bioavailability (%)	T 1/2 (h)	Metabolism and excretion	Protein binding (%)
CBZ	400–1600	4–12	Leukopenia, aplastic anemia, hepatotoxicity, hyponatremia, SJS/TEN	Blocks voltage-dependent Na^+-channels	75–85	5–26	Hepatic epoxidation, conjugation	75
CLB	5–40	0.1–0.3	Sedation, cognitive effects, drowsiness	GABA receptor agonist	80–90	12–60	Hepatic N-demethylation	85
CZP	0.5–4	0.02–0.08	Sedation, cognitive effects, drowsiness	GABA receptor agonist	90	20–80	Hepatic reduction and acetylation	86
FBM	1200–3600	30–100	Hepatic disturbance, SJS, aplastic anemia, insomnia, weight loss	NMDA and Na^+-channel conductance	>90	13–30	Hepatic hydroxylation and conjugation (60%), renal excretion (40%)	20–25
GBP	900–3600	2–20	Weight gain, worsening of seizures	Blocks Ca^+ channels	<65	5–7	Renal excretion without metabolism	None
LCM	200–400	10–20	Dizziness, headache, nausea, diplopia, blurred vision	Slow inactivation of voltage-dependent Na^+-channels	>95	13	Hepatic demethylation, unchanged renal excretion (40%)	<15
LTG	200–600	1–15	Rash, SJS, TEN, DRESS, headache, blood dyscrasia, ataxia	Blocks voltage-dependent Na^+-channels	>95	12–60	Hepatic glucuronidation (without phase 1 reaction), renal excretion (10%)	55
LEV	1000–3000	3–30	Somnolence, asthenia, irritability, psychosis	binding to synaptic vesicle protein 2 (SV2A)	>95	6–8	Partially hydrolyzed in the blood, renal excretion (66%)	None
OXC	900–2400	10–35	Somnolence, headache, diplopia, SJS, hyponatremia	Blocks voltage-dependent Na^+-channels	>95	8–10	Hydroxylation, conjugation	38
PB	30–180	15–40	Rash, hepatotoxicity, impaired cognition, ataxia, mood change	GABA receptor agonist, glutamate antagonist, blocks voltage-dependent Na^+-$Ca+$ channels	80–100	46–136	Hepatic oxidation, glucosidation, hydroxylation, conjugation	45–60
PHT	5 mg/kg	10–20	Blood dyscrasia, hepatitis, SJS, gum hyperplasia, lupuslike reactions, hirsutism	Blocks voltage-dependent Na^+-channels	95	7–42	Hepatic oxidation, hydroxylation, conjugation	85–95
PGB	150–600	2–8	Somnolence, dizziness, ataxia	Binds to Ca^+-channels	90	6	No metabolism, renal excretion	None
PMP	4–12	0.2–1.0	Dizziness, somnolence, fatigue, irritability	AMPA-receptor blocker	100	24–500	Hepatic oxidation, glucuronidation	95
TPM	100–500	2–20	Impaired cognition, hepatotoxicity, weight loss, renal stones	Blocks Na^+-channels, GABA receptor agonist, blocks NMDA receptors	81–95	19–25	Mainly renal excretion without metabolism	13–17

(continued)

Table 9.4 (continued)

AED	Usual dosage (mg/day)	Therapeutic range (mg/l)	Common/ important side effects	Main mechanism of action	Oral bioavailability (%)	T 1/2 (h)	Metabolism and excretion	Protein binding (%)
VGB	200–300	0.8–36	Visual field defects (33%; often irreversible), fatigue, drowsiness	GABA-transaminase inhibitor	80–90	6–8	No metabolism, renal excretion (70%, unchanged)	None
VPA	500–2500	50–100	Hepatotoxicity, thrombo- and neutropenia, aplastic anemia, tremor, weight gain, hair loss, ovarian cystic syndrome	GABA receptor agonist	>95	12–15	Hepatic glucuronidation, oxidation, conjugation	85–95
ZON	200–600	20–30	Somnolence, ataxia, dizziness, renal calculi	Blocks Na^+- and Ca^+-channels	>95	60–70	Hepatic acetylation, glucuronidation (20%), renal excretion (30%)	40–50

Used with permission of Oxford University Press from Bénit and Vecht [159]

efficacy if combined with temozolomide [43, 97–99]. If either levetiracetam or combinations with VPA or lacosamide are insufficiently effective, one can choose lamotrigine for its good tolerability and its potential of synergistic activity with VPA, perampanel for its efficacy and tolerability in refractory partial epilepsy, or zonisamide considering its recent designation as class A agent for the partial epilepsies [73, 88, 89, 100]. For the application of anticonvulsant therapy in daily clinical practice of BTE, see Table 9.4.

Duration of AED therapy depends on the underlying cause of seizures. For seizures associated with metabolic or toxic encephalopathies, we recommend continuing AEDs therapy as long as the underlying cause remains present or can easily recur. In the case of a structural lesion as cause of the epilepsy as with gliomas, we advocate continuing antiepileptic treatment for at least 2 years following seizure control [101, 102]. In patients with long-term good seizure control on polytherapy, it is reasonable to try to gradually taper the patient down to monotherapy.

For treatment recommendations in children, we refer to other reviews [103].

Prophylactic AED Use

It is uncertain whether there is any role for AED prophylaxis in brain tumor patients without a history of seizures. Consensus statements by the American Academy of Neurology and the European Association of Neuro-Oncology (EANO) have advised against long-term AED prophylaxis in newly diagnosed brain tumor patients [71, 75]. Meta-analysis of available studies has not provided evidence in support of AED prophylaxis [104]. A notable exception is that prophylactic AEDs may be considered for the first weeks after surgical resection, given the frequency of immediate postoperative seizures [105–107]. In a study on 121 patients undergoing glioma surgery, despite receiving prophylaxis, 9.1% of patients experienced a seizure within the first postoperative week, and problems with AED tolerability were not uncommon [108]. There is borderline evidence for AED prophylaxis in the peri-operative period [107].

Toxicity

Cognitive Function and AEDs

Overall, AED therapy—and particularly polytherapy—lead to a deterioration of cognitive functioning [109–111]. In a prospective cross-sectional survey in 147 patients with BTE, 54.4% showed cognitive impairment. On multivariate analysis, these impairments were associated with advancing age, lesion laterality, and chemotherapy use [112]. In a group of 156 long-time survivors of low-grade glioma, both the presence of seizures as well as therapy with conventional AEDs correlated with cognitive deterioration on several domains [113, 114]. In another prospective study, the presence of low-grade gliomas, prior radiation therapy (particularly >2 Gy per fraction), and anticonvulsant use were associated with slower psychomotor speed, memory deficits, and attention or executive deficits [115].

In high-grade glioma, data are less convincing that AED use leads to impaired memory [116, 117]. Chemoradiation leads to a diminished brain volume, and in that way patients are probably more prone to factors that lead to cognitive dysfunction [118].

AED polytherapy strongly contributes to cognitive dysfunction. Each added anticonvulsant leads to a further deterioration of cognitive functioning [111]. These effects are enhanced in patients who already have deficits from primary or metastatic brain tumors, brain surgery, and brain tumor therapy [119, 120].

These observations illustrate that in patients with brain tumors, neuropsychological deficits depend on the cumulative effects of previous neurosurgery, radiation therapy, chemotherapy, presence of epilepsy, and AED use [121]. Although the cognitive adverse effects of AEDs are usually mild or moderate, their impact in BTE can be substantial.

In the setting of AED side effects, options include lowering the AED dose or switching to another agent. Importantly, many patients with epilepsy, if forced to choose, would prefer to be free of AED side effects over having complete seizure control [122]. Consequently, a prudent dose reduction is often justified, particularly with partial seizures without loss of consciousness where complete seizure control is not mandatory [123].

Bone Marrow and AEDs

Bone marrow abnormalities may occur as a side effect of several AEDs, and are relatively more common in brain tumors than other epilepsy etiologies [75].

Although hematotoxicity can arise from phenobarbital, phenytoin, carbamazepine, or VPA, it is more common and severe with concurrent use of temozolomide or PCV [42, 124–126].

Aplastic anemia is a rare, though severe complication of AEDs. Its overall incidence is two to six cases in one million, of which about 20% drug-induced [127, 128]. Among AEDs, felbamate is the most frequently implicated with an incidence of 1 in 5000–10,000; for that reason it is rarely utilized. Rare cases have been associated with carbamazepine, lamotrigine, and phenytoin [129]. The odds ratio of inducing aplastic anemia compared to no AED at all is 10.3 for carbamazepine, 3.5 for phenytoin, and 18.2 for VPA [130].

Agranulocytosis occurs rarely, and if present is drug-induced in about 70% of cases. In Europe, the annual incidence of idiosyncratic drug-induced agranulocytosis is between 1.6 and 9.2 cases per 10^6 and in the USA between 2.4 and 15.4 per 10^6, and increases with age [131, 132]. The fatality rate is 7.0%. Carbamazepine is the antiepileptic drug with the highest odds ratio (10.9) and rare cases have been reported with phenytoin and VPA [132].

Thrombocytopenia is seen with VPA and depends on dose-dependent suppression of platelet production in the bone marrow [133]. Nevertheless, it is usually asymptomatic, occurring in 7% of women and 2% of men within the upper therapeutic range of 80–100 ng/ml [133]. At supra-therapeutic levels, thrombocytopenia develops in 14.3% of women at 100–120 ng/ml, and in 16.5% of men at plasma levels of VPA >130 ng/ml. Children are more susceptible, however; platelet levels lower than 100,000 are only seen in 10% of children receiving doses of >70 mg/kg VPA or plasma levels of 160 mg/ml or higher. In two prospective studies in children, lower platelet counts were associated with VPA, though still remaining within the normal range of >100,000 [134–136].

Likewise, VPA may compromise concurrent chemotherapy with temozolomide, PCV and other chemotherapeutic agents [124, 126]. Nevertheless, on multivariate analysis only the use of temozolomide was associated with thrombocytopenia, and in a retrospective study, there was no difference in hematological toxicity in patients taking VPA, levetiracetam or no AED together with temozolomide [126, 137]. If thrombocytopenia develops, discontinuation or reduction of VPA usually promptly rectifies this. In neurosurgical patients, postoperative bleeding or need for transfusions did not differ between patients taking VPA or other anticonvulsants [138, 139].

Skin Reactions and AEDs

Skin reactions associated with AEDs range from mild maculopapular rash or exanthema to potentially life-threatening severe cutaneous adverse reactions (SCAR), including drug reaction with eosinophilia and systemic symptoms (DRESS), Stevens–Johnson syndrome (SJS), and toxic epidermal necrolysis (TEN) [140–142]. One explanation for idiosyncratic hypersensitivity reactions is the presence of an aromatic ring in the chemical structure of a drug leading to arene-oxide intermediates, which are immunogenic through interactions with proteins or cellular macromolecules.

Carbamazepine, phenytoin, phenobarbital, and lamotrigine have an odds ratio of 5.8 for cutaneous hypersensitivity reactions [141, 143]. SJS/TEN has been reported with the use of phenobarbital, phenytoin, carbamazepine, oxcarbazepine, lamotrigine, and zonisamide [144, 145]. Signs include necrosis and blistering of skin and mucosal membranes with a potential mortality varying between 10 and 50% [146].

In BTE, appearance of SJS/TEN has been particularly observed during cranial irradiation with concurrent phenobarbital, phenytoin, carbamazepine, or glucocorticoids [147, 148]. Nevertheless, SCAR is rare in BTE. In a retrospective review of 289 patients receiving radiotherapy and AEDs, only one patient developed SJS [140]. In general epilepsy, use of phenytoin, carbamazepine, or oxcarbazepine strongly increases the risk on SCAR dependent on the expression of certain pharmacogenetic traits, mainly HLA-B 1502 and HLA-A 31:01 alleles [149, 150]. Remarkably, HLA-B 1502 allele carriers taking carbamazepine show a high odds ratio of 58.1 for developing SJS/TEN among Asian populations. HLA-A 31:01 carriers taking carbamazepine have an odds ratio of 13.2 for developing DRESS, independent of populations though with a weaker association of 3.94 for SJS/TEN in Europeans [151]. CYP2C9*3 carriers taking phenytoin show an odds ratio of 11 for developing SCAR [152]. One may consider screening for these alleles in both non-BTE and BTE before prescribing carbamazepine, oxcarbazepine, or phenytoin to prevent severe skin reactions [149, 153].

Drug Interactions with AEDs

Cancer patients commonly undergo intensive treatment including surgery, radiation therapy, and one or more lines of chemotherapy. In addition, patients with gliomas, meningiomas, or brain metastasis often need antiepileptic therapy and almost all require corticosteroids at some point. Almost inevitably, this implies risks of drug–drug interactions (DDIs), with an increased risk in patients with brain tumors in comparison to patients with systemic malignancies (OR > 6) [154]. As antineoplastic drugs often have a narrow therapeutic window close to the maximum tolerated dose (MTD), these interactions can easily result in insufficient antitumor therapy or in drug toxicity. This may have major clinical impact as illustrated by observations of a shorter survival in children with acute lymphoblastic leukemia receiving concurrent EIAEDs [155].

Both pharmacokinetic and pharmacodynamic DDIs occur, though in daily practice existing insights mainly relate to pharmacokinetic effects secondary to up- or downregulation of co-enzymes belonging to the CYP 450 or UGT glucuronidation liver systems. Of a total of 20 CYP isoenzymes, 2C9 and 3A4 cover approximately 60% of all metabolic reactions [156]. Phenytoin, phenobarbital, and carbamazepine, oxcarbazepine and eslicarbazepine represent enzyme inducers, mainly of 2C9, 2C19, and 3A4 together with a number of long-term metabolic effects [157]. Enzyme induction results in faster catabolism of concurrently administered drugs metabolized along the same pathway, including CTDs, TKIs, and glucocorticoids. Eslicarbazepine, oxcarbazepine, perampanel, topiramate, and VPA occasionally produce enzyme inhibition depending on CYP or UGT enzymes involved, leading to toxicity of concomitant drugs unless dose adjustment is applied. Vice versa, therapy with cytotoxic agents and tyrosine kinase inhibitors (TKIs) may similarly affect the pharmacokinetics of concurrent therapy.

More than 50% of glioma patients require more than one AED for seizure control, carrying risks for drug interactions [43, 158, 159]. Although newer generation AEDS have much less enzyme inducing effects compared to the classical AEDs (phenobarbital, phenytoin, carbamazepine), one does not always realize that as drug substrates they are often susceptible to the metabolic effects of other agents including AEDs. With concurrent phenytoin and carbamazepine (acting on 2C9, 2C19, 3A4), the clearance of lamotrigine, oxcarbazepine, pregabalin, tiagabine, and zonisamide increases 1.25–2.0-fold, and that of clobazam 2–3-fold. [160, 161]. Weak inducing effects can occur with the use of eslicarbazepine (3A4, UGT1A1) and lamotrigine (UGT1A4) if combined with drugs metabolized by corresponding co-enzymes. Weak inhibiting effects are seen with eslicarbazepine (2C9, 2C19), oxcarbazepine (2C19), perampanel (2C8, UGT1A9), and topiramate (2C19), often without much clinical impact [162]. VPA is mainly an enzyme inhibitor of UGT1A4, causing a doubling of the AUC of lamotrigine [163]. All these agents principally undergo hepatic metabolism. Highly protein-bound drugs such as phenytoin, VPA, and benzodiazepines including clobazam, clonazepam, and midazolam may cause DDIs because of competition for binding with other strongly protein-bound agents. Gabapentin, levetiracetam, lacosamide, pregabaline, and vigabatrin chiefly undergo renal elimination and thus are much less prone to DDIs.

Drug Interactions of AEDs with Chemotherapeutic Drugs

Temozolomide and bevacizumab, two drugs frequently used in neuro-oncology, neither cause nor are subject to DDIs [164, 165]. However, hematological toxicity of chemotherapeutic drugs (CTDs) may be aggravated by direct toxic effects of VPA on the bone marrow [124–126]. The enzyme-inducing agents carbamazepine, phenytoin, and phenobarbital cause a two- to threefold higher clearance of cyclophosphamide, camptothecin derivatives, taxanes, and topoisomerase II inhibitors with a doubling of their maximum tolerated dose (MTD) [159]. VPA may aggravate thrombocytopenia caused by CTDs via a direct effect on the bone marrow, while its enzyme-inhibiting activity in cancer is mainly limited to temsirolimus. Lomustine combined with VPA may cause hematological toxicity, due to independent though additive effects of both agents on the bone marrow [124, 129]. Cisplatin and high-dose methotrexate lead to lower plasma levels of phenytoin, VPA, tiagabine, and clobazam and other benzodiazepines by competition for protein binding. The enzyme-inhibiting effect of 5-fluorouracil causes a two- to fourfold higher organ exposure to phenytoin and phenobarbital.

Methotrexate, particularly high-dose (HD-MTX), is an essential part of chemotherapy for some leukemias and non-Hodgkin lymphomas including CNS lymphoma. In children with acute leukemia, concomitant use of EIAEDs was associated with worse survival (HR 2.7) and faster clearance of methotrexate and teniposide [155]. Pharmacokinetic studies in primary CNS lymphoma and concurrent EIAEDs result in half the AUC of MTX, possibly depending on altered aldehyde oxidase activity [166].

For clinical practice, it is important to realize that in case of co- or CYP-enzyme dependent conversion/metabolism of a parent drug into its active metabolite, a concurrently given enzyme-inducer not only causes accelerated metabolism of the parent drug, though also enhanced formation of the active metabolite. In this way, the net effect can be enhanced drug activity. Examples are combined use of an EIAED with cyclophosphamide, ifosfamide, and thiotepa [167].

Drug Interactions of AEDs with Tyrosine Kinase Inhibitors and Other Targeted Agents

A number of TKIs have been examined in phase I/II trials on gliomas including pharmacokinetics with concurrent EIAEDs and non-EIAEDs. Together with CYP3A4 inducing AEDs, a twofold higher clearance and corresponding reduction of AUC of TKIs is usually seen. Notably, crizotinib, dasatinib, imatinib, and lapatinib show a substantially faster metabolism with concurrent enzyme inducers [168–170]. For the latter two, organ exposure is about four times lower without dose adjustment, representing a moderate drug interaction. Some TKIs are 3A4 inhibitors with inherent risks of toxicity when combined with other 3A4 substrate drugs such as imatinib and crizotinib, requiring lower dosing of concurrent therapy. Combined use of mTOR inhibitors with EIAEDs reduces systemic exposure to temsirolimus, everolimus, and sirolimus [171, 172].

Drug Interactions of AEDs with Glucocorticoids

Glucocorticoids are frequently employed in cancer. As corticosteroids are CYP3A4 enzyme inducers, they influence the pharmacokinetics of concurrent drugs [173–178]. This explains the observations of more rapid clearance and sub-therapeutic levels of phenytoin with concurrent dexamethasone, with a 1.5–2-fold dose increase of phenytoin necessary to maintain therapeutic plasma levels [176]. Inversely, when steroids are tapered in the setting of a therapeutic phenytoin level, phenytoin concentrations can easily rise to toxic levels if the AED is not lowered correspondingly [178]. Increased phenytoin levels occur occasionally in combination with dexamethasone and have been attributed to competition for protein binding, underscoring the possibility of unexpected DDIs [179, 180]. Vice versa, the inducing effects of phenytoin on the clearance of dexamethasone vary by a factor 3 up to 12 [181]. Overall, the plasma half-life of steroids is approximately halved in the setting of concurrent EIAEDs. The supra-therapeutic corticosteroid doses prescribed in cancer likely explain the rarity of signs of insufficient dosing.

A separate issue is the wide interindividual variability in drug metabolism, which is of multifactorial nature. The activity of CYP enzymes shows high individual variability, including their susceptibility to the effects of drug inducers or inhibitors. Besides, CYP activity depends upon age, sex, and ethnicity as well as on diet and organ factors like hepatic dysfunction [182, 183].

Metabolic Variability

The observations on variability in drug metabolism underscore the need for therapeutic drug monitoring (TDM) by plasma measurement of drug concentrations for the detection of DDIs [162, 182–185]. A position paper of the ILAE has defined when to apply TDM in the daily practice of seizure management [186]. Recommendations include performing plasma drug measurements once a desired clinical response has been achieved based on the variable therapeutic range of an AED, the persistence of seizures, and factors as age, comorbidity, or concomitant therapy. Similar calls for TDM of CTDs and TKIs have been made in systemic cancer [184, 187]. Although many of the TKIs are 3A4 inhibitors, it remains unknown how strongly they affect concurrent therapy. Given the common presence of multidrug regimens in patients with seizures and cancer, routine monitoring of plasma levels of AEDs and of CTDs/TKIs is likely of great value.

Conclusions

Recent years have witnessed a considerable increase in our knowledge of tumor-related epilepsy. In cancer, epilepsy can be the manifestation of a primary brain tumor, metastatic disease, vascular complications, opportunistic infection, surgical complications, or secondary to a variety of antitumor or associated therapies. Often, a single seizure is the presenting symptom of a primary brain tumor and is associated with a better prognosis for survival as opposed to presentation with other neurological symptoms.

Drug-resistant seizures may develop, particularly associated with oligodendrogliomas, occurring in about 40%. Recurrence of seizures following a relatively long period of seizure freedom may herald tumor progression. Surgery, radiotherapy, and chemotherapy all contribute to seizure control.

As regards choice of an AED for symptomatic seizure control, there is no essential difference among the many approved agents for new-onset focal epilepsy to which BTE belongs. The choice mainly depends on the individual characteristics of the patient including age, sex and weight. In neuro-oncology, other important considerations are comorbidities and concomitant therapy including the risk of drug interactions.

Overall, levetiracetam monotherapy is a good first-line AED in BTE. If insufficient, valproic acid or lacosamide can be added. When these combinations are inactive or are associated with side effects, lamotrigine, perampanel, or zonisamide are good alternatives. For a detailed guideline on dose regimens of these AEDs, see Table 9.4.

Neurologic toxicity is a potential side effect of all anticonvulsants, and in neuro-oncology cognitive effects, bone marrow toxicity and skin hypersensitivity reactions are the most prevalent. Unfortunately, as more than 50% of glioma patients require AED polytherapy, these risks are not easily avoidable.

The greatest risk of drug interactions in neuro-oncology arises from the use of the enzyme-inducing AEDs carbamazepine, phenytoin, and phenobarbital. Without appropriate adjustments, this can compromise efficacy of multiple chemotherapeutic drugs including cyclophosphamide, camptothecin derivatives, taxanes, and topoisomerase inhibitors. Likewise, several tyrosine kinase inhibitors including crizotinib, dasatinib, imatinib, and lapatinib are metabolized substantially more rapidly when EIAEDs are administered. Some TKIs are 3A4 inhibitors and thus potentially can produce toxicity if coadministered with other CYP3A4 substrate TKIs, particularly imatinib and crizotinib. The CYP3A4 enzyme-inducing activity of corticosteroids also can influence the pharmacokinetics of concurrent drugs including AEDs. For all these reasons, consensus exists that if possible enzyme-inducing anticonvulsant drugs are rather to be avoided. The large interindividual variability in drug metabolism underscores the need for therapeutic drug monitoring of anticonvulsants, chemotherapeutic and targeted agents for detecting drug interactions and optimally dosing these agents.

References

1. Grewal J, Grewal HK, Forman AD. Seizures and epilepsy in cancer: etiologies, evaluation, and management. Curr Oncol Rep. 2008;10(1):63–71.
2. Singh G, Rees JH, Sander JW. Seizures and epilepsy in oncological practice: causes, course, mechanisms and treatment. J Neurol Neurosurg Psychiatry. 2007;78(4):342–9.
3. Verstappen CCP, Heimans JJ, Hoekman K, Postma TJ. Neurotoxic complications of chemotherapy in patients with cancer—clinical signs and optimal management. Drugs. 2003;63(15):1549–63.
4. Avila EK, Graber J. Seizures and epilepsy in cancer patients. Curr Neurol Neurosci Rep. 2010;10(1):60–7.
5. Lynam LM, Lyons MK, Drazkowski JF, Sirven JI, Noe KH, Zimmerman RS, et al. Frequency of seizures in patients with newly diagnosed brain tumors: a retrospective review. Clin Neurol Neurosurg. 2007;109(7):634–8.
6. Oberndorfer S, Schmal T, Lahrmann H, Urbanits S, Lindner K, Grisold W. The frequency of seizures in patients with primary brain tumors or cerebral metastases. An evaluation from the Ludwig Boltzmann Institute of NeuroOncology and the Department of Neurology, Kaiser Franz Josef Hospital, Vienna. Wien Klin Wochenschr. 2002;114(21–22):911–6.
7. Xue H, Sveinsson O, Tomson T, Mathiesen T. Intracranial meningiomas and seizures: a review of the literature. Acta Neurochir. 2015;157(9):1541–8.
8. Englot DJ, Magill ST, Han SJ, Chang EF, Berger MS, McDermott MW. Seizures in supratentorial meningioma: a systematic review and meta-analysis. J Neurosurg. 2016;124(6):1552–61.
9. Wirsching HG, Morel C, Gmur C, Neidert MC, Baumann CR, Valavanis A, et al. Predicting outcome of epilepsy after meningioma resection. Neuro-Oncol. 2016;18(7):1002–10.
10. Luyken C, Blumcke I, Fimmers R, Urbach H, Elger CE, Wiestler OD, et al. The spectrum of long-term epilepsy-associated tumors: long-term seizure and tumor outcome and neurosurgical aspects. Epilepsia. 2003;44(6):822–30.
11. Blumcke I, Wiestler OD. Gangliogliomas: an intriguing tumor entity associated with focal epilepsies. J Neuropathol Exp Neurol. 2002;61(7):575–84.
12. Compton JJ, Laack NNI, Eckel LJ, Schomas DA, Giannini C, Meyer FB. Long-term outcomes for low-grade intracranial ganglioglioma: 30-year experience from the Mayo Clinic Clinical article. J Neurosurg. 2012;117(5):825–30.
13. Southwell DG, Garcia PA, Berger MS, Barbaro NM, Chang EF. Long-term seizure control outcomes after resection of gangliogliomas. Neurosurgery. 2012;70(6):1406–13.
14. Scheie D, Meling TR, Cvancarova M, Skullerud K, Mork S, Lote K, et al. Prognostic variables in oligodendroglial tumors: a single-institution study of 95 cases. Neuro-Oncol. 2011;13(11):1225–33.
15. Kouwenhoven MCM, Gorlia T, Kros JM, Ibdaih A, Brandes AA, Bromberg JEC, et al. Molecular analysis of anaplastic oligodendroglial tumors in a prospective randomized study: a report from EORTC study 26951. Neuro-Oncol. 2009;11(6):737–46.
16. Chaichana KL, Parker SL, Olivi A, Quinones-Hinojosa A. Long-term seizure outcomes in adult patients undergoing primary resection of malignant brain astrocytomas clinical article. J Neurosurg. 2009;111(2):282–92.
17. Moots PL, Maciunas RJ, Eisert DR, Parker RA, Laporte K, Aboukhalil B. The course of seizure disorders in patients with malifnant gliomas. Arch Neurol. 1995;52(7):717–24.
18. Rosati A, Tomassini A, Pollo B, Ambrosi C, Schwarz A, Padovani A, et al. Epilepsy in cerebral glioma: timing of appearance and histological correlations. J Neurooncol. 2009;93(3):395–400.
19. Zaatreh MM, Spencer DD, Thompson JL, Blumenfeld H, Novotny EJ, Mattson RH, et al. Frontal lobe tumoral epilepsy: clinical, neurophysiologic features and predictors of surgical outcome. Epilepsia. 2002;43(7):727–33.
20. Zaatreh MM, Firlik KS, Spencer DD, Spencer SS. Temporal lobe tumoral epilepsy—characteristics and predictors of surgical outcome. Neurology. 2003;61(5):636–41.
21. Lee JW, Wen PY, Hurwitz S, Black P, Kesari S, Drappatz J, et al. Morphological characteristics of brain tumors causing seizures. Arch Neurol. 2010;67(3):336–42.

22. Engel J Jr, Bragin A, Staba R, Mody I. High-frequency oscillations: what is normal and what is not? Epilepsia. 2009;50(4):598–604.

23. Delgado-Escueta AV, Ward AA Jr, Woodbury DM, Porter RJ. New wave of research in the epilepsies. Adv Neurol. 1986;44:3–55.

24. Chang EF, Potts MB, Keles GE, Lamborn KR, Chang SM, Barbaro NM, et al. Seizure characteristics and control following resection in 332 patients with low-grade gliomas. J Neurosurg. 2008;108(2):227–35.

25. Yuen TI, Morokoff AP, Bjorksten A, D'Abaco G, Paradiso L, Finch S, et al. Glutamate is associated with a higher risk of seizures in patients with gliomas. Neurology. 2012;79(9):883–9.

26. Pallud J, Audureau E, Blonski M, Sanai N, Bauchet L, Fontaine D, et al. Epileptic seizures in diffuse low-grade gliomas in adults. Brain. 2014;137:449–62.

27. de Groot M, Reijneveld JC, Aronica E, Heimans JJ. Epilepsy in patients with a brain tumour: focal epilepsy requires focused treatment. Brain. 2012;135:1002–16.

28. van Breemen MSM, Wilms EB, Vecht CJ. Epilepsy in patients with brain tumours: epidemiology, mechanisms, and management. Lancet Neurol. 2007;6(5):421–30.

29. van Dellen E, Douw L, Hillebrand A, Ris-Hilgersom IH, Schoonheim MM, Baayen JC, et al. MEG network differences between low- and high-grade glioma related to epilepsy and cognition. PLoS One. 2012;7(11):e50122.

30. de Groot M, Toering ST, Boer K, Spliet WGM, Heimans JJ, Aronica E, et al. Expression of synaptic vesicle protein 2A in epilepsy-associated brain tumors and in the peritumoral cortex. Neuro-Oncol. 2010;12(3):265–73.

31. Huang L, You G, Jiang T, Li G, Li S, Wang Z. Correlation between tumor-related seizures and molecular genetic profile in 103 Chinese patients with low-grade gliomas: a preliminary study. J Neurol Sci. 2011;302(1–2):63–7.

32. Prabowo AS, Iyer AM, Veersema TJ, Anink JJ, Schouten-van Meeteren AYN, Spliet WGM, et al. BRAF V600E mutation is associated with mTOR signaling activation in glioneuronal tumors. Brain Pathol. 2014;24(1):52–66.

33. Houillier C, Wang X, Kaloshi G, Mokhtari K, Guillevin R, Laffaire J, et al. IDH1 or IDH2 mutations predict longer survival and response to temozolomide in low-grade gliomas. Neurology. 2010;75(17):1560–6.

34. Liubinas SV, D'Abaco GM, Moffat BM, Gonzales M, Feleppa F, Nowell CJ, et al. IDH1 mutation is associated with seizures and protoplasmic subtype in patients with low-grade gliomas. Epilepsia. 2014;55(9):1438–43.

35. Liang R, Fan Y, Wang X, Mao Q, Liu Y. The significance of IDH1 mutations in tumor-associated seizure in 60 Chinese patients with low-grade gliomas. Sci World J. 2013;2013:403942-.

36. Zhong Z, Wang Z, Wang YY, You G, Jiang T. IDH1/2 mutation is associated with seizure as an initial symptom in low-grade glioma: a report of 311 Chinese adult glioma patients. Epilepsy Res. 2015;109:100–5.

37. Robert SM, Buckingham SC, Campbell SL, Robel S, Holt KT, Ogunrinu-Babarinde T, et al. SLC7A11 expression is associated with seizures and predicts poor survival in patients with malignant glioma. Sci Transl Med. 2015;7(289).

38. Huberfeld G, Vecht CJ. Seizures and gliomas—towards a single therapeutic approach. Nat Rev Neurol. 2016;12(4):204–16.

39. Pallud J, Van Quyen ML, Bielle F, Pellegrino C, Varlet P, Labussiere M, et al. Cortical GABAergic excitation contributes to epileptic activities around human glioma. Sci Transl Med. 2014;6(244).

40. Boer K, Troost D, Timmermans W, Gorter JA, Spliet WGM, Nellist M, et al. Cellular localization of metabotropic glutamate receptors in cortical tubers and subependymal giant cell tumors of tuberous sclerosis complex. Neuroscience. 2008;156(1):203–15.

41. Curatolo P, Moavero R. mTOR inhibitors in tuberous sclerosis complex. Curr Neuropharmacol. 2012;10(4):404–15.

42. Hildebrand J, Lecaille C, Perennes J, Delattre JY. Epileptic seizures during follow-up of patients treated for primary brain tumors. Neurology. 2005;65(2):212–5.

43. Kerkhof M, Dielemans JCM, van Breemen MS, Zwinkels H, Walchenbach R, Taphoorn MJ, et al. Effect of valproic acid on seizure control and on survival in patients with glioblastoma multiforme. Neuro-Oncol. 2013;15(7):961–7.

44. Ruda R, Bello L, Duffau H, Soffietti R. Seizures in low-grade gliomas: natural history, pathogenesis, and outcome after treatments. Neuro-Oncol. 2012;14:55–64.

45. Englot DJ, Berger MS, Barbaro NM, Chang EF. Factors associated with seizure freedom in the surgical resection of glioneuronal tumors. Epilepsia. 2012;53(1):51–7.

46. Blonski M, Taillandier L, Herbet G, Maldonado IL, Beauchesne P, Fabbro M, et al. Combination of neoadjuvant chemotherapy followed by surgical resection as a new strategy for WHO grade II gliomas: a study of cognitive status and quality of life. J Neurooncol. 2012;106(2):353–66.

47. Thom M, Bluemcke I, Aronica E. Long-term epilepsy-associated tumors. Brain Pathol. 2012;22(3):350–79.

48. Pignatti F, van den Bent M, Curran D, Debruyne C, Sylvester R, Therasse P, et al. Prognostic factors for survival in adult patients with cerebral low-grade glioma. J Clin Oncol. 2002;20(8):2076–84.

49. Englot DJ, Berger MS, Barbaro NM, Chang EF. Predictors of seizure freedom after resection of supratentorial low-grade gliomas A review. J Neurosurg. 2011;115(2):240–4.

50. Mirsattari SM, Chong JJR, Hammond RR, Megyesi JF, Macdonald DR, Lee DH, et al. Do epileptic seizures predict outcome in patients with oligodendroglioma? Epilepsy Res. 2011;94(1–2):39–44.

51. Leighton C, Fisher B, Bauman G, Depiero S, Stitt L, Macdonald D, et al. Supratentorial low-grade glioma in adults: An analysis of prognostic factors and timing of radiation. J Clin Oncol. 1997;15(4):1294–301.

52. Stockhammer F, Misch M, Helms H-J, Lengler U, Prall F, von Deimling A, et al. IDH1/2 mutations in WHO grade II astrocytomas associated with localization and seizure as the initial symptom. Seizure-Eur J Epilepsy. 2012;21(3):194–7.

53. Sahm F, Reuss D, Koelsche C, Capper D, Schittenhelm J, Heim S, et al. Farewell to oligoastrocytoma: in situ molecular genetics favor classification as either oligodendroglioma or astrocytoma. Acta Neuropathol. 2014;128(4):551–9.

54. Kerkhof M, Benit C, Duran-Pena A, Vecht CJ. Seizures in oligodendroglial tumors. CNS Oncol. 2015;4(5):347–56.

55. Stark AM, van de Bergh J, Hedderich J, Mehdorn HM, Nabavi A. Glioblastoma: clinical characteristics, prognostic factors and survival in 492 patients. Clin Neurol Neurosurg. 2012;114(7):840–5.

56. Berendsen S, Varkila M, Kroonen J, Seute T, Snijders TJ, Kauw F, et al. Prognostic relevance of epilepsy at presentation in glioblastoma patients. Neuro-Oncol. 2016;18(5):700–6.

57. You G, Sha Z-Y, Yan W, Zhang W, Wang Y-Z, Li S-W, et al. Seizure characteristics and outcomes in 508 Chinese adult patients undergoing primary resection of low-grade gliomas: a clinicopathological study. Neuro-Oncol. 2012;14(2):230–41.

58. Wick W, Menn O, Meisner C, Steinbach J, Hermisson M, Tatagiba M, et al. Pharmacotherapy of epileptic seizures in glioma patients: Who, when, why and how long? Onkologie. 2005;28(8–9):391-396.

59. Englot DJ, Han SJ, Berger MS, Barbaro NM, Chang EF. Extent of surgical resection predicts seizure freedom in low-grade temporal lobe brain tumors. Neurosurgery. 2012;70(4):921–8.

60. van den Bent MJ, Afra D, de Witte O, Ben Hassel M, Schraub S, Hoang-Xuan K, et al. Long-term efficacy of early versus delayed radiotherapy for low-grade astrocytoma and oligodendroglioma in adults: the EORTC 22845 randomised trial. Lancet. 2005;366 (9490):985–90.

61. Warnke PC, Berlis A, Weyerbrock A, Ostertag CB. Significant reduction of seizure incidence and increase of benzodiazepine receptor density after interstitial radiosurgery in low-grade gliomas. Advances in stereotactic and functional neurosurgery 12: Proceedings of the 12th meeting of the European society for stereotactic and functional neurosurgery, Milan, 1996. 1997;12:90–2.

62. Shankar A, Rajshekhar V. Radiological and clinical outcome following stereotactic biopsy and radiotherapy for low-grade insular astrocytomas. Neurol India. 2003;51(4):503–6.

63. Ruda R, Magliola U, Bertero L, Trevisan E, Bosa C, Mantovani C, et al. Seizure control following radiotherapy in patients with diffuse gliomas: a retrospective study. Neuro-Oncol. 2013;15(12):1739–49.

64. Scerrati M, Montemaggi P, Iacoangeli M, Roselli R, Rossi GF. Interstitial brachytherapy for low-grade cerebral gliomas: Analysis of results in a series of 36 cases. Acta Neurochir. 1994;131 (1–2):97–105.

65. Pace A, Vidiri A, Galie E, Carosi A, Telera S, Cianciulli AA, et al. Temozolomide chemotherapy for progressive low-grade glioma: clinical benefits and radiological response. Ann Oncol. 2003;14(12):1722–6.

66. Koekkoek JAF, Dirven L, Heimans JJ, Postma TJ, Vos MJ, Reijneveld JC, et al. Seizure reduction in a low-grade glioma: more than a beneficial side effect of temozolomide. J Neurol Neurosurg Psychiatry. 2015;86(4):366–73.

67. Kaloshi G, Benouaich-Amiel A, Diakite F, Taillibert S, Lejeune J, Laigle-Donadey F, et al. Temozolomide for low-grade gliomas—predictive impact of 1p/19q loss on response and outcome. Neurology. 2007;68(21):1831–6.

68. Sherman JH, Moldovan K, Yeoh HK, Starke RM, Pouratian N, Shaffrey ME, et al. Impact of temozolomide chemotherapy on seizure frequency in patients with low-grade gliomas. J Neurosurg. 2011;114(6):1617–21.

69. Hoang-Xuan K, Capelle L, Kujas M, Taillibert S, Duffau H, Lejeune J, et al. Temozolomide as initial treatment for adults with low-grade oligodendrogliomas or oligoastrocytomas and correlation with chromosome 1p deletions. J Clin Oncol. 2004;22 (15):3133–8.

70. Lebrun C, Fontaine D, Bourg V, Ramaioli A, Chanalet S, Vandenbos F, et al. Treatment of newly diagnosed symptomatic pure low-grade oligodendrogliomas with PCV chemotherapy. Eur J Neurol. 2007;14(4):391–8.

71. Soffietti R, Baumert BG, Bello L, von Deimling A, Duffau H, Frénay M, et al. Guidelines on management of low-grade gliomas: report of an EFNS-EANO Task Force. Eur J Neurol. 2010;17(9):1124–33.

72. Krumholz A, Wiebe S, Gronseth GS, Gloss DS, Sanchez AM, Kabir AA, et al. Evidence-based guideline: management of an unprovoked first seizure in adults report of the guideline development subcommittee of the American Academy of Neurology and the American Epilepsy Society. Neurology. 2015;84 (16):1705–13.

73. Glauser T, Ben-Menachem E, Bourgeois B, Cnaan A, Guerreiro C, Kalviainen R, et al. Updated ILAE evidence review of antiepileptic drug efficacy and effectiveness as initial monotherapy for epileptic seizures and syndromes. Epilepsia. 2013;54(3): 551–63.

74. Karceski S, Morrell MJ, Carpenter D. Treatment of epilepsy in adults: expert opinion, 2005. Epilepsy Behav. 2005;7:S1–64.

75. Glantz MJ, Forsyth PA, Recht LD, Wen PY, Chamberlain MC, Grossman SA, et al. Practice parameter: anticonvulsant prophylaxis in patients with newly diagnosed brain tumors—report of the quality standards subcommittee of the American Academy of Neurology. Neurology. 2000;54(10):1886–93.

76. Maschio M, Dinapoli L, Saveriano F, Pompili A, Carapella CM, Vidiri A, et al. Efficacy and tolerability of zonisamide as add-on in brain tumor-related epilepsy: preliminary report. Acta Neurol Scand. 2009;120(3):210–2.

77. Maschio M, Dinapoli L, Sperati F, Pace A, Fabi A, Vidiri A, et al. Levetiracetam monotherapy in patients with brain tumor-related epilepsy: seizure control, safety, and quality of life. J Neurooncol. 2011;104(1):205–14.

78. Newton HB, Dalton J, Goldlust S, Pearl D. Retrospective analysis of the efficacy and tolerability of levetiracetam in patients with metastatic brain tumors. J Neurooncol. 2007;84(3):293–6.

79. Lim DA, Tarapore P, Chang E, Burt M, Chakalian L, Barbaro N, et al. Safety and feasibility of switching from phenytoin to levetiracetam monotherapy for glioma-related seizure control following craniotomy: a randomized phase II pilot study. J Neurooncol. 2009;93(3):349–54.

80. Mbizvo GK, Dixon P, Hutton JL, Marson AG. Levetiracetam add-on for drug-resistant focal epilepsy: an updated Cochrane Review. Cochrane Database Syst Rev. 2012(9).

81. de Groot M, Douw L, Sizoo EM, Bosma I, Froklage FE, Heimans JJ, et al. Levetiracetam improves verbal memory in high-grade glioma patients. Neuro Oncol. 2013;15(2):216–23.

82. Helmstaedter C, Witt J-A. The effects of levetiracetam on cognition: a non-interventional surveillance study. Epilepsy Behav. 2008;13(4):642–9.

83. Hamed SA. The aspects and mechanisms of cognitive alterations in Epilepsy: The role of antiepileptic medications. CNS Neurosci Ther. 2009;15(2):134–56.

84. Mauro AM, Bomprezzi C, Morresi S, Provinciali L, Formica F, Iacoangeli M, et al. Prevention of early postoperative seizures in patients with primary brain tumors: preliminary experience with oxcarbazepine. J Neurooncol. 2007;81(3):279–85.

85. Maschio M, Dinapoli L, Sperati F, Fabi A, Pace A, Vidiri A, et al. Oxcarbazepine monotherapy in patients with brain tumor-related epilepsy: open-label pilot study for assessing the efficacy, tolerability and impact on quality of life. J Neurooncol. 2012;106(3):651–6.

86. Maschio M, Dinapoli L, Mingoia M, Sperati F, Pace A, Pompili A, et al. Lacosamide as add-on in brain tumor-related epilepsy: preliminary report on efficacy and tolerability. J Neurol. 2011;258(11):2100–4.

87. Saria MG, Corle C, Hu J, Rudnick JD, Phuphanich S, Mrugala MM, et al. Retrospective analysis of the tolerability and activity of lacosamide in patients with brain tumors. J Neurosurg. 2013;118(6):1183–7.

88. Kwan P, Brodie MJ, Laurenza A, FitzGibbon H, Gidal BE. Analysis of pooled phase III trials of adjunctive perampanel for epilepsy: impact of mechanism of action and pharmacokinetics on clinical outcomes. Epilepsy Res. 2015;117:117–24.

89. Lagae L, Villanueva V, Meador KJ, Bagul M, Laurenza A, Kumar D, et al. Adjunctive perampanel in adolescents with inadequately controlled partial-onset seizures: a randomized study evaluating behavior, efficacy, and safety. Epilepsia. 2016;57(7):1120–9.

90. Brodie MJ, Sills GJ. Combining antiepileptic drugs-rational polytherapy? Seizure-Eur J Epilepsy. 2011;20(5):369–75.

91. French JA, Faught E. Rational polytherapy. Epilepsia. 2009;50:63–8.

92. Kaminski RM, Matagne A, Patsalos PN, Klitgaard H. Benefit of combination therapy in epilepsy: a review of the preclinical evidence with levetiracetam. Epilepsia. 2009;50(3):387–97.

93. Otoul C, Arrigo C, van Rijckevorsel K, French JA. Meta-analysis and indirect comparisons of levetiracetam with other second-generation antiepileptic drugs in partial epilepsy. Clin Neuropharmacol. 2005;28(2):72–8.

94. Bodalia PN, Grosso AM, Sofat R, MacAllister RJ, Smeeth L, Dhillon S, et al. Comparative efficacy and tolerability of anti-epileptic drugs for refractory focal epilepsy: systematic review and network meta-analysis reveals the need for long term comparator trials. Br J Clin Pharmacol. 2013;76(5):649–67.

95. Weston J, Shukralla A, McKay AJ, Marson AG. Lacosamide add-on therapy for partial epilepsy. Cochrane Database Syst Rev. 2015(6).

96. Helmstaedter C, Witt J-A. The longer-term cognitive effects of adjunctive antiepileptic treatment with lacosamide in comparison with lamotrigine and topiramate in a naturalistic outpatient setting. Epilepsy Behav. 2013;26(2):182–7.

97. Krauze AV, Myrehaug SD, Chang MG, Holdford DJ, Smith S, Shih J, et al. A phase 2 study of concurrent radiation therapy, temozolomide, and the histone deacetylase inhibitor valproic acid for patients with glioblastoma. Int J Radiat Oncol Biol Phys. 2015;92(5):986–92.

98. Redjal N, Reinshagen C, Le A, Walcott BP, McDonnell E, Dietrich J, et al. Valproic acid, compared to other antiepileptic drugs, is associated with improved overall and progression-free survival in glioblastoma but worse outcome in grade II/III gliomas treated with temozolomide. J Neurooncol. 2016;127(3):505–14.

99. Vecht CJ, Kerkhof M, Duran-Pena A. Seizure prognosis in brain tumors: new insights and evidence-based management. Oncologist. 2014;19(7):751–9.

100. Brodie MJ, Yuen AWC. Lamotrigine substitution study: evidence for synergism with sodium valproate? Epilepsy Res. 1997;26(3):423–32.

101. Strozzi I, Nolan SJ, Sperling MR, Wingerchuk DM, Sirven J. Early versus late antiepileptic drug withdrawal for people with epilepsy in remission. Cochrane Database Syst Rev. 2015;2:CD001902-CD.

102. Beghi E, Giussani G, Grosso S, Iudice A, La Neve A, Pisani F, et al. Withdrawal of antiepileptic drugs: guidelines of the Italian league against epilepsy. Epilepsia. 2013;54:2–12.

103. Wheless JW, Clarke DF, Carpenter D. Treatment of pediatric epilepsy: Expert opinion, 2005. J Child Neurol. 2005;20:S1–56.

104. Sirven JI, Wingerchuk DA, Drazkowsici JF, Lyons MK, Zimmerman RS. Seizure prophylaxis in patients with brain tumors: a meta-analysis. Mayo Clin Proc. 2004;79(12):1489–94.

105. Pulman J, Greenhalgh J, Marson AG. Antiepileptic drugs as prophylaxis for post-craniotomy seizures. Cochrane Database Syst Rev. 2013;2:CD007286-CD.

106. Kong X, Guan J, Yang Y, Li Y, Ma W, Wang R. A meta-analysis: do prophylactic antiepileptic drugs in patients with brain tumors decrease the incidence of seizures? Clin Neurol Neurosurg. 2015;134:98–103.

107. Weston J, Greenhalgh J, Marson AG. Antiepileptic drugs as prophylaxis for post-craniotomy seizures. Cochrane Database Syst Rev. 2015(3).

108. Iuchi T, Hasegawa Y, Kawasaki K, Sakaida T. Epilepsy in patients with gliomas: Incidence and control of seizures. J Clin Neurosci. 2015;22(1):87–91.

109. Rahmann A, Stodieck S, Husstedt IW, Evers S. Pre-attentive cognitive processing in epilepsy—a pilot study on the impact of epilepsy type and anti-epileptic treatment. Eur Neurol. 2002;48(3):146–52.

110. Phabphal K, Kanjanasatien J. Montreal cognitive assessment in cryptogenic epilepsy patients with normal mini-mental state examination scores. Epileptic Disorders. 2011;13(4):375–81.

111. Witt JA, Elger CE, Helmstaedter C. Impaired verbal fluency under topiramate—evidence for synergistic negative effects of epilepsy, topiramate, and polytherapy. Eur J Neurol. 2013;20(1):130–7.

112. Zucchella C, Bartolo M, Di Lorenzo C, Villani V, Pace A. Cognitive impairment in primary brain tumors outpatients: a prospective cross-sectional survey. J Neurooncol. 2013;112(3):455–60.

113. Correa DD, DeAngelis LM, Shi W, Thaler HT, Lin M, Abrey LE. Cognitive functions in low-grade gliomas: disease and treatment effects. J Neurooncol. 2007;81(2):175–84.

114. Klein M, Engelberts NHJ, van der Ploeg HM, Trenite D, Aaronson NK, Taphoorn MJB, et al. Epilepsy in low-grade gliomas: the impact on cognitive function and quality of life. Ann Neurol. 2003;54(4):514–20.

115. Klein M, Heimans JJ, Aaronson NK, van der Ploeg HM, Grit J, Muller M, et al. Effect of radiotherapy and other treatment-related factors on mid-term to long-term cognitive sequelae in low-grade gliomas: a comparative study. Lancet. 2002;360(9343):1361–8.

116. Klein M, Taphoorn MJB, Heimans JJ, van der Ploeg HM, Vandertop WP, Smit EF, et al. Neurobehavioral status and health-related quality of life in newly diagnosed high-grade glioma patients. J Clin Oncol. 2001;19(20):4037–47.

117. Johnson DR, Sawyer AM, Meyers CA, O'Neill BP, Wefel JS. Early measures of cognitive function predict survival in patients with newly diagnosed glioblastoma. Neuro-Oncology. 2012;14(6):808–16.

118. Prust M, Kalpathy-Cramer J, Poloskova P, Jafari-Khouzani K, Gerstner E, Dietrich J. Neuroimaging of treatment associated neurotoxicity in glioblastoma patients. Neuro-Oncol. 2013;15:108–108.

119. Taphoorn MJB, Klein M. Cognitive deficits in adult patients with brain tumors. Lancet Neurol. 2004;3(3):159–68.

120. Klein M. Neurocognitive functioning in adult WHO grade II gliomas: impact of old and new treatment modalities. Neuro-Oncol. 2012;14:17–24.

121. Klein M, Heimans JJ, Aaronson NK, Postma TJ, Muller M, van der Ploeg HM, et al. Impaired cognitive functioning in low-grade glioma patients: relationship to tumor localisation, radiotherapy and the use of anticonvulsants. Ned Tijdschr Geneeskd. 2004;148(44):2175–80.

122. Witt J-A, Elger CE, Helmstaedter C. Which drug-induced side effects would be tolerated in the prospect of seizure control? Epilepsy Behav. 2013;29(1):141–3.

123. Specchio LM, Beghi E. Should antiepileptic drugs be withdrawn in seizure-free patients? CNS Drugs. 2004;18(4):201–12.

124. Bourg V, Lebrun C, Chichmanian RM, Thomas P, Frenay M. Nitroso-urea-cisplatin-based chemotherapy associated with valproate: increase of haematologic toxicity. Ann Oncol. 2001;12(2):217–9.

125. Weller M, Gorlia T, Cairncross JG, van den Bent MJ, Mason W, Belanger K, et al. Prolonged survival with valproic acid use in the EORTC/NCIC temozolomide trial for glioblastoma. Neurology. 2011;77(12):1156–64.

126. Simo M, Velasco R, Graus F, Verger E, Gil M, Pineda E, et al. Impact of antiepileptic drugs on thrombocytopenia in glioblastoma patients treated with standard chemoradiotherapy. J Neurooncol. 2012;108(3):451–8.

127. Kaufman DW, Kelly JP, Anderson T, Harmon DC, Shapiro S. Evaluation of case reports of aplastic anemia among patients treated with Felbamate. Epilepsia. 1997;38(12):1265–9.

128. Montane E, Ibanez L, Vidal X, Ballarin E, Puig R, Garcia N, et al. Epidemiology of aplastic anemia: a prospective multicenter study. Haematol-Hematol J. 2008;93(4):518–23.

129. Verrotti A, Scaparrotta A, Grosso S, Chiarelli F, Coppola G. Anticonvulsant drugs and hematological disease. Neurol Sci. 2014;35(7):983–93.

130. Handoko KB, Souverein PC, van Staa TP, Meyboom RHB, Leufkens HGM, Egberts TCG, et al. Risk of aplastic anemia in patients using antiepileptic drugs. Epilepsia. 2006;47(7):1232–6.

131. Federici L, Weitten T, Alt M, Blaison G, Zamfir A, Audhuy B, et al. Idiosyncratic drug-induced agranulocytosis. Presse Med. 2008;37(9):1327–33.

132. Andres E, Zimmer J, Affenberger S, Federici L, Alt M, Maloisel F. Idiosyncratic drug-induced agranulocytosis: update of an old disorder. Eur J Intern Med. 2006;17(8):529–35.

133. Nasreddine W, Beydoun A. Valproate-induced thrombocytopenia: a prospective monotherapy study. Epilepsia. 2008;49(3):438–45.

134. Delgado MR, Riela AR, Mills J, Browne R, Roach ES. Thrombocytopenia secondary to high valproate levels in children with epilsepsy. J Child Neurol. 1994;9(3):311–4.

135. Koese G, Arhan E, Unal B, Ozaydin E, Guven A, Sayli TR. Valproate-associated coagulopathies in children during short-term treatment. J Child Neurol. 2009;24(12):1493–8.

136. Koenig S, Gerstner T, Keller A, Teich M, Longin E, Dempfle C-E. High incidence of vaproate-induced coagulation disorders in children receiving valproic acid: a prospective study. Blood Coag Fibrinol. 2008;19(5):375–82.

137. Tinchon A, Oberndorfer S, Marosi C, Gleiss A, Geroldinger A, Sax C, et al. Haematological toxicity of valproic acid compared to levetiracetam in patients with glioblastoma multiforme undergoing concomitant radio-chemotherapy: a retrospective cohort study. J Neurol. 2015;262(1):179–86.

138. Gerstner T, Teich M, Bell N, Longin E, Dempfle C-E, Brand J, et al. Valproate-associated coagulopathies are frequent and variable in children. Epilepsia. 2006;47(7):1136–43.

139. Psaras T, Will BE, Schoeber W, Rona S, Mittelbronn M, Honegger JB. Quantitative assessment of postoperative blood collection in brain tumor surgery under valproate medication. Zentralbl Neurochir. 2008;69(4):165–9.

140. Mamon HJ, Wen PY, Burns AC, Loeffler JS. Allergic skin reactions to anticonvulsant medications in patients receiving cranial radiation therapy. Epilepsia. 1999;40(3):341–4.

141. Arif H, Buchsbaum R, Weintraub D, Koyfman S, Salas-Humara C, Bazil CW, et al. Comparison and predictors of rash associated with 15 antiepileptic drugs. Neurology. 2007;68(20):1701–9.

142. Schlienger RG, Shear NH. Antiepileptic drug hypersensitivity syndrome. Epilepsia. 1998;39:S3–7.

143. Handoko KB, van Puijenbroek EP, Bijl AH, Hermens WAJJ, Rijkom JEFZ-v, Hekster YA, et al. Influence of chemical structure on hypersensitivity reactions induced by antiepileptic drugs—the role of the aromatic ring. Drug Saf. 2008;31(8):695–702.

144. Rzany B, Correia O, Kelly JP, Naldi L, Auquier A, Stern R, et al. Risk of Stevens-Johnson syndrome and toxic epidermal necrolysis during first weeks of antiepileptic therapy: a case-control study. Lancet. 1999;353(9171):2190–4.

145. Mockenhaupt M, Messenheimer J, Tennis P, Schlingmann J. Risk of Stevens-Johnson syndrome and toxic epidermal necrolysis in new users of antiepileptics. Neurology. 2005;64(7):1134–8.

146. Roujeau JC, Kelly JP, Naldi L, Rzany B, Stern RS, Anderson T, et al. Medication use and the risk of Stevens-Johnson syndrome or toxic epidermal necrolysis. N Engl J Med. 1995;333(24):1600–7.

147. Delattre JY, Safai B, Posner JB. Erythema multiforme and Stevens-Johnson syndrome in patients receiving cranial irradiation and phenytoin. Neurology. 1988;38(2):194–8.

148. Micali G, Linthicum K, Han N, West DP. Increased risk of erythema multiforme major with combination anticonvulsant and radiation therapies. Pharmacotherapy. 1999;19(2):223–7.

149. Yip VL, Marson AG, Jorgensen AL, Pirmohamed M, Alfirevic A. HLA genotype and carbamazepine-induced cutaneous adverse drug reactions: a systematic review. Clin Pharmacol Ther. 2012;92(6):757–65.

150. Tolou-Ghamari Z, Zare M, Habibabadi JM, Najafi M-R. Antiepileptic drugs: a consideration of clinical and biochemical outcome in patients with epilepsy. Int J Prev Med. 2013;4(Suppl 2):S330–7.

151. Genin E, Chen DP, Hung SI, Sekula P, Schumacher M, Chang PY, et al. HLA-A*31:01 and different types of carbamazepine-induced severe cutaneous adverse reactions: an international study and meta-analysis. Pharmacogenomics J. 2014;14(3):281–8.

152. Chung W-H, Chang W-C, Lee Y-S, Wu Y-Y, Yang C-H, Ho H-C, et al. Genetic variants associated with phenytoin-related severe cutaneous adverse reactions. Jama-J Am Med Assoc. 2014;312(5):525–34.

153. Man CBL, Kwan P, Baum L, Yu E, Lau KM, Cheng ASH, et al. Association between HLA-B*1502 allele and antiepileptic drug-induced cutaneous reactions in han Chinese. Epilepsia. 2007;48(5):1015–8.

154. Riechelmann RP, Tannock IF, Wang L, Saad ED, Taback NA, Krzyzanowska MK. Potential drug interactions and duplicate prescriptions among cancer patients. J Natl Cancer Inst. 2007;99(8):592–600.

155. Relling MV, Pui CH, Sandlund JT, Rivera GK, Hancock ML, Boyett JM, et al. Adverse effect of anticonvulsants on efficacy of chemotherapy for acute lymphoblastic leukaemia. Lancet. 2000;356(9226):285–90.

156. Zanger UM, Klein K, Thomas M, Rieger JK, Tremmel R, Kandel BA, et al. Genetics, epigenetics, and regulation of drug-metabolizing cytochrome P450 enzymes. Clin Pharmacol Ther. 2014;95(3):258–61.

157. Brodie MJ, Mintzer S, Pack AM, Gidal BE, Vecht CJ, Schmidt D. Enzyme induction with antiepileptic drugs: cause for concern? Epilepsia. 2013;54(1):11–27.

158. van Breemen MSM, Rijsman RM, Taphoorn MJB, Walchenbach R, Zwinkels H, Vecht CJ. Efficacy of anti-epileptic drugs in patients with gliomas and seizures. J Neurol. 2009;256(9):1519–26.

159. Benit C, Vecht C. Seizures and cancer: drug interactions of anticonvulsants with chemotherapeutic agents, tyrosine-kinase inhibitors and glucocorticoids. Neuro-Oncol Pract. 2016;3(4):245–60.

160. Johannessen Landmark C, Johannessen SI, Tomson T. Host factors affecting antiepileptic drug delivery-pharmacokinetic variability. Advanced Drug Deliv Rev. 2012;64(10):896–910.

161. de Leon J, Spina E, Diaz FJ. Clobazam therapeutic drug monitoring: a comprehensive review of the literature with proposals to improve future studies. Ther Drug Monit. 2013;35(1):30–47.

162. Patsalos PN. Drug interactions with the newer antiepileptic drugs (AEDs)-part 1: pharmacokinetic and pharmacodynamic interactions between AEDs. Clin Pharmacokinet. 2013;52(11):927–66.

163. Gidal BE, Sheth R, Parnell J, Maloney K, Sale M. Evaluation of VPA dose and concentration effects on lamotrigine pharmacokinetics: implications for conversion to lamotrigine monotherapy. Epilepsy Res. 2003;57(2–3):85–93.

164. Gilbert MR, Armstrong TS. Management of patients with newly diagnosed malignant primary brain tumors with a focus on the evolving role of temozolomide. Ther Clin Risk Manag. 2007;3 (6):1027–33.

165. Maschio M, Albani F, Jandolo B, Zarabla A, Contin M, Dinapoli L, et al. Temozolomide treatment does not affect topiramate and oxcarbazepine plasma concentrations in chronically treated patients with brain tumor-related epilepsy. J Neurooncol. 2008;90(2):217–21.

166. Ferreri AJM, Guerra E, Regazzi M, Pasini F, Arnbrosetti A, Pivnik A, et al. Area under the curve of methotrexate and creatinine clearance are outcome-determining factors in primary CNS lymphomas. Br J Cancer. 2004;90(2):353–8.

167. van Erp NP, Gelderblom H, Guchelaar H-J. Clinical pharmacokinetics of tyrosine kinase inhibitors. Cancer Treat Rev. 2009;35(8):692–706.

168. Mao J, Johnson TR, Shen Z, Yamazaki S. Prediction of crizotinib-midazolam interaction using the Simcyp population-based simulator: comparison of CYP3A time-dependent inhibition between human liver microsomes versus hepatocytes. Drug Metab Dispos. 2013;41(2):343–52.

169. Wen PY, Yung WKA, Lamborn KR, Dahia PL, Wang Y, Peng B, et al. Phase I/II study of imatinib mesylate for recurrent malignant gliomas: North American brain tumor consortium study 99-08. Clin Cancer Res. 2006;12(16):4899–907.

170. Thiessen B, Stewart C, Tsao M, Kamel-Reid S, Schaiquevich P, Mason W, et al. A phase I/II trial of GW572016 (lapatinib) in recurrent glioblastoma multiforme: clinical outcomes, pharmacokinetics and molecular correlation. Cancer Chemother Pharmacol. 2010;65(2):353–61.

171. Kuhn JG, Chang SM, Wen PY, Cloughesy TF, Greenberg H, Schiff D, et al. Pharmacokinetic and tumor distribution characteristics of temsirolimus in patients with recurrent malignant glioma. Clin Cancer Res. 2007;13(24):7401–6.

172. Mason WP, MacNeil M, Kavan P, Easaw J, Macdonald D, Thiessen B, et al. A phase I study of temozolomide and everolimus (RAD001) in patients with newly diagnosed and progressive glioblastoma either receiving or not receiving enzyme-inducing anticonvulsants: an NCIC CTG study. Invest New Drugs. 2012;30(6):2344–51.

173. Bartoszek M, Szefler SJ. Corticosteroid therapy in adolescent patients. J Adolesc Health. 1987;8(1):84–91.

174. Chalk JB, Ridgeway K, Brophy TRO, Yelland JDN, Eadie MJ. Phenytoin impairs the bioavailability of dexamethasone in neurological and neurosurgical patients. J Neurol Neurosurg Psychiatry. 1984;47(10):1087–90.

175. Wong DD, Longenecker RG, Liepman M, Baker S, Lavergne M. Phenytoin-dexamethasone: a possible drug–drug interaction. Jama-J Am Med Assoc. 1985;254(15):2062–3.

176. Gattis WA, May DB. Possible interaction involving phenytoin, dexamethasone, and antineoplastic agents: a case report and review. Ann Pharmacother. 1996;30(5):520–6.

177. McCune JS, Hawke RL, LeCluyse EL, Gillenwater HH, Hamilton G, Ritchie J, et al. In vivo and in vitro induction of human cytochrome P4503A4 by dexamethasone. Clin Pharmacol Ther. 2000;68(4):356–66.

178. Lackner TE. Interaction of dexamethasone with phenytoin. Pharmacotherapy. 1991;11(4):344–7.

179. Lawson GJ, Chakraborty J, Dumasia MC, Baylis EM. Methylprednisolone hemisuccinate and metabolites in urine from patients receiving high-dose corticosteroid therapy. Ther Drug Monit. 1992;14(1):20–6.

180. Vecht CJ, Wagner GL, Wilms EB. Interactions between antiepileptic and chemotherapeutic drugs. Lancet Neurol. 2003;2(7):404–9.

181. Matoulkova P, Pavek P, Maly J, Vlcek J. Cytochrome P450 enzyme regulation by glucocorticoids and consequences in terms of drug interaction. Expert Opin Drug Metab Toxicol. 2014;10 (3):425–35.

182. Johannessen Landmark C, Baftiu A, Tysse I, Valso B, Larsson PG, Rytter E, et al. Pharmacokinetic variability of four newer antiepileptic drugs, lamotrigine, levetiracetam, oxcarbazepine, and topiramate: a comparison of the impact of age and comedication. Therapeutic Drug Monit. 2012;34(4):440–5.

183. Italiano D, Perucca E. Clinical pharmacokinetics of new-generation antiepileptic drugs at the extremes of age: an update. Clin Pharmacokinet. 2013;52(8):627–45.

184. Yu H, Steeghs N, Nijenhuis CM, Schellens JHM, Beijnen JH, Huitema ADR. Practical guidelines for therapeutic drug monitoring of anticancer tyrosine kinase inhibitors: focus on the pharmacokinetic targets. Clin Pharmacokinet. 2014;53(4):305–25.

185. de Wit D, Guchelaar H-J, den Hartigh J, Gelderblom H, van Erp NP. Individualized dosing of tyrosine kinase inhibitors: are we there yet? Drug Discovery Today. 2015;20(1):18–36.

186. Patsalos PN, Berry DJ, Bourgeois BFD, Cloyd JC, Glauser TA, Johannessen SI, et al. Antiepileptic drugs—best practice guidelines for therapeutic drug monitoring: a position paper by the subcommission on therapeutic drug monitoring, ILAE commission on therapeutic strategies. Epilepsia. 2008;49(7):1239–76.

187. Paci A, Veal G, Bardin C, Leveque D, Widmer N, Beijnen J, et al. Review of therapeutic drug monitoring of anticancer drugs part 1-Cytotoxics. Eur J Cancer. 2014;50(12):2010–9.

188. Kerkhof M, Vecht CJ. Seizure characteristics and prognostic factors of gliomas. Epilepsia. 2013;54 Suppl 9:12–7.

189. Lieu AS, Howng SL. Intracranial meningiomas and epilepsy: incidence, prognosis and influencing factors. Epilepsy Res. 2000;38(1):45–52.

Lisa R. Rogers

Introduction

In a large retrospective autopsy study of 3426 systemic cancer patients, stroke was identified in 14.6% of patients, second only to metastasis as the most common CNS pathology. Hemorrhages and ischemic lesions were present in equal numbers. Overall, more than half the patients had significant clinical symptomatology associated with the cerebrovascular disorder, more often in hemorrhages than infarctions [1]. More recent clinical prospective and retrospective studies describe the CNS vascular complications of new antineoplastic treatments and also provide additional information on the risk of stroke in cancer patients, the most sensitive methods for determining the etiology, and the results for stroke and stroke prevention.

The largest prospective study of stroke in cancer patients is a Swedish cohort of 820,491 cancer patients followed for first hospitalization for hemorrhagic or ischemic stroke, as compared to patients without cancer. The overall risk of hemorrhagic and ischemic stroke during the first six months after cancer diagnosis was 2.2 and 1.6, respectively. The risk decreased rapidly, but remained elevated even ten years after cancer diagnosis [2].

A recent clinical retrospective study of intracranial hemorrhages in cancer patients identified 208 intracerebral and 46 subarachnoid hemorrhages. The majority of patients (68%) had systemic solid tumors, and equal numbers were hematopoietic and primary brain tumors. Intratumoral hemorrhage and coagulopathy accounted for the majority of hemorrhages. Hypertension was a rare cause. The prognosis was similar to intracranial hemorrhage in the general population [3]. In a clinical retrospective review of ischemic strokes in 96 cancer patients, the cancers were most commonly lung, brain, and prostate. The most common cause was embolism, due partially to hypercoagulability. Atherosclerosis was the cause in less than 25% [4]. In children with cancer, the prevalence of stroke is approximately 1%, with an equal distribution of hemorrhagic and ischemic strokes [5]. The most common underlying cancers are leukemia and primary brain tumors.

Stroke can also rarely be the presenting sign of cancer. In a retrospective review of 5106 patients admitted for ischemic stroke, Taccone et al. [6] identified less than 1% to have a previously undiagnosed malignancy. The principal mechanisms of stroke in the cancer patients were nonbacterial thrombotic endocarditis (NBTE), diffuse intravascular coagulation, and atherosclerosis. The most frequent neoplasms were lung and breast cancer.

The prognosis of cancer-related CNS hemorrhage varies widely, depending upon the etiology. No detailed retrospective or prospective studies of prognosis are available. The prognosis of patients with ischemic stroke varies depending on the activity of cancer. In a retrospective review of ischemic stroke patients (4918) admitted to a university hospital, 300 were identified to have cancer that was inactive in 227 patients and active in 73 patients. Stroke patients with active cancer were significantly younger than those without active cancer, had more severe strokes, more frequently had cryptogenic strokes, and more often had infarcts in multiple vascular territories of the brain. In-hospital mortality was significantly higher in patients with active cancer (21.9% vs. 5.2%) [7].

In determining the etiology of stroke in the cancer patient, various factors must be considered. Traditional cerebrovascular risk factors seen in the general population such as age, hypertension, coronary artery disease, hypercholesterolemia, tobacco use, diabetes, and family history of stroke should be assessed, but cancer patients more often have stroke as a cancer-related event, in which the malignancy directly or indirectly contributes to the cerebrovascular insult. Thus, additional consideration must be given to the causes of stroke that are unique to the cancer patient. A detailed investigation

L.R. Rogers (✉)
Department of Neurology, University Hospitals Cleveland Medical Center, 11100 Euclid Avenue, Cleveland, OH 44106, USA
e-mail: lisa.rogers1@uhhospitals.org

© Springer International Publishing AG 2018
D. Schiff et al. (eds.), *Cancer Neurology in Clinical Practice*,
DOI 10.1007/978-3-319-57901-6_10

and precise diagnosis of cerebrovascular disorders in cancer patients are critical because early recognition of stroke may allow the cancer patient access to surgical or medical interventions to improve the clinical outcome. In addition, secondary stroke prevention therapies are guided by the etiology of the cerebrovascular event. Lastly, the diagnostic evaluation in young or cryptogenic stroke patients may lead to the first recognition of an underlying malignancy.

This chapter will explore the etiologies of stroke within the oncologic population and discuss their diagnosis and management.

Stroke Due to Central Nervous System Tumor

Intratumoral Parenchymal Hemorrhage

Hemorrhage into brain tumors, both metastatic and primary, is reported to account for 1–10% of all intracranial hemorrhages [8–10]. The variation in reported frequency is due, in part, to the method of diagnosis; some hemorrhages are clinically silent and identified only on imaging or at autopsy. Metastatic tumors are more often associated with hemorrhage than are primary tumors, including hemorrhage as the initial manifestation of CNS tumor.

The most common metastatic brain tumors associated with bleeding are melanoma, lung, renal cell, breast, thyroid, hepatocellular cancer and choriocarcinoma [3, 10, 11]. Hemorrhage associated with metastatic tumors can occur in any location in the cerebral hemispheres, brain stem, or cerebellum and may be single or multiple. In some instances, notably malignant melanoma and other angioinvasive tumors, the diagnosis of brain metastasis is established only at hematoma resection demonstrating microscopic malignant cells.

The most common primary CNS tumors associated with intratumoral hemorrhage are glial tumors, especially glioblastoma, and germ cell tumors. Figure 10.1a, b shows the macroscopic and microscopic features of a fatal intratumoral hemorrhage into a GBM. Oligodendrogliomas are particularly prone to hemorrhage because of the delicate retiform capillaries associated with them [12]. Hemorrhage into meningioma is relatively uncommon and occurs most often in patients who are less than 30 or more than 70 years of age, located in the convexity or ventricle, and of fibrous histology [13]. Intratumoral hemorrhages are also reported infrequently in association with a wide variety of other primary brain tumors, including medulloblastoma, choroid plexus papilloma, schwannoma, ependymoma, pineal region tumors, and lymphoma.

The most common clinical symptoms in patients with intratumoral hemorrhage are headache, nausea, vomiting, obtundation, seizures, and focal neurologic deficits, similar to hemorrhages of other etiology. The symptoms may be acute or subacute. Bleeding may be spontaneous or associated with predisposing factors such as head trauma, hypertension, coagulopathy, shunting procedures, surgery, and anticoagulation [3]. Various pathophysiologic processes unique to the tumor also contribute to intratumoral hemorrhage, including overexpression of vascular endothelial growth factor and matrix metalloproteinases, endothelial proliferation, rapid tumor growth, vessel necrosis, and compression or invasion of adjacent parenchymal vessel walls by tumor [14, 15].

Imaging findings on brain CT or MR scan that suggest neoplastic hemorrhage include early edema, an indentation appearing on the hematoma surface that enhances with administration of contrast, delayed hemorrhage evolution and early perihemorrhage enhancement [16, 17].

Treatment is directed to the underlying tumor and may include surgical resection followed by radiation therapy and medical therapies appropriate to the histology. Patient outcome after intratumoral hemorrhage is related to the specific histological malignancy of the tumor and extent of the systemic cancer. There appears to be a higher risk of

(a)   **(b)**

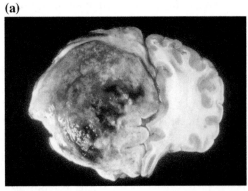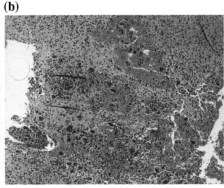

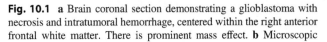

Fig. 10.1 a Brain coronal section demonstrating a glioblastoma with necrosis and intratumoral hemorrhage, centered within the right anterior frontal white matter. There is prominent mass effect. **b** Microscopic image in this patient at autopsy reveals fibrillary and giant cells, with intervening areas of hemorrhage (H&E ×200)

recurrent hemorrhage if the tumor is incompletely excised or if metastases recur.

Hemorrhage into pituitary adenomas (pituitary apoplexy) is a unique and rare disorder, often accompanied by infarction of the pituitary gland. It can be life-threatening because of corticotropin and thyroid hormone deficiency. The most common presenting symptom is headache, followed by visual field abnormalities and cranial nerve palsies. MRI is superior to CT in establishing the diagnosis. MRI typically shows an intra-and suprasellar expanding mass with T1 and T2 signal intensities consistent with the evolution of blood products. Enhancement is usually faint. Thickening of the sphenoid sinus mucosa is highly indicative of pituitary apoplexy [18].

A recent retrospective review from the Mayo Clinic identified 87 cases of pituitary apoplexy, mostly male, with a mean age of 51 years. Only 25% had a known pituitary adenoma. The most common associated factor was hypertension (39%). Long-term outcome was good, although most patients required long-term hormonal placement [19]. There are no controlled studies to prove a benefit of surgical decompression; observation, with replacement of hormones as clinically indicated, is appropriate in many patients.

Neoplastic Subdural Hemorrhage

Subdural hematomas and hygromas are common etiologies for cerebrovascular disease in cancer patients, comprising 12.6% of all strokes and 25.8% of hemorrhagic lesions identified at autopsy within this population [1]. Overall, subdural hemorrhages related to dural metastasis are less common than those related to coagulopathy or trauma in cancer patients [20]. Neoplastic subdural hemorrhages occur more commonly in patients with solid, rather than hematological tumors, and in particular with tumors metastatic from prostate, lung, or breast cancer primaries [20, 21].

Neoplastic infiltration of the dura results from hematogenous spread of tumor into the dural vessels or from direct extension of skull metastasis. Proposed mechanisms for the occurrence of subdural hematoma with dural metastasis include hemorrhage directly into the dural tumor, hemorrhage secondary to dilatation and rupture of the inner dural capillaries/venules/veins due to outer vessel layer obstruction by tumor, and in rare cases, dural tumor production of a hemorrhagic effusion.

Acute and subacute subdural hemorrhages are more common than are chronic. Graus et al. [1] reported that one-quarter of their 53 autopsied subdural hematoma patients with cancer were symptomatic. Clinical manifestations in the oncologic population differ little from the general population. The most common clinical symptoms are altered mental status, headache, and lethargy. Focal neurological deficits and seizures may also be present.

Acute or chronic subdural hematomas and skull metastases are generally easily visualized with both CT and MRI. Contrast studies are helpful in revealing skull or dural enhancement. Histologic examination of the dura with biopsy or cytologic studies of the subdural fluid may be necessary to confirm the tumoral origin of the subdural hematoma. Figure 10.2a–c shows the imaging and subdural fluid cytology findings in a patient with dural metastasis from lung cancer [22].

(a)   **(b)**   **(c)**

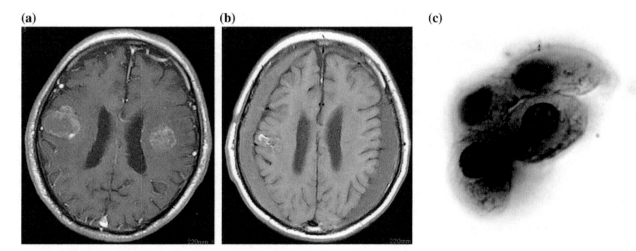

Fig. 10.2 a Brain magnetic resonance image taken on admission shows bilateral masses in the brain. **b** Brain magnetic resonance image taken on deterioration of symptoms shows bilateral crescent-shaped isointensity lesions and a shrunken brain mass. **c** Adenocarcinoma cells detected in hematoma fluid (*All* Used with permission of Elsevier from Hata et al. [22])

Treatment of dural metastasis-associated hemorrhage is palliative and includes drainage of subdural fluid and radiation therapy.

Neoplastic Infiltration of Cerebral Vessels

Venous Infiltration

Thrombosis of cerebral veins or dural sinuses is a rare event in any patient population, including those with cancer. Cerebral venous thrombosis accounted was diagnosed in only 0.3% of neurological consultations in cancer patients over a four year period at Memorial Sloan-Kettering Cancer Center [23].

The most common cause of cerebral venous thrombosis in cancer patients is a coagulopathy associated with hematologic tumors. Invasion or compression of dural sinuses or cortical veins by tumor occurs most commonly in solid tumors that are metastatic to the dura, skull, or rarely, the leptomeninges [23, 24].

The most common vein affected by metastasis is the superior sagittal sinus. Headache is the most frequent presenting symptom of venous thrombosis. This may be accompanied by focal neurological deficits, encephalopathy, or seizures when there is adjacent venous infarction. Occasionally patients present with an isolated intracranial hypertension syndrome, with headache that may be accompanied by visual disturbances associated with papilledema or abducens palsy. When due to neoplastic vessel compression or invasion, neurologic symptoms from venous thrombosis often develop subacutely, in contrast to the thrombosis associated with coagulopathy, in which symptom onset is typically acute [23].

Brain CT or MRI scanning with contrast may reveal a lack of contrast within the sagittal sinus because of the thrombosis, a finding known as the "empty delta sign" but this is uncommon. Overall MRI is superior to CT in detecting venous thrombosis. The sensitivity increases with the concomitant use of MRA and MRV. MRI can also demonstrate parenchymal abnormalities of venous infarction or hemorrhage, and identify adjacent tumor.

When venous occlusion is due to tumor compression or infiltration, the clinical course is generally progressive and antineoplastic therapy to treat the tumor may be indicated. Therapeutic options include tumor resection, radiation, or systemic therapy. The use of anticoagulation or thrombolysis has not been studied in this setting.

Arterial Infiltration

Neoplastic infiltration of arterial vessels has been reported to cause both hemorrhagic and ischemic strokes. Cerebral tumor embolization can result in aneurysm or pseudoaneurysm formation and subsequent aneurysm rupture produces intracerebral and/or subarachnoid hemorrhage. A recent literature review of neoplastic cerebral aneurysms identified 96 published cases. Cardiac myxoma was the most common underlying tumor (60%), choriocarcinoma was next most common (26%) and other malignant tumors accounted for 13.5%. Hemorrhage was universal in choriocarcinoma, less common in other malignant tumors (84.6%) and uncommon in myxoma (19.6%) [25]. Figure 10.3a–c shows multiple brain hemorrhages in a patient with ruptured neoplastic pseudoaneurysms associated with metastatic choriocarcinoma. The diagnosis of neoplastic aneurysm can be made by cerebral arteriography. Neoplastic aneurysms are typically small in size and are often located in distal cerebral arterial branches, in contrast to saccular aneurysms which arise in proximal cerebral arteries. Those from cardiac myxoma are usually multiple, whereas those from malignant tumors are usually single. The prognosis is poor in tumors other than cardiac myxoma. A second, less common, mechanism of aneurysm formation is secondary invasion of nearby vessels by parenchymal brain metastases [26].

Ischemic stroke has also been associated with infiltration of arteries by tumor in the leptomeninges [27, 28]. Patients experiencing ischemia secondary to leptomeningeal metastasis present with abrupt, focal neurological deficits alone or in addition to the typical clinical features of leptomeningeal tumor. Angiography may reveal focal arteriolar narrowing at the base of the brain, over the cerebral convexities, or both. Figure 10.4 demonstrates the angiographic findings in a patient with diffuse leptomeningeal dissemination of glioblastoma. Biopsy showed that leptomeningeal tumor caused vascular narrowing by vessel encasement, vascular wall invasion, and thrombosis [28].

Hematologic Malignancies

Myeloproliferative disorders are acquired clonal disorders characterized by the proliferation of bone marrow myeloid cells. Among these, polycythemia vera and essential thrombocythemia are the most common to be associated with systemic and neurologic thrombotic complications, including cerebral infarction, TIA and venous thrombosis. Risk factors for thrombosis include those associated with the underlying disease, including increased white blood cell counts, vascular cell activation, endothelial dysfunction, and plasmatic risk factors, such as increased plasma viscosity, reduced levels of protein S, increased thrombin generation and standard stroke risk factors such as increased age, previous thrombotic events, smoking, hypertension, diabetes, dyslipidemia and obesity for arterial events. Oral contraceptives and pregnancy/puerperium) may contribute to venous thrombosis. Primary prevention includes antiplatelet therapy for arterial thrombosis and anticoagulation for venous thrombosis [29]. Of interest, cerebral thromboembolic complications frequently occur during the two years

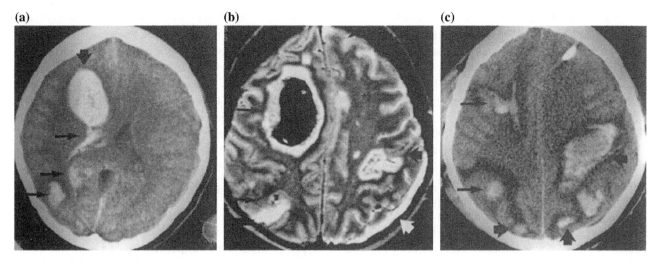

Fig. 10.3 Intracerebral hemorrhages due to metastatic choriocarcinoma with pseudoaneurysm formation. **a** Computed tomography on day 20 shows right frontal (*large arrow*) and right parietal hemorrhages with extension to the lateral ventricle (*small arrows*). **b** Magnetic resonance imaging on day 25 shows a new left posterior frontal hemorrhage (*large black arrow*) and left parieto-occipito-temporal subdural hematoma (*large white arrow*) and old right frontal and parietal hemorrhages (*small arrows*). **c** Computed tomography on day 29 shows increase in the left frontal hemorrhage and new occipital hemorrhages (*large arrows*) and old right temporal and parietal hemorrhages (*small arrows*) (*All* Used with permission of John Wiley and Sons from Kalafut et al. [131])

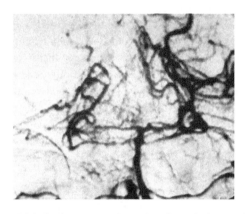

Fig. 10.4 Digital subtraction angiography of vertebral artery injection performed in the anteroposterior projection shows multiple zones of irregularity and narrowing involving the basilar artery, bilateral posterior cerebral arteries, bilateral superior cerebellar arteries and bilateral anterior inferior cerebellar arteries (Used with permission from Herman et al. [28])

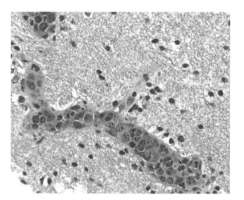

Fig. 10.5 Brain biopsy in a patient with confusion and multiple enhancing parenchymal lesions on brain MRI reveals intravascular lymphoma (H&E ×400)

preceding the diagnosis of a myeloproliferative disorder [30]. Cytoreductive treatment of blood hyperviscosity by phlebotomy or chemotherapy substantially reduces thrombotic events and improves survival.

Hyperleukocytosis (>100,000 WBC/mm^3) is a rare presentation of acute lymphoblastic leukemia (ALL). It can also occur in patients with acute and chronic myelogenous leukemias. It typically occurs during blast crisis and results in leukostasis, the plugging of blood vessels by blasts, most commonly in the lung and brain. Coalescence of cells forms leukemic nodules and can be complicated by brain hemorrhage, typically located in the white matter. Clinical signs include focal neurologic deficits and encephalopathy. Brain MRI findings in hyperleukocytosis are rarely reported; one well-characterized case demonstrated multiple hemorrhages and nonhemorrhagic changes on T1- and T2-weighted images with delayed enhancement and restricted diffusion [31]. It is rapidly fatal if not treated. Emergency treatments include hydration, cytoreduction, prevention of tumor lysis, leukapheresis and brain radiation therapy [32, 33].

Intravascular lymphomatosis (IVL) is a rare variant of non-Hodgkin's lymphoma characterized by a proliferation of lymphoma cells within small caliber blood vessels, with a predilection for the skin and CNS. Figure 10.5 is a brain biopsy depiction of IVL pathology. IVL patients with neurologic involvement most commonly present with subacute progressive multifocal cerebral infarcts and/or a rapidly progressive encephalopathy accompanied by fever. Other sites, such as lung, spleen, and bone marrow may also be involved. In a meta-analysis of the literature between 1962 and 2011, Fonkem et al. [34] identified 740 published cases. The median age was 64 years. The majority (88%) were of B cell origin.

Brain MRI typically demonstrates multiple lesions, most commonly in the cerebral hemispheres. Early diffusion changes that follow the typical time course noted in ischemic events can be observed. Noninvasive and catheter angiography may demonstrate a vasculitis-like appearance [35]. Because the diagnosis is difficult to establish from clinical symptoms, there is often a delay in diagnosis or lack of diagnosis during life. Historically, the majority of cases have been diagnosed postmortem. The most effective therapy is not known, but reports indicate that chemotherapy and rituximab or radiotherapy can stabilize the clinical course.

Tumor Embolus

Ischemic stroke secondary to tumor embolism is rare. In the series by Graus et al. [1] only two patients had tumor emboli identified as the etiology of infarction. Most reported cases of tumor embolic stroke result from intracardiac tumors. The majority of the tumors arise from the left side of the heart. They are most often benign. In a large recent series of resected primary cardiac tumors, myxoma was the most common histology (72.6%). Fibromas and sarcomas were rare, 6.9 and 6.4% respectively. Ten percent of patients with intracardiac tumor experienced a stroke [36].

Cerebral TIA or infarction may also occur from tumor emboli arising from tumors metastatic to the heart. Cardiac metastasis usually occurs in the presence of widely metastatic disease. In an autopsy study of 95 patient with cardiac metastases, the underlying cancers, in descending order, were of lung, lymphoma, breast, leukemia, gastric, melanoma, liver and colon origin [37, 38]. Figure 10.6a–d shows the head CT, echocardiography and brain pathology of cerebral embolism from a cardiac metastatic tumor.

As in other embolic strokes, neurological symptoms are typically sudden and infarction may be preceded by TIA. History and physical examination findings of cardiac dysfunction such as limb edema, dyspnea, arrhythmias, peripheral vascular emboli, and precordial murmurs are helpful in identifying a cardiac tumor. Echocardiography is a reliable means of diagnosing cardiac tumors and may suggest the histology. Transesophageal echocardiogram is superior to transthoracic echocardiography in evaluating atrial tumors. False negative echocardiograms have been reported in cardiac neoplasm patients; cardiac MRI and CT can be useful in this situation. Tissue diagnosis involves obtaining a pathological specimen through endomyocardial biopsy or surgical resection of the tumor.

Primary or metastatic lung cancers can also produce TIA or cerebral infarction from a tumor embolus that accesses the pulmonary venous system and then passes through the left heart chambers to the cerebral vasculature. Cerebral infarction that is identified in the peri-operative period after lung cancer biopsy or resection should suggest embolization of a tumor fragment [39]. Patients with tumor embolic ischemia should be followed with surveillance brain imaging to observe for tumor growth.

Stroke Due to Remote Effects of Tumor: Hyper- and Hypocoagulopathies

Hypercoagulability and Thrombosis

Abnormalities of the coagulation system are very common in the cancer patient, and there is a high propensity for thrombosis of venous or arterial vessels, especially in widely disseminated solid tumors and in glioblastoma. Venous thromboembolism (VTE) and disseminated intravascular coagulation complicate the course in a significant percentage of patients, depending on the histology. Increases of coagulation factors V, VIII, IX, and XI are often documented in malignancy. Markers of coagulation activation are frequently elevated, including prothrombin fragment 1.2, thrombin antithrombin complex, fibrin degradation products, and D-dimers. Also consistent with a consumptive coagulopathy is the frequent finding of increased fibrinogen and platelet turnover.

Schwarzbach et al. [40] documented the presence of hypercoagulation as a cause of stroke in cancer patients, especially those with significantly elevated D-dimer levels, as compared with controls, and in the absence of conventional stroke risk factors. A hypercoagulable state can result in intravascular thrombosis as well as sterile platelet-fibrin deposition on cardiac valves termed nonbacterial thrombotic endocarditis (NBTE). In comparing the sensitivity of transthoracic and transesophageal echocardiograms, a retrospective review of 654 consecutive cancer patients in whom infectious or noninfectious endocarditis was suspected confirmed the diagnosis of endocarditis in 45 patients (75%). TEE was significantly more sensitive in detecting endocarditis: in 21 of 22 cases, TEE examinations were diagnostic and 16 (42%) of 38 patients with initially nondiagnostic TTE studies had the diagnosis confirmed by TEE study. Vegetations were larger in patients with culture positive endocarditis than in patients without culture positive infection [41].

In a study to determine the frequency of cardioembolic findings in 51 consecutive patients with cancer referred for

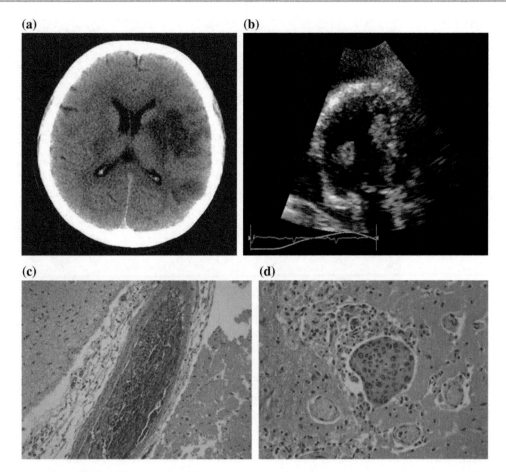

Fig. 10.6 Imaging and histologic findings in a patient with multifocal stroke from tumor emboli. **a** Head computed tomography demonstrating a left frontal lobe hypodensity consistent with middle cerebral artery territory infarction. **b** Transthoracic echocardiogram with apical 3-chamber view showing 2 large mobile echodensities attached to the septum and inferolateral wall of the left ventricle (*V*). **c** Frontal lobe arteriole occluded by moderately differentiated squamous cell carcinoma. Recent infarction is present surrounding the embolus, with disintegration, vacuolization, and pyknosis of neurons (hematoxylin-eosin, original magnification ×20). **d** Tumor embolus of squamous cell carcinoma occluding a cerebellar vessel. Small areas of infarction surround the embolus, with proliferation of capillaries and macrophages (hematoxylin-eosin, original magnification ×40) (*All Used with permission of American Medical Association from Navi et al. [38]. All rights reserved*)

TEE evaluation of cerebrovascular events, 18% had NBTE and 47 and 55% had definite and definite or probable cardiac sources of embolism, respectively [42]. Singhal et al. [43] compared the MRI findings in patients with infectious endocarditis and NBTE. Patients with NBTE uniformly had multiple, widely distributed, small (<10 mm) and large (>30 mm) infarctions (Fig. 10.7a–c), whereas patients with infectious endocarditis had a variety of stroke patterns including a single lesion, territorial infarction, and disseminated punctate lesions, and numerous small, medium or large lesions in multiple territories.

Venous Occlusions

Cerebral venous thrombosis can occur from direct tumor invasion or compression of the dural sinuses (reviewed above), but more commonly occurs from a hypercoagulable state induced by a neoplasm or chemotherapy. A systemic coagulopathy is the most common cause of cerebral venous thrombosis in patients with hematologic malignancies, especially ALL or lymphoma after treatment with L-asparaginase [23]. Steroids may contribute to the development of thrombosis.

The clinical presentation is similar to patients without cancer who develop sinus thrombosis, and includes headache, vomiting, papilledema, and seizures. Focal neurological signs or encephalopathy may also occur if there is associated cerebral infarction or hemorrhage. Imaging characteristics are reviewed above, but in the instance of coagulation-related venous thrombosis, no skull or dural tumor is identified [44]. Spontaneous resolution or recanalization of nonmetastatic sinus thrombosis can occur, especially early in the course of cancer and its treatment. When

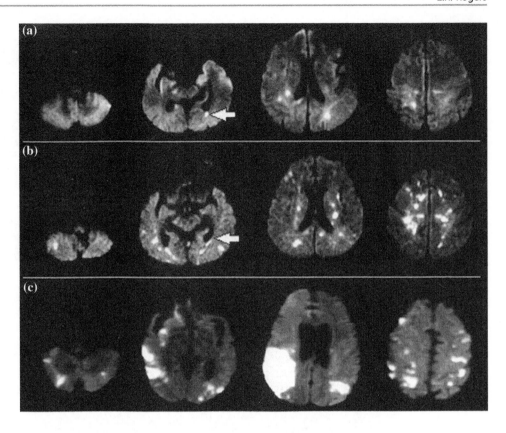

the thrombus is symptomatic and persistent, treatment should be considered. Two randomized clinical trials have studied the benefits and risks of anticoagulation in patients without cancer who develop sinus thrombosis. A small trial of intravenous unfractionated heparin found a benefit; a larger trial of low molecular weight heparin found only a nonsignificant trend to benefit [45, 46]. The safety of anticoagulation in ALL patients has been reported in small numbers of patients [47, 48]. Small series also document the benefit of endovascular thrombectomy and thrombolysis [49, 50]. The safety and efficacy of these latter treatments in the cancer population has not been established.

Arterial Occlusions

Cerebral arterial occlusions constitute a major source of morbidity in cancer patients. The most common cause for thrombotic arterial occlusions in cancer-associated thrombophilia is NBTE (see above) Vegetations are most commonly located on the aortic and mitral valves. NBTE is significantly more common in cancer patients than in patients without malignancy; it occurs most commonly in adenocarcinoma patients, especially pancreatic cancer [51, 52]. Mucin-producing adenocarcinomas, of which many are pancreatic, are strongly associated with NBTE [53]. Rarely, NBTE is the presenting sign of cancer.

The mechanism of cerebral TIA or infarction in NBTE is small vessel thrombosis as a result of intravascular thrombosis or embolization of a sterile vegetation to brain vessels [54]. Systemic thromboembolism, both venous and arterial, may be a clue to NBTE in a cancer patient with cerebral ischemia. However, one-third of patients have only neurologic symptomatology [52]. The diagnosis may be difficult to suspect on clinical grounds alone, because NBTE can result in signs of encephalopathy caused by multiple small vascular thrombosis. In other patients, sudden focal neurological symptoms of TIA or stroke suggest embolization. The majority of patients with NBTE have only mildly abnormal coagulation parameters. The diagnosis of NBTE is most often rendered in vivo by echocardiographic detection of valvular vegetations. Transesophageal echocardiography is more sensitive than transthoracic. Both neuroimaging and autopsy studies show that cerebral infarcts may be multiple and sometimes have a hemorrhagic component. Cerebral angiography typically discloses multiple vessel branch occlusions, commonly in the middle cerebral artery territory [52].

Appropriate treatment of NBTE includes treatment directed to the underlying cause for the coagulation disorder, such as the neoplasm or sepsis if this coexists. There are no prospective studies of anticoagulation in NBTE; however, individual case reports and retrospective cases series suggest that anticoagulation with heparin appears to reduce ischemic

Fig. 10.8 MRI, focal T2 hyperintensities involving all lobes in Case 1, most prominently left occipital lobe in Case 2 (*All* Used with permission of Springer Science from Bernardo et al. [56])

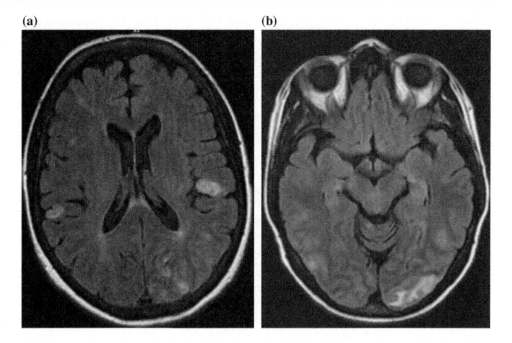

(a) (b)

symptomatology in some patients [52]. The potential benefits of anticoagulation should be weighed cautiously against the potential risks of hemorrhage in the cancer patient with NBTE-associated stroke.

Mucin-Positive Adenocarcinoma-Associated Hypercoaguability

Mucin-producing adenocarcinomas are associated with arterial ischemic stroke both in association with, and independently of, NBTE. A 1989 study examined patients with mucinous adenocarcinoma and systemic and cerebral ischemia [55]. Widely disseminated metastases were present in all cases. Varying sizes of cerebral infarctions were found, including disseminated microinfarcts in all patients and large or small/moderate sized infarcts in most. Ischemia affected widespread areas of the CNS, including the cerebral hemispheres, cerebellum, brainstem, basal ganglia, spinal cord, and dorsal spinal roots. Petechial and small hemorrhages were also relatively common. In each of the cases in this series, intravascular mucin was noted within central nervous system capillaries and small arteries on pathological examination.

The mechanism of hypercoagulability in mucin-secreting adenocarcinoma is still not fully understood. Mucin itself may be prothrombotic, the mucin-producing tumor cells may be prothrombotic, or both [56]. There may also be fat emboli in association with mucin [57]. At present, the diagnosis of mucin-positivity is only reliably made pathologically, typically at autopsy. Treatment of the underlying malignancy is the only known method to reduce further cerebrovascular

events. Cautious anticoagulation has been suggested in the setting of ischemic stroke and mucin-positive neoplasm, but this therapy is unproven. Figure 10.8 shows multifocal bilateral ischemia visualized on MRI in two patients with breast cancer in whom intravascular mucin was identified pathologically.

Combined Hypercoaguability/Bleeding Diathesis

Normal physiologic hemostasis involves a balance between thrombus formation and thrombolysis [58]. Disseminated intravascular coagulation (DIC) is characterized by widespread activation of coagulation, with resulting production of fibrin clot formation and thrombotic occlusion of small and medium size vessels. Formation of thrombi leads to consumption of endogenous coagulation factors, platelets, and anticoagulant factors such as Protein S, Protein C, and antithrombin, increasing a risk for bleeding [59]. Acute DIC is most commonly observed in acute promyelocytic leukemia (APML) because of a unique constellation of factors associated with the leukocytes [60]. Other risk factors for acute DIC are pancreatic and other mucin-producing solid tumors, age >60 years, male gender, breast cancer, tumor necrosis, and advanced stage disease [61]. Patients may present with symptoms and signs of excessive hypercoaguability, uncontrolled hemorrhage, or both simultaneously. In aPML, brain hemorrhage is often fatal. Acute, or uncompensated, DIC occurs most frequently with hematogenous malignancies such as the acute leukemias, and is less frequent with solid tumors. Acute DIC typically presents with clinically significant bleeding with concomitant thrombosis. Bleeding from venipuncture sites and surgical wounds may be seen, as well as diffuse mucosal, skin, or retroperitoneal hemorrhage. Central nervous system hemorrhage is a significant and potentially fatal complication, especially in acute promyelocytic leukemia (APML) Laboratory findings in acute DIC include thrombocytopenia, prolonged PT and aPTT, low fibrinogen, elevated D dimer and microangiopathic changes on the peripheral blood smear.

Chronic DIC develops when blood is continuously or intermittently exposed to smaller amounts of procoagulant substances. The coagulation factors and platelets are consumers, but production is able to compensate. Thrombosis generally predominates over bleeding. Chronic DIC more often manifests as thrombosis, rather than bleeding, although either or both hematologic dyscrasias are possible. Chronic DIC has been reported in the clinical settings of NBTE and mucin-positive adenocarcinoma-associated thrombosis. Patients in chronic DIC typically present with deep venous thrombosis and pulmonary thromboembolism, although some may also develop arterial ischemia. Coagulation tests may be normal or show mild thrombocytopenia, mild prolongation of PT and aPTT, and normal or slightly elevated fibrinogen. D dimer is often elevated.

No prospective clinical trials address the optimal treatment for chronic or acute DIC associated with symptomatic cerebral thrombosis or hemorrhage. Treatment of the cancer is fundamental to successful long-term therapy. Anticoagulants, by interrupting the coagulation cascade, are of theoretical benefit. Unfractionated and low molecular weight heparins have appeared beneficial in small, uncontrolled cohorts but have not been definitively evaluated in controlled clinical trials [62]. Direct thrombin inhibitors are promising but unvalidated in controlled trials [59].

Bleeding Diathesis/Hemorrhage

Primary Fibrinolysis

Primary fibrinolysis is characterized by systemic activation of plasmin or direct fibrinogen degradation. Intracranial hemorrhage may result from primary fibrinolysis in association with acute DIC early in the course of APML. Primary fibrinolysis, without DIC, has been observed in some leukemias and solid tumors, especially prostate cancer. Cerebrovascular complications are rare in this setting. Treatment consists of administering cryoprecipitate or fresh frozen plasma. Epsilon-aminocaproic acid or tranexamic acid may also be given [63].

Thrombocytopenia

Thrombocytopenia is not uncommon in the cancer population and poses a risk for intracranial hemorrhage

Thrombocytopenia-associated cerebral hemorrhage in oncology patients can be secondary to extensive marrow infiltration by tumor, peripheral destruction of platelets due to tumor-associated hypersplenism, under-production of platelets due to radiation- or chemotherapy-induced toxicity, DIC, autoimmune dysfunction, and/or microangiopathic hemolytic anemia. Cancer-associated hemolytic anemia is a Coombs-negative hemolytic anemia. A review of published cases published in 2012 reported 154 cases associated with solid cancer and 14 cases with lymphoma. The majority of the cancers were metastatic. The prognosis is poor. Treatment includes antitumor treatment and plasma exchange or fresh frozen plasma; the latter was rarely effective, except in prostate cancer patients [64].

Immune-mediated peripheral platelet destruction is rarely seen with solid tumors, but has been reported with lymphoproliferative disorders such as Hodgkin's disease, chronic lymphocytic leukemia, and low-grade lymphoma [65]. Diagnosis is difficult but may be supported by the acute onset of thrombocytopenia, large platelet size, elevated megakaryocyte count, and increased platelet-associated immunoglobulin. Treatment may include corticosteroids, immunoglobulin infusions, plasmapheresis, antineoplastic therapy directed at the specific underlying malignancy, vincristine, danazol, and immunoabsorption with staphylococcal protein A.

Thrombotic thrombocytopenic purpura (TTP) is a syndrome of target organ dysfunction due to marked platelet aggregation in the microcirculation that can be induced both by cancer and by chemotherapeutic treatment [66]. Thrombotic thrombocytopenic purpura is characterized by severe thrombocytopenia, a microangiopathic hemolytic anemia, and renal failure (hemolytic-uremic syndrome) Intracerebral hemorrhage and cerebral infarction are potentially disastrous events that may complicate the course of patients with TTP. Platelet aggregates in TTP most commonly occlude the arterioles and capillaries in the brain, heart, kidneys, and adrenal glands. Clinically, purpuric rash, fever, and neurological and renal symptoms are common. Laboratory studies demonstrate severe hemolytic anemia, thrombocytopenia, and schistocytosis. Thrombotic thrombocytopenic purpura can be differentiated from DIC by the absence of a coagulopathy. In cancer patients, TTP is most commonly seen with gastric adenocarcinoma, followed by breast, colon, and small cell lung carcinoma. Treatment options include corticosteroids, plasma exchange, immunoabsorption with staphylococcal protein A, platelet inhibitor drugs, vincristine, and splenectomy. Platelet transfusions are reserved for situations of documented bleeding. Mortality in TTP without treatment is 90–100%. With appropriate treatment, mortality decreases to 10%.

Sequelae of Cancer Treatment

In addition to cancer and its associated coagulopathies as a cause of stroke, ischemic or hemorrhagic strokes can result from certain diagnostic procedures, radiation therapy, surgical therapy, endovascular treatments, or chemotherapy.

Cancer Therapy: Radiation

Radiation-Induced Vasculopathy

A variety of delayed vasculopathies can complicate therapeutic radiation to the brain or neck. Pathologic studies demonstrate that radiotherapy produces a sequence of vascular changes characterized by initial damage to endothelial cells, followed by thickening of the intimal layer, cellular degeneration, and hyaline transformation. Stenosis and occlusion of medium and large vessels leading to ischemic infarction is the most common sequela, but lacunar infarction, primary intracerebral hemorrhage, moyamoya changes resulting in ischemia or hemorrhage, and the formation of cerebral aneurysms and pseudoaneurysms also occur [67, 68].

Several large scale studies, particularly those from the Childrens Cancer Study Group (CCSG) describe the risk of stroke in pediatric cancer survivors (alive ≥ five years), especially those with brain tumors and those with leukemia who received cranial radiation therapy. The rate of first occurrence of late-occurring stroke was determined in leukemia (*n* = 4828) and brain tumor survivors (*n* = 1871) as compared with a group of a random sample of cancer survivor siblings (*n* = 3846). The rate for leukemia survivors was 57.9 per 100,000 person-years and the relative risk for stroke, as compared with the sibling comparison group, was 6.4. In brain tumor survivors, the rate was 267.6 per 100,000 person-years and the relative risk was 29. Mean cranial radiation therapy dose ≥30 Gy was associated with an increased risk in both leukemia and brain tumor survivors in a dose-dependent fashion, with the highest risk after doses of ≥50 Gy [69].

The CCSG also recently identified that among childhood cancer survivors with stroke, there is a risk of recurrent stroke, especially those receiving ≥50 Gy cranial radiation therapy. The risk persists for decades after the first stroke: the ten-year cumulative incidence of late recurrent stroke was 21% overall and 33% for those treated with high dose cranial radiation therapy. Hypertension also independently predicted recurrent stroke in this population [70].

Single institution studies also confirm and characterize the risk of stroke in survivors of pediatric brain tumors and that location of tumor influences the risk. Multivariate and logistic regression analysis in one study showed that children treated with cranial radiation therapy and those with optic pathway gliomas had the highest risk of nonperioperative stroke [71]. Treatment of tumors close to the circle of Willis, especially optic pathway gliomas and the prepontine cistern, were associated with the highest risk in another study [72]. Location of tumor is also important in adult patients. Aizer and coworkers [73] recently identified that radiation therapy administered to primary brain tumors near the circle of Willis was associated with an increased risk of death secondary to cerebrovascular disease as compared to radiation to distant sites. Adults irradiated for pituitary adenomas (especially males) are also at risk for delayed stroke and TIA [74].

A recent literature review between 1978 and 2013 identified 46 patients with 69 intracranial aneurysms within the irradiated field. The mean age at radiation exposure was 34 years and the mean lag time between radiation and diagnosis was 12 years (range, 4 months to 50 years). Aneurysms were saccular in 83%, fusiform in 9, and 9% were considered pseudo-aneurysms. Just over half of the aneurysms presented with hemorrhage [75]. Aneurysms can develop after radiosurgical treatment as well as external beam radiation [76]. There is a high rate of rupture in radiation-induced aneurysms and they are associated with significant morbidity and mortality. Treatment includes surgery or endovascular treatment [77].

Another vascular abnormality that can develop after cranial radiation therapy is a cavernous malformation, reported predominantly in pediatric patients radiated for leukemia, primary brain tumor, and within the setting of hematopoietic stem cell transplantation. They are more common after whole brain than reduced-field radiation [78] and typically develop several years after radiation [79, 80]. Most cavernous malformations are detected incidentally, as seen in Fig. 10.9. In symptomatic patients, the most common presenting symptom is seizure. Roughly one third have hemorrhage and may require surgery [81]. The clinical behavior can be more aggressive when chemotherapy is administered, especially methotrexate [82]. Spinal cord cavernous malformations are also reported within the field of spine radiation therapy [83].

Telangiectasias are smaller vascular malformations that can be observed on MRI after brain radiation therapy administered in childhood. Among 90 children who were followed for at least six months after brain radiation, telangiectasias were observed in at least one area in 18 (20%) patients. The frequency was similar following low dose and high dose radiation. The number of lesions increased on followup of ten years [84].

A literature review of moyamoya syndrome diagnosed after brain radiation therapy from 1967 to 2002 identified 54 patients. Patients with neurofibromatosis 1 and those who received radiation to the parasellar region at a young age (<5 years) were found to be the most susceptible. The

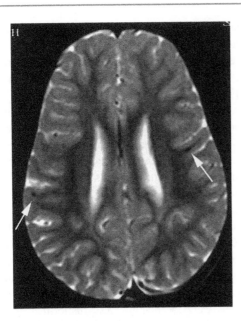

Fig. 10.9 Transverse T2-weighted spin-echo MR images (3000/100) obtained in 20-month-old girl with telangiectasia. Image obtained 4 years after completion of radiation therapy shows two telangiectatic foci (*arrows*) in the left frontal lobe and right parietal lobe (Used with permission of RSNA from Koike et al. [79])

incidence increases with time, with half of cases occurring within four years of radiation and 95% occurring within 12 years [85].

Radiotherapy can produce or accelerate atherosclerosis and it is a causative factor in transient or permanent cerebral ischemia in some patients radiated for head and neck cancer. Because of the radiation treatment portals, extensive areas of the common carotid artery and its branches in the neck are radiated. In a report of stroke in patients younger than 60 years of age who received therapeutic neck radiation for head and neck tumors, Dorresteijn and coworkers reported a 12% 15-year cumulative risk of stroke [86]. In a well-characterized retrospective study, Dorth and coworkers [87] found that 14% of head and neck cancer patients treated with neck radiotherapy had evidence of carotid stenosis at four years as compared to 4.2% in the general population.

The degree to which conventional stroke risk factors, such as hypertension, dyslipidemia, smoking history, and diabetes in head and neck patients also contribute to carotid stenosis is debated. Among 50 patients radiated for head and neck cancer, and comparing carotid artery stenosis and plaque formation between the radiated and non-radiated side, Gujral and coworkers [88] determined that traditional vascular risk factors do not play a significant role in radiation-induced carotid atherosclerosis. A summary of published studies in which the rate of extracranial carotid stenosis was compared between neck cancer patients who received radiation and those who did not (controls) includes 1070 patients. The incidence of severe extracranial carotid stenosis is significantly higher among those who received radiation. Like others, the authors recommend that irradiated patients be closely monitored with periodic carotid ultrasound [89].

Survivors of childhood Hodgkin's disease are also at risk for stroke if they receive mantle radiation exposure. In these patients cerebral ischemia may be related to carotid artery disease or to cardiac valve disease with embolism [90].

Stroke-like migraine attacks after radiation (SMART syndrome) is a rare syndrome occurring within years of brain radiation and is characterized by the occurrence of cerebral symptoms and signs associated with migraine headaches and cortical enhancement on brain MRI. The mechanism is not known, but is speculated to be a delayed manifestation of vascular injury. It typically has a good prognosis, but a recent report indicates that not all patients recover [91].

For symptomatic or high grade post-radiation carotid stenosis revascularization procedures may be indicated. The superiority of endarterectomy versus stenting is controversial. Sano et al. [92] reported that, by comparison, carotid endartectomy is safer. However, Cam et al. [93] reported that stenting is safe and durable. A recent multi-institutional comparison of carotid artery stenting for radiation therapy-associated carotid artery stenosis (43 patients) with non-irradiated patients found no difference in morbidity, revascularization, and restenosis [94].

In head and neck cancer patients, arterial injury due to surgery and radiation therapy may also present as arterial rupture (carotid blow-out). Post-radiation rupture of the carotid artery typically occurs within 2–16 weeks after radical neck surgery and radiation therapy. Rupture may be associated with other local treatment-related complications, such as infection, sloughing of the skin flaps and orocutaneous fistulas. Carotid blowout is a life threatening complication that requires surgical intervention. Brinjikji and Cloft [95] reviewed 2003–2011 data from the Nationwide Inpatient Sample and among 1218 patients who underwent endovascular treatment for carotid blowout; 89% underwent embolization procedures and 11% underwent carotid stenting. Hemiplegia rates were higher in stented patients than embolization (3.8% vs. 1.4%). The mortality rate was similar.

Cancer Therapy: Effects of Surgery

Direct Effects of Surgery

A rare complication of biopsy or removal of a primary or metastatic lung cancer is a peri-or postoperative cerebral infarction due to the release of tumor emboli [96]. It is important to monitor such patients with tumor embolic infarction for the subsequent development of a mass lesion associated with tumor growth [97]. Stroke is also a potential complication of advanced head and neck cancer resection because of the necessity to remove tumor in close proximity to the cervical carotid artery. However, the incidence of this complication has significantly declined in recent years. A recent retrospective study of 14,387 patients undergoing neck dissection found that the 30-day incidence of ischemic stroke was 0.7%, similar to matched patients undergoing thoracic surgery and colectomy. Factors independently associated with a higher risk of stroke within 30 days following neck dissection were standard stroke risk factors: age above 75 years, diabetes, hypertension, or prior stroke [98]. Resection of brain tumors is also associated with adverse effects on blood vessels.

The largest study of surgically-related cerebral infarction and hemorrhage in patients undergoing resection of malignant brain tumors is obtained from the Nationwide Inpatient Sample. Among 16,530 such patients undergoing tumor resection, the most common surgical complication was cerebral infarction, with an estimated incidence of 16.3/1000 cases. The second most common complication was brain hemorrhage or hematoma, with an incidence of 10.3/1000 cases. Because of the nature of data collection by ICD9 codes, it is not possible to determine if the diagnosis of infarction or hemorrhage/hematoma was based on incidental postoperative imaging findings or associated with neurological deficits. However, infarctions and hemorrhage/hematoma were associated with an increase of in-hospital mortality by 9-fold and 3-fold, respectively, suggesting that many of them were symptomatic [99].

Immediate post-operative diffusion-weighted MRI sequences often reveal changes of cerebral ischemia in patients undergoing removal of brain tumors. In recent years, the clinical significance of these imaging changes, particularly after glioma surgery, has been recognized. Rather than simply cortical or subcortical structural damage of eloquent brain tissue from surgery, Gempt et al. [100] demonstrated that peri- or postoperative ischemic lesions play a crucial role in the development of surgery-related motor deficits.

A matched case-control study assessing new postoperative deficits as compared to no deficits in patients undergoing resection of WHO grade 2–4 gliomas identified that postoperative neurological deficits were associated with peritumoral infarction and that volumes of DWI abnormalities were larger in those with deficits than those without. Peri-tumoral infarctions were more common and were larger in patients with acquired deficits after glioma surgery compared to glioma patients without deficits when assessed by early postoperative DWI [101]. Longitudinal followup of the post-operative ischemic lesions shows that the diffusion-weighted abnormality typically resolves and is replaced by contrast enhancement, ultimately demonstrating encephalomalacia at long-term follow up [102]. The early enhancement can be confused with tumor progression and

correlation with the immediate postoperative DWI changes can assist in the differential. Figure 10.10a–d shows the evolution of diffusion-weighted MRI abnormalities following resection of a low-grade glioma.

Diffusion-weighted changes associated with new postoperative deficits have also been reported after resection of brain metastasis. Ischemic lesions were more common in patients who had been treated with brain radiation as compared with those without. Presence of such lesions was significantly associated with transient or permanent neurological deficits [103].

Immediate post-operative areas of brain ischemia can also be identified outside the area of a resected brain tumor and the mechanism for this is not known. Tumor biopsy or resection can also be complicated by hemorrhage. Hemorrhage may also be remote from the site of surgery, most commonly cerebellar hemorrhage following supratentorial tumor surgery. Potential mechanisms include arterial hypertension, coagulation disorders, overdrainage of cerebrospinal fluid, disturbances of venous drainage associated with head position, and unrelated vascular lesions [104].

Other rare vascular complications of surgery for brain tumors include cerebral venous thrombosis, cerebral vasospasm especially following resection of base of skull tumors, and PRES following resection of posterior fossa tumors in children [105, 106].

Endovascular Treatment: Associated Stroke

Selective intra-arterial infusion of blood–brain barrier disruption and antineoplastic agents is a treatment approach for selected cerebral malignancies that can be complicated by ischemic stroke [107]. Catheter-administered embolization to occlude the vascular supply to meningiomas is very effective in obliterating blood supply but carries a small risk of cerebral infarction and hemorrhage [108, 109].

Cancer Therapy: Chemotherapy and Other Antineoplastics

Hypercoagulability and Thrombocytopenia

Antineoplastic chemotherapy, including single or multiagent chemotherapy, hormonal therapy, and hematopoietic growth factors can produce a hypercoagulable state in cancer patients and contribute to cerebral arterial and venous thrombosis [110]. Physiologic investigations in patients treated with chemotherapeutic agents have documented activation of the coagulation pathway, suppression of natural anticoagulants, suppression of natural fibrinolysis, and injury to vascular endothelium. Thrombocytopenia, TTP, DIC, and microangiopathic hemolytic anemia have all been linked to chemotherapeutic agents. Postulated mechanisms for antineoplastic drug-related thrombophilia include release of

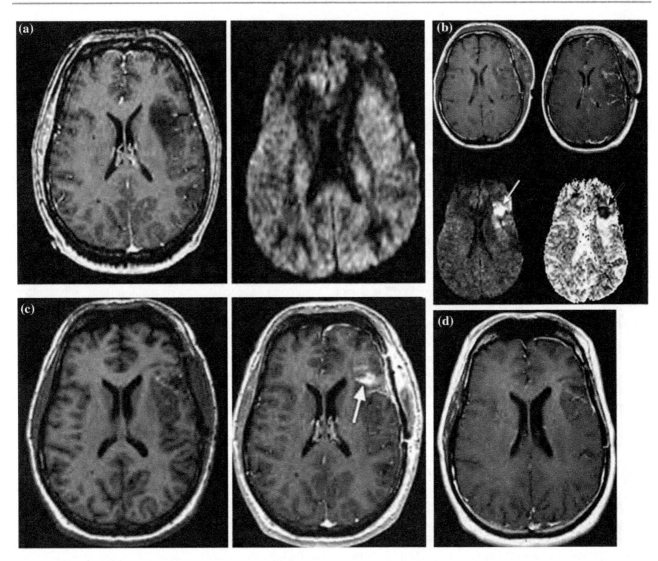

Fig. 10.10 Neuroimages obtained in a 27-year-old man with a left frontal Grade II fibrillary astrocytoma. **a** Axial T1-weighted MR image (*left*) and diffusion-weighted trace image (*right*) revealing a left frontal nonenhancing mass with no evidence of reduced diffusion. **b** Unenhanced and contrast-enhanced T1-weighted images (*upper*) obtained immediately postoperatively. Diffusion-weighted trace image and an ADC map (*lower*) demonstrating a new area of reduced diffusion (*arrows*) in the anterior surgical bed. **c** Two MR images obtained at the 1-month follow-up examination depicting the emergence of new contrast enhancement (*arrow*) corresponding to the area of reduced diffusion seen on the diffusion weighted image obtained immediately postoperatively. **d** An MR image obtained at the 3-month follow-up examination (*All* Used with permission from Smith et al. [102])

procoagulants and cytokines from injured tumor cells, direct drug toxicity to vascular endothelium, direct induction of monocyte or malignant cell tissue factor, and decrease in physiological anticoagulants.

Among individual chemotherapeutic agents associated with stroke, L-asparaginase is one of the most well-known. L-asparaginase is an enzymatic inhibitor of protein synthesis that is used in combination with other chemotherapeutic agents in the treatment of acute lymphoblastic leukemia and some other lymphoid malignancies [111, 112]. The reduction in protein synthesis produced by L-asparaginase not only inhibits growth of leukemic neoplasms, but also decreases liver production of multiple plasma proteins

involved in hemostasis. Strokes associated with L-asparaginase induction therapy may present as dural sinus thrombosis, cortical or capsular infarction, or intracerebral hemorrhage. Venous thrombosis is most common.

The incidence of stroke in patients treated with L-asparaginase induction therapy has ranged in different series from 0.9 to 2.9%. Stroke tends to occur shortly after induction treatment. The clinical presentation varies depending on the location and type of stroke. The precise mechanism for L-asparaginase-associated thrombosis stroke is unclear, although L-asparaginase has been shown to diminish antithrombin III, protein C, protein S, factor XI, factor IX, and fibrinogen, and to increase PT/PTT and platelet aggregability. Coagulation factors return to normal within 7–10 days after therapy. Therapies for L-asparaginase-associated strokes, depending on the clinical situation, vary widely and may include fresh frozen plasma, heparin, cryoprecipitate, platelet transfusion, aspirin, and surgery for hematoma drainage.

Stroke has also been associated with a variety of other chemotherapeutic agents. 5-fluorouracil therapy, alone and in combination with cisplatin, methotrexate, and cyclophosphamide, has been associated with acquired protein C deficiency and stroke. Acute stroke and acquired protein C deficiency has also been reported following cisplatin therapy without 5-fluorouracil. Stroke has been associated with paclitaxel, shortly after administration and in breast cancer survivors after adjuvant chemotherapy and radiation [113].

Granulocyte colony-stimulating factor (G-CSF) and granulocyte-macrophage colony-stimulating factor (GM-CSF) have been associated with venous and arterial thrombosis, possibly by enhancing aggregation and binding of neutrophils to vascular endothelium. A meta-analysis of 52 reported series found an incidence of venous and arterial thrombosis of 4.2% with GM-CSF and 1.2% with G-CSF.

Bevacizumab, a monoclonal antibody that binds to and inhibits the biologic activity of vascular endothelial growth factor (VEGF), is approved for treatment of metastatic colon carcinoma, nonsmall cell lung carcinoma, and recurrent glioblastoma. The most significant toxicities of this agent are systemic thrombosis or hemorrhage, including deep venous thrombosis, myocardial infarction, and hemoptysis. Imatinib mesylate administration for leukemia is rarely associated with subdural hemorrhage [114].

The posterior reversible encephalopathy syndrome (PRES) is increasingly recognized as a neurological complication of cytotoxic chemotherapies and targeted agents used to treat cancer, including brain tumors. It is also a known complication of uncontrolled hypertension, preeclampsia, sepsis, and adverse effect of immunosuppressive drugs used in organ and stem cell transplant. The mechanism of PRES is controversial; it is primarily thought to be a result of endothelial injury leading to impaired autoregulation and vasoconstriction. Characteristic neurological signs commonly include headache, generalized seizures, encephalopathy, sometimes progressing to coma or alteredvision (typically cortical blindness or hemianopia). The onset may be acute or subacute.

The basic PRES pattern resembles the brain watershed zones, with the cortex and subcortical and deep white matter involved to varying degrees. Figure 10.11a, b shows extensive bilateral cerebral hemisphere signal intensity abnormality and abnormal cerebral angiography in a patient with PRES [115].

The largest review of PRES in cancer patients includes 31 patients from Memorial Sloan-Kettering Cancer Center. A retrospective review of the clinical signs of PRES in cancer patients identified that most patients had active cancer at the time of diagnosis. The disorder occurred more commonly in women. Symptoms included confusion, headache, and visual disturbance. More than half of the patients experienced a seizure at onset. 13% had a severely depressed level of consciousness. The majority of patients experienced resolution of neurologic symptoms at the median of 7.5 days [116].

Treatment for PRES includes aggressive supportive care, and antiepileptic drugs and aggressive antihypertensive therapy when seizures or hypertension are present. Rechallenge with the suspected antineoplastic drug is safe in some patients and can be considered if indicated.

Cardiomyopathy

Cardiomyopathy is a well-known complication of anthracycline chemotherapy, occurring in up to 20% or more of patients. Other chemotherapeutic agents less commonly associated with cardiotoxicity include cyclophosphamide, ifosfamide, cisplatin, carmustine, busulfan, and mitomycin. Cardiac arterial or muscle damage can also occur from chest radiation, especially in the treatment of breast cancer [117, 118]. Severe cardiomyopathy with reduced flow in the cardiac chambers permits thrombus formation and cardioembolic stroke. In patients presenting with cerebral cardioembolism, long-term anticoagulation may be recommended for secondary prevention.

Infection and Stroke

Patients with immunosuppression due to cancer, especially leukemia and lymphoma patients, or to the effects of antineoplastic therapy are at increased risk for infection-related stroke. Mechanisms include sepsis-induced DIC, bacterial endocarditis, and angioinvasive microorganisms. Intravascular fungal hyphae can be associated with thrombus formation, contributing to parenchymal ischemia. In the autopsy series by Graus et al. [1], the majority of patients with septic infarction were symptomatic with seizures, focal neurological deficits, and encephalopathy.

The most common fungal infection in cancer patients is Aspergillus, typically arising from the lungs or paranasal sinuses. Cerebral aspergillosis typically presents with large multifocal lesions showing isointense to low signal intensity on T2-weighted images, often with areas of high signal on T1-weighted images due to hemorrhage and reduced diffusion. Irregular parenchymal contrast enhancement can be present in association with infarction [119, 120]. Figure 10.12a–e demonstrates ischemic changes on brain MRI in a patient with Aspergillosis in whom intravascular

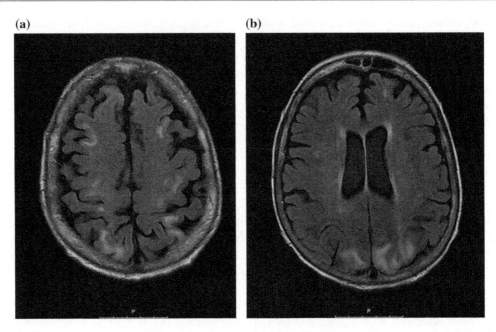

Fig. 10.11 FLAIR MRI in a patient with PRES associated with bevacizumab treatment shows the typical subcortical white matter hyperintensities throughout both cerebral hemispheres (**a**), more prominent posteriorly (**b**)

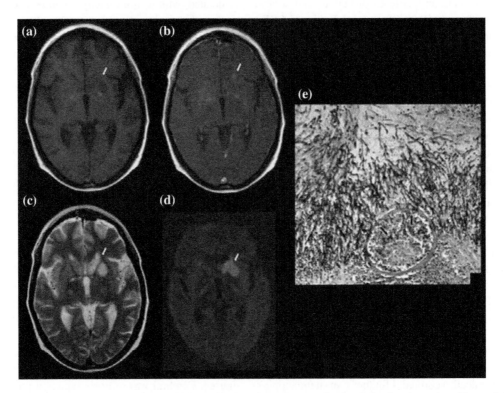

Fig. 10.12 **a** 43-year-old woman (patient 2), aspergillosis manifestation: basal ganglia. **a, b** Unenhanced (**a**) T1-weighted image without pathological signal changes and (**b**) ce T1-weighted image with faint contrast uptake near caudate nuclei on the *left-hand side* as an expression of subacute ischemic lesion (*arrow*). **c** T2-weighted image: lesion with high signal intensity (*arrow*). **d** DWI: very high signal intensity on reflecting infarction (*arrow*). **e** Histopathology: extended parenchymal infiltration by the branched hyphal forms of aspergillus with penetration (*arrows*) of vascular wall and resulting thrombosis (*All Used with permission of John Wiley and Sons from Gabelmann et al.* [120])

hyphae contributing to thrombosis were identified. Mucormycosis is characterized by frontal lobe lesions with markedly reduced diffusion [121]. Paranasal sinusitis due to Mucor species can be complicated by mycotic aneurysms in the adjacent internal carotid artery. Treatment of fungal infection is often unsuccessful and the prognosis of CNS fungal infection is poor.

Anticoagulation-Induced Hemorrhage

Systemic venous thromboembolism (VTE) is common patients with a primary brain tumor as well as patients with systemic cancer. The potential risk of intracranial hemorrhage in patients with a primary or metastatic brain tumor who are treated with anticoagulation for VTE must be assessed with the benefit. In a review of the outcome of anticoagulation for VTE in brain tumor patients, Jo et al. [122] found that therapeutic anticoagulation, particularly low molecular weight heparin, followed by secondary prophylaxis is generally safe. In glioma patients treated with bevacizumab who are anticoagulated for VTE, there is a slight increase in the rate and severity of intracranial hemorrhage, as compared to bevacizumab-treated patients not receiving anticoagulation [123], but this small risk may compare favorably to the potential lack of benefit and risk of complications from inferior vena cava filters when deciding on individual patient management.

Bone Marrow Transplant

A retrospective study of the neurologic complications of 425 patients who underwent bone marrow transplant (BMT) (310 allogeneic, 115 autologous) for leukemia identified 11% with CNS complications, most commonly hemorrhage, metabolic encephalopathy and CNS infections. Eleven of 16 hemorrhages were subdural hematomas (69%), which were more frequent in autologous (8%) than in allogeneic (0.6%) BMT and in patients with acute myelogenous leukemia (AML), as opposed to other leukemias. Eight of 11 subdural hematomas occurred in AML patients receiving autologous BMT. Platelet refractoriness correlated with an increased risk of subdural hematoma [124]. Subdural hematomas can often be managed conservatively [125, 126]. Intraparenchymal hemorrhage has also been identified at autopsy following BMT and is associated with a high mortality rate [127].

PRES is most common during the early post-transplant period of hematopoietic cell transplant (HCT) but the risk continues because of the use of cyclosporine, tacrolimus, or other immune suppressants. This is followed by a risk of Aspergillosis with vascular invasion during the next several months. A thrombotic microangiopathy, which may affect the CNS, occurs in up to 6% of patients following BMT [128, 129]. Contributing factors include the administration of cyclosporine, graft-versus-host disease, irradiation, intensive conditioning chemotherapy, and infection. Rare cases of NBTE-associated stroke have also been reported following bone marrow transplantation.

Miscellaneous

Granulomatous angiitis is a rare condition that can be associated with Hodgkin lymphoma. Therapy directed to the lymphoma typically treats the angiitis [130].

Conclusion

A diverse array of pathophysiologic processes predispose to stroke in patients with cancer. A systematic evaluation will often disclose the type, location, and proximate cause of stroke, allowing classification among the specific etiologies of cerebral infarction and hemorrhage reviewed in this chapter. Accurate diagnosis will guide acute intervention and secondary prevention treatment. All physicians who encounter patients with cancer should be cognizant of the risk of cerebrovascular disease within the oncology population, and include stroke in the differential diagnosis of any alteration in central nervous system function.

References

1. Graus F, Rogers LR, Posner JB. Cerebrovascular complications in patients with cancer. Medicine. 1985;64:16–35.
2. Zoller B, Sundquist JJ, Sundquist K. Risk of haemorrhagic and ischemic stroke in patients with cancer: a nationwide follow-up study from Sweden. Eur J Cancer. 2012;48:1875–83.
3. Navi BB, Reichman JS, Berlin D, et al. Intracerebral and subarachnoid hemorrhage in patients with cancer. Neurology. 2010;74:494–501.
4. Cestari DM, Weine DM, Panageas KS, et al. Stroke in patients with cancer: Incidence and etiology. Neurology. 2004;62:2025–30.
5. Noji C, Cohen K, Jordan LC. Hemorrhagic and ischemic stroke in children with cancer. Pediatr Neurol. 2013;49:1875–83.
6. Taccone FS, Jeangette SM, Blecic SA. First-ever stroke as initial presentation of systemic cancer. J Stroke Cerebrovasc Dis. 2008;17:169–74.
7. Kneihsl M, Enzinger C, Wunsch G, et al. Poor short-term outcome in patients with ischaemic stroke and active cancer. J Neurol. 2016;263:150–6.
8. Schrader B, Barth H, Lang EW. Spontaneous intracranial haematomas caused by neoplasms. Acta Neurochir (Wien). 2000;142:979–85.
9. Abraham NA, Prayson RA. The role of histopathologic examination of intracranial blood clots removed for hemorrhage of unknown etiology: a clinical pathologic analysis of 31 cases. Ann Diagn Pathol. 2000;4:361–6.
10. Yuguang L, Meng L, Shugan Z, et al. Intracranial tumoural haemorrhage—a report of 58 cases. J Clin Neurosci. 2002;9:637–9.
11. Jiang XB, Ke C, Zhang GH, et al. Brain metastases from hepatocellular carcinoma: clinical features and prognostic factors. BMC Cancer. 2012;12:49.

12. Liwnicz BH, Wu SZ, Tew JM. The relationship between the capillary structure and hemorrhage in gliomas. J Neurosurg. 1987;66:536–41.

13. Bosnjak R, Derham C, Popović M, Ravnik J. Spontaneous intracranial meningioma bleeding: clinicopathological features and outcome. J Neurosurg. 2005;103:473–84.

14. Katz JM, Segal AZ. Incidence and etiology of cerebrovascular disease in patients with malignancy. Curr Atheroscler Rep. 2005;7:280–8.

15. Jung S, Moon K-S, Jung T-Y, et al. Possible pathophysiological role of vascular endothelial growth factor (VEGF) and matrix metalloproteinases (MMPs) in metastatic brain tumor-associated intracerebral hemorrhage. J Neurooncol. 2006;76:257–63.

16. Atlas SW, Grossman RI, Gomori JM, et al. Hemorrhagic intracranial malignant neoplasms: spin-echo MR imaging. Radiology. 1987;164:71–7.

17. Kamel H, Navi BB, Hemphill C. A rule to identify patients who require magnetic resonance imaging after intracerebral hemorrhage. Neurocrit Care. 2013;1:59–63.

18. Boellis A, diNapoli A, Romano A, Bozzao A. Pituitary apoplexy: an update on clinical and imaging features. Insights Imaging. 2014;5:753–62.

19. Singh TD, Valizadeh N, Meyer FB, Atkinson JL, Erickson D, Rabinstein AA. Management and outcomes of pituitary apoplexy. J Neurosurg. 2015;122:1450–7.

20. Reichman J, Singer S, Navi B, et al. Subdural hematoma in patients with cancer. Neurosurgery. 2012;71:74–9.

21. Laigle-Donadey F, Taillibert S, Mokhtari K, et al. Dural metastases. J Neurooncol. 2005;75:57–61.

22. Hata A, Fujita S, Katakami N, Sakai C, Imai Y. Bilateral subdural hematoma associated with central nervous system metastasis from lung cancer. J Thorac Oncol. 2011;6:207–8.

23. Raizer JJ, DeAngelis LM. Cerebral sinus thrombosis diagnosed by MRI and MR venography in cancer patients. Neurology. 2000;54:1222–6.

24. Oda N, Sakugawa M, Bessho A, et al. Cerebral venous sinus thrombosis concomitant with leptomeningeal carcinomatosis, in a patient with epidermal growth factor receptor-mutated lung cancer. Oncol Lett. 2014;8:2489–92.

25. Zheng J, Zhang J. Neoplastic cerebral aneurysm from metastatic tumor: a systematic review of clinical and treatment characteristics. Clin Neurol Neurosurg. 2015;128:107–11.

26. Nomura R, Yoshida D, Kim K, Kobayashi S, Teramoto A. Intracerebral hemorrhage caused by a neoplastic aneurysm from pleomorphic lung carcinoma. Neurol Med Chir (Tokyo). 2009;49:33–6.

27. Gutmann DH, Cantor CR, Piacente GJ, McCluskey LF. Cerebral vasculopathy and infarction in a woman with carcinomatous meningitis. J Neurooncol. 1990;9:183–5.

28. Herman C, Kupsky WJ, Rogers L, Duman R, Moore P. Leptomeningeal dissemination of malignant glioma simulating cerebral vasculitis. Stroke. 1995;26:2366–70.

29. Artoni A, Bucciarelli P, Martinelli I. Cerebral thrombosis and myeloproliferative neoplasms. Curr Neurol Neurosci Rep. 2014;14:496.

30. Enblom A, Lindskog E, Hasselbalch H, et al. High rate of abnormal blood values and vascular complications before diagnosis of myeloproliferative neoplasms. Eur J Intern Med. 2015;26:344–7.

31. Koenig MK, Sitton CW, Wang M, Slopis JM. Central nervous system complications of blastic hyperleukocytosis in childhood acute lymphoblastic leukemia: diagnostic and prognostic implications. J Child Neurol. 2008;23:1347–52.

32. Pham HP, Schwartz J. How we approach a patient with symptoms of leukostasis requiring emergent leukocytapheresis. Transfusion. 2015;55:2306–11.

33. Ferro A, Jabbour SK, Taunk NK, et al. Cranial irradiation in adults diagnosed with acute myelogenous leukemia presenting with hyperleukocytosis and neurologic dysfunction. Leuk Lymphoma. 2014;55:105–9.

34. Fonkem E, Lok E, Robison D, Gautam S, Wong ET. The natural history of intravascular lymphomatosis. Cancer Med. 2014;3:1010–24.

35. Baehring JM, Henchcliffe C, Ledezma CH, Fulbright R, Hochberg FH. Intravascular lymphoma: magnetic resonance imaging correlates of disease dynamics within the central nervous system. J Neurol Neurosurg Psychiatry. 2005;76:540–4.

36. Dias RR, Fernandes F, Ramires FJ, Mady C, Albuquerque CP, Jatene FB. Mortality and embolic potential of cardiac tumors. Arq Bras Cardiol. 2014;103:13–8.

37. Abraham KP, Reddy V, Gattuso P. Neoplasms metastatic to the heart: review of 3314 consecutive autopsies. Am J Cardiovasc Pathol. 1990;3:195–8.

38. Navi BB, Kawaguchi K, Hriljac I, et al. Multifocal stroke from tumor emboli. Arch Neurol. 2009;66:1174–5.

39. Spaulding R, Koumoundouros T, Parker JC. Metastatic undifferentiated pleomorphic sarcoma causing intraoperative stroke. Ann Clin Lab Sci. 2013;43:172–5.

40. Schwarzbach CJ, Schaefer A, Ebert A, et al. Stroke and cancer: the importance of cancer-associated hypercoagulation as a possible stroke etiology. Stroke. 2012;43:3029–34.

41. Yusuf SW, Ali SS, Swafford J, et al. Culture-positive and culture-negative endocarditis in patients with cancer: a retrospective observational study, 1994–2004. Medicine (Baltimore). 2006;85:86–94.

42. Merkler AE, Navi BB, Singer S, et al. Diagnostic yield of echocardiography in cancer patients with ischemic stroke. J Neurooncol. 2015;123:115–21.

43. Singhal AB, Topcuoglu MA, Buonanno FS. Acute ischemic stroke patterns in infective and nonbacterial thrombotic endocarditis: a diffusion-weighted magnetic resonance imaging study. Stroke. 2002;33:1267–73.

44. Lafitte F, Boukobza M, Guichard JP, et al. MRI and MRA for diagnosis and follow-up of cerebral venous thrombosis. Clin Radiol. 1997;52:672–9.

45. Einhaupl KM, Villringer A, Meister W, et al. Heparin treatment in sinus venous thrombosis. Lancet. 1991;338:597–600.

46. De Bruijn SF, Stam J. Randomized, placebo-controlled trial of anticoagulant treatment with low-molecular-weight heparin for cerebral sinus thrombosis. Stroke. 1999;304:484–8.

47. Santoro N, Giordano P, Del Vecchio GC, et al. Ischemic stroke in children treated for acute lymphoblastic leukemia. A retrospective study. J Pediatr Hematol Oncol. 2005;27:153–7.

48. Ranta S, Tuckuviene R, Makipernaa A, et al. Cerebral venous thromboses in children with acute lymphoblastic leukaemia—a multicenter study from the Nordic Society of Paediatric Haematology and Oncology. Br J Haematol. 2015;4:547–52.

49. Choudhri O, Feroze A, Marks MP, Do HM. Endovascular management of cerebral venous sinus thrombosis. Neurosurg Focus. 2014;37(Suppl 1):1.

50. Viegas LD, Stolz E, Canhão P, Ferro JM. Systemic thrombolysis for cerebral venous and dural sinus thrombosis: a systematic review. Cerebrovasc Dis. 2014;37:43–50.

51. Gonzalez Quintela A, Candela MJ, Vidal C, et al. Nonbacterial thrombotic endocarditis in cancer patients. Acta Cardiol. 1991;46:1–9.

52. Rogers LR, Cho E, Kempin S, et al. Cerebral infarction from nonbacterial thrombotic endocarditis. Am J Med. 1987;83:746–58.
53. Min KW, Gyorkey F, Sato C. Mucin-producing adenocarcinomas and nonbacterial thrombotic endocarditis: pathogenic role of tumor mucin. Cancer. 1980;45:2374–82.
54. Biller J, Challa VR, Toole JF, et al. Nonbacterial thrombotic endocarditis: a neurologic perspective of clinicopathologic correlations of 99 patients. Arch Neurol. 1982;39:95–8.
55. Amico L, Caplan LR, Thomas C. Cerebrovascular complications of mucinous cancers. Neurology. 1989;39:522–6.
56. Bernardo MC, Menke J, Scheithauer B, et al. Intravascular mucinosis: a rare cause of cerebral infarction. Acta Neuropathol. 2011;121:785–8.
57. Towfighi J, Simmonds MA, Davidson EA. Mucin and fat emboli in mucinous carcinomas. Cause of hemorrhagic cerebral infarcts. Arch Pathol Lab Med. 1983;107:646–9.
58. Arkel YS. Thrombosis and cancer. Semin Oncol. 2000;27:362–74.
59. Levi M, ten Cate H. Disseminated intravascular coagulation. N Engl J Med. 1999;341:586–92.
60. Mantha S, Tallman M, Soff GA. What's new in the pathogenesis of the coagulopathy in acute promyelocytic leukemia? Curr Opin Hematol. 2016;23(2):121–6.
61. Sallah S, Wan JY, Nguyen NP, et al. Disseminated intravascular coagulation in solid tumors: clinical and pathologic study. Thromb Haemost. 2011;86:828–33.
62. Sakuragawa N, Hasegawa H, Maki M, et al. Clinical evaluation of low-molecular-weight–heparin (FR-860) on disseminated intravascular coagulation (DIC): a multicenter co-operative, double-blind trial in comparison with heparin. Thromb Res. 1993;72:475–500.
63. Avvisati G, ten Cate JW, Buller HR, et al. Tranexamic acid for control of hemorrhage in acute promyelocytic leukaemia. Lancet. 1989;2:122–4.
64. Lechner K, Obermeier HL. Cancer-related microangiopathic hemolytic anemia: clinical and laboratory features in 168 reported cases. Medicine (Baltimore). 2012;91:195–205.
65. Kaden BR, Rosse WF, Hauch TW. Immune thrombocytopenia in lymphoproliferative diseases. Blood. 1979;53:545–51.
66. Gordon LI, Kwaan HC. Thrombotic microangiopathy manifesting as thrombotic thrombocytopenic purpura/hemolytic uremic syndrome in the cancer patient. Semin Thromb Hemost. 1999;25:217–21.
67. Omura M, Aida N, Sakido K, et al. Large intracranial vessel occlusive vasculopathy after radiation therapy in children: clinical features and usefulness of magnetic resonance imaging. Int J Radiat Oncol Biol Phys. 1997;38:241–9.
68. Fouladi M, Langston J, Mulhern R, et al. Silent lacunar lesions detected by magnetic resonance imaging of children with brain tumors: a late sequela of therapy. J Clin Oncol. 2000;18:824–31.
69. Bowers DC, Liu Y, Leisenring W, et al. Late-occurring stroke among long-term survivors of childhood leukemia and brain tumors: a report from the Childhood Cancer Survivor Study. J Clin Oncol. 2006;24:5277–82.
70. Fullerton HJ, Stratton K, Mueller S, et al. Recurrent stroke in childhood cancer survivors. Neurology. 2015;85:1–9.
71. Bowers DC, Mulne AF, Reisch JS, et al. Nonperioperative strokes in children with central nervous system tumors. Cancer. 2002;94:1094–101.
72. Campen CJ, Kranick SM, Kasner SE, et al. Cranial irradiation increases risk of stroke in pediatric brain tumor survivors. Stroke. 2012;43:3035–40.
73. Aizer AA, Du R, Wen PY, Arvold ND. Radiotherapy and death from cerebrovascular disease in patients with primary brain tumors. J Neurooncol. 2015;124:291–7.
74. Van Varsseveld NC, van Bunderen CC, Ubachs DH, et al. Cerebrovascular events, secondary intracranial tumors, and mortality after radiotherapy for nonfunctioning pituitary adenomas: a subanalysis from the Dutch national registry of growth hormone treatment in adults. J Clin Endocrinol Metabl. 2015;100:1104–12.
75. Nanney AD, El Tecle NE, El Ahmadieh TY, et al. Intracranial aneurysms in previously irradiated fields: literature review and case report. World Neurosurg. 2014;81:511–9.
76. Kellner CP, McDowell MM, Connolly ES Jr, Sisti MB, Lavine SD. Late onset aneurysm development following radiosurgical obliteration of a cerebellopontine angle meningioma. BMJ Case Rep. 2014; 14. pii: bcr2014011206.
77. Matsumoto H, Minami H, Yamaura I, Oshida Y. Radiation-induced cerebal aneurysm treated with endovascular coil embolization. INR. 2014;20:448–53.
78. Li L, Mugikara AS, Kumabe T, et al. A comparative study of the extent of cerebral microvascular injury following whole-brain irradiation versus reduced-field irradiation in long-term survivors of intracranial germ cell tumors. Radiother Oncol. 2015;117:302–7.
79. Koike S, Aida N, Hata M, Fujita K, Ozawa Y, Inoue T. Asymptomatic radiation-induced telangiectasia in children after cranial irradiation: frequency, latency, and dose relation. Radiology. 2004;230:93–9.
80. Singla A, Brace O'Neill JE, Smith E, Scott RM. Cavernous malformations of the brain after treatment for acute lymphocytic leukemia: presentation and long-term follow-up. J Neurosurg Pediatr. 2013;11:127–32.
81. Nimjee SM, Powers CJ, Bulsara KR. Review of the literature on de novo formation of cavernous malformations of the central nervous system after radiation therapy. Neurosurg Focus. 2006;21:e4.
82. Di Giannatale A, Morana G, Rossi A, et al. Naural history of cavernous malformations in children with brain tumors treated with radiotherapy and chemotherapy. J Neurooncol. 2014;117:311–20.
83. Yoshino M, Morita A, Shibahara J, Kirino T. Radiation-induced spinal cord cavernous malformation. Case report. J Neurosurg. 2005;102(Suppl 1):101–4.
84. Koike T, Yanagimachi N, Ishiguro H, et al. High incidence of radiation-induced cavernous hemangioma in long-term survivors who underwent hematopoietic stem cell transplantation with radiation therapy during childhood or adolescence. Biol Blood Marrow Transplant. 2012;18:1090–8.
85. Desai SS, Paulino AC, Mai WY, Teh BS. Radiation-induced moyamoya syndrome. Int J Radiat Oncol Biol Phys. 2006;65:1222–7.
86. Dorresteijn LD, Kappelle AC, Boogerd W, et al. Increased risk of ischemic stroke after radiotherapy on the neck in patients younger than 60 years. J Clin Oncol. 2002;20:282–8.
87. Dorth JA, Patel PR, Broadwater G, Brizel DM. Incidence and risk factors of significant carotid artery stenosis in asymptomatic survivors of head and neck cancer after radiotherapy. Head Neck. 2014;36:215–9.
88. Gujral DM, Shah BN, Chahal NS, et al. Do traditional risk stratification models for cerebrovascular events apply in irradiated head and neck cancer patients? QJM. 2016;109(6):383–9.
89. Bashar K, Healy D, Clarke-Moloney M, et al. Effects of neck radiation therapy on extra-cranial carotid arteries atherosclerosis disease prevalence: systematic review and a meta-analysis. PLoS ONE. 2014;9:e110389.
90. Bowers DC, McNeil DE, Liu Y, et al. Stroke as a late treatment effect of Hodgkin's disease: a report from the childhood cancer survivor study. J Clin Oncol. 2005;23:6508–15.

91. Black DF, Morris JM, Lindell EP, et al. Stroke-like migraine attacks after radiation therapy (SMART) syndrome is not always completely reversible. AJNR. 2013;34:2298–303.

92. Sano N, Satow T, Maruyama D, et al. Carotid endarterectomy carries less risk than stenting in patients with radiation-induced carotid stenosis. J Vasc Surg. 2015;62:370–7.

93. Cam A, Shishehbor MH, Bajaj NS, et al. Outcomes of carotid stenting in patients with previous neck radiation. Catheter Cardiovasc Interv. 2013;82:689–95.

94. Ravin RA, Gottlieb A, Pasternac K, et al. Carotid artery stenting may be performed safely in patients with radiation therapy-associated carotid stenosis without increased restenosis or target lesion revascularization. JVS. 2015;62:624–30.

95. Brinjikji W, Cloft HJ. Outcomes of endovascular occlusion and stenting in the treatment of carotid blowout. Interv Neuroradiol. 2015;21:543–7.

96. Brown DV, Faber LP, Tuman KJ. Perioperative stroke caused by arterial tumor embolism. Anesth Analg. 2004;98:806–9.

97. Cho Y, Hida Y, Kaga K, Kato H, Iizuka M, Kondo S. Brain metastases secondary to tumor emboli from primary lung cancer during lobectomy. Ann Thorac Surg. 2008;86:312–3.

98. MacNeil SD, Liu K, Garg AX, Tam S, et al. A population-based study of 30-day incidence of ischemic stroke following surgical neck dissection. Medicine (Baltimore). 2015;94:e1106.

99. Garza-Ramos RDl, Kerezoudis P, Tarmago RJ, et al. Surgical complications following malignant brain tumor surgery: an analysis of 2002–2011 data. Clin Neurol Neurosurg. 2015;140:6–10.

100. Gempt J, Gerhardt J, Toth V, et al. Postoperative ischemic changes following brain metastasis resection as measured by diffusion-weighted magnetic resonance imaging. J Neurosurg. 2013;119:1395–400.

101. Jakola AS, Berntsen EM, Christensen P, et al. Surgically acquired deficits and diffusion weighted MRI changes after glioma resection—a matched case-control study with blinded neuroradiological assessment. J Neurosurg. 2013;119:829–36.

102. Smith JS, Cha S, Mayo MC, et al. Serial diffusion–weighted magnetic resonance imaging in cases of glioma: distinguishing tumor recurrence from postresection injury. J Neurosurg. 2005;103:428–38.

103. Gempt J, Krieg SM, Hüttinger S, et al. Postoperative ischemic changes after glioma resection identified by diffusion-weighted magnetic resonance imaging and their association with intraoperative motor evoked potentials. J Neurosurg. 2013;119:829–36.

104. Friedman JA, Piepgras DG, Duke DA, et al. Remote cerebellar hemorrhage after supratentorial surgery. Neurosurgery. 2001;49:1327–40.

105. Keiper GL, Sherman JD, Tomsick TA, et al. Dural sinus thrombosis and pseudotumor cerebri: unexpected complications of suboccitpital craniotomy and translabyrinthine craniectomy. J Neurosurg. 1999;91:192–7.

106. Quarante LH, Mena-Bernal JH, Martin BP, et al. Posterior reversible encephalopathy syndrome (PRES): a rare condition after resection of posterior fossa tumors: two new cases and review of the literature. Childs Nerv Syst. 2016;32(5):857–63.

107. Burkhardt JK, Riina HA, Shin BJ, Moliterno JA, Hofstetter CP, Boockvar JA. Intra-arterial chemotherapy for malignant gliomas: a critical analysis. Interv Neuroradiol. 2011;17:286–95.

108. Kallmes DF, Evans AJ, Kaptain GJ, et al. Hemorrhagic complications in embolization of a meningioma: case report and review of the literature. Neuroradiology. 1997;39:877–80.

109. Shah A, Choudhari O, Jung H, Li G. Preoperative endovascular embolization of meningiomas: update on therapeutic options. Neurosurg Focus. 2015;38:e7.

110. Lee AY, Levine MN. The thrombophilic state induced by therapeutic agents in the cancer patient. Semin Thromb Hemost. 1999;25:137–45.

111. Bushman JE, Palmierir D, Whinna HC, et al. Insight into the mechanism of asparaginase-induced depletion of antithrombin III in treatment of childhood acute lymphoblastic leukemia. Leuk Res. 2000;24:559–65.

112. Gugliotta L, Mazzucconi MG, Leone G, et al. Incidence of thrombotic complications in adult patients with acute lymphoblastic leukaemia receiving l-aspariginase during induction therapy: a retrospective study. Eur J Haematol. 1992;49:63–6.

113. Koppelmans V, Vernooij MW, Boogerd W, et al. Prevalence of cerebral small-vessel disease in long-term breast cancer survivors exposed to both adjuvant radiotherapy and ehemotherapy. J Clin Oncol. 2015;33:588–93.

114. Patel SB, Gojo I, Tidwell ML, Sausvile EA, Baer MR. Subdural hematomas in patients with Philadelphia chromosome-positive acute lymphoblastic leukemia receiving imatinib mesylate in conjunction with systemic and intrathecal chemotherapy. Leuk Lymphoma. 2011;52:1011–4.

115. Bartynski WS. Posterior reversible encephalopathy syndrome, part 1: fundamental imaging and clinical features. AJNR Am J Neuroradiol. 2008;29:1036–42.

116. Singer S, Grommes C, Reiner AS, Rosenblum MK, DeAngelis LM. Posterior reversible encephalopathy syndrome in patients with cancer. Oncologist. 2015;20:806–11.

117. Hamo CE, Bloom MW. Getting to the heart of the matter: an overview of cardiac toxicity related to cancer therapy. Clin Med Insights Cardiol. 2015;9(Suppl 2):47–51.

118. Bloom MW, Hamo CE, Cardinale D, et al. Cancer therapy-related cardiac dysfunction and heart failure: part 1: definitions, pathophysiology, risk Factors, and imaging. Circ Heart Fail. 2016;9:e002661.

119. Dietrich U, Hettmann M, Maschke M, et al. Cerebral aspergillosis: comparison of radiological and neuropathologic findings in patients with bone marrow transplantation. Eur Radiol. 2001;11:1242–9.

120. Gabelmann A, Klein S, Kern W, et al. Relevant imaging findings of cerebral aspergillosis on MRI: a retrospective case-based study in immunocompromised patients. Eur J Neurol. 2007;14:548–55.

121. Starkey J, Moritani T, Kirby P. MRI of CNS fungal infections: review of aspergillosis to histoplasmosis and everything in between. Clin Neuroradiol. 2014;24:217–30.

122. Jo JT, Schiff D, Perry JR. Thrombosis in brain tumors. Semin Thromb Hemost. 2014;40:325–31.

123. Norden AD, Bartolomeo J, Tanaka S, et al. Safety of concurrent bevacizumab therapy and anticoagulation in glioma patients. J Neurooncol. 2012;106:121–5.

124. Coplin WM, Cochran MS, Levine SR, et al. Stroke after bone marrow transplantation: frequency, aetiology and outcome. Brain. 2001;124:1043–51.

125. Graus F, Saiz A, Sierra J, et al. Neurologic complications of autologous and allogeneic bone marrow transplantation in patients with leukemia: a comparative study. Neurology. 1996;46:1004–9.

126. Colosimo M, McCarthy N, Jayasinghe R, et al. Diagnosis and management of subdural haematoma complicating bone marrow transplantation. Bone Marrow Transplant. 2000;25:549–52.

127. Bleggi-Torres LF, Werner B, Gasparetto EL, et al. Intracranial hemorrhage following bone marrow transplantation: an autopsy study of 58 patients. Bone Marrow Transplant. 2002;29:29–32.

128. Paquette RL, Tran L, Landaw EM. Thrombotic microangiopathy following allogeneic bone marrow transplantation is associated with intensive graft-versus-host disease prophylaxis. Bone Marrow Transplant. 1998;22:351–7.

129. Pettitt AR, Clark RE. Thrombotic microangiopathy following bone marrow transplantation. Bone Marrow Transplant. 1994;14:495–504.

130. Le Guennec L, Roos-Weil D, Mokhtari K, et al. Granulomatous angiitis of the CNS revealing a Hodgkin lymphoma. Neurology. 2013;80:323–4.

131. Kalafut M, Vinuela F, Saver JL, et al. Multiple cerebral pseudoaneurysms and hemorrhages: the expanding spectrum of metastatic cerebral choriocarcinoma. J Neuroimaging. 1998;8:44–7.

Elevated Intracranial Pressure and Hydrocephalus in Brain Tumor Patients

Matthew E. Shuman and Mark D. Johnson

Introduction

Caring for brain tumor patients can be a complex undertaking that requires the simultaneous consideration of numerous factors. Although attention must be paid to treatment of the tumor itself, it is also important to address brain tumor-associated processes that can contribute to the development of neurological deficits or poor survivorship. Elevated intracranial pressure (ICP) and hydrocephalus are tumor-associated phenomena that are frequently observed in brain tumor patients. Left untreated, these factors can lead to significant functional disability or loss of life. Thus, it is imperative that healthcare practitioners be cognizant of the signs, symptoms, physiology, and treatment of elevated ICP and hydrocephalus so that appropriate therapeutic interventions can be initiated. Effective management of ICP and hydrocephalus can improve quality of life and prolong the survival of brain tumor patients.

ICP in Brain Tumor Patients

The cranial vault is an enclosed and environmentally controlled space that is designed to protect the components of the central nervous system. It contains three major components: brain tissue, blood, and cerebrospinal fluid (CSF) [1]. Together, these three components completely fill the intracranial space. An increase in any one of these three components will lead to an increase in ICP [1, 2]. For example, blood is pumped into the cranial vault during each

M.E. Shuman
Department of Neurosurgery, Brigham and Women's Hospital, 60 Fenwood Road, Boston, MA 02115, USA
e-mail: meshuman@partners.org

M.D. Johnson (✉)
Department of Neurological Surgery, University of Massachusetts Medical School and UMass Memorial Hospital, University Campus, 55 Lake Avenue North, Worcester, MA 01655, USA
e-mail: mark.johnson3@umassmemorial.org

cardiac cycle. Because the cranium is a confined space, the entry of blood generates a wave of ICP elevation that is related in part to the cardiac-induced change in blood pressure [3]. The normal range for ICP in humans is roughly 5–15 cm of water [1, 2, 4]. The difference between the ICP and the mean arterial pressure (MAP) is the cerebral perfusion pressure (CPP) [1, 2]. CPP is the pressure gradient that drives cerebral blood flow into the cranium [5].

The central nervous system contains a pool of CSF within it, and it is also bathed in CSF, the total volume of which is about 150 cc [4, 6–8]. CSF is produced by the choroid plexus, which is located in the lateral, third, and fourth ventricles [4, 8]. A significant component of the CSF is also produced within the brain interstitium [4]. The adult human brain produces roughly 10–15 cc of CSF/hour [6]. CSF that is produced in the lateral ventricles flows into the third ventricle through the bilateral foramina of Monro. From the third ventricle, it passes through the aqueduct of Sylvius into the fourth ventricle. It then passes from the fourth ventricle through the foramen of Magendie and the bilateral foramina of Luschka into the subarachnoid space where it percolates through the basal cisterns and flows over the brain convexity [4, 6, 8]. Anatomic studies have revealed that the subarachnoid space not only covers the surface of the brain but also extends along the arterial vasculature through the brain proper. The CSF passes through these paravascular subarachnoid spaces, mixes with the interstitial fluid, and is then reabsorbed by the venous system [9] or by recently discovered intracranial lymphatic channels [10, 11].

Studies indicate that the CSF serves several important functions in the nervous system. It is an important vehicle for the distribution of growth factors and other proteins that are important for CNS development [7, 8, 12]. The CSF has also been shown to play a role in the removal of waste products from the brain [7–9]. Because the paravascular subarachnoid membranes are discontinuous, they allow the paravascular CSF to intermix with the interstitial fluid as it flows through the brain prior to being reabsorbed. In this way, the CSF is thought to remove metabolites from the interstitial space [4, 6–9]. The CSF also acts as a shock absorber, blunting the effects of acceleration and deceleration events on the brain and spinal cord [7, 13]. In addition, the CSF opposes the increase in ICP generated by the heart. Each cardiac contraction produces an influx of blood into the cranial vault and a consequent increase in ICP that can be readily observed with intracranial pressure monitors. As blood is pumped into this space, CSF exits the cranial vault via the foramen magnum. This pulsatile egress of CSF counteracts the increase in ICP generated during each cardiac cycle. If this compensatory outflow of CSF is blocked (as occurs in Chiari I malformations), cardiac-induced elevations of ICP are magnified [14]. Because of the key role that the CSF plays in the dynamic regulation of intracranial pressure (ICP), alterations in CSF flow often lead to elevated ICP [4].

Physiological Effects of Elevated ICP

Under normal conditions, the brain ensures an adequate flow of blood by altering the resistance of cerebral blood vessels in response to moderate changes in blood pressure [15]. Thus, cerebral blood flow is determined in part by cerebrovascular resistance and by cerebral perfusion pressure or CPP, which is the difference between mean arterial pressure (MAP) and ICP (i.e., CPP = MAP-ICP) [1, 2]. Marked elevations in ICP decrease CPP and decrease cerebral blood flow. In extreme cases, ICP can exceed MAP and cerebral blood flow can cease altogether [16].

In addition to decreased cerebral blood flow, compartmentalized elevations in ICP can generate pressure gradients that cause shifts in the anatomic position of the nervous system with catastrophic results. Such compartmentalization commonly develops when large tumors occur in the supratentorial or infratentorial compartments, or when there is an obstruction to CSF flow [17]. For example, increased pressure originating in the supratentorial or infratentorial compartments can lead to downward or upward axial brain herniation, respectively, that results in tissue destruction, neurological injury or even death [16–18].

Signs and Symptoms of Elevated ICP

Because severe elevations in ICP can lead to ischemic injury, herniation or even death, it is critical that healthcare practitioners recognize the symptoms and signs of elevated ICP in patients with central nervous system tumors. One of the earliest and most common signs of elevated ICP is headache [19]. These headaches can be localized or generalized in nature, and are often worse in the morning. In fact,

headaches caused by elevated ICP are often made worse by lying down and relieved by being upright [20]. This is thought to result from the decreased effect of gravity on venous drainage from the head and from mobilization of fluid in the lower extremities (and the consequent increased blood return to the heart and brain) that occur when supine [21]. The increase in cerebral blood flow augments intracerebral fluid volume and further elevates ICP. Thus, brain tumor patients who present with chronic headaches, especially morning headaches that improve in the upright position, should be evaluated for elevated ICP.

Patients with elevated ICP may also experience recurrent nausea or vomiting. In addition, patients with chronically elevated ICP can develop visual deficits [20, 22]. This is usually due to the development of papilledema (swelling and elevation of the optic disc). Left untreated, this condition can lead to permanent optic nerve injury and blindness [22].

In cases of extreme elevations in ICP, hypertension and bradycardia (the Cushing reflex) may occur [23]. In addition, extreme elevations in ICP can lead to altered mental status or episodes of loss of consciousness. These symptoms are a warning sign that permanent neurological injury or even death is imminent [24]. When brain tumor patients present with altered mental status, episodes of bradycardia and hypertension, or loss of consciousness, an urgent assessment of whether elevated ICP is a contributor should be made and steps should be taken immediately to ameliorate the situation if needed. The use of an intracranial pressure monitor or a ventriculostomy to measure ICP while treatments are administered can be a useful tool in managing the ICP effectively in critical situations. Even in cases where the ICP is sustained at levels greater than 40 cm of water, patients can experience a good functional outcome as long as the CPP is maintained at an acceptable level, i.e., CPP greater than 60 mm of water [25].

Increased Tumor Volume and Edema as Causes of Elevated ICP

One consequence of the fact that the cranium is a rigid, confined space is that brain tumors must grow within this confined space. As the growing tumor mass crowds brain tissues and fluids that are normally present within the intracranial space, elevations in ICP result [26]. Under such circumstances, neurological deficits may result from damage caused by direct tissue compression by the tumor. However, elevations in ICP caused by the added volume of the tumor mass can also lead to decreased cerebral blood flow and ischemic injury, independent of direct tissue compression [27, 28].

Tumors that secrete angiogenic factors such as VEGF can produce blood vessels in the brain that have an incompetent blood–brain barrier [29]. These abnormal vessels lack the extensive tight junctions that are present in the normal cerebral vasculature and, as a result, proteins and other constituents from the blood can leak into the extracellular space [30, 31]. This tumor-associated vasogenic edema, along with the increased blood volume associated with perfusion of the tumor, increases the intracranial fluid volume and elevates ICP.

Obstructive Hydrocephalus and Elevated ICP

In addition to mass effect from tumor tissue, increased blood volume, and the elaboration of vasogenic edema, tumors in the brain can alter the production, flow or absorption of the CSF. A relatively common cause of tissue compression and elevated ICP in brain tumor patients is the obstruction of CSF flow due to tumor growth [32]. Such obstruction leads to an accumulation of CSF that compresses the surrounding brain and elevates ICP. Obstruction can occur within the ventricular system or, alternatively, it can be caused by ventricular compression. Tumors can cause obstruction from within the body of the ventricles or at the foramen of Monro, the aqueduct of Sylvius or the foramina of Luschka or Magendie [33, 34]. Tumors that frequently occur in the lateral or third ventricles and cause obstructive hydrocephalus [35, 36] include neurocytomas, subependymal giant cell astrocytomas and subependymomas (lateral and third ventricles), meningiomas (atria of lateral ventricles), colloid cysts and septal gliomas (foramen of Monro), craniopharyngiomas (third ventricle), and gliomas (lateral and

third ventricles) [34]. Intraventricular tumors that commonly cause obstructive hydrocephalus in the fourth ventricle include choroid plexus papillomas (Fig. 11.1a, b) and choroid plexus carcinomas, meningiomas [37], glioneuronal tumors [38], medulloblastomas, epidermoids, ependymomas [39] and subependymomas. Metastases can obstruct CSF flow anywhere within the ventricular system.

Brain tumors can also cause obstructive hydrocephalus by compressing the ventricular system from the outside. This may occur in either the supratentorial or infratentorial compartments, although obstruction due to external ventricular compression in the posterior fossa is most common [40]. In the supratentorial compartment, ventricular compression leading to obstructive hydrocephalus usually occurs at the level of the aqueduct of Sylvius and involves tectal gliomas [41] or pineal region tumors [42]. Posterior fossa tumors often cause obstructive hydrocephalus by compressing the fourth ventricle [43]. Included among these are pilocytic astrocytomas, medulloblastomas, hemangioblastomas, subependymomas, schwannomas, and metastases (Fig. 11.2).

Communicating Hydrocephalus and ICP

In addition to obstructive hydrocephalus, brain tumors can also cause communicating hydrocephalus. This may involve several different mechanisms. For example, vestibular schwannomas can present with communicating hydrocephalus, as indicated by the fact that imaging studies show no evidence of ventricular compression and that the

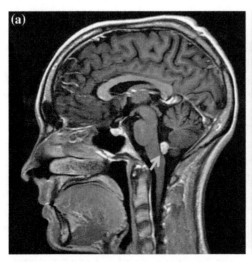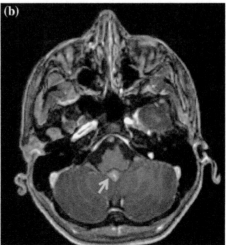

Fig. 11.1 Obstructive hydrocephalus due to an intraventricular mass. Contrast-enhanced sagittal (**a**) and axial (**b**) T1-weighted *images* showing an enhancing lesion (*arrows*) occluding the outflow of the fourth ventricle. The patient was a 20-year-old woman who presented with clinical signs of obstructive hydrocephalus and elevated ICP, including chronic severe headaches, nausea, and intermittent episodes of decreased consciousness. Surgical resection of the lesion lead to a complete resolution of symptoms, with an associated slight decrease in ventricular size. Pathology revealed a choroid plexus papilloma

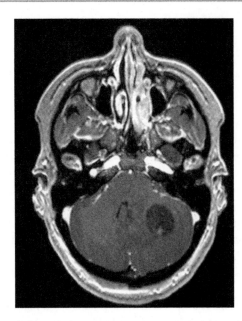

Fig. 11.2 Obstructive hydrocephalus due to external compression of the ventricular system by tumor. Contrast-enhanced axial T1-weighted magnetic resonance image showing a cystic lesion with an enhancing nodule compressing the fourth ventricle from the outside. The patient presented with signs of obstructive hydrocephalus and elevated ICP, including severe morning headaches, nausea, and vomiting. Resection of the lesion lead to a complete resolution of symptoms. Pathology revealed a cerebellar hemangioblastoma

hydrocephalus persists after tumor resection [44, 45]. Although the mechanism underlying hydrocephalus in these cases is uncertain, some investigators have postulated that proteins secreted by the tumor decrease CSF absorption [44, 46, 47]. Choroid plexus tumors (i.e., choroid plexus papilloma and choroid plexus carcinoma) can also cause communicating hydrocephalus [48]. In part, this appears to be the result of an increase in CSF production, a unique property of tumors arising from the choroid plexus [8].

Communicating hydrocephalus can also be caused by infiltration of the meninges by tumor cells, a phenomenon known as leptomeningeal carcinomatosis or carcinomatous meningitis. Tumor cells reach the meninges by dissemination through the CSF [49]. Such meningeal involvement by tumor cells is thought to decrease CSF absorption, leading to hydrocephalus and elevated ICP. Carcinomatous meningitis has been estimated to occur in 3–8% of all cancer patients [49–52]. The two most common cancers involved are breast cancer and lung cancer [44, 53, 54]. In one study, 70% of patients with carcinomatous meningitis had one of these two types of cancer [53]. There is some evidence that piecemeal resection of brain metastases is associated with an increased risk of leptomeningeal dissemination of cancer when compared to en bloc resection of metastases or radiosurgery [55, 56]. This is presumably the result of spillage of cancerous cells into the CSF.

Presenting symptoms and signs of carcinomatous meningitis include headache, nausea, vomiting, cranial nerve palsy, motor dysfunction, mental confusion, transient episodes of loss of consciousness, and enlarged ventricles [49, 53, 57]. In addition to the history and physical examination, several diagnostic tests can be useful in identifying patients with carcinomatous meningitis. Because carcinomatous meningitis causes a communicating hydrocephalus, a lumbar puncture can be performed safely. The ICP is usually elevated. In addition, the CSF obtained from patients with carcinomatous meningitis often contains malignant cells on cytology, and it may also contain less glucose and more protein than the CSF of healthy patients [54, 58]. However, CSF cytology produces a false negative diagnosis in roughly 10% of patients with carcinomatous meningitis [49]. A useful adjunct to CSF analysis for the diagnosis of carcinomatous meningitis is contrast-enhanced MRI [50, 51, 59, 60]. In patients with carcinomatous meningitis, contrast-enhanced MRI may show diffuse meningeal enhancement or enhancing pial nodules scattered widely over the surface of the nervous system [44, 50, 51, 60]. Often (but not always), ventricular enlargement is present as well, and transependymal flow of CSF may be seen on T2-weighted images (Fig. 11.3a, b).

Normal Pressure Hydrocephalus in Brain Tumor Patients

Patients who have central nervous system tumors or who have received radiation and/or chemotherapy for such tumors can develop a form of communicating hydrocephalus that is not associated with severe elevations in ICP. This form of communicating hydrocephalus, called normal pressure hydrocephalus (NPH), is characterized by enlarged cerebral ventricles, gait difficulty, incontinence, and dementia. Although some investigators have reported increased ICP pulsatility in NPH, these patients do not display sustained elevations of ICP [61]. Consequently, they do not develop symptoms of elevated ICP such as headache, nausea, vomiting, decreased consciousness, or herniation.

The incidence of NPH among brain cancer patients is not known, in part because the disorder often goes unrecognized or is misdiagnosed as effects of tumor progression or direct effects of treatment on neuronal function. Inamasu and colleagues reported that 5 of 50 consecutive patients (10%) who underwent treatment for supratentorial malignant glioma developed communicating hydrocephalus [62]. A larger retrospective study of 124 patients who underwent surgery, radiation, and chemotherapy for glioblastoma identified 7 patients (5.6%) who subsequently underwent shunt placement for communicating hydrocephalus [63].

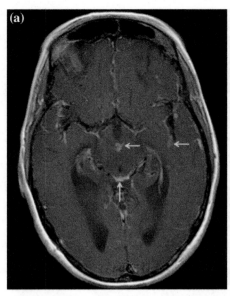
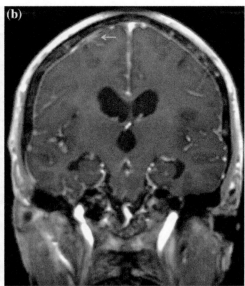

Fig. 11.3 Carcinomatous meningitis. **a** Contrast-enhanced axial T1-weighted magnetic resonance image showing enlarged ventricles and diffuse meningeal enhancement (*arrows*) in a 54-year-old woman with a history of metastatic breast cancer and malignant cells on CSF cytology. She presented with morning headaches, nausea and vomiting. **b** Coronal contrast-enhanced axial T1-weighted magnetic resonance image showing enlarged ventricles and meningeal enhancement (*arrow*) from the same patient as in (**a**)

The mechanisms underlying the development of NPH after brain tumor treatment are poorly understood. Entry into the ventricle at the time of surgery and high CSF protein levels were found to be significant predictors of the development of communicating hydrocephalus in patients with GBM [63]. Fischer and colleagues also reported a statistically significant correlation between ventricular opening at the time of surgery and the development of communicating hydrocephalus after treatment for GBM [64]. In addition, an association between radiation and the development of hydrocephalus has been reported [65, 66]. Shunt placement after therapy-induced hydrocephalus improved symptoms and quality of life in these patients [63, 65].

The gait difficulty seen in NPH is characterized by imbalance and gait apraxia [67]. Patients typically are not weak, even though they may have difficulty rising from a seated position, initiating movement or regulating the amplitude and timing of their movements. The cognitive dysfunction of NPH has multiple components, but is most notable for deficits in executive functioning, visuospatial processing and the ability to encode new memories [68]. Together, these deficits suggest impairment of frontal, parietal and temporal lobe function.

The diagnosis of NPH should be considered in patients who present with slowly progressive gait difficulty, dementia and incontinence [69]. Cranial imaging shows evidence of ventricular enlargement in most cases (Fig. 11.4a, b). The diagnosis of NPH can be confirmed by a trial of CSF drainage to determine whether symptoms improve. Although a high volume (greater than 30 cc) lumbar puncture can lead to immediate improvement, studies indicate that this test is unreliable because of a high frequency of false negatives [70]. The high false negative rate of high volume lumbar puncture for NPH diagnosis occurs largely because many patients require several days of CSF drainage before symptoms improve. Consequently, many practitioners utilize an extended trial of lumbar CSF drainage over several days to increase the likelihood that an accurate assessment of the effect of CSF drainage on NPH symptoms is obtained [69].

Medical Management of Elevated ICP in Brain Tumor Patients

One of the most commonly used and most effective approaches to decreasing elevated ICP caused by vasogenic edema is the use of glucocorticoids such as dexamethasone [71, 72]. Dexamethasone activates glucocorticoid receptors in the nucleus of cells to increase the expression and activation of tight junction proteins in cerebral vessels. Thus, dexamethasone decreases ICP by reducing blood–brain barrier incompetence and decreasing vasogenic edema [71]. However, the long-term use of dexamethasone is limited by its many (and sometimes serious) side effects. These include weight gain, ulcers, aseptic necrosis of the hip, osteopenia, muscle weakness, psychosis, and others [73].

Fig. 11.4 Normal pressure hydrocephalus. **a** Sagittal T1 and axial FLAIR images showing enlarged ventricles in a 66-year-old woman with a history of whole brain radiotherapy for treatment of metastatic breast cancer with brain metastases. The patient presented with inability to walk, incontinence, and dementia. However, she did not have headaches or other symptoms of elevated ICP. **b** Plain skull film and head CT images showing shunt placement in the same patient as shown in (**a**). After shunt placement, the patient's incontinence and dementia resolved and she regained the ability to walk independently

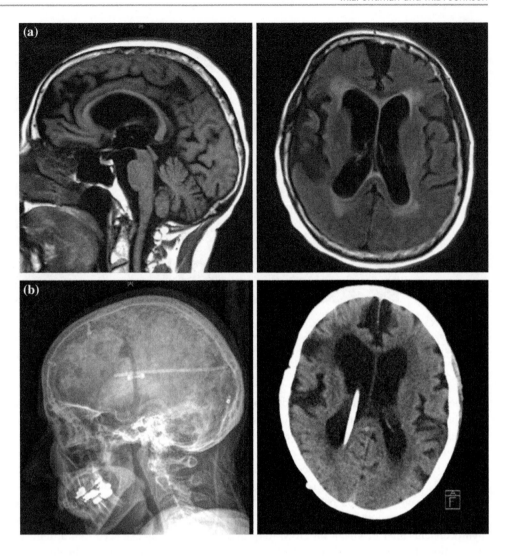

A recent addition to the armamentarium of treatments used to decrease elevated ICP caused by vasogenic edema is the anti-VEGF antibody, bevacizumab [72]. This antibody neutralizes the activity of tumor-secreted VEGF, which is a primary angiogenic stimulus for the generation of leaky blood vessels in many types of brain tumors. Bevacizumab has been shown to decrease cerebral edema by "normalizing" leaky vessels, thereby decreasing mass effect and reducing ICP [74]. By reducing vasogenic edema due to tumor or radiation necrosis [75], bevacizumab has become a useful alternative to dexamethasone for controlling ICP.

Tumor Resection and Radiation for Treatment of Elevated ICP in Brain Tumor Patients

The long-term goal of ICP management in many brain tumor patients can be achieved by tumor removal. This has the combined benefits of cytoreduction, decreased mass effect and restoration of CSF pathway patency. All of these effects contribute to normalizing the ICP. Certain tumors such as tectal gliomas or intraparenchymal brainstem tumors are rarely resected, largely because of their location in particularly sensitive regions of the brain [41, 76]. In such cases, a CSF diversion procedure such as ventricular shunt placement or endoscopic third ventriculostomy may be warranted.

For some patients, however, removal of the tumor does not lead to a complete resolution of the elevated ICP, even though the obstruction to CSF flow has been relieved. The reasons for this are not always clear, although venous sinus thrombosis [77], radiation necrosis with persistent edema [75], or persistent hydrocephalus are most often responsible. Hypotheses regarding the underlying mechanisms of persistent hydrocephalus after tumor resection include elevated protein in the CSF or treatment-associated inflammation of the meninges which leads to occlusion of the CSF absorption pathways. In such cases, ventricular shunt placement for CSF diversion may be warranted.

For radiation-sensitive tumors causing obstructive hydrocephalus such as germinomas or papillary tumors of the pineal region, surgical resection of the lesion may not be necessary to relieve the obstruction [78, 79]. Radiation can cause rapid regression of these tumors, thereby relieving the obstruction of CSF flow. Radiation can also rapidly and effectively reduce the size and mass effect associated with lymphomas [80]. Thus, this group of tumors is generally not surgically resected.

In many cases involving brain tumor patients who present with elevated ICP, however, radiation should be used cautiously. Radiation-induced cytotoxicity can actually contribute to brain edema and further elevate ICP [81]. In cases where significant ventricular compression is already present (e.g., in the posterior fossa), radiation can increase brain swelling, worsen mass effect and even precipitate obstructive hydrocephalus [82]. Thus, many radiation oncologists advocate treating brain edema and decreasing mass effect via the use of steroids, surgical resection or shunt placement prior to initiating radiation therapy.

Treatment of Hydrocephalus in Brain Tumor Patients

The treatment of hydrocephalus in brain tumor patients consists primarily of surgical removal of the obstructive lesion, performance of endoscopic third ventriculostomy (ETV) to bypass an obstructive lesion that cannot be removed, or placement of a shunt for CSF diversion. As mentioned previously, tumor resection to reopen blocked CSF pathways is performed whenever possible, as this allows for therapeutic tumor removal and may avoid the need for a permanent CSF diversion procedure. ETV or placement of a ventriculostomy may be performed to divert the CSF before or during the operative procedure when appropriate [43, 83]. The ventriculostomy can then be weaned under controlled conditions postoperatively in order to ensure that the obstructive hydrocephalus has resolved. Occasionally, hydrocephalus and elevated ICP persist despite resection of the tumor, and shunt placement or ETV is necessary [44, 45].

In most cases of hydrocephalus, shunt placement leads to a rapid improvement in symptoms. Indeed, shunt placement can be a life-saving procedure in brain tumor patients with elevated ICP or mass effect due to hydrocephalus. Because it

frequently alleviates the NPH symptoms of gait difficulty, dementia and incontinence, shunt placement can lead to a significant improvement in the quality of life for both brain tumor patients and their caregivers.

Although CSF drainage provides relief of hydrocephalus-associated symptoms in patients with carcinomatous meningitis, the overall prognosis for patients with this disorder remains very poor. Literature estimates of median survival for untreated patients range from 4 to 6 weeks [49, 54]. With treatment, median survival time increases to 3–6 months [49–51, 57]. Survival of patients with carcinomatous meningitis is usually determined by the site and extent of systemic disease. In one study involving 122 carcinomatous meningitis patients, liver metastases were associated with the worst prognosis [57].

Therapeutic approaches to the treatment of carcinomatous meningitis include high dose systemic or intrathecal chemotherapy and/or radiation to symptomatic disease sites [49, 50, 84]. The most commonly used chemotherapeutic agents for intraventricular therapy include methotrexate, cytarabine, and thio-TEPA [50, 51]. Ventriculoperitoneal shunts (VPS) have also been used in patients with carcinomatous meningitis and hydrocephalus [84–87]. One study demonstrated that the use of a CSF reservoir system in combination with shunt placement led to better outcomes than the use of the reservoir system alone [84]. Other studies have also demonstrated the effectiveness of shunt placement as a palliative measure in this patient population [86, 87].

Conclusion

Here we have reviewed the origins, presentation, and treatment of elevated ICP and hydrocephalus in brain tumor patients. Large tumor volume, vasogenic edema, obstructive hydrocephalus, communicating hydrocephalus, and carcinomatous meningitis can all lead to mass effect and elevated ICP. Although we discussed each of these factors separately, they are often found in combination. For example, patients with large tumors and mass effect can develop vasogenic edema and obstructive hydrocephalus that contributes to elevated ICP (Fig. 11.5a–d). Treatment strategies in such situations are often combinatorial. The plan for which treatments to use and in what order varies, depending upon the specific details of each case. Consequently, neurooncologists, radiation oncologists and neurosurgeons must work collaboratively to formulate an optimal treatment plan for each patient.

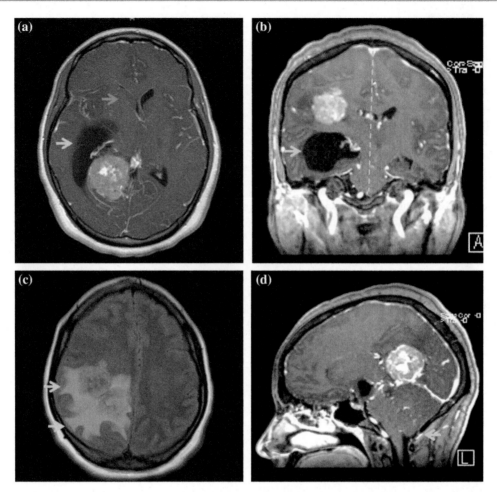

Fig. 11.5 An intraventricular tumor with vasogenic edema and mass effect leading to obstructive hydrocephalus and elevated ICP. T1-weighted contrast-enhanced magnetic resonance images in the axial (**a**), coronal (**b**) and sagittal (**d**) planes, and T2-FLAIR magnetic resonance image in the axial plane (**c**) showing a large intraventricular meningioma in the atrium of the right lateral ventricle. **a**, **b** The tumor has significant mass effect on the surrounding brain and causes midline shift (*blue arrow*) as well as obstructive hydrocephalus of the right temporal horn of the lateral ventricle (*yellow arrow*). The *yellow dotted line* in (**b**) identifies the midline. **c** T2-FLAIR MR image

demonstrates significant vasogenic edema (*yellow arrows*) that contributes to the mass effect of the lesion. **d** The sagittal T1-weighted contrast-enhanced magnetic resonance image shows crowding of the posterior fossa with descent of the cerebellar tonsils (*arrow*) secondary to elevated ICP and mass effect in the supratentorial compartment. The patient presented with chronic headaches and a syncopal episode. She was initially treated with dexamethasone, followed by debulking of the tumor. The obstructive hydrocephalus persisted, and a shunt was placed into the temporal horn of the right lateral ventricle with complete resolution of her symptoms

References

1. Hawthorne C, Piper I. Monitoring of intracranial pressure in patients with traumatic brain injury. Front Neurol. 2014;5:121.
2. Dunn L. Raised intracranial pressure. J Neurol Neurosurg Psychiatry. 2002;73(Suppl 1):i23–7.
3. Di Ieva A, Schmitz EM, Cusimano MD. Analysis of intracranial pressure: past, present, and future. Neuroscientist. 2013;19:592–603.
4. Sakka L, Coll G, Chazal J. Anatomy and physiology of cerebrospinal fluid. Eur Ann Otorhinolaryngol Head Neck Dis. 2011;128(6):309–16.
5. Kirkman MA, Smith M. Intracranial pressure monitoring, cerebral perfusion pressure estimation, and ICP/CPP-guided therapy: a standard of care or optional extra after brain injury? Br J Anaesth. 2014;112:35–46.
6. Brinker T, Stopa E, Morrison J, Klinge P. A new look at cerebrospinal fluid circulation. Fluids Barriers CNS. 2014;11:10.
7. Spector R, Robert Snodgrass S, Johanson CE. A balanced view of the cerebrospinal fluid composition and functions: focus on adult humans. Exp Neurol. 2015;273:57–68.
8. Damkier HH, Brown PD, Praetorius J. Cerebrospinal fluid secretion by the Choroid Plexus. Physiol Rev. 2013;93:1847–92.
9. Jessen NA, Munk AS, Lundgaard I, Nedergaard M. The glymphatic system: a Beginner's guide. Neurochem Res. 2015;40(12):2583–99.
10. Aspelund A, Antila S, Proulx ST, Karlsen TV, Karaman S, Detmar M, Wiig H, Alitalo K. A dural lymphatic vascular system that drains brain interstitial fluid and macromolecules. J Exp Med. 2015;212:991–9.
11. Louveau A, Smirnov I, Keyes TJ, Eccles JD, Rouhani SJ, Peske JD, Derecki NC, Castle D, Mandell JW, Lee KS, Harris TH,

Kipnis J. Structural and functional features of central nervous system lymphatic vessels. Nature. 2015;523:337–41.

12. Lehtinen MK, Zappaterra MW, Chen X, Yang YJ, Hill AD, Lun M, Maynard T, Gonzalez D, Kim S, Ye P, D'Ercole AJ, Wong ET, LaMantia AS, Walsh CA. The cerebrospinal fluid provides a proliferative niche for neural progenitor cells. Neuron. 2011;69:893–905.

13. Magram G, Liakos AM. The CSF accumulator: its role in the central nervous system and implications for advancing hydrocephalus shunt technology. Pediatr Neurosurg. 1997;26:236–46.

14. Chang HS, Nakagawa H. Hypothesis on the pathophysiology of syringomyelia based on simulation of cerebrospinal fluid dynamics. J Neurol Neurosurg Psychiatry. 2003;74:344–7.

15. Czosnyka M, Brady K, Reinhard M, Smielewski P, Steiner LA. Monitoring of cerebrovascular autoregulation: facts, myths, and missing links. Neurocrit Care. 2009;10:373–86.

16. Dennis LJ, Mayer SA. Diagnosis and management of increased intracranial pressure. Neurol India. 2001;49(Suppl 1):S37–50.

17. Zierski J. Blood flow in brain structures during increased ICP. Acta Neurochir Suppl (Wien). 1987;40:95–116.

18. Silbergeld DL, Rostomily RC, Alvord EC Jr. The cause of death in patients with glioblastoma is multifactorial: clinical factors and autopsy findings in 117 cases of supratentorial glioblastoma in adults. J Neurooncol. 1991;10(2):179–85.

19. Graff-Radford SB, Schievink W. High-pressure headaches, low-pressure syndromes, and CSF leaks: diagnosis and management. Headache. 2014;54:394–401.

20. Göbel H, Göbel C, Heinze A. Headache from increased cerebrospinal fluid pressure. Schmerz. 2012;26:331–40 quiz 341.

21. Petersen LG, Petersen JC, Andresen M, Secher NH, Juhler M. Postural influence on intracranial and cerebral perfusion pressure in ambulatory neurosurgical patients. Am J Physiol Regul Integr Comp Physiol. 2016;310(1):R100–4.

22. Passi N, Degnan AJ, Levy LM. MR imaging of papilledema and visual pathways: effects of increased intracranial pressure and pathophysiologic mechanisms. AJNR Am J Neuroradiol. 2013;34:919–24.

23. Agrawal A, Timothy J, Cincu R, Agarwal T, Waghmare LB. Bradycardia in neurosurgery. Clin Neurol Neurosurg. 2008;110:321–7.

24. Ziai WC, Melnychuk E, Thompson CB, Awad I, Lane K, Hanley DF. Occurrence and impact of intracranial pressure elevation during treatment of severe intraventricular hemorrhage. Crit Care Med. 2012;40(5):1601–8.

25. Young JS, Blow O, Turrentine F, Claridge JA, Schulman A. Is there an upper limit of intracranial pressure in patients with severe head injury if cerebral perfusion pressure is maintained? Neurosurg Focus. 2003;15(6):E2.

26. Lee EL, Armstrong TS. Increased intracranial pressure. Clin J Oncol Nurs. 2008;12:37–41.

27. Jantzen JP. Prevention and treatment of intracranial hypertension. Best Pract Res Clin Anaesthesiol. 2007;21:517–38.

28. Singhi SC, Tiwari L. Management of intracranial hypertension. Indian J Pediatr. 2009;76(5):519–29.

29. Donnem T, Hu J, Ferguson R, et al. Vessel co-option in primary human tumors and metastases: an obstacle to effective anti-angiogenic treatment? Cancer Med. 2013;2:427–36.

30. Papadopoulos MC, Saadoun S, Binder DK, Manley GT, Krishna S, Verkman AS. Molecular mechanisms of brain tumor edema. Neuroscience. 2004;129:1011–20.

31. Rosenberg GA, Yang Y. Vasogenic edema due to tight junction disruption by matrix metalloproteinases in cerebral ischemia. Neurosurg Focus. 2007;22(5):E4.

32. Yadav YR, Mukerji G, Shenoy R, Basoor A, Jain G, Nelson A. Endoscopic management of hypertensive intraventricular haemorrhage with obstructive hydrocephalus. BMC Neurol. 2007;7:1.

33. Schroeder HW. Intraventricular tumors. World Neurosurg. 2013;79(Suppl 2):S17.e15-9.

34. Roth J, Ram Z, Constantini S. Endoscopic considerations treating hydrocephalus caused by basal ganglia and large thalamic tumors. Surg Neurol Int. 2015;6:56.

35. Baroncini M, Peltier J, Le Gars D, Lejeune JP. Tumors of the lateral ventricle. Review of 284 cases. Neurochirurgie. 2011;57:170–9.

36. Fenchel M, Beschorner R, Naegele T, Korn A, Ernemann U, Horger M. Primarily solid intraventricular brain tumors. Eur J Radiol. 2012;81:e688–96.

37. Zhang BY, Yin B, Li YX, Wu JS, Chen H, Wang XQ, Geng DY. Neuroradiological findings and clinical features of fourth-ventricular meningioma: a study of 10 cases. Clin Radiol. 2012;67(5):455–60.

38. Zhang J, Babu R, McLendon RE, Friedman AH, Adamson C. A comprehensive analysis of 41 patients with rosette-forming glioneuronal tumors of the fourth ventricle. J Clin Neurosci. 2013;20(3):335–41.

39. Hayashi T, Inamasu J, Kanai R, Sasaki H, Shinoda J, Hirose Y. Clinical, histological, and genetic features of fourth ventricle ependymoma in the elderly. Case report. Neurol Med Chir (Tokyo). 2012;52:611–6.

40. Albright L, Reigel DH. Management of hydrocephalus secondary to posterior fossa tumors. J Neurosurg. 1977;46:52–5.

41. Igboechi C, Vaddiparti A, Sorenson EP, Rozzelle CJ, Tubbs RS, Loukas M. Tectal plate gliomas: a review. Childs Nerv Syst. 2013;29:1827–33.

42. Gaillard F, Jones J. Masses of the pineal region: clinical presentation and radiographic features. Postgrad Med J. 2010;86: 597–607.

43. Schmid UD, Seiler RW. Management of obstructive hydrocephalus secondary to posterior fossa tumors by steroids and subcutaneous ventricular catheter reservoir. J Neurosurg. 1986;65 (5):649–53.

44. Al Hinai Q, Zeitouni A, Sirhan D, et al. Communicating hydrocephalus and vestibular schwannomas: etiology, treatment, and long-term follow-up. J Neurol Surg Part B Skull Base. 2013;74:68–74.

45. Tanaka Y, Kobayashi S, Hongo K, Tada T, Sato A, Takasuna H. Clinical and neuroimaging characteristics of hydrocephalus associated with vestibular schwannoma. J Neurosurg. 2003;98 (6):1188–93.

46. Bloch J, Vernet O, Aubé M, Villemure JG. Non-obstructive hydrocephalus associated with intracranial schwannomas: hyperproteinorrhachia as an etiopathological factor? Acta Neurochir (Wien). 2003;145:73–8.

47. Fukuda M, Oishi M, Kawaguchi T, Watanabe M, Takao T, Tanaka R, Fujii Y. Etiopathological factors related to hydrocephalus associated with vestibular schwannoma. Neurosurgery. 2007;61:1186–93.

48. Pencalet P, Sainte-Rose C, Lellouch-Tubiana A, Kalifa C, Brunelle F, Sgouros S, Meyer P, Cinalli G, Zerah M, Pierre-Kahn A, Renier D. Papillomas and carcinomas of the choroid plexus in children. J Neurosurg. 1998;88:521–8.

49. Grossman SA, Krabak MJ. Leptomeningeal carcinomatosis. Cancer Treat Rev. 1999;25:103–19.

50. Chamberlain MC. Neoplastic meningitis. Oncologist. 2008;13 (9):967–77.

51. DeAngelis LM. Current diagnosis and treatment of leptomeningeal metastasis. J Neurooncol. 1998;38:245–52.

52. Norris LK, Grossman SA, Olivi A. Neoplastic meningitis following surgical resection of isolated cerebellar metastasis: a potentially preventable complication. J Neurooncol. 1997;32: 215–23.

53. Jearanaisilp S, Sangruji T, Danchaivijitr C, Danchaivijitr N. Neoplastic meningitis: a retrospective review of clinical presentations, radiological and cerebrospinal fluid findings. J Med Assoc Thai. 2014;97:870–7.

54. Little JR, Dale AJ, Okazaki H. Meningeal carcinomatosis. Clinical manifestations. Arch Neurol. 1974;30:138–43.

55. Suki D, Abouassi H, Patel AJ, Sawaya R, Weinberg JS, Groves MD. Comparative risk of leptomeningeal disease after resection or stereotactic radiosurgery for solid tumor metastasis to the posterior fossa. J Neurosurg. 2008;108(2):248–57.

56. Suki D, Hatiboglu MA, Patel AJ, Weinberg JS, Groves MD, Mahajan A, Sawaya R. Comparative risk of leptomeningeal dissemination of cancer after surgery or stereotactic radiosurgery for a single supratentorial solid tumor metastasis. Neurosurgery. 2009;64(4):664–74.

57. Amer MH, Al-Sarraf M, Baker LH, Vaitkevicius VK. Malignant melanoma and central nervous system metastases: incidence, diagnosis. Treat Surv Cancer. 1978;42:660–8.

58. Freilich RJ, Krol G, DeAngelis LM. Neuroimaging and cerebrospinal fluid cytology in the diagnosis of leptomeningeal metastasis. Ann Neurol. 1995;38:51–7.

59. Schumacher M, Orszagh M. Imaging techniques in neoplastic meningiosis. J Neurooncol. 1998;38(2–3):111–20.

60. Sze G, Soletsky S, Bronen R, Krol G. MR imaging of the cranial meninges with emphasis on contrast enhancement and meningeal carcinomatosis. AJR Am J Roentgenol. 1989;153(5):1039–49.

61. Eide PK, Sorteberg W. Diagnostic intracranial pressure monitoring and surgical management in idiopathic normal pressure hydrocephalus: a 6-year review of 214 patients. Neurosurgery. 2010;66:80–91.

62. Inamasu J, Nakamura Y, Saito R, Kuroshima Y, Mayanagi K, Orii M, Ichikizaki K. Postoperative communicating hydrocephalus in patients with supratentorial malignant glioma. Clin Neurol Neurosurg. 2003;106:9–15.

63. Montano N, D'Alessandris QG, Bianchi F, Lauretti L, Doglietto F, Fernandez E, Maira G, Pallini R. Communicating hydrocephalus following surgery and adjuvant radiochemotherapy for glioblastoma. J Neurosurg. 2011;115:1126–30.

64. Fischer CM, Neidert MC, Péus D, Ulrich NH, Regli L, Krayenbühl N, Woernle CM. Hydrocephalus after resection and adjuvant radiochemotherapy in patients with glioblastoma. Clin Neurol Neurosurg. 2014;120:27–31.

65. Thiessen B, DeAngelis LM. Hydrocephalus in radiation leukoencephalopathy: results of ventriculoperitoneal shunting. Arch Neurol. 1998;55:705–10.

66. Perrini P, Scollato A, Cioffi F, Mouchaty H, Conti R, Di Lorenzo N. Radiation leukoencephalopathy associated with moderate hydrocephalus: intracranial pressure monitoring and results of ventriculoperitoneal shunting. Neurol Sci. 2002;23:237–41.

67. Adams RD, Fisher CM, Hakim S, Ojemann RG, Sweet WH. Symptomatic occult hydrocephalus with "normal" cerebrospinal-fluid pressure a treatable syndrome. N Engl J Med. 1965;273:117–26.

68. Bugalho P, Alves L, Miguel R, Ribeiro O. Profile of cognitive dysfunction and relation with gait disturbance in normal pressure hydrocephalus. Clin Neurol Neurosurg. 2014;118:83–8.

69. Relkin N, Marmarou A, Klinge P, Bergsneider M, Black PM. Diagnosing idiopathic normal-pressure hydrocephalus. Neurosurgery. 2005;57:S1–3.

70. Wikkelso C, Hellstrom P, Klinge PM, Tans JT, Europen iNPH Multicentre Study Group. The European iNPH multicentre study on the predictivevalues of resistance to CSF outflow and the CSF tap test in patients with idiopathic normal pressure hydrocephalus. J Neurol Neurosurg Psychiatry. 2013;84:562–8.

71. Kaal EC, Vecht CJ. The management of brain edema in brain tumors. Curr Opin Oncol. 2004;16:593–600.

72. Schiff D, Lee EQ, Nayak L, Norden AD, Reardon DA, Wen PY. Medical management of brain tumors and the sequelae of treatment. Neuro Oncol. 2015;17:488–504.

73. Dietrich J, Rao K, Pastorino S, Kesari S. Corticosteroids in brain cancer patients: benefits and pitfalls. Expert Rev Clin Pharmacol. 2011;4:233–42.

74. Jain RK. Antiangiogenic therapy for cancer: current and emerging concepts. Oncology (Williston Park). 2005;19(4 Suppl 3):7–16.

75. Lubelski D, Abdullah KG, Weil RG, Marko NF. Bevacizumab for radiation necrosis following treatment of high grade glioma: a systematic review of the literature. J Neurooncol. 2013;115:317–22.

76. Kaye EC, Baker JN, Broniscer A. Management of diffuse intrinsic pontine glioma in children: current and future strategies for improving diagnosis. CNS Oncol. 2014;3:421–31.

77. Masuhr F, Einhäupl K. Treatment of cerebral venous and sinus thrombosis. Front Neurol Neurosci. 2008;23:132–43.

78. Patel SK, Tomei KL, Christiano LD, Baisre A, Liu JK. Complete regression of papillary tumor of the pineal region after radiation therapy: case report and review of the literature. J Neurooncol. 2012;107:427–34.

79. Gupta R, Songara A. Management of dual intracranial germinoma by radiotherapy alone. J Pediatr Neurosci. 2015;10:38–40.

80. Brastianos PK, Batchelor TT. Primary central nervous system lymphoma: overview of current treatment strategies. Hematol Oncol Clin North Am. 2012;26:897–916.

81. Na A, Haghigi N, Drummond KJ. Cerebral radiation necrosis. Asia Pac J Clin Oncol. 2014;10:11–21.

82. Wolff R, Karlsson B, Dettmann E, Bottcher HD, Seifert V. Pretreatment radiation induced oedema causing acute hydrocephalus after radiosurgery for multiple cerebellar metastases. Acta Neurochir (Wien). 2003;145:691–6.

83. El-Ghandour NM. Endoscopic third ventriculostomy versus ventriculoperitoneal shunt in the treatment of obstructive hydrocephalus due to posterior fossa tumors in children. Childs Nerv Syst. 2011;27:117–26.

84. Lin N, Dunn IF, Glantz M, Allison DL, Jensen R, Johnson MD, Friedlander RM, Kesari S. Benefit of ventriculoperitoneal cerebrospinal fluid shunting and intrathecal chemotherapy in neoplastic meningitis: a retrospective, case-controlled study. J Neurosurg. 2011;115:730–6.

85. Gonda DD, Kim TE, Warnke PC, Kasper EM, Carter BS, Chen CC. Ventriculoperitoneal shunting versus endoscopic third ventriculostomy in the treatment of patients with hydrocephalus related to metastasis. Surg Neurol Int. 2012;3:97.

86. Omuro AM, Lallana EC, Bilsky MH, DeAngelis LM. Ventriculoperitoneal shunt in patients with leptomeningeal metastasis. Neurology. 2005;64:1625–7.

87. Lee SH, Kong DS, Seol HJ, Nam DH, Lee JI. Ventriculoperitoneal shunt for hydrocephalus caused by central nervous system metastasis. J Neurooncol. 2011;104:545–51.

Cognitive Dysfunction, Mood Disorders, and Fatigue as Complications of Cancer

Jörg Dietrich and Michael W. Parsons

Neurocognitive Dysfunction in Cancer Patients

Introduction

Neurocognitive function is frequently altered in cancer patients, regardless of whether patients are treated for brain cancer or systemic malignancies. Multiple factors can contribute to impairment of cognitive function, including the type and location of the tumor, growth pattern of the malignancy, and cancer-directed therapies (e.g., chemotherapy, radiation therapy, and biologic agents). In addition, several medications (e.g., pain medications, anti-epileptic drugs, and corticosteroids), comorbidities (e.g., anemia, lung, renal, or liver disease), preexisting neurological deficits, mood alterations, and fatigue can influence neurocognitive function.

To make matters even more complex, these factors may influence each other. For example, chronic fatigue and depression can interfere with cognitive functioning, and neurocognitive impairment can in turn contribute to symptoms of fatigue and depressed mood.

It therefore can be difficult to delineate the precise contribution and relevance of each of these factors in clinical practice, posing a significant challenge to patient management (Fig. 12.1).

As disruption in neurocognitive function can be a major cause of impaired quality of life, attention to these symptoms and consideration of possible therapeutic interventions

directed to improve neurocognitive deficits have become increasingly important in clinical oncology and cancer survivorship. Importantly, a specific neurocognitive deficit (e.g., impaired short-term memory or executive dysfunction) might result in varying degrees of disability in a given patient, depending on the individual's baseline cognitive function, cognitive reserve, and on how such deficits interfere with a patient's ability to perform social and professional activities. Therefore, patient evaluation and choice of therapeutic intervention must be individually tailored to the patient's perceived deficits and specific needs and evaluated in the context of the patient's personal and professional life.

Tumor Effects on Neurocognitive Function

Impairment or change in neurocognitive function is usually dependent on the location, size, type, and biology of the underlying tumor [1–4]. Accounting for all of these factors, it has been hypothesized that cognitive dysfunction in brain tumor patients is the result of a whole brain network disturbance [5, 6]. Tumor-associated complications, such as cerebral edema, seizures, or use of anti-seizure medications are also known to influence neurocognitive performance [5, 7–10].

The current literature suggests that neurocognitive deficits are frequently evident *prior to* tumor directed therapies in brain tumor patients [4, 11]. For instance, neurocognitive dysfunction was present in 90% of patients with frontal or temporal gliomas *prior to* any therapeutic intervention, with impairment of memory and attention in 60% and executive dysfunction in 78% of patients [12].

The influence of tumor pathology and degree of malignancy on neurocognitive function remains poorly understood. Interestingly, impairment of attention and executive dysfunction are considered unfavorable prognostic markers in patients with high-grade gliomas [13]. It is conceivable that neurocognitive and behavioral deficits more easily result from rapidly growing malignant brain tumors than from

J. Dietrich (✉)
Department of Neurology, Harvard Medical School,
Massachusetts General Hospital, 55 Fruit Street, Yawkey 9E,
Boston, MA 02114, USA
e-mail: dietrich.jorg@mgh.harvard.edu

M.W. Parsons
Burkhardt Brain Tumor Center and Section of Neuropsychology,
Cleveland Clinic, 9500 Euclid Avenue P-57, Cleveland,
OH 44195, USA
e-mail: parsonm2@ccf.org

© Springer International Publishing AG 2018
D. Schiff et al. (eds.), *Cancer Neurology in Clinical Practice*,
DOI 10.1007/978-3-319-57901-6_12

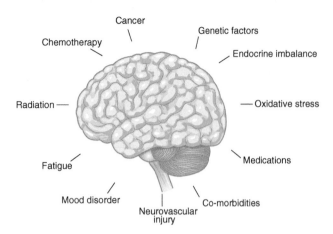

Fig. 12.1 Multifactorial etiology of cognitive dysfunction in cancer patients

low-grade or benign tumors, in which long-term compensatory mechanisms might play a role in the maintenance of cognitive function [3, 14–16]. However, other studies have not revealed a correlation between cognitive performance and degree of malignancy. For instance, Kayl and Meyers were unable to identify a significant difference in cognitive performance between glioblastoma and anaplastic astrocytoma patients, accounting for patient age, gender, education, tumor location, and tumor volume [17].

The development of specific neurocognitive deficits depends on the location of the tumor within specific brain regions. For example, tumors that affect the dominant hemisphere and fronto-temporal region are likely to cause disruption in language function, including verbal learning, memory, and speech [3]. Nondominant hemispheric tumors are more likely to result in impairment of nonverbal speech, visual-spatial, and visual-perceptual functions [1, 18].

Frontal lobe tumors commonly cause executive dysfunction and personality changes, including a lack of motivation, spontaneity, and impaired social judgment. Parietal lobe tumors commonly result in difficulties with spatial orientation, and tumors in the occipital lobes can cause visual-perceptive deficits. Neurocognitive and mood disorders have also been described in patients with cerebellar tumors [19–23] and brainstem lesions [24], supporting the notion that the cerebellum has important functions in neural network systems relevant to higher cognitive function.

Treatment Effects on Neurocognitive Function

Radiation Therapy

Cranial radiation therapy is well known to cause neurocognitive deficits [25–29]. Radiation can result in progressive cognitive decline in both children [30–33] and adults [25, 34–36]. The effects of cranial radiation have been best studied in patients treated with whole brain radiation therapy (WBRT) (e.g., [37]), though emerging data reveal that focal and stereotactic radiosurgery (SRS) can also result in structural brain changes and significant functional morbidity in a subset of patients [38, 39].

In general, risk factors for developing radiation related central nervous system toxicity include age (with neurotoxic complications more likely to occur at age <5 years and >60 years), a fractionation dose of >2 Gy, cumulative radiation dose, volume of brain irradiated, shorter overall treatment time, concurrent or subsequent use of chemotherapy, and preexisting cerebrovascular risk factors [25, 40–42]. In addition, genetic factors are likely to play a role in tissue vulnerability to radiation [43–45].

Cognitive dysfunction has been reported in up to 85% of patients treated with cranial radiation therapy [42]. A wide range of reported incidences is conceivably explained by differences in patient populations, treatment variables, and study methodology.

Radiation-induced neurotoxicity usually follows a progressive pattern, and long-term survivors are at particular risk to demonstrate cognitive decline, such as children treated with prophylactic cranial radiation for childhood leukemia [46]. The use of concurrent or sequential chemotherapy can increase the incidence and severity of radiation-induced toxicity [25]. For example, patients with primary central nervous system lymphoma (PCNSL) treated with whole brain radiation and subsequent chemotherapy are at particular risk for profound cognitive impairment; imaging findings can demonstrate brain volume loss and leukoencephalopathy [47]. Recent studies also revealed a surprisingly high degree of early onset and progressive brain atrophy in glioblastoma patients treated with combined standard temozolomide chemotherapy and focal brain radiation [39].

In general, radiation-induced neurotoxicity has been categorized in three phases: an acute, early delayed, and late-delayed reaction [42, 48].

In the acute phase, symptoms occur within days to weeks of therapy and are usually characterized by development of fatigue, subacute neurological decline, and worsening of preexisting deficits, which fortunately is reversible in most patients with supportive management. Symptoms are likely the result of inflammatory mechanisms, vascular toxicity, blood–brain barrier disruption, and cerebral edema [49, 50].

Early delayed neurotoxic symptoms occur within weeks to several months of treatment. Symptoms mainly consist of fatigue, inattention, and short-term memory impairment. Neurocognitive testing may demonstrate slowed information-processing speed, word and memory retrieval deficits, diminished executive function, and impaired fine motor dexterity [25, 51–53], suggesting impairment of orbito-frontal and fronto-temporal network systems.

Early delayed neurotoxic symptoms are thought to be related to radiation-induced transient demyelination [54].

Late-delayed side effects occur months to years after radiation and are mostly irreversible and progressive. Deficits in memory, attention, concentration, and executive dysfunction are frequently reported [55]. Most patients will demonstrate mild to moderate cognitive impairment, but only infrequently are these associated with abnormal imaging findings [56]. However, in more severe cases of late-delayed radiation toxicity, patients will develop progressive cognitive decline [27], and imaging and histopathological studies may demonstrate focal necrosis, leukoencephalopathy, and global brain atrophy [47, 57–62]. The current data suggest that nonspecific diffuse white matter changes can be seen on MRI in nearly all patients receiving doses of 20 Gy or higher who survive more than one year [63]. The risk of white matter changes following WBRT is higher in patients with baseline white matter changes [64].

Concerns regarding delayed radiation-induced neurotoxic adverse effects in long-term survivors have stimulated a contentious debate on the preferential use of SRS, WBRT, or a combination of both in patients with brain metastases [65]. One of the main questions is whether patients with a limited number of brain metastases should be treated with either WBRT or with SRS [66, 67]. With comparable survival data in patients treated with either modality, the benefit of WBRT has been challenged especially in patients with limited number of cerebral metastases and in light of more pronounced neurocognitive deficits (e.g., learning and memory decline) following WBRT [63, 67].

WBRT has also been shown to impact *patient-reported* quality of life. A large multi-institutional study of patients with one to three brain metastases revealed that WBRT, when added to SRS, was associated with more pronounced decline in patient-reported cognitive functioning at one year compared with patients that were treated with SRS alone [68]. Other studies using prophylactic cranial radiation in lung cancer patients revealed similar results [69].

Partial brain radiation may also have negative long-term effects on neurocognitive function, even though the risk of developing neurotoxicity is lower than with whole brain radiation therapy [70, 71]. Nevertheless, cognitive dysfunction, including impaired executive function, poor attention, and reduced information processing, can result in significant impairment of quality of life and overall performance in long-term survivors, such as in patients with low-grade gliomas [72, 73].

The precise mechanisms of chronic radiation toxicity are not entirely understood but likely include chronic inflammatory responses and damage to various neuroglial cell types, including neural progenitor cells and myelin producing cells [74–77]. Disruption of adult hippocampal neurogenesis has been identified as one of the relevant physiological processes driving cognitive decline following cranial irradiation [78].

There have been increasing efforts to minimize the negative impact of radiation on germinal zones of the brain. For instance, in a phase II multicenter study (RTOG 0933) Gondi and colleagues demonstrated preservation of cognitive function with conformal avoidance of the hippocampus during WBRT in patients with brain metastases [79]. In addition, pharmacological interventions have been explored to improve cognitive function in patients treated with cranial radiation [80]. For instance, the acetylcholinesterase inhibitor donezepil has shown promise to improve executive function and memory performance in both childhood brain tumor survivors [81], and cognitive function, quality of life, and mood in adult brain cancer patients treated with cranial irradiation [82]. Moreover, Brown and colleagues demonstrated in a recent randomized, double blind, placebo-controlled clinical trial that memantine, an NMDA receptor antagonist, was associated with delayed onset and improved cognitive function in adult patients treated with whole brain radiotherapy for brain metastases [83].

Chemotherapy

Chemotherapy can result in cognitive dysfunction, which has been most convincingly demonstrated in patients treated for non-CNS malignancies. The most frequently described neurocognitive problems include difficulties with memory, learning, attention, concentration, information-processing speed, organization, and executive function (Fig. 12.2).

Interestingly, neurocognitive deficits may be of *delayed onset* and can be progressive even years after cessation of anticancer therapy. Neurocognitive adverse effects from chemotherapy have long been recognized as a disturbing problem in long-term survivors of childhood cancer [27–29,

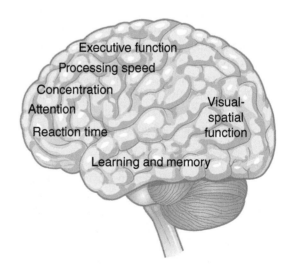

Fig. 12.2 Cognitive domains commonly affected by cancer therapy

84, 85]. Similarly, studies in adult cancer patients have demonstrated that chemotherapy-associated cognitive dysfunction is more common than previously anticipated [42, 86–97].

Incidences of chemotherapy-associated cognitive dysfunction range from 15 to 95% [89, 93, 98, 99]. This wide range of reported incidences has been attributed to the use of different neuropsychological tests with varying degrees of sensitivities to detect cognitive deficits, differences in study design (retrospective vs. prospective design, longitudinal versus cross-sectional analysis, etc.), and different patient populations studied.

Cognitive impairment has been demonstrated in patients treated for various solid cancer types [100–104]. The most compelling data exist in breast cancer patients, showing that approximately 20–40% of breast cancer patients have cognitive deficits on post-treatment evaluation [93, 97, 105–113]. Long-term evaluation of patients examined 1–2 years after treatment with high-dose chemotherapy demonstrated that cognitive impairment is notable in approximately 30–60% of patients [87, 107, 114].

While some patients experience neurocognitive deficits only transiently during and immediately after chemotherapy, symptoms may persist in other patients for years and can cause considerable decline in quality of life, preventing affected individuals to return to their previous level of academic, occupational, or social activities [115]. A recent study of nearly 200 breast cancer survivors who had undergone adjuvant chemotherapy more than 21 years prior found deficits in verbal memory, processing speed, executive functioning, and psychomotor speed when compared with a healthy reference group [116].

Neurocognitive adverse effects have been observed with virtually all categories of chemotherapeutic agents (Table 12.1) [26, 93, 117–119], including antimetabolites (e.g., cytosine arabinoside, 5-fluorouracil, and methotrexate), DNA cross-linking agents (e.g., nitrosureas and cisplatin), mitotic inhibitors (e.g., vincristine), and anti-hormonal agents (e.g., tamoxifen). Some agents, such as methotrexate and carmustine (BCNU), are well known to cause cognitive deficits and leukoencephalopathy, especially when administered at high doses, intrathecally, or in combination with cranial radiotherapy [120–123]. However, imaging abnormalities on MRI only infrequently correlate with the degree of cognitive deficits [124, 125].

Experimental studies have revealed insights into the underlying mechanisms of cognitive dysfunction in cancer patients. Chemotherapy-induced damage to neural progenitor cells required for neurogenesis, gliogenesis, and white matter integrity throughout life has been identified as an important etiologic factor [78, 126–132], and has offered a

Table 12.1 Chemotherapeutic agents associated with cognitive dysfunction in cancer patients

Chemotherapeutic agent
• ACNU/CCNU/BCNU (Nitrosureas)
• Carmofur
• Cisplatin
• Corticosteroids
• Cyclophosphamide
• Cytosine arabinoside (Ara-C)
• Dacarbazine
• Fludarabine
• 5-Fluorouracil (5-FU)
• Ifosfamide
• Interferon
• Levamisole
• Methotrexate

compelling explanation for delayed and progressive neurotoxic effects of chemotherapy.

Importantly, chemotherapeutic agents can affect brain function through direct cytotoxic effects or indirectly through vascular injury, pro-oxidative changes, and immune-mediated inflammation [29, 47, 133–138]. However, the etiology of cognitive dysfunction during and following chemotherapy is likely multifactorial. Risk factors of cognitive decline include timing of chemotherapy, combination of chemotherapy with radiation therapy, and patient age. Metabolic alterations, hormonal imbalance, fatigue, the level of cognitive function prior to treatment and other medical comorbidities have also been shown to influence the manifestation of cognitive symptoms [2, 42, 96]. In addition, certain genetic risk factors have been identified to modulate the degree of cognitive dysfunction. For instance, polymorphisms that influence the efficiency of DNA-repair mechanisms and drug efflux pump systems may expose certain individuals to a higher risk of developing central nervous system toxicity [139–149].

Diagnostic Considerations

The application of a comprehensive testing battery to capture the full range of neurocognitive and psychological function can be time consuming and may be difficult to administer in a demanding oncology practice. In general, assessment of neurocognitive function requires reliable, quantifiable, and valid measures sensitive to cognitive and quality of life deficits in cancer patients. Longitudinal assessment of the patient's self-perception of cognitive function is equally

Table 12.2 Neurocognitive testing battery

Neurocognitive domain	Typical neuropsychological tests
Motor dexterity/speed	Lafayette grooved pegboard test[a]
Visuospatial perception	Benton judgment of line orientation
	Block design subtest of the WAIS-IV
Language	Boston naming test
	Vocabulary subtest of the WAIS-IV
	Category fluency test
Information processing speed	Trail making test A[a]
	Digit symbol subtest of the WAIS-IV
Working memory/attention	Digit span subtest of the WAIS-IV
	Paced auditory serial addition test
Recent/episodic memory	Hopkins verbal learning test[a]
	Brief visuospatial memory test
	Wechsler memory scales-IV
Executive function	Controlled oral word association[a]
	Trail making test B[a]
	Wisconsin card sorting test

[a]Included in RTOG and NCCTG (now NRG and Alliance) clinical trials batteries [152]

important for patient management. Testing strategies that closely relate to real-life situations during which cognitive deficits readily manifest are considered most relevant. It has been an ongoing effort to develop guidelines regarding selection of neuropsychological tests for efficient and comprehensive assessment of cognitive function that can be uniformly applied to cancer patients and allow for comparable data analysis [97, 150–152].

Neuropsychological evaluations are conducted to assess a range of cognitive functions. The neuropsychologist chooses tests that are relevant to the cognitive concerns of the patient, family, or physician and interprets test performance, facilitating care for the patient's cognitive and behavioral symptoms (Table 12.2). The application of a comprehensive testing battery to capture the full range of neurocognitive and psychological function can be time consuming and may be difficult to administer in a multi-site clinical trial. A brief neurocognitive testing battery conceptualized to evaluate memory, visual motor function, executive function, motor dexterity, verbal fluency, and functional independence has been successfully used in several clinical trials by the Radiation Therapy Oncology Group (RTOG) and North Central Cancer Treatment Group (NCCTG). This testing battery has been shown to be sensitive to important cognitive symptoms, time efficient, and easy to administer [153]. Assessment of cognitive function, Quality of Life, and functional status has been shown to provide clinically relevant information in clinical trials assessment of novel treatment strategies [154, 155]. An improved understanding of neurocognitive sequelae is integral part of clinical management and allows clinicians, caregivers, and patients' families to address important needs of cancer patients.

Collectively, rigorous neurocognitive evaluation using standardized testing batteries will be important for optimal management of cancer patients. In addition, the identification of biomarkers to identify and monitor chemotherapy-associated cognitive changes remains an important objective of ongoing investigations. Recent translational imaging studies using structural MRI, functional MRI, and PET imaging have identified compelling evidence for chemotherapy-related brain damage [155, 156]. Advanced neuroimaging studies are therefore likely to increasingly complement future patient evaluation and neurocognitive assessment in cancer patients.

Treatment Considerations

There are currently no standard therapies for patients who experience cognitive symptoms following chemotherapy. While some agents have shown promising results in pilot studies, larger prospective and randomized clinical trials are missing and definite treatment guidelines have so far not been established. Increasing our understanding of the detailed mechanisms underlying cognitive dysfunction in cancer patients will be most relevant to develop

Table 12.3 Treatment strategies for cancer therapy-associated cognitive dysfunction

Agent or intervention	References	Study population
Methylphenidate (Ritalin®, Novartis, Basel, Switzerland)	[157–161]	Breast cancer, ovarian cancer, childhood cancer, brain tumors, melanoma
Modafinil (Provigil®, Cephalon, Frazer, PA, USA)	[162, 163]	Breast cancer
Donepezil (Aricept®)	[82, 164]	Small cell lung cancer and brain cancer
Erythropoietin (Procrit®, Janssen Biotech, Horsham, PA, USA; Aranesp®, Amgen, Thousand Oaks, CA, USA)	[115, 165–169]	Breast cancer, lung cancer, ovarian cancer, endometrial cancer, brain cancer and hematological cancer
Neurocognitive rehabilitation	[170]	Breast cancer
Meditation	[172]	Various cancer types
Exercise	[160, 173, 174]	Breast cancer and melanoma
Sleep regulation	[175]	Various cancer types

neuroprotective therapies. Therapeutic interventions currently include strategies to either prevent side effects or to minimize the severity of symptoms.

Table 12.3 highlights some therapeutic interventions that have shown a potential clinical benefit in treatment of cancer therapy-associated neurocognitive side effects. For instance, psychostimulants such as methylphenidate [157–161] and modafinil [162, 163] are promising agents for treatment of cancer therapy-related cognitive dysfunction. In addition, donepezil—a reversible acetylcholinesterase inhibitor used to treat Alzheimer's type dementia—has shown to improve cognitive function, mood, and quality of life in patients with brain and small cell lung cancer [82, 164].

Optimal management of fatigue, mood disorders, and other comorbidities (e.g., treatment of anemia) needs to be an integral part of patient management [115, 165–169]. Cognitive and behavioral intervention strategies used in patients with stroke and traumatic brain injury may also be employed in patients with chemotherapy-associated cognitive dysfunction [170]. These interventions often focus on compensatory strategies, stress management, energy conservation, and psycho-education. External memory aids (e.g., memory notebooks, pagers) have been among the most widely used interventions [171]. Other non-pharmacological interventions include meditation [172], exercise [160, 173, 174], and regulation of sleep [175].

Mood and Other Psychiatric Disorders in Cancer Patients

Introduction

Cancer patients have a high risk of developing mood alterations or other psychiatric illness [176]. Depression, anxiety, adjustment disorder, neurobehavioral, and neurocognitive changes are common and collectively affect the majority of cancer patients [177, 178].

Moreover, nonspecific emotional distress through the combined impact of social, psychological, and religious or spiritual stressors is highly prevalent in cancer patients, ranging from approximately 15–45% [179]. The National Comprehensive Cancer Network recommends screening for mood and psychiatric illness routinely in all cancer patients [180], and some guidelines for patient evaluation have been released (e.g., [181, 182]).

Psychiatric and Neurobehavioral Symptoms in Brain Tumor Patients

Among all cancer patients, brain tumor patients are considered at highest risk of developing neuropsychiatric symptoms during their course of disease [183, 184]. Quality of life studies have identified a high degree of depression, anxiety, and reduced family functioning in brain tumor patients [185].

Notably, changes in *mood, cognition, behavior, and personality* can be the initial sign or symptom of a tumor of the central nervous system [186]. In addition, neuropsychiatric conditions can occur as a consequence of cancer treatment, including cranial irradiation [187], chemotherapy [119, 188, 189], and various other medications (e.g., corticosteroids) [190–193]. Therefore, clinicians need to be aware of neuropsychiatric symptoms in brain tumor patients at time of diagnosis and throughout their course of the disease in order to recognize symptoms early and to initiate appropriate treatment as soon as possible. For instance, more than 90% of patients with high-grade gliomas reported symptoms of depression prior to and up to six months after surgery [194].

Neuropsychiatric symptoms are usually *nonspecific* in terms of tumor localization, and also do not strictly correlate with the type or the degree of malignancy [194, 195]. Brain tumors in frontal and temporal brain regions may produce varying degrees of neurobehavioral changes, including mood alterations, impaired judgment, inattentiveness, irritability, memory deficits, and frank dementia [196–198]. Patients with tumors affecting the corpus callosum, cingulate gyrus and deep and midline brain areas frequently demonstrate neurobehavioral symptoms, personality changes and affective disorders, reported in up to 90% of patients [199]. Psychotic symptoms (e.g., paranoid delusions) can be part of the presentation [198]. Tumors affecting the cerebellum and neural pathways within the cerebellar network system may also produce neurocognitive deficits, psychotic symptoms, and mood alterations [200].

Psychiatric and Neurobehavioral Symptoms in Patients with Cancer Outside the Nervous System

The prevalence of mood alterations is significantly higher in cancer patients when compared to the general population. Approximately 10–50% of cancer patients are considered to have some emotional distress or depression [176, 201, 202].

Cancer patients frequently report some degree of anxiety. Anxiety can have several etiologies in cancer patients and can occur alongside or independent of a mood alteration. As physical, psychological, or cognitive symptoms can be the lead manifestation of anxiety, the diagnosis can be challenging [182, 203]. Depression and anxiety are significantly more common in patients with advanced illness, poorly controlled pain, physical deficits, younger cancer patients, and prior history of affective disorders [202, 204–206].

Interestingly, the presence of mood alterations has been associated with poor survival in cancer patients [207–209]. Studying the connection between mood and emotional state on the one hand and the immune system and tumor behavior on the other hand has been an increasingly relevant topic in the field of psychoneuroimmunology [209, 210].

Making matters even more complex, there appears to be a high level of discordance between patient and physician-reported affective disorders, such as depression [194, 211], posing a challenge to the optimal management of cancer patients. In general, a patient's perception of mood alterations is considered higher when compared with the clinician's perception. This discordance and underestimation from side of the health care professionals may result in insufficient treatment of patients with such symptoms.

Treatment of cancer patients with adjustment disorder, anxiety, depression, or other psychiatric illness is similar to management of non-cancer patients. Pharmacological and non-pharmacological interventions, such as cognitive-behavioral therapy, supportive psychotherapy, psychosocial interventions, and support groups have been used successfully in cancer patients [212–214].

The choice of a specific intervention or medication will depend on several factors, including the predominant symptoms, comorbid medical conditions, and potential side effect profiles. For instance, a psychostimulant (e.g., methylphenidate or modafinil) may be a reasonable choice as a monotherapy, or in combination with a less sedating antidepressant (e.g., SSRI) for a fatigued cancer patient with depression.

A multidisciplinary team approach will be essential for optimal patient management. A detailed discussion on possible therapeutic interventions is beyond the scope of this book chapter but can be found elsewhere (e.g., [215, 216]).

Fatigue in Cancer Patients

Introduction

Fatigue is a major reason of impaired quality of life in cancer patients [217–219]. Fatigue can be associated with the cancer itself [220], or specific kinds of treatment, such as radiation or chemotherapy [221]. Fatigue is usually described as a permanent and distressing sense of tiredness that is not significantly relieved by rest or sleep. Patients may perceive fatigue as physical (e.g., generalized muscle weakness), or mental (e.g., decreased motivation and lack of energy), or a combination of both.

Prevalence and Epidemiology

The majority of cancer patients experience fatigue during their course of disease [222]. The current literature suggests a prevalence of fatigue in over 60% of patients [223, 224]. In patients with a diverse group of underlying cancers, fatigue was present in 50–75% of patients at time of diagnosis, but was even more common throughout their course of treatment, including chemotherapy or radiation, affecting up to 93–95% of patients [224]. While the majority of patients report significant fatigue during active therapy [225], fatigue can persist for years after cancer treatment completion and can be a major cause of chronic morbidity in long-term survivors [220]. Notably, chronic fatigue in cancer survivors has been increasingly recognized and occurs at a prevalence ranging from 15 to 50% [226–235].

Etiology and Mechanisms

Given the complexity of potential causes, fatigue is considered multifactorial in origin in most cancer patients (Table 12.4). For instance, it is well known that specific

Table 12.4 Possible factors to cause or contribute to fatigue in cancer patients

Cancer and cancer therapy related factors	• Tumor and brain area involved
	• Surgery
	• Radiation therapy
	• Chemotherapy
	• Biologics and molecular-targeted therapies
	• Hormonal therapy
Comorbidities and cancer associated conditions	• Sleep dysregulation
	• Mood disorder
	• Anxiety
	• Pain
	• Electrolyte imbalance
	• Liver dysfunction
	• Renal disease
	• Thyroid dysfunction
	• Diabetes mellitus
	• Cardiopulmonary disease
	• Anemia
	• Infections
	• Rheumatological disease
	• Neurological disease
Psychosocial factors	• Personal and emotional stressors
Medications	• Antiepileptic drugs
	• Opiates
	• Anxiolytics
	• Cardiac medications
	• Hypnotics
	• Analgesics
Constitutional factors	• Behavioral factors (eating behavior, lack of exercise, alcohol and other substance abuse)
	• Obesity or anorexia

comorbidities, such as anemia, liver, or renal disease, cause fatigue [236]. In addition, many medications, mood-related issues, pain, sleep dysfunction, lifestyle patterns, cognitive deficits, and psychological stressors are associated with fatigue [237–239].

This issue is particularly relevant in the management of brain tumor patients, in whom mood dysfunction, cognitive impairment, sleep alterations, and fatigue appear to coexist and correlate with each other, causing significant impairment of quality of life in affected patients [240].

The pathophysiological mechanisms that induce chronic fatigue remain poorly understood. Possible causal factors include physical conditions, mood and cognitive dysfunction, metabolic and neuroendocrine factors, and an increase in circulatory inflammatory cytokines [241]. A chronic inflammatory state has been recognized as one major etiological factor in the manifestation of chronic fatigue during cancer treatment or in the post-treatment phase [220]. Specifically, TNF-α signaling has been identified as a likely contributor to chemotherapy-induced fatigue in breast cancer patients [238]. In addition, alterations of sympathetic and parasympathetic nervous system activity have been identified as a possible cause of cancer-related fatigue [242, 243]. However, given a considerable variability of fatigue in cancer patients, various other factors unrelated to treatment, or the underlying disease, appear to influence the degree of fatigue in individual patients. Modulators of fatigue include genetic factors [241], metabolic, behavioral, and lifestyle factors [244, 245], mood-related issues [231], or psychological factors [232, 246] (Table 12.4).

Patient Evaluation

Every patient managed for cancer during the active treatment or post-treatment phase should be evaluated for symptoms of fatigue [247]. Several questionnaires are used and have been validated to assess symptoms and severity of fatigue in cancer patients [237, 248–250]. With the increasing awareness of the high prevalence of fatigue among cancer patients, evaluation and management of fatigue has become an important aspect of supportive care in oncology and survivorship. Several guidelines have been published from expert groups, including the American Society of Clinical Oncology and the National Comprehensive Cancer Network, recommending screening for fatigue at the initial visit, during active treatment, and in the post-treatment setting [251, 252]. A multidisciplinary team approach is necessary in most patients to rule out and treat conditions that might be unrelated to cancer but possibly to treatment, such as endocrine dysfunction (e.g., thyroid disease), medical comorbidities (such as anemia), untreated depression, or sleep disorders [206].

Treatment and Management

Any comorbidity or treatable condition possibly contributing to the manifestation of fatigue will need to be addressed and treated as the initial step in patient management (Table 12.4). For instance, correction of an underlying anemia or thyroid dysfunction [253] and treatment of depression or sleep disorder [254] need to be integral part of patient management.

A variety of therapeutic interventions, evaluated in randomized controlled clinical trials, have resulted in improvement of chronic fatigue in cancer patients. Treatment interventions shown to have clinical benefit include pharmacological interventions (e.g., psychostimulants such as methylphenidate and modafinil) [161, 255], and non-pharmacological interventions [252, 256], such as relaxation techniques [257–259], acupuncture [260], meditation [172, 261, 262], lifestyle interventions [263–266], and physical exercise [217, 252, 267–271]. In addition, strategies aiming at a reduction of psychosocial stressors may involve lifestyle modifications and can improve symptoms of fatigue [252, 272–275].

Collectively, management of fatigue requires identification and treatment of comorbidities and several conditions known to cause fatigue [276]. The complexity of potential etiological factors in cancer-related fatigue underscores the importance of an individualized and multi-disciplinary team approach in patient management. Both pharmacological and non-pharmacological interventions have shown promise to improve fatigue-related symptoms and increase quality of life in cancer patients.

Acknowledgements J.D. has been supported by a Paul Calabresi Career Development Award for Clinical Oncology, the Stephen E. and Catherine Pappas Cancer Research Foundation Award, the American Academy of Neurology Foundation, the American Cancer Society, and the National Institute of Health. JD received generous philanthropic support from the Sheila McPhee and Ronald Tawil family foundations.

References

1. Wefel JS, Kayl AE, Meyers CA. Neuropsychological dysfunction associated with cancer and cancer therapies: a conceptual review of an emerging target. Br J Cancer. 2004;90(9):1691–6.
2. Wefel JS, Witgert ME, Meyers CA. Neuropsychological sequelae of non-central nervous system cancer and cancer therapy. Neuropsychol Rev. 2008;18(2):121–31.
3. Noll KR, Sullaway C, Ziu M, Weinberg JS, Wefel JS. Relationships between tumor grade and neurocognitive functioning in patients with glioma of the left temporal lobe prior to surgical resection. Neuro Oncol. 2015;17(4):580–7.
4. Wu AS, Witgert ME, Lang FF, Xiao L, Bekele BN, Meyers CA, et al. Neurocognitive function before and after surgery for insular gliomas. J Neurosurg. 2011;115(6):1115–25.
5. Heimans JJ, Reijneveld JC. Factors affecting the cerebral network in brain tumor patients. J Neurooncol. 2012;108(2):231–7.
6. Derks J, Reijneveld JC, Douw L. Neural network alterations underlie cognitive deficits in brain tumor patients. Curr Opin Oncol. 2014;26(6):627–33.
7. Shields LB, Choucair AK. Management of low-grade gliomas: a review of patient-perceived quality of life and neurocognitive outcome. World Neurosurg. 2014;82(1–2):e299–309.
8. Guerrini R, Rosati A, Giordano F, Genitori L, Barba C. The medical and surgical treatment of tumoral seizures: current and future perspectives. Epilepsia. 2013;54(Suppl 9):84–90.
9. van Breemen MS, Wilms EB, Vecht CJ. Epilepsy in patients with brain tumours: epidemiology, mechanisms, and management. Lancet Neurol. 2007;6(5):421–30.
10. Bosma I, Vos MJ, Heimans JJ, Taphoorn MJ, Aaronson NK, Postma TJ, et al. The course of neurocognitive functioning in high-grade glioma patients. Neuro Oncol. 2007;9(1):53–62.
11. Racine CA, Li J, Molinaro AM, Butowski N, Berger MS. Neurocognitive function in newly diagnosed low-grade glioma patients undergoing surgical resection with awake mapping techniques. Neurosurgery. 2015;77(3):371–9 (discussion 9).
12. Tucha O, Smely C, Preier M, Lange KW. Cognitive deficits before treatment among patients with brain tumors. Neurosurgery. 2000;47(2):324–33 (discussion 33–4).
13. Johnson DR, Sawyer AM, Meyers CA, O'Neill BP, Wefel JS. Early measures of cognitive function predict survival in patients with newly diagnosed glioblastoma. Neuro Oncol. 2012;14 (6):808–16.
14. Duffau H, Mandonnet E, Gatignol P, Capelle L. Functional compensation of the claustrum: lessons from low-grade glioma surgery. J Neuro Oncol. 2007;81(3):327–9.

15. Rosenberg K, Liebling R, Avidan G, Perry D, Siman-Tov T, Andelman F, et al. Language related reorganization in adult brain with slow growing glioma: fMRI prospective case-study. Neurocase. 2008;14(6):465–73.

16. Krieg SM, Sollmann N, Hauck T, Ille S, Foerschler A, Meyer B, et al. Functional language shift to the right hemisphere in patients with language-eloquent brain tumors. PLoS ONE. 2013;8(9): e75403.

17. Kayl AE, Meyers CA. Does brain tumor histology influence cognitive function? Neuro Oncol. 2003;5(4):255–60.

18. Gott PS. Cognitive abilities following right and left hemispherectomy. Cortex. 1973;9(3):266–74 (A journal devoted to the study of the nervous system and behavior).

19. Gottwald B, Wilde B, Mihajlovic Z, Mehdorn HM. Evidence for distinct cognitive deficits after focal cerebellar lesions. J Neurol Neurosurg Psychiatry. 2004;75(11):1524–31.

20. Schmahmann JD, Sherman JC. The cerebellar cognitive affective syndrome. Brain J Neurol. 1998;121(Pt 4):561–79.

21. Riva D, Giorgi C. The cerebellum contributes to higher functions during development: evidence from a series of children surgically treated for posterior fossa tumours. Brain J Neurol. 2000;123(Pt 5):1051–61.

22. Schmahmann JD, Weilburg JB, Sherman JC. The neuropsychiatry of the cerebellum—insights from the clinic. Cerebellum. 2007;6(3):254–67.

23. Ronning C, Sundet K, Due-Tonnessen B, Lundar T, Helseth E. Persistent cognitive dysfunction secondary to cerebellar injury in patients treated for posterior fossa tumors in childhood. Pediatr Neurosurg. 2005;41(1):15–21.

24. D'Aes T, Marien P. Cognitive and affective disturbances following focal brainstem lesions: a review and report of three cases. Cerebellum. 2015;14(3):317–40.

25. Crossen JR, Garwood D, Glatstein E, Neuwelt EA. Neurobehavioral sequelae of cranial irradiation in adults: a review of radiation-induced encephalopathy. J Clin Oncol. 1994;12 (3):627–42.

26. Keime-Guibert F, Napolitano M, Delattre JY. Neurological complications of radiotherapy and chemotherapy. J Neurol. 1998;245(11):695–708.

27. DeAngelis LM, Delattre JY, Posner JB. Radiation-induced dementia in patients cured of brain metastases. Neurology. 1989;39(6):789–96.

28. Duffner PK. Long-term effects of radiation therapy on cognitive and endocrine function in children with leukemia and brain tumors. Neurologist. 2004;10(6):293–310.

29. Perry A, Schmidt RE. Cancer therapy-associated CNS neuropathology: an update and review of the literature. Acta Neuropathol. 2006;111(3):197–212.

30. Edelstein K, Spiegler BJ, Fung S, Panzarella T, Mabbott DJ, Jewitt N, et al. Early aging in adult survivors of childhood medulloblastoma: long-term neurocognitive, functional, and physical outcomes. Neuro Oncol. 2011;13(5):536–45.

31. Roman DD, Sperduto PW. Neuropsychological effects of cranial radiation: current knowledge and future directions. Int J Radiat Oncol Biol Phys. 1995;31(4):983–98.

32. Anderson VA, Godber T, Smibert E, Weiskop S, Ekert H. Cognitive and academic outcome following cranial irradiation and chemotherapy in children: a longitudinal study. Br J Cancer. 2000;82(2):255–62.

33. Moore BD 3rd, Copeland DR, Ried H, Levy B. Neurophysiological basis of cognitive deficits in long-term survivors of childhood cancer. Arch Neurol. 1992;49(8):809–17.

34. Abayomi OK. Pathogenesis of irradiation-induced cognitive dysfunction. Acta Oncol. 1996;35(6):659–63.

35. Surma-aho O, Niemela M, Vilkki J, Kouri M, Brander A, Salonen O, et al. Adverse long-term effects of brain radiotherapy in adult low-grade glioma patients. Neurology. 2001;56 (10):1285–90.

36. Laack NN, Brown PD. Cognitive sequelae of brain radiation in adults. Semin Oncol. 2004;31(5):702–13.

37. Tallet AV, Azria D, Barlesi F, Spano JP, Carpentier AF, Goncalves A, et al. Neurocognitive function impairment after whole brain radiotherapy for brain metastases: actual assessment. Radiat Oncol. 2012;7:77.

38. Gondi V, Hermann BP, Mehta MP, Tome WA. Hippocampal dosimetry predicts neurocognitive function impairment after fractionated stereotactic radiotherapy for benign or low-grade adult brain tumors. Int J Radiat Oncol Biol Phys. 2013;85 (2):348–54.

39. Prust MJ, Jafari-Khouzani K, Kalpathy-Cramer J, Polaskova P, Batchelor TT, Gerstner ER, et al. Standard chemoradiation for glioblastoma results in progressive brain volume loss. Neurology. 2015;85(8):683–91.

40. Lee AW, Kwong DL, Leung SF, Tung SY, Sze WM, Sham JS, et al. Factors affecting risk of symptomatic temporal lobe necrosis: significance of fractional dose and treatment time. Int J Radiat Oncol Biol Phys. 2002;53(1):75–85.

41. Lawrence YR, Li XA, el Naqa I, Hahn CA, Marks LB, Merchant TE, et al. Radiation dose-volume effects in the brain. Int J Radiat Oncol Biol Phys. 2010;76(3 Suppl):S20–7.

42. Dietrich J, Monje M, Wefel J, Meyers C. Clinical patterns and biological correlates of cognitive dysfunction associated with cancer therapy. Oncologist. 2008;13(12):1285–95.

43. Andreassen CN, Alsner J. Genetic variants and normal tissue toxicity after radiotherapy: a systematic review. Radiother Oncol J Eur Soc Ther Radiol Oncol. 2009;92(3):299–309.

44. West CM, Barnett GC. Genetics and genomics of radiotherapy toxicity: towards prediction. Genome Med. 2011;3(8):52.

45. Barnett GC, West CM, Dunning AM, Elliott RM, Coles CE, Pharoah PD, et al. Normal tissue reactions to radiotherapy: towards tailoring treatment dose by genotype. Nat Rev Cancer. 2009;9(2):134–42.

46. Krull KR, Zhang N, Santucci A, Srivastava DK, Krasin MJ, Kun LE, et al. Long-term decline in intelligence among adult survivors of childhood acute lymphoblastic leukemia treated with cranial radiation. Blood. 2013;122(4):550–3.

47. Lai R, Abrey LE, Rosenblum MK, DeAngelis LM. Treatment-induced leukoencephalopathy in primary CNS lymphoma: a clinical and autopsy study. Neurology. 2004;62(3): 451–6.

48. Sheline GE. Radiation therapy of brain tumors. Cancer. 1977;39 (2 Suppl):873–81.

49. Rubin P, Gash DM, Hansen JT, Nelson DF, Williams JP. Disruption of the blood-brain barrier as the primary effect of CNS irradiation. Radiother Oncol J Eur Soc Ther Radiol Oncol. 1994;31(1):51–60.

50. Behin A, Delattre JY. Complications of radiation therapy on the brain and spinal cord. Semin Neurol. 2004;24(4):405–17.

51. Meyers CA, Geara F, Wong PF, Morrison WH. Neurocognitive effects of therapeutic irradiation for base of skull tumors. Int J Radiat Oncol Biol Phys. 2000;46(1):51–5.

52. Gregor A, Cull A, Traynor E, Stewart M, Lander F, Love S. Neuropsychometric evaluation of long-term survivors of adult brain tumours: relationship with tumour and treatment parameters. Radiother Oncol J Eur Soc Ther Radiol Oncol. 1996;41 (1):55–9.

53. Armstrong CL, Gyato K, Awadalla AW, Lustig R, Tochner ZA. A critical review of the clinical effects of therapeutic irradiation

damage to the brain: the roots of controversy. Neuropsychol Rev. 2004;14(1):65–86.

54. Wong CS, Van der Kogel AJ. Mechanisms of radiation injury to the central nervous system: implications for neuroprotection. Mol Interv. 2004;4(5):273–84.

55. Strother DR. Tumors of the central nervous system. In: Pizzo PPA, Poplack DG, editors. Principles and practice of pediatric oncology. Philadelphia: Lippincott, Williams and Wilkins; 2002. p. 751–824.

56. Dropcho EJ. Central nervous system injury by therapeutic irradiation. Neurol Clin. 1991;9(4):969–88.

57. Oppenheimer JH, Levy ML, Sinha U, el-Kadi H, Apuzzo ML, Luxton G, et al. Radionecrosis secondary to interstitial brachytherapy: correlation of magnetic resonance imaging and histopathology. Neurosurgery. 1992;31(2):336–43.

58. Morris JG, Grattan-Smith P, Panegyres PK, O'Neill P, Soo YS, Langlands AO. Delayed cerebral radiation necrosis. Q J Med. 1994;87(2):119–29.

59. Chong VE, Fan YF. Radiation-induced temporal lobe necrosis. AJNR Am J Neuroradiol. 1997;18(4):784–5.

60. Fouladi M, Chintagumpala M, Laningham FH, Ashley D, Kellie SJ, Langston JW, et al. White matter lesions detected by magnetic resonance imaging after radiotherapy and high-dose chemotherapy in children with medulloblastoma or primitive neuroectodermal tumor. J Clin Oncol. 2004;22(22):4551–60.

61. Constine LS, Konski A, Ekholm S, McDonald S, Rubin P. Adverse effects of brain irradiation correlated with MR and CT imaging. Int J Radiat Oncol Biol Phys. 1988;15 (2):319–30.

62. Dietrich J, Klein JP. Imaging of cancer therapy-induced central nervous system toxicity. Neurol Clin. 2014;32(1):147–57.

63. Monaco EA 3rd, Faraji AH, Berkowitz O, Parry PV, Hadelsberg U, Kano H, et al. Leukoencephalopathy after whole-brain radiation therapy plus radiosurgery versus radiosurgery alone for metastatic lung cancer. Cancer. 2013;119(1):226–32.

64. Sabsevitz DS, Bovi JA, Leo PD, Laviolette PS, Rand SD, Mueller WM, et al. The role of pre-treatment white matter abnormalities in developing white matter changes following whole brain radiation: a volumetric study. J Neurooncol. 2013;114(3):291–7.

65. Sneed PK, Suh JH, Goetsch SJ, Sanghavi SN, Chappell R, Buatti JM, et al. A multi-institutional review of radiosurgery alone vs. radiosurgery with whole brain radiotherapy as the initial management of brain metastases. Int J Radiat Oncol Biol Phys. 2002;53(3):519–26.

66. Soffietti R, Ruda R, Trevisan E. Brain metastases: current management and new developments. Curr Opin Oncol. 2008;20 (6):676–84.

67. McDuff SG, Taich ZJ, Lawson JD, Sanghvi P, Wong ET, Barker FG 2nd, et al. Neurocognitive assessment following whole brain radiation therapy and radiosurgery for patients with cerebral metastases. J Neurol Neurosurg Psychiatry. 2013;84 (12):1384–91.

68. Soffietti R, Kocher M, Abacioglu UM, Villa S, Fauchon F, Baumert BG, et al. A European organisation for research and treatment of cancer phase III trial of adjuvant whole-brain radiotherapy versus observation in patients with one to three brain metastases from solid tumors after surgical resection or radiosurgery: quality-of-life results. J Clin Oncol. 2013;31(1):65–72.

69. Gondi V, Paulus R, Bruner DW, Meyers CA, Gore EM, Wolfson A, et al. Decline in tested and self-reported cognitive functioning after prophylactic cranial irradiation for lung cancer: pooled secondary analysis of radiation therapy oncology group randomized trials 0212 and 0214. Int J Radiat Oncol Biol Phys. 2013;86(4):656–64.

70. Correa DD, DeAngelis LM, Shi W, Thaler HT, Lin M, Abrey LE. Cognitive functions in low-grade gliomas: disease and treatment effects. J Neurooncol. 2007;81(2):175–84.

71. Kiehna EN, Mulhern RK, Li C, Xiong X, Merchant TE. Changes in attentional performance of children and young adults with localized primary brain tumors after conformal radiation therapy. J Clin Oncol. 2006;24(33):5283–90.

72. Klein M, Heimans JJ, Aaronson NK, van der Ploeg HM, Grit J, Muller M, et al. Effect of radiotherapy and other treatment-related factors on mid-term to long-term cognitive sequelae in low-grade gliomas: a comparative study. Lancet. 2002;360(9343):1361–8.

73. Douw L, Klein M, Fagel SS, van den Heuvel J, Taphoorn MJ, Aaronson NK, et al. Cognitive and radiological effects of radiotherapy in patients with low-grade glioma: long-term follow-up. Lancet Neurol. 2009;8(9):810–8.

74. Belka C, Budach W, Kortmann RD, Bamberg M. Radiation induced CNS toxicity–molecular and cellular mechanisms. Br J Cancer. 2001;85(9):1233–9.

75. Noble M, Dietrich J. Intersections between neurobiology and oncology: tumor origin, treatment and repair of treatment-associated damage. Trends Neurosci. 2002;25(2):103–7.

76. Monje ML, Palmer T. Radiation injury and neurogenesis. Curr Opin Neurol. 2003;16(2):129–34.

77. Fike JR, Rola R, Limoli CL. Radiation response of neural precursor cells. Neurosurg Clin N Am. 2007;18(1):115–27.

78. Monje M, Dietrich J. Cognitive side effects of cancer therapy demonstrate a functional role for adult neurogenesis. Behav Brain Res. 2012;227(2):376–9.

79. Gondi V, Pugh SL, Tome WA, Caine C, Corn B, Kanner A, et al. Preservation of memory with conformal avoidance of the hippocampal neural stem-cell compartment during whole-brain radiotherapy for brain metastases (RTOG 0933): a phase II multi-institutional trial. J Clin Oncol. 2014;32(34):3810–6.

80. Attia A, Page BR, Lesser GJ, Chan M. Treatment of radiation-induced cognitive decline. Curr Treat Options Oncol. 2014;15 (4):539–50.

81. Castellino SM, Tooze JA, Flowers L, Hill DF, McMullen KP, Shaw EG, et al. Toxicity and efficacy of the acetylcholinesterase (AChe) inhibitor donepezil in childhood brain tumor survivors: a pilot study. Pediatr Blood Cancer. 2012;59(3):540–7.

82. Shaw EG, Rosdhal R, D'Agostino RB Jr, Lovato J, Naughton MJ, Robbins ME, et al. Phase II study of donepezil in irradiated brain tumor patients: effect on cognitive function, mood, and quality of life. J Clin Oncol. 2006;24(9):1415–20.

83. Brown PD, Pugh S, Laack NN, Wefel JS, Khuntia D, Meyers C, et al. Memantine for the prevention of cognitive dysfunction in patients receiving whole-brain radiotherapy: a randomized, double-blind, placebo-controlled trial. Neuro Oncol. 2013;15(10):1429–37.

84. Butler RW, Haser JK. Neurocognitive effects of treatment for childhood cancer. Ment Retard Dev Disabil Res Rev. 2006;12 (3):184–91.

85. Alvarez JA, Scully RE, Miller TL, Armstrong FD, Constine LS, Friedman DL, et al. Long-term effects of treatments for childhood cancers. Curr Opin Pediatr. 2007;19(1):23–31.

86. van Dam FS, Schagen SB, Muller MJ, Boogerd W, vd Wall E, Droogleever Fortuyn ME, et al. Impairment of cognitive function in women receiving adjuvant treatment for high-risk breast cancer: high-dose versus standard-dose chemotherapy. J Natl Cancer Inst. 1998;90(3):210–8.

87. Schagen SB, van Dam FS, Muller MJ, Boogerd W, Lindeboom J, Bruning PF. Cognitive deficits after postoperative adjuvant chemotherapy for breast carcinoma. Cancer. 1999;85(3):640–50.

88. Brezden CB, Phillips KA, Abdolell M, Bunston T, Tannock IF. Cognitive function in breast cancer patients receiving adjuvant chemotherapy. J Clin Oncol. 2000;18(14):2695–701.

89. Ahles TA, Saykin A. Cognitive effects of standard-dose chemotherapy in patients with cancer. Cancer Invest. 2001;19 (8):812–20.

90. Schagen SB, Muller MJ, Boogerd W, Rosenbrand RM, van Rhijn D, Rodenhuis S, et al. Late effects of adjuvant chemotherapy on cognitive function: a follow-up study in breast cancer patients. Ann Oncol. 2002;13(9):1387–97.

91. Anderson-Hanley C, Sherman ML, Riggs R, Agocha VB, Compas BE. Neuropsychological effects of treatments for adults with cancer: a meta-analysis and review of the literature. J Int Neuropsychol Soc. 2003;9(7):967–82.

92. Tannock IF, Ahles TA, Ganz PA, Van Dam FS. Cognitive impairment associated with chemotherapy for cancer: report of a workshop. J Clin Oncol. 2004;22(11):2233–9.

93. Wefel JS, Lenzi R, Theriault RL, Davis RN, Meyers CA. The cognitive sequelae of standard-dose adjuvant chemotherapy in women with breast carcinoma: results of a prospective, randomized, longitudinal trial. Cancer. 2004;100(11):2292–9.

94. Schagen SB, Muller MJ, Boogerd W, Mellenbergh GJ, van Dam FS. Change in cognitive function after chemotherapy: a prospective longitudinal study in breast cancer patients. J Natl Cancer Inst. 2006;98(23):1742–5.

95. Hurria A, Rosen C, Hudis C, Zuckerman E, Panageas KS, Lachs MS, et al. Cognitive function of older patients receiving adjuvant chemotherapy for breast cancer: a pilot prospective longitudinal study. J Am Geriatr Soc. 2006;54(6):925–31.

96. Ahles TA, Saykin AJ. Candidate mechanisms for chemotherapy-induced cognitive changes. Nat Rev Cancer. 2007;7(3):192–201.

97. Vardy J, Wefel JS, Ahles T, Tannock IF, Schagen SB. Cancer and cancer-therapy related cognitive dysfunction: an international perspective from the Venice cognitive workshop. Ann Oncol. 2008;19(4):623–9.

98. Moleski M. Neuropsychological, neuroanatomical, and neurophysiological consequences of CNS chemotherapy for acute lymphoblastic leukemia. Arch Clin Neuropsychol. 2000;15 (7):603–30.

99. Shilling V, Jenkins V, Morris R, Deutsch G, Bloomfield D. The effects of adjuvant chemotherapy on cognition in women with breast cancer-preliminary results of an observational longitudinal study. Breast. 2005;14(2):142–50.

100. Jansen CE, Miaskowski C, Dodd M, Dowling G, Kramer J. A metaanalysis of studies of the effects of cancer chemotherapy on various domains of cognitive function. Cancer. 2005;104(10):2222–33.

101. Grosshans DR, Meyers CA, Allen PK, Davenport SD, Komaki R. Neurocognitive function in patients with small cell lung cancer: effect of prophylactic cranial irradiation. Cancer. 2008;112 (3):589–95.

102. Cherrier MM, Aubin S, Higano CS. Cognitive and mood changes in men undergoing intermittent combined androgen blockade for non-metastatic prostate cancer. Psycho Oncol. 2009;18(3):237–47.

103. Hess LM, Chambers SK, Hatch K, Hallum A, Janicek MF, Buscema J, et al. Pilot study of the prospective identification of changes in cognitive function during chemotherapy treatment for advanced ovarian cancer. J Supp Oncol. 2010;8(6):252–8.

104. Wefel JS, Vidrine DJ, Marani SK, Swartz RJ, Veramonti TL, Meyers CA, et al. A prospective study of cognitive function in men with non-seminomatous germ cell tumors. Psycho Oncol. 2014;23(6):626–33.

105. Meyers CA, Abbruzzese JL. Cognitive functioning in cancer patients: effect of previous treatment. Neurology. 1992;42 (2):434–6.

106. Matsuda T, Takayama T, Tashiro M, Nakamura Y, Ohashi Y, Shimozuma K. Mild cognitive impairment after adjuvant

107. Wefel JS, Saleeba AK, Buzdar AU, Meyers CA. Acute and late onset cognitive dysfunction associated with chemotherapy in women with breast cancer. Cancer. 2010;116(14):3348–56.

108. Heflin LH, Meyerowitz BE, Hall P, Lichtenstein P, Johansson B, Pedersen NL, et al. Cancer as a risk factor for long-term cognitive deficits and dementia. J Natl Cancer Inst. 2005;97(11):854–6.

109. Roe CM, Behrens MI, Xiong C, Miller JP, Morris JC. Alzheimer disease and cancer. Neurology. 2005;64(5):895–8.

110. Wefel JS, Meyers CA. Cancer as a risk factor for dementia: a house built on shifting sand. J Natl Cancer Inst. 2005;97 (11):788–9.

111. Hermelink K, Untch M, Lux MP, Kreienberg R, Beck T, Bauerfeind I, et al. Cognitive function during neoadjuvant chemotherapy for breast cancer: results of a prospective, multicenter, longitudinal study. Cancer. 2007;109(9):1905–13.

112. Vardy J, Rourke S, Tannock IF. Evaluation of cognitive function associated with chemotherapy: a review of published studies and recommendations for future research. J Clin Oncol. 2007;25 (17):2455–63.

113. Jansen CE, Dodd MJ, Miaskowski CA, Dowling GA, Kramer J. Preliminary results of a longitudinal study of changes in cognitive function in breast cancer patients undergoing chemotherapy with doxorubicin and cyclophosphamide. Psycho Oncol. 2008;17(12):1189–95.

114. Hutchinson AD, Hosking JR, Kichenadasse G, Mattiske JK, Wilson C. Objective and subjective cognitive impairment following chemotherapy for cancer: a systematic review. Cancer Treat Rev. 2012;38(7):926–34.

115. Joly F, Rigal O, Noal S, Giffard B. Cognitive dysfunction and cancer: which consequences in terms of disease management? Psycho Oncol. 2011;20(12):1251–8.

116. Koppelmans V, Breteler MM, Boogerd W, Seynaeve C, Gundy C, Schagen SB. Neuropsychological performance in survivors of breast cancer more than 20 years after adjuvant chemotherapy. J Clin Oncol. 2012;30(10):1080–6.

117. Dropcho EJ. Neurotoxicity of cancer chemotherapy. Semin Neurol. 2004;24(4):419–26.

118. Minisini A, Atalay G, Bottomley A, Puglisi F, Piccart M, Biganzoli L. What is the effect of systemic anticancer treatment on cognitive function? Lancet Oncol. 2004;5(5):273–82.

119. Dietrich J, Wen P. Neurologic complications of chemotherapy. In: Schiff D, Kesari S, Wen P, editors. Cancer neurology in clinical practice. 2nd ed. Totowa, New Jersey: Humana Press Inc.; 2008. p. 287–326.

120. Shapiro WR, Chernik NL, Posner JB. Necrotizing encephalopathy following intraventricular instillation of methotrexate. Arch Neurol. 1973;28(2):96–102.

121. Bashir R, Hochberg FH, Linggood RM, Hottleman K. Pre-irradiation internal carotid artery BCNU in treatment of glioblastoma multiforme. J Neurosurg. 1988;68(6):917–9.

122. Rosenblum MK, Delattre JY, Walker RW, Shapiro WR. Fatal necrotizing encephalopathy complicating treatment of malignant gliomas with intra-arterial BCNU and irradiation: a pathological study. J Neurooncol. 1989;7(3):269–81.

123. Newton HB. Intra-arterial chemotherapy of primary brain tumors. Curr Treat Options Oncol. 2005;6(6):519–30.

124. Fliessbach K, Helmstaedter C, Urbach H, Althaus A, Pels H, Linnebank M, et al. Neuropsychological outcome after chemotherapy for primary CNS lymphoma: a prospective study. Neurology. 2005;64(7):1184–8.

125. Neuwelt EA, Guastadisegni PE, Varallyay P, Doolittle ND. Imaging changes and cognitive outcome in primary CNS

lymphoma after enhanced chemotherapy delivery. AJNR Am J Neuroradiol. 2005;26(2):258–65.

126. Dietrich J, Han R, Yang Y, Mayer-Proschel M, Noble M. CNS progenitor cells and oligodendrocytes are targets of chemotherapeutic agents in vitro and in vivo. J Biol. 2006;5(7):22.

127. Han R, Yang YM, Dietrich J, Luebke A, Mayer-Proschel M, Noble M. Systemic 5-fluorouracil treatment causes a syndrome of delayed myelin destruction in the central nervous system. J Biol. 2008;7(4):12.

128. Seigers R, Schagen SB, Beerling W, Boogerd W, van Tellingen O, van Dam FS, et al. Long-lasting suppression of hippocampal cell proliferation and impaired cognitive performance by methotrexate in the rat. Behav Brain Res. 2008;186(2):168–75.

129. Winocur G, Vardy J, Binns MA, Kerr L, Tannock I. The effects of the anti-cancer drugs, methotrexate and 5-fluorouracil, on cognitive function in mice. Pharmacol Biochem Behav. 2006;85(1):66–75.

130. Fardell JE, Vardy J, Logge W, Johnston I. Single high dose treatment with methotrexate causes long-lasting cognitive dysfunction in laboratory rodents. Pharmacol Biochem Behav. 2010;97(2):333–9.

131. Seigers R, Schagen SB, Van Tellingen O, Dietrich J. Chemotherapy-related cognitive dysfunction: current animal studies and future directions. Brain Imaging Behav. 2013;7(4):453–9.

132. Dietrich J, Prust M, Kaiser J. Chemotherapy, cognitive impairment and hippocampal toxicity. Neuroscience. 2015;309:224–32.

133. Mahaley MS Jr, Whaley RA, Blue M, Bertsch L. Central neurotoxicity following intracarotid BCNU chemotherapy for malignant gliomas. J Neurooncol. 1986;3(4):297–314.

134. Hook CC, Kimmel DW, Kvols LK, Scheithauer BW, Forsyth PA, Rubin J, et al. Multifocal inflammatory leukoencephalopathy with 5-fluorouracil and levamisole. Ann Neurol. 1992;31(3):262–7.

135. Kaya E, Keskin L, Aydogdu I, Kuku I, Bayraktar N, Erkut MA. Oxidant/antioxidant parameters and their relationship with chemotherapy in Hodgkin's lymphoma. J Int Med Res. 2005;33(6):687–92.

136. Papageorgiou M, Stiakaki E, Dimitriou H, Malliaraki N, Notas G, Castanas E, et al. Cancer chemotherapy reduces plasma total antioxidant capacity in children with malignancies. Leuk Res. 2005;29(1):11–6.

137. Kennedy DD, Ladas EJ, Rheingold SR, Blumberg J, Kelly KM. Antioxidant status decreases in children with acute lymphoblastic leukemia during the first six months of chemotherapy treatment. Pediatr Blood Cancer. 2005;44(4):378–85.

138. Noble M, Mayer-Proschel M, Li Z, Dong T, Cui W, Proschel C, et al. Redox biology in normal cells and cancer: restoring function of the redox/Fyn/c-Cbl pathway in cancer cells offers new approaches to cancer treatment. Free Radic Biol Med. 2015;79:300–23.

139. Chen Y, Lomnitski L, Michaelson DM, Shohami E. Motor and cognitive deficits in apolipoprotein E-deficient mice after closed head injury. Neuroscience. 1997;80(4):1255–62.

140. Hoffmeyer S, Burk O, von Richter O, Arnold HP, Brockmoller J, Johne A, et al. Functional polymorphisms of the human multidrug-resistance gene: multiple sequence variations and correlation of one allele with P-glycoprotein expression and activity in vivo. Proc Natl Acad Sci USA. 2000;97(7):3473–8.

141. Ahles TA, Saykin AJ, Noll WW, Furstenberg CT, Guerin S, Cole B, et al. The relationship of APOE genotype to neuropsychological performance in long-term cancer survivors treated with standard dose chemotherapy. Psycho Oncol. 2003;12(6):612–9.

142. McAllister TW, Ahles TA, Saykin AJ, Ferguson RJ, McDonald BC, Lewis LD, et al. Cognitive effects of cytotoxic cancer chemotherapy: predisposing risk factors and potential treatments. Current Psychiatr Rep. 2004;6(5):364–71.

143. Okcu MF, Selvan M, Wang LE, Stout L, Erana R, Airewele G, et al. Glutathione S-transferase polymorphisms and survival in primary malignant glioma. Clin Cancer Res. 2004;10(8):2618–25.

144. Muramatsu T, Johnson DR, Finch RA, Johnson LK, Leffert JJ, Lin ZP, et al. Age-related differences in vincristine toxicity and biodistribution in wild-type and transporter-deficient mice. Oncol Res. 2004;14(7–8):331–43.

145. Jamroziak K, Balcerczak E, Cebula B, Kowalczyk M, Panczyk M, Janus A, et al. Multi-drug transporter MDR1 gene polymorphism and prognosis in adult acute lymphoblastic leukemia. Pharmacol Rep. 2005;57(6):882–8.

146. Linnebank M, Pels H, Kleczar N, Farmand S, Fliessbach K, Urbach H, et al. MTX-induced white matter changes are associated with polymorphisms of methionine metabolism. Neurology. 2005;64(5):912–3.

147. Krajinovic M, Robaey P, Chiasson S, Lemieux-Blanchard E, Rouillard M, Primeau M, et al. Polymorphisms of genes controlling homocysteine levels and IQ score following the treatment for childhood ALL. Pharmacogenomics. 2005;6(3):293–302.

148. Largillier R, Etienne-Grimaldi MC, Formento JL, Ciccolini J, Nebbia JF, Ginot A, et al. Pharmacogenetics of capecitabine in advanced breast cancer patients. Clin Cancer Res. 2006;12(18):5496–502.

149. Fishel ML, Vasko MR, Kelley MR. DNA repair in neurons: so if they don't divide what's to repair? Mutat Res. 2007;614(1–2):24–36.

150. Abrey LE, Batchelor TT, Ferreri AJ, Gospodarowicz M, Pulczynski EJ, Zucca E, et al. Report of an international workshop to standardize baseline evaluation and response criteria for primary CNS lymphoma. J Clin Oncol. 2005;23(22):5034–43.

151. Correa DD, Maron L, Harder H, Klein M, Armstrong CL, Calabrese P, et al. Cognitive functions in primary central nervous system lymphoma: literature review and assessment guidelines. Ann Oncol. 2007;18(7):1145–51.

152. Krull KR, Okcu MF, Potter B, Jain N, Dreyer Z, Kamdar K, et al. Screening for neurocognitive impairment in pediatric cancer long-term survivors. J Clin Oncol. 2008;26(25):4138–43.

153. Meyers CA, Hess KR, Yung WK, Levin VA. Cognitive function as a predictor of survival in patients with recurrent malignant glioma. J Clin Oncol. 2000;18(3):646–50.

154. Herman MA, Tremont-Lukats I, Meyers CA, Trask DD, Froseth C, Renschler MF, et al. Neurocognitive and functional assessment of patients with brain metastases: a pilot study. Am J Clin Oncol. 2003;26(3):273–9.

155. Kaiser J, Bledowski C, Dietrich J. Neural correlates of chemotherapy-related cognitive impairment. Cortex. 2014;54:33–50 (A journal devoted to the study of the nervous system and behavior).

156. Horky LL, Gerbaudo VH, Zaitsev A, Plesniak W, Hainer J, Govindarajulu U, et al. Systemic chemotherapy decreases brain glucose metabolism. Ann Clin Trans Neurol. 2014;1(10):788–98.

157. Lower EE, Fleishman S, Cooper A, Zeldis J, Faleck H, Yu Z, et al. Efficacy of dexmethylphenidate for the treatment of fatigue after cancer chemotherapy: a randomized clinical trial. J Pain Symptom Manage. 2009;38(5):650–62.

158. Conklin HM, Khan RB, Reddick WE, Helton S, Brown R, Howard SC, et al. Acute neurocognitive response to methylphenidate among survivors of childhood cancer: a randomized, double-blind, cross-over trial. J Pediatr Psychol. 2007;32(9):1127–39.

159. Mulhern RK, Khan RB, Kaplan S, Helton S, Christensen R, Bonner M, et al. Short-term efficacy of methylphenidate: a

randomized, double-blind, placebo-controlled trial among survivors of childhood cancer. J Clin Oncol. 2004;22(23):4795–803.

160. Schwartz AL, Thompson JA, Masood N. Interferon-induced fatigue in patients with melanoma: a pilot study of exercise and methylphenidate. Oncol Nurs Forum. 2002;29(7):E85–90.

161. Meyers CA, Weitzner MA, Valentine AD, Levin VA. Methylphenidate therapy improves cognition, mood, and function of brain tumor patients. J Clin Oncol. 1998;16(7):2522–7.

162. Kohli S, Fisher SG, Tra Y, Adams MJ, Mapstone ME, Wesnes KA, et al. The effect of modafinil on cognitive function in breast cancer survivors. Cancer. 2009;115(12):2605–16.

163. Lundorff LE, Jonsson BH, Sjogren P. Modafinil for attentional and psychomotor dysfunction in advanced cancer: a double-blind, randomised, cross-over trial. Palliat Med. 2009;23(8):731–8.

164. Jatoi A, Kahanic SP, Frytak S, Schaefer P, Foote RL, Sloan J, et al. Donepezil and vitamin E for preventing cognitive dysfunction in small cell lung cancer patients: preliminary results and suggestions for future study designs. Supp Care Cancer. 2005;13(1):66–9.

165. Jacobsen PB, Garland LL, Booth-Jones M, Donovan KA, Thors CL, Winters E, et al. Relationship of hemoglobin levels to fatigue and cognitive functioning among cancer patients receiving chemotherapy. J Pain Symptom Manage. 2004;28(1):7–18.

166. Heras P, Argyriou AA, Papapetropoulos S, Karagiannis S, Argyriou K, Mitsibounas D. The impact of weekly dosing of epoetin alfa on the haematological parameters and on the quality of life of anaemic cancer patients. Eur J Cancer Care. 2005;14(2):108–12.

167. O'Shaughnessy JA, Vukelja SJ, Holmes FA, Savin M, Jones M, Royall D, et al. Feasibility of quantifying the effects of epoetin alfa therapy on cognitive function in women with breast cancer undergoing adjuvant or neoadjuvant chemotherapy. Clin Breast Cancer. 2005;5(6):439–46.

168. Massa E, Madeddu C, Lusso MR, Gramignano G, Mantovani G. Evaluation of the effectiveness of treatment with erythropoietin on anemia, cognitive functioning and functions studied by comprehensive geriatric assessment in elderly cancer patients with anemia related to cancer chemotherapy. Crit Rev Oncol Hematol. 2006;57(2):175–82.

169. Iconomou G, Koutras A, Karaivazoglou K, Kalliolias GD, Assimakopoulos K, Argyriou AA, et al. Effect of epoetin alpha therapy on cognitive function in anaemic patients with solid tumours undergoing chemotherapy. Eur J Cancer Care. 2008;17(6):535–41.

170. Ferguson RJ, Ahles TA, Saykin AJ, McDonald BC, Furstenberg CT, Cole BF, et al. Cognitive-behavioral management of chemotherapy-related cognitive change. Psycho Oncol. 2007;16(8):772–7.

171. Evans JJ, Wilson BA, Needham P, Brentnall S. Who makes good use of memory aids? Results of a survey of people with acquired brain injury. J Int Neuropsychol Soc. 2003;9(6):925–35.

172. Biegler KA, Chaoul MA, Cohen L. Cancer, cognitive impairment, and meditation. Acta Oncol. 2009;48(1):18–26.

173. Hsieh CC, Sprod LK, Hydock DS, Carter SD, Hayward R, Schneider CM. Effects of a supervised exercise intervention on recovery from treatment regimens in breast cancer survivors. Oncol Nurs Forum. 2008;35(6):909–15.

174. Mitchell SA. Cancer-related fatigue: state of the science. PM & R J Injury Funct Rehabil. 2010;2(5):364–83.

175. Berger AM. Update on the state of the science: sleep-wake disturbances in adult patients with cancer. Oncol Nurs Forum. 2009;36(4):E165–77.

176. Derogatis LR, Morrow GR, Fetting J, Penman D, Piasetsky S, Schmale AM, et al. The prevalence of psychiatric disorders among cancer patients. JAMA. 1983;249(6):751–7.

177. Kathol RG, Mutgi A, Williams J, Clamon G, Noyes R Jr. Diagnosis of major depression in cancer patients according to four sets of criteria. Am J Psychiatr. 1990;147(8):1021–4.

178. Chochinov HM. Depression in cancer patients. Lancet Oncol. 2001;2(8):499–505.

179. Strong V, Waters R, Hibberd C, Rush R, Cargill A, Storey D, et al. Emotional distress in cancer patients: the Edinburgh Cancer Centre symptom study. Br J Cancer. 2007;96(6):868–74.

180. Distress management. Clinical practice guidelines. J Natl Compr Cancer Netw JNCCN. 2003;1(3):344–74.

181. Jacobsen PB, Donovan KA, Trask PC, Fleishman SB, Zabora J, Baker F, et al. Screening for psychologic distress in ambulatory cancer patients. Cancer. 2005;103(7):1494–502.

182. Andersen BL, DeRubeis RJ, Berman BS, Gruman J, Champion VL, Massie MJ, et al. Screening, assessment, and care of anxiety and depressive symptoms in adults with cancer: an American Society of Clinical Oncology guideline adaptation. J Clin Oncol. 2014;32(15):1605–19.

183. Pringle AM, Taylor R, Whittle IR. Anxiety and depression in patients with an intracranial neoplasm before and after tumour surgery. Br J Neurosurg. 1999;13(1):46–51.

184. Mainio A, Hakko H, Niemela A, Koivukangas J, Rasanen P. Depression and functional outcome in patients with brain tumors: a population-based 1-year follow-up study. J Neurosurg. 2005;103(5):841–7.

185. Weitzner MA, Meyers CA. Cognitive functioning and quality of life in malignant glioma patients: a review of the literature. Psycho Oncol. 1997;6(3):169–77.

186. Madhusoodanan S, Danan D, Moise D. Psychiatric manifestations of brain tumors: diagnostic implications. Expert Rev Neurother. 2007;7(4):343–9.

187. Proctor SJ, Kernaham J, Taylor P. Depression as component of post-cranial irradiation somnolence syndrome. Lancet. 1981;1(8231):1215–6.

188. Holland J, Fasanello S, Onuma T. Psychiatric symptoms associated with L-asparaginase administration. J Psychiatr Res. 1974;10(2):105–13.

189. Adams F, Quesada JR, Gutterman JU. Neuropsychiatric manifestations of human leukocyte interferon therapy in patients with cancer. JAMA. 1984;252(7):938–41.

190. Stiefel FC, Breitbart WS, Holland JC. Corticosteroids in cancer: neuropsychiatric complications. Cancer Invest. 1989;7(5):479–91.

191. Gaudreau JD, Gagnon P, Harel F, Roy MA, Tremblay A. Psychoactive medications and risk of delirium in hospitalized cancer patients. J Clin Oncol. 2005;23(27):6712–8.

192. Gaudreau JD, Gagnon P, Roy MA, Harel F, Tremblay A. Opioid medications and longitudinal risk of delirium in hospitalized cancer patients. Cancer. 2007;109(11):2365–73.

193. Dietrich J, Rao K, Pastorino S, Kesari S. Corticosteroids in brain cancer patients: benefits and pitfalls. Expert Rev Clin Pharmacol. 2011;4(2):233–42.

194. Litofsky NS, Farace E, Anderson F, Jr., Meyers CA, Huang W, Laws ER, Jr. Depression in patients with high-grade glioma: results of the Glioma outcomes project. Neurosurgery. 2004;54(2):358–66 (discussion 66–7).

195. Gupta RK, Kumar R. Benign brain tumours and psychiatric morbidity: a 5-years retrospective data analysis. Aust NZ J Psychiatr. 2004;38(5):316–9.

196. Belyi BI. Mental impairment in unilateral frontal tumours: role of the laterality of the lesion. Int J Neurosci. 1987;32(3–4):799–810.

197. Cummings JL. Dementia: a clinical approach. Stoneham, MA: Butterworth-Heinemann; 1992.

198. Price T, Lovell MR. Neuropsychiatric aspects of brain tumors. Yudovsky SC, Hales RE, editors. Washington, D.C.: American Psychiatric Publishing; 2002.

199. Nasrallah HA, McChesney CM. Psychopathology of corpus callosum tumors. Biol Psychiat. 1981;16(7):663–9.

200. Schmahmann JD. Disorders of the cerebellum: ataxia, dysmetria of thought, and the cerebellar cognitive affective syndrome. J Neuropsychiatr Clin Neurosci. 2004;16(3):367–78.

201. Massie MJ. Prevalence of depression in patients with cancer. J Natl Cancer Inst Monogr. 2004;32:57–71.

202. Walker J, Hansen CH, Martin P, Symeonides S, Ramessur R, Murray G, et al. Prevalence, associations, and adequacy of treatment of major depression in patients with cancer: a cross-sectional analysis of routinely collected clinical data. Lancet Psychiatr. 2014;1(5):343–50.

203. Holland JC. Anxiety and cancer: the patient and the family. J Clin Psychiatr. 1989;50(Suppl):20–5.

204. Bukberg J, Penman D, Holland JC. Depression in hospitalized cancer patients. Psychosom Med. 1984;46(3):199–212.

205. Meyers CA. Neurocognitive dysfunction in cancer patients. Oncology (Williston Park). 2000;14(1):75–9 (discussion 9, 81–2, 5).

206. Valentine AD, Meyers CA. Cognitive and mood disturbance as causes and symptoms of fatigue in cancer patients. Cancer. 2001;92(6 Suppl):1694–8.

207. Mainio A, Tuunanen S, Hakko H, Niemela A, Koivukangas J, Rasanen P. Decreased quality of life and depression as predictors for shorter survival among patients with low-grade gliomas: a follow-up from 1990 to 2003. Eur Arch Psychiatry Clin Neurosci. 2006;256(8):516–21.

208. Mainio A, Hakko H, Niemela A, Koivukangas J, Rasanen P. Gender difference in relation to depression and quality of life among patients with a primary brain tumor. Eur Psychiatr J Assoc Eur Psychiatrists. 2006;21(3):194–9.

209. Steel JL, Geller DA, Gamblin TC, Olek MC, Carr BI. Depression, immunity, and survival in patients with hepatobiliary carcinoma. J Clin Oncol. 2007;25(17):2397–405.

210. Irwin MR. Depression and risk of cancer progression: an elusive link. J Clin Oncol. 2007;25(17):2343–4.

211. Ell K, Sanchez K, Vourlekis B, Lee PJ, Dwight-Johnson M, Lagomasino I, et al. Depression, correlates of depression, and receipt of depression care among low-income women with breast or gynecologic cancer. J Clin Oncol. 2005;23(13):3052–60.

212. Spiegel D, Bloom JR, Yalom I. Group support for patients with metastatic cancer. A randomized outcome study. Arch Gen Psychiatr. 1981;38(5):527–33.

213. Davis BD, Fernandez F, Adams F, Holmes V, Levy JK, Lewis D, et al. Diagnosis of dementia in cancer patients. Cognitive impairment in these patients can go unrecognized. Psychosomatics. 1987;28(4):175–9.

214. Williams S, Dale J. The effectiveness of treatment for depression/depressive symptoms in adults with cancer: a systematic review. Br J Cancer. 2006;94(3):372–90.

215. Akechi T, Okuyama T, Onishi J, Morita T, Furukawa TA. Psychotherapy for depression among incurable cancer patients. Cochrane Database Syst Rev. 2008;2:CD005537.

216. Ostuzzi G, Matcham F, Dauchy S, Barbui C, Hotopf M. Antidepressants for the treatment of depression in people with cancer. Cochrane Database Syst Rev. 2015;6:CD011006.

217. Cella D, Peterman A, Passik S, Jacobsen P, Breitbart W. Progress toward guidelines for the management of fatigue. Oncology (Williston Park). 1998;12(11A):369–77.

218. Barsevick A, Frost M, Zwinderman A, Hall P, Halyard M. I'm so tired: biological and genetic mechanisms of cancer-related fatigue. Qual Life Res Int J Qual Life Aspects Treat Care Rehabil. 2010;19(10):1419–27.

219. Dagnelie PC, Pijls-Johannesma MC, Lambin P, Beijer S, De Ruysscher D, Kempen GI. Impact of fatigue on overall quality of life in lung and breast cancer patients selected for high-dose radiotherapy. Ann Oncol. 2007;18(5):940–4.

220. Bower JE. Cancer-related fatigue–mechanisms, risk factors, and treatments. Natl Rev Clin Oncol. 2014;11(10):597–609.

221. Mock V. Evidence-based treatment for cancer-related fatigue. J Natl Cancer Inst Monogr. 2004;32:112–8.

222. Stone P, Richardson A, Ream E, Smith AG, Kerr DJ, Kearney N. Cancer-related fatigue: inevitable, unimportant and untreatable? Results of a multi-centre patient survey. Cancer Fatigue Forum. Ann Oncol 2000;11(8):971–5.

223. Pelletier G, Verhoef MJ, Khatri N, Hagen N. Quality of life in brain tumor patients: the relative contributions of depression, fatigue, emotional distress, and existential issues. J Neurooncol. 2002;57(1):41–9.

224. Stasi R, Abriani L, Beccaglia P, Terzoli E, Amadori S. Cancer-related fatigue: evolving concepts in evaluation and treatment. Cancer. 2003;98(9):1786–801.

225. Schmidt ME, Chang-Claude J, Vrieling A, Heinz J, Flesch-Janys D, Steindorf K. Fatigue and quality of life in breast cancer survivors: temporal courses and long-term pattern. J Cancer Surviv Res Pract. 2012;6(1):11–9.

226. Sprauten M, Haugnes HS, Brydoy M, Kiserud C, Tandstad T, Bjoro T, et al. Chronic fatigue in 812 testicular cancer survivors during long-term follow-up: increasing prevalence and risk factors. Ann Oncol. 2015;26(10):2133–40.

227. Jones JM, Olson K, Catton P, Catton CN, Fleshner NE, Krzyzanowska MK, et al. Cancer-related fatigue and associated disability in post-treatment cancer survivors. J Cancer Surviv Res Pract. 2016;10(1):51–61.

228. Seland M, Holte H, Bjoro T, Schreiner T, Bollerslev J, Loge JH, et al. Chronic fatigue is prevalent and associated with hormonal dysfunction in long-term non-Hodgkin lymphoma survivors treated with radiotherapy to the head and neck region. Leuk Lymphoma. 2015;56(12):3306–14.

229. Husson O, Mols F, van de Poll-Franse L, de Vries J, Schep G, Thong MS. Variation in fatigue among 6011 (long-term) cancer survivors and a normative population: a study from the population-based PROFILES registry. Supp Care Cancer. 2015;23(7):2165–74.

230. Sawka AM, Naeem A, Jones J, Lowe J, Segal P, Goguen J, et al. Persistent posttreatment fatigue in thyroid cancer survivors: a scoping review. Endocrinol Metab Clin North Am. 2014;43 (2):475–94.

231. Wang XS, Zhao F, Fisch MJ, O'Mara AM, Cella D, Mendoza TR, et al. Prevalence and characteristics of moderate to severe fatigue: a multicenter study in cancer patients and survivors. Cancer. 2014;120(3):425–32.

232. Daniels LA, Oerlemans S, Krol AD, Creutzberg CL, van de Poll-Franse LV. Chronic fatigue in Hodgkin lymphoma survivors and associations with anxiety, depression and comorbidity. Br J Cancer. 2014;110(4):868–74.

233. Oerlemans S, Mols F, Issa DE, Pruijt JH, Peters WG, Lybeert M, et al. A high level of fatigue among long-term survivors of non-Hodgkin's lymphoma: results from the longitudinal population-based PROFILES registry in the south of the Netherlands. Haematologica. 2013;98(3):479–86.

234. Berger AM, Gerber LH, Mayer DK. Cancer-related fatigue: implications for breast cancer survivors. Cancer. 2012;118(8 Suppl):2261–9.

235. Andrykowski MA, Donovan KA, Laronga C, Jacobsen PB. Prevalence, predictors, and characteristics of off-treatment fatigue in breast cancer survivors. Cancer. 2010;116(24):5740–8. 236.

236. Swain MG. Fatigue in chronic disease. Clin Sci (Lond). 2000;99 (1):1–8.

237. Portenoy RK, Itri LM. Cancer-related fatigue: guidelines for evaluation and management. Oncologist. 1999;4(1):1–10.

238. Bower JE, Ganz PA, Irwin MR, Kwan L, Breen EC, Cole SW. Inflammation and behavioral symptoms after breast cancer treatment: do fatigue, depression, and sleep disturbance share a common underlying mechanism? J Clin Oncol. 2011;29 (26):3517–22.

239. Clanton NR, Klosky JL, Li C, Jain N, Srivastava DK, Mulrooney D, et al. Fatigue, vitality, sleep, and neurocognitive functioning in adult survivors of childhood cancer: a report from the childhood cancer survivor study. Cancer. 2011;117 (11):2559–68.

240. Fox SW, Lyon D, Farace E. Symptom clusters in patients with high-grade glioma. J Nurs Sch. 2007;39(1):61–7.

241. Saligan LN, Olson K, Filler K, Larkin D, Cramp F, Yennurajalingam S, et al. The biology of cancer-related fatigue: a review of the literature. Supp Care Cancer. 2015;23(8):2461–78.

242. Fagundes CP, Murray DM, Hwang BS, Gouin JP, Thayer JF, Sollers JJ 3rd, et al. Sympathetic and parasympathetic activity in cancer-related fatigue: more evidence for a physiological substrate in cancer survivors. Psychoneuroendocrinology. 2011;36 (8):1137–47.

243. Crosswell AD, Lockwood KG, Ganz PA, Bower JE. Low heart rate variability and cancer-related fatigue in breast cancer survivors. Psychoneuroendocrinology. 2014;45:58–66.

244. Zeller B, Loge JH, Kanellopoulos A, Hamre H, Wyller VB, Ruud E. Chronic fatigue in long-term survivors of childhood lymphomas and leukemia: persistence and associated clinical factors. J Pediatr Hematol Oncol. 2014;36(6):438–44.

245. Rogers LQ, Markwell SJ, Courneya KS, McAuley E, Verhulst S. Physical activity type and intensity among rural breast cancer survivors: patterns and associations with fatigue and depressive symptoms. J Cancer Surviv Res Pract. 2011;5(1):54–61.

246. Corbett T, Devane D, Walsh JC, Groarke A, McGuire BE. Protocol for a systematic review of psychological interventions for cancer-related fatigue in post-treatment cancer survivors. Syst Rev. 2015;4:174.

247. Mock V, Atkinson A, Barsevick A, Cella D, Cimprich B, Cleeland C, et al. NCCN practice guidelines for cancer-related fatigue. Oncology (Williston Park). 2000;14(11A):151–61.

248. Jacobsen PB. Assessment of fatigue in cancer patients. J Natl Cancer Inst Monogr. 2004;32:93–7.

249. Radbruch L, Strasser F, Elsner F, Goncalves JF, Loge J, Kaasa S, et al. Fatigue in palliative care patients—an EAPC approach. Palliat Med. 2008;22(1):13–32.

250. Mortimer JE, Barsevick AM, Bennett CL, Berger AM, Cleeland C, DeVader SR, et al. Studying cancer-related fatigue: report of the NCCN scientific research committee. J Natl Compr Cancer Netw JNCCN. 2010;8(12):1331–9.

251. Dy SM, Lorenz KA, Naeim A, Sanati H, Walling A, Asch SM. Evidence-based recommendations for cancer fatigue, anorexia, depression, and dyspnea. J Clin Oncol. 2008;26(23):3886–95.

252. Bower JE, Bak K, Berger A, Breitbart W, Escalante CP, Ganz PA, et al. Screening, assessment, and management of fatigue in adult survivors of cancer: an American Society of clinical oncology clinical practice guideline adaptation. J Clin Oncol. 2014;32(17):1840–50.

253. Bohlius J, Tonia T, Nuesch E, Juni P, Fey MF, Egger M, et al. Effects of erythropoiesis-stimulating agents on fatigue- and anaemia-related symptoms in cancer patients: systematic review and meta-analyses of published and unpublished data. Br J Cancer. 2014;111(1):33–45.

254. Howell D, Oliver TK, Keller-Olaman S, Davidson JR, Garland S, Samuels C, et al. Sleep disturbance in adults with cancer: a systematic review of evidence for best practices in assessment and management for clinical practice. Ann Oncol. 2014;25 (4):791–800.

255. Mucke M, Cuhls H, Peuckmann-Post V, Minton O, Stone P, Radbruch L. Pharmacological treatments for fatigue associated with palliative care. Cochrane Database Syst Rev. 2015;5: CD006788.

256. Lotfi-Jam K, Carey M, Jefford M, Schofield P, Charleson C, Aranda S. Nonpharmacologic strategies for managing common chemotherapy adverse effects: a systematic review. J Clin Oncol. 2008;26(34):5618–29.

257. Yuen HK, Mitcham M, Morgan L. Managing post-therapy fatigue for cancer survivors using energy conservation training. J Allied Health. 2006;35(2):121E–39E (Epub 2006/07/01).

258. Barsevick AM, Dudley W, Beck S, Sweeney C, Whitmer K, Nail L. A randomized clinical trial of energy conservation for patients with cancer-related fatigue. Cancer. 2004;100(6):1302–10.

259. Hoffman CJ, Ersser SJ, Hopkinson JB, Nicholls PG, Harrington JE, Thomas PW. Effectiveness of mindfulness-based stress reduction in mood, breast- and endocrine-related quality of life, and well-being in stage 0 to III breast cancer: a randomized, controlled trial. J Clin Oncol. 2012;30(12):1335–42.

260. Mao JJ, Xie SX, Farrar JT, Stricker CT, Bowman MA, Bruner D, et al. A randomised trial of electro-acupuncture for arthralgia related to aromatase inhibitor use. Eur J Cancer. 2014;50(2):267–76.

261. Cramer H, Rabsilber S, Lauche R, Kummel S, Dobos G. Yoga and meditation for menopausal symptoms in breast cancer survivors-a randomized controlled trial. Cancer. 2015;121 (13):2175–84.

262. Bower JE, Crosswell AD, Stanton AL, Crespi CM, Winston D, Arevalo J, et al. Mindfulness meditation for younger breast cancer survivors: a randomized controlled trial. Cancer. 2015;121 (8):1231–40.

263. Smits A, Smits E, Lopes A, Das N, Hughes G, Talaat A, et al. Body mass index, physical activity and quality of life of ovarian cancer survivors: time to get moving? Gynecol Oncol. 2015;139 (1):148–54.

264. Koutoukidis DA, Knobf MT, Lanceley A. Obesity, diet, physical activity, and health-related quality of life in endometrial cancer survivors. Nutr Rev. 2015;73(6):399–408.

265. George SM, Alfano CM, Neuhouser ML, Smith AW, Baumgartner RN, Baumgartner KB, et al. Better postdiagnosis diet quality is associated with less cancer-related fatigue in breast cancer survivors. J Cancer Surviv Res Pract. 2014;8(4):680–7.

266. Ligibel J. Lifestyle factors in cancer survivorship. J Clin Oncol. 2012;30(30):3697–704.

267. Fong DY, Ho JW, Hui BP, Lee AM, Macfarlane DJ, Leung SS, et al. Physical activity for cancer survivors: meta-analysis of randomised controlled trials. BMJ. 2012;344:e70.

268. Tian L, Lu HJ, Lin L, Hu Y. Effects of aerobic exercise on cancer-related fatigue: a meta-analysis of randomized controlled trials. Supp Care Cancer. 2016;24(2):969–83.

269. Lopes-Junior LC, Bomfim EO, Nascimento LC, Nunes MD, Pereira-da-Silva G, Lima RA. Non-pharmacological interventions to manage fatigue and psychological stress in children and adolescents with cancer: an integrative review. Eur J Cancer Care. 2016;25(6):921–35.

270. Meneses-Echavez JF, Gonzalez-Jimenez E, Ramirez-Velez R. Effects of supervised exercise on cancer-related fatigue in breast cancer survivors: a systematic review and meta-analysis. BMC Cancer. 2015;15:77.

271. Meneses-Echavez JF, Gonzalez-Jimenez E, Ramirez-Velez R. Supervised exercise reduces cancer-related fatigue: a systematic review. J Physiother. 2015;61(1):3–9.

272. Reinertsen KV, Cvancarova M, Loge JH, Edvardsen H, Wist E, Fossa SD. Predictors and course of chronic fatigue in long-term breast cancer survivors. J Cancer Surviv Res Pract. 2010;4 (4):405–14.

273. Guest DD, Evans EM, Rogers LQ. Diet components associated with perceived fatigue in breast cancer survivors. Eur J Cancer Care. 2013;22(1):51–9.

274. Schmitz KH, Neuhouser ML, Agurs-Collins T, Zanetti KA, Cadmus-Bertram L, Dean LT, et al. Impact of obesity on cancer survivorship and the potential relevance of race and ethnicity. J Natl Cancer Inst. 2013;105(18):1344–54.

275. Zick SM, Sen A, Han-Markey TL, Harris RE. Examination of the association of diet and persistent cancer-related fatigue: a pilot study. Oncol Nurs Forum. 2013;40(1):E41–9.

276. Cancer-related fatigue. Clinical practice guidelines in oncology. J Natl Compr Cancer Netw JNCCN. 2003;1(3):308–31.

Paraneoplastic Syndromes of the Nervous System as Complications of Cancer

13

Myrna R. Rosenfeld and Josep Dalmau

Introduction

In patients with cancer the development of neurological symptoms usually represents metastatic involvement of the nervous system or complications secondary to coagulopathy, infection, metabolic and nutritional deficits, and toxic effects of cancer therapy [1]. A neurologic disorder is defined as paraneoplastic when none of the above causes are detected or when specific cancer-related immunological mechanisms are involved. Paraneoplastic neurologic disorders are important for several reasons. They may affect any part of the central and peripheral nervous system and mimic other neurologic complications of cancer. The paraneoplastic disorder usually develops before the presence of a cancer is known and its prompt recognition may help to uncover the neoplasm. The neurologic symptoms are often severe and can result in the patient's death. Early intervention with oncologic and immunotherapy may result in stabilization or improvement of neurologic symptoms although the potential for improvement depends on the type of syndrome and associated immune responses [2, 3].

Frequency and Pathogenesis

It is estimated that less than 1% of patients with cancer develop clinically symptomatic paraneoplastic neurologic syndromes, but the frequency varies with the type of cancer.

For example, while 10–30% of patients with plasma cell dyscrasias or thymoma develop paraneoplastic neurologic symptoms, far less than 1% of patients with breast or ovarian cancer develop these disorders.

Most paraneoplastic neurologic disorders appear to be mediated by immunological mechanisms. The occurrence of serum and cerebrospinal (CSF) antibodies that target proteins selectively expressed by the tumor and nervous system has suggested a mechanism whereby the tumor expression of neuronal proteins triggers an anti-tumor immune response that cross-reacts with the nervous system. In general, the efficacy of the immune response against the tumor is limited or not sustained enough to control its growth, but the effects on the nervous system are prominent.

In some antibody-associated paraneoplastic syndromes, the accompanying cytotoxic T-cell mechanisms appear to be the main pathogenic effectors [4, 5]. The autoantigens of these disorders are usually intracellular, and the associated antibodies are detectable in serum and CSF of the patients. Although not directly pathogenic, these antibodies may play an ancillary role in enhancing the immune response [6]. The detection of these antibodies, also known as paraneoplastic or onconeuronal antibodies (Table 13.1), forms part of the diagnostic tests that confirm the paraneoplastic nature of the neurologic disorder and directs the search of the underlying tumor. In contrast, there are antibody-associated paraneoplastic syndromes in which the humoral immune response plays a dominant pathogenic role [7, 8]. These include the autoimmune encephalitis syndromes and some disorders of the neuromuscular junction and peripheral nerves that associate with antibodies to proteins of the neuronal cell surface, the synapse or the neuromuscular junction (further referred to as cell surface antibodies). In general these syndromes are more responsive to immunotherapies and for some syndromes, patients can have complete or near complete recoveries with treatment [9].

Several other paraneoplastic disorders, including inflammatory neuropathies or myopathies, are likely immune

M.R. Rosenfeld (✉)
Institut d'Investigació Biomèdica August Pi i Sunyer (IDIBAPS), CELLEX, Neuroimmunology, P3A, c/Casanova 143, 08036 Barcelona, Catalonia, Spain
e-mail: mrrosenf@clinic.ub.es

J. Dalmau
Hospital Clínic, Institució Catalana de Recerca i Estudis Avançats (ICREA), Institut d'Investigació Biomèdica August Pi i Sunyer (IDIBAPS), CELLEX, Neuroimmunology, P3A, c/Casanova 143, 08036 Barcelona, Catalonia, Spain
e-mail: jdalmau@clinic.ub.es

© Springer International Publishing AG 2018
D. Schiff et al. (eds.), *Cancer Neurology in Clinical Practice*,
DOI 10.1007/978-3-319-57901-6_13

Table 13.1 Paraneoplastic antibodies*

Antibody	Associated cancer	Syndrome
Anti-Hu	SCLC, other	Encephalomyelitis, sensory neuronopathy
Anti-Yo	Gynecological, breast	Cerebellar degeneration
Anti-Ri	Breast, gynecological, SCLC	Cerebellar ataxia, opsoclonus, brainstem encephalitis
Anti-Tr/DNER	Hodgkin's lymphoma	Cerebellar degeneration
Anti-CV2/CRMP5	SCLC, thymoma, other	Encephalomyelitis, striatal encephalitis (chorea), cerebellar degeneration, uveitis, peripheral neuropathy
Anti-Ma proteins[a]	Testicular germ-cell tumors and other neoplasms	Limbic, diencephalic (hypothalamic) and upper brainstem encephalitis; rarely cerebellar degeneration
Anti-amphiphysin	Breast, SCLC	Stiff-man syndrome, encephalomyelitis
Anti-recoverin	Retinopathy	SCLC
Anti-bipolar cells of the retina[b]	Retinopathy	Melanoma

*The detection of these antibodies confirms the paraneoplastic nature of the neurologic disorder

[a]Antibodies limited to Ma2 (also called anti-Ta antibodies) usually associate with limbic and brainstem encephalitis and germ-cell tumors. Antibodies directed at Ma1 and Ma2 usually associate with brainstem encephalitis, cerebellar degeneration and several types of cancer (lung, breast, ovary, among others)

[b]Antibodies to other retinal proteins such as transducin-β, rhodopsin, and arrestin among others have also been described in some patients with melanoma and retinopathy. The diagnostic value of these antibodies is unclear

mediated and associate with infiltrates of mononuclear cells, cytotoxic T-cells, or deposits of IgG and complement in the involved nerve or muscle [10, 11]. Patients with these disorders have a variety of antibodies that when present support the diagnosis of the inflammatory process. In general these antibodies do not serve as surrogate markers of paraneoplasia. However, recent reports show that patients with dermatomyositis and antibodies to TF1γ are more likely to have an associated cancer compared to patients without these antibodies suggest that the immune classification of these disorders is evolving [12].

In addition to immune-mediated mechanisms, there are other paraneoplastic causes of neurologic dysfunction, including competition between the tumor and nervous system for substrates (e.g., glucose), inappropriate secretion of hormones or cytokines by tumor cells (e.g., anti-diuretic hormone), among others. This chapter focuses on the syndromes that occur in association with immune-mediated mechanisms.

Diagnosis of Paraneoplastic Neurologic Disorders: General Concepts

There are four clinical features that complicate the diagnosis of most paraneoplastic neurologic disorders, (1) the frequent presentation of neurologic symptoms before the diagnosis of the cancer, (2) the occurrence of similar syndromes without a cancer association, (3) the absence of well characterized antibodies in a variable proportion of patients, and (4) the small size of the associated tumors, which are usually difficult to demonstrate at the time of neurologic symptom presentation [13].

Presentation of Symptoms

The majority of paraneoplastic neurologic syndromes develop rapidly in a matter of days or weeks. Patients who develop syndromes of the central nervous system often describe prodromic gastrointestinal or upper respiratory tract symptoms resembling a viral illness that is followed by the neurologic symptoms. Most patients with syndromes affecting the central nervous system have CSF abnormalities such as pleocytosis, increased protein concentration, oligoclonal bands, and elevated IgG index that suggest an inflammatory or immune-mediated process.

In about 60% of patients, the paraneoplastic neurologic disorder develops before the presence of a tumor is known. There are a few exceptions such as the paraneoplastic retinopathy that affects patients with melanoma ("melanoma-associated retinopathy"); patients with this disorder usually have a history of metastatic melanoma [14].

Syndromes Similar to Paraneoplastic Disorders May Occur Without a Cancer Association

Although some syndromes are more frequently associated with cancer than others, all paraneoplastic syndromes have a counterpart that may occur without a cancer association. The disorders that are frequent paraneoplastic manifestations of cancer include limbic encephalitis, opsoclonus-myoclonus, subacute cerebellar degeneration of the elderly, Lambert-Eaton myasthenic syndrome (LEMS), encephalomyelitis, sensory neuronopathy, cancer-associated retinopathy, and melanoma-associated retinopathy [13]. A patient presenting with any of these syndromes should raise suspicion of a paraneoplastic etiology. For some syndromes the age of the patient can be an important clue to whether the disorder is likely paraneoplastic. For example, acute or subacute cerebellar symptoms in an adult are more likely to be paraneoplastic than in children, in whom other etiologies are much more frequent. Young women with anti-N-methyl-D-aspartate (NMDA) receptor encephalitis are much more likely to have an associated tumor than children or older patients with this disorder [9].

Antibodies and Paraneoplastic Neurologic Disorders

The antibodies that are associated with paraneoplastic neurologic disorders can be divided into two broad categories. There are the paraneoplastic (or onconeuronal) antibodies that when detected almost always indicate that the neurologic disorder is a paraneoplastic manifestation of cancer (Table 13.1). The other category comprises the cell surface antibodies. These antibodies associate with neurologic syndromes that occur with or without a cancer association, such as the antibodies against voltage-gated calcium channels (VGCC) in the Lambert-Eaton myasthenic syndrome.

The probability of detecting an antibody characteristic of a paraneoplastic syndrome depends on the type of cancer association. For example, older women with cerebellar degeneration associated with breast or gynecologic cancers almost always harbor anti-Yo antibodies, but if another tumor is involved other antibodies or no antibodies will be identified. Most paraneoplastic syndromes of the peripheral nervous system do not associate with paraneoplastic antibodies. Only a few sensorimotor neuropathies develop in association with anti-CV2/CRMP5 antibodies or anti-Hu, the latter suggesting a neuronopathy caused by dorsal root ganglia dysfunction, rather than a peripheral neuropathy [15, 16].

When testing for antibodies it is important to be aware that some antibodies may be detected at low titers in the serum of patients with or without cancer or neurologic findings [17]. These low titer serum antibodies have not been shown to have clinical relevance and should not mislead the differential diagnosis away from other non-paraneoplastic causes of the patients' complaints. Additionally, for the paraneoplastic syndromes that affect the central nervous system and dorsal root ganglia, antibody titers are higher in the CSF than the serum and in some cases, serum may be negative; therefore, evaluation of the CSF should be undertaken when making the initial diagnosis [18].

Tumors Associated with Paraneoplastic Disorders

At the time of neurologic symptom presentation the tumors of many patients are usually small and confined to a single organ or to the regional lymph nodes. The combined use of CT and PET imaging uncovers occult tumors in approximately 80% of cases; the remaining 20% require close follow-up with repeat studies [19–22]. Ultimately, 90% of all tumors associated with paraneoplastic disorders are diagnosed within the first year of neurologic symptom development.

The detection of specific antibodies often helps in the selection of diagnostic tests, directing the search of the tumor to a few organs. For some syndromes, such as anti-Ma2 encephalitis associated with germ-cell neoplasms of the testis, CT and PET studies can be negative, but ultrasound often reveals the neoplasm or abnormalities that associate with the neoplasm (e.g., microcalcifications). In men younger than 50 with anti-Ma2-associated encephalitis but without a clinically detectable tumor, studies have shown that in most instances a microscopic tumor was present at orchiectomy [23, 24]. The tumors involved in paraneoplastic neurologic syndromes are most commonly malignant, either carcinomas or less frequently lymphoma or leukemia. However, some disorders are associated with benign tumors such as mature cystic teratomas (dermoid cysts) [25]. In these cases PET studies are often negative and other studies such as CT, MRI, and pelvic or vaginal ultrasound for detecting ovarian teratoma should be pursued [26].

Specific Paraneoplastic Neurologic Disorders

Paraneoplastic Limbic Encephalitis

This disorder is characterized by mood disturbances, seizures, and short-term memory loss [27]. The outcome is variable; the disorder may stabilize leaving the patient with severe anterograde memory deficits, may progress causing profound deficits of behavior and cognition leading to frank dementia, or may resolve. In two thirds of the patients, the CSF shows mild pleocytosis, increased proteins, intrathecal synthesis of IgG, and oligoclonal bands. The typical MRI findings include uni- or bilateral mesial temporal lobe abnormalities that are best seen on T2-weighted images, and infrequently contrast enhance (Fig. 13.1a, b) [28]. However, the MRI may be normal despite evidence of temporal lobe dysfunction demonstrated by EEG or hypermetabolism sometimes detected by PET [29]. The EEG may reveal that patients with unexplained low level of consciousness are in status epilepticus. Neurological symptoms usually precede

Fig. 13.1 a, b MRI findings in limbic encephalitis. Axial (**a**) and coronal (**b**) MRI fluid-attenuated inversion recovery (FLAIR) sequences from a patient with anti-Hu associated limbic encephalitis. Note the bilateral medial temporal lobe hyperintensities that are considered characteristic of most cases of limbic encephalitis. Similar findings occur with other immune-mediated limbic encephalitis, paraneoplastic or not, and with some viral encephalitis

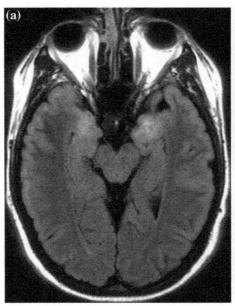
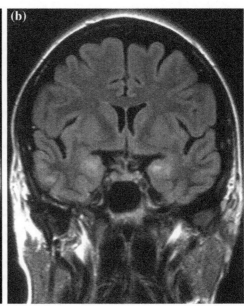

the diagnosis of the tumor. The tumors most frequently involved are lung cancer, usually small-cell lung cancer (SCLC) and tumors of the testes and breast [27].

The pathological findings in most paraneoplastic limbic encephalitis associated to paraneoplastic (onconeuronal) antibodies include perivascular and interstitial inflammatory infiltrates, neuronal loss, and microglial proliferation that predominate in the limbic system (hippocampus, amygdala, hypothalamus, and insular and cingulate cortex). In addition, the majority of patients have variable involvement of other areas of the nervous system, mainly the brainstem [30].

There are several immune responses that may associate with limbic encephalitis. Patients with anti-Hu antibodies often have limbic encephalitis as part of a multifocal encephalomyelitis [31, 32]. Similarly the limbic encephalitis associated with CV2/CRMP5 antibodies rarely stays confined to the limbic system and these patients often have additional sensorimotor neuropathy, cerebellar ataxia, chorea, uveitis, and optic neuritis [15]. Anti-Ma2 antibodies are most commonly found in young men who develop limbic encephalitis in association with hypothalamic and brainstem dysfunction and a tumor of the testis [23]. A classic syndrome of limbic encephalitis is uncommonly found in association with antibodies to amphiphysin.

Several of the autoimmune encephalitis syndromes associated with cell surface antibodies manifest primarily as limbic encephalitis. These include anti-alpha-amino-3-hydroxy-5-methyl-4-isoxazolepropionic acid receptor (AMPAR), gamma-amino-butyric acid B receptor [(GABA (B)], leucine-rich, glioma-inactivated 1 (LGI1), and metabotropic glutamate receptor 5 (mGluR5) antibody associated disorders. These antibodies are markers of the neurologic disorder and the suspicion that the disorder is paraneoplastic

should be based on the presence of cancer risk factors and the specific immune response. For example, AMPAR encephalitis (discussed further later in this chapter) is paraneoplastic in about 70% of cases (usually cancer of the lung, breast, or thymus) while less than 10% of LGI1 encephalitis cases are paraneoplastic (usually thymoma).

Detection of antibodies to VGKC had been considered as a characteristic marker of limbic encephalitis but these antibodies are not specific and have been reported in patients with a variety of syndromes including neurodegenerative and nonimmune diseases [33, 34]. Most patients reported with VGKC antibodies and typical limbic encephalitis were likely cases of LGI1 encephalitis [35].

When associated with antibodies to intracellular antigens limbic encephalitis is usually poorly responsive to treatment. The exception is the encephalitis associated with Ma2 antibodies for which treatment of the tumor and immunotherapy results in improvement in about one third of cases. The limbic encephalitis associated with the autoimmune encephalitis syndromes and antibodies to the neuronal cell surface are much more treatment responsive (tumor directed and immunotherapy) [36].

Paraneoplastic Cerebellar Degeneration

The presenting symptoms of this disorder are dizziness, nausea, blurry or double vision, oscillopsia, and gait difficulties. Associated with these symptoms, or occurring after a few days, the patient develops truncal and limb ataxia, dysarthria, and dysphagia. At examination, patients usually have down-beating nystagmus [37]. This clinical picture is similar for most types of paraneoplastic cerebellar

Fig. 13.2 a–d Studies in a patient with anti-Yo associated cerebellar degeneration. **a** corresponds to a normal FDG-PET obtained when the patient had anti-Yo associated cerebellar degeneration for 2 years. **b** is an FDG-PET obtained 3 years later (5 years after neurologic symptom presentation) showing a hypermetabolic abnormality in the right axillary lymph nodes (*arrow*). **c** shows the patient's anti-Yo antibodies immunolabeling a section of rat cerebellum (note the characteristic Purkinje cell reactivity of the anti-Yo antibodies). **d** shows that the neoplastic cells from the lymph node (identified by PET) react with the anti-Yo antibodies of the patient (*brown cells*). **c** and **d** Avidin-biotin-peroxidase, ×400

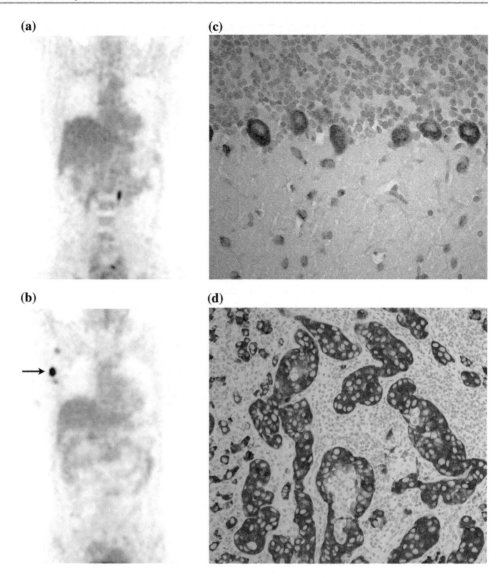

degeneration, irrespective of the type of cancer or antibody association, although the course of the disease may be different depending upon the associated immune response [38]. In general, neurologic symptoms precede the tumor diagnosis. The CSF usually shows pleocytosis, increased proteins, intrathecal synthesis of IgG, and oligoclonal bands. In the early stages of the disease, brain MRI is usually normal, but after several months may show global cerebellar atrophy.

There is a strong association between the development of specific anti-neuronal antibodies and the type of tumor associated with the paraneoplastic cerebellar disorder (Fig. 13.2a–d). These include SCLC and anti-Hu antibodies [32, 39], ovarian or breast cancer and anti-Yo antibodies [40], Hodgkin's lymphoma and anti-Tr/DNER antibodies [41], and breast, ovarian, or SCLC cancer and anti-Ri antibodies (Table 13.1) [42, 43]. Furthermore, the presence of anti-Hu antibodies is usually associated with symptoms indicating involvement of other areas of the nervous system

(i.e., encephalomyelitis and sensory neuronopathy) [31]. The presence of anti-Ri antibodies is associated with opsoclonus or other abnormalities of ocular motility, including nystagmus, abnormal visual tracking, and abnormal vestibulo–ocular reflexes in 70% of the patients; these patients may also develop laryngeal spasms.

Symptoms of paraneoplastic cerebellar dysfunction may occur without the presence of anti-neuronal antibodies. In this case, the tumors more frequently involved are non-Hodgkin's lymphoma and lung cancer (non-SCLC and SCLC) [39, 44]. A subset of patients with SCLC without anti-Hu antibodies develops antibodies against VGCC [45]. These antibodies are similar to those associated with LEMS and some patients develop symptoms of both cerebellar dysfunction and LEMS.

Pathological studies show diffuse loss of Purkinje cells accompanied by degeneration of the dentate and olivary nuclei, and long tracts of the spinal cord. These findings can be associated with mild or prominent lymphocytic infiltrates [46, 47]. When present, the inflammatory infiltrates usually involve the deep cerebellar nuclei in addition to the brainstem and other areas of the nervous system, suggesting that the cerebellum is the main target of a multifocal encephalomyelitis.

Treatment of the tumor and immunosuppressants do not usually affect the course of the cerebellar disorder although there are a few reports of responses to tumor treatment and immunotherapies [48–50].

Paraneoplastic Encephalomyelitis

This disorder describes patients with cancer who develop multifocal neurological deficits and signs of inflammation involving two or more areas of the nervous system, including brain, cerebellum, brainstem, spinal cord, dorsal root ganglia, and autonomic ganglia [46]. This gives rise to a mixture of symptoms derived from limbic encephalitis, cerebellar degeneration, brainstem encephalitis, and myelitis along with sensory deficits and autonomic dysfunction.

Symptoms of paraneoplastic brainstem encephalitis can include diplopia, dysarthria, dysphagia, internuclear or supranuclear gaze abnormalities, facial numbness, and sub-acute hearing loss. The spinal cord symptoms usually result from an inflammatory degeneration of the lower motor neurons [51]. Symptoms of autonomic dysfunction may include gastrointestinal paresis and pseudo-obstruction, orthostatic hypotension, cardiac arrhythmias among others (see discussion later in this chapter).

Several paraneoplastic immunities can associate with encephalomyelitis or multifocal encephalitis including the ones discussed next.

Anti-Hu

Patients with anti-Hu antibodies frequently develop encephalomyelitis in association with sensory neuronopathy secondary to dorsal root ganglia involvement; the tumor most frequently involved is SCLC [31, 32, 52, 53]. Other antineuronal antibodies that occur less frequently (sometimes in combination with anti-Hu) include, anti-CV2/CRMP5 and anti-amphiphysin [54, 55].

Anti-CV2/CRMP5

The encephalomyelitis associated with anti-CV2/CRMP5 antibodies may affect any of the areas indicated above along with the striatum (chorea), uvea (uveitis), and peripheral nerves, resulting in a mixed axonal demyelinating sensori-motor neuropathy [15, 56, 57]. The tumors more frequently associated are SCLC and thymoma.

Paraneoplastic disorders associated with anti-CV2/CRMP5 or anti-Hu are in general poorly responsive to treatment of the tumor or immunotherapies, including

plasma exchange, intravenous immunoglobulins (IVIg) or cyclophosphamide. However, successful treatment of the tumor and prompt immunotherapy directed at the cytotoxic T-cell response (e.g., IVIg and cyclophosphamide) may result in stabilization or partial improvement of symptoms [3].

Anti-Ma Proteins

The encephalitis of patients with immunity to Ma proteins is more restricted to the limbic system, hypothalamus, brainstem, and cerebellum than the encephalomyelitis associated with other antibodies [58]. These patients may present with classical limbic encephalitis or severe hypokinesis and hypophonesis (pseudomutism) with relative preservation of cognitive functions [59]. Supranuclear ocular paresis is common, usually affecting vertical gaze more than horizontal gaze leading some patients to be incorrectly diagnosed with progressive supranuclear palsy. The tumors more frequently associated are germ-cell neoplasms of the testis and non-SCLC [23]. About 35% of patients with anti-Ma2 associated encephalitis respond to treatment; the neurological improvement is usually partial and predominantly occurs in young men with successfully treated testicular neoplasms [2].

Autoimmune Encephalitis with Cell Surface Antibodies

This group of encephalitic disorders occurs in association with antibodies located on the neuronal cell surface or related to the synaptic junction. The syndromes vary according to the associated immune response and include a variety of complex neuropsychiatric symptoms such as deficits of memory, behavior, cognition, psychosis, seizures, movement disorders, or coma. As the antibodies are pathogenic their removal often results in improvement although relapses occur at a variable rate based on the syndrome. The autoimmune encephalitis syndromes in which a paraneoplastic etiology is relatively frequent are discussed next; other syndromes are rarely or not known to be associated with cancer.

NMDAR Encephalitis

This disorder usually affects young women and children ($\sim$80% of patients), but can also affect male and older individuals [9]. Many patients have a viral-like prodrome followed by the development of prominent psychiatric symptoms (bizarre behavior, hallucinations), seizures, orofacial and limb dyskinesias, dystonia, and decreased level of consciousness that within days or weeks progresses to include autonomic or breathing instability requiring intensive care and ventilator support. Partial syndromes such as patients with predominant psychiatric symptoms or abnormal movements, and less severe phenotypes can occur, although virtually all patients develop several elements of the syndrome.

All patients have IgG antibodies against the GluN1 subunit of the NMDAR (Fig. 13.3a–c) [60]. At presentation these antibodies are always present in the CSF but were shown to be absent in the serum of 13% of patients, supporting the importance of CSF analyses at initial diagnosis [18]. These antibodies should not be confused with other IgG antibodies that target other subunits of the NMDAR or those of the IgM or IgA subtypes that are unrelated to NMDAR encephalitis. Other CSF findings often include a lymphocytic pleocytosis sometimes with increased proteins and/or oligoclonal bands. About one third of patients have increased signal on MRI T2 or fluid-attenuated inversion recovery (FLAIR) sequences involving the cortical or subcortical brain regions, and at times the cerebellar cortex [60].

The likelihood of an underlying tumor, most commonly a teratoma of the ovary, is age-dependent ($\sim$40% in patients $\geq$14 years; <10% in patients <14 years) while tumors in children and men are uncommon [9].

The treatment for all of the autoimmune encephalitis is based on experience with NMDAR encephalitis that is the most frequent of these disorders and centers on immunosuppression. This includes corticosteroids, IVIg, or plasmapheresis, either alone or in combination as first-line treatments and rituximab and/or cyclophosphamide as second-line agents. Identification and treatment of an accompanying tumor is important as it appears to associate with better outcome and decreased risk of relapses [9].

AMPAR Encephalitis

This disorder primarily affects middle-aged women. Some patients present with the subacute onset of confusion, memory loss, seizures, and psychiatric symptoms consistent with limbic encephalitis that may be associated with prominent psychiatric features, whereas other cases present with rapidly progressive abnormal behaviors similar to acute psychosis [61–63]. About 70% of cases are paraneoplastic with tumors of the thymus, lung, and breast more commonly associated [62]. Interestingly, patients with AMPAR antibody associated encephalitis as with other autoimmune encephalitis often have other autoantibodies such as thyroid peroxide or ANA antibodies suggesting an underlying propensity to develop autoimmunity. The CSF findings are similar to NMDAR encephalitis and there are cases in which antibodies are only present in CSF [62]. MRI findings are seen in many but not all patients and in about half are limited to increased T2 or FLAIR signal in the medial temporal lobes; in other patients the MRI may show increased signal in cortical regions [63].

GABA(B)R Encephalitis

Patients with antibodies to GABA(B)R develop symptoms of limbic encephalitis including memory loss, confusion, and hallucinations with seizures that can be difficult to control [64]. A few patients have been reported with additional findings including ataxia, opsoclonus-myoclonus,

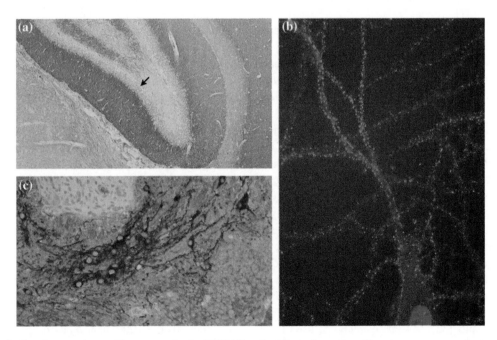

Fig. 13.3 a–c Studies in a patient with paraneoplastic NMDAR encephalitis and ovarian teratoma. **a** shows the CSF reactivity of a patient with anti-NMDAR antibodies with a sagittal section of rat hippocampus; the immunolabeling is mainly concentrated in the inner aspect of the molecular layer adjacent to the dentate gyrus (*arrow*). **b** shows that the antibody reactivity is with the cell surface and dendrites of neurons (the picture corresponds to a culture of rat hippocampal neurons immunolabeled with the patient's antibodies). **c** shows that the teratoma of the patient contains immature neurons; these are demonstrated with MAP2 labeling, a specific marker of neurons and dendrites. **a** avidin-biotin-peroxidase, ×50; **b** immunofluorescence ×800; **c** avidin-biotin-peroxidase, ×400

autonomic dysfunction and hypoventilation, and prominent psychiatric symptoms [65].

The disorder equally affects men and women and about half of the cases are paraneoplastic with SCLC or other neuroendocrine lung tumors most common. Patients with an associated cancer are older than those without a tumor (median age of 67.7 vs. 39 years) and in these cases the neurologic symptoms usually predate the cancer diagnosis [65].

Paraneoplastic Sensory Neuronopathy

This disorder is characterized by progressive sensory loss involving lower and upper extremities, trunk, and face. The sensory deficits are frequently accompanied by painful paresthesias and dysesthesias. This and the frequent asymmetric presentation of symptoms may lead to the diagnosis of radiculopathy or multineuropathy [66, 67]. At presentation, vibration and joint position sensations may be more affected than nociceptive sensation. The sensory loss causes disorganization of movement resulting in sensory ataxia and pseudoathetoid movements. Some patients develop sensorineural hearing loss. Paraneoplastic sensory neuronopathy frequently develops in association with encephalomyelitis and autonomic dysfunction (see paraneoplastic encephalomyelitis). In more than 80% of the patients, the sensory neuronopathy precedes the diagnosis of the tumor, usually a SCLC [31].

Nerve conduction studies demonstrate small amplitude or absent sensory nerve action potentials. Motor nerve and F-wave studies are usually normal, with no signs of denervation unless there is involvement of the spinal motor neurons in the setting of encephalomyelitis. Some patients develop motor conduction abnormalities as a result of a mixed axonal and demyelinating neuropathy that accompanies the degeneration of dorsal root ganglia neurons [68, 69].

Pathological studies show an inflammatory, probably immune-mediated degeneration of the neurons of the dorsal root ganglia, and equivalent ganglia of cranial nerves (e.g., Gasserian ganglia) [70]. Other findings include atrophy of the posterior nerve roots, axonal degeneration, and secondary degeneration of the posterior columns of the spinal cord. Mild inflammatory infiltrates can be found in peripheral nerves and sometimes muscle [66].

Paraneoplastic sensory neuronopathy rarely responds to immunotherapies, including plasma exchange, IVIg, and immunosuppressants [32]. In some patients the use of steroids may result in partial improvement of symptoms [71]. Efforts should be directed toward prompt identification and treatment of the tumor.

Paraneoplastic Opsoclonus-Myoclonus (POM)

POM usually affects infants younger than 4 years of age (median age, 18 months) and often presents with staggering and falling along with body jerks, ataxia, refusal to walk or sit, opsoclonus, irritability, and sleep problems that may contribute to episodes of rage [72, 73]. Nearly 50% of children with POM have neuroblastoma, and about 2% of children with this tumor develop opsoclonus. Neurologic symptoms may precede or develop after the diagnosis of neuroblastoma.

POM frequently responds to treatment of the tumor and immunotherapy that may include corticosteroids, adrenocorticotrophic hormone, IVIg, cyclophosphamide, and rituximab [74]. The sleep disturbances and episodes of rage often respond to trazodone; however, residual psychomotor deficits, behavioral and sleep disturbances are common [72, 73, 75]. Patients with POM have a better tumor prognosis than patients without paraneoplastic symptoms.

In adults, POM develops in association with truncal ataxia resulting in gait difficulty and frequent falls. In more than half of the patients, POM precedes the diagnosis of the tumor, usually a SCLC [76]. Patients with breast cancer may harbor anti-Ri antibodies (see paraneoplastic cerebellar degeneration) although most patients are antibody negative [42, 77]. The clinical course of paraneoplastic opsoclonus is worse than that of idiopathic opsoclonus. Paraneoplastic opsoclonus may respond to immunotherapy or IVIg, but symptom improvement depends on successful treatment of the tumor [78]. If the tumor is not treated, neurologic symptoms often progress to a severe encephalopathy resulting in the patients' death. In addition to treatment of the tumor and IVIg, there are reported clinical responses to depletion of serum IgG using protein-A columns, clonazepam, valproic acid, and thiamine [79].

There is a recent description of a POM syndrome occurring in a subgroup of young women within the context of a brainstem-cerebellar syndrome associated with ovarian teratoma [80]. The majority of these patients had full recovery with tumor treatment and immunotherapy; one patient who did not have tumor treatment improved with immunotherapy. Antibodies to intracellular or cell surface neuronal proteins were not detected in these patients.

Paraneoplastic Stiff-Person Syndrome

This disorder is characterized by fluctuating rigidity of the axial musculature with superimposed spasms. Rigidity primarily affects the lower trunk and legs, but it can extend to the shoulders, upper limbs, neck, and less frequently muscles of the face. Symptoms may be limited to one extremity (stiff-limb syndrome). Spasms are often precipitated by voluntary movement, emotional upset, and auditory and somesthetic stimuli. Typically, the rigidity disappears during sleep or following general anesthesia, suggesting dysfunction at the spinal or supraspinal level [81]. Electrophysiologic studies show continuous activity of motor units in the stiffened muscles that considerably improve after treatment with diazepam.

The disorder can occur as a paraneoplastic manifestation of cancer (usually breast or SCLC) but about 85% of cases are idiopathic [82]. Patients with paraneoplastic stiff-person syndrome tend to be older than non-paraneoplastic cases and to have asymmetric and distal distribution of symptoms often with cervical involvement, spinal myoclonus, and pruritus [83, 84].

The serum and CSF of patients with paraneoplastic stiff-person syndrome may contain antibodies to amphiphysin and these patients usually have breast or SCLC [83–85]. Amphiphysin antibodies are not syndrome specific and have been described in encephalitis, neuropathy, and myelopathy [83]. In patients without cancer the major autoantigen is glutamic acid decarboxylase 65 (GAD65) sometimes found in association with antibodies to GABA (A) receptor; 70% of these patients develop type I diabetes and other autoimmune diseases [83, 86, 87].

In addition to stiff-person syndrome, paraneoplastic rigidity and spasms can occur in patients with extensive encephalomyelitis or focal myelitis [88]. Some of these patients harbor anti-Ri antibodies [89]. Patients with progressive encephalomyelitis, rigidity and myoclonus (PERM) often have antibodies to the alpha 1 subunit of the glycine receptor (GlyR) [90–92]. These cases are rarely associated with cancer (Hodgkin's lymphoma, thymoma). Serum GlyR antibodies are not specific to PERM as they have been described in patient with SPS without features of PERM as well as in patients with various disorders, including optic neuritis or multiple sclerosis [92, 93].

Histopathological abnormalities found in stiff-person syndrome ranges from normal to include mild perivascular lymphocyte infiltration and loss of motor neurons and interneurons in the anterior horns of the spinal cord [94–96].

Improvement of stiff-person syndrome can be obtained with IVIg and GABA-enhancing drugs, such as diazepam, clonazepam, gabapentin, or baclofen, but sustained improvement usually requires treatment of the tumor and steroids [97, 98]. Patients with PERM and glycine receptor antibodies can respond with good outcome to immunotherapy [99].

Motor Neuron Dysfunction

The occurrence of motor neuron disease as a paraneoplastic syndrome is controversial. Two systematic reviews of the literature concluded that there was not an increased incidence of cancer among patients with amyotrophic lateral

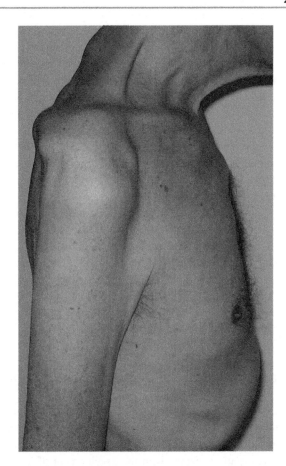

Fig. 13.4 Severe neurogenic muscle atrophy in a patient with SCLC and anti-Hu-associated myelitis. The initial neurologic symptom of this patient was flaccid motor weakness selectively involving the upper extremities and neck extension. After eight weeks he was unable to move the upper extremities. These symptoms associated with fasciculations and loss of reflexes in the arms. Cranial nerves, strength and reflexes in the lower extremities were normal. The picture demonstrates widespread atrophy of the muscles of the neck and shoulder

sclerosis (ALS) while a recent report using data from 16 population-based cancer registries found an elevated risk of death from ALS in survivors of melanoma and tongue cancer [100–102]. About 20% of patients with anti-Hu antibody associated encephalomyelitis and sensory neuronopathy develop symptoms resembling ALS due to predominant involvement of the spinal cord (Fig. 13.4) [31, 51]. Patients with lymphoma rarely develop subacute, progressive, painless, and often asymmetrical lower motor neuron dysfunction. Upper motor signs are absent, fasciculations are rare and the bulbar muscles are usually spared contrasting this syndrome with typical ALS [103, 104].

Paraneoplastic Sensorimotor Neuropathy

Many patients with advanced malignancy develop a peripheral neuropathy that is usually mild, with little impact on quality of life [105]. The cause of these neuropathies is multifactorial, including metabolic abnormalities, nutritional deficits, and toxic effects of chemotherapy and biologic therapies (e.g., cisplatin, paclitaxel, docetaxel, vinca alkaloids, thalidomide, and bortezomib, among others) [106].

There is a group of sensorimotor neuropathies that develop a few months before or by the time a malignancy is discovered. Symptoms may present in a subacute or acute fashion and are usually progressive. In most cases the neuropathy is part of other processes such as encephalomyelitis, mononeuritis multiplex, or acute or chronic inflammatory demyelinating polyneuropathy [107]. Antibody studies are negative except for patients with SCLC who may have CV2/CRMP5 antibodies and less commonly Hu antibodies [108]. Pathological studies usually show axonal degeneration with frequent inflammatory infiltrates, although some patients have predominant demyelinating findings. The latter are more likely to respond to corticosteroids and IVIg than the axonal neuropathies.

Paraneoplastic Vasculitis of Nerve and Muscle

This disorder is a nonsystemic vasculitic neuropathy that involves nerve, muscle, or both and has been reported in association with solid tumors and lymphoma [109–111]. The onset is usually subacute with the development of a painful symmetric or asymmetric sensorimotor polyneuropathy, or less frequently mononeuritis multiplex. The course is progressive. The erythrocyte sedimentation rate is usually elevated and the CSF shows a high protein content. Electrophysiological studies show a diffuse asymmetric axonal polyneuropathy or multifocal mononeuropathy [112]. Nerve biopsy studies show intramural and perivascular inflammatory infiltrates, usually without necrotizing vasculitis. The inflammatory infiltrates are mainly composed of CD8+ T-cells [113].

Paraneoplastic vasculitis of nerve and muscle often responds to treatment of the tumor, corticosteroids, and cyclophosphamide [109].

Sensorimotor Polyneuropathy Associated with Malignant Monoclonal Gammopathies

The malignancies that are associated with monoclonal gammopathies or M proteins include multiple myeloma and osteosclerotic myeloma, which are typically associated with IgG or IgA M proteins, and Waldenström's macroglobulinemia, B-cell lymphoma, and chronic B-cell lymphocytic leukemia, which are associated with IgM M proteins.

Multiple Myeloma

The current leading cause of peripheral neuropathy in multiple myeloma is iatrogenic and due to direct nerve toxicity of the drugs used for tumor treatment (e.g., vincristine, thalidomide, bortezomib, among others). Paraneoplastic neuropathies do occur in about 10% of patients with neurologic symptoms usually preceding the myeloma diagnosis. The neuropathy is most often sensorimotor and slowly progressive. Treatment of the myeloma rarely improves the neuropathy. Amyloid deposition is a cause of neuropathy in some patients [114, 115]. In patients with amyloid-associated neuropathy, symptoms are similar to those with distal axonal sensorimotor neuropathy, but frequently include atypical features, such as pain, carpal tunnel syndrome, a clinical picture of multiple mononeuropathy, and autonomic dysfunction. Treatment is aimed at the myeloma but even when successful, the neuropathy often persists [116].

Osteosclerotic Myeloma/POEMS Syndrome

This is an unusual form of myeloma characterized by single or multiple plasmacytomas that manifest as sclerotic bone lesions. These lesions involve ribs, vertebrae, pelvic bones, and proximal long bones, and usually spare skull and distal extremities [117]. All or some features of the POEMS syndrome (*p*olyneuropathy, *o*rganomegaly, *e*ndocrinopathy, *M* component, and *s*kin changes) may be present and it is under debate if there is a true distinction between osteosclerotic myeloma and POEMS [118]. More than 50% of patients with sclerotic myeloma develop a peripheral neuropathy, often before the tumor diagnosis that resembles a chronic demyelinating polyradiculoneuropathy with motor predominance and high CSF protein content [119]. However, compared to CIDP, there is no macrophage-associated demyelination, and levels of vascular endothelial growth factor (VEGF) in serum are commonly quite elevated [120]. Focal treatment of the sclerotic lesions with resection or radiation therapy, the use of prednisone alone or in combination with melphalan, or lenalidomide with or without dexamethasone often results in neurologic improvement [121, 122]. Patients with widespread lesions or rapidly progressive neuropathy may respond to peripheral blood stem cell transplant [123].

Waldenström's Macroglobulinemia

Symptoms of peripheral neuropathy occur in about 45% of these patients, and in approximately 10% the deficits are severe [124]. The cause of the neuropathy are heterogeneous and include axonal neuropathies related to amyloid, cryoglobulinemia, tumor infiltration, and vasculitis and demyelinating neuropathies related to antibodies against myelin-associated glycoprotein (MAG), sulphatide or various gangliosides [125, 126]. The neuropathy associated with IgM anti-MAG is characterized by progressive distal sensorimotor deficits, with predominant involvement of vibration sense, sometimes with postural tremor, pseudoathetosis, and progressive gait dysfunction.

Electrophysiologic studies demonstrate slow conduction velocities and prolonged distal motor and sensory latencies, compatible with a demyelinating neuropathy. Pathology studies show widening between lamellae of myelin sheaths due to intercalation of anti-MAG antibodies [127]. The neuropathy associated with anti-sulphatide antibodies is predominantly axonal.

Treatment should be directed at the Waldenström's macroglobulinemia. Patients with demyelinating neuropathy and IgM anti-MAG M proteins may respond to plasma exchange, IVIg, or rituximab [128]. However, most patients require aggressive treatment with chemotherapeutic agents such as chlorambucil, cyclophosphamide, or fludarabine [129, 130]. Responses to rituximab with or without fludarabine or cyclophosphamide have been reported [131, 132].

Paraneoplastic Autonomic Dysfunction

This disorder usually develops in association with other paraneoplastic syndromes, such as encephalomyelitis or LEMS. Symptoms often precede the detection of the tumor, usually a SCLC. The autonomic dysfunction may result from adrenergic or cholinergic nerve dysfunction at the pre- or, most frequently, postganglionic level [133, 134]. There are three disorders that can be life threatening: esophageal and gastrointestinal dysmotility with intestinal pseudoobstruction, cardiac dysrhythmias, and orthostatic hypotension. Other accompanying symptoms may include dry mouth, erectile, and sphincter dysfunction. Because autonomic dysfunction can be the presentation of encephalomyelitis, testing for anti-Hu antibodies should be considered in some patients [135, 136]. About one third of patients with anti-CV2/CRMP5 will have manifestations of autonomic neuropathy [56]. There is another subgroup of patients with autonomic neuropathy who develop antibodies to the ganglionic acetylcholine receptor [137]; these antibodies may occur in patients with or without cancer, and their detection suggests that symptoms may improve with immunotherapy [138].

Lambert–Eaton Myasthenic Syndrome

LEMS is a disorder of the neuromuscular junction characterized by impaired acetylcholine release from the presynaptic motor terminal [139]. Symptoms include fatigue, leg weakness, muscle aches, and vague parasthesias. Dry mouth and other symptoms of autonomic dysfunction are common [140]. Cranial nerve involvement tends to be mild and transient, usually described as transient diplopia. Neurologic examination shows proximal weakness in the legs more than the arms and depressed reflexes, sometimes accompanied by eyelid ptosis and sluggishly reactive pupils. After brief muscle contraction, reflexes may potentiate. Similarly, after brief exercise strength may improve.

Routine nerve conduction studies show small amplitude compound muscle action potentials (CMAP) [141]. At slow rates of repetitive nerve stimulation (2–5 Hz), a decremental response of greater than 10% is seen; at fast rates (20 Hz or greater) or after maximal voluntary muscle contraction, facilitation occurs and there is an incremental response of at least 100%.

LEMS is associated with cancer in 50–70% of patients, most commonly SCLC. LEMS can also occur in conjunction with other paraneoplastic syndromes, such as paraneoplastic cerebellar degeneration or encephalomyelitis [39, 142]. Patients with paraneoplastic LEMS tend to be men older than 50 years of age while non-paraneoplastic LEMS occurs over a much wider age group with a slight female predominance [143]. Neurologic symptoms typically precede or coincide with the diagnosis of the tumor. In one study 91% of SCLCs were detected within 3 months of LEMS onset and 96% within 1 year [144]. Patients diagnosed with SCLC beyond 2 years of the LEMS diagnosis often had inadequate initial cancer screening. The Dutch-English LEMS Tumor Association Prediction (DELTA-P) score can be used at initial diagnosis to predict those patients with a high risk of having an associated SCLC [143]. Additionally, about 65% of patients with LEMS and SCLC have serum antibodies to SOX1 [145].

LEMS results from an antibody mediated attack against the presynaptic VGCC which results in decreased release of acetylcholine vesicles during depolarization. The detection of antibodies to P/Q-type VGCC is used as a serologic test for LEMS [146]. About 90% of LEMS patients have these antibodies regardless of whether the disorder is paraneoplastic or not [146].

Therapies for LEMS include treatment of the associated cancer, medication to increase the release of acetylcholine, and immunotherapy with the majority of patients having neurological improvement. The drug of choice is 3,4-diaminopyridine which is well tolerated and results in improvement of 80% of patients [147]. Long-term immunosuppression with prednisone alone or combined with azathioprine or cyclosporine should be considered in patients who remain symptomatic after controlling the tumor [148–150]. Immunomodulation with IVIg or plasma exchange is usually effective but the benefits are short lasting [148, 151, 152].

Paraneoplastic Peripheral Nerve Hyperexcitability

Paraneoplastic peripheral nerve hyperexcitability (PNH), also known as paraneoplastic neuromyotonia or Isaacs syndrome, is characterized by spontaneous and continuous muscle fiber activity of peripheral nerve origin [153]. Symptoms include muscle cramps, weakness, difficulty in muscle relaxation, carpopedal spasms, and sometimes excessive sweating. The involved muscles show undulating myokymia and may be hypertrophic [154]. EMG shows fibrillation, fasciculation, and doublet, triplet or multiplet single unit discharges that have a high intraburst frequency [155]. This abnormal activity continues during sleep and general anesthesia, is abolished by curare, and may be reduced or abolished by peripheral nerve block [153, 156].

Approximately 25% of patients with PNH develop central nervous system dysfunction characterized by changes in mood, hallucinations, and sleep dysfunction or in some cases typical limbic encephalitis. The combination of PNH and central nervous system involvement is called Morvan's syndrome. About 30–50% of cases of Morvan's syndrome are paraneoplastic with thymoma the most commonly associated tumor; patients with thymoma may have additional symptoms of myasthenia gravis [157].

About 80% of patients with Morvan's have antibodies that were previously identified as targeting the voltage-gated potassium channel (called anti-VGKC antibodies) [158]. It is now known that these antibodies do not target the VGKC but rather another protein in the VGKC-complex called contactin-associated protein-2 (Caspr2) [159, 160]. In contrast, isolated PNH rarely associates with Caspr2 or other antibodies [161]. Antibodies to other unidentified targets in the VGKC-complex have been found in some patients and are of unclear clinical significance.

Neuromyotonia often improves with sodium channel-blocking agents such as phenytoin, carbamazepine and lamotrigine. Plasma exchange can provide transient benefit for patients with severe symptoms although immunosuppression (corticosteroids, azathioprine) may be required for prolonged responses [162]. There are reports of marked improvement with oncologic treatment [163, 164].

Dermatomyositis

Dermatomyositis (DM) is a multi-system inflammatory myopathy. The classic skin manifestations include purplish discoloration of the eyelids (heliotrope rash) with edema, and erythematous, scaly lesions over the knuckles. The presence of necrotic skin ulcerations and pruritus appears to occur more frequently when the DM is paraneoplastic than without a cancer association [165].

DM occurs more often in women at a 2:1 ratio and about 30% of cases are paraneoplastic [166]. The risk of developing cancer is highest within the first 3 years of DM onset although the cancer diagnosis may precede or be concurrent with the DM diagnosis [167, 168]. In women the most common tumors are ovarian and breast cancer, and in men, lung and gastrointestinal cancer. In an Asian population there was an over-representation of nasopharyngeal carcinoma [169]. An association with cancer has not been demonstrated in childhood DM.

Clinical, electromyographic, and pathological findings of DM are similar in patients with and without cancer. Patients typically present with proximal muscle weakness of subacute onset and elevated levels of muscle enzymes. Electromyographic features include short, small, polyphasic motor unit potentials, fibrillations, sharp waves, insertional irritability, and high-frequency repetitive discharges [170]. The muscle biopsy shows degeneration, regeneration, necrosis, phagocytosis, and an interstitial mononuclear infiltrate [171, 172]. Neck flexors and pharyngeal and respiratory muscles are commonly involved; their dysfunction may result in aspiration and hypoventilation and contribute to death. Reflexes and sensory exam are normal. There is a subset of DM patients who develop cutaneous involvement without clinically evident myopathy (amyopathic dermatomyositis); MRI studies may show subclinical muscle involvement [173].

A variety of autoantibodies have been described in patients with DM. Studies suggest that antibodies to transcription intermediary factor 1γ (TIFγ) and/or nuclear matrix protein (NXP2) are useful markers of a paraneoplastic origin of the DM [174–176]. In one study, at least one of these two antibodies was present in 83% of patients with cancer-associated DM, compared with 51% of patients without cancer [177].

Other than treatment of the underlying cancer, the general approach to treatment of DM is the same whether paraneoplastic or not. Corticosteroids and methotrexate are the most commonly used medications while IVIg and/or cyclosporine are used in refractory or intolerant patients [11]. Other immunomodulatory treatments reported as useful in severe, refractory cases include mycophenolate mofetil, tacrolimus, and rituximab [178, 179].

Patients with graft versus host disease (GVHD) may develop symptoms that resemble those associated with DM. Treatment with cyclosporine or tacrolimus in association with corticosteroids often results in improvement [180, 181].

Acute Necrotizing Myopathy

Patients with this disorder develop subacute or less commonly acute muscle pain and symmetric proximal weakness, associated with high levels of serum creatine kinase. The disorder evolves rapidly to generalized weakness, which involves pharyngeal and respiratory muscles, often leading to death in a few weeks. Several types of tumors are involved including SCLC, cancer of the gastrointestinal tract (stomach, colon, gall bladder, pancreas), breast, kidney and prostate [182]. Muscle biopsy shows prominent necrosis with little or absent inflammation and macrophages that are seen around the necrotic fibers [183, 184]. In cancer patients, the differential diagnosis should include chemotherapy and cytokine-induced (IL-2, interferon-α) rhabdomyolysis [185]. In one series of eight patients, three who had cancer, all patients improved with prolonged immunotherapy, mostly high-dose prednisone and IVIg [184]. One patient with SCLC and severe weakness from biopsy proven necrotizing myopathy had marked improvement over 3 months with tumor treatment (chemoradiation) in the absence of immunotherapy [186].

References

1. Posner JB. Neurologic complications of cancer. Philadelphia: F. A.Davis Company; 1995.
2. Dalmau J, Graus F, Villarejo A, Posner JB, Blumenthal D, Thiessen B, et al. Clinical analysis of anti-Ma2-associated encephalitis. Brain. 2004;127(Pt 8):1831–44.
3. Vernino S, O'Neill BP, Marks RS, O'Fallon JR, Kimmel DW. Immunomodulatory treatment trial for paraneoplastic neurological disorders. Neuro-oncol. 2004;6(1):55–62.
4. Darnell RB, Posner JB. Paraneoplastic syndromes involving the nervous system. N Engl J Med. 2003;349(16):1543–54.
5. Rousseau A, Benyahia B, Dalmau J, Connan F, Guillet JG, Delattre JY, et al. T cell response to Hu-D peptides in patients with anti-Hu syndrome. J Neurooncol. 2005;71(3):231–6.
6. Blachere NE, Orange DE, Santomasso BD, Doerner J, Foo PK, Herre M, et al. T cells targeting a neuronal paraneoplastic antigen mediate tumor rejection and trigger CNS autoimmunity with humoral activation. Eur J Immunol. 2014;44(11):3240–51.
7. Fukunaga H, Engel AG, Lang B, Newsom-Davis J, Vincent A. Passive transfer of Lambert-Eaton myasthenic syndrome with IgG from man to mouse depletes the presynaptic membrane active zones. Proc Natl Acad Sci USA. 1983;80(24):7636–40.
8. Planaguma J, Leypoldt F, Mannara F, Gutierrez-Cuesta J, Martin-Garcia E, Aguilar E, et al. Human N-methyl D-aspartate receptor antibodies alter memory and behaviour in mice. Brain. 2015;138(Pt 1):94–109.
9. Titulaer MJ, McCracken L, Gabilondo I, Armangue T, Glaser C, Iizuka T, et al. Treatment and prognostic factors for long-term outcome in patients with anti-NMDA receptor encephalitis: an observational cohort study. Lancet Neurol. 2013;12(2):157–65.
10. Luo YB, Mastaglia FL. Dermatomyositis, polymyositis and immune-mediated necrotising myopathies. Biochim Biophys Acta. 2015;1852(4):622–32.
11. Dalakas MC, Hohlfeld R. Polymyositis and dermatomyositis. Lancet. 2003;362(9388):971–82.
12. Ghirardello A, Bassi N, Palma L, Borella E, Domeneghetti M, Punzi L, et al. Autoantibodies in polymyositis and dermatomyositis. Curr Rheumatol Rep. 2013;15(6):335.
13. Graus F, Delattre JY, Antoine JC, Dalmau J, Giometto B, Grisold W, et al. Recommended diagnostic criteria for paraneoplastic neurological syndromes. J Neurol Neurosurg Psychiatry. 2004;75(8):1135–40.
14. Keltner JL, Thirkill CE, Yip PT. Clinical and immunologic characteristics of melanoma-associated retinopathy syndrome: eleven new cases and a review of 51 previously published cases. J Neuroophthalmol. 2001;21(3):173–87.
15. Antoine JC, Honnorat J, Camdessanche JP, Magistris M, Absi L, Mosnier JF, et al. Paraneoplastic anti-CV2 antibodies react with peripheral nerve and are associated with a mixed axonal and demyelinating peripheral neuropathy. Ann Neurol. 2001;49(2):214–21.
16. Kuntzer T, Antoine JC, Steck AJ. Clinical features and pathophysiological basis of sensory neuronopathies (ganglionopathies). Muscle Nerve. 2004;30(3):255–68.
17. Monstad SE, Knudsen A, Salvesen HB, Aarseth JH, Vedeler CA. Onconeural antibodies in sera from patients with various types of tumours. Cancer Immunol Immunother. 2009;58(11):1795–800.
18. Gresa-Arribas N, Titulaer MJ, Torrents A, Aguilar E, McCracken L, Leypoldt F, et al. Antibody titres at diagnosis and during follow-up of anti-NMDA receptor encephalitis: a retrospective study. Lancet Neurol. 2014;13(2):167–77.
19. Younes-Mhenni S, Janier MF, Cinotti L, Antoine JC, Tronc F, Cottin V, et al. FDG-PET improves tumour detection in patients with paraneoplastic neurological syndromes. Brain. 2004; 127(Pt 10):2331–8.
20. Rees JH, Hain SF, Johnson MR, Hughes RA, Costa DC, Ell PJ, et al. The role of [18F]fluoro-2-deoxyglucose-PET scanning in the diagnosis of paraneoplastic neurological disorders. Brain. 2001;124(Pt 11):2223–31.
21. McKeon A, Apiwattanakul M, Lachance DH, Lennon VA, Mandrekar JN, Boeve BF, et al. Positron emission tomography-computed tomography in paraneoplastic neurologic disorders: systematic analysis and review. Arch Neurol. 2010; 67(3):322–9.
22. Titulaer MJ, Soffietti R, Dalmau J, Gilhus NE, Giometto B, Graus F, et al. Screening for tumours in paraneoplastic syndromes: report of an EFNS task force. Eur J Neurol. 2011;18(1):19–e3.
23. Mathew RM, Vandenberghe R, Garcia-Merino A, Yamamoto T, Landolfi JC, Rosenfeld MR, et al. Orchiectomy for suspected microscopic tumor in patients with anti-Ma2-associated encephalitis. Neurology. 2007;68(12):900–5.
24. Hoffmann LA, Jarius S, Pellkofer HL, Schueller M, Krumbholz M, Koenig F, et al. Anti-Ma and anti-Ta associated paraneoplastic neurological syndromes: 22 newly diagnosed patients and review of previous cases. J Neurol Neurosurg Psychiatry. 2008;79(7):767–73.
25. Vitaliani R, Mason W, Ances B, Zwerdling T, Jiang Z, Dalmau J. Paraneoplastic encephalitis, psychiatric symptoms, and hypoventilation in ovarian teratoma. Ann Neurol. 2005; 58(4):594–604.
26. Dalmau J, Tuzun E, Wu HY, Masjuan J, Rossi JE, Voloschin A, et al. Paraneoplastic anti-N-methyl-D-aspartate receptor encephalitis associated with ovarian teratoma. Ann Neurol. 2007;61(1):25–36.
27. Gultekin SH, Rosenfeld MR, Voltz R, Eichen J, Posner JB, Dalmau J. Paraneoplastic limbic encephalitis: Neurological symptoms, immunological findings, and tumor association in 50 patients. Brain. 2000;123(Pt 7):1481–94.
28. Lawn ND, Westmoreland BF, Kiely MJ, Lennon VA, Vernino S. Clinical, magnetic resonance imaging, and electroencephalographic findings in paraneoplastic limbic encephalitis. Mayo Clin Proc. 2003;78(11):1363–8.

29. Ances BM, Vitaliani R, Taylor RA, Liebeskind DS, Voloschin A, Houghton DJ, et al. Treatment-responsive limbic encephalitis identified by neuropil antibodies: MRI and PET correlates. Brain. 2005;128(Pt 8):1764–77.

30. Corsellis JA, Goldberg GJ, Norton AR. "Limbic encephalitis" and its association with carcinoma. Brain. 1968;91(3):481–96.

31. Dalmau J, Graus F, Rosenblum MK, Posner JB. Anti-Hu–associated paraneoplastic encephalomyelitis/sensory neuronopathy. A clinical study of 71 patients. Medicine (Baltimore). 1992;71(2):59–72.

32. Graus F, Keime-Guibert F, Rene R, Benyahia B, Ribalta T, Ascaso C, et al. Anti-Hu-associated paraneoplastic encephalomyelitis: analysis of 200 patients. Brain. 2001; 124(Pt 6):1138–48.

33. Paterson RW, Zandi MS, Armstrong R, Vincent A, Schott JM. Clinical relevance of positive voltage-gated potassium channel (VGKC)-complex antibodies: experience from a tertiary referral centre. J Neurol Neurosurg Psychiatry. 2014;85(6):625–30.

34. Fujita K, Yuasa T, Watanabe O, Takahashi Y, Hashiguchi S, Adachi K, et al. Voltage-gated potassium channel complex antibodies in Creutzfeldt-Jakob disease. J Neurol. 2012;259(10): 2249–50.

35. Lai M, Huijbers MG, Lancaster E, Graus F, Bataller L, Balice-Gordon R, et al. Investigation of LGI1 as the antigen in limbic encephalitis previously attributed to potassium channels: a case series. Lancet Neurol. 2010;9(8):776–85.

36. Bataller L, Kleopa KA, Wu GF, Rossi JE, Rosenfeld MR, Dalmau J. Autoimmune limbic encephalitis in 39 patients: immunophenotypes and outcomes. J Neurol Neurosurg Psychiatry. 2007;78(4):381–5.

37. Peterson K, Rosenblum MK, Kotanides H, Posner JB. Paraneoplastic cerebellar degeneration. I. A clinical analysis of 55 anti-Yo antibody-positive patients. Neurology. 1992;42(10): 1931–7.

38. Shams'ili S, Grefkens J, De Leeuw B, van den Bent M, Hooijkaas H, van der Holt B, et al. Paraneoplastic cerebellar degeneration associated with antineuronal antibodies: analysis of 50 patients. Brain. 2003;126(Pt 6):1409–18.

39. Mason WP, Graus F, Lang B, Honnorat J, Delattre JY, Valldeoriola F, et al. Small-cell lung cancer, paraneoplastic cerebellar degeneration and the Lambert-Eaton myasthenic syndrome. Brain. 1997;120(Pt 8):1279–300.

40. Rojas-Marcos I, Rousseau A, Keime-Guibert F, Rene R, Cartalat-Carel S, Delattre JY, et al. Spectrum of paraneoplastic neurologic disorders in women with breast and gynecologic cancer. Medicine (Baltimore). 2003;82(3):216–23.

41. Bernal F, Shams'ili S, Rojas I, Sanchez-Valle R, Saiz A, Dalmau J, et al. Anti-Tr antibodies as markers of paraneoplastic cerebellar degeneration and Hodgkin's disease. Neurology. 2003;60(2):230–4.

42. Luque FA, Furneaux HM, Ferziger R, Rosenblum MK, Wray SH, Schold SC, et al. Anti-Ri: an antibody associated with paraneoplastic opsoclonus and breast cancer. Ann Neurol. 1991;29(3): 241–51.

43. Sutton IJ, Barnett MH, Watson JD, Ell JJ, Dalmau J. Paraneoplastic brainstem encephalitis and anti-Ri antibodies. J Neurol. 2002;249(11):1597–8.

44. Sabater L, Bataller L, Carpentier AF, Aguirre-Cruz ML, Saiz A, Benyahia B, et al. Protein kinase Cgamma autoimmunity in paraneoplastic cerebellar degeneration and non-small-cell lung cancer. J Neurol Neurosurg Psychiatry. 2006;77(12):1359–62.

45. Graus F, Lang B, Pozo-Rosich P, Saiz A, Casamitjana R, Vincent A. P/Q type calcium-channel antibodies in paraneoplastic cerebellar degeneration with lung cancer. Neurology. 2002;59(5): 764–6.

46. Henson RA, Hoffman HL, Urich H. Encephalomyelitis with carcinoma. Brain. 1965;88(3):449–64.

47. Verschuuren J, Chuang L, Rosenblum MK, Lieberman F, Pryor A, Posner JB, et al. Inflammatory infiltrates and complete absence of Purkinje cells in anti-Yo-associated paraneoplastic cerebellar degeneration. Acta Neuropathol (Berl). 1996;91(5): 519–25.

48. Widdess-Walsh P, Tavee JO, Schuele S, Stevens GH. Response to intravenous immunoglobulin in anti-Yo associated paraneoplastic cerebellar degeneration: case report and review of the literature. J Neurooncol. 2003;63(2):187–90.

49. Shams'ili S, de Beukelaar J, Gratama JW, Hooijkaas H, van den Bent M, van't Veer V, et al. An uncontrolled trial of rituximab for antibody associated paraneoplastic neurological syndromes. J Neurol. 2006;253(1):16–20.

50. Yeo KK, Walter AW, Miller RE, Dalmau J. Rituximab as potential therapy for paraneoplastic cerebellar degeneration in pediatric Hodgkin disease. Pediatr Blood Cancer. 2012;58(6): 986–7.

51. Forsyth PA, Dalmau J, Graus F, Cwik V, Rosenblum MK, Posner JB. Motor neuron syndromes in cancer patients. Ann Neurol. 1997;41(6):722–30.

52. Lucchinetti CF, Kimmel DW, Lennon VA. Paraneoplastic and oncologic profiles of patients seropositive for type 1 antineuronal nuclear autoantibodies. Neurology. 1998;50(3):652–7.

53. Sillevis SP, Grefkens J, De Leeuw B, van den BM, van Putten W, Hooijkaas H, et al. Survival and outcome in 73 anti-Hu positive patients with paraneoplastic encephalomyelitis/sensory neuronopathy. J Neurol. 2002;249(6):745–53.

54. Honnorat J, Antoine JC, Derrington E, Aguera M, Belin MF. Antibodies to a subpopulation of glial cells and a 66 kDa developmental protein in patients with paraneoplastic neurological syndromes. J Neurol Neurosurg Psychiatry. 1996;61(3):270–8.

55. Dropcho EJ. Antiamphiphysin antibodies with small-cell lung carcinoma and paraneoplastic encephalomyelitis. Ann Neurol. 1996;39(5):659–67.

56. Yu Z, Kryzer TJ, Griesmann GE, Kim KK, Benarroch EE, Lennon VA. CRMP-5 neuronal autoantibody: Marker of lung cancer and thymoma related autoimmunity. Ann Neurol. 2001; 49(2):146–54.

57. Vernino S, Tuite P, Adler CH, Meschia JF, Boeve BF, Boasberg P, et al. Paraneoplastic chorea associated with CRMP-5 neuronal antibody and lung carcinoma. Ann Neurol. 2002;51(5):625–30.

58. Rosenfeld MR, Eichen J, Wade D, Posner JB, Dalmau J. Molecular and clinical diversity in paraneoplastic immunity to Ma proteins. Ann Neurol. 2001;50(3):339–48.

59. Matsumoto L, Yamamoto T, Higashihara M, Sugimoto I, Kowa H, Shibahara J, et al. Severe hypokinesis caused by paraneoplastic anti-Ma2 encephalitis associated with bilateral intratubular germ-cell neoplasm of the testes. Mov Disord. 2007;22(5):728–31.

60. Dalmau J, Gleichman AJ, Hughes EG, Rossi JE, Peng X, Lai M, et al. Anti-NMDA-receptor encephalitis: case series and analysis of the effects of antibodies. Lancet Neurol. 2008;7(12):1091–8.

61. Lai M, Hughes EG, Peng X, Zhou L, Gleichman AJ, Shu H, et al. AMPA receptor antibodies in limbic encephalitis alter synaptic receptor location. Ann Neurol. 2009;65(4):424–34.

62. Graus F, Boronat A, Xifro X, Boix M, Svigelj V, Garcia A, et al. The expanding clinical profile of anti-AMPA receptor encephalitis. Neurology. 2010;74(10):857–9.

63. Hoftberger R, van Sonderen A, Leypoldt F, Houghton D, Geschwind M, Gelfand J, et al. Encephalitis and AMPA receptor antibodies: novel findings in a case series of 22 patients. Neurology. 2015;84(24):2403–12.

64. Lancaster E, Lai M, Peng X, Hughes E, Constantinescu R, Raizer J, et al. Antibodies to the GABA(B) receptor in limbic encephalitis with seizures: case series and characterisation of the antigen. Lancet Neurol. 2010;9(1):67–76.

65. Hoftberger R, Titulaer MJ, Sabater L, Dome B, Rozsas A, Hegedus B, et al. Encephalitis and GABAB receptor antibodies: novel findings in a new case series of 20 patients. Neurology. 2013;81(17):1500–6.

66. Denny-Brown D. Primary sensory neuropathy with muscular changes associated with carcinoma. J Neurol Neurosurg Psychiatry. 1948;11(2):73–87.

67. Chalk CH, Windebank AJ, Kimmel DW, McManis PG. The distinctive clinical features of paraneoplastic sensory neuronopathy. Can J Neurol Sci. 1992;19(3):346–51.

68. Oh SJ, Gurtekin Y, Dropcho EJ, King P, Claussen GC. Anti-Hu antibody neuropathy: a clinical, electrophysiological, and pathological study. Clin Neurophysiol. 2005;116(1):28–34.

69. Camdessanche JP, Antoine JC, Honnorat J, Vial C, Petiot P, Convers P, et al. Paraneoplastic peripheral neuropathy associated with anti-Hu antibodies. A clinical and electrophysiological study of 20 patients. Brain. 2002;125(Pt 1):166–75.

70. Wanschitz J, Hainfellner JA, Kristoferitsch W, Drlicek M, Budka H. Ganglionitis in paraneoplastic subacute sensory neuronopathy: a morphologic study. Neurology. 1997;49(4):1156–9.

71. Oh SJ, Dropcho EJ, Claussen GC. Anti-Hu-associated paraneoplastic sensory neuropathy responding to early aggressive immunotherapy: report of two cases and review of literature. Muscle Nerve. 1997;20(12):1576–82.

72. Russo C, Cohn SL, Petruzzi MJ, de Alarcon PA. Long-term neurologic outcome in children with opsoclonus-myoclonus associated with neuroblastoma: a report from the Pediatric Oncology Group. Med Pediatr Oncol. 1997;28(4):284–8.

73. Pranzatelli MR, Tate ED, Dukart WS, Flint MJ, Hoffman MT, Oksa AE. Sleep disturbance and rage attacks in opsoclonus-myoclonus syndrome: response to trazodone. J Pediatr. 2005; 147(3):372–8.

74. Pranzatelli MR, Tate ED, Travelstead AL, Barbosa J, Bergamini RA, Civitello L, et al. Rituximab (anti-CD20) adjunctive therapy for opsoclonus-myoclonus syndrome. J Pediatr Hematol Oncol. 2006;28(9):585–93.

75. Koh PS, Raffensperger JG, Berry S, Larsen MB, Johnstone HS, Chou P, et al. Long-term outcome in children with opsoclonus-myoclonus and ataxia and coincident neuroblastoma. J Pediatr. 1994;125(5 Pt 1):712–6.

76. Anderson NE, Budde-Steffen C, Rosenblum MK, Graus F, Ford D, Synek BJ, et al. Opsoclonus, myoclonus, ataxia, and encephalopathy in adults with cancer: a distinct paraneoplastic syndrome. Medicine. 1988;67(2):100–9.

77. Sabater L, Xifro X, Saiz A, Alberch J, Graus F. Analysis of antibodies to neuronal surface antigens in adult opsoclonus-myoclonus. J Neuroimmunol. 2008;196(1–2):188–91.

78. Bataller L, Graus F, Saiz A, Vilchez JJ. Clinical outcome in adult onset idiopathic or paraneoplastic opsoclonus-myoclonus. Brain. 2001;124(Pt 2):437–43.

79. Batchelor TT, Platten M, Hochberg FH. Immunoadsorption therapy for paraneoplastic syndromes. J Neurooncol. 1998;40(2): 131–6.

80. Armangue T, Titulaer MJ, Sabater L, Pardo-Moreno J, Gresa-Arribas N, Barbero-Bordallo N, et al. A novel treatment-responsive encephalitis with frequent opsoclonus and teratoma. Ann Neurol. 2014;75(3):435–41.

81. Espay AJ, Chen R. Rigidity and spasms from autoimmune encephalomyelopathies: stiff-person syndrome. Muscle Nerve. 2006;34(6):677–90.

82. Brown P, Marsden CD. The stiff man and stiff man plus syndromes. J Neurol. 1999;246(8):648–52.

83. Pittock SJ, Lucchinetti CF, Parisi JE, Benarroch EE, Mokri B, Stephan CL, et al. Amphiphysin autoimmunity: paraneoplastic accompaniments. Ann Neurol. 2005;58(1):96–107.

84. Murinson BB, Guarnaccia JB. Stiff-person syndrome with amphiphysin antibodies: distinctive features of a rare disease. Neurology. 2008;71(24):1955–8.

85. De Camilli P, Thomas A, Cofiell R, Folli F, Lichte B, Piccolo G, et al. The synaptic vesicle-associated protein amphiphysin is the 128- kD autoantigen of Stiff-Man syndrome with breast cancer. J Exp Med. 1993;178(6):2219–23.

86. Solimena M, Folli F, Aparisi R, Pozza G, De Camilli P. Autoantibodies to GABA-ergic neurons and pancreatic beta cells in stiff-man syndrome. N Engl J Med. 1990;322(22):1555–60.

87. Raju R, Rakocevic G, Chen Z, Hoehn G, Semino-Mora C, Shi W, et al. Autoimmunity to GABAA-receptor-associated protein in stiff-person syndrome. Brain. 2006;129(Pt 12):3270–6.

88. Ishii A, Hayashi A, Ohkoshi N, Matsuno S, Shoji S. Progressive encephalomyelitis with rigidity associated with anti-amphiphysin antibodies. J Neurol Neurosurg Psychiatry. 2004;75(4):661–2.

89. Casado JL, Gil-Peralta A, Graus F, Arenas C, Lopez JM, Alberca R. Anti-Ri antibodies associated with opsoclonus and progressive encephalomyelitis with rigidity. Neurology. 1994; 44(8):1521–2.

90. Hutchinson M, Waters P, McHugh J, Gorman G, O'Riordan S, Connolly S, et al. Progressive encephalomyelitis, rigidity, and myoclonus: a novel glycine receptor antibody. Neurology. 2008;71(16):1291–2.

91. Mas N, Saiz A, Leite MI, Waters P, Baron M, Castano D, et al. Anti-glycine receptor encephalomyelitis with rigidity. J Neurol Neurosurg Psychiatry. 2011;82:1399–401.

92. McKeon A, Martinez-Hernandez E, Lancaster E, Matsumoto JY, Harvey RJ, McEvoy KM, et al. Glycine receptor autoimmune spectrum with stiff-man syndrome phenotype. JAMA Neurol. 2013;70(1):44–50.

93. Gresa-Arribas N, Arino H, Martinez-Hernandez E, Petit-Pedrol M, Sabater L, Saiz A, et al. Antibodies to inhibitory synaptic proteins in neurological syndromes associated with glutamic acid decarboxylase autoimmunity. PLoS ONE. 2015;10(3): e0121364.

94. Ishizawa K, Komori T, Okayama K, Qin X, Kaneko K, Sasaki S, et al. Large motor neuron involvement in Stiff-man syndrome: a qualitative and quantitative study. Acta Neuropathol (Berl). 1999;97(1):63–70.

95. Warich-Kirches M, von BP, Treuheit T, Kirches E, Dietzmann K, Feistner H, et al. Stiff-man syndrome: possible autoimmune etiology targeted against GABA-ergic cells. Clin Neuropathol. 1997;16(4):214–9.

96. Saiz A, Minguez A, Graus F, Marin C, Tolosa E, Cruz-Sanchez F. Stiff-man syndrome with vacuolar degeneration of anterior horn motor neurons. J Neurol. 1999;246(9):858–60.

97. Folli F, Solimena M, Cofiell R, Austoni M, Tallini G, Fassetta G, et al. Autoantibodies to a 128-kD synaptic protein in three women with the stiff-man syndrome and breast cancer. N Engl J Med. 1993;328(8):546–51.

98. Dalakas MC, Fujii M, Li M, Lutfi B, Kyhos J, McElroy B. High-dose intravenous immune globulin for stiff-person syndrome. N Engl J Med. 2001;345(26):1870–6.

99. Stern W, Howard R, Chalmers RM, Woodhall MR, Waters P, Vincent A, et al. Glycine receptor antibody mediated Progressive Encephalomyelitis with Rigidity and Myoclonus (PERM): a rare but treatable neurological syndrome. Pract Neurol. 2014;14(2): 123–7.

100. Barron KD, Rodichok LD. Cancer and disorders of motor neurons. In: Rowland LP, editor. Human motor neuron diseases. New York: Raven Press; 1982. p. 267–72.

101. Rosenfeld MR, Posner JB. Paraneoplastic motor neuron disease. In: Rowland LP, editor. Advances in neurology, volume 56: amyotrophic lateral sclerosis and other motor neuron diseases. New York: Raven Press; 1991. p. 445–59.

102. Freedman DM, Curtis RE, Daugherty SE, Goedert JJ, Kunci RW, Tucker MA. The association between cancer and amyotrophic lateral sclerosis. Cancer Causes Control. 2013;24(1):55–60.

103. Schold SC, Cho ES, Somasundaram M, Posner JB. Subacute motor neuronopathy: a remote effect of lymphoma. Ann Neurol. 1979;5:271–87.

104. Younger DS, Rowland LP, Latov N, Hays AP, Lange DJ, Sherman W, et al. Lymphoma, motor neuron diseases, and amyotrophic lateral sclerosis. Ann Neurol. 1991;29(1):78–86.

105. Croft PB, Urich H, Wilkinson M. Peripheral neuropathy of sensorimotor type associated with malignant disease. Brain. 1967;90(1):31–66.

106. Park SB, Goldstein D, Krishnan AV, Lin CS, Friedlander ML, Cassidy J, et al. Chemotherapy-induced peripheral neurotoxicity: a critical analysis. CA Cancer J Clin. 2013;63(6):419–37.

107. Antoine JC, Mosnier JF, Absi L, Convers P, Honnorat J, Michel D. Carcinoma associated paraneoplastic peripheral neuropathies in patients with and without anti-onconeural antibodies. J Neurol Neurosurg Psychiatry. 1999;67(1):7–14.

108. Honnorat J, Cartalat-Carel S, Ricard D, Camdessanche JP, Carpentier AF, Rogemond V, et al. Onco-neural antibodies and tumour type determine survival and neurological symptoms in paraneoplastic neurological syndromes with Hu or CV2/CRMP5 antibodies. J Neurol Neurosurg Psychiatry. 2009;80(4):412–6.

109. Oh SJ. Paraneoplastic vasculitis of the peripheral nervous system. Neurol Clin. 1997;15(4):849–63.

110. Choi HS, Kim DH, Yang SN, Sung HJ, Choi SJ. A case of paraneoplastic vasculitic neuropathy associated with gastric cancer. Clin Neurol Neurosurg. 2013;115(2):218–21.

111. Vasku M, Papathemelis T, Maass N, Meinhold-Heerlein I, Bauerschlag D. Endometrial carcinoma presenting as vasculitic sensorimotor polyneuropathy. Case Rep Obstet Gynecol. 2011;2011:968756.

112. Zivkovic SA, Ascherman D, Lacomis D. Vasculitic neuropathy–electrodiagnostic findings and association with malignancies. Acta Neurol Scand. 2007;115(6):432–6.

113. Matsumuro K, Izumo S, Umehara F, Arisato T, Maruyama I, Yonezawa S, et al. Paraneoplastic vasculitic neuropathy: immunohistochemical studies on a biopsied nerve and post-mortem examination. J Intern Med. 1994;236(2):225–30.

114. Ropper AH, Gorson KC. Neuropathies associated with paraproteinemia. N Engl J Med. 1998;338(22):1601–7.

115. Kelly JJ Jr. The electrodiagnostic findings in peripheral neuropathy associated with monoclonal gammopathy. Muscle Nerve. 1983;6(7):504–9.

116. Matsuda M, Gono T, Morita H, Katoh N, Kodaira M, Ikeda S. Peripheral nerve involvement in primary systemic AL amyloidosis: a clinical and electrophysiological study. Eur J Neurol. 2011;18(4):604–10.

117. Kelly JJ Jr, Kyle RA, Miles JM, Dyck PJ. Osteosclerotic myeloma and peripheral neuropathy. Neurology. 1983;33(2):202–10.

118. Dispenzieri A. POEMS syndrome: update on diagnosis, risk-stratification, and management. Am J Hematol. 2012;87(8):804–14.

119. Nasu S, Misawa S, Sekiguchi Y, Shibuya K, Kanai K, Fujimaki Y, et al. Different neurological and physiological profiles in POEMS syndrome and chronic inflammatory demyelinating polyneuropathy. J Neurol Neurosurg Psychiatry. 2012;83(5):476–9.

120. Nobile-Orazio E, Terenghi F, Giannotta C, Gallia F, Nozza A. Serum VEGF levels in POEMS syndrome and in immune-mediated neuropathies. Neurology. 2009;72(11):1024–6.

121. Dispenzieri A, Kyle RA, Lacy MQ, Rajkumar SV, Therneau TM, Larson DR, et al. POEMS syndrome: definitions and long-term outcome. Blood. 2003;101(7):2496–506.

122. Zagouri F, Kastritis E, Gavriatopoulou M, Sergentanis TN, Psaltopoulou T, Terpos E, et al. Lenalidomide in patients with POEMS syndrome: a systematic review and pooled analysis. Leuk Lymphoma. 2014;55(9):2018–23.

123. Dispenzieri A, Moreno-Aspitia A, Suarez GA, Lacy MQ, Colon-Otero G, Tefferi A, et al. Peripheral blood stem cell transplantation in 16 patients with POEMS syndrome, and a review of the literature. Blood. 2004;104(10):3400–7.

124. Levine T, Pestronk A, Florence J, Al Lozi MT, Lopate G, Miller T, et al. Peripheral neuropathies in Waldenstrom's macroglobulinaemia. J Neurol Neurosurg Psychiatry. 2006;77(2):224–8.

125. Dimopoulos MA, Panayiotidis P, Moulopoulos LA, Sfikakis P, Dalakas M. Waldenstrom's macroglobulinemia: clinical features, complications, and management. J Clin Oncol. 2000;18(1):214–26.

126. Viala K, Stojkovic T, Doncker AV, Maisonobe T, Lenglet T, Bruneteau G, et al. Heterogeneous spectrum of neuropathies in Waldenstrom's macroglobulinemia: a diagnostic strategy to optimize their management. J Peripher Nerv Syst. 2012;17(1):90–101.

127. Vital C, Vallat JM, Deminiere C, Loubet A, Leboutet MJ. Peripheral nerve damage during multiple myeloma and Waldenstrom's macroglobulinemia: an ultrastructural and immunopathologic study. Cancer. 1982;50(8):1491–7.

128. Pestronk A, Florence J, Miller T, Choksi R, Al-Lozi MT, Levine TD. Treatment of IgM antibody associated polyneuropathies using rituximab. J Neurol Neurosurg Psychiatry. 2003;74(4):485–9.

129. Latov N. Prognosis of neuropathy with monoclonal gammopathy. Muscle Nerve. 2000;23(2):150–2.

130. Weide R, Heymanns J, Koppler H. The polyneuropathy associated with Waldenstrom's macroglobulinaemia can be treated effectively with chemotherapy and the anti-CD20 monoclonal antibody rituximab. Br J Haematol. 2000;109(4):838–41.

131. Lunn MP, Nobile-Orazio E. Immunotherapy for IgM anti-myelin-associated glycoprotein paraprotein-associated peripheral neuropathies. Cochrane Database Syst Rev. 2012;5:CD002827.

132. Gruson B, Ghomari K, Beaumont M, Garidi R, Just A, Merle P, et al. Long-term response to rituximab and fludarabine combination in IgM anti-myelin-associated glycoprotein neuropathy. J Peripher Nerv Syst. 2011;16(3):180–5.

133. Koike H, Tanaka F, Sobue G. Paraneoplastic neuropathy: wide-ranging clinicopathological manifeations. Curr Opin Neurol. 2011;24(5):504–10.

134. Fagius J, Westerberg C-E, Olsson Y. Acute pandysautonomia and severe sensory deficit with poor clinical recovery. A clinical, neurophysiological and pathological case study. J Neurol Neurosurg Psychiatry. 1983;46(8):725–33.

135. Lennon VA, Sas DF, Busk MF, Scheithauer B, Malagelada JR, Camilleri M, et al. Enteric neuronal autoantibodies in pseudoobstruction with small- cell lung carcinoma. Gastroenterology. 1991;100(1):137–42.

136. Condom E, Vidal A, Rota R, Graus F, Dalmau J, Ferrer I. Paraneoplastic intestinal pseudo-obstruction associated with high

titres of Hu autoantibodies. Virchows Archiv A Pathol Anat. 1993;423(6):507–11.

137. McKeon A, Lennon VA, Lachance DH, Fealey RD, Pittock SJ. Ganglionic acetylcholine receptor autoantibody: oncological, neurological, and serological accompaniments. Arch Neurol. 2009;66(6):735–41.

138. Schroeder C, Vernino S, Birkenfeld AL, Tank J, Heusser K, Lipp A, et al. Plasma exchange for primary autoimmune autonomic failure. N Engl J Med. 2005;353(15):1585–90.

139. Elmqvist D, Lambert EH. Detailed analysis of neuromuscular transmission in a patient with the myasthenic syndrome sometimes associated with bronchogenic carcinoma. Mayo Clinic Proc. 1968;43(10):689–713.

140. Titulaer MJ, Wirtz PW, Kuks JB, Schelhaas HJ, van der Kooi AJ, Faber CG, et al. The Lambert-Eaton myasthenic syndrome 1988-2008: a clinical picture in 97 patients. J Neuroimmunol. 2008;15(201–202):153–8.

141. AAEM Quality Assurance Committee, American Association of Electrodiagnostic Medicine. Practice parameter for repetitive nerve stimulation and single fiber EMG evaluation of adults with suspected myasthenia gravis or Lambert-Eaton myasthenic syndrome: summary statement. Muscle Nerve. 2001;24(9):1236–8.

142. Nagashima T, Mizutani Y, Kawahara H, Maguchi S, Terayama Y, Shinohara T, et al. Anti-Hu paraneoplastic syndrome presenting with brainstem-cerebellar symptoms and Lambert-Eaton myasthenic syndrome. Neuropathology. 2003;23(3):230–8.

143. Titulaer MJ, Maddison P, Sont JK, Wirtz PW, Hilton-Jones D, Klooster R, et al. Clinical Dutch-English Lambert-Eaton Myasthenic syndrome (LEMS) tumor association prediction score accurately predicts small-cell lung cancer in the LEMS. J Clin Oncol. 2011;29(7):902–8.

144. Titulaer MJ, Wirtz PW, Willems LN, van Kralingen KW, Smitt PA, Verschuuren JJ. Screening for small-cell lung cancer: a follow-up study of patients with Lambert-Eaton myasthenic syndrome. J Clin Oncol. 2008;26(26):4276–81.

145. Titulaer MJ, Klooster R, Potman M, Sabater L, Graus F, Hegeman IM, et al. SOX antibodies in small-cell lung cancer and Lambert-Eaton myasthenic syndrome: frequency and relation with survival. J Clin Oncol. 2009;27(26):4260–7.

146. Motomura M, Lang B, Johnston I, Palace J, Vincent A, Newsom-Davis J. Incidence of serum anti-P/O-type and anti-N-type calcium channel autoantibodies in the Lambert-Eaton myasthenic syndrome. J Neurol Sci. 1997;147(1):35–42.

147. Keogh M, Sedehizadeh S, Maddison P. Treatment for Lambert-Eaton myasthenic syndrome. Cochrane Database Syst Rev. 2011;(2):CD003279.

148. Newsom-Davis J. Lambert-Eaton myasthenic syndrome. Rev Neurol (Paris). 2004;160(2):177–80.

149. Vedeler CA, Antoine JC, Giometto B, Graus F, Grisold W, Hart IK, et al. Management of paraneoplastic neurological syndromes: report of an EFNS task force. Eur J Neurol. 2006;13(7):682–90.

150. Maddison P, Lang B, Mills K, Newsom-Davis J. Long term outcome in Lambert-Eaton myasthenic syndrome without lung cancer. J Neurol Neurosurg Psychiatry. 2001;70(2):212–7.

151. Rich MM, Teener JW, Bird SJ. Treatment of Lambert-Eaton syndrome with intravenous immunoglobulin. Muscle Nerve. 1997;20(5):614–5.

152. Bain PG, Motomura M, Newsom-Davis J, Misbah SA, Chapel HM, Lee ML, et al. Effects of intravenous immunoglobulin on muscle weakness and calcium-channel autoantibodies in the Lambert-Eaton myasthenic syndrome. Neurology. 1996;47(3):678–83.

153. Isaacs H. A syndrome of continuous muscle-fibre activity. J Neurol Neurosurg Psychiatry. 1961;24(4):319–25.

154. Hart IK, Maddison P, Newsom-Davis J, Vincent A, Mills KR. Phenotypic variants of autoimmune peripheral nerve hyperexcitability. Brain. 2002;125(Pt 8):1887–95.

155. Maddison P, Mills KR, Newsom-Davis J. Clinical electrophysiological characterization of the acquired neuromyotonia phenotype of autoimmune peripheral nerve hyperexcitability. Muscle Nerve. 2006;33(6):801–8.

156. Newsom-Davis J, Mills KR. Immunological associations of acquired neuromyotonia (Isaac's syndrome). Report of five cases and literature review. Brain. 1993;116(Pt 2):453–69.

157. Hart IK, Waters C, Vincent A, Newland C, Beeson D, Pongs O, et al. Autoantibodies detected to expressed K+ channels are implicated in neuromyotonia. Ann Neurol. 1997;41(2):238–46.

158. Irani SR, Pettingill P, Kleopa KA, Schiza N, Waters P, Mazia C, et al. Morvan syndrome: clinical and serological observations in 29 cases. Ann Neurol. 2012;72(2):241–55.

159. Lancaster E, Huijbers MG, Bar V, Boronat A, Wong A, Martinez-Hernandez E, et al. Investigations of Caspr2, an autoantigen of encephalitis and neuromyotonia. Ann Neurol. 2011;69(2):303–11.

160. Irani SR, Alexander S, Waters P, Kleopa KA, Pettingill P, Zuliani L, et al. Antibodies to Kv1 potassium channel-complex proteins leucine-rich, glioma inactivated 1 protein and contactin-associated protein-2 in limbic encephalitis. Morvan's syndrome and acquired neuromyotonia. Brain. 2010;133 (9):2734–48.

161. Rubio-Agusti I, Perez-Miralles F, Sevilla T, Muelas N, Chumillas MJ, Mayordomo F, et al. Peripheral nerve hyperexcitability: a clinical and immunologic study of 38 patients. Neurology. 2011;76(2):172–8.

162. Skeie GO, Apostolski S, Evoli A, Gilhus NE, Illa I, Harms L, et al. Guidelines for treatment of autoimmune neuromuscular transmission disorders. Eur J Neurol. 2010;17(7):893–902.

163. Fukushima K, Sato T, Mitsuhashi S, Kaneko K, Yazaki M, Matsuda M, et al. Isaacs' syndrome associated with myasthenia gravis, showing remission after cytoreductive surgery of pleural recurrence of thymoma. Neuromuscul Disord. 2006;16(11):763–5.

164. Abou-Zeid E, Boursoulian LJ, Metzer WS, Gundogdu B. Morvan syndrome: a case report and review of the literature. J Clin Neuromuscul Dis. 2012;13(4):214–27.

165. Mahe E, Descamps V, Burnouf M, Crickx B. A helpful clinical sign predictive of cancer in adult dermatomyositis: cutaneous necrosis. Arch Dermatol. 2003;139(4):539.

166. Zampieri S, Valente M, Adami N, Biral D, Ghirardello A, Rampudda ME, et al. Polymyositis, dermatomyositis and malignancy: a further intriguing link. Autoimmun Rev. 2010;9(6):449–53.

167. Fardet L, Dupuy A, Gain M, Kettaneh A, Cherin P, Bachelez H, et al. Factors associated with underlying malignancy in a retrospective cohort of 121 patients with dermatomyositis. Medicine (Baltimore). 2009;88(2):91–7.

168. Madan V, Chinoy H, Griffiths CE, Cooper RG. Defining cancer risk in dermatomyositis. Part I. Clin Exp Dermatol. 2009;34(4):451–5.

169. Liu WC, Ho M, Koh WP, Tan AW, Ng PP, Chua SH, et al. An 11-year review of dermatomyositis in Asian patients. Ann Acad Med Singap. 2010;39(11):843–7.

170. Iaccarino L, Ghirardello A, Bettio S, Zen M, Gatto M, Punzi L, et al. The clinical features, diagnosis and classification of dermatomyositis. J Autoimmun. 2014;48–49:122–7.

171. Bohan A, Peter JB. Polymyositis and dermatomyositis (second of two parts). N Engl J Med. 1975;292(8):403–7.

172. Bohan A, Peter JB. Polymyositis and dermatomyositis (first of two parts). N Engl J Med. 1975;292(7):344–7.

173. Lam WW, Chan H, Chan YL, Fung JW, So NM, Metreweli C. MR imaging in amyopathic dermatomyositis. Acta Radiol. 1999;40(1):69–72.

174. Targoff IN, Mamyrova G, Trieu EP, Perurena O, Koneru B, O'Hanlon TP, et al. A novel autoantibody to a 155-kd protein is associated with dermatomyositis. Arthritis Rheum. 2006;54(11): 3682–9.

175. Trallero-Araguas E, Rodrigo-Pendas JA, Selva-O'Callaghan A, Martinez-Gomez X, Bosch X, Labrador-Horrillo M, et al. Usefulness of anti-p155 autoantibody for diagnosing cancer-associated dermatomyositis: a systematic review and meta-analysis. Arthritis Rheum. 2012;64(2):523–32.

176. Ichimura Y, Matsushita T, Hamaguchi Y, Kaji K, Hasegawa M, Tanino Y, et al. Anti-NXP2 autoantibodies in adult patients with idiopathic inflammatory myopathies: possible association with malignancy. Ann Rheum Dis. 2012;71(5):710–3.

177. Fiorentino DF, Chung LS, Christopher-Stine L, Zaba L, Li S, Mammen AL, et al. Most patients with cancer-associated dermatomyositis have antibodies to nuclear matrix protein NXP-2 or transcription intermediary factor 1gamma. Arthritis Rheum. 2013;65(11):2954–62.

178. Nalotto L, Iaccarino L, Zen M, Gatto M, Borella E, Domenighetti M, et al. Rituximab in refractory idiopathic inflammatory myopathies and antisynthetase syndrome: personal experience and review of the literature. Immunol Res. 2013; 56(2–3):362–70.

179. Choy EH, Hoogendijk JE, Lecky B, Winer JB. Immunosuppressant and immunomodulatory treatment for dermatomyositis and polymyositis. Cochrane Database Syst Rev. 2005;(3):CD003643.

180. Arin MJ, Scheid C, Hubel K, Krieg T, Groth W, Haerrmann G. Chronic graft-versus-host disease with skin signs suggestive of dermatomyositis. Clin Exp Dermatol. 2006;31(1):141–3.

181. Couriel DR, Beguelin GZ, Giralt S, De LM, Hosing C, Kharfan-Dabaja MA, et al. Chronic graft-versus-host disease manifesting as polymyositis: an uncommon presentation. Bone Marrow Transplant. 2002;30(8):543–6.

182. Levin MI, Mozaffar T, Al-Lozi MT, Pestronk A. Paraneoplastic necrotizing myopathy: clinical and pathological features. Neurology. 1998;50(3):764–7.

183. Grable-Esposito P, Katzberg HD, Greenberg SA, Srinivasan J, Katz J, Amato AA. Immune-mediated necrotizing myopathy associated with statins. Muscle Nerve. 2010;41(2):185–90.

184. Bronner IM, Hoogendijk JE, Wintzen AR, van der Meulen MF, Linssen WH, Wokke JH, et al. Necrotising myopathy, an unusual presentation of a steroid-responsive myopathy. J Neurol. 2003;250(4):480–5.

185. Anderlini P, Buzaid AC, Legha SS. Acute rhabdomyolysis after concurrent administration of interleukin-2, interferon-alfa, and chemotherapy for metastatic melanoma. Cancer. 1995;76(4):678–9.

186. Vu HJ, Pham D, Makary R, Nguyen T, Shuja S. Paraneoplastic necrotizing myopathy presenting as severe muscle weakness in a patient with small-cell lung cancer: successful response to chemoradiation therapy. Clin Adv Hematol Oncol. 2011;9(7): 557–6.

Neurologic Complications of Radiation Therapy

14

Damien Ricard, Thomas Durand, Arnault Tauziède-Espariat,
Delphine Leclercq, and Dimitri Psimaras

Introduction

Radiation therapy (RT) has a key role in oncology but is associated with significant, sometimes life-threatening neurotoxicity. The development of new techniques (such as radiosurgery or brachytherapy) has widened the indications of RT to more benign lesions (e.g., trigeminal neuralgia or vascular malformations), and has increased rates of long-term survivors who may develop late toxicity. Thus, complications of RT have garnered increasing interest. Neural tissue tolerance depends on several currently well-defined factors such as volume, total dose, dose per fraction, and duration of irradiation. In addition, other factors that may increase the risk of radiation-induced toxicity are older age, concurrent diseases (such as diabetes, vascular diseases), adjuvant chemotherapy, and probably genetic predisposition [1–3]. The adverse neurological effects of radiotherapy are usually classified according to the time course in relation to irradiation and include acute disorders (days to weeks), early-delayed complications (1–6 months) and late-delayed

D. Ricard (✉)
Department of Neurology, Hôpital d'Instruction des Armées Percy, 101 boulevard Henri Barbusse, 92140 Clamart, France
e-mail: damien.ricard@m4x.org

T. Durand
UMR MD4 8257 Cognition and Action Group, 45 Rue Des Saints Peres, 75005 Paris, France
e-mail: durand.thomas@live.fr

A. Tauziède-Espariat
Laboratory of Neuropathology, Sainte-Anne Hospital, 1, rue Cabanis, 75014 Paris, France
e-mail: a.tauziede-espariat@ch-sainte-anne.fr

D. Leclercq
Department of Neuroradiology, Pitié Salpêtrière Hospital, 47-83 Bd de l'Hôpital, 75013 Paris, France
e-mail: del.leclercq@gmail.com

D. Psimaras
Department of Neurology, Pitié Salpêtrière Hospital, 47 Bd de l'Hôpital, 75013 Paris, France
e-mail: dimitri.psimaras@aphp.fr

© Springer International Publishing AG 2018
D. Schiff et al. (eds.), *Cancer Neurology in Clinical Practice*,
DOI 10.1007/978-3-319-57901-6_14

complications (more than 6 months) (Table 14.1). Radiation damage may be direct to the central or peripheral nervous system or secondary to vascular or endocrine lesions, or to the development of a radiation-induced tumor.

Sequelae of Radiation Therapy to the Brain

Acute Encephalopathy

Acute encephalopathy usually appears within 2 weeks after the beginning of cranial RT, often a few hours after delivery of the first fraction. The patient presents with nausea and vomiting, drowsiness, headache, dysarthria, and a worsening of pre-existing neurological deficits, sometimes associated with fever. T2 hyperintensities on MRI may be seen according to a recent case report [4]. The clinical course is usually favorable, but herniation and death have been reported in patients with large tumors who have already presented with intracranial hypertension (e.g., with multiple metastases, posterior fossa, or intraventricular tumors). Large doses per fraction (usually >3 Gy/fraction) are the main risk factor: Young et al. [5] reported acute radiation damage in 50% of patients with brain metastases treated with 15 Gy in two fractions to the whole brain, and Hindo et al. [6] reported four deaths within 48 h of a 10 Gy RT given in one fraction. As these large doses are no longer in use, this syndrome is rarely seen. However, a minor form of this condition occurs in many patients, consisting of nausea and moderate headache occurring within hours following cranial irradiation. The pathophysiology of acute complications supposedly results from radiation-induced blood–brain barrier (BBB) disruption, resulting in a rise in intracranial pressure [7]. Steroids may help in preventing or limiting the consequences of acute encephalopathy, especially in patients with large primary or secondary brain tumors or with considerable edema particularly at risk of herniation. In such patients, daily doses of steroids of at least 16 mg

Table 14.1 Main neurological complications of radiotherapy

Site	Acute complication (<4 weeks after RT)	Early-delayed complications (1–6 month after RT)	Late-delayed complications (>6 month after RT)
Brain	• Acute encephalopathy	• Somnolence syndrome • Worsening of pre-existing symptoms • Transient cognitive impairments • Subacute rhombencephalitis	• Focal brain radionecrosis • Cognitive impairment and leukoencephalopathy • Secondary brain tumors
Spinal cord		• Lhermitte's sign	• Focal spinal radionecrosis • Progressive myelopathy • Spinal hemorrhage
Cranial nerves		• Transient hearing loss • Anosmia • Ageusia	• Hearing loss • Visual loss • Lower cranial nerves palsies
Peripheral nerves	• Paresthesiae	• Brachial or lumbosacral plexopathy (transient)	• Brachial or lumbosacral plexopathy • Malignant nerve sheath tumors • Lower motor neuron syndrome

dexamethasone should be prescribed 48–72 h before the first fraction; a limited dose per fraction (2 Gy or less per fraction) is also recommended in this situation [8, 9]. An encouraging double-blind randomized placebo-controlled trial has demonstrated in 44 patients that *Boswellia serrata* derived from Indian frankincense may protect against radiotherapy-induced acute edema [10]. To prevent this complication, surgical debulking should ideally be carried out before starting RT treatment.

Early-Delayed Complications of RT

Several early-delayed clinical patterns have been described (Table 14.1). They occur 2 weeks to 6 months after RT. The pathophysiology is thought to a transient demyelinating process triggered by BBB disruption and/or selective oligodendrocyte dysfunction.

Somnolence Syndrome

This condition was first described in the late 1920s in children receiving low-dose RT for scalp ringworm. Several studies reported cases of children who developed somnolence syndrome 5–8 weeks after prophylactic cranial RT for leukemia [11, 12]; other reports have shown that it also occurs in adults. The incidence of somnolence syndrome varies greatly (with figures ranging from 8 [12] to 84% [13]); this difference is related to various factors including tumor type, radiation dose, fractionation, and diagnostic criteria [14]. Prominent symptoms include drowsiness, somnolence, nausea, and anorexia. Headache and/or fever may also be reported. Friends or family often notice irritability, attentional deficits, and short-term memory impairment. The clinical severity of this complication is variable, with extremes ranging from minimal disorders to sleeping >20 h/day [12]. MRI studies are not contributory.

Electroencephalographic abnormalities include nonspecific diffuse slow waves [14]. Most studies report a monophasic course of symptoms, usually with a favorable outcome within a few weeks. However, a prospective study of 19 adults treated for primary brain tumors with cranial RT (45–55 Gy) reported a biphasic pattern of symptoms with two critical periods (from the 11th to the 21st day and from the 31st to the 35th day) following RT [15]. Furthermore, in this study, an accelerated fractionation led to significantly more severe drowsiness and fatigue than a conventional scheme. Some authors advocate the use of steroids during and after radiotherapy as prophylactic or symptomatic treatment [16]. A prospective double-blind randomized trial in leukemic children found that a dose of 4 mg/m^2 of dexamethasone during cranial radiotherapy reduced the incidence of somnolence syndrome (17.6% vs. 64.3%) as compared to a dose of 2 mg/m^2 [17].

Worsening of Pre-existing Symptoms, or Tumor Pseudoprogression

In patients under treatment for malignant brain tumors, a worsening of pre-existing neurological focal deficits leads to concerns of tumor progression, especially when observed in association with features of the somnolence syndrome and with transitory cognitive impairment. This complication arises within 6 weeks to 3 months after RT, and is clinically impossible to differentiate from progressive disease. Neuroimaging may be normal or show edema and increased contrast enhancement within the tumor bed, a situation that does not allow this syndrome to be differentiated from tumor recurrence and explains why inclusion of patients in experimental regimens for "recurrence" is not indicated during this period [18]; it is worthwhile noting that this radiological pattern can also be associated with no clinical worsening. Pseudoprogression rates can reach 20% after concomitant temozolomide and radiotherapy regimen used to treat glioblastoma and may be associated with better long-term tumor control tumor [19]. Improvement usually follows within a few weeks or months and a follow-up MR scan will commonly show spontaneous regression within 4–8 weeks (Fig. 14.1a–h). As in the somnolence syndrome, the treatment relies upon supportive care with steroids. Improvements in imaging techniques such as magnetic resonance spectroscopy (MRS) and perfusion may help in distinguishing between pseudoprogression and true progression with signs such as subependymal spread of the enhancing lesion [20] but is limited by the fact that residual tumor is often still present within the irradiated area [21].

Transient Cognitive Decline

A transient cognitive decline can be observed within the first 6 months after cranial RT, mainly affecting attention and recent memory, and may sometimes be associated with a somnolence syndrome. Armstrong et al. [22] prospectively followed 5 patients treated for primary brain tumors: memory impairment was conspicuous in all patients 1.5 months after focal cranial RT (43–63 Gy), but complete regression was observed after 2.5–10.5 months.

In another prospective study by Vigliani et al. [23] comparing 17 patients treated with focal cranial RT (54 Gy) for good prognosis gliomas and 14 matched control patients who did not undergo RT, 36% of the patients had a significant early-delayed impairment of their reaction test, with a return to normal baseline performance 12 months after RT. This test result was correlated with their occupational status: 69% of the patients could not work at 6 months, whereas 73% had continued or resumed their job at 1 year.

A recent study [24] investigated the cognitive status and radiological abnormalities during the first months after radiochemotherapy in 39 high-grade glioma patients. Seventy per cent of patients experienced cognitive stability or improvement whereas 30% declined. However, 80% of the decliners showed tumor progression during the following 4 months. The authors could not demonstrate a clear association between cognitive impairments and post-treatment radiographic changes in this study. Hahn et al. [25] showed a dose-dependent correlation between metabolism decrease in brain areas treated with >40 Gy and performances in problem solving and cognitive flexibility during the first 6 months after radiotherapy for CNS tumors.

However, transient cognitive decline is not always observed [26–28] and seems to vary according to patient and mental function involved. In our experience, informing patients about the possible difficulty in returning to a normal life (particularly work) at least during the first 6 months following radiotherapy is useful. Brain irradiation patterns limiting the hippocampal dose may limit subacute cognitive decline in brain and head and neck tumor patients [29, 30]. Although severe and, in some cases, persistent early-delayed

symptoms have been occasionally reported [31], it is of note that transient cognitive impairment does not appear to be a clear-cut predictive factor for subsequent development of long-term cognitive disorders.

Subacute Rhombencephalitis

Distinct from brainstem radionecrosis, which occurs later, early-delayed subacute rhombencephalitis may be observed 1–3 months after RT using portals involving the brainstem, as for ocular, pituitary, or head and neck tumors. The clinical picture includes ataxia, dysarthria, diplopia, and/or nystagmus as well as auditory loss. In some cases, the cerebrospinal fluid analysis shows inflammatory changes. MRI may demonstrate white matter abnormalities appearing as grossly round or more extensive T1-weighted hypointensities and T2-weighted hyperintensities affecting the brain stem and cerebellar peduncles; the lesions may enhance after gadolinium injection [32, 33]. The condition usually improves progressively over a few weeks to months, either spontaneously or with steroids, but coma and death have been reported in rare cases [34, 35].

Late-Delayed Complications of RT

Two principal delayed complications may follow RT, usually after more than 6 months: focal radionecrosis and mild-to-severe cognitive impairment associated with leucoencephalopathy. These adverse effects may occasionally be delayed many years.

Focal Brain Radionecrosis

Focal radionecrosis constitutes a challenging complication of radiation therapy because it appears as a bulky contrast-enhancing lesion often mimicking tumor recurrence and its functional consequences can be devastating. This complication may occur not only in patients who received focal RT for a primary or metastatic brain tumor but also in patients without brain lesions with a history of RT for extraparenchymal lesions, in whom normal brain was included in the radiation field (e.g., head and neck or pituitary tumors, meningiomas, skull osteosarcomas). A classic example is the bilateral medial temporal lobe necrosis that results from RT for pituitary or nasopharyngeal tumors (Fig. 14.2a–d). This once frequent complication of conventional RT has become rare over the last 20 years, as a consequence of the generalized use of safer radiation protocols. It has been shown that the upper limits of a "safe dose" were defined by a total dose of 55–60 Gy administered to a focal field with fractions of 1.8–2 Gy per day [36]. The chief risk factors are age at radiation and concurrent chemotherapy with a 5-year toxicity ranging from 27 to 37% in patients with nasopharyngeal carcinomas [37]. The focal delivery of

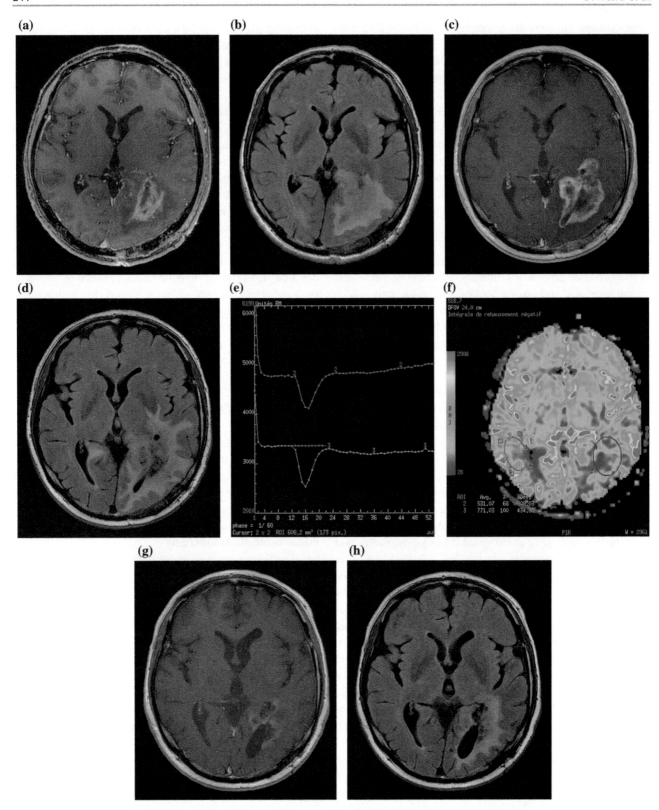

Fig. 14.1 **a–h** Tumor "pseudoprogression". A 59-year-old patient treated by surgery followed by radiochemotherapy for a left temporo-occipital glioblastoma. 2 months after the end of radiochemotherapy, MRI suggested tumor progression based on the increased tumor volume. The tumor volume decreased 3 months later. **a** Postsurgery axial T1 gadolinium. **b** Postsurgery axial T2 FLAIR. **c** 2 months post-radiochemotherapy axial T1 gadolinium. **d** 2 months post-radiochemotherapy axial T2 FLAIR. **e** 2 months post-radiochemotherapy perfusion-weighted curves showed an absence of neoangiogenesis. **f** 2 months post-radiochemotherapy axial perfusion-weighted image. **g** 5 months post-radiochemotherapy axial T1 gadolinium. **h** 5 months post-radiochemotherapy axial T2 FLAIR

Fig. 14.2 a–d Bi-temporal radionecrosis. **a** 69-year-old patient treated for a clival chordoma with radiotherapy (20 fractions of 1.8 Gy with tomotherapy and 21 fractions of 1.8 Gy with proton therapy). 3 years later, the patient developed memory impairment. **a** Axial T1 gadolinium shows large heterogeneous contrast-enhanced lesion in each temporal lobe. **b** Axial T2 FLAIR is suggestive of perilesionnal edema. **c** Axial T2* shows some microbleeds. **d** Axial perfusion-weighted image indicates no neo-angiogenesis

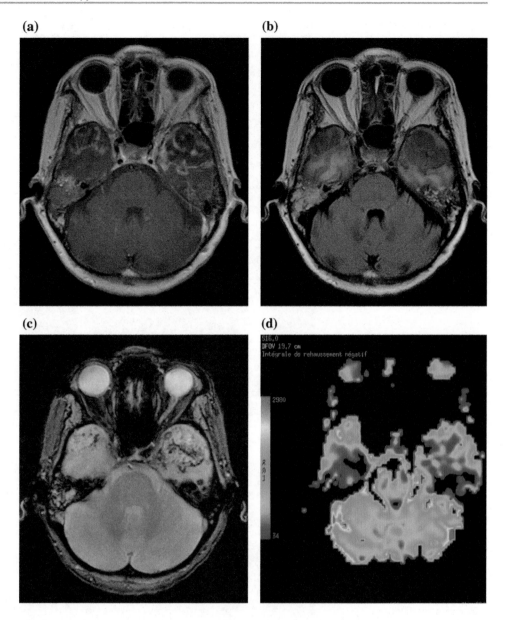

a single large radiation fraction during "radiosurgery" may also lead to focal necrosis of the brain adjacent to the irradiated lesion [38]. In arteriovenous malformations (AVM), the incidence of brain necrosis ranges from <5 to 20% of cases, with location and volume found to be the main risk factors [39–41] with an individual and unpredictable sensitivity to ionizing radiation [42]. After standard RT, radiation necrosis generally occurs within 1–2 years [43], but it has been observed after several decades. As described above, shorter latencies (as short as 3 months) have also been reported, especially in patients treated with interstitial brachytherapy [44] or radiosurgery.

Histopathologically, focal brain radionecrosis is characterized by prominent vascular damages including vascular fibrosis/hyalinization with luminal stenosis, thrombosis, hemorrhage, fibrinous exudates, telangiectasias, and

fibrinoid vascular necrosis (Fig. 14.3a–d) [45]. These features are associated with edema of brain parenchyma due to disruptions in the blood–brain barrier and parenchymal necrosis. Other common histopathological findings are calcifications, histiocytic infiltrates, and hyalinized and dilated blood vessels with enlargement of parenchymal Virchow–Robin spaces (Fig. 14.4a–d) [45]. The brain parenchyma often contains dystrophic neurons and reactive astrocytes that may be very atypical with pleomorphism and bizarre nuclei [45]. Those changes may raise the differential diagnosis of radiation-induced glioma. Nevertheless, those findings are not associated with high mitotic index or high MIB-1 labeling index as a tumor would have.

The pathophysiology of focal brain radionecrosis is not well understood. Kamiryo et al. [46] followed changes in the rat brain within one year of radiation at doses of 50, 75, and

Fig. 14.3 a–d Focal brain radionecrosis. Histopathological findings of focal brain radionecrosis. **a** Hyperplasia of thickened and hyalinized vessels (HES, 60× magnification). **b** Telangiectatic proliferation of vessels with hemorrhage and some inflammatory cells (HES, 70× magnification). **c** Hyaline necrosis with ghostly vessels (HES, 70× magnification). **d** Pallor of the white matter due to loss of myelin (HES, 40× magnification)

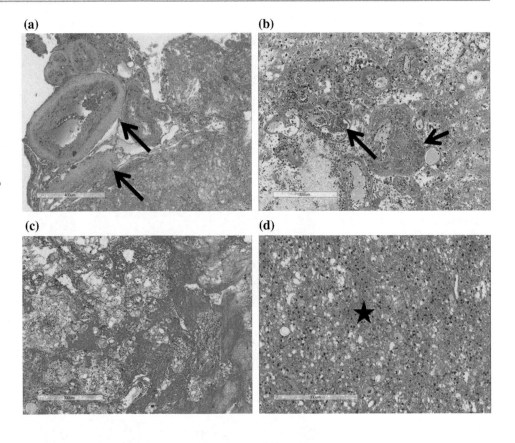

Fig. 14.4 a–d Focal brain radionecrosis. Histopathological findings of focal brain radionecrosis. **a** Calcifications (HES, 60× magnification). **b** histiocytic inflammation (HES, 70× magnification). **c** Enlargement of Virchow-Robin spaces (HES, 70× magnification). **d** Gliosis in the adjacent white matter with dystrophic astrocytes (HES, 100× magnification)

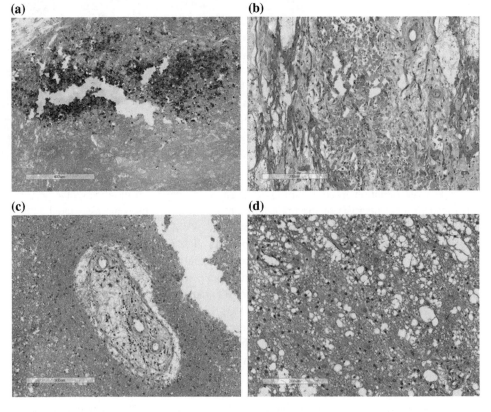

120 Gy mimicking therapeutic radiosurgery. The authors observed time- and dose-dependent changes. The first lesions to appear were morphological changes in astrocytes followed by vasodilation and fibrin deposition in capillary walls for all the studied doses. BBB leakage (Blue Evans permeability assay) was observed only after 75 and 120 Gy and necrosis only after 120 Gy.

An earlier study by Calvo et al. [47] focused on radiation-induced damage in the choroid plexus of the rat brain after a single dose of 17.5–25 Gy. They observed early morphological changes in the epithelial cells, followed by interstitial fibrosis associated with degenerative changes of arterioles and thrombi. Severity of lesions was dose and time-dependent. The same authors showed that necrosis was more frequent and occurred earlier in the fimbria than in the internal capsule and corpus callosum. They found a correlation between the incidence of necrosis in the white matter seen after a latent interval of 26 weeks and earlier changes in the vasculature such as blood vessel dilatation, blood vessel wall thickening, endothelial cell nuclear enlargement, and hypertrophy of perivascular astrocytes suggesting a continuous long-lasting mechanism induced by irradiation. Necrosis would be a consequence of ischemia secondary to blood vessel damage. At the molecular level, VEGF seems to play a pivotal role in the endothelial cell loss [48]. This progressive loss would eventually lead to overt necrosis [49]. Despite these findings, several points argue against a purely ischemic model: first, neurons are very sensitive to ischemia and should be prominently damaged if the lesion was primarily vascular whereas neurons are in fact largely spared during radionecrosis [50]. Second, vascular damage is not always present in radionecrosis [51]. Other cellular mechanisms may be involved and perpetuate vascular damage or contribute to edema, gliosis, and demyelination in the brain, such as upregulation of diverse adhesion molecules [52], production of cytokines [53, 54] or cumulative oxidative stress in endothelial cells.

Patients may experience seizures (first symptom in about 50% of cases), intracranial hypertension and/or focal neurological deficits [55–57]. Such symptoms closely mimic tumor recurrence or progression. Diagnosing radiation necrosis is often a challenge. In many cases, CT and MR scans show a tumor-like pattern, often indistinguishable from tumor progression or recurrence [58]. White matter FLAIR hyperintense lesions are the first imaging manifestation of focal brain radionecrosis. Contrast-enhanced lesions develop after white matter hyperintensities; their appearance changes with size, with an increasing tendency to necrosis with increasing size. Cysts are the least frequent and develop in the late stage of brain focal radionecrosis, always arising from a contrast-enhanced lesion that has undergone necrosis [59]. As diagnostic assessment based on clinical and standard neuroimaging data is difficult, many studies have tried to address the problem of noninvasive differentiation between tumor recurrence/progression and radionecrosis. Positron emission tomography (PET) with ^{18}F-fluorodeoxyglucose [60] or 18F-Dopa [61] or ^{11}C-methionine, single photon emission computed tomography (SPECT) with [201]thallium or marked methoxy-isobutyl-isonitrile (99mTc-MIBI) [62] and the use of 3-[(123)I]iodo-alpha-methyl-l-tyrosine (IMT) [63, 64] have been used to assess the nature of the lesions. In typical cases, radionecrosis is characterized by hypometabolism and tumoral growth by hypermetabolism but results have been obtained on small series and standardization of detection thresholds is still awaited among teams [65]. The development of magnetic resonance spectroscopy (MRS) may help [66] as spectral analysis of necrosis areas shows an overall, harmonious decrease of metabolite peaks, and a possible increase of lipids corresponding to cellular necrosis; no lactate peak is observed [67, 68]. However, none of these techniques offers 100% sensitivity or specificity [69, 70]. One of the reasons for limitations is the frequent co-existence of radiation-induced necrosis with viable tumor tissue within the same area, a situation that obviously renders clear-cut distinction impossible [8, 65]. In some cases, angiography may provide further information, with an avascular mass seen in patients with radionecrosis; however, the risks and benefits of this procedure must be carefully weighed. While neuropathological examination remains the standard of diagnosis [71], even pathological analysis may be difficult because of the frequent mixture of both residual/recurrent tumor and radiation necrosis within the lesion [45].

Focal radionecrosis is sometimes spontaneously reversible even in the setting of a contrast-enhancing lesion [59]. Nevertheless, resection of a necrotic mass is often the best treatment in symptomatic cases. Steroids are generally used, with possible long-term improvement [8]; steroid dependence does occur. Other treatments have been reported in this setting, but their efficacy has not yet been addressed in large studies: anticoagulants have been prescribed by Glantz et al. [72] in 8 glioma patients (7 with histological evidence of necrosis) after the failure of steroids, leading to improvement in 5 patients. In our experience, anticoagulants have been somewhat disappointing. Some authors have advocated the use of hyperbaric oxygen (HBO) , with the rationale that HBO increases the tissue pO2 and enhances angiogenesis. Chuba et al. [73] treated 10 patients with CNS radionecrosis (biopsy-proven by biopsy in 8) with 100% oxygen for 90–120 min/session for at least 20 sessions. All patients stabilized or improved initially, and the 6 surviving patients showed durable improvement after 3–36 months. However, most patients were given steroids, and the respective effect of each treatment is not clear. HBO treatment was also reported to improve radionecrosis due to radiosurgery [74, 75]. The possible role of HBO in radiation-induced neurotoxicity needs to be evaluated in prospective trials [76]. Other drugs or combinations such as pentoxifylline, alpha-tocopherol [77], low-iron diet, desferrioxamine, and pentobarbital [1] have also been proposed occasionally without definite evidence of efficacy. The usefulness of radioprotective agents such as difluoromethylornithine (DMO) [78], U-74389G (a 21 aminosteroid) [79], or others [80–83], in reducing the risk of necrosis have been proved efficient in preclinical studies and request confirmation in clinical trials. There are increasing data about short-course bevacizumab therapy used for cerebral radiation necrosis, with symptomatic positive effects in case reports, small case series and one 14-patient randomized double-blind study [84]. Tye et al. [85] reviewed 16 publications from 2007 to 2012, including 71 cases where bevacizumab was administered for the treatment of focal brain radiation necrosis; 97% of the patients showed radiographic improvement and 79% improved performance status after treatment with bevacizumab. Bevacizumab is thus recommended in the second line setting following corticosteroids.

Cognitive Dysfunction and Leukoencephalopathy

Late-delayed cognitive impairment covers a wide continuum of patterns ranging from mild dysfunction to severe (and sometimes fatal) dementia, and has become an important concern over the last 20 years. The impact (and awareness) of this complication has grown because of both a better assessment of cognition and quality of life in clinical practice and the growing population of long-term survivors with tumor stability or remission.

Attributing all cognitive dysfunction to RT alone would result in a considerable overestimate of the incidence of radiation-induced sequelae. Cognitive impairment may be the consequence of complex interactions [3, 86, 87] between pre-existing cognitive abnormalities (especially in the case of brain tumors), brain tumor growth, concomitant treatments (such as chemotherapy, antiepileptic [88] or psychotropic drugs), paraneoplastic encephalomyelitis, and endocrine dysfunction. In practice, this should lead to an individualized workup in patients with potential radiation-induced cognitive impairment, but also to a careful and critical interpretation of the higher cognitive dysfunction rates found in the literature. Although high-dose per fraction (>2 Gy) is an important risk factor for induced cognitive impairments, decreases in cognitive function are also observed with small daily radiation doses [89].

Studies suggest that RT alone plays a more limited role in cognitive decline when using modern radiation techniques and fractionation schedules [27, 90, 91, 92]. Nevertheless, several factors have been clearly linked to an increased risk of radiation-induced cognitive impairment: (i) *Advancing age at brain irradiation*: several studies have demonstrated that demented patients were clearly older (55–60 years) than non-demented patients (<45 year old) [93–96]; (ii) *Large radiation doses*, particularly when fractions over 2 Gy are used; (iii) *Large irradiated brain volume*: this factor may also increase the risk of cognitive impairment; the rate of RT-induced cognitive dysfunction [94, 95, 97, 98] may be as high as 50% in patients receiving whole brain radiotherapy (WBRT), whereas the precise incidence of cognitive impairment after focal brain radiotherapy is difficult to assess because of contradictory figures in the literature; (iv) *Combined treatment*: the incidence of dementia in patients treated with combined RT and chemotherapy ranges from 4 to 63%. Methotrexate (MTX) is clearly implicated in combined toxicity; neurotoxic by itself, it is responsible for frequent cognitive dysfunction when associated with RT. In children, most studies to date have concluded that the combination of cranial irradiation and intrathecal MTX was associated with declines in both IQ and achievement scores [99]. In adults treated with WBRT (40 Gy + 14 Gy boost) and a combination of intravenous and intrathecal MTX for CNS lymphoma, the incidence of severe progressive cognitive impairment increases with age, reaching 83% in patients over 60 years [96, 100, 101, 102]. The timing of MTX chemotherapy is important because the cognitive dysfunction rate is higher whenever MTX is prescribed during or after RT. This drug should therefore be given before irradiation. Data regarding the neurotoxicity of other combinations are sparse, but agents such as nitrosourea, cisplatin, etoposide, cytarabine, or actinomycin D are also suspected to increase radiation-induced cognitive toxicity. Multidrug regimens or high-dose chemotherapy combined with WBRT are probably associated with a higher risk of neurotoxicity [103]. Although there is a continuum between mild-to-moderate cognitive impairment and severe fatal dementia, we will consider the two conditions separately.

Radiation-Induced Mild-to-Moderate Cognitive Impairment

Mild-to-moderate cognitive dysfunction is more frequent in long-term survivors than frank dementia. The features of this condition are incompletely defined, as results vary across studies, likely attributable to neuropsychological evaluation procedures, duration of follow-up and population discrepancies [104]. Thus, the incidence of cognitive decrement related to radiation is difficult to evaluate. With anaplastic oligodendrogliomas and oligoastrocytomas, Habets et al. [92] reported that 30% of 32 progression-free patients were severely and 44% mildly impaired 2.5 years after initial chemoradiotherapy treatment. The most affected domains were psychomotor functions, attention and working memory, but these domains also manifested high interindividual variability. Further more, executive functioning and information speed processing were often weak, with results ranging from normal to pathologic. In another study, Douw et al. [89] explored the cognitive status of 65 low-grade glioma patients after a long-term follow-up (mean of 12 years, range 6–28 years) and observed that 53% of the patients who received radiotherapy were impaired in at least 5/18 neuropsychological test versus 27% in the patients who did not had radiotherapy. The most impaired functions were attention, executive functions, and information speed processing. Thus, radiation-induced cognitive impairment mainly affects attention, executive functioning, and information speed processing, while intellectual functions are generally preserved on neuropsychological evaluations [3, 86]. Nevertheless, most patients have to decrease or even discontinue their professional activities. These functions involve fontal corticosubcortical networks on which atrophy of white matter lesions can be observed. At this stage, CT scan may be abnormal, showing periventricular hypodensities, an increase in the normal interface between white and gray matter, and ventricular enlargement. However, there seems to be no correlation between CT scan abnormalities and the degree of cognitive impairment. MRI shows variable degrees of T2-weighted hyperintensities in the white matter but the functional correlate is not clear [24]. Fractional anisotropy may prove an interesting biomarker in normal-appearing white matter of patients treated with brain radiotherapy [105].

The course of radiation-related cognitive decline is difficult to predict: some patients deteriorate slowly while the majority apparently remain stable. Progression to dementia is seldom reported. There is no recognized treatment for this syndrome, although some authors have advocated the use of methylphenidate [106–108], anticholinesterase drugs [109, 110], memantine [111], or modafinil [108, 112, 113] for symptomatic relief. Psychological interventions may be useful [114, 115], as well as other non-pharmacological interventions like hyperbaric oxygen therapy [116], but solid replicated results are lacking. Day et al. [117] reviewed the randomized controlled trials that evaluated interventions aiming to reduce impairment related to cranial irradiation; they concluded there was a beneficial effect of donepezil and memantine despite limited studies.

Attempts to prevent cognitive impairment with potential neuroprotective agents or treatment methods have been made. Randomized trials have demonstrated that use of Motexafin Gadolinium (MGd) may protect against cognitive decline following whole brain radiation on cognition [118–120], though this effect may be related to this agent's suppression of tumor growth. Phase 2 data suggest hippocampal sparing during radiation may prevent memory loss from fractionated radiotherapy for brain metastases [30, 121]. Sparing of other structures critical to cognitive

functions (e.g., corpus callosum, frontal lobes, posterior fossa) might result in reducing neurotoxicity but unfortunately dose–response data are missing [122].

Other agents have been proposed for a potential neuroprotective effect, including erythropoietin (EPO) [123–125], lithium [126], and free-radical scavengers such as amifostine or angiotensin-converting enzyme inhibitors (ACEi) [127, 128].

Radiation-Induced Dementia

The incidence of this devastating complication varies widely in the literature (from 0% to more than 60%) according to the series. In a large review of several studies comprising 748 adult patients, the incidence of severe cognitive impairment compatible with dementia was at least 12.3% [129]. More recent studies and clinical practice are more reassuring [96, 130].

A "subcortical dementia" pattern that probably reflects the consequences of diffuse white matter injury characterizes the clinical picture.

The histopathological lesions of this radiation-induced leukoencephalopathy are similar to focal brain radionecrosis, consisting of well-demarcated areas of disseminated white matter necrosis (Fig. 14.5), myelin pallor and axonal alterations (which appear swollen and fragmented with calcifications), spongiosis, histiocytic inflammation, white matter gliosis, fibrotic thickening of small blood vessels in the deep white matter (Fig. 14.6), and atherosclerosis of the large vessels. Its pathogenesis remains unclear. Due to the difficulty in obtaining human tissue, histopathological studies of irradiated brains in human are scarce. However, a few

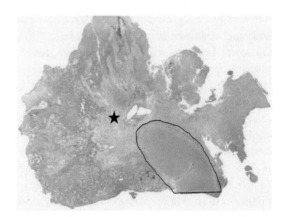

Fig. 14.5 Radiation-induced leukoencephalopathy. Histopathological findings of radiation-induced leukoencephalopathy showing well-defined limitation between the areas of necrosis (*asterisk*) and preserved brain parenchyma (*surrounded zone*) (HES, 25× magnification)

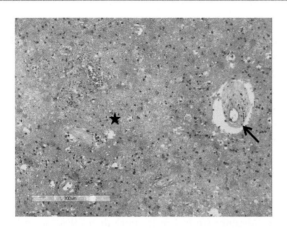

Fig. 14.6 Radiation-induced leukoencephalopathy. Histopathological findings of radiation-induced leukoencephalopathy showing pallor of the white matter (*asterisk*) associated with gliosis and fibrotic thickening of small blood vessels (*arrow*) (HES, 80× magnification)

autopsy studies in adults and children are available and show similar features of vascular and demyelinating lesions at light microscopic level. Lai et al. [131] studied the brain of 5 adult patients with primary CNS lymphoma who were in complete remission but who died after combined modality therapy with WBRT and chemotherapy. The MRI showed cerebral atrophy, ventricular dilatation, and white matter hyperintensity on FLAIR and T2 images. Occasional enhancing lesions were observed. The histopathological lesions were myelin and axonal loss, spongiosis, gliosis in white matter, fibrotic thickening of small blood vessels in the deep white matter and atherosclerosis of the large vessels in the circle of Willis. All patients but one were older than 60, and symptoms of neurotoxicity developed within 3 months of completion of treatment. Another autopsy study included 34 children with gliomas, 22 of whom had undergone CNS radiation therapy [132]. Causes of death were not detailed in this study and cognitive status of children before they died was unknown. Lesions such as demyelination, focal necrosis, cortical atrophy, endothelial proliferation, vascular thrombosis, vascular thickening were more frequently observed in irradiated brains, whereas neuronal degeneration, cerebral edema, and gliosis were common in both irradiated and unirradiated brains. Demyelination was observed at all time points from 6 months but was more common 9+ months after radiotherapy. Vascular changes were a late effect of radiation injury. Panagiotakos et al. [133] performed an original and extensive study on human normal and irradiated white matter brain samples from surgical biopsies of peritumoral glial tissue. Samples from irradiated patients exhibited persistent loss of oligoprogenitors starting as early as 2 months after radiation, whereas the decline of more mature oligodendrocytes only started beyond a year after irradiation. Early and transitory

endothelial cell loss was noted. Myelin sheaths showed signs of degradation. Signs suggesting axonal damage were only seen long after irradiation. Neuronal cell bodies seemed to be spared from radiation injury.

Because histological examination usually shows both vascular lesions and demyelination, vessels and glial cells have often been considered as the primary target of postirradiation leukoencephalopathy [134]. A short discussion of the main aspects of the pathophysiology of RT-related injuries follows.

Vascular Damage

Transient disruption of the blood–brain barrier, possibly initiated by sphingomyelinase-mediated endothelial apoptosis, is observed in animal models [45, 135, 136]. Thus, a cascade could be initiated at the time of irradiation, producing gradual cell loss throughout the clinically silent period. At the molecular level, VEGF seems to play a pivotal role in the endothelial cell loss [48]. This progressive loss would eventually lead to overt necrosis [49]. Despite these findings, several points argue against a purely ischemic model: first, neurons are very sensitive to ischemia and should be prominently damaged if the lesion was primarily vascular whereas neurons are in fact largely spared during radiation-induced leukoencephalopathy [50]. Second, vascular damage is not always present in animal models [51]. Other cellular mechanisms may be involved and perpetuate vascular damage or contribute to edema, gliosis, and demyelination in the brain, such as upregulation of diverse adhesion molecules [52], production of cytokines [53, 54] or cumulative oxidative stress in endothelial cells.

Oligodendrocytes

The demyelinating lesions observed after RT underscore the putative role of oligodendrocytes as a target of radiation damage. Oligodendrocytes are responsible for the production of the myelin sheath in the CNS and derive from progenitor cells such as O2A. CNS radiation induces depletion of oligodendrocytes and suppresses, at least transiently, the production of oligodendrocytes progenitors [137–139], possibly through a p53-dependent pathway [140–142]. However, the contribution of demyelination to tissue destruction remains questionable since severely demyelinating conditions such as multiple sclerosis do not lead to overt necrosis [50].

Other CNS Cell Types

Several studies have focused on the potential role of neurons, astrocytes, and microglia in the development of

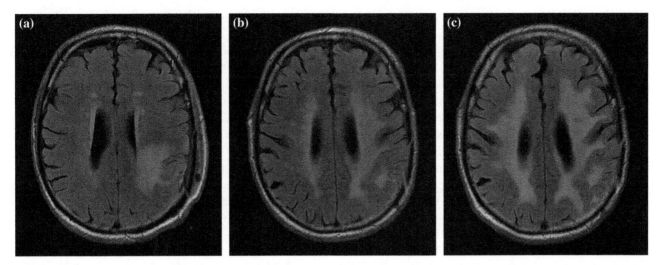

Fig. 14.7 a–c   Radiationo-induced   leukoencephalopathy. A 67-year-old patient treated with partial surgery followed by radiochemotherapy for a left parietal glioblastoma. MRI shows progressive signs of leukoencephalopathy with periventricular diffuse white mater hyperintensities and cortical atrophy. **a** Axial T2 FLAIR after surgery and before radiochemotherapy. **b** Axial T2 FLAIR 5 months after radiotherapy. **c** Axial T2 FLAIR 15 months after radiotherapy showing a progressive increase

radiation-induced lesions, either as primary targets or through alterations of their regulatory capacity [143–145]. Particularly noteworthy is the possible role of microglia [146] that may enhance radiation injury through persistent oxidative stress [147]. Radiation damage to the subventricular zone, a tissue containing glial and neural stem cells, was reported more than 40 years ago [148]. Others studies have found a dose-dependent reduction of neural stem cells of the subependyma after irradiation in this region [149, 150]. Their implication in radiation injury thus seems probable but remains to be elucidated. As a whole, the development of radiation injury is complex, and results from interactions between vascular cells and oligodendrocytes, as well as neural stem cells and the physiological responses of these cells to injury.

Patients present with progressive memory and attention deficits, intellectual loss, gait abnormalities, emotional lability, apathy, and fatigue [151]. The absence of hallucinations or delirium and the very unusual. Occurrence of aphasia, agnosia, or apraxia (deficits suggesting cortical involvement) are important clinical features for narrowing the differential diagnosis, especially in elderly patients. Depression is frequent, but antidepressants do not improve cognitive function. Eventually, patients may develop gait ataxia, incontinence, and sometimes a picture of akinetic mutism. Nonspecific features such as seizures, pyramidal or extrapyramidal signs, or tremor are also frequently encountered in the course of the disease. Neuroimaging always shows diffuse white matter lesions, best seen on MRI as T2-weighted hyperintensities, associated with cortical and subcortical atrophy as well as ventricular enlargement

(Fig. 14.7a–c). When performed, the lumbar puncture usually shows normal-to-moderately elevated (<1 g/l) CSF protein levels.

No specific treatment is currently able to cure radiation-induced dementia. However, as the clinical features are similar to those of normal pressure hydrocephalus, some authors have advocated ventriculoperitoneal shunting; this procedure does improve the quality of life in a few selected patients [96, 152, 153]. In our experience, cognitive and gait-oriented rehabilitation are usually helpful.

Deterioration occurs in about 80% of cases, leading to death; stabilization is possible (18% of cases). Lasting improvement is exceptional. Death generally occurs within 1–48 months after the onset of the disorder [154].

Other Long-Term Direct Brain Parenchyma Radiation-Induced Lesions

Recent advances in high-grade gliomas treatment have increased the awareness that progressive lesions on MRI do not always mean tumor recurrence [18]. Importantly, the possibility of pseudoprogression is not entirely restricted to the early post-radiochemotherapy period [155].

It has also been suggested that post-radiation cortical vasculopathy might lead to the occurrence of non-epileptic reversible neurological symptoms, which have been described as the SMART syndrome (Stroke-like Migraine Attacks after Radiation Therapy) [156]. SMART syndrome is clinically defined by episodic cephalalgia with transient focal neurological deficit mimicking migraine aura years after radiation for brain tumor. Interestingly, these symptoms are associated with transient dramatic cortical gadolinium enhancement of the affected cerebral hemisphere [156, 157] (Fig. 14.8a–c).

Approximately half of patients with brain tumors develop seizures during the course of their illness [158], and the occurrence of a first seizure or the recurrence of epilepsy after prolonged seizure control is frequently associated with tumor relapse. However, brain tumor-related seizures can also result in transient MRI abnormalities that can wrongly suggest tumor progression. This phenomenon has recently been described and called peri-ictal pseudoprogression (PIPG) [159].

Recently, 5 patients sharing some common features, including a remote history of whole brain irradiation in young to middle age, acute but long-lasting (4–24 days) impaired consciousness (Glasgow Coma Scale score 3–10), and clinical improvement after high-dose steroids were reported [160]. Vigilance impairment rapidly progressed to coma within 24–72 h. All patients required intermediate or intensive care. Other neurologic signs and symptoms included motor deficits and aphasia, headache, and visual hallucinations. Several consecutive EEG recordings performed during the acute phase showed bilateral/diffuse slow abnormalities in all patients, with unilateral predominance. MRI showed multiple bilateral areas of subcortical patchy enhancement and focal leptomeningeal enhancement. These were resolved at a follow-up MRI performed 5–8 months later. This syndrome was termed ALERT, for acute late onset leukoencephalopathy after radiotherapy.

Radiation-Induced Brain Tumors

The precise role of RT in the development of a tumor in any given case is difficult to determine, in great part because these tumors lack distinctive features compared to unirradiated patients. However, data from animal and epidemiological studies indicate that irradiated patients or animals are more likely to develop a second brain tumor than would be expected [161].

Several large studies have assessed the relative risk of developing a radiation-induced tumor. A study of 10,834 patients treated with low-dose cranial and cervical irradiation for *Tinea capitis* (mean dose to neural tissue: 1.5 Gy) found a relative risk of developing a tumor of 6.9; the risk for glioma was 2.6 [162].

In another study of 10,106 survivors of childhood cancers [163], the relative risk of developing a secondary CNS tumor was 7. Most other studies have found similar results [164, 165]. However, the risk is probably higher in patients treated for acute lymphoblastic leukemia (ALL) : a large retrospective cohort study of 9720 children [166] found a relative risk of developing a nervous system tumor as high as 22. In another setting, a large study on second brain tumors in 426 patients with pituitary adenoma treated with surgery and radiotherapy showed a 2.4% risk at 20 years [165].

Criteria for a radiation-induced tumor include: (a) long interval between radiotherapy and the occurrence of the second tumor (the mean onset delay is 12 years, with cases ranging from 1 to 40 years); (b) tumor growth within the radiation portal or at its margins; (c) a different histological

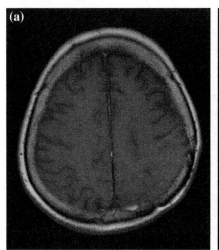 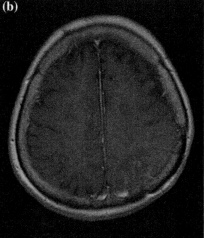 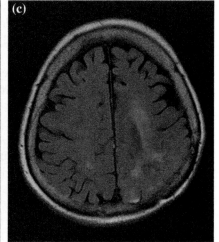

Fig. 14.8 a–c SMART syndrome. 72 year old patient treated for a high-grade glioma with radiochemotherapy (30*2 Gy). 7 years after the treatment, the patient presented with transitory cephalalgias, motor deficit and right hemiparesis. **a** Axial T1. **b** Axial T1 with gadolinium injection showing contrast-enhancing nodular pericortical lesions. **c** Axial T2 FLAIR showing focal white mater hyperintensity

subtype. After stereotactic radiosurgery, radiation-induced neoplasms are extremely rare, with only four reported cases [167]. Three types of tumors have been reported to be linked with cranial irradiation: meningioma in about 70% of cases, glioma in 20%, and sarcoma in fewer than 10%.

More than 900 cases [168] of radiation-induced meningiomas have been reported dating back to 1953 [169]; female predominance is less prominent than in spontaneous meningiomas [170]. The risk of occurrence correlates with radiation dose: low-dose RT induced a relative risk of 9.5 in one study [162], whereas high-dose RT was linked to a relative risk of 37 [164]. The tumor emerges after a long latency period: a review found extremes ranging from 2 to 63 years (mean 18.7 years) after high-dose RT [171].

Histopathologically, the most frequent subtypes are meningothelial and transitional (Fig. 14.9a–c), followed by fibroblastic and angioblastic [172], but other meningioma variants have been described after irradiation including metaplastic meningiomas (xanthomatous, myxomatous) [173, 174], chordoid meningiomas [175].

In the majority of cases, radiation-associated meningiomas are benign, multiple, and recurrent (World Health Organization grade I) [168, 176]. Nevertheless, atypical (grade II) or anaplastic (grade III) meningiomas have been also frequently reported. They evidence features of malignancy (Fig. 14.10a, b) such as nuclear pleomorphism with great variation in nuclear size, shape and chromatin density,

high cellularity, increased mitotic figures, atypia and necrotic changes [168, 172, 177, 178] and high MIB-1 labeling index. Other nonspecific findings include numerous multinucleated and giant cells, thickened blood vessels and vacuolated nuclear inclusions [168]. Radiation-induced meningiomas are sporadic.

Cytogenetic studies have been performed in some radiation-induced meningiomas and showed numerous genetic alterations such as loss of 1p and 7p chromosomes [179], loss of 22q12.2 [175], loss or deletion on choromosome 6 [180]. Indeed, these chromosomal alterations evoked by radiation accelerate loss of cellular control mechanisms and earlier expression of the neoplastic phenotype [181, 182]. Radiation-induced gliomas are much less frequent. Since 1960, about 120 cases have been reported in the English literature [183, 184]; fewer than half of these were glioblastomas. In the group of patients treated with RT for acute leukemia, multifocality occurred in 20% of cases. The median delay of onset ranges from 6 to 9 years [184]. It is well recognized that radiation-induced gliomas in children are high grade [185]. Among these radiation-induced gliomas, all histopathological subtypes have been reported: high-grade tumors such as glioblastoma, anaplastic astrocytoma or oligodendroglioma (Fig. 14.10a, b), but more rarely low-grade tumors such as grade II diffuse astrocytomas [186]. Gliosarcoma, characterized by mixed glial and mesenchymal elements (Fig. 14.11a–c), is a classical

Fig. 14.9 a–c Radiation-induced meningiomas. Histopathological findings of a case of radiation-induced meningioma. **a** High cellular proliferation compound of meningothelial cells with small foci of necrosis (*asterisk*) (HES, 130× magnification). **b** Pleomorphic tumoral cells with prominent nucleoli and mitosis (*arrow*) (HES, 300× magnification). **c** High MIB-1 labeling index (120× magnification)

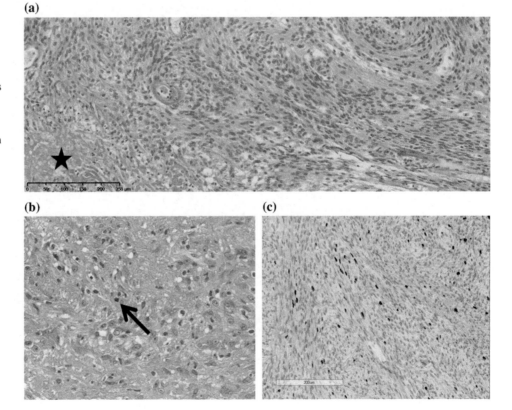

(a)

(b)

(c)

Fig. 14.10 a,
b Radiation-induced
oligodendroglioma.
Histopathological findings of a
case of radiation-induced
oligodendroglioma with signs of
malignity. **a** High cellular
proliferation with endothelial
proliferation (*arrows*) and
necrosis (*asterisk*) (HES,
50× magnification).
b Oligodendroglial proliferation
with pleomorphism, atypia, and
numerous mitoses (*arrows*) (HES,
200× magnification)

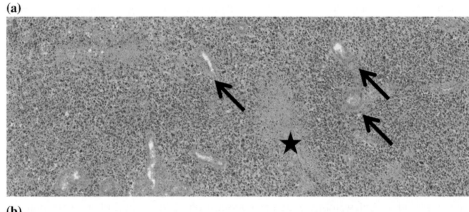

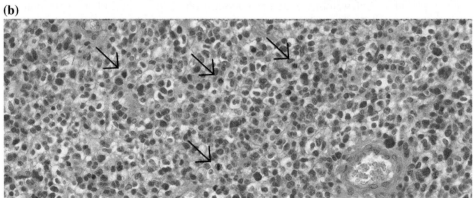

Fig. 14.11 a–
c Radiation-induced gliosarcoma.
Histopathological findings of a
case of radiation-induced
gliosarcoma. a High cellular
proliferation compound of
pleomorphic cells with a spindle
cell component (HES,
90× magnification). **b** GFAP
immunoreactivity in a subset of
tumor cells
(180× magnification).
c Expression of vimentin in
spindle tumor cells
(130× magnification)

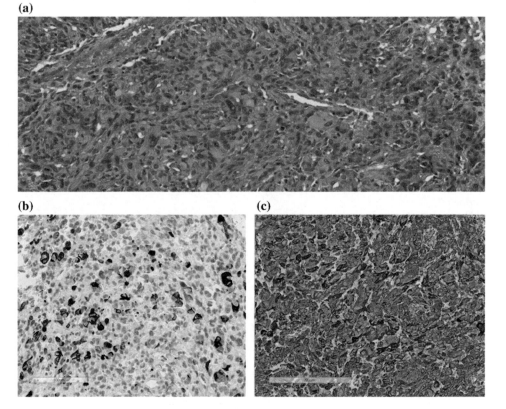

radiation-induced glioma and may result from the sarcomatous transformation of an irradiated glioma [187, 188]. The tumorigenesis of radiation-induced gliomas seems to be multifactorial, resulting from the impairment of cellular immunity, immunosuppressive effects of radiation and direct cellular effects of this treatment [189]. Few series have studied molecular changes in radiation-induced gliomas. It appears these tumors manifest similar alterations of *PTEN, EGFR,* and *TP53* alterations to sporadic gliomas [190] but do not depend upon classical molecular pathway implicated in gliomagenesis such as *IDH1/2* mutations [191], except when they result from the sarcomatous transformation of an irradiated glioma [187]. Moreover, most of the reported cases of malignant transformation of pilocytic astrocytomas (WHO grade I) received prior radiation therapy [192].

The prognosis of these tumors is poor: intrinsic resistance to treatment as well as previously received aggressive therapies substantially limit available therapies.

Fewer than 40 cases of sarcomas have been reported to date, including several histological types (e.g., meningiosarcomas, neurofibrosarcomas) [161].

Radiation-Induced Vasculopathy

Distinct from radionecrosis, in which severe lesions of the arterioles and capillaries constitute a cardinal feature, radiation (particularly of tumors near the central arterial circulation) can induce other types of vascular damage leading to stroke or intracerebral hemorrhage and must be considered as comorbidity predictive of stroke [193].

Large and Medium Intra- and Extracranial Artery Injury

An arteriopathy affecting the large cervical blood vessels, especially the carotid artery [194], is a recognized complication of cervical radiation therapy, usually administered for lymphomas or head and neck cancers. Intracranial vessels may also be affected. The main early-delayed vascular complication is carotid rupture [195, 196], which usually follows a few weeks after cervical RT and surgery for head and neck tumors. Associated skin lesions such as necrosis or wound infection are common. The outcome of this exceptional complication is very poor.

Late-delayed complications are more frequent, and generally occur many years after RT (median time approximately 20 years for extracranial, 7 years for intracranial artery lesions). The lesions are similar to those induced by atherosclerosis, but are often located in unusual places for common atherosclerosis and occur in an accelerated fashion. It has been observed that the larger the diameter of an irradiated artery, the longer the latency between RT and the onset of vasculopathy, a fact that

might explain the shorter latency of RT-induced vasculopathy in children. Shorter latencies have also been reported with interstitial radiotherapy [197]. The dose required to induce vascular lesions usually exceeds 50 Gy, but the type of radiation, fractionation, and portal differs greatly from one case to another. The lesions consist of one or more stenoses or occlusions in the arteries included within the radiation portal. The diagnosis, suspected when a cervical murmur is heard in the immediate vicinity of radiation-induced skin lesions, relies upon magnetic resonance angiography, ultrasound examination, and arteriography. The treatment is similar to that of usual atherosclerotic lesions; in the event of carotid stenoses, endarterectomy may be appropriate. However, surgery may be more difficult than in unirradiated patients because of vascular fibrosis and skin lesions, with higher postoperative risk of infection or wound healing problems. In other patients, antiplatelet agents may be prescribed if there is no contraindication. Some authors have advocated lowering serum cholesterol levels to prevent the development of such lesions in patients at risk [193, 194, 198].

Radiation-Induced Vasculopathy with Moyamoya Pattern

Intracranial vasculopathy leading to a progressive occlusive disease and a moyamoya pattern (characterized by abnormal anastomoses and netlike blood vessels) accounting for focal seizures, strokes, or transient ischemic attacks may follow intracranial irradiation, especially in very young children. This complication is particularly frequent in children treated for optic chiasm glioma, a condition often associated with neurofibromatosis type 1 (NF-1, which is a risk factor for vasculopathy itself). It may also occur with other tumors such as brainstem glioma and craniopharyngioma [199]. In a series [200] of 69 childrens (11 with NF-1) treated for optic pathway glioma with RT (median dose 55 Gy), 13 (19%) developed clinical and radiological signs of vasculopathy after a median latency of 36 months. The strong association between NF-1 and moyamoya is one of the reasons why radiation has been replaced with chemotherapy in younger children [130]. The treatment focuses on preventing further strokes through surgical revascularization techniques; calcium blockers such as flunarizine have been advocated by some authors [201–204]. The role of antiplatelet agents has not been defined in this setting.

Silent Lacunar Lesions

A report [205] described a rare pattern of silent cerebral lacunes occurring in children treated for brain tumors. In this study reviewing 524 consecutive children, 5 of 421 treated with RT and chemotherapy had lacunes. Median age at tumor diagnosis and RT administration was 4.5 years old, and lacunes developed after a median latency of 2 years (ranging from 0.26 to 6 years). This pattern was associated with no further clinical deficit or neuropsychological impairment when compared to patients without lacunes. This condition is probably linked to delayed radiation-induced capillary and small vessel lesions.

Radiation-Induced Cavernomas, Angiomatous Malformations, and Aneurysms

Brain vascular malformations such as telangiectasiae and cavernomas [170, 206, 207] have been rarely observed following RT (Fig. 14.12a–c). Ocular telangiectasiae may also occur [208]. When present, their main risk is intracranial bleeding. Several cases of multiple radiation-induced cavernous angiomas have also been reported [209], occurring 18 months to 23 years after RT.

Histopathologically, radiation-induced cavernomas do not differ from sporadic or familial cavernomas (Fig. 14.13 a–c), and are characterized by juxtaposition of abnormal vessels showing thick walls and conspicuous fibrin deposits [210]. This vascular malformation is often accompanied by gliosis, numerous macrophages and calcifications [210]. The pathogenesis of radiation-induced cavernomas remains unclear. Indeed, those cavernomas may exist before radiation and hemorrhage in response to the radiation [207, 211].

Finally, fewer than 15 cases of radiation-induced intracranial aneurysms have been described in the literature [212, 213]. The median age of the patients was 37.5 years (ranging from 11 to 65 years) with a latency of 10 months to 21 years; there was no correlation between the onset of aneurysm and the radiation dose. This represents a rare but severe problem, as rupture is always possible; 6 of 9 aneurysmal ruptures proved fatal. An enlarging aneurysm can also mimic tumor recurrence. Aneurysms are sometimes detected preclinically with standard imaging procedures for tumors (CT scan and MRI) [214], and particular attention should be drawn to evaluating the onset of such lesions during imaging follow-up. When an aneurysm is detected on CT or MR scan, or if the clinical history strongly suggests its presence, cerebral angiography is required for delineation.

Endocrine Dysfunction

Frequently underestimated [130, 131, 215], endocrine disorders can be the consequence of direct irradiation of a gland (e.g., the thyroid gland, with about 50% of patients developing hypothyroidism within 20 years following radiotherapy for Hodgkin disease or certain head and neck cancers) or result from hypothalamic–pituitary dysfunction secondary to cranial irradiation (several authors believe that the hypothalamus is more radiosensitive than the pituitary gland) [216]. We will focus on the second type of disorder, which can be induced by cerebral or nasopharyngeal tumor irradiation.

There is a positive correlation between radiation dose and the incidence of endocrine complications. In a prospective study on 268 patients treated with different brain RT schemes Littley and colleagues found that the incidence of TSH deficiency was 9% after treatment with 20 Gy, 22% with 35–37 Gy, and 52% with 42–45 Gy 5 years after RT [217]. Hormonal deficits can appear at any time after RT but may arise more rapidly in patients treated with higher radiation doses [218].

In children, varied endocrine deficits may result from cranial RT (administered for brain tumors or during prophylactic irradiation in acute lymphoblastic leukemia).

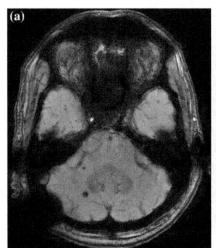
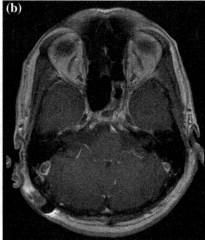
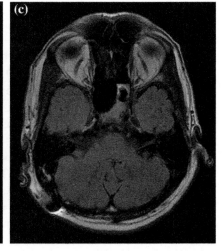

Fig. 14.12 **a–c** Radiation-induced cavernomas. A 46-year-old patient treated with chemotherapy and radiotherapy 22 years previously for an anaplastic astrocytoma. MRI shows cavernomas in the cerebellum. **a** Axial SWAN sequence showing 2 cerebellar carvernomas. **b** Axial T1 with gadolinium injection. **c** Axial T2 FLAIR

Fig. 14.13 a–
c Radiation-induced cavernoma.
Histopathological findings in a
case of radiation-induced
cavernoma. **a** Juxtaposition of
abnormal vessels showing thick
walls (*arrows*) (HES,
50× magnification).
b Calcifications (*asterisk*) (HES,
50× magnification). **c** Expression
of CD34 by endothelial cells
(50× magnification)

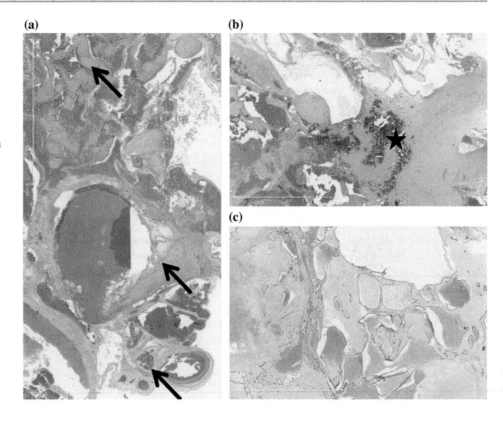

Growth hormone (GH) is usually the first and in many cases the only anterior pituitary deficit in young patients. This complication affects approximately 50% of children treated with prophylactic cranial RT for acute lymphoblastic leukemia [219].

According to a Danish study of 73 children treated with RT for a primary brain tumor (not involving the hypothalamo-pituitary axis directly) and with a long follow-up (median 15 years), 80% of patients manifested growth hormone deficiency; the median biological effective dose (BED) in the hypothalamo-pituitary area was higher in GH-deficient children than in patients without GH deficiency [220]. Administration of GH is recommended in children with growth hormone deficiency; however, as GH has no effect on vertebral bodies, long-term survivors acquire a typical "spiderlike" physical appearance with long extremities and short trunk [130]. Subtle central hypothyroidism is common in children and should be treated with thyroxine replacement therapy in order to limit the potential for thyroid carcinoma as well as to improve longitudinal growth [221, 222].

In adults, a study [223] evaluating 31 long-term brain tumor survivors followed 1.5–11 years after RT with a mean total dose of 62.3 Gy compared with 31 matched controls found hypothalamic hypothyroidism in 26% of patients, hypothalamic hypogonadism in 32% of patients, hyperprolactinemia in 29% of patients and panhypopituitarism in one patient. Low adrenal hormone levels were found in most patients, but without apparent clinical consequence. In the control group, only 6% had a baseline hormonal concentration outside the normal range. None of the controls had two or more hormonal abnormalities, while 42% of the patients had multiple deficits. Only 23% of patients had normal thyroid, gonadal and adrenal baseline levels; this result is consistent with an earlier study reporting hypothalamic–pituitary dysfunction in 10 of 13 (77%) long-term survivors irradiated for supratentorial low-grade glioma [224]. Another study of patients treated for nasopharyngeal cancer found secondary hypothyroidism in 27% of cases (of hypothalamic origin in 19% and pituitary origin in 8%) [225].

The neurological consequences of severe hypothyroidism are well known, including encephalopathy, cerebellar ataxia, pseudomyotonia, and sometimes peripheral neuropathy. Increased CSF protein is also usual. All these abnormalities may be misleading if the correct diagnosis is not considered.

Secondary hypogonadism is an important concern, especially in male patients, responsible for decreased libido and sometimes impotence impacting negatively on quality of life. Hyperprolactinemia of hypothalamic origin is a notable concern in women who develop oligomenorrhea and galactorrhea [226]; in men, it may result in gynecomastia and decreased libido.

Follow-up consultations provide an opportunity for regular clinical endocrine evaluations; the precise biological follow-up scheme is debated and is adapted according to the emerging deficits, but long-term assessment should be the rule. The treatment of hormonal deficits lies in replacement therapy, and usually leads to an improvement in the patient's condition. Bromocriptine has been utilized with success in patients with symptomatic hyperprolactinemia [161].

Sequelae of Radiotherapy to the Spinal Cord

Radiation for the treatment of spinal cord tumors, Hodgkin disease, mediastinal, or head and neck cancers may eventuate in spinal cord damage. Early descriptions in the 1940s [227] were followed by numerous descriptions of post-radiation myelopathy delineating the main clinical patterns: early-delayed myelopathy and several types of late-delayed complications including progressive myelopathy, lower motor neuron disorder, and spinal hemorrhage. There is no clear clinical or experimental evidence of acute spinal cord toxicity due to RT, and a sudden worsening during radiation should lead to a search for intratumoral hemorrhage or tumor progression [8].

Early-Delayed (Transient) Radiation Myelopathy

The onset of this complication occurs from 6 weeks to 6 months after RT, and improvement follows in most cases within 2–9 months [228], though persistence of the symptoms for a longer time is possible in rare cases. It usually follows radiation to the cervical or thoracic spinal cord. After mantle RT for Hodgkin disease, early-delayed myelopathy occurs in 15% of cases [229]. Another study reported a global incidence of 3.6% (40 cases among 1112 patients receiving 30 Gy or more). The incidence was 8% in patients receiving 50 Gy or more, 3% after doses of 45–49.9 Gy, 4% after doses of 40–44.9 Gy, and 2% after doses of 30–39.9 Gy. The risk was also increased with a fraction size >2 Gy [230].

The clinical pattern first described by Esik et al. [231] generally consists of Lhermitte's phenomenon triggered by neck flexion, and is characterized by brief unpleasant sensations of numbness, tingling, and/or often electric-like feelings from the neck to the spine and extremities. No MRI abnormalities are associated with this condition. This symptom is nonspecific, and other causes should be considered in a patient with cancer [232] including chemotherapy (cisplatin or docetaxel), spinal tumor, vitamin B12 deficiency, herpes zoster, or even multiple sclerosis (which may be aggravated by radiation).

The presumed pathophysiology of early-delayed myelopathy is transient demyelination, probably secondary to a loss of oligodendroglial cells following RT [233, 234]. There is no specific treatment for this condition, and none is required, as recovery occurs in most cases. Early-delayed radiation myelopathy is not predictive of evolution to the much more serious progressive myelopathy.

Late-Delayed Radiation-Induced Spinal Cord Disorders

Spinal radionecrosis (Fig. 14.14a–c) (with features similar to its cerebral counterpart), progressive myelopathy, and spinal hemorrhage have been described as late complications of spinal radiation.

Progressive Myelopathy, or Delayed Radiation Myelopathy (DRM)

This complication occurs 6 months to 10 years after exposure to RT. Risk factors include advancing age, large radiation doses and fractions, previous irradiation especially in childhood, and large portals involving thoracic or lumbar spinal cord [228]. Chemotherapy may increase the risk of delayed radiation myelopathy [235]. The generally accepted tolerance for the spinal cord is 45 Gy in 22–25 daily fractions, with a risk <1% for a dose of 50 Gy increasing to 5% for a dose of 60 Gy delivered in 1.8–2 Gy fractions [236, 237].

No histological study in humans has been reported. Radiation of the rat spinal cord leads to progressive abnormalities in the white matter beginning at 19 weeks for doses greater than 17 Gy. The spinal cord of paralyzed animals showed areas of necrosis and demyelination, but neither gross vascular lesion nor inflammatory infiltrate was found [48]. Occasional vessel dilation was observed.

Delayed radiation myelopathy may begin abruptly or, more often, in a progressive way; patients complain of sensory and/or motor deficits leading to para- or tetraparesis. A typical initial clinical presentation is a Brown–Sequard syndrome, consisting of a motor deficit associated with ipsilateral sensory loss affecting tactile, vibration, and passive movement sense on one side, and contralateral sensory loss affecting temperature and pain sensory modalities. In some patients, a transverse myelopathy develops with bilateral leg weakness and sensory loss up to the irradiated region. Some patients also experience pain. Bladder and bowel sphincter as well as diaphragmatic dysfunction (in upper cervical spinal cord lesions) are possible. The evolution of delayed radiation myelopathy varies; in some patients the symptoms stabilize, while in others they progress to a complete deficit.

The diagnosis of delayed radiation myelopathy implies—as was underlined as early as 1961 by Pallis et al. [238]—that the site of the main lesion is within the radiation-exposed area of the spinal cord and that all other potential causes of myelopathy have been carefully reviewed and eliminated.

Fig. 14.14 **a–c** Spinal radionecrosis. 52 year old patient treated with radiochemotherapy (40 Gy in 16 fractions) 29 years earlier for Hodgkin deases. **a** Axial T1 with fat saturation showing intramedullary hyperintensity. **b** Sagittal T1. **c** Sagittal T1 gadolinium showing contrast enhancement

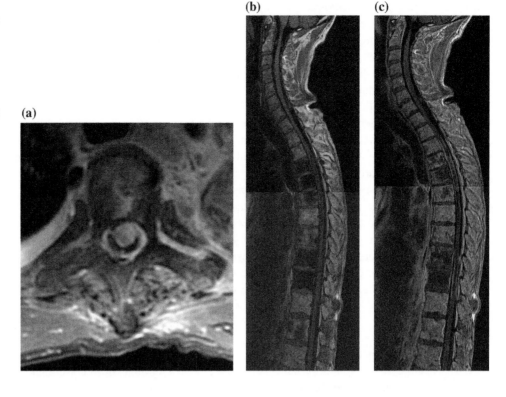

Spinal cord MRI is helpful, though nonspecific. The initial description of Wang and colleagues [239, 240] has been confirmed in several subsequent studies [241–243]: the initial MRI may be normal if performed during the first weeks of the disease, but a slightly delayed examination usually reveals a swollen cord with T1-weighted hypointensity and T2-weighted hyperintensity. Lesions enhance in about 50% of cases after gadolinium injection (Fig. 14.14a–c) [244, 245]. In contrast, late examinations, performed years after the onset of the disease, may show spinal cord atrophy without any signal abnormality; a case of cystic formation in late-delayed radiation myelopathy has also been reported. Moderately elevated protein is the most common finding in the CSF but lacks any specificity. If performed, somatosensory evoked potentials show changes correlated to the extent of the lesions, whereas spinal conduction velocity is decreased.

Corticosteroids may improve some patients, probably because of their action on the inflammatory and edematous components of the disorder; however, patients often become steroid-dependent and only a few experience long-term improvements. There is no current proven long-term treatment for delayed radiation myelopathy. However, Angibaud and colleagues reported the efficacy of hyperbaric oxygen in stabilizing or improving 6 out of 9 patients with DRM [246], and Calabro and workers reported a similar case [247]. Anticoagulation has also been tried, with improvement in one patient with myelopathy treated for >3 months with full anticoagulation and stabilization in another treated with coumarin [72]. Two case reports suggested that bevacizumab might be of benefit [248] in radiation-induced myelopathy.

Late-Delayed Spinal Hematoma

This rare complication has only been described in a few cases, following spinal radiotherapy by 6–30 years, and occurring within the radiation portal but outside the location of the primary tumor [249]; acute-onset leg weakness and back pain rapidly lead to para- or tetraparesis. The diagnosis relies on MRI demonstration of hemorrhage.

Spontaneous symptom resolution is possible, but new episodes may occur later. There is no proven effective treatment for this condition. Avoidance of aspirin or nonsteroid anti-inflammatory agents is prudent. Radiation-induced telangiectasias with secondary hemorrhage may be the culprit.

Sequelae of Radiotherapy on the Cranial Nerves

Apart from acute reversible radiation toxicity, all cranial nerves may be involved in late-delayed radiation-induced complications if included in the radiation portal (usually during the treatment of neck and head tumors). These complications are rare, probably arising in fewer than 5% of cases after conventional radiotherapy (70, 2 Gy per daily fraction) [250]. Modern intensity modulation radiation therapy protocols likely reduce this rate further [251]. Cranial nerve dysfunction occurs during the first five years post-radiation therapy [251]. Large daily radiation fractions increase this risk, which can reach 47% with a median follow-up of 7.6 years with a median equivalent dose in 2 Gy fractions of 94 Gy in nasophayngeal carcinoma patients [252]. Thus radiosurgery also puts cranial nerves at risk. Based upon results of a phase III study including nasopharyngeal carcinoma patients, concomitant chemotherapy has also been described as a risk factor of cranial nerve toxicity [250]. Moreover, a study in brain tumor survivors found that 17% of patients developed neurosensory impairment and that RT exposure greater than 50 Gy to the posterior fossa was associated with a higher likelihood of developing any hearing impairment [253]. The principal complications are described below for each cranial nerve.

Olfactory Nerve Injury

Olfactory dysfunction is rare but classically reported with radiotherapy [254–256]. This may be due to direct acute stimulation of the olfactory neurons. Anosmia has also been described in some patients [257], often associated with taste disorders [258].

Optic Neuropathy

Visual impairment from radiation-induced optic neuropathy is uncommon but disabling. Complication data for radiotherapy-induced optic nerve and chiasm injury have been reported for several external beam radiation delivery systems, including fractionated photons, stereotactic radiosurgery, protons and carbon ions [259]. The interval between radiotherapy and the development of visual symptoms is generally <3 years [260]. The toxic total dose and fractions for the optic nerve and chiasm depend on the tumor treated and have been recently reviewed [259]. In radiosurgery, 8 Gy has been proposed as a limit for optic nerve tolerance [261]. Probably facilitated by pre-existing factors (e.g., diabetes), optic neuropathy may occur 6 months to 14 years after radiation therapy for orbital, pituitary, or suprasellar tumors [262]. Optic neuropathy can also overshadow the prognosis of patients treated with high-energy electron beam therapy for age-related macular degeneration in up to 19% of cases [263].

The classical pattern consists of progressive or sometimes acute-onset visual loss, leading to monocular or binocular blindness with optic atrophy [264]. This disorder is painless. In the case of anterior lesions, the ocular fundus usually shows papilledema and prepapillary and premacular hemorrhage, sometimes associated with radiation-induced retinal lesions. In contrast, fundoscopy may be normal if the lesions are posterior. In those cases, brain MRI may be useful, demonstrating enlargement of the optic nerve and chiasm (Fig. 14.15a, b).

Demyelination, axonal loss, gliosis, and modifications of the vessel walls characterize these lesions histologically; endothelial cell loss has been stressed in this setting, with more significant abnormalities in patients treated with high-dose (55–70 Gy) compared with those treated with low-dose (10 Gy or less) radiation therapy [265]. These lesions are irreversible in many patients. Corticosteroids and anticoagulants [266] have been advocated in chiasmatic

(a)   **(b)**

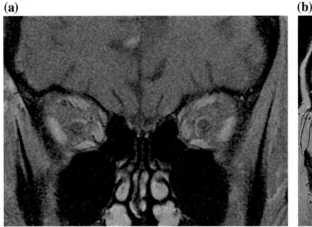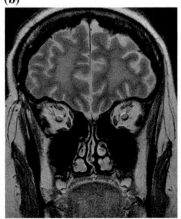

Fig. 14.15 **a**, **b** Perichiasmal radionecrosis. A 51-year-old patient treated with radiochemotherapy (40 Gy in 20 fractions) 4 years previously for a primary cerebral lymphoma. The patient developed bilateral blindness. MRI suggests perichiasmal radionecrosis. **a** Coronal T1 with fat saturation showing atrophy of the chiasm. **b** Coronal T2 showing hyperintensity in both optic nerve

lesions, with inconsistent results, while the use of hyperbaric oxygen in optic neuropathy remains controversial [267–269]. Optic nerve sheath fenestration has been attempted with some success in a few patients [270].

Angiotensin-converting enzyme inhibitors (ACEi) might have a protective role of the optic nerve independently of its antihypertensive effect. ACEi given 2 weeks after stereotaxic brain irradiation of rats significantly reduced radiation-induced optic neuropathy electrophysiologically in terms of the visual evoked potential response to light and morphologically in terms of quantitative changes in myelin contents and axons in the optic nerves and chiasm [271].

Three-dimensional radiotherapy seems to enable the delivery of radiation of tumors with a lower toxicity than conventional radiotherapy to the optic pathway [272].

Ocular Motor Nerve Injury

Rarely reported, the involvement of ocular motor nerves may be associated with optic neuropathy. The most frequent of these palsies affects the abducens nerve [8]. Transient ocular motor palsies have been reported following radiation schemes focused on the pituitary tract, but permanent palsies have also been described after radiation therapy of nasopharyngeal carcinoma. Possible regression suggests that a demyelinating process may be involved, rather than progressive fibrosis.

Neuromyotonia is a late-delayed complication occurring several years after RT to the sella turcica or the cavernous sinus region, characterized by spontaneous spasms of the eye muscles, responsible for episodes of transitory painless diplopia, usually lasting a few seconds; these episodes can occur up to several times an hour [273]. Membrane stabilizers such as phenytoin or carbamazepine may improve this disorder. Radiation-induced hyperexcitability of the nerve fibers may underlie the pathophysiology.

Trigeminal Nerve Dysfunction

Involvement of the trigeminal nerve is quite rare. Neuromyotonia in trigeminal distribution is exceptionally encountered; treatment with carbamazepine is effective in this condition [274, 275]. After gamma knife radiosurgery for trigeminal neuralgia, the main reported complication to this day is mild facial numbness occurring in 2.7–14% of patients [276–278]. Trigeminal neuropathy can also result from radiosurgery for vestibular schwannoma [279, 280] or external beam radiotherapy with endocavitary boost for nasopharyngeal cancer [252].

Facial Nerve Injury

The different branches of the facial nerve are not equally affected by radiation. Taste dysfunction is usual and many patients complain of ageusia, a symptom that may be permanent in up to 50% of patients irradiated with 50–60 Gy for head and neck tumors [281]. However, taste disturbances are a common feature in cancer patients, and chemotherapy may play a part [282].

Motor deficit is almost never the consequence of fractionated RT and should lead to look for tumoral invasion [8]. In contrast, radiosurgery has been reported to account for possible facial palsy; however, the relatively high initial figures of facial weakness after treatment for vestibular schwannoma [283, 284] seems to have decreased markedly, currently under 5% of cases [278, 280, 285]. Pre-existing pathological conditions such as multiple sclerosis may be a risk factor of facial palsy after gamma knife treatment of intracranial tumor [286].

Acoustic Nerve Dysfunction

Acute damage to the cochlea may be responsible for usually reversible complaints of high-frequency hearing loss and tinnitus. Otitis media can also be responsible for an early-delayed hearing loss. Following RT by a few weeks; this condition results from obliteration of the eustachian tube by edema and mucosal vasodilatation.

The diagnosis is often easy, as otoscopic examination reveals fluid behind the tympanic membrane. Usually spontaneously regressive, otitis media can require myringotomy in some cases for symptom alleviation. In most cases, relief can be obtained by prescribing nasal vasoconstriction agents.

Late-delayed hearing loss might result from lesions to the organ of Corti with subsequent acoustic nerve atrophy; however, a report underlines the relative resistance of the organ of Corti to radiation [287]. The precise histological pattern of these disorders is not known; however, the labyrinth has been shown to be damaged in previous studies [287, 288].

We have observed long-term progressive hearing loss with several external beam radiation delivery systems, including fractionated photons, stereotactic radiosurgery, protons and carbon ions in 10+ year survivors.

The consequences of radiosurgery for vestibular schwannoma on hearing have been better assessed over the last few years [285–287, 289, 290]. In one report [291], 14% of patients with measurable hearing before treatment became deaf after radiosurgery (median follow-up 49 months), and

42% of patients had an elevation of their pure tone threshold of 20 dB or more. The risk factors for hearing loss in this study included neurofibromatosis type 2 (NF-2), history of prior surgical resection, and tumor size. This risk is also associated with the volume of the irradiated tumor [292].

Lower Cranial Nerve Involvement

These nerves (glossopharyngeal, vagus, spinal accessory, and hypoglossal nerves) can be damaged after high-dose head or neck radiation therapy [252]. Complications occur earlier with larger radiation doses and typically arise months to years after the treatment. The dose delivered to the superior pharyngeal constrictor has also been shown to be a risk factor of lower cranial neuropathies [293]. The pathophysiology is likely radiation fibrosis. Cranial nerve palsies may accompany skull base osteoradionecrosis after radiotherapy for nasopharyngeal carcinoma [294]. The hypoglossal nerve is the most commonly involved lower cranial nerve [295] the patient may present with unilateral, often asymptomatic tongue paralysis [296–298], or with bilateral and disabling paralysis. This complication may occur many years after RT [297].

Long-standing paralysis is responsible for tongue atrophy, with asymmetry that may be associated with fatty infiltration or edema-like changes on MRI [299, 300]. Paralysis of the vagus nerve leads to unilateral paralysis of the vocal cord and of the palate, responsible for difficulties in swallowing [301]. Horner's syndrome may be associated with these disorders, resulting from injury to the sympathetic fibers [8]. Lesions of the spinal accessory nerve lead to shoulder drop which is easily diagnosed during the clinical examination. Patients may also present with multiple lower cranial nerve palsies [252, 253, 302].

Consequences of RT on the Extracranial Nerves

Brachial and lumbosacral plexopathies are some of the most common and disabling complications of RT on the peripheral nervous system, and can have a similar presentation to neoplastic infiltration of the plexus. Differentiating between these two entities is often a challenge, even with modern imaging techniques.

Brachial Plexopathy

Brachial plexopathy results from RT to the supraclavicular, infraclavicular or axillary regions, usually for lung, breast or head and neck cancers, and sometimes Hodgkin disease.

Improvements in the delivery of radiation therapy have led to a decrease in the incidence of brachial plexopathy: in the 1950s, with a dose of 60 Gy in 5 Gy/fraction, the incidence of brachial plexopathy was 66%; in the 1960s–1970s 45–50 Gy in 4 Gy/fraction resulted in brachial plexopathy incidence of 50%; in the 1980s, 42–45 Gy in 3 Gy/fraction yielded an incidence of 10–15% [303, 304]. In addition to total dose and fraction size, the incidence of brachial plexopathy depends upon the size of the radiotherapy field and use concomitant chemotherapy. Thus, the incidence is significantly higher when the axillary dose exceeds 50 Gy and chemotherapy is administered [305]. Doses of 2.2–2.5 Gy per fraction delivered to a total dose of 34–40 Gy have a brachial plexopathy risk of <1% [306].

Generally, radiation damage to the brachial plexus manifests as three different syndromes: early-delayed reversible plexopathy, late-delayed progressive plexopathy, and acute ischemic plexopathy.

Early-Delayed Brachial Plexopathy

This complication occurs within the first 6 months after RT and usually follows a transient and reversible course. Its incidence is less than 2% after radiation for breast cancer [305]. The initial clinical pattern includes pain (60% of cases, moderate, spontaneous, or after movement), paresthesias and a distal motor deficit; amyotrophy and fasciculations may be present at later stages. Neurological signs recover, often completely, after 12 months; Pierce and workers showed that 80% of patients present a transient and mild course, resolving within 1 year [305]. The pathophysiology of this condition is not fully understood; direct radiation toxicity to Schwann cells inducing demyelination has been hypothesized [307].

Late-Delayed Brachial Plexopathy

Radiation-induced brachial plexopathy (RIBP) is a progressive radiation injury with fibrosis [308]. In a study of 140 patients with breast cancer (with supraclavicular lymph node irradiation to a total dose of 60 Gy in 3 fractions), Bajrovic and workers described the long-standing risk of this complication [309] The annual incidence of brachial plexopathy was 2.9% for mild deficits and 0.8% for severe deficits within a 20-year follow-up period. The incidence may be higher in patients with apical lung cancer treated with radiotherapy (and often concomitant chemotherapy), RIBP's incidence may reach 6.2% when the total dose exceeds 78 Gy [310].

The pathophysiology is unclear and may have biphasic components: during the first phase, direct radiation damage to the nerves may cause electrophysiological and histopathological changes; later, injury to the small vessels with elastosis and fibrosis around the atrophic nerves may account for severe nerve injury [311].

The median time to RIBP's appearance is 40 months (and up to 20 years) [312]. The disorder is progressive and is characterized by hand paresthesias (typically, pins, needles, or numbness of the thumb and other fingers) followed several months or years after by weakness of shoulder, arm and hand muscles. The disorder usually begins in the upper plexus and may progress to a pan plexopathy that paralyzes the entire extremity. Early loss of reflexes, amyotrophy, lymphedema, pain and palpable induration in the supraclavicular fossa are also observed.

The differential diagnosis must necessarily include neoplastic invasion of the brachial plexus. Several features help differentiate RIBP from neoplastic brachial plexopathy. Tumor recurrence is more likely to involve the lower trunk of the plexus and is more often associated with severe pain and Horner syndrome than RIBP [313, 314]. MRI of the brachial plexus (with and without gadolinium) and PET scans (positron emission neoplasm) are very helpful to differentiate tumor infiltration from RIBP and can detect active neoplasm in the region of the plexus (Fig. 14.16) [314, 315], Electrodiagnostic studies can also help, particularly if they demonstrate myokymia, present in up to 60% of patients with RIBP [314].

Treatment of RIBP is challenging. The optimal approach is prevention by reducing total radiation dose, dose per fraction and radiotherapy volume every time is possible and in particular in patients with serious comorbidities. Surgical

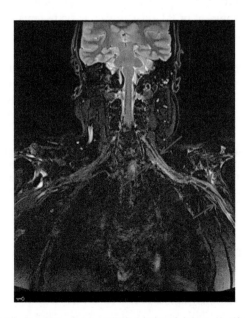

Fig. 14.16 Brachial plexus radiation-induced injury. A 69-year-old patient treated withy radiochemotherapy 35 years ago for breast cancer with a supraclavicular radiation field. She developed pain and motor deficit in her left hand. Coronal STIR MRI shows focal involvement of brachial plexus corresponding to radiation fields, suggesting a post-radiation injury [Courtesy of Dr. Christophe Vandendries (Paris)]

treatment (most commonly neurolysis) can preserve the functionality of limbs [316] but often worsens sensory and motor functions [317] and is not commonly utilized. There is no convincing evidence for the benefit of hyperbaric oxygen and anticoagulants [303]. Combined treatment with pentoxifylline, tocopherol and clodronate is currently under study in France (NCT01291433). Pain management is often the chief concern for clinicians. Pain is usually treated with non-opioid analgesics, tricyclic antidepressants, and/or anticonvulsants. Steroids can also be helpful. Physiotherapy should also be considered.

Ischemic Late-Delayed Brachial Plexopathy

Sudden late-delayed brachial plexopathy has been reported following occlusion of the subclavian artery and can occur years after RT to the breast [318] The plexopathy is painless, acute in onset and nonprogressive (but irreversible).

Lumbosacral Plexopathy

Far less common than brachial plexopathy, lumbosacral plexopathy may follow pelvic or lower abdomen cancer (uterus, ovary, testis, rectum, or lymphoma) irradiation.

Early-Delayed Lumbosacral Plexopathy

As with brachial plexopathies, an early-delayed, generally transient lumbosacral plexopathy is possible but very rare. It usually begins within 6 months after RT, with a typical pattern of distal bilateral paresthesias of the lower limbs. Motor deficit and impaired bowel/bladder function are rarely described [319]. Clinical examination is generally normal, and improvement follows within 3–6 months. Brydoy and workers [320] described a transient lumbosacral plexopathy following L-field (12th thoracic up to 5th lumbar vertebrae) RT for testicular cancer after relatively low RT doses (median total dose of 25 Gy). Seven of 316 patients presented with bilateral paresthesia in the 6 months after RT, reversible within 3 months. Weakness lasting at least one year has been noted in 4 other patients, ranging from 3–9 years, after a total dose of 36–40 Gy. Isolated cases have been reported after pelvic or lumbar RT with a dose of 45–55 Gy [319].

Late-Delayed Lumbosacral Plexopathy (or Radiculoplexopathy)

This disorder is essentially motor, suggesting a predominant anatomical lesion in the anterior horn cell of the spinal cord or the proximal nerve roots rather than the plexus. Several cases have even been described presenting like a lower motor neuron syndrome [321–325]. The onset arises 1–25 years after lymphoma, testicular or pelvic cancer radiation [303] with a median time to appearance less than 7 years [326].

Progressive, usually asymmetric but bilateral motor deficit of the lower limbs characterize the clinical picture. Muscle atrophy and fasciculations may be associated. Physical examination confirms a flaccid motor deficit and areflexia, but no sensory loss appears during the early stages. Sensory deficit may appear after several years, as may sphincter disturbance characterized by lack of bladder sensation and incontinence [324]. Pain is generally mild or absent. Motor deficits typically worsen slowly. The patient may stabilize after several months or years [327].

Diagnosis of this late disorder requires neuroradiological examination to rule out tumor invasion or narrowing of the lumbar canal. Lumbar MRI can also show abnormalities in vertebral bodies and nodular meningeal enhancing lesions that can mimic leptomeningeal metastases but often correspond to late radiation abnormalities or even vascular dilatations or cavernomas [324, 328]. As this disorder often has a pure motor form, the main differential diagnosis is amyotrophic lateral sclerosis; electromyography can be a helpful tool.

Radiation-Induced Peripheral Neuropathy

When segments of peripheral nerves lie within the radiation field, those nerves may develop delayed progressive sensory and motor deficits. Although rare, isolated mononeuropathies have been reported, generally in the lower limbs (femoral, sciatic or pudendal nerves) [329–332] and rarely in the upper limbs [333].

Radiation-Induced Malignant Peripheral Nerve Sheath Tumors

The most common post-radiation neoplasm is the malignant peripheral nerve sheath tumor (MPNST) ; rarely, schwannomas, or neurofibromas arise [334, 335].

MPNST refers to tumors previously termed malignant neurilemmona, malignant schwannoma and neurofibrosarcoma. It is well recognized that prior RT increases the risk of MPNST [336–339]. The most common preceding neoplasms were testicular seminoma, Hodgkin lymphoma, thyroid carcinoma, breast cancer or medulloblastoma. MPNSTs most frequently develop in extremities and trunk rather than in the head and neck nerves. Patients with neurofibromatosis type 1 (NF-1) have an increased risk of developing this complication [340].

Presenting signs and symptoms depend on tumor location. Pain is typically prominent and is followed by the development of a sensorimotor deficit. MRI reveals a tumor mass in the affected area. Confirmatory biopsy or resection should proceed initiation of other therapy.

Dropped Head Syndrome and Camptocormia

Dropped head syndrome (DHS) is a potential late-delayed complication of RT. To date 45 patients with DHS have been described [341]. These patients usually develop weakness of neck extensors developing less than 15 years after RT involving the cervical region; most cases are reported in Hodgkin lymphoma. Clinical examination reveals an amyotrophic deficit of neck muscles, often extending to other muscles innervated by upper cervical roots, without any impairment of sensation. The differential diagnoses include myasthenia gravis, amyotrophic lateral sclerosis, Parkinson disease, and inflammatory myopathies. The mechanism and precise location (nerve or muscle) of the causative lesions are unclear.

The use of wide radiation fields including many spinal segments with paraspinal muscles and the thoracolumbar spine involved can lead to camptocormia [342], an involuntary forward flexion of the thoracolumbar spine, rarely seen after radiation treatment.

Conclusion

Radiation therapy remains one of the most efficient treatments of cancer and will probably become, through the development of new irradiation techniques, a standard option for treating some nonmalignant diseases. Familiarity with its potential risks is thus essential in order to prevent complications when possible as well as to be able to inform the patients of their possible onset. The development of RT-related neurotoxicity remains largely unpredictable, and seems to depend on yet to be discovered individual predispositions. As progress has been made in understanding the pathophysiology of radiation-induced injury and in determining "safe" doses over the past few decades, many complications have become rarer than a few years ago.

Acknowledgements The authors of this third edition chapter would like to thank the authors of this chapter in the previous (second) edition (Daisy Chi, MD, Anthony Béhin, MD, and Jean-Yves Delattre, MD), as this newly revised and updated chapter relies on their fine work.

References

1. New P. Radiation injury to the nervous system. Curr Opin Neurol. 2001;14:725–34.
2. Swennen MH. Delayed radiation toxicity after focal or whole brain radiotherapy for low-grade glioma. J Neurooncol. 2004;66:333–9.
3. Soussain C, Ricard D, Fike JR, et al. CNS complications of radiotherapy and chemotherapy. Lancet. 2009;374:1639–51.

4. Madani O, Bompaire F, Mokhtari K, Sanson M, Ricard D. Acute demyelination secondary to radiation therapy in a patient with glioma. Presse Med. 2014;43:1139–43.

5. Young DF, Posner JB, Chu F, et al. Rapid-course radiation therapy of cerebral metastases: results and complications. Cancer. 1974;34:1069–76.

6. Hindo WA, DeTrana FA III, Lee MS, et al. Large dose increment irradiation in treatment of cerebral metastases. Cancer. 1970;26:138–41.

7. Phillips PC, Delattre JY, Berger CA, et al. Early and progressive increases in regional brain capillary permeability following single and fractionated-dose cranial radiation in rat. Neurology. 1987;37 (Suppl. 1):301.

8. Posner JB. Side effects of radiation therapy. In: Posner JB, editor. Neurologic complications of cancer. Philadelphia: F.A. Davis Company; 1995. p. 311–37.

9. Keime–Guibert F, Napolitano M, Delattre JY. Neurological complications of radiotherapy and chemotherapy. J Neurol. 1998;245:695–708.

10. Kirste S, Treier M, Wehrle SJ, et al. Boswellia serrata acts on cerebral edema in patients irradiated for brain tumors: a prospective, randomized, placebo-controlled, double-blind pilot trial. Cancer. 2011;117:3788–95.

11. Freeman JE, Johnston PG, Voke JM. Somnolence after prophylactic cranial irradiation in children with acute lymphoblastic leukaemia. Br Med J. 1973;4:523–5.

12. Littman P, Rosenstock J, Gale G, et al. The somnolence syndrome in leukemic children following reduced daily dose fractions of cranial radiation. Int J Radiat Oncol Biol Phys. 1984;10:1851–3.

13. Ch'ien LT, Aur RJ, Stagner S et al. Long-term neurological implications of somnolence syndrome in children with acute lymphocytic leukemia. Ann Neurol. 1980;8:273–7.

14. Chow E, Davis L, Holden L, et al. Prospective assessment of patient-rated symptoms following whole brain radiotherapy for brain metastases. J Pain Symptom Manage. 2005;30:18–23.

15. Faithfull S, Brada M. Somnolence syndrome in adults following cranial irradiation for primary brain tumors. Clin Oncol. 1998;10:250–4.

16. Mandell LR, Walker RW, Steinherz P, et al. Reduced incidence of the somnolence syndrome in leukemic children with steroid coverage during prophylactic cranial radiation therapy: results of a pilot study. Cancer. 1989;63:1975–8.

17. Uzal D, Ozyar E, Hayran M, et al. Reduced incidence of the somnolence syndrome after prophylactic cranial irradiation in children with acute lymphoblastic leukemia. Radiother Onco. 1998;48:29–32.

18. Brandsma D, Stalpers L, Taal W, et al. Clinical features, mechanisms, and management of pseudoprogression in malignant gliomas. Lancet Oncol. 2008;9:453–61.

19. Brandes AA, Tosoni A, Spagnolli F, Frezza G, Leonardi M, Calbucci F, Franceschi E. Disease progression or pseudoprogression after concomitant radiochemotherapy treatment: Pitfalls in neurooncology. Neuro Oncol. 2008;26:2192–7.

20. Young RJ, Gupta A, Shah AD, et al. Potential utility of conventional MRI signs in diagnosing pseudoprogression in glioblastoma. Neuology. 2011;76:1918–24.

21. Melquizo-Gavilanes I, Bruner JM, Guha-Thakurta N, et al. Characterization of pseudoprogression in patients with glioblastoma: is histology the gold standard? J Neurooncol. 2015;123:141–50.

22. Armstrong CL, Ruffer J, Corn B, et al. Biphasic patterns of memory deficits following moderate-dose partial-brain irradiation: neuropsychologic outcome and proposed mechanisms. J Clin Oncol. 1995;13:2263–71.

23. Vigliani MC, Sichez N, Poisson M, et al. A prospective study of cognitive functions following conventional radiotherapy for supratentorial gliomas in young adults: 4-year results. Int J Radiat Oncol Biol Phys. 1996;35:527–33.

24. Froklage FE, Oosterbaan LJ, Sizoo EM, et al. Central neurotoxicity of standard treatment in patients with newly-diagnosed high-grade glioma: a prospective longitudinal study. J Neurooncol. 2014;116:387–94.

25. Hahn CA, Zhou SM, Raynor R, et al. Dose-dependent effects of radiation therapy on cerebral blood flow, metabolism, and neurocognitive dysfunction. Int J Radiat Oncol Biol Phys. 2009;73(4):1082–7.

26. Hilverda K, Bosma I, Heimans JJ, et al. Cognitive functioning in glioblastoma patients during radiotherapy and temozolomide treatment: initial findings. J Neurooncol. 2010;97:89–94.

27. Correa DD, Shi W, Thaler HT, et al. Longitudinal cognitive follow-up in low grade gliomas. J Neurooncol. 2008;86:321–7.

28. Correa DD, Rocco-Donovan M, DeAngelis LM, et al. Prospective cognitive follow-up in primary CNS lymphoma patients treated with chemotherapy and reduced-dose radiotherapy. J Neurooncol. 2009;91:315–21.

29. Kazda T, Jancalek R, Pospisil P, et al. Why and how to spare the hippocampus during brian radiotherapy: the developing role of hippocampal avoidance in cranila radiotherapy. Radiat Oncol. 2014;9:139.

30. Gondi V, Pugh SL, Tome WA, et al. Preservation of memory with conformal avoidance of the hippocampal neural stem-cell compartment during whole-brain radiotherapy for brain metastases (RTOG 0933): a phase II multi-institutional trial. J Clin Oncol. 2014;32(34):3810–6.

31. Chak LY, Zatz LM, Wasserstein P, et al. Neurologic dysfunction in patients treated for small cell carcinoma of the lung: a clinical and radiological study. Int J Radiat Oncol Biol Phys. 1986;12:385–9.

32. Creange A, Felten D, Kiesel I, et al. Leucoencéphalopathie subaiguë du rhombencéphale après radiothérapie hypophysaire. Rev Neurol (Paris). 1994;150:704–8.

33. Song T, Liang BL, Huang SQ et al. Magnetic resonance imaging manifestations of radiation injury in brain stem and cervical spinal cord of nasopharyngeal carcinoma patients after radiotherapy. Ai Zheng. 2005;24:357–61 [Abstract].

34. Lampert P, Tom MI, Rider WD. Disseminated demyelination of the brain following Co60 radiation. Arch Pathol. 1959;68:322–30.

35. Ochi S, Takahashi Y, Yokoyama S. Fulminating midbrain irradiation injury of pediatric brain tumor. No To Shinke. 2005; 57:800–5 [Abstract].

36. Marks JE, Baglan RJ, Prassad SC, Blank WF. Cerebral radionecrosis: incidence and risk in relation to dose, time, fractionation and volume. Int J Radiat Oncol Biol Phys. 1981;7:243–52.

37. Lee AW, Ng WT, Hung WM, et al. Major late toxicities after conformal radiotherapy for nasopharyngeal carcinoma-patient- and treatment-related risk factors. Int J Radiat Oncol Biol Phys. 2009;73(4):1121–8.

38. Telera S, Fabi A, Pace A, et al. Radionecrosis induced by stereotactic radiosurgery of brain metastases: results of surgery and outcome of disease. J Neurooncol. 2013;113:313–25.

39. Flickinger JC, Kondziolka D, Lunsford LD, et al. Development of a model to predict permanent symptomatic postradiosurgery injury for arteriovenous malformation patients. Arteriovenous Malformation Radiosurgery Study Group. Int J Radiat Oncol Biol Phys. 2000;46:1143–8.

40. Schlienger M, Atlan D, Lefkopoulos D, et al. Linac radiosurgery for cerebral arteriovenous malformations: results in 169 patients. Int J Radiat Oncol Biol Phys. 2000;46:1135–42.

41. Miyawaki L, Dowd C, Wara W, et al. Five-year results of LINAC radiosurgery for arteriovenous malformations: outcome for large AVMS. Int J Radiat Oncol Biol Phys. 1999;44:1089–106.

42. Malone S, Raaphorst GP, Gray R, et al. Enhanced in vitro radiosensitivity of skin fibroblasts in two patients developing brain necrosis following AVM radiosurgery: a new risk factor with potential for a predictive assay. Int J Radiat Oncol Biol Phys. 2000;47:185–9.

43. Morris GM, Coderre JA, Micca PL, et al. Central nervous system tolerance to boron neutron capture therapy with p-boronophenylalanine. Br J Cancer. 1997;76:1623–9.

44. Oppenheimer JH, Levy ML, Sinha U, et al. Radionecrosis secondary to interstitial brachytherapy: correlation of magnetic resonance imaging and histopathology. Neurosurgery. 1992;31:336–43.

45. Perry A, Schmidt RE. Cancer therapy–associated CNS neuropathology: an update and review of the literature. Acta Neuropathol (Berl). 2006;111:197–212.

46. Kamiryo T, Kassell NF, Thai QA, Lopes MB, Lee KS, Steiner L. Histological changes in the normal rat brain after gamma irradiation. Acta Neurochir. 1996;138:451–9.

47. Calvo W, Hopewell JW, Reinhold HS, Yeung TK. Radiation induced damage in the choroid plexus of the rat brain: a histological evaluation. Neuropathol Appl Neurobiol. 1986;12:47–61.

48. Nordal RA, Nagy A, Pintilie M, Wong CS. Hypoxia and hypoxia-inducible factor-1 target genes in central nervous system radiation injury: a role for vascular endothelial growth factor. Clin Cancer Res. 2004;10:3342–53.

49. Coderre JA, Morris GM, Micca PL, et al. Late effects of radiation on the central nervous system: role of vascular endothelial damage and glial stem cell survival. Radiat Res. 2006;166:495–503.

50. Tofilon PJ, Fike JR. The radioresponse of the central nervous system: a dynamic process. Radiat Res. 2000;153:357–70.

51. Schultheiss TE, Kun LE, Ang KK, et al. Radiation response of the central nervous system. Int J Radiat Oncol Biol Phys. 1995;31:1093–112.

52. Quarmby S, Kumar P, Kumar S. Radiation-induced normal tissue injury: role of adhesion molecules in leukocyte–endothelial cell interactions. Int J Cancer. 1999;82:385–95.

53. Eissner G, Kohlhuber F, Grell M, et al. Critical involvement of transmembrane tumor necrosis factor-alpha in endothelial programmed cell death mediated by ionizing radiation and bacterial endotoxin. Blood. 1995;86:4184–93.

54. Daigle JL, Hong JH, Chiang CS, et al. The role of tumor necrosis factor signaling pathways in the response of murine brain to irradiation. Cancer Res. 2001;61:8859–65.

55. Van Effenterre R, Boch AL. Radionécrose du chiasma. Neurochirurgie. 1993;39:75–84.

56. Coghlan KM, Magennis P. Cerebral radionecrosis following the treatment of parotid tumors: a case report and review of the literature. Int J Oral Maxillofac Surg. 1999;28:50–2.

57. Cirafisi C, Verderame F. Radiation-induced rhombencephalopathy. Ital J Neurol Sci. 1999;20:55–8.

58. Kumar AJ, Leeds NE, Fuller GN, et al. Malignant gliomas: MR imaging spectrum of radiation therapy–and chemotherapy-induced necrosis of the brain after treatment. Radiology. 2000;217:377–84.

59. Wang YX, King AD, Zhou H, et al. Evolution of radiation-induced brain injury: MR imaging-based study. Radiology. 2010;254:210–8.

60. Janus TJ, Kim EE, Tilbury R, et al. Use of [18F]fluorodeoxyglucose positron emission tomography in patients with primary malignant brain tumors. Ann Neurol. 1993;33:540–8.

61. Karunanithi S, Sharma P, Kumar A, et al. 18F-FDOPA PET/CT for detection of recurrence in patients with glioma: prospective comparison with 18F-FDG PET/CT. Eur J Nucl Med Mol Imaging. 2013;40:1025–35.

62. Lamy-Lhullier C, Dubois F, Blond S, et al. Intérêt de la tomoscintigraphie cérébrale au sestamibi marqué au technétium dans le diagnostic différentiel récidive tumorale-radionécrose des tumeurs gliales sus-tentorielles de l'adulte. Neurochirurgie. 1999;45:110–7.

63. Henze M, Mohammed A, Schlemmer H, et al. Detection of tumor progression in the follow–up of irradiated low-grade astrocytomas: comparison of 3–[123I]iodo–alpha–methyl-l-tyrosine and 99mTc–MIBI SPET. Eur J Nucl Med Mol Imaging. 2002;29:1455–61.

64. Matheja P, Weckesser M, Rickert Ch, et al. I-123-Iodo-alpha-methyl tyrosine SPECT in nonparenchymal brain tumors. Nuklearmedizin. 2002;41:191–6.

65. Jain R, Narang J, Sundgren PM, et al. Treatment induced necrosis versus recurrent/progressing brain tumor: going beyond the boundaries of conventional morphologic imaging. J Neurooncol. 2010;100:17–29.

66. Galanaud D, Nicoli F, Figarella-Branger D, et al. MR spectroscopy of brain tumors. J Radiol. 2006;87:822–32.

67. Schlemmer HP, Bachert P, Herfarth KK, et al. Proton MR spectroscopic evaluation of suspicious brain lesions after stereotactic radiotherapy. AJNR Am J Neuroradiol. 2001;22:1316–24.

68. Lichy MP, Bachert P, Hamprecht F et al. Application of (1)H MR spectroscopic imaging in radiation oncology: choline as a marker for determining the relative probability of tumor progression after radiation of glial brain tumors. Rofo. 2006;178:627–33 [Abstract].

69. Ricci PE, Karis JP, Heiserman JE, et al. Differentiating recurrent tumor from radiation necrosis: time for re-evaluation of positron emission tomography? AJNR Am J Neuroradiol. 1998;19:407–13.

70. Matheja P, Rickert C, Weckesser M, et al. Scintigraphic pitfall: delayed radionecrosis: case illustration. J Neurosurg. 2000;92:732.

71. Forsyth PA, Kelly PJ, Cascino TL, et al. Radiation necrosis or glioma recurrence: is computer-assisted stereotactic biopsy useful? J Neurosurg. 1995;82:436–44.

72. Glantz MJ, Burger PC, Friedman AH, et al. Treatment of radiation-induced nervous system injury with heparin and warfarin. Neurology. 1994;44:2020–7.

73. Chuba PJ, Aronin P, Bhambhani K, et al. Hyperbaric oxygen therapy for radiation-induced brain injury in children. Cancer. 1997;80:2005–12.

74. Leber KA, Eder HG, Kovac H, et al. Treatment of cerebral radionecrosis by hyperbaric oxygen therapy. Stereotact Funct Neurosurg. 1998;70:229–36.

75. Kohshi K, Imada H, Nomoto S, et al. Successful treatment of radiation-induced brain necrosis by hyperbaric oxygen therapy. J Neurol Sci. 2003;209:115–7.

76. Feldmeier JJ, Hampson NB. A systematic review of the literature reporting the application of hyperbaric oxygen prevention and treatment of delayed radiation injuries: an evidence based approach. Undersea Hyperb Med. 2002;29:4–30 [Abstract].

77. Chan AS, Cheung MC, Law SC, et al. Phase II study of alpha-tocopherol in improving the cognitive function of patients with temporal lobe radionecrosis. Cancer. 2004;100:398–404.

78. Fike JR, Gobbel GT, Marton LJ, et al. Radiation brain injury is reduced by the polyamine inhibitor alpha-difluoromethylornithine. Radiat Res. 1994;138:99–106.

79. Kondziolka D, Mori Y, Martinez AJ, et al. Beneficial effects of the radioprotectant 21-aminosteroid U-74389G in a radiosurgery

rat malignant glioma model. Int J Radiat Oncol Biol Phys. 1999;44:179–84.

80. Guelman LR, Zorilla Z, Rios H, et al. GM1 ganglioside treatment protects against long-term neurotoxic effects of neonatal X-irradiation on cerebellarcortex cytoarchitecture and motor functions. Brain Res. 2000;858:303–11.

81. Guelman LR, Zorrilla Zubilete MA, Rios H, et al. WR–2721 (amifostine, ethyol) prevents motor and morphological changes induced by neonatal X-irradiation. Neurochem Int. 2003;42:385–91.

82. Sasse AD, Clark LG, Sasse EC, et al. Amifostine reduces side effects and improves complete response rate during radiotherapy: results of a meta-analysis. Int J Radiat Oncol Biol Phys. 2006;64:784–91.

83. Lyubimova N, Coultas P, Yuen K, et al. In vivo radioprotection of mouse brain endothelial cells by Hoechst 33342. Br J Radiol. 2001;74:77–82.

84. Levin VA, Bidaut L, Hou P, et al. Randomized double-blind placebo-controlled trial of bevacizumab therapy for radiation necrosis of the central nervous system. Int J Radiat Oncol Biol Phys. 2011;79:1487–95.

85. Tye K, Engelhard HH, Slavin KV, et al. An analysis of radiation necrosis of the central nervous system treated with bevacizumab. J Neurooncol. 2014;117:321–7.

86. Scoccianti S, Detti B, Cipressi S, et al. Changes in neurocognitive functioning and quality of life in adult patients with brain tumors treated with radiotherapy. J Neurooncol. 2012;108:291–308.

87. Taphoorn MJ, Klein M. Cognitive deficits in adult patients with brain tumors. Lancet Neurol. 2004;3:159–68.

88. Klein M, Engelberts NH, van der Ploeg HM, et al. Epilepsy in low-grade gliomas: the impact on cognitive function and quality of life. Ann Neurol. 2003;54:514–20.

89. Douw L, Klein M, Fagel SSAA, et al. Cognitive and radiological effects of radiotherapy in patients with low-grade glioma: long-term follow-up. Lancet Neurol. 2009;8:810–8.

90. Armstrong CL, Hunter JV, Ledakis GE, et al. Late cognitive and radiographic changes related to radiotherapy: initial prospective findings. Neurology. 2002;59:40–8.

91. Correa DD, DeAngelis LM, Shi W, et al. Cognitive functions in low-grade gliomas: disease and treatment effects. J Neurooncol. 2007;81:175–84.

92. Habets EJ, Taphoorn MJ, Nederend S, et al. Health-related quality of life and cognitive functioning in long-term anaplastic oligodendroglioma and oligoastrocytoma survivors. J Neurooncol. 2014;116(1):161–8.

93. Asai A, Matsutani M, Kohno T, et al. Subacute brain atrophy after radiation therapy for malignant brain tumor. Cancer. 1989;63:1962–74.

94. Imperato JP, Paleologos NA, Vick NA. Effects of treatment on long-term survivors with malignant astrocytomas. Ann Neurol. 1990;28:818–22.

95. Vigliani MC, Duyckaerts C, Delattre JY. Radiation-induced cognitive dysfunction in adults. In: Vecht CJ, editor. Handbook of clinical neurology, vol. 23. Amsterdam: Elsevier Science; 1997. p. 371–88.

96. Omuro AM. Delayed neurotoxicity in primary central nervous system lymphoma. Arch Neurol. 2005;62:1595–600.

97. Fisher B, Seiferheld W, Schultz C, et al. Secondary analysis of Radiation Therapy Oncology Group study (RTOG) 9310: an intergroup phase II combined modality treatment of primary central nervous system lymphoma. J Neurooncol. 2005;74:201–5.

98. Archibald YM, Lunn D, Ruttan LA, et al. Cognitive functioning in long-term survivors of high-grade glioma. J Neurosurg. 1994;80:247–53.

99. Duffner PK. Long-term effects of radiation on cognitive and endocrine function in children with leukemia and brain tumors. Neurologist. 2004;10:293–310.

100. DeAngelis LM, Yahalom J, Thaler HT, et al. Combined modality therapy for primary CNS lymphoma. J Clin Oncol. 1992;10:635–43.

101. Abrey LE, Yahalom J, DeAngelis LM. Treatment for primary CNS lymphoma: the next step. J Clin Oncol. 2000;18:3144–50.

102. Doolittle ND, Korfel A, Lubow MA, et al. Long-term cognitive function, neuroimaging, and quality of life in primary CNS lymphoma. Neurology. 2013;81:84–92.

103. Wassenberg MW, Bromberg JE, Witkamp TD, et al. White matter lesions and encephalopathy in patients treated for primary central nervous system lymphoma. J Neurooncol. 2001;52:73–80.

104. Armstrong CL, Corn BW, Ruffer JE, et al. Radiotherapeutic effects on brain function: double dissociation of memory systems. Neuropsychiatry Neuropsychol Behav Neurol. 2000;13:101–11.

105. Palmer SL, Glass JO, Li Y, et al. White matter integrity is associated with cognitive processing in patients treated for a posterior fossa brain tumor. Neuro Oncol. 2012;14:1185–93.

106. Meyers CA, Weitzner MA, Valentine AD, et al. Methylphenidate therapy improves cognition, mood, and function of brain tumor patients. J Clin Oncol. 1998;16:2522–7.

107. Butler JM Jr, Case LD, Atkins et al. A phase III, double-blind, placebo-controlled prospective randomized clinical trial of d-threo-methylphenidate HCI in brain tumor patients receiving radiation therapy. Int J Radiat Oncol Biol Phys. 2007;69 (5):1496–501.

108. Gehring K, Patwardhan SY, Collins R, et al. A randomized trial on the efficacy of methylphenidate and modafinil for improving cognitive functioning and symptoms in patients with a primary brain tumor. J Neurooncol. 2012;107(1):165–74.

109. Shaw EG, Rosdhal R, D'Agostino RB Jr, et al. Phase II study of donepezil in irradiated brain tumor patients: effect on cognitive function, mood, and quality of life. J Clin Oncol. 2006;24:1415–20 [Abstract].

110. Rapp SR, Case D, Peiffer A, et al. Donepezil for irradiated brain tumor survivors: a phase III randomized placebo-controlled clinical trial. J Clin Oncol. 2015;33(15):1653–9.

111. Brown PD, Pugh S, Laack NN, et al. Memantine for the prevention of cognitive dysfunction in patients receiving whole-brain radiotherapy: a randomized, double-blind, placebo-controlled trial. Neuro-Oncol. 2013;15(10):1429–37.

112. Kaleita TA, Wellisch DK, Graham CA, et al. Pilot study of madafinil for treatment of neurobehavioral dysfunction and fatigue in adult patients with brain tumors. J Clin Oncol. 2006;24(18S):1503.

113. Boele FW, Douw L, de Groo M, et al. The effect of modafinil on fatigue, cognitive functioning, and mood in primary brain tumor patients: a multicenter randomized controlled trial. Neuro Oncol. 2013;15(10):1420–8.

114. Gehring K, Sitskoorn MM, Cm Gundy, et al. Cognitive rehabilitation in patients with gliomas: a randomized, controlled trial. J Clin Oncol. 2009;27(22):3712–22.

115. Locke DE, Cerhan JH, Wu W, et al. Cognitive rehabilitation and problem-solving to improve quality of life of patients with primary brain tumors: a pilot study. J Support Oncol. 2008;6 (8):383–91.

116. Schellart NA, Reits D, van der Kleij AJ, Stalpers LJ. Hyperbaric oxygen treatment improved neuropsychologic performance in brain tumor patients after neurosurgery and radiotherapy: a preliminary report. Cancer. 2011;117(15):3434–44.

117. Day J, Zienius K, Gehring K, et al. Interventions for preventing and ameliorating cognitive deficits in adults treated with cranial irradiation. Cochrane Database Syst Rev. 2014;12:CD011335.

118. Mehta MP, Shapiro WR, Phan SC, et al. Motexafin gadolinium combined with prompt whole brain radiotherapy prolongs time to neurologic progression in non-small-cell lung cancer patients with brain metastases: results of a phase III trial. Int J Radiat Oncol Biol Phys. 2009;73(4):1069–76.

119. Meyers CA, Smith JA, Bezjak A, et al. Neurocognitive function and progression in patients with brain metastases treated with whole brain radiation and motexafin gadolinium: results of a randomized phase III trial. J Clin Oncol. 2004;22:157–65.

120. Mehta MP, Rodrigus P, Terhaard CH, et al. Survival and neurologic outcomes in a randomized trial of motexafin gadolinium and whole-brain radiation therapy in brain metastases. J Clin Oncol. 2003;21(13):2529–36.

121. Gondi V, Hermann BP, Mehta MP, et al. Hippocampal dosimetry predicts neurocognitive function impairment after fractionated stereotactic radiotherapy for benign or low-grade adult brain tumours. Int J Radiat Oncol Biol Phys. 2012;85(2):348–54.

122. Peiffer AM, Leyrer CM, Greene-Schloesser DM, et al. Neuroanatomical target theory as a predictive model for radiation-induced cognitive decline. Neurology. 2013;80(8):747–53.

123. Senzer N. Rationale for a phase III study of erythropoietin as a neurocognitive protectant in patients with lung cancer receiving prophylactic cranial irradiation. Semin Oncol. 2002;29:47–52.

124. Smith RE Jr. Erythropoietic agents in the management of cancer patients. Part 2: studies on their role in neuroprotection and neurotherapy. J Support Oncol. 2004;2(1):39–49.

125. Genc S, Koroglu TF, Genc K. Erythropoietin as a novel neuroprotectant. Restaur Neurol Neurosci. 2004;22(2):105–19.

126. Khasraw M, Ashley D, Wheeler G, Berk M. Using lithium as a neuroprotective agent in patients with cancer. BMC Med. 2012;10:131.

127. Robbins ME, Diz DI. Pathogenic role of the renin-angiotensin system in modulating radiation-induced late effects. Int J Radiat Oncol Biol Phys. 2006;64:6–12.

128. Robbins ME, Zhao W, Garcia-Espinosa MA, Diz DI. Renin-angiotensin system blokers and modulation of radiation-induced brain injury. Curr Drug Target. 2010;11(11):1413–22.

129. Crossen JR, Garwood D, Glatstein E, et al. Neurobehavioral sequelae of cranial irradiation in adults: a review of radiation-induced encephalopathy. J Clin Oncol. 1994;12:627–42.

130. Mulhern RK, Merchant TE, Gajjar A, et al. Late neurocognitive sequelae in survivors of brain tumors in childhood. Lancet Oncol. 2004;5:399–408.

131. Lai R, Abrey LE, Rosenblum MK, DeAngelis LM. Treatment-induced leukoencephalopathy in primary CNS lymphoma: a clinical and autopsy study. Neurology. 2004;62:451–6.

132. Oi S, Kokunai T, Ijichi A, Matsumoto S, Raimondi AJ. Radiation-induced brain damage in children–histological analysis of sequential tissue changes in 34 autopsy cases. Neurol Med Chir. 1990;30:36–42.

133. Panagiotakos G, Alshamy G, Chan B, Abrams R, Greenberg E, Saxena A, Bradbury M, Edgar M, Gutin P, Tabar V. Long-term impact of radiation on the stem cell and oligodendrocyte precursors in the brain. PLoS ONE. 2007;2:e588.

134. Belka C, Budach W, Kortmann RD, et al. Radiation-induced CNS toxicity: molecular and cellular mechanisms. Br J Cancer. 2001;85:1233–9.

135. Li YQ, Chen P, Haimovitz-Friedman A, et al. Endothelial apoptosis initiates acute blood–brain barrier disruption after ionizing radiation. Cancer Res. 2003;63:5950–6.

136. Lyubimova N, Hopewell JW. Experimental evidence to support the hypothesis that damage to vascular endothelium plays the primary role in the development of late radiation-induced CNS injury. Br J Radiol. 2004;77:488–92.

137. Van der Maazen RWM, Berhagen I, Kleiboer BJ, et al. Radiosensitivity of glial progenitor cells of the perinatal and adult rat optic nerve studied by an in vitro clonogenic assay. Radiother Oncol. 1991;20:258–64.

138. Van der Maazen RWM, Kleiboer BJ, Berhagen I et al. Irradiation in vitro discriminates between different O-2A progenitor cell subpopulations in the perinatal central nervous system of rats. Radiat Res. 1991;128:64–72 [Abstract].

139. Van der Maazen RWM, Kleiboer BJ, Berhagen I, et al. Repair capacity of adult rat glial progenitor cells determined by an in vivo clonogenic assay after in vitro or in vivo fractionated irradiation. Int J Radiat Biol. 1993;63:661–6.

140. Chow BM, Li YQ, Wong CS. Radiation-induced apoptosis in the adult central nervous system is p53-dependent. Cell Death Differ. 2000;7:712–20.

141. Atkinson SL, Li YQ, Wong CS. Apoptosis and proliferation of oligodendrocyte progenitor cells in the irradiated rodent spinal cord. Int J Radiat Oncol Biol Phys. 2005;62:535–44.

142. Hornsey S, Myers R, Coultas PG, et al. Turnover of proliferative cells in the spinal cord after X-irradiation and its relation to time-dependent repair of radiation damage. Br J Radiol. 1981;54:1081–5.

143. Enokido Y, Araki T, Tanaka K, et al. Involvement of p53 in DNA strand break-induced apoptosis in postmitotic CNS neurons. Eur J Neurosci. 1996;8:1812–21.

144. Gobbel GT, Bellinzona M, Vogt AR, et al. Response of postmitotic neurons to X-irradiation: implications for the role of DNA damage in neuronal apoptosis. J Neurosci. 1998;18:147–55.

145. Chiang CS, McBride WH, Withers HR. Radiation-induced astrocytic and microglial responses in mouse brain. Radiother Oncol. 1993;29:60–8.

146. Thomas WE. Brain macrophages: evaluation of microglia and their function. Brain Res Rev. 1992;B17:61–74.

147. Rola R, Zou Y, Huang TT, Fishman K, Baure J, Rosi S, Milliken H, Limoli CL, Fike JR. Lack of extracellular superoxide dismutase (EC-SOD) in the microenvironment impacts radiation-induced changes in neurogenesis. Free Radic Biol Med. 2007;42:1133–45.

148. Hopewell JW, Cavanagh JB. Effects of X-irradiation on the mitotic activity of the subependymal plate of rats. Br J Radiol. 1972;45:461–5.

149. Tada E, Yang E, Gobbel GT, Lamborn KR, et al. Long-term impairment of subependymal repopulation following damage by ionizing irradiation. Exp Neurol. 1999;160:66–77.

150. Bellinzona M, Gobbel GT, Shinohara C, et al. Apoptosis is induced in the subependyma of young adult rats by ionizing irradiation. Neurosci Lett. 1996;208:163–6.

151. Brown PD, Buckner JC, O'Fallon JR, et al. Effects of radiotherapy on cognitive function in patients with low-grade glioma measured by the Folstein Mini-Mental State Examination. J Clin Oncol. 2003;21:2519–24.

152. Thiessen B, DeAngelis LM. Hydrocephalus in radiation leukoencephalopathy: results of ventriculoperitoneal shunting. Arch Neurol. 1998;55:705–10.

153. Perrini P, Scollato A, Cioffi F, et al. Radiation leukoencephalopathy associated with moderate hydrocephalus: intracranial pressure monitoring and results of ventriculoperitoneal shunting. Neurol Sci. 2002;23:237–41.

154. DeAngelis LM, Delattre JY, Posner JB. Radiation-induced dementia in patients cured of brain metastases. Neurology. 1989;39:789–96.

155. Wen PY, Macdonald DR, Reardon DA, et al. Updated response assessment criteria for high-grade gliomas: response assessment in neuro-oncology working group. J Clin Oncol. 2010;28:1963–72.

156. Shuper A, Packer RJ, Vezina LG, et al. 'Complicated migraine-like episodes' in children following cranial irradiation and chemotherapy. Neurology. 1995;45:1837–40.

157. Kerklaan JP, Lycklama a Nijeholt GJ, Wiggenraad RG, et al. SMART syndrome: a late reversible complication after radiation therapy for brain tumors. J Neurol. 2011;258:1098–104.

158. Ruda R, Trevisan E, Soffietti R. Epilepsy and brain tumors. Curr Opin Oncol. 2010;22:611–20.

159. Rheims S, Ricard D, van den Bent M, et al. Peri-ictal pseudoprogression in patients with brain tumor. Neuro Oncol. 2011;13:775–82.

160. Di Stefano AL, Berzero G, Vitali P, et al. Acute late-onset encephalopathy after radiotherapy: an unusual life-threatening complication. Neurology. 2013;81:1014–7.

161. Kleinschmidt-Demasters BK, Kang JS, Lillehei KO. The burden of radiation-induced central nervous system tumors: a single institutions experience. J Neuropathol Exp Neurol. 2006;65:204–16.

162. Ron E, Modan B, Boice JD Jr, et al. Tumors of the brain and nervous system after radiotherapy in childhood. N Engl J Med. 1988;319:1033–9.

163. Hawkins MM, Draper GJ, Kingston JE. Incidence of second primary tumors among childhood cancer survivors. Br J Cancer. 1987;56:339–47.

164. Brada M, Ford D, Ashley S, et al. Risk of second brain tumor after conservative surgery and radiotherapy for pituitary adenoma. BMJ. 1992;304:1343–6.

165. Minniti G, Traish D, Ashley S, et al. Risk of second brain tumor after conservative surgery and radiotherapy for pituitary adenoma: update after further 10 years. J Clin Endocrinol Metab. 2005;90:800–4.

166. Neglia JP, Meadows AT, Robison LL, et al. Second neoplasms after acute lymphoblastic leukemia in childhood. N Engl J Med. 1991;325:1330–6.

167. Muracciole X, Cowen D, Regis J. Radiosurgery and brain radio-induced carcinogenesis: update. Neurochirurgie. 2004;50:414–20.

168. Godlewski B, Drummond KJ, Kaye AH. Radiation-induced meningiomas after high-dose cranial irradiation. J Clin Neurosci. 2012;19(12):1627–35.

169. Mann I, Yates PC, Ainslie JP. Unusual case of double primary orbital tumor. Br J Ophthalmol. 1953;37(12):758–62.

170. Amirjamshidi A, Abbassioun K. Radiation-induced tumors of the central nervous system occurring in childhood and adolescence: four unusual lesions in three patients and a review of the literature. Childs Nerv Syst. 2000;16:390–7.

171. Strojan P, Popovic M, Jereb B. Secondary intracranial meningiomas after high-dose cranial irradiation: report of five cases and review of the literature. Int J Radiat Oncol Biol Phys. 2000;48:65–73.

172. Rubinstein AB, Shalit MN, Cohen ML, et al. Radiation-induced cerebral meningioma: a recognizable entity. J Neurosurg. 1984;61(5):966–71.

173. Ijiri R, Tanaka Y, Hara M, Sekido K. Radiation-associated xanthomatous meningioma in a child. Childs Nerv Syst. 2000;16 (5):304–8.

174. Starshak RJ. Radiation-induced meningioma in children: report of two cases and review of the literature. Pediatr Radiol. 1996;26 (8):537–41.

175. Elbabaa SK, Gokden M, Crawford JR, et al. Radiation-associated meningiomas in children: clinical, pathological, and cytogenetic characteristics with a critical review of the literature. J Neurosurg Pediatr. 2012;10(4):281–90.

176. Musa BS, Pople IK, Cummins BH. Intracranial meningiomas following irradiation: a growing problem? Br J Neurosurg. 1995;9:629–37.

177. Tashima T, Fukui M, Nishio S, et al. Radiation-induced meningiomas and their proliferative activity. Cytokinetic study usingbromodeoxyuridine. Acta Neurochir. 1990;102(1–2):69–72.

178. Kolles H, Niedermayer I, Schmitt C, et al. Triple approach for diagnosis and grading of meningiomas: histology, morphometry of ki-67/Feulgen strainings, and cytogenetics. Acta Neurochir (Wien). 1995;137(3–4):174–81.

179. Rajcan-Separovic E, Maguire J, Loukianova T, et al. Loss of 1p and 7p in radiation-induced meningiomas identified by comparative genomic hybridization. Cancer Genet Cytogene. 2003;144:6–11.

180. Al-Mefty O, Topsakal C, Pravdenkova S, et al. Radiation-induced meningiomas: clinical, pathological, cytokinetic, and cytogenetic characteristics. J Neurosurg. 2004;100(6).

181. Salvati M, Cervoni L, Puzzilli F, et al. High-dose radiation-induced meningiomas. Surg Neurol. 1997;47(5):435–41.

182. Dörr W, Herrmann T. Cancer induction by radiotherapy: dose dependence and spatial relationship to irradiated volume. J Radiol Prot. 2002;22(3A):A117–21.

183. Mack EE. Radiation-induced tumors. In: Berger MS, Wilson CB, editors. The gliomas. Philadelphia: WB Saunders; 1999. p. 724–35.

184. Salvati M, Frati A, Russo N, et al. Radiation-induced gliomas: report of 10 cases and review of the literature. Surg Neurol. 2003;60:60–7.

185. Makidono A, Kobayashi N, Saida Y. Metachronous gliomas following cranial irradiation for mixed germ cell tumors. Childs Nerv Syst. 2009;25(6):713–8.

186. You SH, Lyu CJ, Kim DS, Suh CO. Second primary brain tumors following cranial irradiation for pediatric solid brain tumors. Childs Nerv Syst. 2013;29(10):1865–70.

187. Hiniker A, Hagenkord JM, Powers MP, et al. Gliosarcoma arising from an oligodendroglioma (oligosarcoma). Clin Neuropathol. 2013;32(3):165–70.

188. Perry JR, Ang LC, Bilbao JM, Muller PJ. Clinicopathologic features of primary and postirradiation cerebral gliosarcoma. Cancer. 1995;75(12):2910–8.

189. Riffaud L, Bernard M, Lesimple T, Morandi X. Radiation-induced spinal cord glioma subsequent to treatment of Hodgkin's disease: case report and review. J Neurooncol. 2006;76(2).

190. Brat DJ, James CD, Jedlicka AE, et al. Molecular genetic alterations in radiation-induced astrocytomas. Am J Pathol. 1999;154:1431–8.

191. Lee D, Kang SY, Suh YL, et al. Clinicopathologic and genomic features of gliosarcomas. J Neurooncol. 2012;107(3):643–50.

192. Jager B, Schuhmann MU, Schober R, et al. Induction of gliosarcoma and atypical meningioma 13 years after radiotherapy of residual pilocytic astrocytoma in childhood. Pediatr Neurosurg. 2008;44(2):153–8.

193. Aizer AA, Du R, Wen PY, Arvold ND. Radiotherapy and death from cerebrovascular disease in patients with primary brain tumors. J Neurooncol. 2015;124:291–7.

194. Murros KE, Toole JF. The effect of radiation on carotid arteries: a review article. Arch Neurol. 1989;46:449–55.

195. Gupta S. Radiation-induced carotid artery blow out: a case report. Acta Chir Belg. 1994;94:299–300.

196. McCready RA, Hyde GL, Bivins BA, et al. Radiation-induced arterial injuries. Surgery. 1983;93:306–12.

197. Bernstein M, Lumley M, Davidson G, et al. Intracranial arterial occlusion associated with high-activity iodine-125 brachytherapy for glioblastoma. J Neurooncol. 1993;17:253–60.

198. Werner MH, Burger PC, Heinz ER, et al. Intracranial atherosclerosis following radiotherapy. Neurology. 1988;38:1158–60.

199. Bitzer M, Topka H. Progressive cerebral occlusive disease after radiation therapy. Stroke. 1995;26:131–6.

200. Grill J, Couanet D, Cappelli C, et al. Radiation-induced cerebral vasculopathy in children with neurofibromatosis and optic pathway glioma. Ann Neurol. 1999;45:393–6.

201. Suzuki Y, Negoro M, Shibuya M, et al. Surgical treatment for pediatric moyamoya disease: use of the superficial temporal artery for both areas supplied by the anterior and middle cerebral arteries. Neurosurgery. 1997;40:324–9.

202. Dauser RC, Tuite GF, McCluggage CW. Dural inversion procedure for moyamoya disease: technical note. J Neurosurg. 1997;86:719–23.

203. Ross IB, Shevell MI, Montes JL, et al. Encephaloduroarteriosynangiosis (EDAS) for the treatment of childhood moyamoya disease. Pediatr Neurol. 1994;10:199–204.

204. Kim SK, Wang KC, Kim IO, et al. Combined encephaloduroarteriosynangiosis and bifrontal encephalogaleo(periosteal)synangiosis in pediatric moyamoya disease. Neurosurgery. 2002;50:88–96.

205. Fouladi M, Langston J, Mulhern R, et al. Silent lacunar lesions detected by magnetic resonance imaging of children with brain tumors: a late sequela of therapy. J Clin Oncol. 2000;18:824–31.

206. Baumgartner JE, Ater JL, Ha CS, et al. Pathologically proven cavernous angiomas of the brain following radiation therapy for pediatric brain tumors. Pediatr Neurosurg. 2003;39:201–7.

207. Heckl S, Aschoff A, Kunze S. Radiation-induced cavernous hemangiomas of the brain: a late effect predominantly in children. Cancer. 2002;94:3285–91.

208. Mauget-Faysse M, Vuillaume M, Quaranta M, et al. Idiopathic and radiation-induced ocular telangiectasia: the involvement of the ATM gene. Invest Ophthalmol Vis Sci. 2003;44:3257–62.

209. Novelli PM, Reigel DH, Langham GP, et al. Multiple cavernous angiomas after high-dose whole-brain radiation therapy. Pediatr Neurosurg. 1997;26:322–5.

210. Fukushima S, Narita Y, Miyakita Y, et al. A case of more than 20 years survival with glioblastoma, and development of cavernous angioma as a delayed complication of radiotherapy. Neuropathology. 2013;33(5):576–81.

211. Larson JJ, Ball WS, Bove KE, et al. Formation of intracerebral cavernous malformations after radiation treatment for central nervous system neoplasia in children. J Neurosurg. 1998;88(1):51–6.

212. Jensen FK, Wagner A. Intracranial aneurysm following radiation therapy for medulloblastoma: a case report and review of the literature. Acta Radiol. 1997;38:37–42.

213. Louis E, Martin-Duverneuil N, Carpentier AF, et al. Anévrysme post-radique de la carotide intra–caverneuse. Rev Neurol (Paris). 2003;159:319–22.

214. Azzarelli B, Moore J, Gilmor R, et al. Multiple fusiform intracranial aneurysms following curative radiation therapy for suprasellar germinoma: case report. J Neurosurg. 1984;61:1141–5.

215. Constine LS, Woolf PD, Cann D, et al. Hypothalamic-pituitary dysfunction after radiation for brain tumors. N Engl J Med. 1993;328:87–94.

216. Littley MD, Shalet SM, Beardwell CG. Radiation and hypothalamic-pituitary function. Baillieres Clin Endocrinol Metab. 1990;4:147–75.

217. Littley MD, Shalet SM, Beardwell CG, et al. Radiation-induced hypopituitarism is dose-dependent. Clin Endocrinol (Oxf). 1989;31:363–73.

218. Clayton PE, Shalet SM. Dose dependency of time of onset of radiation-induced growth hormone deficiency. J Pediatr. 1991;118:226–8.

219. Rappaport R, Brauner R. Growth and endocrine disorders secondary to cranial irradiation. Pediatr Res. 1989;25:561–7.

220. Schmiegelow M, Lassen S, Poulsen HS, et al. Cranial radiotherapy of childhood brain tumors: growth hormone deficiency and its relation to the biological effective dose of irradiation in a large population based study. Clin Endocrinol (Oxf). 2000;53:191–7.

221. Stevens G, Downes S, Ralston A. Thyroid dose in children undergoing prophylactic cranial irradiation. Int J Radiat Oncol Biol Phys. 1998;42:385–90.

222. Livesey EA, Hindmarsh PC, Brook CGD, et al. Endocrine disorders following treatment of childhood brain tumors. Br J Cancer. 1990;61622–5.

223. Arlt W, Hove U, Muller B, et al. Frequent and frequently overlooked: treatment-induced endocrine dysfunction in adult long-term survivors of primary brain tumors. Neurology. 1997;49:498–506.

224. Taphoorn MJ, Heimans JJ, van der Veen EA, et al. Endocrine functions in long-term survivors of low-grade supratentorial glioma treated with radiation therapy. J Neurooncol. 1995;25:97–102.

225. Samaan NA, Vieto R, Schultz PN, et al. Hypothalamic, pituitary and thyroid dysfunction after radiotherapy to the head and neck. Int J Radiat Oncol Biol Phys. 1982;8:1857–67.

226. Petterson T, MacFarlane IA, Foy PM, et al. Hyperprolactinemia and infertility following cranial irradiation for brain tumors: successful treatment with bromocriptine. Br J Neurosurg. 1993;7:571–4.

227. Ahlbom H. Results of radiotherapy of hypopharyngeal cancer at Radium-Hemmet, Stockholm. Acta Radio. 1941;22:155–71.

228. Rampling R, Symonds P. Radiation myelopathy. Curr Opin Neurol. 1998;11:627–32.

229. Word JA, Kalokhe UP, Aron BS, et al. Transient radiation myelopathy (L'hermitte's sign) in patients with Hodgkin's disease treated by mantle irradiation. Int J Radiat Oncol Biol Phys. 1980;6:1731–3.

230. Fein DA, Marcus RB Jr, Parsons JT, et al. L'hermitte's sign: incidence and treatment variables influencing risk after irradiation of the cervical spinal cord. Int J Radiat Oncol Biol Phys. 1993;27:1029–33.

231. Esik O, Csere T, Stefanits K, et al. A review on radiogenic L'hermitte's sign. Pathol Oncol Res. 2003;9:115–20.

232. Lewanski CR, Sinclair JA, Stewart JS. L'hermitte's sign following head and neck radiotherapy. Clin Oncol (R Coll Radiol). 2000;12:98–103.

233. Li YQ, Jay V, Wong CS. Oligodendrocytes in the adult rat spinal cord undergo radiation-induced apoptosis. Cancer Res. 1996;56:5417–22.

234. Lengyel Z, Reko G, Majtenyi K, et al. Autopsy verifies demyelination and lack of vascular damage in partially reversible radiation myelopathy. Spinal Cord. 2003;41:577–85.

235. Chao MW, Wirth A, Ryan G, et al. Radiation myelopathy following transplantation and radiotherapy for non-Hodgkin's lymphoma. Int J Radiat Oncol Biol Phys. 1998;41:1057–61.

236. Schultheiss TE, Stephens LC. Invited review: permanent radiation myelopathy. Br J Radiol. 1992;65:737–53.

237. Sahgal A, Ma L, Gibbs I, et al. Spinal cord tolerance for stereotactic body radiotherapy. Int J Radiat Oncol Biol Phys. 2010;77:548–53.

238. Pallis CA, Louis S, Morgan RL. Radiation myelopathy. Brain. 1961;84(460–47):9.

239. Wang PY, Shen WC, Jan JS. MR imaging in radiation myelopathy. AJNR Am J Neuroradiol. 1992;13:1049–55.

240. Wang PY, Shen WC, Jan JS. Serial MRI changes in radiation myelopathy. Neuroradiology. 1995;37:374–7.

241. Yasui T, Yagura H, Komiyama M, et al. Significance of gadolinium-enhanced magnetic resonance imaging in differentiating spinal cord radiation myelopathy from tumor: case report. J Neurosurg. 1992;77:628–31.

242. Komachi H, Tsuchiya K, Ikeda M, et al. Radiation myelopathy: a clinicopathological study with special reference to correlation between MRI findings and neuropathology. J Neurol Sci. 1995;132:228–32.

243. Koehler PJ, Verbiest H, Jager J, et al. Delayed radiation myelopathy: serial MR-imaging and pathology. Clin Neurol Neurosurg. 1996;98:197–201.

244. Michikawa M, Wada Y, Sano M, et al. Radiation myelopathy: significance of gadolinium-DTPA enhancement in the diagnosis. Neuroradiology. 1991;33:286–9.

245. Alfonso ER, De Gregorio MA, Mateo P, et al. Radiation myelopathy in over-irradiated patients: MR imaging findings. Eur Radiol. 1997;7:400–4.

246. Angibaud G, Ducasse JL, Baille G, et al. Potential value of hyperbaric oxygenation in the treatment of post-radiation myelopathies. Rev Neurol (Paris). 1995;151:661–6.

247. Calabro F, Jinkins JR. MRI of radiation myelitis: a report of a case treated with hyperbaric oxygen. Eur Radiol. 2000;10:1079–84.

248. Chamberlain MC, Eaton KD, Fink J. Radiation-induced myelopathy: treatment with bevacizumab. Arch Neurol. 2011;68:1608–9.

249. Allen JC, Miller DC, Budzilovich GN, et al. Brain and spinal cord hemorrhage in long-term survivors of malignant pediatric brain tumors: a possible late effect of therapy. Neurology. 1991;41:148–50.

250. Chen Y, Sun Y, Liang SB, et al. Progress report of randomized trial comparing long-term survival and late toxicity of concurrent chemoradiotherapy with adjuvant chemotherapy versus radiotherapy alone in patients with stage III to IVB nasopharyngeal carcinoma from endemic regions of china. Cancer. 2013;119:2230–8.

251. Zheng Y, Han F, Xiao W, et al. Analysis of late toxicity in nasopharyngeal carcinoma patients treated with intensity modulated radiation therapy. Radiat Oncol. 2015;10:17.

252. Schinagl DA, Marres HA, Kappelle AC, et al. External beam radiotherapy with endocavitary boost for nasopharyngeal cancer: treatment results and late toxicity after extended follow-up. Int J Radiat Oncol Biol Phys. 2010;78:689–95.

253. Packer RJ, Gurney JG, Punyko JA, et al. Long-term neurologic and neurosensory sequelae in adult survivors of a childhood brain tumor: childhood cancer survivor study. J Clin Oncol. 2003;21:3255–61.

254. Bramerson A, Nyman J, Nordin S, Bende M. Olfactory loss after head and neck cancer radiation therapy. Rhinology. 2013;51:206–9.

255. Veyseller B, Ozucer B, Degirmenci N, et al. Olfactory bulb volume and olfactory function after radiotherapy in patients with nasopharyngeal cancer. Auris Nasus Larynx. 2014;41:436–40.

256. Grande A, Kano H, Bowden G, et al. Gamma knife radiosurgery of olfactory groove meningiomas provides a method to preserve subjective olfactory function. J Neurooncol. 2014;116:577–83.

257. Harrabi SB, Adeberg S, Welzel T, et al. Long term results after fractionated stereotactic radiotherapy (FSRT) in patients with craniopharyngioma: maximal tumor control with minimal side effects. Radiat Oncol. 2014;9:203.

258. Qiu Q, Chen S, Meng C, et al. Observation on the changes in nasopharyngeal carcinoma patients' olfactory before and after radiotherapy. Lin Chuang Er Bi Yan Hou Ke Za Zhi. 2001;15:57–8 [Abstract].

259. Mayo C, Martel MK, Marks LB, et al. Radiation dose-volume effects of optic nerves and chiasm. Int J Radiat Oncol Biol Phys. 2010;76(3 suppl):S28–35.

260. Danesh-Meyer HV. Radiation-induced optic neuropathy. J Clin Neurosci. 2008;15:95–100.

261. Tishler RB, Loeffler JS, Lunsford LD, et al. Tolerance of cranial nerves of the cavernous sinus to radiosurgery. Int J Radiat Oncol Biol Phys. 1993;27:215–21.

262. Lessell S. Friendly fire: neurogenic visual loss from radiation therapy. J Neuroophthalmol. 2004;24:243–50.

263. Valanconny C, Koenig F, Benchaboune M, et al. Complications de la radiothérapie des néovaisseaux de la dégénérescence maculaire liée à l'âge. J Fr Ophtalmol. 2000;23:151–7.

264. Piquemal R, Cottier JP, Arsene S, et al. Radiation-induced optic neuropathy 4 years after radiation: report of a case followed up with MRI. Neuroradiology. 1998;40:439–41.

265. Levin LA, Gragoudas ES, Lessell S. Endothelial cell loss in irradiated optic nerves. Ophthalmology. 2000;107:370–4.

266. Indaram M, Ali FS, Levin MH. In search of a treatment for radiation-induced optic neuropathy. Curr Treat Options Neurol. 2015;17(1):325. doi: 10.1007/s11940-014-0325-2. PubMed PMID: 25398466.

267. Borruat FX, Schatz NJ, Glaser JS, et al. Visual recovery from radiation-induced optic neuropathy. The role of hyperbaric oxygen therapy. J Clin Neuroophthalmol. 1993;13:98–101.

268. Roden D, Bosley TM, Fowble B, et al. Delayed radiation injury to the retrobulbar optic nerves and chiasm. Clinical syndrome and treatment with hyperbaric oxygen and corticosteroids. Ophthalmology. 1990;97:346–51.

269. Boschetti M, De Lucchi M, Giusti M, et al. Partial visual recovery from radiation-induced optic neuropathy after hyperbaric oxygen therapy in a patient with Cushing disease. Eur J Endocrinol. 2006;154:813–8.

270. Mohamed IG, Roa W, Fulton D, et al. Optic nerve sheath fenestration for a reversible optic neuropathy in radiation oncology. Am J Clin Oncol. 2000;23:401–5.

271. Kim JH, Brown SL, Kolozsvary A, Jenrow KA, Ryu S, Rosenblum ML, Carretero OA. Modification of radiation injury by ramipril, inhibitor of angiotensin-converting enzyme, on optic neuropathy in the rat. Radiat Res. 2004;161:137–42.

272. Kamian S, Kazemian A, Esfahani M, et al. Comparison of three-dimensional vs. conventional radiotherapy in saving optic tract in paranasal sinus tumors. J BUON. 2010;15:281–4.

273. Lessell S, Lessell IM, Rizzo JF III. Ocular neuromyotonia after radiation therapy. Am J Ophthalmol. 1986;102:766–70.

274. Marti-Fabregas J, Montero J, Lopez-Villegas D, et al. Post-irradiation neuromyotonia in bilateral facial and trigeminal nerve distribution. Neurology. 1997;48:1107–9.

275. Diaz JM, Urban ES, Schiffman JS, et al. Post-irradiation neuromyotonia affecting trigeminal nerve distribution: an unusual presentation. Neurology. 1992;42:1102–4.

276. Maesawa S, Salame C, Flickinger JC, et al. Clinical outcomes after stereotactic radiosurgery for idiopathic trigeminal neuralgia. J Neurosurg. 2001;94:14–20.

277. Rogers CL, Shetter AG, Fiedler JA, et al. Gamma knife radiosurgery for trigeminal neuralgia: the initial experience of The Barrow Neurological Institute. Int J Radiat Oncol Biol Phys. 2000;47:1013–9.

278. Combs SE, Thilmann C, Debus J, et al. Long-term outcome of stereotactic radiosurgery (SRS) in patients with acoustic neuromas. Int J Radiat Oncol Biol Phys. 2006;64:1341–7.

279. McClelland S 3rd, Gerbi BJ, Higgins PD, Orner JB, Hall WA. Safety and efficacy of fractionated stereotactic radiotherapy for acoustic neuromas. J Neurooncol. 2008;86:191–4.

280. Benghiat H, Heyes G, Nightingale P, et al. Linear accelerator stereotactic radiosurgery for vestibular schwannomas: a UK series. Clin Oncol (R Coll Radiol). 2014;26:309–15.

281. Giese WL, Kinsella TJ. Radiation injury to peripheral and cranial nerves. In: Gutin PH, Leibel SA, Sheline GE, editors. Radiation injury to the nervous system. New York: Raven Press; 1991. p. 383–403.

282. DeWys WD, Walters K. Abnormalities of taste sensation in cancer patients. Cancer. 1975;36:1888–96.

283. Noren G, Greitz D, Hirsch A, et al. Gamma knife surgery in acoustic tumors. Acta Neurochir Suppl (Wien). 1993;58:104–7.

284. Foote RL, Coffey RJ, Swanson JW, et al. Stereotactic radiosurgery using the gamma knife for acoustic neuromas. Int J Radiat Oncol Biol Phys. 1995;32:1153–60.

285. Selch MT, Pedroso A, Lee SP, et al. Stereotactic radiotherapy for the treatment of acoustic neuromas. J Neurosurg. 2004;101:362–72.

286. Lowell D, Tatter SB, Bourland JD, et al. Toxicity of gamma knife radiosurgery in the treatment of intracranial tumors in patients with collagen vascular diseases or multiple sclerosis. Int J Radiat Oncol Biol Phys. 2011;81:e519–24.

287. Gibb AG, Loh KS. The role of radiation in delayed hearing loss in nasopharyngeal carcinoma. J Laryngol Otol. 2000;114:139–44.

288. McDonald LW, Donovo MP, Plantz RG. Radiosensitivity of the vestibular apparatus of the rabbit. Radiat Res. 1966;27:510–1.

289. Kondziolka D, Lunsford LD, McLaughlin MR, et al. Long-term outcomes after radiosurgery for acoustic neuromas. N Engl J Med. 1998;339:1426–33.

290. Niranjan A, Lunsford LD, Flickinger JC, et al. Dose reduction improves hearing preservation rates after intracanalicular acoustic tumor radiosurgery. Neurosurgery. 1999;45:753–62.

291. Ito K, Shin M, Matsuzaki M, et al. Risk factors for neurological complications after acoustic neurinoma radiosurgery: refinement from further experiences. Int J Radiat Oncol Biol Phys. 2000;48:75–80.

292. Milligan BD, Pollock BE, Foote RL, Link MJ. Long-term tumor control and cranial nerve outcomes following gamma knife surgery for larger-volume vestibular schwannomas. J Neurosurg. 2012;116:598–604.

293. Awan MJ, Mohamed AS, Lewin JS, et al. Late radiation-associated dysphagia (late-RAD) with lower cranial neuropathy after oropharyngeal radiotherapy: a preliminary dosimetric comparison. Oral Oncol. 2014;50:746–52.

294. Huang XM, Zheng YQ, Zhang XM, et al. Diagnosis and management of skull base osteoradionecrosis after radiotherapy for nasopharyngeal carcinoma. Laryngoscope. 2006;116:1626–31.

295. Berger PS, Bataini JP. Radiation-induced cranial nerve palsy. Cancer. 1977;40:152–5.

296. Cheng VS, Schultz MD. Unilateral hypoglossal nerve atrophy as a late complication of radiation therapy of head and neck carcinoma: a report of four cases and a review of the literature on peripheral and cranial nerve damages after radiation therapy. Cancer. 1975;35:1537–44.

297. Johnston EF, Hammond AJ, Cairncross JG. Bilateral hypoglossal palsies: a late complication of curative radiotherapy. Can J Neurol Sci. 1989;16:198–9.

298. Kang MY, Holland JM, Stevens KR Jr. Cranial neuropathy following curative chemotherapy and radiotherapy for carcinoma of the nasopharynx. J Laryngol Otol. 2000;114:308–10.

299. King AD, Ahuja A, Leung SF, et al. MR features of the denervated tongue in radiation-induced neuropathy. Br J Radiol. 1999;72:349–53.

300. King AD, Leung SF, Teo P, et al. Hypoglossal nerve palsy in nasopharyngeal carcinoma. Head Neck. 1999;21:614–9.

301. Stern Y, Marshak G, Shpitzer T, et al. Vocal cord palsy: possible late complication of radiotherapy for head and neck cancer. Ann Otol Rhinol Laryngol. 1995;104:294–6.

302. Takimoto T, Saito Y, Suzuki M, et al. Radiation-induced cranial nerve palsy: hypoglossal nerve and vocal cord palsies. J Laryngol Otol. 1991;105:44–5.

303. Delanian S, Lefaix JL, Pradat PF. Radiation-induced neuropathy in cancer survivors. Radiother Oncol. 2012;105:273–82.

304. Stubblefield MD, Keole N. Upper body pain and functional disorders with breast cancer. PM R. 2014;6:170–83.

305. Pierce SM, Recht A, Lingos TI, et al. Long-term radiation complications following conservative surgery (CS) and radiation therapy (RT) in patients with early stage breast cancer. Int J Radiat Oncol Biol Phys. 1992;23:915–23.

306. Galecki J, Hicer-Grzenkowicz J, Grudzien-Kowalska M, et al. Radiation-induced brachial plexopathy and hypofractionated regimens in adjuvant irradiation of patients with breast cancer: a review. Acta Oncol. 2006;45:280–4.

307. Vega F, Davila L, Delattre JY, et al. Experimental carcinomatous plexopathy. J Neurol. 1993;240:54–8.

308. Owen JB, Coia LR, Hanks GE. Recent patterns of growth in radiation therapy facilities in the United States: a patterns of care study report. Int J Radiat Oncol Biol Phys. 1992;24:983–6.

309. Bajrovic A, Rades D, Fehlauer F, et al. Is there a life-long risk of brachial plexopathy after radiotherapy of supraclavicular lymph nodes in breast cancer patients? Radiother Oncol. 2004;71:297–301.

310. Eblan MJ, Corradetti MN, Lukens JN, et al. Brachial plexopathy in apical non-small cell lung cancer treated with definitive radiation: dosimetric analysis and clinical implications. Int J Radiat Oncol Biol Phys. 2013;85:175–81.

311. Gillette EL, Mahler PA, Powers BE, et al. Late radiation injury to muscle and peripheral nerves. Int J Radiat Oncol Biol Phys. 1995;31:1309–18.

312. Pradat PF, Poisson M, Delattre JY. Neuropathies radiques. Rev Neurol (Paris). 1994;150:664–77.

313. Kori SH, Foley KM, Posner JB. Brachial plexus lesions in patients with cancer: 100 cases. Neurology. 1981;31:45–50.

314. Jaeckle KA. Neurologic manifestations of neoplastic and radiation-induced plexopathies? Semin Neurol. 2010;30:254–62.

315. Stubblefield MD, Custodio CM. Upper-extermity pain disorders in breast cancer. Arch Phys Med Rehabil. 2006;87(3 suppl):S96–9.

316. LeQuang C. Postirradiation lesions of the brachial plexus. Results if surgical treatment. Hand Clin. 1989;5:23–32.

317. Dropcho EJ. Neurotoxicity of radiation therapy. Neurol Clin. 2010;28:217–34.

318. Gerard JM, Franck N, Moussa Z, et al. Acute ischemic brachial plexus neuropathy following radiation therapy. Neurology. 1989;39:450–1.

319. Dahele M, Davey P, Reingold S, Shun Wong C. Radiation-induced lumbo-sacral plexopathy (RILSP): an important enigma. Clin Oncol (R coll Radiol). 2006;18:427–8.

320. Brydoy M, Storstein A, Dahl O. Transient neurological adverse effects following low dose radiation therapy for early stage testicular seminoma. Radiother Oncol. 2007;82:137–44.

321. Maier JG, Perry RH, Saylor W, et al. Radiation myelitis of the dorsolumbar spinal cord. Radiology. 1969;93:153–60.

322. Feistner H, Weissenborn K, Münte TF, et al. Post-irradiation lesions of the caudal roots. Acta Neurol Scand. 1989;80:277–81.

323. Lamy C, Mas JL, Varet B, et al. Post-radiation lower motor neuron syndrome presenting as monomelic amyotrophy. J Neurol Neurosurg Psychiatry. 1991;54:648–9.

324. Bowen J, Gregory R, Squier M, et al. The post-irradiation lower motor neuron syndrome neuronopathy or radiculopathy? Brain. 1996;119(Pt 5):1429–39.

325. Wohlgemuth WA, Rottach K, Jaenke G, et al. Radiogenic amyotrophy: cauda equina lesion as a late radiation sequel. Nervenarz. 1998;69:1061–65 [Abstract].

326. Pieters RS, Niemierko A, Fullerton BC, Munzenrider JE. Cauda equine tolerance to high-dose fractionated irradiation. Int J Radiat Oncol Biol Phys. 2006;64:251–7.

327. Thomas JE, Cascino TL, Earle JD. Differential diagnosis between radiation and tumor plexopathy of the pelvis. Neurology. 1985;35:1–7.

328. Ducray F, Guillevin R, Psimaras D, et al. Postradiation lumbosacral radiculopathy with spinal root cavernomas mimicking carcinomatous meningitis. Neuro Oncol. 2008;10:1035–9.

329. Mendes DG, Nawalkar RR, Eldar S. Post-irradiation femoral neuropathy. A case report. J Bone Joint Surg Am. 1991;73:137–40.

330. Pradat PF, Bouche P, Delanian S. Sciatic nerve moneuropathy: an unusual late effect of radiotherapy. Muscle Nerve. 2009;40:872–4.

331. Gikas PD, Hanna SA, Aston W, et al. Post-radiation sciatic neuropathy: a case report and review of the littérature. World J Surg Oncol. 2008;6:130.

332. Elahi F, Callahan D, Greenlee J, Dann TL. Pudental entrapment neuropathy: a rare complication of pelvic radiation therapy. Pain Physician. 2013;16:E793–7.

333. Padua L, Paciello N, Aprile I, et al. Damage to peripheral nerves following radiotherapy at the wrist. J Neurol. 2000;247:313–4.

334. Zadeh G, Buckle C, Shannon P, et al. Radiation induced peripheral nerve tumors: case series and review of the literature. J Neurooncol. 2007;83(2):205–12.

335. Lohmeyer JA, Kimming B, Gocht A, et al. Combined manifestation of a neurofibroma and a nerve sheath ganglion in the ulnar nerve after radiotherapy in early childhood. J Last Reconstr Aesthet Surg. 2007;60:1338–41.

336. Adamson DC, Cummings TJ, Friedman AH. Malignant peripheral nerve sheath tumor of the spine after radiation therapy for Hodgkin's lymphoma. Clin Neuropathol. 2004;23:245–55.

337. Braunstein S, Nakamura JL. Radiotherapy-induced malignancies: review of clinical features, pathobiology, and evolving approaches for mitigating risk. Front Oncol. 2013;3:73.

338. Van den Belt-Dusebout AW, de Wit R, Gietema JA, et al. Treatment-specific risks of second malignancies and cardiovascular disease in 5-years survivors of testicular cancer. J Clin Oncol. 2007;25:4370–8.

339. Lau D, Moon DH, Park P, et al. Radiation-induced intradural malignant peripheral nerve sheath tumor of the cauda equine with diffuse leptomeningeal metastasis. J Neurosurg Spine. 2014;21:719–26.

340. Ducatman BS, Scheithauer BW. Postirradiation neurofibrosarcoma. Cancer. 1983;51:1028–33.

341. Seidel C, Kuhnt T, Kortmann DD, Hering K. Radiation-induced camptocormia and dropped head syndrome: review and case report of radiation-induced movement disorders. Strahlenther Onkol. 2015;191:765–70.

342. Psimaras D, Maisonobe T, Delanian S, et al. Late onset radiation-induced comptocormia. J Neurol. 2011;258:1723–5.

Neurological Complications of Chemotherapy

15

Craig A. Vargo, Leslie A. Ray, and Herbert B. Newton

Abbreviations	
CNS	Central nervous system
PNS	Peripheral nervous system
BBB	Blood–brain barrier
IT	Intrathecal
IV	Intravenous
HSCT	Hematopoietic stem cell transplant
IA	Intra-arterial
CLL	Chronic lymphocytic leukemia
EEG	Electroencephalography
BCNU	Carmustine
CCNU	Lomustine
Methyl-CCNU	Semustine
ACNU	Nimustine
CSF	Cerebrospinal fluid
CML	Chronic myelogenous leukemia
AED	Anti-epileptic drug
MTX	Methotrexate
Ara-C	Cytosine arabinoside
SIADH	Syndrome of inappropriate antidiuretic hormone
MAO	Monoamine oxidase
CT	Computed topography
MRI	Magnetic resonance imaging
DPD	Dihydropyrimidine dehydrogenase
5-FU	Fluorouracil
ALL	Acute lymphoblastic leukemia
PML	Progressive multifocal leukoencephalopathy

C.A. Vargo · L.A. Ray
Department of Pharmacy, The James Cancer Hospital, The Ohio State University, 460 W. 10th Ave., Columbus, OH 43210, USA
e-mail: craig.vargo@osumc.edu

L.A. Ray
e-mail: leslie.ray@osumc.edu

H.B. Newton (✉)
Neuro-Oncology Center, Florida Hospital Cancer Institue & Florida Hospital Orlando, 2501 N. Orange Avenue, Orlando, FL 32804, USA
e-mail: Herbert.Newton.MD@FLHosp.org

© Springer International Publishing AG 2018
D. Schiff et al. (eds.), *Cancer Neurology in Clinical Practice*,
DOI 10.1007/978-3-319-57901-6_15

PRES	Posterior reversible encephalopathy syndrome
RBC	Red blood cell
AML	Acute myeloid leukemia
HDAC	Histone deacetylase
MDS	Myelodysplastic syndrome
GnRH	Gonadotropin-releasing hormone
ITP	Immune thrombocytopenia

Introduction

Neurotoxicity from chemotherapy is a common and likely dose-limiting toxicity of cancer therapy. Several chemotherapy agents can cause distinct neurological side effects and there are often limited treatment options for these toxicities. With significant advances in all modalities of oncology care through advances in therapy, as well as new combinations of therapy, overall survival has increased and major toxicities, such as bone marrow toxicity, can be controlled. Due to these advances the neurologic complications of chemotherapy are being observed in higher frequency. Chemotherapy can cause peripheral neurotoxicity, with peripheral neuropathy being the most commonly manifested toxicity. Central neurotoxicity can vary from patient to patient with respect to symptoms and severity. These toxicities can be due to direct toxic effects to neural tissues (e.g., vascular injury and ischemia), or secondary to systemic causes (e.g., electrolyte disturbances, hepatotoxicity).

The vinca alkaloids, taxanes, platinums, and proteasome inhibitors are the most common agents to cause peripheral neuropathy. Peripheral neuropathy is generally dose-dependent and persistent, with symptoms potentially lasting for months to years after therapy is discontinued. Unfortunately, therapies for prevention or treatment of peripheral neuropathy are controversial, with positive and negative results being reported.

Despite the protective role of the blood–brain barrier (BBB), many chemotherapeutic agents have the ability to cause central neurotoxic side effects. Methotrexate, ifosfamide, and cytarabine are known for their central neurotoxic effects. This toxicity can range from fatigue and headache to cognitive deficits, seizures, cerebellar dysfunction, and psychiatric syndromes. These toxicities can cause significant treatment-related morbidity and even mortality in some cases. The symptoms may have an acute, subacute, or delayed presentation. Symptoms of CNS toxicity vary widely from patient to patient, causing mild, transient, and reversible effects in some and more severe, chronic, and progressive dysfunction in others.

Intrathecal (IT) chemotherapy can be used for the treatment of primary or metastatic brain tumors and forgoes the protective role of the BBB. Toxicities of IT chemotherapy can cause symptoms of aseptic meningitis with methotrexate or cytarabine, and death if vinca alkaloids are inadvertently administered intrathecally.

It is essential for oncologists and other clinicians providing care for patients with cancer to be aware of the potential neurotoxicity associated with chemotherapy agents. They must also be able to recognize the various syndromes when they arise as the differential diagnosis can be broad, including metastatic tumor spread, opportunistic infections, metabolic disturbances, paraneoplastic syndromes, and neurotoxicity from other medications or modalities of cancer therapy. This chapter will review the central and peripheral neurotoxicity associated with conventional chemotherapy drugs, hormonal therapies, and supportive medications used in cancer therapy. Tables 15.1 and 15.2 provide an overview of the central and peripheral neurotoxicity associated with conventional chemotherapy agents.

Alkylating Agents

Nitrogen Mustards

Mechlorethamine

Mechlorethamine is the original nitrogen mustard, which inhibits DNA and RNA syntheses by producing interstrand and intrastrand cross-links in DNA. It is used in lymphomas and malignant effusions. When used at conventional intravenous (IV) doses, mechlorethamine does not cause neurotoxicity. When used in high-dose IV regimens, such as preparation for bone marrow transplantation (BMT), the drug has been reported to cause encephalopathy, headache, and seizures [1, 2]. The symptom onset is usually within a

Table 15.1 Chemotherapy drugs that can cause central neurotoxicity

Acute or subacute encephalopathy

Methotrexate	Cisplatin	Vinca alkaloids
Mechlorethamine	Procarbazine	Cytosine Arabinoside (Ara-C)
Fludarabine	Gemcitabine	Hydroxyurea
Pentostatin	Chlorambuicil	Thiotepa (high dose)
Ifosfamide	Hexamethylmelamine	Cyclophosphamide
Etoposide	Paclitaxel	Docetaxel
Doxorubicin (IT administration)	Mitotane	L-Asparaginase

Chronic encephalopathy

Methotrexate	Cytosine Arabinoside (Ara-C) (IT administration)	5-Fluorouracil
Carmustine (IA or high-dose IV administration)	Ifosfamide	Fludarabine
Cisplatin (IA administration)	–	–

Seizures

Methotrexate	Cisplatin	Vinca alkaloids
Mechlorethamine	Nitrosoureas (IA or intracavitary administration)	Chlorambuicil (overdose only)
Hexamethylmelamine	Cyclophosphamide	5-Fluorouracil
Cytosine arabinoside (Ara-C)	Fludarabine	Gemcitabine
Pentostatin	Dacarbazine	Temozolomide
Ifosfamide	Etoposide	Paclitaxel
Docetaxel	L-asparaginase	–

Headache

Methotrexate (IT administration)	5-Fluorouracil	Cytosine arabinoside (Ara-C) (IT administration)
Cladribine	Gemcitabine	Hydroxyurea
Dacarbazine	Temozolomide	Nitrosoureas (i.e., BCNU) (IA administration)
Mechlorethamine	Procarbazine	Thiotepa (IT administration)
Hexamethylmelamine	Retinoids	Etoposide
Topotecan	Mitomycin C	L-Asparaginase
Thalidomide	Lenalidomide	Pomalidomide
Octreotide	Mitotane	–

Cerebrovascular complications

Cisplatin	Doxorubicin (IA administration)	Mitomycin C
L-Asparaginase	–	–

Visual loss

Fludarabine	Cisplatin (IA and high-dose IV administration)	Carmustine (BCNU) (IA and high-dose administration)
Retinoids	Chlorambucil	Vinca alkaloids
Paclitaxel	Mitotane	–

Data derived and updated from Cavaliere and Schiff [189], Newton [3], and Hammack [414]

Abbreviations: *IA* Intra-arterial, *IT* Intrathecal, *IV* Intravenous

Table 15.2 Chemotherapy drugs that can cause peripheral neurotoxicity

Sensory neuropathy

Cisplatin	Carboplatin	Oxaliplatin
Vinca alkaloids	Taxanes	Bortezomib
Carfilzomib	Ixabepilone	Thalidomide
Lenalidomide	Pomalidomide	–

Motor neuropathy

Oxaliplatin	Vinca alkaloids	Taxanes
Bortezomib	Ixabepilone	Thalidomide
Lenalidomide	Pomalidomide	–

Autonomic neuropathy

Vinca alkaloids	Bortezomib	Thalidomide
Lenalidomide	Pomalidomide	–

Data derived and updated from Cavaliere and Schiff [189] and from Hammack [414]

few days of treatment; spontaneous recovery is typical. Mechlorethamine has also been administered during intra-arterial (IA) chemotherapy for treatment of recurrent gliomas in the 1950s and 1960s, but was associated with significant cerebral edema, seizure activity, focal neurological deficits, and encephalopathy [3].

Chlorambucil

Chlorambucil is an orally administered nitrogen mustard interfering with DNA replication and RNA transcription by cross-linking DNA strands, used in the treatment of chronic lymphocytic leukemia (CLL), Hodgkin's lymphoma, and non-Hodgkin's lymphomas. Rarely, seizures may occur. A history of nephrotic syndrome and high-dose chlorambucil pulses are risk factors for chlorambucil-induced seizures [4, 5]. Ocular toxicities including retinal edema and hemorrhage, as well as keratitis, have been described [6]. Uncommon central neurotoxicities include agitation, ataxia, confusion, drug fever, hallucinations, encephalopathy, and myoclonus [7, 8]. PNS toxicity of chlorambucil includes neuropathy, tremor, and myoclonia [9, 10].

Cyclophosphamide

Cyclophosphamide is a prodrug that requires activation in the liver. Antineoplastic properties are derived from cross-linking DNA strands and decreasing DNA synthesis. It is frequently used in combination chemotherapy regimens for many solid and hematologic tumors. Neurotoxicity is uncommon, especially compared to ifosfamide, but may present during high-dose IV infusions used for hematopoietic stem cell transplant. Toxicity at these doses includes a mild, reversible encephalopathy with dizziness, blurred vision, and confusion. Posterior reversible encephalopathy has also been described [11].

Ifosfamide

Ifosfamide is an alkylating agent structurally similar to cyclophosphamide that is used for treatment of many solid and hematopoietic tumors, known to frequently cause CNS toxicity. Central neurotoxicity occurs in 10–30% of all patients that receive high-dose IV ifosfamide treatment [12–15]. The toxicity is more likely to occur when IV therapy is continuous over several days or given in a large bolus dose, as opposed to fractionated schedules. Other risk factors include low serum albumin [12, 13], renal dysfunction [12, 13], use of the antiemetic aprepitant [16–19], underlying brain disease [20], concurrent phenobarbital treatment [21], previous neurotoxicity with ifosfamide [12], and prior cisplatin therapy [12, 13]. Accumulation of chloroacetaldehyde, a metabolite of ifosfamide, is thought to cause the encephalopathy. Neurotoxicity can occur hours to days into the treatment and the majority of patients do not require treatment; the encephalopathy resolves completely within days [22]. Small studies have used dexmedetomidine, thiamine, and/or methylene blue as treatment of prevention of ifosfamide-induced encephalopathy [23–26]. The most common symptoms include delirium, mutism, visual hallucinations, seizures, focal motor deficits, facial nerve palsy, and aphasia. Cases of death [27, 28] and irreversible neurologic deficits have been reported [22]. Electroencephalography (EEG) generally reveals diffuse, slow-wave activity, without epileptiform discharges. Other neurotoxicity with ifosfamide is typically described in the setting of encephalopathy but includes seizures [29, 30], ataxia [29], neuropathy [31], extrapyramidal symptoms [32, 33], and cranial nerve dysfunction [13].

Melphalan

Melphalan inhibits DNA and RNA syntheses by creating cross-links in DNA. It is used in multiple myeloma, ovarian cancer, and as a conditioning regimen for autologous hematopoietic stem cell transplantation. Neurotoxicity is uncommon, although cases of encephalopathy and seizures have been reported [34–36].

Bendamustine

Bendamustine is a nitrogen mustard derivative that causes single- and double-strand breaks leading to cell death. It is used in the treatment of chronic lymphocytic leukemia (CLL) and non-Hodgkin's lymphoma. Neurotoxicity is uncommon with fatigue, headache, vertigo, anxiety, and depression described [37, 38].

Estramustine

Estramustine, a nitrogen mustard linked to estradiol, has both antiandrogen and anti-microtubular effects. It is mainly used for refractory prostate cancer and is not associated with significant CNS toxicity. Trials report uncommon neurotoxicity such as lethargy, insomnia, emotional lability, anxiety, and headache [39]. Approximately 25% of patients experienced a thromboembolic event [40]. Rare cases of thrombotic microangiopathy with cerebral infarction have been described [41].

Nitrosoureas

The nitrosoureas are a class of drugs that alkylate DNA and RNA, and include carmustine (BCNU), lomustine (CCNU), semustine (methyl-CCNU), nimustine (ACNU), fotemustine, and streptozotocin. They are all very lipid soluble and have excellent penetration of the BBB, with CSF drug levels approximately 15–30% of simultaneous plasma levels. Nitrosoureas are used predominantly for the treatment of high-grade gliomas, melanoma, lymphoma, and in conditioning regimens for allogeneic hematopoietic stem cell transplantation. When used at conventional IV doses, the incidence of CNS toxicity is minimal. High-dose BCNU has been associated with optic neuropathy and leukoencephalopathy in rare cases [42].

CNS toxicity is more likely to occur when nitrosoureas are administered to the brain via the IA route [3]. IA BCNU and ACNU have been used for the treatment of high-grade gliomas, with a high incidence of cerebral and ocular toxicity. Ocular toxicity included acute orbital pain during drug infusion, along with optic neuropathy and retinal injury. These symptoms could be mitigated with supra-ophthalmic delivery of the drug. Cerebral symptoms could include focal or generalized seizures, encephalopathy, coma, focal weakness, and stroke. In some patients this constellation of symptoms and signs can be caused by necrotizing leukoencephalopathy, a relatively uncommon and occasionally fatal complication of IA BCNU [43]. Concurrent irradiation increases the risk for development of the syndrome [43]. The onset of symptoms is often delayed after drug administration, up to 6 months in some cases. Neuroimaging usually demonstrates prominent edema in the ipsilateral hemisphere; gyral enhancement may be present. Pathological evaluation reveals focal necrosis and mineralizing axonopathy in the affected hemisphere. The mechanism of injury remains unknown but, similar to methotrexate, may be related to a combination of a direct neurotoxic effect of the drug and endothelial damage.

BCNU is also administered to brain tumor patients in wafer form, implanted directly into the resection cavity [44]. In general, there is only a mild risk of neurotoxicity in this setting, with the potential for increased cerebral edema, seizure activity, and new focal neurological deficits after BCNU wafer placement.

Alkyl Sulfonates

Busulfan

Busulfan is a non-cell-cycle-specific alkylating agent that interferes with DNA replication and transcription of RNA. It is used as an oral treatment for chronic myelogenous leukemia (CML) and IV in hematopoietic stem cell transplant conditioning regimens. Busulfan is known to cross the BBB easily with a CSF-to-plasma ration of 1:1. Seizures have been reported with IV busulfan and with high-dose oral busulfan [45–47]. The seizures usually appear within 48 h of drug administration. Seizures are more common in adults compared to children [48]. When busulfan is used as a conditioning regimen for transplant, prophylactic anticonvulsant therapy should be initiated (e.g., phenytoin, levetiracetam, benzodiazepines, or valproic acid) prior to treatment. It should be noted that phenytoin increases busulfan clearance by greater than 15% and doses should be adjusted accordingly. Busulfan should be used with caution in patients predisposed to seizures, history of seizures, head trauma, or with other medications associated with inducing seizures. Dimethylacetamide is the solvent in IV busulfan and has been associated with hallucinations, somnolence, lethargy, and confusion. Other neurotoxic side effects of busulfan include insomnia, fever, anxiety, headache, chills, vertigo, depression, confusion, delirium, encephalopathy, and cerebral hemorrhage [49].

Triazines

Dacarbazine

Dacarbazine causes DNA double-strand breaks leading to cell apoptosis. It is commonly used in Hodgkin's lymphoma, melanoma, and many sarcoma histologies. Seizures, encephalopathy, and dementia have rarely been reported [50]. Mild neurotoxicy, such as headache and fatigue, are more common and self-limiting.

Temozolomide

Temozolomide is a prodrug that is converted to the active alkylating metabolite MTIC. It is used in the treatment of Ewing's sarcoma, melanoma, and many types of brain tumors including astrocytoma and glioblastoma. Central neurotoxicity appears to be very uncommon, with reports of seizures and exacerbation of focal neurological deficits [51]. However, it is difficult to differentiate if these symptoms might be related to the underlying brain tumor, the medication, or a combination of both. Transient neurological deterioration may occur in the early stages of therapy in glioma patients and has been referred to as "tumor flare" syndrome, "treatment effect," and tumor "pseudoprogression" [52, 53]. The incidence of tumor "pseudoprogression" ranges from 28 to 66% in glioblastoma patients and typically occurs within 3 months post-completion of temozolomide and concurrent radiation [53]. Neuroimaging shows an increased area of contrast enhancement and enlargement of noncontrast T2/FLAIR hyperintensities surrounding the enhancement. Treatment of "pseudoprogression" may include corticosteroids, bevacizumab, or watchful waiting with short-interval brain MRI depending on the extent radiological changes and neurological symptoms.

Ethylenimines

Thiotepa

Thiotepa is an alkylating agent that produces DNA cross-links leading to inhibition of DNA, RNA, and protein syntheses. It is used for ovarian cancer, intracavitary effusions, intrathecally for leptomeningeal metastases, intravesically for bladder cancer, and at high doses for hematopoietic stem cell transplant in patients with active CNS malignancy. It readily crosses the BBB [54]. Thiotepa may cause chills, vertigo, fatigue, fever, and headache. Intrathecal use can cause similar toxicity to that of MTX and Ara-C including a mild, reversible aseptic meningitis and, in rare cases, a transient or persistent myelopathy [55–57]. Neurotoxicity from thiotepa is significantly increased in patients with previous CNS radiation [58]. CNS toxicity is rare at conventional IV doses. High doses of thiotepa IV have been associated with neurotoxicity in the form of encephalopathy, including fatal encephalopathy [59].

Hexamethylmelamine (Altretamine)

Hexamethylmelamine structurally resembles an alkylating agent but has demonstrated activity in tumors resistant to classic alkylating agents. Its mechanism is not fully understood, but it is thought to bind and damage DNA. It is used for recurrent ovarian cancer [60]. The parent drug does not readily cross the BBB, but the metabolites readily enter the CNS. Peripheral neuropathy with hexamethylmelamine can occur, but the drug has been administered safely to patients with pre-existing neuropathy due to cisplatin [61, 62]. It is recommended that a neurological examination be done routinely before each cycle and throughout treatment. The most common neurotoxic side effects include headache and mild encephalopathy. Less frequent CNS toxicities include seizures, ataxia, tremor, and Parkinsonism. These usually occur in patients receiving high-dose daily treatment, and in most cases are reversible after drug discontinuation [59].

Platinum Compounds

Cisplatin (Cis-Diamminedichloroplatinum (II), CDDP, DDP)

Cisplatin inhibits DNA synthesis by the formation of DNA cross-links. It is utilized in a variety of oncologic and hematologic malignancies. Cisplatin has a wide range of neurotoxicity including peripheral neuropathy, ototoxicity, vestibulopathy, and encephalopathy.

The peripheral neuropathy associated with cisplatin is a sensory peripheral neuropathy. This typically begins developing at a cumulative dose of 300 mg/m^2. Once a cumulative dose of 500–600 mg/m^2 has been achieved, almost all patients have evidence ofperipheral neuropathy [63–65]. Increasing the dose intensity of cisplatin therapy has been shown not to increase the severity of the peripheral neuropathy [66]. There is significant variance among patients in the susceptibility of peripheral neuropathy [64, 67, 68], thought to be due to genetic polymorphisms in the enzymes responsible for cisplatin metabolism [69, 70].

Cisplatin-induced peripheral neuropathy is an axonal neuropathy that affects large myelinated sensory fibers [63, 67, 71, 72]. The major site of damage is the dorsal root ganglion [73], where cisplatin promotes alterations in cell-cycle kinetics leading to induction of apoptosis [74]. Oxidative stress and mitochondrial dysfunction may also trigger neuronal apoptosis and could also play a role in cisplatin-induced peripheral neuropathy [75–77].

Symptomatology of cisplatin-induced peripheral neuropathy includes numbness, paresthesias, and pain. Normally these symptoms begin bilaterally in the toes and fingers, spreading proximally to the arms and legs. Pinprick, temperature sensation, and motor strength are usually intact or less severely affected compared to proprioception and reflexes [63]. Nerve conduction studies exhibit sensory axonal damage, with decreased amplitude of sensory nerve action potentials and prolonged sensory latencies [78].

After discontinuation, cisplatin-induced peripheral neuropathy worsens in 30% of patients [71, 72], and symptoms may even begin after therapy is discontinued. A large study in patients with testicular cancer found that peripheral neuropathy remained detectable on long-term follow-up (i.e., greater than 5 years) in approximately 20% of patients, and caused significant symptoms in 10% of patients [65]. Once developed, there is no effective therapy to reverse the neuropathy and treatment is aimed at controlling symptoms. Over time, the peripheral neuropathy improves but full recovery is often not observed.

High-frequency sensorineural hearing loss with tinnitus is a dose-dependent toxicity of cisplatin [79]. This has been reported with both intravenous and rarely with intraperitoneal use [80]. Cisplatin-induced ototoxicity occurs from damage to the outer hair cells in the organ of Corti and the vascularized epithelium in the lateral wall of the cochlea [81, 82]. Ototoxicity occurs in approximately 15–20% of patients receiving cisplatin, and early detection with audiometry is vital to prevention as there is no consensus on pharmacologic agents to prevent or treat this toxicity.

The most frequent neurotoxic side effects of cisplatin involve the peripheral nervous system. However, central nervous system toxicity can also be very significant in selected patients, and will depend on the dose and route of administration (i.e., IV vs. IA). Seizures and diffuse encephalopathy are the most common forms of CNS toxicity associated with cisplatin [83–85], yet still rarely occur (Fig. 15.1a, b). This occurs due to acute injury to neural tissues, metabolic abnormalities, or a combination of both. Hypomagnesaemia is common in patients receiving cisplatin, noted in 55–60% of patients. It is caused by impaired magnesium reabsorption in the proximal renal tubules [86]. Both seizure activity and encephalopathy can occur in the setting of hypomagnesaemia, along with diffuse muscle weakness, depending on the severity of the magnesium deficit. Patients are also at risk for hyponatremia, which can result from the syndrome of inappropriate antidiuretic hormone (SIADH), excessive hydration with hypotonic fluids during cisplatin infusion, or severe cisplatin-induced emesis [87]. In rare cases, especially those with intracranial space-occupying lesions, excessive hydration during cisplatin therapy can result in cerebral edema, somnolence, seizure activity, and tonsillar herniation [88]. Lhermitte's phenomenon, manifesting as paresthesias in the back and extremities with neck flexion can be seen in patients receiving cisplatin. This is most likely caused from transient demyelination of the posterior columns [89]. Lhermitte's phenomenon is self-limiting after drug discontinuation [90, 91]. Encephalopathy may occur as a direct toxic effect during IV treatment, but is even more common during IA infusion [3, 92]. Other symptoms that can arise during or within hours to days of IV cisplatin include stroke, seizures, cortical blindness, retinal toxicity, dysphasia, and focal motor deficits. The neurological injury usually resolves without specific intervention and may not recur with subsequent cycles of cisplatin. In patients with stroke, angiography may reveal branch occlusion or, in some cases, be completely normal. The cause of cisplatin-induced stroke remains unclear; possible mechanisms include vasospasm in the setting of hypomagnesaemia, coagulopathy, and drug-induced endothelial injury.

Intra-arterial cisplatin is associated with a broad range of CNS neurological complications, including encephalopathy, confusional states, seizures, stroke, chronic leukoencephalopathy, and ocular toxicity [3, 92]. The ocular injury

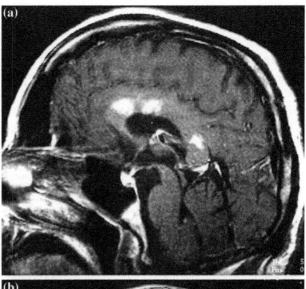

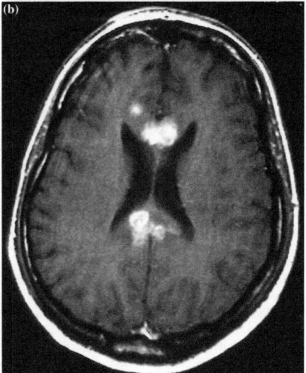

Fig. 15.1 **a, b** Acute cisplatin toxicity. The MRI with sagittal (**a**) and axial (**b**) T1-weighted and gadolinium enhanced sequences shows multiple small hemorrhages and small necrotic cysts with minor focal contrast enhancement and small edema restricted to the corpus callosum. The 38-year-old developed significant lethargy and confusion after the second cycle of cisplatin chemotherapy (cisplatin, ifosfamide, and etoposide) for testicular cancer (Generously provided by Dr. Patrick Wen, Dana-Farber Cancer Institute, Boston, MA.)

can manifest as optic neuropathy and/or retinopathy, and may include retinal infarcts. The risk for ocular toxicity is reduced if the catheter is advanced beyond the origin of the ophthalmic artery. However, supra-ophthalmic delivery of cisplatin has been associated with more frequent and severe neurological toxicity.

Carboplatin

Carboplatin is a platinum alkylating agent that covalently binds to DNA-producing interstrand DNA cross-links. It is used in many different solid and hematologic malignancies, as well as in high doses for hematopoietic stem cell transplant. Peripheral neuropathy and CNS toxicity are uncommon when carboplatin is given at conventional dosing. A severe neuropathy can develop with higher than standard dose carboplatin, in the setting of hematopoietic cell transplantation [93]. Reversible posterior leukoencephalopathy has been described with carboplatin [94] and retinal toxicity after IA administration [95], along with stroke-like symptoms [96] and cortical blindness [97]. The incidence of neuropathy is lower than with cisplatin [98]. Carboplatin, via the IA route, has been used for the treatment of primary or metastatic brain tumors and appears to have less neurotoxicity compared to cisplatin [3].

Oxaliplatin

Oxaliplatin forms cross-links in DNA leading to inhibition of DNA replication and transcription. It is commonly used in colorectal cancer, gastric cancer, esophageal cancer, pancreatic cancer, and types of lymphomas. Peripheral neuropathy is common with oxaliplatin and comprises two distinct syndromes. The first is an acute peripheral neurotoxicity that can appear during or shortly after the first couple of infusions. The second is a cumulative sensory neuropathy, with distal loss of sensation and dysesthesias. Oxaliplatin-induced peripheral neuropathy is extremely common with greater than 85% of patients affected [99].

Acute symptoms are more frequently observed at single doses ≥ 130 mg/m^2 than with doses ≤ 85 mg/m^2 [100]. Typical symptoms include cold intolerance with discomfort swallowing cold beverages, throat discomfort, sensitivity to touching cold items, paresthesias and dysesthesias of the hands, feet, and perioral region, and muscle cramps. Prolonging the infusion time from 2 to 6 h decreases the incidence of acute neuropathy including pseudolaryngospasm [101].

General consensus has been that oxaliplatin-induced acute neuropathy resolves after two to three days; a more recent report suggests that it may not completely resolve between oxaliplatin doses with every two-week dosing [102]. Symptoms are typically most severe with the first cycle but recur with each cycle. In subsequent cycles, the severity of the acute neuropathy is approximately half as severe compared to the first cycle and maintains that severity throughout treatment [102].

The mechanism of oxaliplatin-induced acute peripheral neuropathy has been postulated to be a result of chelation of calcium by oxalate, a metabolite of oxaliplatin. This causes a transient activation of disinhibited peripheral nerve voltage-gated calcium-dependent sodium channels, causing hyperexcitability of peripheral nerves [103, 104]. As patients progress through therapy, acute changes in axonal excitability seem to become less pronounced. This is likely due to chronic nerve dysfunction and sensory loss that mask the acute effects at higher cumulative doses [105]. Calcium and magnesium supplementations for treatment and prevention are controversial. Several studies have shown benefit [106–108] while others, including a prospective phase III study, were not able to show benefit [109, 110].

The second distinct oxaliplatin-induced peripheral neuropathy is a cumulative sensory neuropathy. It is dose-limiting with a late onset comparable to that of cisplatin. It presents as a symmetric distal axonal neuropathy without motor involvement, and with rare autonomic involvement. The mechanism of this neuropathy is similar to cisplatin. Oxaliplatin forms fewer platinum-DNA adducts compared to cisplatin, and thus is slightly less neurotoxic [111]. Other rare manifestations of neurotoxicity include urinary retention and Lhermitte's phenomenon in patients receiving high cumulative oxaliplatin doses [112, 113]. Reversible posterior leukoencephalopathy has also been reported [114–116].

Other Alkylating Agents

Procarbazine-HCL (*N*-Methylhydrazine)

Procarbazine is a prodrug that is activated in the liver. It inhibits transmethylation of methionine into transfer RNA and thus inhibits DNA, RNA, and protein syntheses. It penetrates the BBB and is used for the treatment of lymphomas and brain tumors. Procarbazine can cause a mild reversible encephalopathy at normal doses (100 mg/m^2 for 14 days every 28 days). At this dose it may also rarely cause psychosis and stupor [117]. The incidence of encephalopathy may be higher in patients receiving higher doses for gliomas [118]. In addition, due to its weak activity as an MAO inhibitor, procarbazine can cause hypertensive encephalopathy, headache, and delirium when administered in combination with sympathomimetic agents or after consumption of tyramine-containing foods.

Antimetabolites

5-Fluorouracil (5-FU)

5-FU is a pyrimidine analog metabolite that interferes with DNA and RNA syntheses. It is a prodrug that inhibits thymidylate synthetase, depleting thymidine triphosphate, which is a necessary component of DNA synthesis. It is used in many oncologic settings including breast cancer, colon cancer, rectal cancer, pancreatic cancer, gastric cancer, and others.

5-FU rarely causes an acute cerebellar syndrome manifesting as acute onset of ataxia, dysmetria, dysarthria, and nystagmus [119, 120]. It can develop weeks to months after the initiation of therapy. 5-FU is known to readily cross the BBB and has been found to have the highest concentration in the cerebellum, potentially explaining the acute cerebellar syndrome. Clinical investigations with CT, MRI, and CSF evaluation are generally unremarkable. 5-FU should be discontinued if patients experience cerebellar toxicity and over time signs and symptoms usually resolve completely. Encephalopathy has also been described with 5-FU chemotherapy [121–124]. In these cases, elevated serum ammonia levels without evidence of decompensated liver have been observed. Risk factors associated with encephalopathy include renal dysfunction, weight loss, and constipation.

Other rare neurologic side effects of 5-FU include seizure [125], peripheral neuropathy [126], a parkinsonian syndrome [127], cerebrovascular disorders [128], focal dystonia [129], eye movement abnormalities [130], and optic neuropathy [131]. Approximately 3–5% of the general population has a deficiency in the enzyme responsible for 5-FU metabolism, dihydropyrimidine dehydrogenase (DPD) [132, 133]. Patients with a DPD deficiency are at increased risk of developing severe neurologic toxicity, including cerebellar toxicity [134].

The biochemical basis of 5-FU neurotoxicity remains unknown [125, 135]. Pathological examination of the brains of patients with 5-FU neurotoxicity is usually benign, with minimal if any abnormality. Numerous theories have been proposed, including blockade of the Kreb's cycle by fluoroacetate, a by-product of 5-FU catabolism that is able to inhibit the Kreb's cycle enzyme aconitase. Another proposal suggests that the drug may induce neurological toxicity via an acute deficiency of thiamine, since 5-FU is able to block the production of thiamine phosphate, the active form of the vitamin [136].

The differential diagnosis of 5-FU neurotoxicity is broad, and covers a wide range of disease processes, including cerebellar metastases, paraneoplastic cerebellar syndromes, vertebrobasilar ischemia, and intoxication by other medications.

Capecitabine

Capecitabine is an oral prodrug that is converted to fluorouracil in the liver and tissue. It is commonly used in breast cancer, colorectal cancer, and many other malignancies. Neurotoxicity includes fatigue, paresthesia, lethargy, neuropathy, headache, insomnia, vertigo, depression, and mood changes [137–139]. A subacute encephalopathy is rare with symptoms of confusion, memory loss, and white matter changes on MRI [140, 141]. Symptoms resolve within days following discontinuation of therapy. Cranial MRI showed some nonspecific white matter changes [140], while other reports detail more pronounced white matter changes on MRI in patients with capcitabine-induced encephalopathy [140, 141]. Pure syndromes causing only encephalopathy or a cerebellar syndrome have also been described [142, 143].

Mercaptopurine

Mercaptopurine is used in the maintenance phase for acute lymphoblastic leukemia. It is a purine antagonist that inhibits DNA and RNA syntheses. Neurotoxicity is rare and mainly includes fatigue. Cases of drug fever have been reported [144].

Cytosine Arabinoside (Ara-C, Cytarabine)

Cytosine arabinoside (Ara-C) is a pyrimidine analog that is phosphorylated within tumor cells into aracytidine triphosphate (Ara-CTP), the active moiety that inhibits DNA polymerase. It is commonly used in multi-agent chemotherapy regimens for the treatment of leukemia and lymphoma, as well as for carcinomatous meningitis. Central neurotoxicity from Ara-C is usually noted in the context of high-dose IV therapy (≥ 3 g/m^2 every 12 h $\times$ 4–6 days), and typically presents with a subacute, pancerebellar syndrome [145–147]. In most cases, the onset of symptoms is within hours to days of completion of the infusion but can rarely occur during the infusion. The size of an individual dose may be more important than the cumulative dose of the drug. Patients with renal failure are at increased risk of developing the syndrome. The decrease in use of high-dose Ara-C in patients with renal dysfunction has led to a decrease in the incidence of cerebellar syndrome [148]. Symptoms include dysarthria, dysmetria, ataxia, nystagmus, and dysdiadochokinesia. Signs of cerebral dysfunction, such as somnolence, altered mentation, headache, and seizures [149], can also be noted in some patients. Symptoms usually resolve after complete discontinuation of Ara-C.

MRI shows T2/FLAIR hyperintensities, with white matter abnormalities and cerebellar atrophy almost resembling reversible posterior leukoencephalopathy [150] (Fig. 15.2). CSF analysis is usually unremarkable and EEG may show slowing. On neuropathological examination, the most common findings are cerebellar cortical atrophy and Purkinje cell loss.

Other central neurotoxic effects of IV Ara-C include Horner's syndrome, parkinsonism [151], and anosmia [152, 153]. Peripheral neurotoxicy is rare. Neuropathies have been described with high doses [154–156] but are most commonly described in the setting of other neurotoxic agents [157, 158]. Demyelinating [152, 159], axonal [160], and fatal cases of neuropathy [158, 160] have been reported.

Intrathecal use of Ara-C can produce a mild chemical meningitis, similar to methotrexate [161]. Myelopathy [162, 163], seizure [149], papilledema [164], and locked-in syndrome [165] have been associated with intrathecal use. Neurotoxicity is more common with the liposomal, sustained-release preparation of Ara-C (i.e., DepoCyt®, Sigma-Tau Pharmaceuticals, Gaithersburg, MD), and can recur with subsequent doses of the drug. Dexamethasone prophylaxis should be used in all patients receiving IT liposomal Ara-C to decrease the incidence and severity of chemical meningitis. Rarely, seizures, and confusional syndromes occur with IT usage.

Floxuridine

Floxuridine is catabolized to fluorouracil after IA administration, inhibiting thymidylate synthetase and interrupting

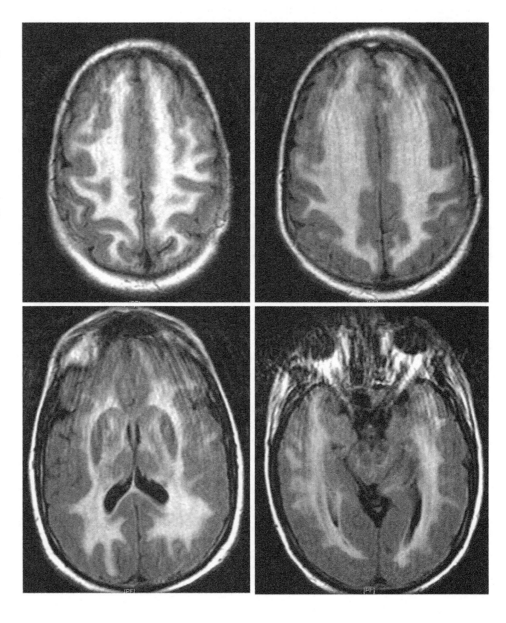

Fig. 15.2 Leukoencephalopathy after high-dose Ara-C and idarubicin. The axial MRI reveals extensive and diffuse T2/FLAIR air hyperintensities affecting bilateral subcortical white matter consistent with diffuse leukoencephalopathy. Two years earlier, this 44-year-old patient received chemotherapy with cytosine arabinoside/idarubicin and bone marrow transplant for AML. The patient became increasingly symptomatic with progressive cognitive impairment and recurrent falls (Generously provided by Dr. Patrick Wen, Dana-Farber Cancer Institute, Boston, MA.)

DNA and RNA synthesis. It is administered intra-arterially for hepatic metastases from colorectal cancer. Due to the local administration, neurotoxicity is rare.

Fludarabine

Fludarabine inhibits DNA synthesis by blocking DNA polymerase and ribonucleotide reductase, leading to cell apoptosis. It is mainly used in chronic lymphocytic leukemia (CLL) . Serious neurotoxicity has been observed at higher than recommended doses (up to 96 mg/m^2/day for 5–7 days) including delayed blindness, coma, and death [166]. After high-dose fludarabine, neurotoxicity generally appeared from 21 to 60 days following the last dose of fludarabine, and has been reported as early as 7 days and as late as 225 days after treatment. At the standard dose of 40 mg/m^2, severe neurotoxicity is observed in less than 1% of patients [167]. Other neurotoxicity including agitation, coma, confusion, and seizure has been reported with standard CLL doses [167].

Reports of fludarabine neurotoxicity have relied on brain CT or have described MRI abnormalities without detail [166–171]. One series of three patients describes variable, ill-defined, mildly hyperintense lesions on the periventricular and periarterial cerebral white matter on T2 and FLAIR sequences with restricted diffusion but no enhancement. The MRI abnormalities were minimal compared to the profound clinical deficits of the patients. Abnormalities reportedly increased in intensity and size over time, further emphasizing the point that fludarabine neurotoxicity appears to be delayed with progressive lesions many weeks after drug cessation [172].

Progressive multifocal leukoencephalopathy (PML) has been reported with the use of fludarabine [173–180] (Fig. 15.3a–d). The majority of these patients had received previous chemotherapy and/or other concurrent chemotherapy. The onset of PML may be within a few weeks or can be delayed up to one year [167, 170]. PML may be confused with fludarabine neurotoxicity as described above; however, imaging should differentiate the two. PML lesions involve the subcortical white matter and do not show restricted diffusion with lesion size correlating with clinical symptoms. Both PML and fludarabine neurotoxicity generally lack enhancement and mass effect.

Neuropathological examination shows multifocal demyelination and necrosis [169, 173].

Gemcitabine

Gemcitabine, a pyrimidine antimetabolite, inhibits DNA synthesis by inhibition of DNA polymerase and ribonucleotide reductase. It is used in breast, lung, ovarian, pancreatic, cervical, bladder, sarcoma, and head and neck cancer. Posterior reversible encephalopathy syndrome (PRES) has been reported both with single-agent and with combination chemotherapy [181–184]. PRES may manifest with blindness, confusion, headache, hypertension, lethargy, seizure, and other visual and neurologic disturbances. Therapy should be discontinued if PRES is confirmed. Other neurotoxicity includes drowsiness and paresthesias. Peripheral neurotoxicity can occur, with studies showing that approximately 20% of patients treated with gemcitabine experience sensory neuropathy; however, it should be noted that in these studies gemcitabine was administered with oxaliplatin [185, 186].

Hydroxyurea

Hydroxyurea is an antimetabolite that inhibits ribonucleotide reductase thus halting the cell cycle at the G1/S phase. For sickle cell anemia, hydroxyurea increased red blood cell (RBC) hemoglobin F levels, RBC water content, deformability of sickled cells, and alters the adhesion of RBCs to endothelium. It is used for chronic myelocytic leukemia, in solid tumors in conjunction with radiation, and sickle cell anemia. Significant neurotoxicity is rare with only scattered reports of mild encephalopathy and headaches [187].

Methotrexate (Amethopterin, MTX)

Methotrexate (MTX) is an antimetabolite drug that inhibits the enzyme dihydrofolate reductase. This inhibition prevents the conversion of folic acid into tetrahydrofolate, and inhibits DNA synthesis in the S phase of the cell cycle. MTX is often used for systemic malignancies such as leukemia, lymphoma, and sarcoma, and is also the most effective chemotherapeutic agent for primary CNS lymphoma [188]. The drug does not cross the BBB very well, as it is highly ionized and somewhat hydrophobic. Therefore, CNS toxicity is uncommon unless MTX is administered IV at high doses or via the IT route. MTX-induced neurotoxicity can be divided into acute (during or within hours of administration), subacute (days to weeks after administration), and chronic (months to years after administration) effects.

Acute/Subacute Effects

After IT administration, MTX induces a chemical meningitis in approximately 10% of patients [189, 190]. Symptoms include headache, stiff neck, photophobia, and low-grade fever, arising within hours of drug administration and potentially lasting for days. CSF analysis will typically demonstrate a mild pleocytosis, with no evidence of a viral

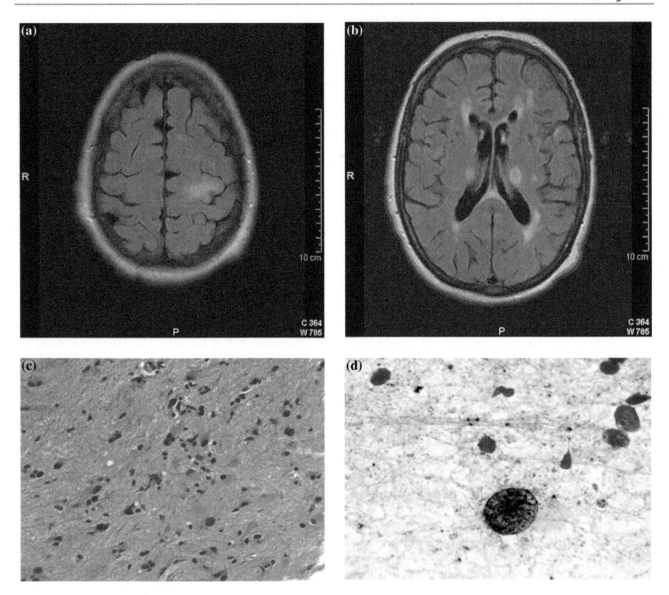

Fig. 15.3 **a–d** This 78-year-old woman with an 8-year history of CLL developed slowly progressive right hemiparesis and hand twitching over several months. She had received rituximab and fludarabine within one year of onset of these symptoms. FLAIR MR sequences demonstrated multiple hyperintense lesions (**a**, **b**). Brain biopsy revealed prominent gliosis with scattered cells with enlarged nuclei and stippled, rim-like chromatin patter suggestive of viral inclusions (**c**). Immunohistochemistry for JC virus showed positive staining of these cells (**d**) (Generously provided by Dr. David Schiff, University of Virginia, Charlottessville, VA.)

and/or bacterial process. The reaction appears to be idiosyncratic, does not usually recur with subsequent cycles of IT treatment, and does not seem to be dose-related. Oral corticosteroids or hydrocortisone along with the MTX may decrease the severity and incidence of chemical meningitis. The symptoms are usually self-limiting and require no treatment. Patients that have had an acute reaction to IT MTX do not appear to be predisposed to developing a late or chronic effect of the drug.

Less common acute and subacute side effects of IT and systemic MTX include seizures, encephalopathy, transient focal neurologic deficits, and transverse myelopathy [189, 190]. Seizures rarely occur as an acute toxicity after IT administration and are self-limiting. The most extensive experience with this complication has been in pediatric patients receiving IT MTX for treatment of acute leukemia [191]. Acute and subacute encephalopathy can occur in the setting of high-dose IV MTX ($3–12.5 \text{ g/m}^2$; 2.5–15% of patients), most often administered in combination with other chemotherapy agents for CNS lymphoma [188]. The clinical presentation typically includes somnolence, the acute onset of focal signs such as hemiparesis, dysphasia, dysarthria, and occasional seizure activity. Brain CT and MRI may demonstrate transient white matter abnormalities, or can be normal in some cases (Fig. 15.4). One report discussed the use of MRI within 1 h of onset of the syndrome. This revealed bilateral, symmetrical restricted diffusion involving white matter of the cerebral hemispheres, without evidence of vasospasm or perfusion defect [192]. The authors suggested that transient cytotoxic edema in the white matter was the likely mechanism of MTX-induced neurotoxicity. EEG evaluation usually reveals an abnormal study, with diffuse slowing of the background. The syndrome is not likely to correlate with serum or CSF MTX concentrations, and symptoms can occasionally recur with subsequent courses of treatment. In most cases, there is complete resolution of the clinical and imaging abnormalities but, rarely, a chronic leukoencephalopathy can be noted. Transverse myelopathy can occur after IT MTX, often within hours to weeks of administration of the drug [190, 193]. In most cases, the toxicity develops after the patient has received multiple doses of MTX. The clinical examination reveals bilateral leg weakness, pain, spasticity, sensory loss, bladder dysfunction, and gait difficulty. MRI of the spinal cord may be normal or show T2 high signal abnormalities with patchy enhancement [194]. Pathological examination is often unrevealing, although one case has been reported with vacuolar degeneration and necrosis, without inflammation [195]. The symptoms improve after drug discontinuation but the extent of improvement is variable [196]. Accidental overdosage of IT MTX is extremely uncommon, with cases describing no neurologic injury [197] and others reporting severe reactions to overdosage, with rapidly progressive encephalopathy and death [198]. Potential treatment options for patients with an overdose of IT MTX include CSF drainage, ventriculo-lumbar perfusion, and administration of IT carboxypeptidase-G2, an enzyme that hydrolyzes MTX into inactive metabolites [199, 200].

Chronic Effects

Chronic and/or late side effects of IT and IV MTX occur at least six months after initial drug administration [189, 190]. The most common chronic effect is a leukoencephalopathy, which is well described in children with acute leukemia, but can also occur in adults [201]. In children, the clinical presentation includes progressive learning disorders, developmental delay, memory loss, gait difficulty, and urinary incontinence. These symptoms are similar in adults, with confusion and memory loss that often progresses to dementia, as well as somnolence, irritability, impaired vision, dysphasia, seizures, and ataxia. Imaging with CT and MR reveals diffuse white matter damage, cortical atrophy, ventricular enlargement, and punctate areas of calcification within the basal ganglia and deep white matter (Fig. 15.5). In addition, asymptomatic patients who have only received high-dose IV or IT MTX may demonstrate similar, but much milder, damage to the white matter on imaging studies.

The leukoencephalopathy is most likely to occur after combination treatment with high-dose IV MTX, IT MTX, and cranial irradiation (45%), with a much lower incidence following high-dose MTX and/or IT MTX alone (2% or less) [190, 202]. Neurotoxicity is especially enhanced when the patient receives irradiation before the administration of MTX (Fig. 15.6). The mechanisms underlying this synergistic toxicity remain unclear. It may be due to a radiation-induced increase in the permeability of the BBB, reduced clearance of MTX from the CSF, increased passage of MTX into the white matter through the ependymal–brain

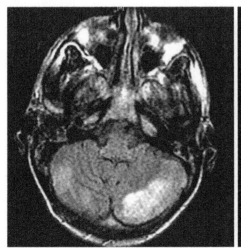
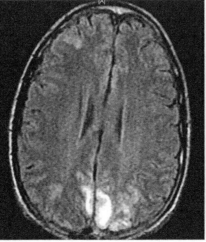
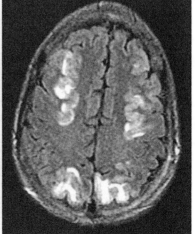

Fig. 15.4 Acute methotrexate toxicity. The axial MRI shows bihemispheric T2/FLAIR hyperintensities with frontal and occipital accentuation after intrathecal methotrexate injection in a 19-year old with AML. The patient developed mental status changes and confusion 1–2 h after methotrexate injection (Generously provided by Dr. Patrick Wen, Dana-Farber Cancer Institute, Boston, MA.)

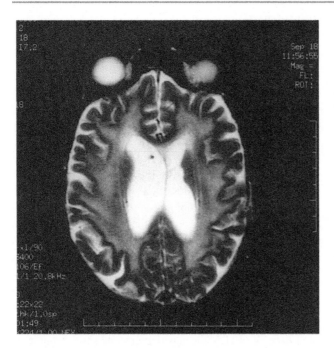

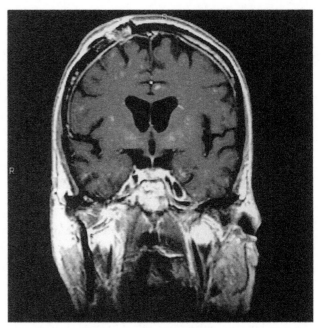

Fig. 15.5 Leukoencephalopathy. A 75-year-old woman with primary central nervous system lymphoma was treated with CHOP, ten doses of intraventricular methotrexate, and fractionated whole brain radiotherapy (5040 cGy in 28 fractions). Her tumor responded and never recurred. Three years later, she noted moderate short-term memory deficits and gait unsteadiness. MRI (axial T2-weighted image) demonstrated extensive periventricular white matter changes. The patient's dementia progressed, and she developed rigidity and mutism prior to her death one year later (Generously provided by Dr. Patrick Wen, Dana-Farber Cancer Institute, Boston, MA.)

Fig. 15.6 Disseminated necrotizing leukoencephalopathy. This 44-year-old man with Burkitt's lymphoma developed progressive lethargy and subsequent coma weeks after receiving fractionated radiotherapy to the skull base and eight doses of intraventricular methotrexate for lymphomatous involvement of the right cavernous sinus. Multiple CSF exams demonstrated no leptomeningeal lymphoma despite his neurologic deterioration. Persistent vegetative state ensued, and he died 2 months later from systemic relapse. MRI (coronal, T1 with gadolinium) demonstrated multiple scattered punctate foci and abnormal signal, particularly in the deep gray nuclei, with contrast enhancement. Postmortem analysis revealed multiple discrete, microscopic foci of demyelination, axonal loss, and necrosis distributed in a random manner throughout the white matter and gray/white interface. The foci contained a moderate to large number of CD68-immunoreactive foamy macrophages and a scant number of perivascular lymphocytes. Although there was no evidence of dural lymphoma, there was no leptomeningeal tumor identified (Generously provided by Dr. Patrick Wen, Dana-Farber Cancer Institute, Boston, MA.)

barrier, and potential direct cellular toxicity caused by irradiation [190]. Neuropathological changes are most notable around the periventricular white matter and deep centrum semiovale, and include demyelination, multifocal white matter necrosis, astrocytosis, dystrophic calcification of deep cerebral vessels, and axonal damage. Inflammatory cellular infiltration is typically not present.

Pemetrexed

Pemetrexed acts as an antifolate by disrupting folate-dependent metabolic processes essential for cell replication. It is indicated in the treatment of pleural mesothelioma and non-small cell lung cancer. It has little associated neurotoxicity. Fatigue is a dose-limiting toxicity and depression has been rarely reported [203].

Pralatrexate

Pralatrexate is an antifolate analog used for cutaneous and peripheral T-cell lymphoma. It competes for the folate-binding site to inhibit dihydrofolate reductase and

therefore inhibits DNA, RNA, and protein syntheses. Fatigue is the only CNS complication that has been reported [204, 205].

Nelarabine

Nelarabine is a prodrug that incorporates into DNA of leukemic blasts and inhibits DNA synthesis inducing cell apoptosis. It is used in the treatment of T-cell acute lymphoblastic leukemia (ALL) . When first studied, a higher dose was utilized that produced significant neurotoxicity. In phase II trials, 40–72% of patients have had neurotoxicity of any grade attributed to nelarabine, and 15–20% had severe neurotoxicity [206–208]. CNS toxicity can manifest in numerous ways including somnolence, vertigo, headache, hypoesthesia, ataxia, confusion, depressed level of consciousness, seizure, motor dysfunction, amnesia, gait disorders, sensory loss, aphasia, encephalopathy, etc. One series described three patients post-stem-cell transplant that developed irreversible paresthesias and muscle weakness in both lower extremities after neutrophil engraftment [209].

Dosing should occur on alternate days to decrease neurotoxicity, as early studies found that daily administration can result in 72% of patients experiencing some form of neurotoxicity [210]. A demyelination syndrome similar to Guillain-Barre syndrome, with an ascending peripheral neuropathy, has also been reported [206]. Neurologic toxicity may not fully resolve even after treatment cessation. Studies have shown that concurrent or previous intrathecal chemotherapy or crainospinal irradiation increase the risk of nelarabine-induced neurotoxicity [211].

Many antimetobolite chemotherapy agents cause neurotoxicity, and the mechanism for nelarabine-induced neurotoxicity remains unknown. CNS consequences of abnormal purine metabolism can occur in patients with a purine nucleoside phophorylase deficiency that is associated with spasticity and other neurologic abnormalities [212, 213]. Cytotoxic ara-GTP, the prodrug of nelarabine, has been postulated to be in high concentrations in brain and nerve tissue due to the high levels of deoyguanosine kinase activity. Further studies are needed to determine the risk factors and pathogenesis of nelarabine-induced neurotoxicity.

Clofarabine

Clofarabine is a purine nucleoside analog used for acute lymphoblastic leukemia (ALL). Hemorrhage, including intracranial hemorrhage, has been seen due to the profound thrombocytopenia that is associated with therapy. CNS toxicity includes headache, chills, fatigue, anxiety, irritability, lethargy, agitation, mental status changes, and confusion [214, 215].

Thioguanine (6-TG)

Thioguanine is a purine analog that incorporates into DNA and RNA blocking the synthesis of purine nucleotides. It is used in the treatment of pediatric patients with ALL. No central or peripheral neurotoxicity has been reported.

Cladribine (2-Chlorodeoxyadenosine)

Cladribine is a purine nucleoside analog that incorporates into DNA and results in DNA strand breaks, shutting down DNA synthesis and repair. It is utilized in the treatment of hairy cell leukemia. Cladribine is associated with dose-related neurologic toxicity including irreversible paraparesis and quadriparesis. This was reported with continuous infusion or higher doses (4–9 times conventional dosing), but may still rarely occur at the normal dose. This neurotoxicity may be delayed and present as progressive, irreversible weakness. Diagnostics with electromyography and nerve conduction studies are consistent with demyelinating disease. Treatment with cladribine is also associated with fever with or without neutropenia. Other central neurotoxicity includes fatigue, headache, dizziness, insomnia, and anxiety. Cases of confusion and progressive multifocal leukoencephalopathy have also been reported [216].

Pentostatin (2'-Deoxycoformycin)

Pentostatin is a purine antimetabolite that inhibits adenosine deaminase. The anti-tumor effects occur due to a reduction in purine metabolism which blocks DNA synthase and ultimately leads to cell death. It is used in hairy cell leukemia. Phase I dose findings studies showed increased neurotoxicity at higher doses (5–30 mg/m^2/day for 1–5 days) [217]. Toxicity included somnolence, lethargy, and one case of fatal coma. CNS toxicity was described as delayed onset and prolonged lasting as long as three weeks. Neurotoxicity is infrequent when used within the typical dose range. Ocular toxicity has also been reported as blurred vision, photophobia, and retinopathy [217, 218].

Anti-Tumor Antibiotics

Anthracyclines

Doxorubicin, Daunorubicin, Epirubicin, Idarubicin

Doxorubicin and daunorubicin are anthracycline antibiotics that bind nucleic acids, disrupting the structural integrity of DNA, and are used for the treatment of numerous hematologic and solid malignancies. Following IV infusion, neither drug penetrates the BBB to any significant degree; central neurotoxicity has not been reported. Doxorubicin when administered with cyclosporine has resulted in neurological symptoms and coma [219]. However, when administered IA for brain tumors, doxorubicin has been linked to cerebral infarcts and hemorrhagic necrosis [220]. Inadvertent IT injection of either drug can lead to an acute or subacute ascending myelopathy and encephalopathy, which can be fatal [221].

Epirubicin is an anthracycline known to inhibit DNA and RNA syntheses by intercalating between DNA base pairs used in breast cancer, gastric cancer, and types of sarcoma.

Neurotoxicity is rare though studies have reported lethargy and fever.

Idarubicin is mainly used in the treatment of acute myeloid leukemia (AML) . Like other anthracyclines, it inhibits DNA and RNA syntheses by intercalation between DNA base pairs. Neurotoxicity is rare with headache and seizure described. All anthracyclines can cause arrhythmias and cardiomyopathies that can lead to cerebrovascular complications.

Other Anti-Tumor Antibiotics

Dactinomycin

Dactinomycin is used in testicular cancer, gestational trophoblastic neoplasm, and several types of sarcomas. It intercalates DNA inhibiting DNA, RNA, and protein syntheses. Neurotoxicity is rare including fatigue, lethargy, and malaise [222, 223].

Bleomycin Sulfate

Bleomycin acts by directly binding to DNA, leading to both single- and double-strand breaks, as well as inhibiting RNA and protein synthesis. Bleomycin is utilized in the treatment of testicular cancer, and Hodgkin's lymphoma. Generally, neurotoxicity is uncommon. An idiosyncratic reaction has been reported in 1% of lymphoma patients treated with bleomycin that is similar to anaphylaxis, but can include symptoms of confusion, fever, and chills along with other non-CNS toxicity. Cerebral infarction has been described following the combination of bleomycin and cisplatin [224].

Mitomycin C

Mitomycin acts as an alkylating agent by producing DNA cross-links and therefore inhibiting DNA and RNA syntheses. It is used for gastric and pancreatic cancer. It is only known to cause central neurotoxicity in the context of mitomycin-induced disseminated intravascular coagulation and thrombotic microangiopathy, which can lead to headaches and other CNS complications [225].

Mitoxantrone

Mitoxantrone has a mechanism similar to anthracyclines by intercalating into DNA, resulting in cross-links and strand breaks. It is utilized in the treatment of acute myeloid leukemia (AML) and multiple sclerosis. Like anthracyclines, neurotoxicity is uncommon with headache, anxiety, depression, and seizures reported [226]. Radiculopathy and myelopathy have been reported following intrathecal administration [227].

Topoisomerase Inhibitors

Topoisomerase I Inhibitors

Topotecan

Topotecan is a topoisomerase I inhibitor and derives its activity from binding to topoisomerase I and stabilizing the cleavable complex so that relegation of the cleaved DNA strand cannot occur. It is used in cervical, ovarian, small cell lung cancer, and sarcoma. Neurotoxicity is rare with fatigue and headache reported [228, 229].

Irinotecan (CPT-11)

Irinotecan is a topoisomerase I inhibitor resulting in the prevention of re-ligation of single-strand breaks in DNA during DNA synthesis. It is used in colon, lung, cervical, ovarian, pancreatic, glioblastoma, and skin cancer. Irinotecan has been associated with nonspecific dizziness and insomnia, as well as occasional episodes of dysarthria, either alone or in combination with other drugs. The dysarthria resolves after discontinuation of the drug.

Topoisomerase II Inhibitors

Etoposide (VP-16)

Etoposide, a topoisomerase II inhibitor, delays transit of cells through the S phase and arrests cells in late S or early G2 phase, halting the cell cycle and leading to apoptosis. Etoposide is commonly used in lung cancer, testicular cancer, hematopoietic stem cell transplant, and mobilization. Neurotoxicity is uncommon, with rare reports of peripheral neuropathy, transient cortical blindness, and optic neuritis. Hypersensitivity reactions can occur during the infusion that can manifest with chills, fever, and loss of consciousness. It is important to note that the injectable formulation contains ethanol (approximately 33% v/v) and may contribute to neurotoxicity due to ethanol toxicity, especially at higher doses used for stem cell mobilization. Rarely, confusion, papilledema, somnolence, worsening motor deficits, and seizures have been described [230].

Teniposide (VM-26)

Teniposide (VM-26) is a topoisomerase II inhibitor that induces single- and double-strand breaks in DNA and DNA–protein cross-links. Teniposide is used in refractory acute lymphoblastic leukemia (ALL). It is highly protein bound and poorly penetrates the BBB. Hypersensitivity reactions can occur and include chills and fever. Acute CNS depression has been reported with high IV dosing [231]. Like in etoposide, there is an ethanol component to the diluent used in the medication, which can cause acute ethanol toxicity leading to CNS depression.

Mitotic Inhibitors

Paclitaxel

Paclitaxel is a semisynthetic derivative of the Western yew tree. It is a microtubule-inhibiting compound that is widely used in solid tumors, including breast and ovarian cancer. Paclitaxel stabilizes microtubules leading to mitotic arrest and apoptosis in dividing cells. The neurotoxicity of paclitaxel is manifested by a motor and sensory polyneuropathy [232]. The major manifestations are burning paresthesias of the hands and feet, as well as loss of reflexes. The main risk factor that contributes to the peripheral neuropathy is cumulative dose of approximately 1000 mg/m^2 [233]. Paclitaxel may induce peripheral neuropathy after the first cycle of treatment with higher doses (>250 mg/m^2) [234]. Paclitaxel also causes a motor neuropathy affecting proximal muscles [234].

There are conflicting data regarding the impact of the dosing schedule on paclitaxel-induced peripheral neuropathy. Studies have reported less neuropathy with weekly paclitaxel [235, 236], while others have found no difference [237]. The length of infusion has also been studied with conflicting results. Studies have found that increasing the infusion from 3 to 24 h decreases the incidence of neuropathy [238], while others did not find a difference in rates of severe neuropathy [239].

Less common paclitaxel neurotoxicity includes perioral numbness, autonomic neuropathies [232], seizure [240], transient encephalopathy [240, 241], and phantom limb pain [242]. There are reports of transient scintillating scotomas and occasional visual loss [243]. An acute pain syndrome associated with paclitaxel has been described. It is characterized by severe arthralgias and myalgias with numbness and tingling, beginning one to two days after treatment and lasting four to five days. Recent data suggest that this is a form of an acute neuropathy rather than a joint and/or muscle disorder [244–246].

Protein-Bound Paclitaxel

Protein-bound paclitaxel is an albumin-bound paclitaxel that promotes microtubule assembly and stabilizes the microtubules interfering with the mitotic phase and inhibiting cell replication. It is used in metastatic breast cancer, non-small cell lung cancer, and pancreatic adenocarcinoma. Like paclitaxel, this formulation commonly produces a sensory neuropathy. Rarely, autonomic neuropathy and cranial nerve palsy have been described [247]. Other neurotoxicity includes fatigue, headache, decreased visual acuity, optic nerve damage, and depression [248, 249].

Docetaxel

Docetaxel is derived from the needles of the European yew tree. Like paclitaxel, docetaxel promotes the assembly of microtubules and inhibits the depolymerization of tubulin which stabilizes the mircotubules, inhibiting DNA, RNA, and protein synthesis. It is commonly used in breast, non-small cell lung, prostate cancer, and sarcomas. Docetaxel, like paclitaxel, causes both sensory and motor neuropathies, although both occur less frequently in comparison to paclitaxel [236]. Peripheral neurotoxicity is directly related to the cumulative docetaxel dose with the threshold being approximately 400 mg/m^2 [233]. A phase III trial in women with breast cancer patients used a dose of docetaxel of 100 mg/m^2 every three weeks. The onset of moderate to severe neuropathy occurred at a median cumulative dose of 371 mg/m^2 [250].

There are conflicting data as to the effect of the administration schedule on docetaxel-induced peripheral neuropathy. A trial in breast cancer patients compared docetaxel 75 mg/m^2 every three weeks to 35 mg/m^2 weekly and rates of severe peripheral neuropathy were higher with every three-week docetaxel administration (10% vs. 5%) [251]. Conversely, a meta-analysis of randomized trials in non-small cell lung cancer comparing the two dosing regimens found similar rates of moderate to severe peripheral neuropathy with both schedules (2.5% with every three-week administration versus 3% with weekly administration) [252]. Docetaxel has also been associated with Lhermitte's phenomenon [253].

Cabazitaxel

Cabazitaxel is a taxane derivative that acts as a microtubule inhibitor by stabilizing microtubules and thus inhibiting tumor proliferation. It is used in castration-resistant prostate cancer. Central nervous system toxicity includes fatigue, vertigo, and headache [254]. Peripherally, cabazitaxel can cause peripheral neuropathy but a recent report indicated that there is significantly less peripheral neuropathy compared to docetaxel [255].

Eribulin

Eribulin is a non-taxane microtubule inhibitor used for metastatic breast cancer. It inhibits the growth phase of the microtubule by inhibiting the formation of mitotic spindles, thus arresting the cell cycle. Centrally, eribulin can cause fatigue, headache, depression, dizziness, insomnia, and myasthenia. 35% of patients report peripheral neuropathy, with 8% reporting severe neuropathy symptoms. The peripheral neuropathy associated with eribulin may be prolonged and lasts greater than one year in approximately 5% of patients [256–258].

Ixabepilone

Ixabepilone is a microtubuluar stabilizing agent that promotes tubulin polymerization and stabilizing the microtubular function, arresting the cell cycle, and inducing apoptosis. It is approved for metastatic breast cancer. The diluent of ixabepilone contains ethanol and patients should be cautioned about performing tasks that require alertness after treatment. Headache, vertigo, and insomnia have also been reported.

Peripheral sensory neuropathy is common (up to 63% of patients) and dose-limiting. The peripheral neuropathy typically occurs during the first three cycles of therapy. A peripheral motor neuropathy can also occur in approximately 10% of patients. Small studies have shown that ixabepilone exposure induces a dose-dependent toxicity on small sensory fibers and progression axonal loss where mitochondria appear to bear the cumulative toxic effect [259]. Cases of autonomic neuropathy have also been reported [260, 261].

Vincristine, Vinblastine, Vinorelbine

Vincristine binds to tubulin and inhibits microtubule formation arresting the cell at metaphase causing cell apoptosis. It is widely used in both solid and hematologic malignancies. Vincristine has poor penetration of the BBB and therefore is not commonly associated with central neurotoxicity. Mental status changes, depression, confusion, and insomnia rarely occur. These neurotoxicities occur more frequently in the presence of other neurotoxic agents and spinal cord irradiation. Ataxia, coma, dizziness, headache, seizures, and vertigo may also occur. Cranial nerve dysfunction manifesting as auditory damage, extraocular muscle impairment, laryngeal muscle impairment, paralysis, paresis, vestibular damage, and vocal cord paralysis can also occur.

The dose-limiting toxicity of vincristine is an axonal neuropathy. Vincristine disrupts the microtubules within the axons and interferes with axonal transport [262, 263]. These neuropathies include both sensory and motor fibers, with small sensory fibers being especially affected. Almost all patients treated with vincristine with have signs and symptoms of neuropathy. Early neuropathy manifests as paresthesias in the fingers and feet with or without pain. These symptoms develop at a cumulative dose of approximately 30–50 mg [264] but may occur after the first dose. Symptoms may also appear after the medication has been discontinued. Like other chemotherapy-induced peripheral neuropathy, the neuropathy improves over time but may not completely resolve. Risk factors for severe vincristine neuropathies include age, nutritional status, prior irradiation to peripheral nerves, concomitant hematopoietic colony-stimulating factors [265], use of azole antifungal agents or other CYP3A4 inhibitors [266, 267], and those with pre-existing neurologic conditions such as Charcot–Marie–Tooth syndrome [268, 269], and high-dose liposomal vincristine [270].

Autonomic neuropathies are common in patients who are treated with vincristine and may precede paresthesias or loss of deep tendon reflexes. Abdominal pain and constipation occur in almost 50% of patients; paralytic ileus can occur rarely [262]. Vincristine may also cause focal mononeuropathies, at times involving the cranial nerves [271], with the oculomotor nerve most commonly affected. Other nerves may be involved include recurrent laryngeal nerve, optic nerve, facial nerve, and the auditory nerve. Vincristine may also cause retinal damage and night blindness, and patients may experience jaw and/or parotid pain.

Vincristine can rarely cause inappropriate secretion of antidiuretic hormone (SIADH), resulting in hyponatremia, confusion, and seizures [272]. Other rare neurotoxicities include seizures [273], reversible posterior leukoencephalopathy [274, 275], transient cortical blindness [276], ataxia, athetosis, and parkinsonism.

Liposomal vincristine is approved for acute lymphoblastic leukemia and can also cause significant peripheral neuropathy [277–279]. Vincristine and liposomal vincristine are not interchangeable. With both agents intrathecal administration is associated with ascending myelopathy, coma, and death [280–282]. Pathological analysis after IT administration demonstrates diffuse necrosis in the brain and spinal cord in regions exposed to the CSF.

Vinblastine is used in many lymphomas, mycosis fungoides, testicular cancer, and Kaposi sarcoma. Vinblastine-induced peripheral neuropathy is less severe than that of vincristine, but occurs in the majority of patients. Vinorelbine is utilized in the treatment of lung and breast cancer. It is associated with mild distal neuropathy, mainly paresthesias in approximately 20% of patients. Severe neuropathies are rare and most often manifest in patients with prior paclitaxel exposure [283, 284].

Proteasome Inhibitors

Bortezomib

Bortezomib reversibly inhibits the 26S proteasome activating signaling cascades leading to cell-cycle arrest and apoptosis. It is used in multiple myeloma as well as many lymphomas and amyloidosis. Peripheral neuropathy is the major dose-limiting toxicity associated with bortezomib [285–287]. Peripheral neuropathy manifests early, normally within the first course of therapy, and generally worsens through the fifth cycle. After five cycles of therapy the peripheral neuropathy does not seem to worsen [288]. It is typically reversible within months of discontinuation, but can persist for years or even indefinitely [287, 289, 290].

Many mechanisms of bortezomib-induced peripheral neuropathy have been proposed but the precise mechanism is unclear [288]. It has been shown to cause direct toxicity to the dorsal root ganglion [291]. Bortezomib is able to activate the mitochondrial apoptotic pathway that leads to mitochondrial and endoplasmic reticulum damage potentially playing a role in the peripheral neuropathy [292]. Dysregulation of intracellular calcium and/or neurotrophins has also been shown to be a potential determinant of bortezomib-induced peripheral neuropathy [293, 294].

Bortezomib-induced neurotoxicity manifests as painful sensory neuropathy with dysesthesias of the fingers and toes. On exam, there is distal sensory loss to all modalities and changes in proprioception, with absent or suppressed deep tendon reflexes [286, 295]. Motor neuropathy is less common and manifests as distal weakness in the lower extremities. Autonomic neuropathies have also been described, leading to diarrhea, constipation, and orthostatic hypotension [294, 296, 297]. Demyelinating neuropathies have also been reported [286, 298].

Studies have examined strategies to prevent the incidence and severity of bortezomib peripheral neuropathy. When compared to twice weekly administration, weekly administration of bortezomib resulted in significantly less severe neuropathy and fewer patients discontinued therapy due to neuropathy [299]. Studies have also shown that subcutaneous administration significantly reduces the overall occurrence and severity of peripheral neuropathy compared to intravenous administration [300, 301]. This is thought to be due to the decrease in peak concentrations with subcutaneous dosing compared to intravenous administration. Dose reductions at the onset of peripheral neuropathy have been associated with an improvement or reversal in many patients [285, 289, 294, 302].

Central neurotoxicity with bortezomib is rare but includes headache, fatigue, dizziness, agitation, and insomnia. Reversible posterior leukoencephalopathy has also been described [303–305].

Carfilzomib

Carfilzomib is a second-generation proteasome inhibitor that binds the 20S proteasome, leading to cell-cycle arrest and apoptosis. It is used in refractory multiple myeloma. Peripheral neuropathy can still occur but the incidence and severity seems less than that of bortezomib [306–308]. Centrally, carfilzomib causes fatigue, headache, insomnia, and dizziness.

Histone Deacetylase (HDAC) Inhibitors

Belinostat, Panobinostat, Romidepsin, Vorinostat

Histone deacetylase inhibitors increase acetylation of histone proteins causing cell-cycle arrest and apoptosis. They are used for peripheral and cutaneous T-cell lymphoma as well as multiple myeloma. CNS toxicity is uncommon with fatigue, headache, and dizziness reported [309–312]. Ischemic stroke has been reported with vorinostat [313].

DNA Methylation Inhibitors

Decitabine

Decitabine is a prodrug that incorporates into DNA and causes DNA hypomethylation leading to cell death. It is used in myelodysplastic syndrome (MDS) and acute myelogenous leukemia (AML). Neurotoxicity is uncommon but may include headache, insomnia, dizziness, and fatigue [314, 315].

Azacitidine (5-Azacytidine)

Azacitidine, like decitabine, is a hypomethylating agent, incorporating into DNA, inhibiting DNA methylation, leading to cell death. Azacitidine is used for MDS and AML. Central nervous system toxicities include fatigue, rigors, headache, vertigo, anxiety, depression, insomnia, malaise, and hypoesthesia. Rare reports of hepatic coma [316] and seizure have been described [317, 318].

Miscellaneous Chemotherapy Agents

Thalidomide

Thalidomide is a drug with anti-angiogenesis and immunomodulatory properties, mainly used for the treatment of myeloma and Kaposi's sarcoma. Peripheral neuropathy is a dose-limiting toxicity of thalidomide. Clinically, patients present with symmetric paresthesias and or dysesthesias, with or without sensory loss. Motor neuropathy is also common [319–325]. Neuropathy was more common and severe when high doses were given (greater than 200 mg per day) [326]. With newer dosing regimens peripheral neuropathy is present in about half of patients treated with thalidomide, but the severity of the neuropathy is significantly decreased [322, 327, 328]. Mechanistically, toxic axonopathy and dysregulation of neurotrophin activity may play a role with the pathogenesis of the neuropathy [321, 329].

Central neurotoxicity is generally mild, with varying degrees of somnolence as the most common manifestation. At high doses (i.e., 400 mg/day or above), the somnolence can be quite severe in some patients. Headache can also be noted on occasion. Seizures have been reported, but generally occur in patients with an underlying epileptogenic brain disorder (i.e., brain tumor) [330]. Dizziness [320], tremor [322, 324], and unresponsiveness leading to coma [331] have also been reported.

Lenalidomide

Lenalidomide, a second-generation agent, has immunomodulatory, antiangiogenic, and antineoplastic properties due to multiple mechanisms. It is used in mantle cell lymphoma, multiple myeloma, and myelodysplastic syndromes. Like thalidomide, it can cause peripheral neuropathy but the incidence and severity is significantly less compared to thalidomide [332]. It has been used in patients with pre-existing peripheral neuropathies [333]. Cognitive decline and expressive aphasia have been described with resolution after drug discontinuation [331]. A case of short-term memory loss is also described [331].

Pomalidomide

Pomalidomide is a second-generation agent used to treat refractory multiple myeloma. It has a similar mechanism to that of thalidomide and lenalidomide causing antiangiogenic, immunomodulatory, and antineoplastic effects. In the large phase III trials, peripheral neuropathy was seen in 9% of patients but severe peripheral neuropathy was not observed [334, 335]. A case of dysarthria has been described [331].

Arsenic Trioxide

Arsenic trioxide induces apoptosis and damages and degrades the fusion protein PML–RAR alpha. It is used for acute promyelocytic leukemia. Common CNS toxicity includes fatigue, fever, headache, insomnia, anxiety, tremor, and vertigo. Less common side effects include seizures that occur in 8% of patients. Agitation, coma, and confusion have also been described [336].

Bexarotene

Bexarotene binds and activates the retinoid X receptors, which function as the regulation pathway to express genes which control cell proliferation. It is used in cutaneous T-cell lymphoma. It can cause headache, fever, and insomnia [337].

L-Asparaginase

L-asparagine is an amino acid required for the synthesis of many cellular proteins in normal human cells. Many tumors lack the enzyme L-asparagine synthetase and are unable to synthesize cellular proteins, and therefore require an exogenous supply of the amino acid. L-asparaginase is a bacterial-derived enzyme that hydrolyzes L-asparagine into aspartic acid and ammonia. It is capable of depleting the extracellular supply of L-asparagine, thereby depleting tumor cells of the amino acid and inhibiting protein synthesis [338]. L-asparaginase is a large molecule with poor BBB penetration as negligible CSF levels are noted after an IV infusion. However, even though the drug does not readily cross the BBB it is associated with several forms of central neurotoxicity, including diffuse encephalopathy, cerebral venous thrombosis with venous infarction, and cerebral hemorrhage [339] (Fig. 15.7). The encephalopathy can be acute or subacute and appears to be dose-related. Although the mechanism remains unclear, it may be due to hepatic toxicity and hyperammonemia [340, 341]. Symptoms are variable, and can range from mild lethargy and personality changes to coma. Focal neurological deficits and seizures may also be noted [342]. EEGs usually demonstrate diffuse slowing with triphasic waves. The majority of patients with encephalopathy have elevated levels of ammonia. Improvement in symptoms usually occurs within a few days of discontinuing L-asparaginase. More modern protocols use lower doses of L-asparaginase and are much less likely to induce encephalopathy.

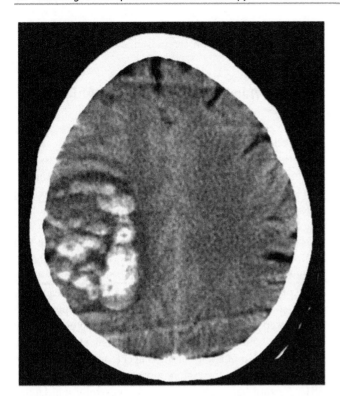

Fig. 15.7 Acute L-Asparaginase toxicity. Intracerebral hemorrhage after cortical vein thrombosis in a 41-year-old female during induction chemotherapy with L-asparaginase for ALL. The patient developed dizziness, left-sided weakness, and headaches. CT imaging (without contrast) revealed a right fronto-parietal hemorrhage. Additional imaging with CT angiography and CT venogram demonstrated the presence of a right cortical vein thrombosis and left vertebral artery occlusion (not shown) (Generously provided by Dr. Darren Volpe, Brigham and Women's Hospital, Boston, MA.)

Cerebrovascular complications related to L-asparaginase can be severe in some patients, but are less common. The drug depletes serum levels of numerous hemostatic factors, including fibrinogen, antithrombin III, protein C, protein S, factors IX and X, and fibrinolytic enzymes. As a result, the serum prothrombin time and partial thromboplastin time are typically elevated during treatment, even in asymptomatic patients [343]. The most common cerebrovascular complication of L-asparaginase is cerebral venous or dural sinus thrombosis, with secondary venous infarction [344–346]. Headache is typically the first symptom, often associated with nausea, emesis, and visual obscuration. Generalized or partial seizures and somnolence can also be noted. Focal neurological deficits and papilledema may be present. Cranial CT and MRI may be able to demonstrate venous infarction adjacent to the thrombosed vein or dural sinus. MRI is more sensitive than CT, especially in conjunction with a magnetic resonance venogram (MRV), which will be able to clearly demonstrate the filling void of the involved sinus. Initial treatment consists of discontinuation of L-asparaginase and therapeutic anticoagulation, if there is no

evidence of hemorrhage. Fresh-frozen plasma may also be of benefit to prevent extension of the thrombus [339]. The pegylated formulation, peg-asparaginase, has a similar neurotoxicity profile as L-asparaginase.

Retinoic Acid

The retinoids, tretinoin and aliretinoin, are synthetic analogs of vitamin A that induce cellular differentiation in tumors such as Kaposi's sarcoma and acute promyelocytic leukemia [347]. All of the retinoids readily cross the BBB. The most common central neurotoxicity is headache, which is seen in approximately 50–80% of patients on higher dose regimens. Headache can be a dose-limiting toxicity of therapy. In most patients, there is no clinical evidence of elevated intracranial pressure. However, a small percentage of these patients develop the syndrome of retinoid-induced pseudotumor cerebri, with symptoms of severe headache and visual impairment [348]. The mechanism of retinoid-induced pseudotumor cerebri is thought to be the reduction of CSF resorption at the level of the arachnoid granulations. Discontinuation of the offending medication will result in resolution of the headaches, even if associated with pseudotumor cerebri. For patients that require continued treatment with retinoids, serial lumbar punctures and CSF drainage may provide benefit. Other less common neurological side effects of retinoids include abnormal color vision, transient visual loss, oculogyric crisis, and ataxia.

Omacetaxane

Omacetaxane is a reversible protein synthesis inhibitor that interferes with chain elongation and inhibits protein synthesis. It is approved for CML and has activity against many known mutations of the disease. Many CNS toxicities have been reported—most commonly fatigue, headache, and insomnia. Less common toxicities include anxiety, agitation, confusion, depression, vertigo, dysphonia, hyperthermia, hypoesthesia, lethargy, mental status changes, and seizures. Peripherally, paresthesias, sciatica, and tremor have been reported [349].

Radium 223 Dichloride

Radium 223 dichloride is a radiopharmaceutical used for the treatment of patients with castration-resistant prostate cancer. It is an alpha particle-emitting isotope that mimics calcium to form complexes with bone to target bone metastases. Radium 223 dichloride has no known neurotoxicity.

Hormonal Agents

Selective Estrogen Receptor Modulators

Tamoxifen
Tamoxifen acts as an antiestrogen by binding the estrogen receptors on tumors and other tissues and decreasing DNA synthesis and inhibiting the effects of estrogen. It is used in hormone receptor positive breast cancer [350]. Tamoxifen can cause ocular effects including retinal vein thrombosis, retinopathy, keratopathy, and color perception changes [351–356]. Rarely encephalopathy can occur [357]. Mood changes, depression, insomnia, headache, dizziness, and fatigue are also described. Tamoxifen is known to increase the risk of thromboembolic events but the risk for stroke was not as high as the risk for deep vein thrombosis or pulmonary embolism [358–361].

Toremifene Citrate
Toremifene is a potent antiestrogen compound that competitively binds to estrogen receptors on tissue and tumors, decreasing the effects of estrogen and decreasing DNA synthesis. It is used in refractory breast cancer. Dizziness, vision changes, fatigue, and depression have been reported [362, 363].

Raloxifene Hydrochloride
Raloxifene acts as a selective estrogen receptor modulator preventing bone loss and blocking estrogen effects in breast and uterine tissues. Raloxifene is utilized in invasive breast cancer risk reduction as well as osteoporosis. It has been associated with increased clotting risk and was shown to increase the risk of fatal stroke [364].

Estrogen Receptor Antagonists

Faslodex
Faslodex is an antiestrogen that acts as a direct estrogen receptor antagonist by binding to estrogen receptors on tumors and other tissues used for metastatic breast cancer. It rarely causes headache and fatigue [365].

Aromatase Inhibitors

Anastrozole, Letrozole, and Exemestane
Anastrozole and letrozole are nonsteroidal aromatase inhibitors that prevent the conversion of androgens to estradiol. Exemestane has a similar mechanism of action but is a steroidal aromatase inhibitor. They are used in hormone receptor positive breast cancer. As a drug class, these medications can cause fatigue, mood changes, somnolence, anxiety, headache, and depression [366–371]. Anastrazole has been associated with cerebral infarction [372].

Gonadotropin-Releasing Hormone (GnRH) Agonists

Goserelin, Leuprolide Acetate, Histrelin
Gonadotropin-releasing hormone (GNRH) agonists, with continuous administration, suppress the release to luteinizing hormone and follicle-stimulating hormone, decreasing testosterone levels in males and estrogen levels in women. They are utilized in the treatment of breast cancer and prostate cancer. As a class, they can cause tumor flare with an initial surge of testosterone or estrogen levels before suppression. This surge can potentially exacerbate symptoms of bone disease, including spinal disease, leading to spinal cord compression. Cases of pituitary apoplexy have been described and are a class effect. Symptoms include headache, vomiting, and visual or mental status changes [373–378]. Neurotoxicity of these agents includes headache, emotional lability, depression, insomnia, and lethargy [379–381]. Seizure has been reported with goserelin and leuprolide acetate therapy [382, 383].

Antiandrogens

Bicalutamide, Flutamide, Nilutamide
Antiandrogens bind to androgen receptors preventing the ability of testosterone to stimulate prostate cancer cell growth. Neurotoxicity is uncommon with all three agents, with headache, neuropathy, confusion, depression, dizziness, and fatigue being described [384]. These medications are hepatotoxic and cases of hepatic encephalopathy have been reported [385, 386]. Vision changes including a delayed adaptation to dark have been reported with nilutamide [387, 388].

Miscellaneous Hormone Agents

Mitotane
Mitotane is an adrenolytic agent which directly leads to adrenal cortical atrophy. It is used for the treatment of inoperable adrenocortical carcinoma and Cushing's syndrome. Central CNS toxicity includes confusion, ataxia, and vertigo [389]. Long-term use, defined as greater than 2 years, may lead to brain damage and/or functional impairment which may be reversible upon drug discontinuation [390]. This neurotoxicity has been associated with plasma concentrations >16 mcg/mL in some cases [391] and >20 mcg/mL in others [390]. Myasthenia due to damage of

neuromuscular junctions, requiring dose reductions or discontinuation, has been observed [392].

Octreotide

Octreotide mimics the natural effects of somatostatin through inhibition of serotonin release and secretion of gastrin, vasoactive intestinal peptide, insulin, glucagon, secretin, motilin, and pancreatic polypeptide. It is used to control the symptoms of carcinoid tumors and to treat diarrhea associated with vasoactive intestinal peptide-secreting tumors. It can cause fatigue, headache, and dizziness. Seizure activity has also been rarely described [393].

Megestrol

Megestrol is a hormonal agent used for advanced breast and ovarian cancer as well as an appetite stimulant for cancer-related anorexia and/or cachexia. It is a synthetic progestin with antiestrogenic properties. Neurotoxicity is not common with headache, insomnia, confusion, depression, and neuropathy rarely being reported [394, 395].

Degarelix

Degarelix acts as a gonadotropin-releasing hormone (GnRH) antagonist by binding GnRH receptors in the anterior pituitary gland decreasing secretion of luteinizing hormone (LH) and follicle stimulation hormone (FSH). This results in a rapid decrease in androgens through a decrease in testosterone production. It is used in prostate cancer. Neurotoxicity is not common with fatigue, headache, chills, dizziness, insomnia, and stroke being reported [396–398].

Enzalutamide

Enzalutamide is a novel pure androgen receptor signaling inhibitor used for prostate cancer. It has been associated with seizures that may occur early or late in therapy with an onset ranging from 1 to 20 months after treatment. Seizures associated with enzalutamide therapy resolve upon therapy cessation [399, 400]. Predisposing factors included seizure history, underlying brain injury with loss of consciousness, TIA within past 12 months, stroke, and brain metastases. It is recommended that enzalutamide be permanently discontinued if seizures develop during therapy. Other CNS toxicity includes fatigue, falling, headache, vertigo, myasthenia, insomnia, anxiety, paresthesias, cauda equine syndrome, altered mental status, hypoesthesia, hallucination, and restless leg syndrome [400].

Abiraterone

Abiraterone irreversibly inhibits CYP 17 inhibiting the conversion of precursors to testosterone. It is used for metastatic prostate cancer. It can cause adrenocortical insufficiency; prednisone is administered along with abiraterone to mitigate this side effect. Neurologically, adrenocortical insufficiency can manifest as weakness, disorientation, fatigue, and dizziness. Insomnia and falling have also been reported [401, 402].

Supportive Care Agents

Dexrazoxane

Dexrazoxane is an intracellular chelating agent used to prevent anthracycline-induced cardiomyopathy as well as for extravasation of anthracyclines. There is little neurotoxicity, with fatigue and fever being described [403].

Rasburicase

Rasburicase is a recombinant urate-oxidase enzyme which converts uric acid to an inactive and soluble metabolite allantoin. It is used for treatment and prevention of hyperurecemia that is seen from tumor lysis in different types of malignancies. Neurotoxicity is rare with headache and fever reported [404].

Glucarpidase

Glucarpidase is a recombinant enzyme which rapidly metabolizes methotrexate into inactive metabolites, quickly reducing methotrexate concentrations. It is utilized for methotrexate toxicity. Neurotoxicity is rare. Glucarpidase has been administered intrathecally for accidental intrathecal methotrexate overdose and was shown to be effective without causing neurotoxicity [196, 197].

Eltrombopag Olamine

Eltrombopag, a thrombopoietin agonist, increases platelet count by activating the human thrombopoietin receptor. It is utilized in chronic immune thrombocytopenia (ITP), hepatitis C-associated thrombocytopenia, and aplastic anemia. Fatigue, headache, insomnia, and dizziness have been reported [405–407].

Filgrastim

Filgrastim is a granulocyte colony-stimulating factor that promotes production, maturation, and activation of neutrophils. It is used in numerous malignancies for prevention of febrile neutropenia, to aid in neutrophil recovery after cytotoxic therapy, and mobilization for stem cell transplant. No known neurotoxic effects have been described.

Sargramostim

Sargramostim is a growth factor that stimulates the proliferation, differentiation, and functional activity of neutrophils, eosinophils, monocytes, and macrophages. It is used to shorten the time of neutropenia post-chemotherapy or hematopoietic stem cell transplant. Neurotoxicity is uncommon with headache and fatigue described.

Palifermin

Palifermin is a recombinant keratinocyte growth factor that induces proliferation, differentiation, and migration of epithelial cells. It has been shown to decrease the oral mucositis associated with hematopoietic stem cell transplant conditioning regimens. Fever, pain, and oral dysesthesias were described in trials [408, 409].

Amifostine

Amifostine is a supportive agent that can be used for cisplatin-induced renal toxicity as well as to reduce the risk of xerostomia from head and neck cancer radiation treatment. Amifostine is a prodrug that is converted to a free thiol metabolite that acts as a free radical scavenger. Anxiety, fatigue, and fever have been reported [410].

Denosumab

Denosumab is a monoclonal antibody that targets nuclear factor kappa ligand (RANKL), which prevents osteoclast formation leading to decreased bone resorption and increased bone mass. It is used for hypercalcemia of malignancy, prevention of skeletal-related events, and treatment of giant cell tumor of the bone. Neurotoxicity is rare but headache and fatigue have been reported [411].

Zolendronic Acid and Pamidronate

Zolendronic acid and pamidronate are bisphosphonates which inhibit bone resorption by inhibiting osteoclastic activity. They are used for hypercalcemia of malignancy and prevention of skeletal-related events in patients with bone metastases. Neurotoxicity is rare with each agent.

Romiplostim

Romiplostim is a thrombopoietin peptide mimetic increasing platelet counts by activating the human TPO receptor. Its main use is in chronic immune thrombocytopenia (ITP). Neurotoxicity includes headache, dizziness, and insomnia. Romiplostim is known to increase the risk of thromboembolic events, but increased stroke risk was not reported in the clinical studies [412, 413].

Conclusion

Chemotherapy-induced neurotoxicity is a common complication of cancer therapy that can result in both peripheral and central nervous system toxicity. Direct and secondary toxicity can occur from these medications, and can result in severe and potentially permanent neurological symptoms. These toxicities can affect the overall cancer therapy as dose-limiting effects, thereby potentially impacting further chemotherapy. Clinicians caring for patients with cancer must recognize the risks of drug-related neurotoxicity, in order to appropriately differentiate them from other potential causes of neurotoxicity associated with cancer.

References

1. Sullivan KM, Storb R, Shulman HM, Shaw CM, Spence A, Beckham C, et al. Immediate and delayed neurotoxicity after mechlorethamine preparation for bone marrow transplantation. Ann Intern Med. 1982;97(2):182–9.
2. Shapiro WR, Young DF. Neurological complications of antineoplastic therapy. Acta Neurol Scand Suppl. 1984;100:125–32.
3. Newton HB. Intra-arterial chemotherapy. In: Newton HB, editor. Handbook of brain tumor chemotherapy. Amsterdam: Academic Press; 2006. p. 247–61.
4. Williams SA, Makker SP, Ingelfinger JR, Grupe WE. Long-term evaluation of chlorambucil plus prednisone in the idiopathic nephrotic syndrome of childhood. N Engl J Med. 1980;302 (17):929–33.
5. Salloum E, Khan KK, Cooper DL. Chlorambucil-induced seizures. Cancer. 1997;79(5):1009–13.
6. Burns LJ. Ocular toxicities of chemotherapy. Semin Oncol. 1992;19(5):492–500.
7. Vandenberg SA, Kulig K, Spoerke DG, Hall AH, Bailie VJ, Rumack BH. Chlorambucil overdose: accidental ingestion of an antineoplastic drug. J Emerg Med. 1988;6(6):495–8.
8. Wyllie AR, Bayliff CD, Kovacs MJ. Myoclonus due to chlorambucil in two adults with lymphoma. Ann Pharmacother. 1997;31(2):171–4.
9. Rai KR, Peterson BL, Appelbaum FR, Kolitz J, Elias L, Shepherd L, et al. Fludarabine compared with chlorambucil as primary therapy for chronic lymphocytic leukemia. New Engl J Med. 2000;343(24):1750–7.
10. Raphael B, Andersen JW, Silber R, Oken M, Moore D, Bennett J, et al. Comparison of chlorambucil and prednisone versus cyclophosphamide, vincristine, and prednisone as initial treatment for chronic lymphocytic leukemia: long-term follow-up of

an Eastern Cooperative Oncology Group randomized clinical trial. J Clin Oncol. 1991;9(5):770–6.

11. Jayaweera JL, Withana MR, Dalpatadu CK, Beligaswatta CD, Rajapakse T, Jayasinghe S, et al. Cyclophosphamide-induced posterior reversible encephalopathy syndrome (PRES): a case report. J Med Case Rep. 2014;8:442.

12. Meanwell CA, Blake AE, Kelly KA, Honigsberger L, Blackledge G. Prediction of ifosfamide/mesna associated encephalopathy. Eur J Cancer Clin Oncol. 1986;22(7):815–9.

13. David KA, Picus J. Evaluating risk factors for the development of ifosfamide encephalopathy. Am J Clin Oncol. 2005;28(3):277–80.

14. Rieger C, Fiegl M, Tischer J, Ostermann H, Schiel X. Incidence and severity of ifosfamide-induced encephalopathy. Anticancer Drugs. 2004;15(4):347–50.

15. Lorigan P, Verweij J, Papai Z, Rodenhuis S, Le Cesne A, Leahy MG, et al. Phase III trial of two investigational schedules of ifosfamide compared with standard-dose doxorubicin in advanced or metastatic soft tissue sarcoma: a European Organisation for Research and Treatment of Cancer Soft Tissue and Bone Sarcoma Group Study. J Clin Oncol. 2007;25(21):3144–50.

16. Durand JP, Gourmel B, Mir O, Goldwasser F. Antiemetic neurokinin-1 antagonist aprepitant and ifosfamide-induced encephalopathy. Ann Oncol. 2007;18(4):808–9.

17. Howell JE, Szabatura AH, Hatfield Seung A, Nesbit SA. Characterization of the occurrence of ifosfamide-induced neurotoxicity with concomitant aprepitant. J Oncol Pharm Pract. 2008;14(3):157–62.

18. Hansen H, Yuen C. Aprepitant-associated ifosfamide neurotoxicity. J Oncol Pharm Pract. 2010;16(2):137–8.

19. Jarkowski A 3rd. Possible contribution of aprepitant to ifosfamide-induced neurotoxicity. Am J Health Syst Pharm Ajhp. 2008;65(23):2229–31.

20. Chastagner P, Sommelet-Olive D, Kalifa C, Brunat-Mentigny M, Zucker JM, Demeocq F, et al. Phase II study of ifosfamide in childhood brain tumors: a report by the French Society of Pediatric Oncology (SFOP). Med Pediatr Oncol. 1993;21(1):49–53.

21. Ghosn M, Carde P, Leclerq B, Flamant F, Friedman S, Droz JP, et al. Ifosfamide/mesna related encephalopathy: a case report with a possible role of phenobarbital in enhancing neurotoxicity. Bull Cancer. 1988;75(4):391–2.

22. Watkin SW, Husband DJ, Green JA, Warenius HM. Ifosfamide encephalopathy: a reappraisal. Eur J Cancer Clin Oncol. 1989;25(9):1303–10.

23. Kupfer A, Aeschlimann C, Wermuth B, Cerny T. Prophylaxis and reversal of ifosfamide encephalopathy with methylene-blue. Lancet. 1994;343(8900):763–4.

24. Pelgrims J, De Vos F, Van den Brande J, Schrijvers D, Prove A, Vermorken JB. Methylene blue in the treatment and prevention of ifosfamide-induced encephalopathy: report of 12 cases and a review of the literature. Br J Cancer. 2000;82(2):291–4.

25. Buesa JM, Garcia-Teijido P, Losa R, Fra J. Treatment of ifosfamide encephalopathy with intravenous thiamin. Clin Cancer Res. 2003;9(12):4636–7.

26. Bernard PA, McCabe T, Bayliff S, Hayes D Jr. Successful treatment of ifosfamide neurotoxicity with dexmedetomidine. J Oncol Pharm Pract. 2010;16(4):262–5.

27. Verdeguer A, Castel V, Esquembre C, Ferris J, Fernandez JM, Ruiz JG. Fatal encephalopathy with ifosfamide/mesna. Pediatr Hematol Oncol. 1989;6(4):383–5.

28. Shuper A, Stein J, Goshen J, Kornreich L, Yaniv I, Cohen IJ. Subacute central nervous system degeneration in a child: an unusual manifestation of ifosfamide intoxication. J Child Neurol. 2000;15(7):481–3.

29. Primavera A, Audenino D, Cocito L. Ifosfamide encephalopathy and nonconvulsive status epilepticus. Can J Neurol Sci. 2002;29(2):180–3.

30. Taupin D, Racela R, Friedman D. Ifosfamide chemotherapy and nonconvulsive status epilepticus: case report and review of the literature. Clin EEG Neurosci. 2014;45(3):222–5.

31. Patel SR, Forman AD, Benjamin RS. High-dose ifosfamide-induced exacerbation of peripheral neuropathy. J Natl Cancer Inst. 1994;86(4):305–6.

32. Anderson NR, Tandon DS. Ifosfamide extrapyramidal neurotoxicity. Cancer. 1991;68(1):72–5.

33. Ames B, Lewis LD, Chaffee S, Kim J, Morse R. Ifosfamide-induced encephalopathy and movement disorder. Pediatr Blood Cancer. 2010;54(4):624–6.

34. Dubey D, Freeman M, Neeley OJ, Carter G. Encephalopathy following melphalan administration. J Chemother. 2017;29(1):45–8.

35. Alayon-Laguer D, Alsina M, Ochoa-Bayona JL, Ayala E. Melphalan culprit or confounder in acute encephalopathy during autologous hematopoietic stem cell transplantation? Case Rep Transplant. 2012;2012:942795.

36. Schuh A, Dandridge J, Haydon P, Littlewood TJ. Encephalopathy complicating high-dose melphalan. Bone Marrow Transplant. 1999;24(10):1141–3.

37. Knauf WU, Lissichkov T, Aldaoud A, Liberati A, Loscertales J, Herbrecht R, et al. Phase III randomized study of bendamustine compared with chlorambucil in previously untreated patients with chronic lymphocytic leukemia. J Clin Oncol. 2009;27(26):4378–84.

38. Moskowitz AJ, Hamlin PA Jr, Perales MA, Gerecitano J, Horwitz SM, Matasar MJ, et al. Phase II study of bendamustine in relapsed and refractory Hodgkin lymphoma. J Clin Oncol. 2013;31(4):456–60.

39. Petrylak DP, Tangen CM, Hussain MH, Lara PN Jr, Jones JA, Taplin ME, et al. Docetaxel and estramustine compared with mitoxantrone and prednisone for advanced refractory prostate cancer. N Engl J Med. 2004;351(15):1513–20.

40. Lubiniecki GM, Berlin JA, Weinstein RB, Vaughn DJ. Thromboembolic events with estramustine phosphate-based chemotherapy in patients with hormone-refractory prostate carcinoma: results of a meta-analysis. Cancer. 2004;101(12):2755–9.

41. Halevy D, Radhakrishnan J, Markowitz G, Appel G. Thrombotic microangiopathies. Crit Care Clin. 2002;18(2):309–20, vi.

42. Shingleton BJ, Bienfang DC, Albert DM, Ensminger WD, Chandler WF, Greenberg HS. Ocular toxicity associated with high-dose carmustine. Arch Ophthalmol. 1982;100(11):1766–72.

43. Rosenblum MK, Delattre JY, Walker RW, Shapiro WR. Fatal necrotizing encephalopathy complicating treatment of malignant gliomas with intra-arterial BCNU and irradiation: a pathological study. J Neurooncol. 1989;7(3):269–81.

44. Raza SM, Pradilla G, Legnani FG, Thai QA, Olivi A, Weingart JD, et al. Local delivery of antineoplastic agents by controlled-release polymers for the treatment of malignant brain tumours. Expert Opin Biol Ther. 2005;5(4):477–94.

45. Caselli D, Rosati A, Faraci M, Podda M, Ripaldi M, Longoni D, et al. Risk of seizures in children receiving busulphan-containing regimens for stem cell transplantation. Biol Blood Marrow Transplant J Am Soc Blood Marrow Transplant. 2014;20(2):282–5.

46. Diaz-Carrasco MS, Olmos R, Blanquer M, Velasco J, Sanchez-Salinas A, Moraleda JM. Clonazepam for seizure prophylaxis in adult patients treated with high dose busulfan. Int J Clin Pharm. 2013;35(3):339–43.

47. Soni S, Skeens M, Termuhlen AM, Bajwa RP, Gross TG, Pai V. Levetiracetam for busulfan-induced seizure prophylaxis in children undergoing hematopoietic stem cell transplantation. Pediatr Blood Cancer. 2012;59(4):762–4.

48. Chan KW, Mullen CA, Worth LL, Choroszy M, Koontz S, Tran H, et al. Lorazepam for seizure prophylaxis during

high-dose busulfan administration. Bone Marrow Transplant. 2002;29(12):963–5.

49. Anderson JE, Appelbaum FR, Schoch G, Gooley T, Anasetti C, Bensinger WI, et al. Allogeneic marrow transplantation for myelodysplastic syndrome with advanced disease morphology: a phase II study of busulfan, cyclophosphamide, and total-body irradiation and analysis of prognostic factors. J Clin Oncol. 1996;14(1):220–6.

50. Paterson AH, McPherson TA. A possible neurologic complication of DTIC. Cancer Treat Rep. 1977;61(1):105–6.

51. Yung WK, Albright RE, Olson J, Fredericks R, Fink K, Prados MD, et al. A phase II study of temozolomide versus procarbazine in patients with glioblastoma multiforme at first relapse. Br J Cancer. 2000;83(5):588–93.

52. Rosenthal MA, Ashley DL, Cher L. Temozolomide-induced flare in high-grade gliomas: a new clinical entity. Intern Med J. 2002;32(7):346–8.

53. Fink J, Born D, Chamberlain MC. Pseudoprogression: relevance with respect to treatment of high-grade gliomas. Curr Treat Options Oncol. 2011;12(3):240–52.

54. Maanen MJ, Smeets CJ, Beijnen JH. Chemistry, pharmacology and pharmacokinetics of N, N', N''-triethylenethiophosphoramide (ThioTEPA). Cancer Treat Rev. 2000;26(4):257–68.

55. Gutin PH, Levi JA, Wiernik PH, Walker MD. Treatment of malignant meningeal disease with intrathecal thioTEPA: a phase II study. Cancer Treat Rep. 1977;61(5):885–7.

56. Gutin PH, Weiss HD, Wiernik PH, Walker MD. Intrathecal N, N', N''-triethylenethiophosphoramide [thio-TEPA (NSC 6396)] in the treatment of malignant meningeal disease: phase I-II study. Cancer. 1976;38(4):1471–5.

57. Comte A, Jdid W, Guilhaume MN, Kriegel I, Piperno-Neumann S, Dieras V, et al. Survival of breast cancer patients with meningeal carcinomatosis treated by intrathecal thiotepa. J Neurooncol. 2013;115(3):445–52.

58. Valteau-Couanet D, Fillipini B, Benhamou E, Grill J, Kalifa C, Couanet D, et al. High-dose busulfan and thiotepa followed by autologous stem cell transplantation (ASCT) in previously irradiated medulloblastoma patients: high toxicity and lack of efficacy. Bone Marrow Transplant. 2005;36(11):939–45.

59. Kokolo MB, Fergusson D, O'Neill J, Tay J, Tinmouth AT, Stewart D, et al. Effectiveness and safety of thiotepa as conditioning treatment prior to stem cell transplant in patients with central nervous system lymphoma. Leuk Lymphoma. 2014;55(12):2712–20.

60. Manetta A, Tewari K, Podczaski ES. Hexamethylmelamine as a single second-line agent in ovarian cancer: follow-up report and review of the literature. Gynecol Oncol. 1997;66(1):20–6.

61. Markman M, Blessing JA, Moore D, Ball H, Lentz SS. Altretamine (hexamethylmelamine) in platinum-resistant and platinum-refractory ovarian cancer: a Gynecologic Oncology Group phase II trial. Gynecol Oncol. 1998;69(3):226–9.

62. Alberts DS, Jiang C, Liu PY, Wilczynski S, Markman M, Rothenberg ML. Long-term follow-up of a phase II trial of oral altretamine for consolidation of clinical complete remission in women with stage III epithelial ovarian cancer in the Southwest Oncology Group. Int J Gynecol Cancer. 2004;14(2):224–8.

63. Argyriou AA, Bruna J, Marmiroli P, Cavaletti G. Chemotherapy-induced peripheral neurotoxicity (CIPN): an update. Crit Rev Oncol/Hematol. 2012;82(1):51–77.

64. Roelofs RI, Hrushesky W, Rogin J, Rosenberg L. Peripheral sensory neuropathy and cisplatin chemotherapy. Neurology. 1984;34(7):934–8.

65. Glendenning JL, Barbachano Y, Norman AR, Dearnaley DP, Horwich A, Huddart RA. Long-term neurologic and peripheral vascular toxicity after chemotherapy treatment of testicular cancer. Cancer. 2010;116(10):2322–31.

66. Hilkens PH, van der Burg ME, Moll JW, Planting AS, van Putten WL, Vecht CJ, et al. Neurotoxicity is not enhanced by increased dose intensities of cisplatin administration. Eur J Cancer. 1995;31A(5):678–81.

67. van der Hoop RG, Vecht CJ, van der Burg ME, Elderson A, Boogerd W, Heimans JJ, et al. Prevention of cisplatin neurotoxicity with an ACTH(4–9) analogue in patients with ovarian cancer. New Engl J Med. 1990;322(2):89–94.

68. van der Hoop RG, van der Burg ME, ten Bokkel Huinink WW, van Houwelingen C, Neijt JP. Incidence of neuropathy in 395 patients with ovarian cancer treated with or without cisplatin. Cancer. 1990;66(8):1697–702.

69. Khrunin AV, Moisseev A, Gorbunova V, Limborska S. Genetic polymorphisms and the efficacy and toxicity of cisplatin-based chemotherapy in ovarian cancer patients. Pharmacogenomics J. 2010;10(1):54–61.

70. Oldenburg J, Kraggerud SM, Brydoy M, Cvancarova M, Lothe RA, Fossa SD. Association between long-term neuro-toxicities in testicular cancer survivors and polymorphisms in glutathione-s-transferase-P1 and -M1, a retrospective cross sectional study. J Transl Med. 2007;5:70.

71. Siegal T, Haim N. Cisplatin-induced peripheral neuropathy. Frequent off-therapy deterioration, demyelinating syndromes, and muscle cramps. Cancer. 1990;66(6):1117–23.

72. von Schlippe M, Fowler CJ, Harland SJ. Cisplatin neurotoxicity in the treatment of metastatic germ cell tumour: time course and prognosis. Br J Cancer. 2001;85(6):823–6.

73. Krarup-Hansen A, Helweg-Larsen S, Schmalbruch H, Rorth M, Krarup C. Neuronal involvement in cisplatin neuropathy: prospective clinical and neurophysiological studies. Brain J Neurol. 2007;130(Pt 4):1076–88.

74. Gill JS, Windebank AJ. Cisplatin-induced apoptosis in rat dorsal root ganglion neurons is associated with attempted entry into the cell cycle. J Clin Investig. 1998;101(12):2842–50.

75. Zhang H, Mizumachi T, Carcel-Trullols J, Li L, Naito A, Spencer HJ, et al. Targeting human 8-oxoguanine DNA glycosylase (hOGG1) to mitochondria enhances cisplatin cytotoxicity in hepatoma cells. Carcinogenesis. 2007;28(8):1629–37.

76. McDonald ES, Windebank AJ. Cisplatin-induced apoptosis of DRG neurons involves bax redistribution and cytochrome c release but not fas receptor signaling. Neurobiol Dis. 2002;9(2):220–33.

77. Scuteri A, Galimberti A, Maggioni D, Ravasi M, Pasini S, Nicolini G, et al. Role of MAPKs in platinum-induced neuronal apoptosis. Neurotoxicology. 2009;30(2):312–9.

78. Daugaard GK, Petrera J, Trojaborg W. Electrophysiological study of the peripheral and central neurotoxic effect of cis-platin. Acta Neurol Scand. 1987;76(2):86–93.

79. Rademaker-Lakhai JM, Crul M, Zuur L, Baas P, Beijnen JH, Simis YJ, et al. Relationship between cisplatin administration and the development of ototoxicity. J Clin Oncol. 2006;24(6):918–24.

80. Nieves L, Currie J, Hoffman J, Sorosky JI. Ototoxicity after intraperitoneal chemotherapy: a case report. Int J Gynecol Cancer. 2007;17(5):1133–5.

81. Brock PR, Knight KR, Freyer DR, Campbell KC, Steyger PS, Blakley BW, et al. Platinum-induced ototoxicity in children: a consensus review on mechanisms, predisposition, and protection, including a new International Society of Pediatric Oncology Boston ototoxicity scale. J Clin Oncol. 2012;30(19):2408–17.

82. Hellberg V, Wallin I, Eriksson S, Hernlund E, Jerremalm E, Berndtsson M, et al. Cisplatin and oxaliplatin toxicity: importance of cochlear kinetics as a determinant for ototoxicity. J Natl Cancer Inst. 2009;101(1):37–47.

83. Markman M. Toxicities of the platinum antineoplastic agents. Expert Opin Drug Saf. 2003;2(6):597–607.

84. Ito Y, Arahata Y, Goto Y, Hirayama M, Nagamutsu M, Yasuda T, et al. Cisplatin neurotoxicity presenting as reversible posterior leukoencephalopathy syndrome. AJNR Am J Neuroradiol. 1998;19(3):415–7.

85. Lyass O, Lossos A, Hubert A, Gips M, Peretz T. Cisplatin-induced non-convulsive encephalopathy. Anticancer Drugs. 1998;9(1):100–4.

86. Lajer H, Daugaard G. Cisplatin and hypomagnesemia. Cancer Treat Rev. 1999;25(1):47–58.

87. Berghmans T. Hyponatremia related to medical anticancer treatment. Support Care Cancer. 1996;4(5):341–50.

88. Walker RW, Cairncross JG, Posner JB. Cerebral herniation in patients receiving cisplatin. J Neurooncol. 1988;6(1):61–5.

89. Walsh TJ, Clark AW, Parhad IM, Green WR. Neurotoxic effects of cisplatin therapy. Arch Neurol. 1982;39(11):719–20.

90. List AF, Kummet TD. Spinal cord toxicity complicating treatment with cisplatin and etoposide. Am J Clin Oncol. 1990;13 (3):256–8.

91. Walther PJ, Rossitch E Jr, Bullard DE. The development of Lhermitte's sign during cisplatin chemotherapy. Possible drug-induced toxicity causing spinal cord demyelination. Cancer. 1987;60(9):2170–2.

92. Newton HB, Page MA, Junck L, Greenberg HS. Intra-arterial cisplatin for the treatment of malignant gliomas. J Neurooncol. 1989;7(1):39–45.

93. Heinzlef O, Lotz JP, Roullet E. Severe neuropathy after high dose carboplatin in three patients receiving multidrug chemotherapy. J Neurol Neurosurg Psychiatry. 1998;64(5):667–9.

94. Vieillot S, Pouessel D, de Champfleur NM, Becht C, Culine S. Reversible posterior leukoencephalopathy syndrome after carboplatin therapy. Ann Oncol. 2007;18(3):608–9.

95. Stewart DJ, Belanger JM, Grahovac Z, Curuvija S, Gionet LR, Aitken SE, et al. Phase I study of intracarotid administration of carboplatin. Neurosurgery. 1992;30(4):512–6; discussion 6–7.

96. Walker RW, Rosenblum MK, Kempin SJ, Christian MC. Carboplatin-associated thrombotic microangiopathic hemolytic anemia. Cancer. 1989;64(5):1017–20.

97. O'Brien ME, Tonge K, Blake P, Moskovic E, Wiltshaw E. Blindness associated with high-dose carboplatin. Lancet. 1992;339(8792):558.

98. Alberts DS. Clinical pharmacology of carboplatin. Semin Oncol. 1990;17(4 Suppl 7):6–8.

99. Argyriou AA, Cavaletti G, Briani C, Velasco R, Bruna J, Campagnolo M, et al. Clinical pattern and associations of oxaliplatin acute neurotoxicity: a prospective study in 170 patients with colorectal cancer. Cancer. 2013;119(2):438–44.

100. Gamelin E, Gamelin L, Bossi L, Quasthoff S. Clinical aspects and molecular basis of oxaliplatin neurotoxicity: current management and development of preventive measures. Semin Oncol. 2002;29 (5 Suppl 15):21–33.

101. Petrioli R, Pascucci A, Francini E, Marsili S, Sciandivasci A, Tassi R, et al. Neurotoxicity of FOLFOX-4 as adjuvant treatment for patients with colon and gastric cancer: a randomized study of two different schedules of oxaliplatin. Cancer Chemother Pharmacol. 2008;61(1):105–11.

102. Pachman DR QR, Seisler DK, et al. Clinical course of patients with oxaliplatin-associated neuropathy: N08CB(Alliance) (abstract). J Clin Oncol. 2014;32(suppl; abstr 3595). http://meetinglibrary.asco.org/content/131813-144. Accessed 27 April 2015.

103. Park SB, Lin CS, Krishnan AV, Goldstein D, Friedlander ML, Kiernan MC. Oxaliplatin-induced neurotoxicity: changes in axonal excitability precede development of neuropathy. Brain J Neurol. 2009;132(Pt 10):2712–23.

104. Grolleau F, Gamelin L, Boisdron-Celle M, Lapied B, Pelhate M, Gamelin E. A possible explanation for a neurotoxic effect of the anticancer agent oxaliplatin on neuronal voltage-gated sodium channels. J Neurophysiol. 2001;85(5):2293–7.

105. Park SB, Lin CS, Krishnan AV, Goldstein D, Friedlander ML, Kiernan MC. Dose effects of oxaliplatin on persistent and transient Na^+ conductances and the development of neurotoxicity. PLoS ONE. 2011;6(4):e18469.

106. Grothey A, Nikcevich DA, Sloan JA, Kugler JW, Silberstein PT, Dentchev T, et al. Intravenous calcium and magnesium for oxaliplatin-induced sensory neurotoxicity in adjuvant colon cancer: NCCTG N04C7. J Clin Oncol. 2011;29(4):421–7.

107. Gamelin L, Boisdron-Celle M, Delva R, Guerin-Meyer V, Ifrah N, Morel A, et al. Prevention of oxaliplatin-related neurotoxicity by calcium and magnesium infusions: a retrospective study of 161 patients receiving oxaliplatin combined with 5-Fluorouracil and leucovorin for advanced colorectal cancer. Clin Cancer Res. 2004;10(12 Pt 1):4055–61.

108. Hochster HS, Grothey A, Childs BH. Use of calcium and magnesium salts to reduce oxaliplatin-related neurotoxicity. J Clin Oncol. 2007;25(25):4028–9.

109. Loprinzi CL, Qin R, Dakhil SR, Fehrenbacher L, Flynn KA, Atherton P, et al. Phase III randomized, placebo-controlled, double-blind study of intravenous calcium and magnesium to prevent oxaliplatin-induced sensory neurotoxicity (N08CB/Alliance). J Clin Oncol. 2014;32(10):997–1005.

110. Grothey A, Hedrick EE, Mass RD, Sarkar S, Suzuki S, Ramanathan RK, et al. Response-independent survival benefit in metastatic colorectal cancer: a comparative analysis of N9741 and AVF2107. J Clin Oncol. 2008;26(2):183–9.

111. Ta LE, Espeset L, Podratz J, Windebank AJ. Neurotoxicity of oxaliplatin and cisplatin for dorsal root ganglion neurons correlates with platinum-DNA binding. Neurotoxicology. 2006;27(6):992–1002.

112. Taieb S, Trillet-Lenoir V, Rambaud L, Descos L, Freyer G. Lhermitte sign and urinary retention: atypical presentation of oxaliplatin neurotoxicity in four patients. Cancer. 2002;94 (9):2434–40.

113. Park SB, Lin CS, Krishnan AV, Goldstein D, Friedlander ML, Kiernan MC. Oxaliplatin-induced lhermitte's phenomenon as a manifestation of severe generalized neurotoxicity. Oncology. 2009;77(6):342–8.

114. Pinedo DM, Shah-Khan F, Shah PC. Reversible posterior leukoencephalopathy syndrome associated with oxaliplatin. J Clin Oncol. 2007;25(33):5320–1.

115. Moris G, Ribacoba R, Gonzalez C. Delayed posterior encephalopathy syndrome following chemotherapy with oxaliplatin and gemcitabine. J Neurol. 2007;254(4):534–5.

116. Skelton MR, Goldberg RM, O'Neil BH. A case of oxaliplatin-related posterior reversible encephalopathy syndrome. Clin Colorectal Cancer. 2007;6(5):386–8.

117. Weiss HD, Walker MD, Wiernik PH. Neurotoxicity of commonly used antineoplastic agents (second of two parts). New Engl J Med. 1974;291(3):127–33.

118. Postma TJ, van Groeningen CJ, Witjes RJ, Weerts JG, Kralendonk JH, Heimans JJ. Neurotoxicity of combination chemotherapy with procarbazine, CCNU and vincristine (PCV) for recurrent glioma. J Neurooncol. 1998;38(1):69–75.

119. Riehl JL, Brown WJ. Acute cerebellar syndrome secondary to 5-fluorouracil therapy. Neurology. 1964;14:961–7.

120. Gottlieb JA, Luce JK. Cerebellar ataxia with weekly 5-fluorouracil administration. Lancet. 1971;1(7690):138–9.

121. Liaw CC, Liaw SJ, Wang CH, Chiu MC, Huang JS. Transient hyperammonemia related to chemotherapy with continuous infusion of high-dose 5-fluorouracil. Anticancer Drugs. 1993;4 (3):311–5.

122. Liaw CC, Wang HM, Wang CH, Yang TS, Chen JS, Chang HK, et al. Risk of transient hyperammonemic encephalopathy in cancer patients who received continuous infusion of 5-fluorouracil with the complication of dehydration and infection. Anticancer Drugs. 1999;10(3):275–81.

123. Nott L, Price TJ, Pittman K, Patterson K, Fletcher J. Hyperammonemia encephalopathy: an important cause of neurological deterioration following chemotherapy. Leuk Lymphoma. 2007;48(9):1702–11.

124. Kikuta S, Asakage T, Nakao K, Sugasawa M, Kubota A. The aggravating factors of hyperammonemia related to 5-fluorouracil infusion–a report of two cases. Auris Nasus Larynx. 2008;35 (2):295–9.

125. Pirzada NA, Ali II, Dafer RM. Fluorouracil-induced neurotoxicity. Ann Pharmacother. 2000;34(1):35–8.

126. Stein ME, Drumea K, Yarnitsky D, Benny A, Tzuk-Shina T. A rare event of 5-fluorouracil-associated peripheral neuropathy: a report of two patients. Am J Clin Oncol. 1998;21(3):248–9.

127. Bergevin PR, Patwardhan VC, Weissman J, Lee SM. Letter: neurotoxicity of 5-fluorouracil. Lancet. 1975;1(7903):410.

128. El Amrani M, Heinzlef O, Debroucker T, Roullet E, Bousser MG, Amarenco P. Brain infarction following 5-fluorouracil and cisplatin therapy. Neurology. 1998;51(3):899–901.

129. Brashear A, Siemers E. Focal dystonia after chemotherapy: a case series. J Neurooncol. 1997;34(2):163–7.

130. Bixenman WW, Nicholls JV, Warwick OH. Oculomotor disturbances associated with 5-fluorouracil chemotherapy. Am J Ophthalmol. 1977;83(6):789–93.

131. Delval L, Klastersky J. Optic neuropathy in cancer patients. Report of a case possibly related to 5 fluorouracil toxicity and review of the literature. J Neurooncol. 2002;60(2):165–9.

132. Morel A, Boisdron-Celle M, Fey L, Soulie P, Craipeau MC, Traore S, et al. Clinical relevance of different dihydropyrimidine dehydrogenase gene single nucleotide polymorphisms on 5-fluorouracil tolerance. Mol Cancer Ther. 2006;5(11):2895–904.

133. van Kuilenburg AB. Dihydropyrimidine dehydrogenase and the efficacy and toxicity of 5-fluorouracil. Eur J Cancer. 2004;40 (7):939–50.

134. Takimoto CH, Lu ZH, Zhang R, Liang MD, Larson LV, Cantilena LR Jr, et al. Severe neurotoxicity following 5-fluorouracil-based chemotherapy in a patient with dihydropyrimidine dehydrogenase deficiency. Clin Cancer Res. 1996;2 (3):477–81.

135. Choi SM, Lee SH, Yang YS, Kim BC, Kim MK, Cho KH. 5-fluorouracil-induced leukoencephalopathy in patients with breast cancer. J Korean Med Sci. 2001;16(3):328–34.

136. Aksoy M, Basu TK, Brient J, Dickerson JW. Thiamin status of patients treated with drug combinations containing 5-fluorouracil. Eur J Cancer. 1980;16(8):1041–5.

137. Bachelot T, Romieu G, Campone M, Dieras V, Cropet C, Dalenc F, et al. Lapatinib plus capecitabine in patients with previously untreated brain metastases from HER2-positive metastatic breast cancer (LANDSCAPE): a single-group phase 2 study. Lancet Oncol. 2013;14(1):64–71.

138. Cassidy J, Clarke S, Diaz-Rubio E, Scheithauer W, Figer A, Wong R, et al. Randomized phase III study of capecitabine plus oxaliplatin compared with fluorouracil/folinic acid plus oxaliplatin as first-line therapy for metastatic colorectal cancer. J Clin Oncol. 2008;26(12):2006–12.

139. Geyer CE, Forster J, Lindquist D, Chan S, Romieu CG, Pienkowski T, et al. Lapatinib plus capecitabine for HER2-positive advanced breast cancer. New Engl J Med. 2006;355(26):2733–43.

140. Formica V, Leary A, Cunningham D, Chua YJ. 5-Fluorouracil can cross brain-blood barrier and cause encephalopathy: should we expect the same from capecitabine? A case report on capecitabine-induced central neurotoxicity progressing to coma. Cancer Chemother Pharmacol. 2006;58(2):276–8.

141. Videnovic A, Semenov I, Chua-Adajar R, Baddi L, Blumenthal DT, Beck AC, et al. Capecitabine-induced multifocal leukoencephalopathy: a report of five cases. Neurology. 2005;65(11):1792–4; discussion 685.

142. Niemann B, Rochlitz C, Herrmann R, Pless M. Toxic encephalopathy induced by capecitabine. Oncology. 2004;66 (4):331–5.

143. Renouf D, Gill S. Capecitabine-induced cerebellar toxicity. Clin Colorectal Cancer. 2006;6(1):70–1.

144. Rehr EL, Swanson KA, Kern JA. Mercaptopurine-induced fever in a patient with Crohn's disease. Ann Pharmacother. 1992;26(7–8):907–9.

145. Herzig RH, Hines JD, Herzig GP, Wolff SN, Cassileth PA, Lazarus HM, et al. Cerebellar toxicity with high-dose cytosine arabinoside. J Clin Oncol. 1987;5(6):927–32.

146. Hwang TL, Yung WK, Estey EH, Fields WS. Central nervous system toxicity with high-dose Ara-C. Neurology. 1985;35 (10):1475–9.

147. Winkelman MD, Hines JD. Cerebellar degeneration caused by high-dose cytosine arabinoside: a clinicopathological study. Ann Neurol. 1983;14(5):520–7.

148. Smith GA, Damon LE, Rugo HS, Ries CA, Linker CA. High-dose cytarabine dose modification reduces the incidence of neurotoxicity in patients with renal insufficiency. J Clin Oncol. 1997;15(2):833–9.

149. Eden OB, Goldie W, Wood T, Etcubanas E. Seizures following intrathecal cytosine arabinoside in young children with acute lymphoblastic leukemia. Cancer. 1978;42(1):53–8.

150. Saito B, Nakamaki T, Nakashima H, Usui T, Hattori N, Kawakami K, et al. Reversible posterior leukoencephalopathy syndrome after repeat intermediate-dose cytarabine chemotherapy in a patient with acute myeloid leukemia. Am J Hematol. 2007;82(4):304–6.

151. Luque FA, Selhorst JB, Petruska P. Parkinsonism induced by high-dose cytosine arabinoside. Mov Disord. 1987;2(3):219–22.

152. Nevill TJ, Benstead TJ, McCormick CW, Hayne OA. Horner's syndrome and demyelinating peripheral neuropathy caused by high-dose cytosine arabinoside. Am J Hematol. 1989;32(4):314–5.

153. Hoffman DL, Howard JR Jr, Sarma R, Riggs JE. Encephalopathy, myelopathy, optic neuropathy, and anosmia associated with intravenous cytosine arabinoside. Clin Neuropharmacol. 1993;16 (3):258–62.

154. Russell JA, Powles RL. Letter: neuropathy due to cytosine arabinoside. BMJ. 1974;4(5945):652–3.

155. Borgeat A, De Muralt B, Stalder M. Peripheral neuropathy associated with high-dose Ara-C therapy. Cancer. 1986;58 (4):852–4.

156. Saito T, Asai O, Dobashi N, Yano S, Osawa H, Takei Y, et al. Peripheral neuropathy caused by high-dose cytosine arabinoside treatment in a patient with acute myeloid leukemia. J Infect Chemother. 2006;12(3):148–51.

157. Powell BL, Capizzi RL, Lyerly ES, Cooper MR. Peripheral neuropathy after high-dose cytosine arabinoside, daunorubicin, and asparaginase consolidation for acute nonlymphocytic leukemia. J Clin Oncol. 1986;4(1):95–7.

158. Osborne WL, Holyoake TL, McQuaker IG, Parker AN. Fatal peripheral neuropathy following FLA chemotherapy. Clin Lab Haematol. 2004;26(4):295–6.

159. Openshaw H, Slatkin NE, Stein AS, Hinton DR, Forman SJ. Acute polyneuropathy after high dose cytosine arabinoside in patients with leukemia. Cancer. 1996;78(9):1899–905.

160. Paul M, Joshua D, Rahme N, Pollard J, Ell J, Gibson J, et al. Fatal peripheral neuropathy associated with axonal degeneration after high-dose cytosine arabinoside in acute leukaemia. Br J Haematol. 1991;79(3):521–3.

161. Baker WJ, Royer GL Jr, Weiss RB. Cytarabine and neurologic toxicity. J Clin Oncol. 1991;9(4):679–93.

162. Dunton SF, Nitschke R, Spruce WE, Bodensteiner J, Krous HF. Progressive ascending paralysis following administration of intrathecal and intravenous cytosine arabinoside. A Pediatric Oncology Group study. Cancer. 1986;57(6):1083–8.

163. Resar LM, Phillips PC, Kastan MB, Leventhal BG, Bowman PW, Civin CI. Acute neurotoxicity after intrathecal cytosine arabinoside in two adolescents with acute lymphoblastic leukemia of B-cell type. Cancer. 1993;71(1):117–23.

164. Jabbour E, O'Brien S, Kantarjian H, Garcia-Manero G, Ferrajoli A, Ravandi F, et al. Neurologic complications associated with intrathecal liposomal cytarabine given prophylactically in combination with high-dose methotrexate and cytarabine to patients with acute lymphocytic leukemia. Blood. 2007;109(8):3214–8.

165. Kleinschmidt-DeMasters BK, Yeh M. "Locked-in syndrome" after intrathecal cytosine arabinoside therapy for malignant immunoblastic lymphoma. Cancer. 1992;70(10):2504–7.

166. Chun HG, Leyland-Jones BR, Caryk SM, Hoth DF. Central nervous system toxicity of fludarabine phosphate. Cancer Treat Rep. 1986;70(10):1225–8.

167. Cheson BD, Vena DA, Foss FM, Sorensen JM. Neurotoxicity of purine analogs: a review. J Clin Oncol. 1994;12(10):2216–28.

168. Von Hoff DD. Phase I clinical trials with fludarabine phosphate. Semin Oncol. 1990;17(5 Suppl 8):33–8.

169. Spriggs DR, Stopa E, Mayer RJ, Schoene W, Kufe DW. Fludarabine phosphate (NSC 312878) infusions for the treatment of acute leukemia: phase I and neuropathological study. Can Res. 1986;46(11):5953–8.

170. Warrell RP Jr, Berman E. Phase I and II study of fludarabine phosphate in leukemia: therapeutic efficacy with delayed central nervous system toxicity. J Clin Oncol. 1986;4(1):74–9.

171. Ding X, Herzlich AA, Bishop R, Tuo J, Chan CC. Ocular toxicity of fludarabine: a purine analog. Expert Rev Ophthalmol. 2008;3(1):97–109.

172. Lee MS, McKinney AM, Brace JR, Santacruz K. Clinical and imaging features of fludarabine neurotoxicity. J Neuro-Ophthalmol. 2010;30(1):37–41.

173. Gonzalez H, Bolgert F, Camporo P, Leblond V. Progressive multifocal leukoencephalitis (PML) in three patients treated with standard-dose fludarabine (FAMP). Hematol Cell Ther. 1999;41(4):183–6.

174. Smolle E, Trojan A, Schuster SJ, Haybaeck J. Progressive multifocal leukoencephalopathy–a case report and review of the literature. In vivo. 2014;28(5):941–8.

175. Lejniece S, Murovska M, Chapenko S, Breiksa B, Jaunmuktane Z, Feldmane L, et al. Progressive multifocal leukoencephalopathy following fludarabine treatment in a chronic lymphocytic leukemia patient. Exp Oncol. 2011;33(4):239–41.

176. Bonavita S, Conforti R, Russo A, Sacco R, Tessitore A, Gallo A, et al. Infratentorial progressive multifocal leukoencephalopathy in a patient treated with fludarabine and rituximab. Neurol Sci. 2008;29(1):37–9.

177. Kiewe P, Seyfert S, Korper S, Rieger K, Thiel E, Knauf W. Progressive multifocal leukoencephalopathy with detection of JC virus in a patient with chronic lymphocytic leukemia parallel to onset of fludarabine therapy. Leuk Lymphoma. 2003;44(10):1815–8.

178. Saumoy M, Castells G, Escoda L, Mares R, Richart C, Ugarriza A. Progressive multifocal leukoencephalopathy in chronic lymphocytic leukemia after treatment with fludarabine. Leuk Lymphoma. 2002;43(2):433–6.

179. Vidarsson B, Mosher DF, Salamat MS, Isaksson HJ, Onundarson PT. Progressive multifocal leukoencephalopathy after fludarabine therapy for low-grade lymphoproliferative disease. Am J Hematol. 2002;70(1):51–4.

180. Cid J, Revilla M, Cervera A, Cervantes F, Munoz E, Ferrer I, et al. Progressive multifocal leukoencephalopathy following oral fludarabine treatment of chronic lymphocytic leukemia. Ann Hematol. 2000;79(7):392–5.

181. Truong QV, Abraham J, Nagaiah G, Newton M, Veltri L. Gemcitabine associated with posterior reversible encephalopathy syndrome (PRES): a case report and review of the literature. Clin Adv Hematol Oncol H&O. 2012;10(9):611–3.

182. Marrone LC, Marrone BF, de la Puerta Raya J, Gadonski G, da Costa JC. Gemcitabine monotherapy associated with posterior reversible encephalopathy syndrome. Case Rep Oncol. 2011;4(1):82–7.

183. Kwon EJ, Kim SW, Kim KK, Seo HS, Kim do Y. A case of gemcitabine and cisplatin associated posterior reversible encephalopathy syndrome. Cancer Res Treat. 2009;41(1):53–5.

184. Russell MT, Nassif AS, Cacayorin ED, Awwad E, Perman W, Dunphy F. Gemcitabine-associated posterior reversible encephalopathy syndrome: MR imaging and MR spectroscopy findings. Magn Reson Imaging. 2001;19(1):129–32.

185. Airoldi M, Cattel L, Passera R, Pedani F, Delprino L, Micari C. Gemcitabine and oxaliplatin in patients with metastatic breast cancer resistant to or pretreated with both anthracyclines and taxanes: clinical and pharmacokinetic data. Am J Clin Oncol. 2006;29(5):490–4.

186. Harder J, Riecken B, Kummer O, Lohrmann C, Otto F, Usadel H, et al. Outpatient chemotherapy with gemcitabine and oxaliplatin in patients with biliary tract cancer. Br J Cancer. 2006;95(7):848–52.

187. Barry M, Clarke S, Mulcahy F, Back D. Hydroxyurea-induced neurotoxicity in HIV disease. Aids. 1999;13(12):1592–4.

188. Green MR, Chowdhary S, Lombardi KM, Chalmers LM, Chamberlain M. Clinical utility and pharmacology of high-dose methotrexate in the treatment of primary CNS lymphoma. Expert Rev Neurother. 2006;6(5):635–52.

189. Cavaliere R, Schiff D. Neurologic toxicities of cancer therapies. Curr Neurol Neurosci Rep. 2006;6(3):218–26.

190. Vezmar S, Becker A, Bode U, Jaehde U. Biochemical and clinical aspects of methotrexate neurotoxicity. Chemotherapy. 2003;49(1–2):92–104.

191. Winick NJ, Bowman WP, Kamen BA, Roach ES, Rollins N, Jacaruso D, et al. Unexpected acute neurologic toxicity in the treatment of children with acute lymphoblastic leukemia. J Natl Cancer Inst. 1992;84(4):252–6.

192. Eichler AF, Batchelor TT, Henson JW. Diffusion and perfusion imaging in subacute neurotoxicity following high-dose intravenous methotrexate. Neuro-oncology. 2007;9(3):373–7.

193. Bates S, McKeever P, Masur H, Levens D, Macher A, Armstrong G, et al. Myelopathy following intrathecal chemotherapy in a patient with extensive Burkitt's lymphoma and altered immune status. Am J Med. 1985;78(4):697–702.

194. McLean DR, Clink HM, Ernst P, Coates R, al Kawi MZ, Bohlega S, et al. Myelopathy after intrathecal chemotherapy. A case report with unique magnetic resonance imaging changes. Cancer. 1994;73(12):3037–40.

195. Clark AW, Cohen SR, Nissenblatt MJ, Wilson SK. Paraplegia following intrathecal chemotherapy: neuropathologic findings and elevation of myelin basic protein. Cancer. 1982;50(1):42–7.

196. Gagliano RG, Costanzi JJ. Paraplegia following intrathecal methotrexate: report of a case and review of the literature. Cancer. 1976;37(4):1663–8.

197. Ettinger LJ, Freeman AI, Creaven PJ. Intrathecal methotrexate overdose without neurotoxicity: case report and literature review. Cancer. 1978;41(4):1270–3.

198. Ettinger LJ. Pharmacokinetics and biochemical effects of a fatal intrathecal methotrexate overdose. Cancer. 1982;50(3):444–50.

199. Adamson PC, Balis FM, McCully CL, Godwin KS, Bacher JD, Walsh TJ, et al. Rescue of experimental intrathecal methotrexate overdose with carboxypeptidase-G2. J Clin Oncol. 1991;9 (4):670–4.

200. Widemann BC, Balis FM, Shalabi A, Boron M, O'Brien M, Cole DE, et al. Treatment of accidental intrathecal methotrexate overdose with intrathecal carboxypeptidase G2. J Natl Cancer Inst. 2004;96(20):1557–9.

201. Price RA, Jamieson PA. The central nervous system in childhood leukemia. II. Subacute leukoencephalopathy. Cancer. 1975;35 (2):306–18.

202. Bleyer WA. Neurologic sequelae of methotrexate and ionizing radiation: a new classification. Cancer Treat Rep. 1981;65(Suppl 1):89–98.

203. Ciuleanu T, Brodowicz T, Zielinski C, Kim JH, Krzakowski M, Laack E, et al. Maintenance pemetrexed plus best supportive care versus placebo plus best supportive care for non-small-cell lung cancer: a randomised, double-blind, phase 3 study. Lancet. 2009;374(9699):1432–40.

204. O'Connor OA, Horwitz S, Hamlin P, Portlock C, Moskowitz CH, Sarasohn D, et al. Phase II-I-II study of two different doses and schedules of pralatrexate, a high-affinity substrate for the reduced folate carrier, in patients with relapsed or refractory lymphoma reveals marked activity in T-cell malignancies. J Clin Oncol. 2009;27(26):4357–64.

205. O'Connor OA, Pro B, Pinter-Brown L, Bartlett N, Popplewell L, Coiffier B, et al. Pralatrexate in patients with relapsed or refractory peripheral T-cell lymphoma: results from the pivotal PROPEL study. J Clin Oncol. 2011;29(9):1182–9.

206. Berg SL, Blaney SM, Devidas M, Lampkin TA, Murgo A, Bernstein M, et al. Phase II study of nelarabine (compound 506U78) in children and young adults with refractory T-cell malignancies: a report from the Children's Oncology Group. J Clin Oncol. 2005;23(15):3376–82.

207. DeAngelo DJ, Yu D, Johnson JL, Coutre SE, Stone RM, Stopeck AT, et al. Nelarabine induces complete remissions in adults with relapsed or refractory T-lineage acute lymphoblastic leukemia or lymphoblastic lymphoma: Cancer and Leukemia Group B study 19801. Blood. 2007;109(12):5136–42.

208. Cohen MH, Johnson JR, Massie T, Sridhara R, McGuinn WD Jr, Abraham S, et al. Approval summary: nelarabine for the treatment of T-cell lymphoblastic leukemia/lymphoma. Clin Cancer Res. 2006;12(18):5329–35.

209. Kawakami M, Taniguchi K, Yoshihara S, Ishii S, Kaida K, Ikegame K, et al. Irreversible neurological defects in the lower extremities after haploidentical stem cell transplantation: possible association with nelarabine. Am J Hematol. 2013;88(10):853–7.

210. Kurtzberg J, Ernst TJ, Keating MJ, Gandhi V, Hodge JP, Kisor DF, et al. Phase I study of 506U78 administered on a consecutive 5-day schedule in children and adults with refractory hematologic malignancies. J Clin Oncol. 2005;23(15):3396–403.

211. Ngo D, Patel S, Kim EJ, Brar R, Koontz MZ. Nelarabine neurotoxicity with concurrent intrathecal chemotherapy: case report and review of literature. J Oncol Pharm Pract. 2015;21 (4):296–300.

212. Rijksen G, Kuis W, Wadman SK, Spaapen LJ, Duran M, Voorbrood BS, et al. A new case of purine nucleoside phosphorylase deficiency: enzymologic, clinical, and immunologic characteristics. Pediatr Res. 1987;21(2):137–41.

213. Stoop JW, Zegers BJ, Hendrickx GF, van Heukelom LH, Staal GE, de Bree PK, et al. Purine nucleoside phosphorylase deficiency associated with selective cellular immunodeficiency. New Engl J Med. 1977;296(12):651–5.

214. Jeha S, Gaynon PS, Razzouk BI, Franklin J, Kadota R, Shen V, et al. Phase II study of clofarabine in pediatric patients with refractory or relapsed acute lymphoblastic leukemia. J Clin Oncol. 2006;24(12):1917–23.

215. Kantarjian H, Gandhi V, Cortes J, Verstovsek S, Du M, Garcia-Manero G, et al. Phase 2 clinical and pharmacologic study of clofarabine in patients with refractory or relapsed acute leukemia. Blood. 2003;102(7):2379–86.

216. Robak T, Jamroziak K, Gora-Tybor J, Stella-Holowiecka B, Konopka L, Ceglarek B, et al. Comparison of cladribine plus cyclophosphamide with fludarabine plus cyclophosphamide as first-line therapy for chronic lymphocytic leukemia: a phase III randomized study by the Polish Adult Leukemia Group (PALG-CLL3 Study). J Clin Oncol. 2010;28(11):1863–9.

217. Major PP, Agarwal RP, Kufe DW. Clinical pharmacology of deoxycoformycin. Blood. 1981;58(1):91–6.

218. Kraut EH, Bouroncle BA, Grever MR. Pentostatin in the treatment of advanced hairy cell leukemia. J Clin Oncol. 1989;7(2):168–72.

219. Barbui T, Rambaldi A, Parenzan L, Zucchelli M, Perico N, Remuzzi G. Neurological symptoms and coma associated with doxorubicin administration during chronic cyclosporin therapy. Lancet. 1992;339(8806):1421.

220. Neuwelt EA, Glasberg M, Frenkel E, Barnett P. Neurotoxicity of chemotherapeutic agents after blood-brain barrier modification: neuropathological studies. Ann Neurol. 1983;14(3):316–24.

221. Mortensen ME, Cecalupo AJ, Lo WD, Egorin MJ, Batley R. Inadvertent intrathecal injection of daunorubicin with fatal outcome. Med Pediatr Oncol. 1992;20(3):249–53.

222. Blatt J, Trigg ME, Pizzo PA, Glaubiger D. Tolerance to single-dose dactinomycin in combination chemotherapy for solid tumors. Cancer Treat Rep. 1981;65(1–2):145–7.

223. Carli M, Pastore G, Perilongo G, Grotto P, De Bernardi B, Ceci A, et al. Tumor response and toxicity after single high-dose versus standard five-day divided-dose dactinomycin in childhood rhabdomyosarcoma. J Clin Oncol. 1988;6(4):654–8.

224. Doll DC, Yarbro JW. Vascular toxicity associated with antineoplastic agents. Semin Oncol. 1992;19(5):580–96.

225. Pisoni R, Ruggenenti P, Remuzzi G. Drug-induced thrombotic microangiopathy: incidence, prevention and management. Drug Saf. 2001;24(7):491–501.

226. Amadori S, Arcese W, Isacchi G, Meloni G, Petti MC, Monarca B, et al. Mitoxantrone, etoposide, and intermediate-dose cytarabine: an effective and tolerable regimen for the treatment of refractory acute myeloid leukemia. J Clin Oncol. 1991;9(7):1210–4.

227. Hall C, Dougherty WJ, Lebish IJ, Brock PG, Man A. Warning against use of intrathecal mitoxantrone. Lancet. 1989;1(8640):734.

228. Eckardt JR, von Pawel J, Pujol JL, Papai Z, Quoix E, Ardizzoni A, et al. Phase III study of oral compared with intravenous topotecan as second-line therapy in small-cell lung cancer. J Clin Oncol. 2007;25(15):2086–92.

229. Herzog TJ, Sill MW, Walker JL, O'Malley D, Shahin M, DeGeest K, et al. A phase II study of two topotecan regimens evaluated in recurrent platinum-sensitive ovarian, fallopian tube or primary peritoneal cancer: a Gynecologic Oncology Group Study (GOG 146Q). Gynecol Oncol. 2011;120(3):454–8.

230. Leff RS, Thompson JM, Daly MB, Johnson DB, Harden EA, Mercier RJ, et al. Acute neurologic dysfunction after high-dose

etoposide therapy for malignant glioma. Cancer. 1988;62(1):32–5.

231. McLeod HL, Baker DK Jr, Pui CH, Rodman JH. Somnolence, hypotension, and metabolic acidosis following high-dose teniposide treatment in children with leukemia. Cancer Chemother Pharmacol. 1991;29(2):150–4.

232. Rowinsky EK, Chaudhry V, Cornblath DR, Donehower RC. Neurotoxicity of taxol. J Nat Cancer Inst Monogr. 1993;15:107–15.

233. Grisold W, Cavaletti G, Windebank AJ. Peripheral neuropathies from chemotherapeutics and targeted agents: diagnosis, treatment, and prevention. Neuro-oncology. 2012;14 Suppl 4:iv45–54.

234. Freilich RJ, Balmaceda C, Seidman AD, Rubin M, DeAngelis LM. Motor neuropathy due to docetaxel and paclitaxel. Neurology. 1996;47(1):115–8.

235. Seidman AD, Berry D, Cirrincione C, Harris L, Muss H, Marcom PK, et al. Randomized phase III trial of weekly compared with every-3-weeks paclitaxel for metastatic breast cancer, with trastuzumab for all HER-2 overexpressors and random assignment to trastuzumab or not in HER-2 nonoverexpressors: final results of Cancer and Leukemia Group B protocol 9840. J Clin Oncol. 2008;26(10):1642–9.

236. Sparano JA, Wang M, Martino S, Jones V, Perez EA, Saphner T, et al. Weekly paclitaxel in the adjuvant treatment of breast cancer. New Engl J Med. 2008;358(16):1663–71.

237. Mauri D, Kamposioras K, Tsali L, Bristianou M, Valachis A, Karathanasi I, et al. Overall survival benefit for weekly vs. three-weekly taxanes regimens in advanced breast cancer: a meta-analysis. Cancer Treat Rev. 2010;36(1):69–74.

238. Smith RE, Brown AM, Mamounas EP, Anderson SJ, Lembersky BC, Atkins JH, et al. Randomized trial of 3-hour versus 24-hour infusion of high-dose paclitaxel in patients with metastatic or locally advanced breast cancer: National Surgical Adjuvant Breast and Bowel Project Protocol B-26. J Clin Oncol. 1999;17(11):3403–11.

239. Eisenhauer EA, ten Bokkel Huinink WW, Swenerton KD, Gianni L, Myles J, van der Burg ME, et al. European-Canadian randomized trial of paclitaxel in relapsed ovarian cancer: high-dose versus low-dose and long versus short infusion. J Clin Oncol. 1994;12(12):2654–66.

240. Perry JR, Warner E. Transient encephalopathy after paclitaxel (Taxol) infusion. Neurology. 1996;46(6):1596–9.

241. Rook J, Rosser T, Fangusaro J, Finlay J. Acute transient encephalopathy following paclitaxel treatment in an adolescent with a recurrent suprasellar germinoma. Pediatr Blood Cancer. 2008;50(3):699–700.

242. Khattab J, Terebelo HR, Dabas B. Phantom limb pain as a manifestation of paclitaxel neurotoxicity. Mayo Clin Proc. 2000;75(7):740–2.

243. Capri G, Munzone E, Tarenzi E, Fulfaro F, Gianni L, Caraceni A, et al. Optic nerve disturbances: a new form of paclitaxel neurotoxicity. J Natl Cancer Inst. 1994;86(14):1099–101.

244. Loprinzi CL, Maddocks-Christianson K, Wolf SL, Rao RD, Dyck PJ, Mantyh P, et al. The Paclitaxel acute pain syndrome: sensitization of nociceptors as the putative mechanism. Cancer J. 2007;13(6):399–403.

245. Loprinzi CL, Reeves BN, Dakhil SR, Sloan JA, Wolf SL, Burger KN, et al. Natural history of paclitaxel-associated acute pain syndrome: prospective cohort study NCCTG N08C1. J Clin Oncol. 2011;29(11):1472–8.

246. Reeves BN, Dakhil SR, Sloan JA, Wolf SL, Burger KN, Kamal A, et al. Further data supporting that paclitaxel-associated acute pain syndrome is associated with development of peripheral neuropathy: North Central Cancer Treatment Group trial N08C1. Cancer. 2012;118(20):5171–8.

247. Minatani N, Kosaka Y, Sengoku N, Kikuchi M, Nishimiya H, Waraya M, et al. A case of facial nerve palsy induced by nab-paclitaxel. Gan to kagaku ryoho Cancer Chemother. 2013;40(12):2375–7.

248. Gradishar WJ, Tjulandin S, Davidson N, Shaw H, Desai N, Bhar P, et al. Phase III trial of nanoparticle albumin-bound paclitaxel compared with polyethylated castor oil-based paclitaxel in women with breast cancer. J Clin Oncol. 2005;23(31):7794–803.

249. Von Hoff DD, Ervin T, Arena FP, Chiorean EG, Infante J, Moore M, et al. Increased survival in pancreatic cancer with nab-paclitaxel plus gemcitabine. New Engl J Med. 2013;369(18):1691–703.

250. Jones SE, Erban J, Overmoyer B, Budd GT, Hutchins L, Lower E, et al. Randomized phase III study of docetaxel compared with paclitaxel in metastatic breast cancer. J Clin Oncol. 2005;23(24):5542–51.

251. Rivera E, Mejia JA, Arun BK, Adinin RB, Walters RS, Brewster A, et al. Phase 3 study comparing the use of docetaxel on an every-3-week versus weekly schedule in the treatment of metastatic breast cancer. Cancer. 2008;112(7):1455–61.

252. Di Maio M, Perrone F, Chiodini P, Gallo C, Camps C, Schuette W, et al. Individual patient data meta-analysis of docetaxel administered once every 3 weeks compared with once every week second-line treatment of advanced non-small-cell lung cancer. J Clin Oncol. 2007;25(11):1377–82.

253. van den Bent MJ, Hilkens PH, Sillevis Smitt PA, van Raaij-van den Aarssen VJ, Bontenbal M, Verweij J. Lhermitte's sign following chemotherapy with docetaxel. Neurology. 1998;50(2):563–4.

254. de Bono JS, Oudard S, Ozguroglu M, Hansen S, Machiels JP, Kocak I, et al. Prednisone plus cabazitaxel or mitoxantrone for metastatic castration-resistant prostate cancer progressing after docetaxel treatment: a randomised open-label trial. Lancet. 2010;376(9747):1147–54.

255. Omlin A, Sartor O, Rothermundt C, Cathomas R, De Bono JS, Shen L, et al. Analysis of side effect profile of alopecia, nail changes, peripheral neuropathy, and dysgeusia in prostate cancer patients treated with docetaxel and cabazitaxel. Clin Genitourin Cancer. 2015;13(4):e205–8.

256. Cortes J, O'Shaughnessy J, Loesch D, Blum JL, Vahdat LT, Petrakova K, et al. Eribulin monotherapy versus treatment of physician's choice in patients with metastatic breast cancer (EMBRACE): a phase 3 open-label randomised study. Lancet. 2011;377(9769):914–23.

257. Cortes J, Vahdat L, Blum JL, Twelves C, Campone M, Roche H, et al. Phase II study of the halichondrin B analog eribulin mesylate in patients with locally advanced or metastatic breast cancer previously treated with an anthracycline, a taxane, and capecitabine. J Clin Oncol. 2010;28(25):3922–8.

258. Vahdat LT, Pruitt B, Fabian CJ, Rivera RR, Smith DA, Tan-Chiu E, et al. Phase II study of eribulin mesylate, a halichondrin B analog, in patients with metastatic breast cancer previously treated with an anthracycline and a taxane. J Clin Oncol. 2009;27(18):2954–61.

259. Ebenezer GJ, Carlson K, Donovan D, Cobham M, Chuang E, Moore A, et al. Ixabepilone-induced mitochondria and sensory axon loss in breast cancer patients. Ann Clin Transl Neurol. 2014;1(9):639–49.

260. Denduluri N, Low JA, Lee JJ, Berman AW, Walshe JM, Vatas U, et al. Phase II trial of ixabepilone, an epothilone B analog, in patients with metastatic breast cancer previously untreated with taxanes. J Clin Oncol. 2007;25(23):3421–7.

261. Lee JJ, Swain SM. Peripheral neuropathy induced by microtubule-stabilizing agents. J Clin Oncol. 2006;24(10): 1633–42.

262. Legha SS. Vincristine neurotoxicity. Pathophysiology and management. Med Toxicol. 1986;1(6):421–7.

263. Casey EB, Jellife AM, Le Quesne PM, Millett YL. Vincristine neuropathy. Clinical and electrophysiological observations. Brain J Neurol. 1973;96(1):69–86.

264. Postma TJ, Benard BA, Huijgens PC, Ossenkoppele GJ, Heimans JJ. Long-term effects of vincristine on the peripheral nervous system. J Neurooncol. 1993;15(1):23–7.

265. Weintraub M, Adde MA, Venzon DJ, Shad AT, Horak ID, Neely JE, et al. Severe atypical neuropathy associated with administration of hematopoietic colony-stimulating factors and vincristine. J Clin Oncol. 1996;14(3):935–40.

266. Teusink AC, Ragucci D, Shatat IF, Kalpatthi R. Potentiation of vincristine toxicity with concomitant fluconazole prophylaxis in children with acute lymphoblastic leukemia. Pediatr Hematol Oncol. 2012;29(1):62–7.

267. Harnicar S, Adel N, Jurcic J. Modification of vincristine dosing during concomitant azole therapy in adult acute lymphoblastic leukemia patients. J Oncol Pharm Pract. 2009;15(3):175–82.

268. Hogan-Dann CM, Fellmeth WG, McGuire SA, Kiley VA. Polyneuropathy following vincristine therapy in two patients with Charcot-Marie-Tooth syndrome. JAMA. 1984;252 (20):2862–3.

269. Naumann R, Mohm J, Reuner U, Kroschinsky F, Rautenstrauss B, Ehninger G. Early recognition of hereditary motor and sensory neuropathy type 1 can avoid life-threatening vincristine neurotoxicity. Br J Haematol. 2001;115(2):323–5.

270. O'Brien S, Schiller G, Lister J, Damon L, Goldberg S, Aulitzky W, et al. High-dose vincristine sulfate liposome injection for advanced, relapsed, and refractory adult Philadelphia chromosome-negative acute lymphoblastic leukemia. J Clin Oncol. 2013;31(6):676–83.

271. Pal PK. Clinical and electrophysiological studies in vincristine induced neuropathy. Electromyogr Clin Neurophysiol. 1999;39 (6):323–30.

272. Robertson GL, Bhoopalam N, Zelkowitz LJ. Vincristine neurotoxicity and abnormal secretion of antidiuretic hormone. Arch Intern Med. 1973;132(5):717–20.

273. Hurwitz RL, Mahoney DH Jr, Armstrong DL, Browder TM. Reversible encephalopathy and seizures as a result of conventional vincristine administration. Med Pediatr Oncol. 1988;16 (3):216–9.

274. Haefner MD, Siciliano RD, Widmer LA, Vogel Wigger BM, Frick S. Reversible posterior leukoencephalopathy syndrome after treatment of diffuse large B-cell lymphoma. Onkologie. 2007;30(3):138–40.

275. Ozyurek H, Oguz G, Ozen S, Akyuz C, Karli Oguz K, Anlar B, et al. Reversible posterior leukoencephalopathy syndrome: report of three cases. J Child Neurol. 2005;20(12):990–3.

276. Byrd RL, Rohrbaugh TM, Raney RB Jr, Norris DG. Transient cortical blindness secondary to vincristine therapy in childhood malignancies. Cancer. 1981;47(1):37–40.

277. Rodriguez MA, Pytlik R, Kozak T, Chhanabhai M, Gascoyne R, Lu B, et al. Vincristine sulfate liposomes injection (Marqibo) in heavily pretreated patients with refractory aggressive non-Hodgkin lymphoma: report of the pivotal phase 2 study. Cancer. 2009;115(15):3475–82.

278. Silverman LB, Stevenson KE, O'Brien JE, Asselin BL, Barr RD, Clavell L, et al. Long-term results of Dana-Farber Cancer Institute ALL Consortium protocols for children with newly diagnosed acute lymphoblastic leukemia (1985–2000). Leukemia. 2010;24(2):320–34.

279. Bedikian AY, Silverman JA, Papadopoulos NE, Kim KB, Hagey AE, Vardeleon A, et al. Pharmacokinetics and safety of Marqibo (vincristine sulfate liposomes injection) in cancer patients with impaired liver function. J Clin Pharmacol. 2011;51(8):1205–12.

280. Bleck TP, Jacobsen J. Prolonged survival following the inadvertent intrathecal administration of vincristine: clinical and electrophysiologic analyses. Clin Neuropharmacol. 1991;14(5):457–62.

281. Bain PG, Lantos PL, Djurovic V, West I. Intrathecal vincristine: a fatal chemotherapeutic error with devastating central nervous system effects. J Neurol. 1991;238(4):230–4.

282. Williams ME, Walker AN, Bracikowski JP, Garner L, Wilson KD, Carpenter JT. Ascending myeloencephalopathy due to intrathecal vincristine sulfate. A fatal chemotherapeutic error. Cancer. 1983;51(11):2041–7.

283. Norris B, Pritchard KI, James K, Myles J, Bennett K, Marlin S, et al. Phase III comparative study of vinorelbine combined with doxorubicin versus doxorubicin alone in disseminated metastatic/recurrent breast cancer: National Cancer Institute of Canada Clinical Trials Group Study MA8. J Clin Oncol. 2000;18 (12):2385–94.

284. Fazeny B, Zifko U, Meryn S, Huber H, Grisold W, Dittrich C. Vinorelbine-induced neurotoxicity in patients with advanced breast cancer pretreated with paclitaxel–a phase II study. Cancer Chemother Pharmacol. 1996;39(1–2):150–6.

285. Richardson PG, Xie W, Jagannath S, Jakubowiak A, Lonial S, Raje NS, et al. A phase 2 trial of lenalidomide, bortezomib, and dexamethasone in patients with relapsed and relapsed/refractory myeloma. Blood. 2014;123(10):1461–9.

286. Badros A, Goloubeva O, Dalal JS, Can I, Thompson J, Rapoport AP, et al. Neurotoxicity of bortezomib therapy in multiple myeloma: a single-center experience and review of the literature. Cancer. 2007;110(5):1042–9.

287. Argyriou AA, Iconomou G, Kalofonos HP. Bortezomib-induced peripheral neuropathy in multiple myeloma: a comprehensive review of the literature. Blood. 2008;112(5):1593–9.

288. Windebank AJ, Grisold W. Chemotherapy-induced neuropathy. J Peripheral Nerv Syst JPNS. 2008;13(1):27–46.

289. Richardson PG, Sonneveld P, Schuster MW, Stadtmauer EA, Facon T, Harousseau JL, et al. Reversibility of symptomatic peripheral neuropathy with bortezomib in the phase III APEX trial in relapsed multiple myeloma: impact of a dose-modification guideline. Br J Haematol. 2009;144(6):895–903.

290. Cavaletti G, Jakubowiak AJ. Peripheral neuropathy during bortezomib treatment of multiple myeloma: a review of recent studies. Leuk Lymphoma. 2010;51(7):1178–87.

291. Cavaletti G, Gilardini A, Canta A, Rigamonti L, Rodriguez-Menendez V, Ceresa C, et al. Bortezomib-induced peripheral neurotoxicity: a neurophysiological and pathological study in the rat. Exp Neurol. 2007;204(1):317–25.

292. Pei XY, Dai Y, Grant S. Synergistic induction of oxidative injury and apoptosis in human multiple myeloma cells by the proteasome inhibitor bortezomib and histone deacetylase inhibitors. Clin Cancer Res. 2004;10(11):3839–52.

293. Landowski TH, Megli CJ, Nullmeyer KD, Lynch RM, Dorr RT. Mitochondrial-mediated disregulation of Ca^{2+} is a critical determinant of Velcade (PS-341/bortezomib) cytotoxicity in myeloma cell lines. Can Res. 2005;65(9):3828–36.

294. Richardson PG, Hideshima T, Anderson KC. Bortezomib (PS-341): a novel, first-in-class proteasome inhibitor for the treatment of multiple myeloma and other cancers. Cancer Control J Moffitt Cancer Cent. 2003;10(5):361–9.

295. Argyriou AA, Cavaletti G, Bruna J, Kyritsis AP, Kalofonos HP. Bortezomib-induced peripheral neurotoxicity: an update. Arch Toxicol. 2014;88(9):1669–79.

296. San Miguel JF, Schlag R, Khuageva NK, Dimopoulos MA, Shpilberg O, Kropff M, et al. Bortezomib plus melphalan and prednisone for initial treatment of multiple myeloma. New Engl J Med. 2008;359(9):906–17.

297. Jagannath S, Barlogie B, Berenson J, Siegel D, Irwin D, Richardson PG, et al. A phase 2 study of two doses of bortezomib in relapsed or refractory myeloma. Br J Haematol. 2004;127(2):165–72.

298. Ravaglia S, Corso A, Piccolo G, Lozza A, Alfonsi E, Mangia-cavalli S, et al. Immune-mediated neuropathies in myeloma patients treated with bortezomib. Clin Neurophysiol. 2008;119 (11):2507–12.

299. Bringhen S, Larocca A, Rossi D, Cavalli M, Genuardi M, Ria R, et al. Efficacy and safety of once-weekly bortezomib in multiple myeloma patients. Blood. 2010;116(23):4745–53.

300. Arnulf B, Pylypenko H, Grosicki S, Karamanesht I, Leleu X, van de Velde H, et al. Updated survival analysis of a randomized phase III study of subcutaneous versus intravenous bortezomib in patients with relapsed multiple myeloma. Haematologica. 2012;97(12):1925–8.

301. Moreau P, Pylypenko H, Grosicki S, Karamanesht I, Leleu X, Grishunina M, et al. Subcutaneous versus intravenous adminis-tration of bortezomib in patients with relapsed multiple myeloma: a randomised, phase 3, non-inferiority study. Lancet Oncol. 2011;12(5):431–40.

302. Treon SP, Hunter ZR, Matous J, Joyce RM, Mannion B, Advani R, et al. Multicenter clinical trial of bortezomib in relapsed/refractory Waldenstrom's macroglobulinemia: results of WMCTG Trial 03-248. Clin Cancer Res. 2007;13(11):3320–5.

303. Nixon NA, Parhar K. Posterior reversible encephalopathy syndrome resulting from repeat bortezomib usage. BMJ Case Rep. 2014. pii: bcr2014204592.

304. Kager LM, Kersten MJ, Kloppenborg RP, Van Oers R, Van den Born BJ. Reversible posterior leucoencephalopathy syndrome associated with bortezomib in a patient with relapsed multiple myeloma. BMJ Case Rep. 2009. doi:10.1136/bcr.06.2009.1926.

305. Ho CH, Lo CP, Tu MC. Bortezomib-induced posterior reversible encephalopathy syndrome: clinical and imaging features. Intern Med. 2014;53(16):1853–7.

306. Vij R, Wang M, Kaufman JL, Lonial S, Jakubowiak AJ, Stewart AK, et al. An open-label, single-arm, phase 2 (PX-171-004) study of single-agent carfilzomib in bortezomib-naive patients with relapsed and/or refractory multi-ple myeloma. Blood. 2012;119(24):5661–70.

307. Siegel DS, Martin T, Wang M, Vij R, Jakubowiak AJ, Lonial S, et al. A phase 2 study of single-agent carfilzomib (PX-171-003-A1) in patients with relapsed and refractory mul-tiple myeloma. Blood. 2012;120(14):2817–25.

308. Jakubowiak AJ, Dytfeld D, Griffith KA, Lebovic D, Vesole DH, Jagannath S, et al. A phase 1/2 study of carfilzomib in combination with lenalidomide and low-dose dexamethasone as a frontline treatment for multiple myeloma. Blood. 2012;120 (9):1801–9.

309. Foss F, Advani R, Duvic M, Hymes KB, Intragumtornchai T, Lekhakula A, et al. A phase II trial of Belinostat (PXD101) in patients with relapsed or refractory peripheral or cutaneous T-cell lymphoma. Br J Haematol. 2015;168(6):811–9.

310. San-Miguel JF, Hungria VT, Yoon SS, Beksac M, Dimopoulos MA, Elghandour A, et al. Panobinostat plus bortezomib and dexamethasone versus placebo plus bortezomib and dexamethasone in patients with relapsed or relapsed and refractory multiple myeloma: a multicentre, randomised, double-blind phase 3 trial. Lancet Oncol. 2014;15(11):1195–206.

311. Sharma S, Witteveen PO, Lolkema MP, Hess D, Gelderblom H, Hussain SA, et al. A phase I, open-label, multicenter study to evaluate the pharmacokinetics and safety of oral panobinostat in patients with advanced solid tumors and varying degrees of renal function. Cancer Chemother Pharmacol. 2015;75(1):87–95.

312. Piekarz RL, Frye R, Prince HM, Kirschbaum MH, Zain J, Allen SL, et al. Phase 2 trial of romidepsin in patients with peripheral T-cell lymphoma. Blood. 2011;117(22):5827–34.

313. Olsen EA, Kim YH, Kuzel TM, Pacheco TR, Foss FM, Parker S, et al. Phase IIb multicenter trial of vorinostat in patients with persistent, progressive, or treatment refractory cutaneous T-cell lymphoma. J Clin Oncol. 2007;25(21):3109–15.

314. Cashen AF, Schiller GJ, O'Donnell MR, DiPersio JF. Multicen-ter, phase II study of decitabine for the first-line treatment of older patients with acute myeloid leukemia. J Clin Oncol. 2010;28 (4):556–61.

315. Kantarjian H, Oki Y, Garcia-Manero G, Huang X, O'Brien S, Cortes J, et al. Results of a randomized study of 3 schedules of low-dose decitabine in higher-risk myelodysplastic syndrome and chronic myelomonocytic leukemia. Blood. 2007;109(1):52–7.

316. Saiki JH, Bodey GP, Hewlett JS, Amare M, Morrison FS, Wilson HE, et al. Effect of schedule on activity and toxicity of 5-azacytidine in acute leukemia: a Southwest Oncology Group Study. Cancer. 1981;47(7):1739–42.

317. Douvali E, Papoutselis M, Vassilakopoulos TP, Papadopoulos V, Spanoudakis E, Tsatalas C, et al. Safety and efficacy of 5-azacytidine treatment in myelodysplastic syndrome patients with moderate and mild renal impairment. Leuk Res. 2013;37 (8):889–93.

318. Kornblith AB, Herndon JE 2nd, Silverman LR, Demakos EP, Odchimar-Reissig R, Holland JF, et al. Impact of azacytidine on the quality of life of patients with myelodysplastic syndrome treated in a randomized phase III trial: a Cancer and Leukemia Group B study. J Clin Oncol. 2002;20(10):2441–52.

319. Mileshkin L, Stark R, Day B, Seymour JF, Zeldis JB, Prince HM. Development of neuropathy in patients with myeloma treated with thalidomide: patterns of occurrence and the role of electrophysiologic monitoring. J Clin Oncol. 2006;24 (27):4507–14.

320. Tosi P, Zamagni E, Cellini C, Plasmati R, Cangini D, Tacchetti P, et al. Neurological toxicity of long-term (>1 yr) thalidomide therapy in patients with multiple myeloma. Eur J Haematol. 2005;74(3):212–6.

321. Plasmati R, Pastorelli F, Cavo M, Petracci E, Zamagni E, Tosi P, et al. Neuropathy in multiple myeloma treated with thalidomide: a prospective study. Neurology. 2007;69(6):573–81.

322. Rajkumar SV, Rosinol L, Hussein M, Catalano J, Jedrzejczak W, Lucy L, et al. Multicenter, randomized, double-blind, placebo-controlled study of thalidomide plus dexamethasone compared with dexamethasone as initial therapy for newly diagnosed multiple myeloma. J Clin Oncol. 2008;26(13):2171–7.

323. Prince HM, Mileshkin L, Roberts A, Ganju V, Underhill C, Catalano J, et al. A multicenter phase II trial of thalidomide and celecoxib for patients with relapsed and refractory multiple myeloma. Clin Cancer Res. 2005;11(15):5504–14.

324. Spencer A, Prince HM, Roberts AW, Prosser IW, Bradstock KF, Coyle L, et al. Consolidation therapy with low-dose thalidomide and prednisolone prolongs the survival of multiple myeloma patients undergoing a single autologous stem-cell transplantation procedure. J Clin Oncol. 2009;27(11):1788–93.

325. Cundari S, Cavaletti G. Thalidomide chemotherapy-induced peripheral neuropathy: actual status and new perspectives with thalidomide analogues derivatives. Mini Rev Med Chem. 2009;9 (7):760–8.

326. Glasmacher A, Hahn C, Hoffmann F, Naumann R, Gold-schmidt H, von Lilienfeld-Toal M, et al. A systematic review of phase-II trials of thalidomide monotherapy in patients with

relapsed or refractory multiple myeloma. Br J Haematol. 2006;132(5):584–93.

327. Facon T, Mary JY, Hulin C, Benboubker L, Attal M, Pegourie B, et al. Melphalan and prednisone plus thalidomide versus melphalan and prednisone alone or reduced-intensity autologous stem cell transplantation in elderly patients with multiple myeloma (IFM 99-06): a randomised trial. Lancet. 2007;370 (9594):1209–18.

328. Hulin C, Facon T, Rodon P, Pegourie B, Benboubker L, Doyen C, et al. Efficacy of melphalan and prednisone plus thalidomide in patients older than 75 years with newly diagnosed multiple myeloma: IFM 01/01 trial. J Clin Oncol. 2009;27 (22):3664–70.

329. Mohty B, El-Cheikh J, Yakoub-Agha I, Moreau P, Harousseau JL, Mohty M. Peripheral neuropathy and new treatments for multiple myeloma: background and practical recommendations. Haematologica. 2010;95(2):311–9.

330. Clark TE, Edom N, Larson J, Lindsey LJ. Thalomid (Thalidomide) capsules: a review of the first 18 months of spontaneous postmarketing adverse event surveillance, including off-label prescribing. Drug Saf. 2001;24(2):87–117.

331. Patel UH, Mir MA, Sivik JK, Raheja D, Pandey MK, Talamo G. Central neurotoxicity of immunomodulatory drugs in multiple myeloma. Hematol Rep. 2015;7(1):5704.

332. Dimopoulos MA, Chen C, Spencer A, Niesvizky R, Attal M, Stadtmauer EA, et al. Long-term follow-up on overall survival from the MM-009 and MM-010 phase III trials of lenalidomide plus dexamethasone in patients with relapsed or refractory multiple myeloma. Leukemia. 2009;23(11):2147–52.

333. Briani C, Torre CD, Campagnolo M, Lucchetta M, Berno T, Candiotto L, et al. Lenalidomide in patients with chemotherapy-induced polyneuropathy and relapsed or refractory multiple myeloma: results from a single-centre prospective study. J Peripheral Nerv Syst JPNS. 2013;18(1):19–24.

334. Richardson PG, Siegel DS, Vij R, Hofmeister CC, Baz R, Jagannath S, et al. Pomalidomide alone or in combination with low-dose dexamethasone in relapsed and refractory multiple myeloma: a randomized phase 2 study. Blood. 2014;123 (12):1826–32.

335. San Miguel J, Weisel K, Moreau P, Lacy M, Song K, Delforge M, et al. Pomalidomide plus low-dose dexamethasone versus high-dose dexamethasone alone for patients with relapsed and refractory multiple myeloma (MM-003): a randomised, open-label, phase 3 trial. Lancet Oncol. 2013;14(11):1055–66.

336. Powell BL, Moser B, Stock W, Gallagher RE, Willman CL, Stone RM, et al. Arsenic trioxide improves event-free and overall survival for adults with acute promyelocytic leukemia: North American Leukemia Intergroup Study C9710. Blood. 2010;116 (19):3751–7.

337. Duvic M, Hymes K, Heald P, Breneman D, Martin AG, Myskowski P, et al. Bexarotene is effective and safe for treatment of refractory advanced-stage cutaneous T-cell lymphoma: multinational phase II-III trial results. J Clin Oncol. 2001;19(9): 2456–71.

338. Verma N, Kumar K, Kaur G, Anand S. L-asparaginase: a promising chemotherapeutic agent. Crit Rev Biotechnol. 2007;27 (1):45–62.

339. Feinberg WM, Swenson MR. Cerebrovascular complications of L-asparaginase therapy. Neurology. 1988;38(1):127–33.

340. Leonard JV, Kay JD. Acute encephalopathy and hyperammonaemia complicating treatment of acute lymphoblastic leukaemia with asparaginase. Lancet. 1986;1(8473):162–3.

341. Foreman NK, Mahmoud HH, Rivera GK, Crist WM. Recurrent cerebrovascular accident with L-asparaginase rechallenge. Med Pediatr Oncol. 1992;20(6):532–4.

342. Hamdan MY, Frenkel EP, Bick R. L-asparaginase-provoked seizures as singular expression of central nervous toxicity. Clin Appl Thromb Hemost. 2000;6(4):234–8.

343. Priest JR, Ramsay NK, Bennett AJ, Krivit W, Edson JR. The effect of L-asparaginase on antithrombin, plasminogen, and plasma coagulation during therapy for acute lymphoblastic leukemia. J Pediatr. 1982;100(6):990–5.

344. Lee JH, Kim SW, Sung Kim J. Sagittal sinus thrombosis associated with transient free protein S deficiency after L-asparaginase treatment: case report and review of the literature. Clin Neurol Neurosurg. 2000;102(1):33–6.

345. Cairo MS, Lazarus K, Gilmore RL, Baehner RL. Intracranial hemorrhage and focal seizures secondary to use of L-asparaginase during induction therapy of acute lymphocytic leukemia. J Pediatr. 1980;97(5):829–33.

346. Priest JR, Ramsay NK, Steinherz PG, Tubergen DG, Cairo MS, Sitarz AL, et al. A syndrome of thrombosis and hemorrhage complicating L-asparaginase therapy for childhood acute lymphoblastic leukemia. J Pediatr. 1982;100(6):984–9.

347. Garattini E, Gianni M, Terao M. Cytodifferentiation by retinoids, a novel therapeutic option in oncology: rational combinations with other therapeutic agents. Vitam Horm. 2007;75:301–54.

348. Visani G, Manfroi S, Tosi P, Martinelli G. All-trans-retinoic acid and pseudotumor cerebri. Leuk Lymphoma. 1996;23(5–6):437–42.

349. Cortes J, Lipton JH, Rea D, Digumarti R, Chuah C, Nanda N, et al. Phase 2 study of subcutaneous omacetaxine mepesuccinate after TKI failure in patients with chronic-phase CML with T315I mutation. Blood. 2012;120(13):2573–80.

350. Gasco M, Argusti A, Bonanni B, Decensi A. SERMs in chemoprevention of breast cancer. Eur J Cancer. 2005;41 (13):1980–9.

351. Ugurlu S, Karagoz A, Altin Ekin M. Ocular findings in breast cancer patients using tamoxifen. Cutan Ocul Toxicol. 2015;34 (1):16–20.

352. Tarafdar S, Lim LT, Collins CE, Ramaesh K. Tamoxifen keratopathy as seen with in-vivo confocal microscopy. Semin Ophthalmol. 2012;27(1–2):27–8.

353. Kaiser-Kupfer MI, Lippman ME. Tamoxifen retinopathy. Cancer Treat Rep. 1978;62(3):315–20.

354. Nayfield SG, Gorin MB. Tamoxifen-associated eye disease. A review. J Clin Oncol. 1996;14(3):1018–26.

355. Pavlidis NA, Petris C, Briassoulis E, Klouvas G, Psilas C, Rempapis J, et al. Clear evidence that long-term, low-dose tamoxifen treatment can induce ocular toxicity. A prospective study of 63 patients. Cancer. 1992;69(12):2961–4.

356. Ashford AR, Donev I, Tiwari RP, Garrett TJ. Reversible ocular toxicity related to tamoxifen therapy. Cancer. 1988;61(1):33–5.

357. Ron IG, Inbar MJ, Barak Y, Stier S, Chaitchik S. Organic delusional syndrome associated with tamoxifen treatment. Cancer. 1992;69(6):1415–7.

358. Davies C, Pan H, Godwin J, Gray R, Arriagada R, Raina V, et al. Long-term effects of continuing adjuvant tamoxifen to 10 years versus stopping at 5 years after diagnosis of oestrogen receptor-positive breast cancer: ATLAS, a randomised trial. Lancet. 2013;381(9869):805–16.

359. Early Breast Cancer Trialists' Collaborative G. Effects of chemotherapy and hormonal therapy for early breast cancer on recurrence and 15-year survival: an overview of the randomised trials. Lancet. 2005;365(9472):1687–717.

360. Ragaz J, Coldman A. Survival impact of adjuvant tamoxifen on competing causes of mortality in breast cancer survivors, with analysis of mortality from contralateral breast cancer, cardiovascular events, endometrial cancer, and thromboembolic episodes. J Clin Oncol. 1998;16(6):2018–24.

361. Goldhaber SZ. Tamoxifen: preventing breast cancer and placing the risk of deep vein thrombosis in perspective. Circulation. 2005;111(5):539–41.

362. Gianni L, Panzini I, Li S, Gelber RD, Collins J, Holmberg SB, et al. Ocular toxicity during adjuvant chemoendocrine therapy for early breast cancer: results from International Breast Cancer Study Group trials. Cancer. 2006;106(3):505–13.

363. International Breast Cancer Study G, Pagani O, Gelber S, Price K, Zahrieh D, Gelber R, et al. Toremifene and tamoxifen are equally effective for early-stage breast cancer: first results of International Breast Cancer Study Group Trials 12–93 and 14–93. Ann Oncol. 2004;15(12):1749–59.

364. Barrett-Connor E, Mosca L, Collins P, Geiger MJ, Grady D, Kornitzer M, et al. Effects of raloxifene on cardiovascular events and breast cancer in postmenopausal women. New Engl J Med. 2006;355(2):125–37.

365. Robertson JF, Llombart-Cussac A, Rolski J, Feltl D, Dewar J, Macpherson E, et al. Activity of fulvestrant 500 mg versus anastrozole 1 mg as first-line treatment for advanced breast cancer: results from the FIRST study. J Clin Oncol. 2009;27 (27):4530–5.

366. Jenkins VA, Ambroisine LM, Atkins L, Cuzick J, Howell A, Fallowfield LJ. Effects of anastrozole on cognitive performance in postmenopausal women: a randomised, double-blind chemo-prevention trial (IBIS II). Lancet Oncol. 2008;9(10):953–61.

367. Kaufmann M, Jonat W, Hilfrich J, Eidtmann H, Gademann G, Zuna I, et al. Improved overall survival in postmenopausal women with early breast cancer after anastrozole initiated after treatment with tamoxifen compared with continued tamoxifen: the ARNO 95 study. J Clin Oncol. 2007;25(19):2664–70.

368. Coates AS, Keshaviah A, Thurlimann B, Mouridsen H, Mauriac L, Forbes JF, et al. Five years of letrozole compared with tamoxifen as initial adjuvant therapy for postmenopausal women with endocrine-responsive early breast cancer: update of study BIG 1-98. J Clin Oncol. 2007;25(5):486–92.

369. Goss PE, Ingle JN, Martino S, Robert NJ, Muss HB, Piccart MJ, et al. A randomized trial of letrozole in postmenopausal women after five years of tamoxifen therapy for early-stage breast cancer. New Engl J Med. 2003;349(19):1793–802.

370. Goss PE, Ingle JN, Ales-Martinez JE, Cheung AM, Chlebowski RT, Wactawski-Wende J, et al. Exemestane for breast-cancer prevention in postmenopausal women. New Engl J Med. 2011;364(25):2381–91.

371. Paridaens RJ, Dirix LY, Beex LV, Nooij M, Cameron DA, Cufer T, et al. Phase III study comparing exemestane with tamoxifen as first-line hormonal treatment of metastatic breast cancer in postmenopausal women: the European Organisation for Research and Treatment of Cancer Breast Cancer Cooperative Group. J Clin Oncol. 2008;26(30):4883–90.

372. Sagara Y, Kosha S, Baba S, Dokiya F, Tamada S, Sagara Y, et al. Adverse events and bone health during anastrozole therapy in postmenopausal Japanese breast cancer patients. Breast Cancer. 2010;17(3):212–7.

373. Eaton HJ, Phillips PJ, Hanieh A, Cooper J, Bolt J, Torpy DJ. Rapid onset of pituitary apoplexy after goserelin implant for prostate cancer: need for heightened awareness. Inter Med J. 2001;31(5):313–4.

374. Ando S, Hoshino T, Mihara S. Pituitary apoplexy after goserelin. Lancet. 1995;345(8947):458.

375. Sasagawa Y, Tachibana O, Nakagawa A, Koya D, Iizuka H. Pituitary apoplexy following gonadotropin-releasing hormone agonist administration with gonadotropin-secreting pituitary adenoma. J Clin Neurosci. 2015;22(3):601–3.

376. Huang TY, Lin JP, Lieu AS, Chen YT, Chen HS, Jang MY, et al. Pituitary apoplexy induced by Gonadotropin-releasing hormone

377. Davis A, Goel S, Picolos M, Wang M, Lavis V. Pituitary apoplexy after leuprolide. Pituitary. 2006;9(3):263–5.

378. Morsi A, Jamal S, Silverberg JD. Pituitary apoplexy after leuprolide administration for carcinoma of the prostate. Clin Endocrinol. 1996;44(1):121–4.

379. Hackshaw A, Baum M, Fornander T, Nordenskjold B, Nicolucci A, Monson K, et al. Long-term effectiveness of adjuvant goserelin in premenopausal women with early breast cancer. J Natl Cancer Inst. 2009;101(5):341–9.

380. Baum M, Hackshaw A, Houghton J, Rutqvist Fornander T, Nordenskjold B, et al. Adjuvant goserelin in pre-menopausal patients with early breast cancer: results from the ZIPP study. Eur J Cancer. 2006;42(7):895–904.

381. Horwitz EM, Bae K, Hanks GE, Porter A, Grignon DJ, Brereton HD, et al. Ten-year follow-up of radiation therapy oncology group protocol 92-02: a phase III trial of the duration of elective androgen deprivation in locally advanced prostate cancer. J Clin Oncol. 2008;26(15):2497–504.

382. Gatti J, Brinker A, Avigan M. Spontaneous reports of seizure in association with leuprolide (lupron depot), goserelin (zoladex implant), and naferelin (synarel nasal spray). Obstet Gynecol. 2013;121(5):1107.

383. Akaboshi S, Takeshita K. A case of atypical absence seizures induced by leuprolide acetate. Pediatr Neurol. 2000;23(3):266–8.

384. Schellhammer P, Sharifi R, Block N, Soloway M, Venner P, Patterson AL, et al. A controlled trial of bicalutamide versus flutamide, each in combination with luteinizing hormone-releasing hormone analogue therapy, in patients with advanced prostate cancer. Casodex Combination Study Group. Urology. 1995;45(5):745–52.

385. Tanvetyanon T, Choudhury AM. Fatal acute tumor lysis syndrome, hepatic encephalopathy and flare phenomenon following combined androgen blockade. J Urol. 2004;171(4):1627.

386. Patel H, Rhee E, Zimmern PE. Hepatic encephalopathy induced by flutamide administered for the treatment of prostatic cancer. J Urol (Paris). 1996;102(3):123–5.

387. Bertagna C, De Gery A, Hucher M, Francois JP, Zanirato J. Efficacy of the combination of nilutamide plus orchidectomy in patients with metastatic prostatic cancer. A meta-analysis of seven randomized double-blind trials (1056 patients). Br J Urol. 1994;73(4):396–402.

388. Dijkman GA, Janknegt RA, De Reijke TM, Debruyne FM. Long-term efficacy and safety of nilutamide plus castration in advanced prostate cancer, and the significance of early prostate specific antigen normalization. International Anandron Study Group. J Urol. 1997;158(1):160–3.

389. Terzolo M, Angeli A, Fassnacht M, Daffara F, Tauchmanova L, Conton PA, et al. Adjuvant mitotane treatment for adrenocortical carcinoma. New Engl J Med. 2007;356(23):2372–80.

390. Lanser JB, van Seters AP, Moolenaar AJ, Haak HR, Bollen EL. Neuropsychologic and neurologic side effects of mitotane and reversibility of symptoms. J Clin Oncol. 1992;10(9):1504.

391. Zancanella P, Pianovski MA, Oliveira BH, Ferman S, Piovezan GC, Lichtvan LL, et al. Mitotane associated with cisplatin, etoposide, and doxorubicin in advanced childhood adrenocortical carcinoma: mitotane monitoring and tumor regression. J Pediatr Hematol Oncol. 2006;28(8):513–24.

392. Kasperlik-Zaluska AA. Clinical results of the use of mitotane for adrenocortical carcinoma. Braz J Med Biol Res. 2000;33 (10):1191–6 (Revista brasileira de pesquisas medicas e biologicas/Sociedade Brasileira de Biofisica [et al]).

393. Hatzipantelis E, Pana ZD, Pavlou E, Balakou E, Tsotoulidou V, Papageorgiou T, et al. Epileptic seizures after octreotide

administration in a 6.5-year-old female with ALL and L-asparaginase associated pancreatitis: a possible drug interaction. Klin Padiatr. 2011;223(6):360–3.

394. Lentz SS, Brady MF, Major FJ, Reid GC, Soper JT. High-dose megestrol acetate in advanced or recurrent endometrial carcinoma: a Gynecologic Oncology Group Study. J Clin Oncol. 1996;14(2):357–61.

395. Loprinzi CL, Michalak JC, Schaid DJ, Mailliard JA, Athmann LM, Goldberg RM, et al. Phase III evaluation of four doses of megestrol acetate as therapy for patients with cancer anorexia and/or cachexia. J Clin Oncol. 1993;11(4):762–7.

396. Crawford ED, Tombal B, Miller K, Boccon-Gibod L, Schroder F, Shore N, et al. A phase III extension trial with a 1-arm crossover from leuprolide to degarelix: comparison of gonadotropin-releasing hormone agonist and antagonist effect on prostate cancer. J Urol. 2011;186(3):889–97.

397. Klotz L, Boccon-Gibod L, Shore ND, Andreou C, Persson BE, Cantor P, et al. The efficacy and safety of degarelix: a 12-month, comparative, randomized, open-label, parallel-group phase III study in patients with prostate cancer. BJU Int. 2008;102 (11):1531–8.

398. Smith MR, Klotz L, Persson BE, Olesen TK, Wilde AA. Cardiovascular safety of degarelix: results from a 12-month, comparative, randomized, open label, parallel group phase III trial in patients with prostate cancer. J Urol. 2010;184(6):2313–9.

399. Scher HI, Beer TM, Higano CS, Anand A, Taplin ME, Efstathiou E, et al. Antitumour activity of MDV3100 in castration-resistant prostate cancer: a phase 1-2 study. Lancet. 2010;375(9724):1437–46.

400. Beer TM, Armstrong AJ, Rathkopf DE, Loriot Y, Sternberg CN, Higano CS, et al. Enzalutamide in metastatic prostate cancer before chemotherapy. New Engl J Med. 2014;371(5):424–33.

401. Attard G, Reid AH, A'Hern R, Parker C, Oommen NB, Folkerd E, et al. Selective inhibition of CYP17 with abiraterone acetate is highly active in the treatment of castration-resistant prostate cancer. J Clin Oncol. 2009;27(23):3742–8.

402. Fizazi K, Scher HI, Molina A, Logothetis CJ, Chi KN, Jones RJ, et al. Abiraterone acetate for treatment of metastatic castration-resistant prostate cancer: final overall survival analysis of the COU-AA-301 randomised, double-blind, placebo-controlled phase 3 study. Lancet Oncol. 2012;13(10):983–92.

403. Marty M, Espie M, Llombart A, Monnier A, Rapoport BL, Stahalova V, et al. Multicenter randomized phase III study of the cardioprotective effect of dexrazoxane (Cardioxane) in advanced/metastatic breast cancer patients treated with anthracycline-based chemotherapy. Ann Oncol. 2006;17 (4):614–22.

404. Coiffier B, Altman A, Pui CH, Younes A, Cairo MS. Guidelines for the management of pediatric and adult tumor lysis syndrome: an evidence-based review. J Clin Oncol. 2008;26(16):2767–78.

405. Bussel JB, Cheng G, Saleh MN, Psaila B, Kovaleva L, Meddeb B, et al. Eltrombopag for the treatment of chronic idiopathic thrombocytopenic purpura. New Engl J Med. 2007;357 (22):2237–47.

406. Cheng G, Saleh MN, Marcher C, Vasey S, Mayer B, Aivado M, et al. Eltrombopag for management of chronic immune thrombocytopenia (RAISE): a 6-month, randomised, phase 3 study. Lancet. 2011;377(9763):393–402.

407. McHutchison JG, Dusheiko G, Shiffman ML, Rodriguez-Torres M, Sigal S, Bourliere M, et al. Eltrombopag for thrombocytopenia in patients with cirrhosis associated with hepatitis C. New Engl J Med. 2007;357(22):2227–36.

408. Henke M, Alfonsi M, Foa P, Giralt J, Bardet E, Cerezo L, et al. Palifermin decreases severe oral mucositis of patients undergoing postoperative radiochemotherapy for head and neck cancer: a randomized, placebo-controlled trial. J Clin Oncol. 2011;29 (20):2815–20.

409. Stiff PJ, Emmanouilides C, Bensinger WI, Gentile T, Blazar B, Shea TC, et al. Palifermin reduces patient-reported mouth and throat soreness and improves patient functioning in the hematopoietic stem-cell transplantation setting. J Clin Oncol. 2006;24(33):5186–93.

410. Brizel DM, Wasserman TH, Henke M, Strnad V, Rudat V, Monnier A, et al. Phase III randomized trial of amifostine as a radioprotector in head and neck cancer. J Clin Oncol. 2000;18 (19):3339–45.

411. Stopeck AT, Lipton A, Body JJ, Steger GG, Tonkin K, de Boer RH, et al. Denosumab compared with zoledronic acid for the treatment of bone metastases in patients with advanced breast cancer: a randomized, double-blind study. J Clin Oncol. 2010;28 (35):5132–9.

412. Bussel JB, Kuter DJ, Pullarkat V, Lyons RM, Guo M, Nichol JL. Safety and efficacy of long-term treatment with romiplostim in thrombocytopenic patients with chronic ITP. Blood. 2009;113 (10):2161–71.

413. Kuter DJ, Bussel JB, Lyons RM, Pullarkat V, Gernsheimer TB, Senecal FM, et al. Efficacy of romiplostim in patients with chronic immune thrombocytopenic purpura: a double-blind randomised controlled trial. Lancet. 2008;371(9610):395–403.

414. Hammack J. Neurologic complications of chemo-therapy and biologic therapies. In: Schiff D, O'Neill BP, editors. Principles of neuro-oncology. New York: McGraw-Hill; 2005. p. 679–710.

Neurological Complications of Targeted Therapies

16

Deborah A. Forst and Patrick Y. Wen

Introduction

As our understanding of the molecular drivers of cancers has grown, drug development in oncology has increasingly shifted from a focus on cytotoxic chemotherapy to the production of targeted agents designed to address specific molecular targets that drive tumor growth. Targeted agents include monoclonal antibodies and antibody–drug conjugates, as well as small molecule inhibitors; they are typically more tolerable than their cytotoxic counterparts, but carry their own unique toxicities [1, 2]. Most targeted therapies are well tolerated from the neurologic standpoint, in part because many of them penetrate across the blood–brain barrier poorly, and serious neurologic complications are fortunately uncommon. In this chapter, we will discuss the neurologic complications that have been described with the use of these targeted therapies, including small molecule inhibitors, antibodies/antibody–drug conjugates, and antiangiogenic agents.

Antiangiogenic Agents

Angiogenesis is an inherent feature of malignant neoplasms, and has been correlated with tumor growth, invasiveness, metastatic potential, and prognosis [3, 4]. The concept of anti-angiogenesis as a potential therapeutic target in cancer treatment was introduced by Judah Folkman more than 40 years ago, and the 1990s saw a boom in the development of anti-angiogenic agents, with primary targets including vascular endothelial growth factor (VEGF) and the vascular

D.A. Forst (✉)
Department of Neuro-Oncology, Massachusetts General Hospital, 55 Fruit Street, Yawkey 9E, Boston, MA 02142, USA
e-mail: dforst@partners.org

P.Y. Wen
Center for Neuro-Oncology, Dana-Farber/Brigham and Women's Cancer Center, 450 Brookline Avenue, Boston, MA 02215, USA
e-mail: pywen@partners.org

© Springer International Publishing AG 2018
D. Schiff et al. (eds.), *Cancer Neurology in Clinical Practice*,
DOI 10.1007/978-3-319-57901-6_16

endothelial growth factor receptor (VEGFR) [5, 6]. This section will discuss the neurologic complications associated with the use of anti-angiogenic agents, including monoclonal antibodies, small molecule inhibitors, and immunomodulatory anti-angiogenic agents (thalidomide and its analogs); this information is summarized in Table 16.1.

Monoclonal Antibodies

Bevacizumab

Bevacizumab is a recombinant, humanized monoclonal antibody against VEGF-A, and is approved by the United States Food and Drug Administration (U.S. FDA) for use in the treatment of metastatic colorectal cancer, advanced nonsquamous non-small cell lung cancer, platinum-resistant ovarian cancer, advanced cervical cancer, metastatic renal cell carcinoma, and recurrent glioblastoma [7]. Although bevacizumab is generally well tolerated, there are a few rare but serious neurologic complications. Use of bevacizumab is associated with an increased rate of intracranial hemorrhage, with incidence ranging from 0.3 to 0.7% in patients with systemic tumors [8, 9]. In patients with brain metastases or primary brain tumors, the incidence is increased and ranges from 0.8 to 3.3%; this is slightly increased from the baseline rate of spontaneous intracranial hemorrhage in patients with these tumors not treated with anti-angiogenic agents (Fig. 16.1) [8, 10, 11]. Patients receiving bevacizumab are thought to have an increased risk of arterial thromboembolic events, including ischemic stroke (Fig. 16.2). In a meta-analysis of 1745 patients with metastatic cancer, treatment with bevacizumab plus chemotherapy in comparison with chemotherapy alone resulted in an increased risk of an arterial thromboembolic event with a hazard ratio of 2.0 and an absolute rate of 5.5 events per 100 person-years. Of 37 patients with thromboembolic events noted in this study, there were 16 cerebrovascular events (stroke or TIA); rates were higher in patients over 65 years old or with a prior

Table 16.1 Neurological complications of antiangiogenic agents

Agent	Therapeutic target(s)/ mechanism of action	Use(s) in cancer treatment	Common neurologic toxicities (≥ 10% of patients)	Rare neurologic toxicities (<10%)
Monoclonal antibodies				
Bevacizumab	VEGF-A	Metastatic colorectal cancer, nonsquamous NSCLC, platinum-resistant ovarian cancer, advanced cervical cancer, metastatic renal cell carcinoma, recurrent glioblastoma	–	Ischemic stroke, intracranial hemorrhage, RPLS, optic neuropathy
Ramucirumab	VEGFR2	Metastatic NSCLC, advanced or metastatic gastric or GE junction cancer	–	Headache, cerebral ischemia, RPLS
Ziv-aflibercept	VGFR-1/2 + IgG1 Fc fusion protein	Metastatic colorectal cancer	Headache	Arterial thrombotic events; RPLS
Tyrosine kinase inhibitors				
Lenvatinib mesylate	VEGFR, FGFR, RET, KIT, PDGFRα	Progressive radioactive iodine-refractory differentiated thyroid cancer	Headache	Cerebrovascular ischemic event, TIA, intracranial hemorrhage, seizures, RPLS
Sorafenib tosylate	VEGFR, PDGFR, Raf kinase, KIT, FLT-3	Renal cell carcinoma, hepatocellular carcinoma, radioactive iodine-refractory thyroid cancer	–	Ischemic stroke
Sunitinib	VEGFR, PDGFR, KIT	Renal cell carcinoma, pancreatic neuroendocrine tumors, imatinib-resistant GIST	–	Ischemic stroke, reversible cognitive dysfunction with extrapyramidal symptoms, RPLS
Pazopanib	VEGFR, PDGFR, FGFR, Itk, c-Fms	Renal cell carcinoma, soft tissue sarcoma	Headache	Stroke, TIA, intracranial hemorrhage, RPLS
Ponatinib	BCR-ABL, VEGFR, PDGFR, FGFR, ephrin receptor, Src family kinases, c-Kit, RET, TIE2, FLT-3	CML, Philadelphia chromosome-positive ALL	Headache, venous and arterial thrombotic events including stroke, peripheral neuropathy	–
Regorafenib	VEGFR, PDGFR, FGFR, TIE2, KIT, RET, RAF1, BRAF, mutant BRAF	Advanced GIST, metastatic colorectal cancer	–	Sensory neuropathy, headache, RPLS, transverse myelopathy
Axitinib	VEGFR	Renal cell carcinoma	–	Arterial thrombotic events, RPLS
Immunomodulatory agents				
Thalidomide	Immune mediating and anti-angiogenic properties	Multiple myeloma	Somnolence, Treatment-emergent peripheral neuropathy (dose-dependent and cumulative)	Reversible altered mental status, worsening of preexisting Parkinson's disease
Lenalidomide	Second-generation thalidomide analog	Multiple myeloma, mantle cell lymphoma, transfusion-dependent anemia in MDS	–	Peripheral neuropathy, reversible cognitive/memory deficits and aphasia
Pomalidomide	Second-generation thalidomide analog	Multiple myeloma	–	Peripheral neuropathy, reversible aphasia

AIDP acute inflammatory demyelinating polyneuropathy, *ALL* acute lymphoblastic leukemia, *ALK* anaplastic lymphoma kinase, *BCR-ABL* breakpoint cluster region-Abelson murine leukemia viral oncogene homolog 1, *BTK* Bruton's tyrosine kinase, *CDK* cyclin-dependent kinase, *c-Fms* colony-stimulating factor 1 receptor , *CLL* chronic lymphocytic leukemia, *CML* chronic myelogenous leukemia, *EGFR* epidermal growth factor receptor, *ER* estrogen receptor, *FLT-3* FMS-like tyrosine kinase 3, *GIST* gastrointestinal stromal tumor, *HDAC* histone deacetylase, *HER* human epidermal growth factor receptor, *JAK* Janus kinase, *MDS* myelodysplastic syndrome, *MEK* mitogen-activated protein kinase kinase, *MPD* myeloproliferative disorder, *mTOR* mammalian target of rapamycin, *NHL* non-Hodgkin lymphoma, *NSCLC* non-small cell lung cancer, *PARP* poly (ADP-ribose) polymerase, *PDGFR* platelet-derived growth factor receptor, *PI3K* phosphoinositide-3-kinase, *RCC* renal cell carcinoma, *RET* REarranged during Transfection, *RPLS* reversible posterior leukoencephalopathy syndrome, *SEGA* subependymal giant cell astrocytoma, *SMO* smoothened, *TIA* transient ischemic attack, *VEGFR* vascular endothelial growth factor receptor

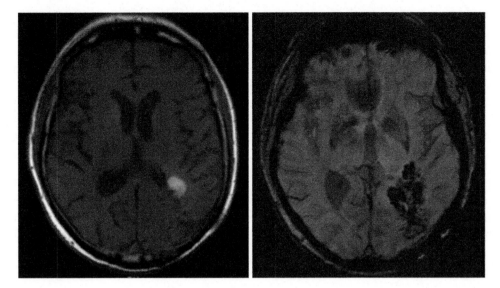

Fig. 16.1 Bevacizumab-related intracranial hemorrhage. MRI of the brain in a 72-year-old man with a *left* parietotemporal glioblastoma on bevacizumab therapy, who was found to have evidence of subacute hemorrhage on MRI. The T1-weighted image on the *left* shows a hyperintense signal abnormality in the *left* posterior periventricular area, consistent with blood. In the susceptibility weighted imaging (SWI) sequence on the *right*, there are hypointense signal changes in the *left* posterior periventricular region, consistent with blood products

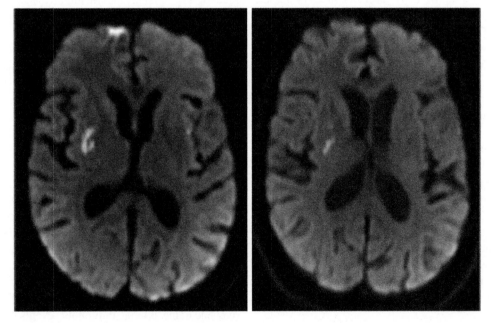

Fig. 16.2 Bevacizumab-related ischemic stroke. MRI of the brain in a 71-year-old woman with a left frontal anaplastic astrocytoma on bevacizumab therapy, who presented with an episode of slurred speech. The diffusion weighted imaging (DWI) sequences show hyperintense signal abnormalities in the right basal ganglia, consistent with acute ischemia. (Image courtesy of Ivana Vodopivec, M.D., Ph.D., Brigham and Women's Hospital.)

arterial thrombotic event. [12]. A retrospective study of recurrent high-grade glioma patients treated with bevacizumab in clinical trials found the incidence of ischemic stroke to be 1.9%, or 0.38 cases per 100 patient-months [13]. Bevacizumab administration also has been associated with the development of the rare clinical-radiologic Posterior Reversible Encephalopathy Syndrome (PRES), also known as the Reversible Posterior Leukoencephalopathy Syndrome (RPLS). This syndrome has been described in association with a variety of medications, including angiogenesis inhibitors, and is characterized by neurological symptoms including headache, visual disturbance, confusion, and seizures, in conjunction with subcortical/white matter abnormalities, including prominent vasogenic edema, especially in the parietal and occipital lobes, on MRI [14, 15]. These symptoms usually resolve with supportive care. Rarely, optic neuropathy has been described in association with bevacizumab, with an incidence of 1.2% in one study [16]. Of note, all of the patients in that study had also received radiation to the brain for glioblastoma, but at doses felt to be safe to the optic nerves; in comparison, the incidence of severe optic neuropathy in patients receiving radiation but not bevacizumab was 0.2% [16]. Another case series reported three patients with glioblastoma previously treated with radiation therapy who developed optic neuropathy following bevacizumab use [17].

Ramucirumab

Ramucirumab is a humanized monoclonal antibody against VEGFR2 and was approved by the FDA in 2014 for the treatment of progressive metastatic non-small cell lung cancer (NSCLC) and for the treatment of advanced or metastatic gastric or gastroesophageal junction cancer. Neurologic complications are rare, and include headache in 9% of patients, arterial thromboembolic events (including cerebrovascular accident, cerebral ischemia, cardiac arrest, myocardial infarction) in 1.7%, and RPLS in <0.1% [18].

Ziv-Aflibercept

Ziv-aflibercept is a recombinant fusion protein comprised of VEGF-binding portions from VEGFR-1 and -2 fused to the Fc portion of the human immunoglobulin IgG1. In August 2012, it received FDA approval for use in combination with 5-fluorouracil, leucovorin and irinotecan (the FOLFIRI regimen) in patients with progressive metastatic colorectal cancer after oxaliplatin therapy. Headache is a common side effect; rare but potentially serious neurologic complications include arterial thrombotic events and RPLS [19].

VEGF Receptor Tyrosine Kinase Inhibitors

Lenvatinib Mesylate

Lenvatinib is an oral inhibitor of VEGFR 1, 2, and 3, as well as an inhibitor of fibroblast growth factor receptors (FGFR) 1, 2, 3, and 4, REarranged during Transfection (RET), KIT, and platelet-derived growth factor receptor alpha (PDGFRα). It was approved by the U.S. FDA in February 2015 for the treatment of locally recurrent or metastatic radioactive iodine-refractory differentiated thyroid cancer. In the Phase III clinical trial, headache was common,

experienced in 27.6% of treated patients versus 6.1% of patients receiving placebo. About 3.6% of patients experienced a serious neurologic complication, including cerebrovascular ischemic event, TIA, intracranial hemorrhage, seizures or RPLS [20].

Sorafenib Tosylate

Sorafenib is a multikinase inhibitor active against numerous targets, including VEGFR-2 and -3, PDGFR, Raf kinase, KIT and FMS-like tyrosine kinase 3 (FLT-3), and is used in the treatment of renal cell carcinoma, hepatocellular carcinoma, and radioactive iodine-refractory thyroid cancer. The most concerning potential neurologic complication associated with sorafenib use is stroke; a meta-analysis of clinical trials using sorafenib and sunitinib found a threefold increased risk of arterial thrombotic events, including ischemic stroke [21].

Sunitinib

Sunitinib is a multikinase inhibitor with targets including VEGFR, PDGFR, and KIT, and is approved for use in metastatic renal cell carcinoma, progressive pancreatic neuroendocrine tumors, and imatinib-resistant gastrointestinal stromal tumor. Sunitinib has been associated with increased risk of ischemic stroke, with threefold increased risk of arterial thrombotic events, including ischemic stroke, in a meta-analysis of clinical trials using sorafenib and sunitinib [21]. A reversible syndrome of cognitive dysfunction has been described, with symptoms including confusion, language problems, extrapyramidal symptoms, and gait abnormalities [22]. RPLS also has been reported in association with sunitinib therapy [23].

Pazopanib

Pazopanib is a multi-tyrosine kinase inhibitor of VEGFR, PDGFR, KIT, fibroblast growth factor receptor (FGFR), interleukin-2 receptor inducible T-cell kinase (Itk), and colony-stimulating factor 1 receptor (c-Fms) that is FDA approved for the treatment of advanced renal cell carcinoma and advanced soft tissue sarcoma. Headache has been in reported in 10–23% of patients; serious adverse events are rare, including arterial thrombotic events [stroke and transient ischemic attack (TIA)] and central nervous system (CNS) hemorrhage (subarachnoid hemorrhage, intracranial hemorrhage) [24–26]. Cases of RPLS also have been described [27–29].

Ponatinib

Ponatinib is an oral multi-target tyrosine kinase inhibitor designed as a pan-BCR-ABL inhibitor but also targeting VEGFR, PDGFR, FGFR, ephrin receptor, Src family kinases, c-Kit, RET, tunica interna endothelial cell kinase 2 (TIE2), and FLT-3 [30]. It received accelerated FDA approval in 2012 for the treatment of patients with chronic myeloid leukemia (CML) or Philadelphia chromosome-positive acute lymphoblastic leukemia, whose disease was resistant or intolerant to prior tyrosine kinase inhibitor therapy [30]. Headache was common in clinical trial participants, and arterial thrombotic events were noted, with cerebrovascular events considered to be at least possibly attributable to the drug in 0.7% of patients in the initial study [31]. Additional data gathered after initial FDA approval showed a high incidence of venous and arterial thrombotic events, some of which were fatal or life-threatening, noted in approximately 24% of patients in the phase II trial and 48% of patients in the phase I trial. This led to temporary suspension of ponatinib marketing and sales by the FDA, a black box warning on the drug, and cancelation of a planned randomized trial of imatinib versus ponatinib [31, 32]. Peripheral neuropathy has been reported in 13% of ponatinib-treated patients (2% grade 3–4) [33].

Regorafenib

Regorafenib is an oral multikinase inhibitor active against VEGFR, PDGFR, FGFR, TIE2, KIT, RET, RAF1, BRAF, and mutant BRAF [34]. It is approved by the U.S. Food and Drug Administration for the treatment of advanced gastrointestinal stromal tumors and previously treated metastatic colorectal cancer. Neurologic side effects are rare; in the colorectal cancer trials, sensory neuropathy was reported in 7% of patients receiving regorafenib (vs. 4% receiving placebo) and headache in 5% of regorafenib patients (vs. 3% with placebo) [34]. There are isolated case reports of RPLS [35] and transverse myelopathy (in a patient previously treated with stereotactic body radiation therapy) [36].

Axitinib

Axitinib is a potent, selective, second-generation inhibitor of VEGFR-1, -2, and -3 [37]. It is FDA approved for the treatment of advanced renal cell carcinoma. Neurologic side effects are rare, but as with other agents of this class, serious adverse effects including arterial thrombotic events and RPLS have been described [38].

Immunomodulatory Anti-angiogenic Agents (Thalidomide and Its Analogs)

Thalidomide

Thalidomide was the first immunomodulatory drug approved for use in multiple myeloma, and has potent immune mediating and antiangiogenic properties [39]. Frequent but mild (grade 1–2) neurologic side effects in the phase II multiple myeloma trial included (at the 200 mg/day dose) somnolence in 34%, tingling or numbness in 12%,

incoordination in 16%, tremors in 10%, and headache in 12% [40]. The most prominent neurologic complication associated with thalidomide use is peripheral neuropathy, which has been reported in 23–70% of patients, and appears to be dose-dependent (worse with doses in excess of 200 mg per day) and cumulative with longer duration of treatment. Length-dependent sensory neuropathy is most commonly reported, and autonomic neuropathy is thought to mediate some thalidomide-related side effects including constipation, orthostatic hypotension, bradycardia and sexual dysfunction; motor symptoms are rare [41]. Other than somnolence, CNS toxicity is uncommon. There is a reported case of thalidomide-induced altered mental status progressing to coma, promptly reversed with drug discontinuation [42]. Thalidomide has also been associated with worsening of preexisting Parkinson's disease [43].

Lenalidomide

Lenalidomide is a second-generation immunomodulatory agent derived from thalidomide, initially approved for use in transfusion-dependent anemia in patients with myelodysplastic syndrome, and subsequently approved for use in multiple myeloma and mantle cell lymphoma. In addition to its immunomodulatory effects, it has direct cytotoxic and antiangiogenic properties [39]. In contrast to thalidomide, lenalidomide is much less neurotoxic; although mild to moderate neuropathy during treatment has been reported, the phase III trial of lenalidomide plus dexamethasone in comparison with lenalidomide alone in relapsed multiple myeloma showed no significant increase in the incidence of peripheral neuropathy in lenalidomide-treated patients [41]. Lenalidomide use rarely has been associated with CNS toxicity, with case reports of reversible cognitive decline, memory problems and expressive language difficulties [42].

Pomalidomide

Pomalidomide is a second-generation thalidomide analog approved for the treatment of progressive multiple myeloma. From the neurologic standpoint, it is generally well tolerated, with 9% of patients experiencing grades 1–2 peripheral neuropathy and no reported cases of grades 3–4 neuropathy in clinical trials [44, 45]. CNS toxicity is uncommon, with one case report of reversible expressive language difficulties associated with pomalidomide use [42].

Small Molecule Inhibitors that Do not Target VEGFR

The growing shift from cytotoxic chemotherapy toward targeted molecular therapy has led to a revolution in drug development, with the rise of many new small molecule drugs designed to inhibit specific cancer targets. This was particularly spurred by the discovery of the BCR-ABL translocation [breakpoint cluster region (BCR)—Abelson murine leukemia viral oncogene homolog 1 (ABL)] as a driver of chronic myeloid leukemia, and the successful use of imatinib, a BCR-ABL inhibitor, to treat these patients [46]. Since then, small molecules have been developed to inhibit varied targets that play a role in oncogenesis in different cancers, many of which are kinase inhibitors. Overall, small molecule inhibitors have relatively few neurologic complications as a class. This section will review the neurologic complications that have been described with treatment using these small molecules, including tyrosine kinase inhibitors, serine/threonine kinase inhibitors, lipid kinase inhibitors, histone deacetylase inhibitors, poly (ADP-ribose) polymerase (PARP) inhibitors, smoothened (SMO) inhibitors, and proteasome inhibitors. This information is summarized in Table 16.2.

Table 16.2 Neurological complications of small molecule inhibitors

Agent	Therapeutic target(s)/ mechanism of action	Use(s) in cancer treatment	Common neurologic toxicities ($\geq$ 10% of patients)	Rare neurologic toxicities (<10%)
Proteasome inhibitors				
Bortezomib	Reversible inhibitor of 26S proteasome	Multiple myeloma; mantle cell lymphoma	Peripheral neuropathy (sensory > autonomic > motor)	RPLS
Carfilzomib	Second-generation proteasome inhibitor	Progressive multiple myeloma	Peripheral neuropathy	–
Tyrosine kinase inhibitors				
Erlotinib Hydrochloride	EGFR	NSCLC	None	Stroke (in combination with gemcitabine)
Gefitinib	EGFR	NSCLC	None	–
Afatinib Dimaleate	EGFR, HER2, HER4	NSCLC	None	–
Lapatinib Ditosylate	EGFR1, HER2	HER2 overexpressing breast cancer	Headache	–
Vandetanib	EGFR, RET, VEGFR2	Medullary thyroid cancer	Headache	Back pain, RPLS, cerebral ischemia, TIA
Crizotinib	ALK, MET, ROS1	ALK-rearranged NSCLC	Visual changes, dizziness	–
Ceritinib	ALK	ALK-rearranged NSCLC	Headache, dizziness	Muscle spasms, dysphonia, tremor, convulsion
Cabozantinib	MET, VEGFR2, RET	Medullary thyroid cancer	Dysphonia, back pain, headache, dizziness	RPLS, hemorrhage, venous and arterial thrombosis
Imatinib	BCR-ABL, PDGFR, c-Fms, c-Kit	CML, ALL, chronic eosinophilic leukemia, dermatofibrosarcoma protuberans, GIST, MDS/MPD, systemic mastocytosis	Headache, muscle spasms	Intraparenchymal hemorrhage, subdural hemorrhage
Nilotinib	BCR-ABL	CML	Headache	Muscle spasm, CNS hemorrhage
Dasatinib	BCR-ABL, SRC family kinases (Lyn, Src)	ALL, CML	Headache	Subdural hemorrhage
Bosutinib	SRC/ABL1	CML	Headache	Muscle spasms
Ponatinib	BCR-ABL, VEGFR, PDGFR, FGFR, ephrin receptor, Src family kinases, c-Kit, RET, TIE2, FLT-3	CML, Philadelphia chromosome-positive ALL	Headache, venous and arterial thrombotic events including stroke, peripheral neuropathy	–

(continued)

Table 16.2 (continued)

Agent	Therapeutic target(s)/ mechanism of action	Use(s) in cancer treatment	Common neurologic toxicities ($\geq 10\%$ of patients)	Rare neurologic toxicities (<10%)
Ibrutinib	BTK	CLL, mantle cell lymphoma, Waldenström's macroglobulinemia	Back pain	Subdural hematoma, confusional state
Ruxolitinib	JAK1 and 2	Polycythemia vera, myelofibrosis	Headache, muscle spasms, dizziness	–
Serine/threonine kinase inhibitors				
Vemurafenib	BRAF	Melanoma	Headache	Facial palsy, AIDP
Dabrafenib	BRAF	Melanoma	–	Headache
Sorafenib	VEGFR, PDGFR, Raf kinase, KIT, FLT-3	Renal cell carcinoma, hepatocellular carcinoma, radioactive iodine-refractory thyroid cancer	–	Ischemic stroke
Trametinib	MEK	Melanoma	–	Ocular toxicity (blurred vision, chorioretinopathy)
Palbociclib	CDK4, CDK6	ER+ metastatic breast cancer	Headache, dizziness, peripheral neuropathy	–
Lipid kinase inhibitors				
Idelalisib	PI3K delta	CLL, follicular B-cell NHL, small lymphocytic lymphoma	Headache	–
Histone deacetylase inhibitors				
Vorinostat	HDAC	Cutaneous T-cell lymphoma	Muscle spasms, headache	–
Belinostat	HDAC	Peripheral T-cell lymphoma	Dizziness, headache	Apraxia
Romidepsin	HDAC	Cutaneous T-cell lymphoma	Headache	–
Panobinostat	HDAC	Multiple myeloma	Headache, dizziness, back pain, peripheral neuropathy	–
mTOR inhibitors				
Everolimus	mTOR	Breast cancer, pancreatic cancer, RCC, SEGA in tuberous sclerosis patients	Convulsions[a], headache	–
Sirolimus	mTOR	Immunosuppression in solid organ transplant, lymphangioleiomyomatosis	–	RPLS
Temsirolimus	mTOR	Advanced RCC	–	CNS hemorrhage
Smoothened inhibitors				
Vismodegib	SMO	Basal Cell Carcinoma	Muscle spasms	–
Sonidegib	SMO	Basal Cell Carcinoma	Muscle spasms, headache	–
PARP inhibitors				
Olaparib	PARP	Ovarian cancer	Headache, peripheral neuropathy	Hemorrhagic stroke

[a]In tuberous sclerosis patients; frequency not increased in comparison with placebo

AIDP acute inflammatory demyelinating polyneuropathy, *ALL* acute lymphoblastic leukemia, *ALK* anaplastic lymphoma kinase, BCR-ABL breakpoint cluster region-Abelson murine leukemia viral oncogene homolog 1, *BTK* Bruton's tyrosine kinase, *CDK* cyclin-dependent kinase, *c-Fms* colony-stimulating factor 1 receptor , *CLL* chronic lymphocytic leukemia, *CML* chronic myelogenous leukemia, *CNS* central nervous system, *EGFR* epidermal growth factor receptor, *ER* estrogen receptor, *FLT-3* FMS-like tyrosine kinase 3, *GIST* gastrointestinal stromal tumor, *HDAC* histone deacetylase, *HER* human epidermal growth factor receptor, *JAK* Janus kinase, *MDS* myelodysplastic syndrome, *MEK* mitogen-activated protein kinase kinase, *MPD* Myeloproliferative disorder, mTOR mammalian target of rapamycin, *NHL* non-Hodgkin lymphoma, *NSCLC* non-small cell lung cancer, *PARP* poly (ADP-ribose) polymerase, *PDGFR* platelet-derived growth factor receptor, *PI3K* phosphoinositide-3-kinase, *RCC* renal cell carcinoma, *RET* REarranged during Transfection, *RPLS* reversible posterior leukoencephalopathy syndrome, *SEGA* subependymal giant cell astrocytoma, *SMO* smoothened, *TIA* transient ischemic attack, *TIE2* tunica interna endothelial cell kinase, *VEGFR* vascular endothelial growth factor receptor

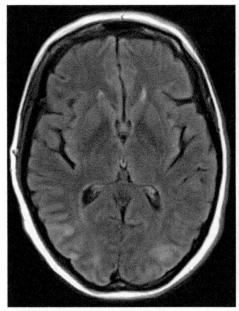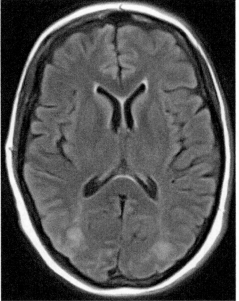

Fig. 16.3 Bortezomib-Induced Posterior Reversible Encephalopathy Syndrome MRI of the brain in a 66-year-old woman recently treated with bortezomib for multiple myeloma, who presented with new onset of seizures. The T2/FLAIR images shown are notable for fairly symmetric cortical and subcortical hyperintense signal abnormalities with a posterior predominance (Image courtesy of Aaron Berkowitz, M. D., Ph.D., Brigham and Women's Hospital.)

Proteasome Inhibitors

Bortezomib

Bortezomib is a reversible inhibitor of the 26S proteasome, and is FDA approved for the treatment of multiple myeloma and patients with mantle cell lymphoma who have received at least one prior therapy [47]. The most significant neurotoxicity associated with bortezomib is treatment-emergent peripheral neuropathy. In studies of treatment-naïve multiple myeloma patients receiving bortezomib, 40–64% of patients experienced peripheral neuropathy, with 14–30% requiring dose decrease or discontinuation; it was the most common reason for drug discontinuation [48]. There is a cumulative dose effect through the first five cycles of treatment, and there has been some suggestion that the route of administration may have an impact, with one study showing significantly decreased incidence of neuropathy with subcutaneous versus intravenous administration [49]. Bortezomib typically causes a painful, length-dependent, axonal sensory neuropathy which is often at least partly reversible upon discontinuation of treatment [47]. Neurologic examination, nerve conduction studies and electromyography are often normal except in severe cases [50]. Constipation and orthostasis, noted in 10–15% of patients receiving bortezomib, are thought to be largely mediated by autonomic neuropathy. Motor nerve involvement is rare [41]. Other than neuropathy, neurologic complications are rare, although isolated cases of bortezomib-induced PRES have been reported (Fig. 16.3) [51, 52].

Carfilzomib

Carfilzomib is a second-generation proteasome inhibitor that is FDA approved as monotherapy for the treatment of progressive multiple myeloma in patients previously on treatment with bortezomib and an immunomodulatory agent, and in combination with lenalidomide and dexamethasone in patients with recurrent multiple myeloma previously treated with one to three other regimens. Carfilzomib has significantly less neurotoxicity than bortezomib; this is felt to be possibly explained by the off-target effects on non-proteasome serine proteases seen with bortezomib but not carfilzomib [53]. In an integrated safety analysis of four phase II clinical trials using single-agent carfilzomib, 84.8% of patients had a history of treatment-related peripheral neuropathy (from bortezomib or thalidomide), with 71.9% of patients with active peripheral neuropathy at the time of trial enrollment (all grades 1 or 2). However, there were infrequent reports of neuropathy as an adverse side effect in these trials, reported in 13.9% of patients overall, the majority of which were grades 1–2 (1.3% of patients experienced grade 3 peripheral neuropathy, all in patients with preexisting grade 1–2 neuropathy at baseline). There was no grade 4 neuropathy and as neuropathy appeared to arise early in treatment, there was no evidence of cumulative toxicity [54].

Tyrosine Kinase Inhibitors

Epidermal Growth Factor Receptor Inhibitors

Erlotinib Hydrochloride

Erlotinib is an EGFR tyrosine kinase inhibitor that is FDA approved for use as first-line treatment of EGFR mutant, metastatic non-small cell lung cancer, as well as for pre-treated advanced or metastatic non-small cell lung cancer. It is also approved for use in conjunction with gemcitabine hydrochloride in the treatment of pancreatic cancer. In the original lung cancer trials, neurologic side effects were uncommon [55]. Death related to stroke was reported in a phase III trial using erlotinib in combination with gemcitabine in patients with advanced pancreatic cancer; this was ultimately attributed to a combination of cancer and treatment-related complications [56].

Gefitinib

The EGFR inhibitor gefitinib received accelerated FDA approval in 2003 for the treatment of locally advanced or metastatic non-small cell lung cancer, based on the use of tumor response rate as a surrogate endpoint for clinical efficacy in clinical trials. In 2005, after follow-up studies failed to show an overall survival benefit, its use in the United States was subsequently limited to patients who were currently or previously benefiting from its use [57]. In 2015, it received additional FDA approval for use in metastatic non-small cell lung cancer with specified epidermal growth factor receptor gene mutations [58]. It remains the more widely used EGFR tyrosine kinase inhibitor in Europe and Asia, and is under ongoing investigation in lung cancer and other malignancies [59]. Gefitinib is well tolerated from the neurologic perspective, with no significant adverse neurologic side effects [60].

Afatinib Dimaleate

Afatinib, an irreversible inhibitor of EGFR, human epidermal growth factor receptor 2 (HER2) and HER4, is FDA approved for the treatment of EGFR mutant, metastatic non-small cell lung cancer. There are no significant neurologic side effects commonly associated with afatinib therapy [61, 62]

Lapatinib Ditosylate

Lapatinib is an oral small molecule HER2 and EGFR1 tyrosine kinase inhibitor. It is FDA approved for use in combination with letrozole or capecitabine in the treatment of patients with HER2 overexpressing breast cancer. Other than headache, neurologic complications are not commonly described [63, 64].

Vandetanib

Vandetanib, an oral selective inhibitor of EGFR, RET and VEGFR2 signaling, is FDA approved for the treatment of unresectable, locally advanced, or metastatic medullary thyroid cancer. In a randomized, double-blind, phase III trial of vandetanib versus placebo in patients with locally advanced or metastatic thyroid cancer, headache was common, noted in 26% of patients, and back pain was experienced by 9% of patients receiving vandetanib (vs. 20% in the placebo arm) [65]. Serious neurologic events were similar to those seen with other anti-VEGF agents, including RPLS and an increased risk of cerebrovascular events (cerebral ischemia or transient ischemic attack were noted in 1.3% of patients in the vandetanib arm and no patients in the control arm) [66].

Anaplastic Lymphoma Kinase (ALK) Inhibitors

Crizotinib

Rearrangements of the ALK gene with the echinoderm microtubule associated protein like 4 (EML4) result in a fusion oncogene EML4-ALK which is present in 3–5% of non-small cell lung cancer. Crizotinib, a small molecule inhibitor of ALK, MET and ROS1 tyrosine kinases, is FDA approved for the treatment of ALK-rearranged non-small cell lung cancer, with clinical trials showing superiority to standard chemotherapy in patients with progressive tumors. It is generally neurologically well tolerated, although visual side effects are common and may include diplopia, photopsia, chromatopsia, blurred vision, impaired vision, and vitreous floaters. Dizziness, generally mild, occurred in about 20% of patients in clinical studies [67, 68].

Ceritinib

In April 2014, certinib, an oral, small molecule tyrosine kinase inhibitor of ALK, received accelerated FDA approval for the treatment of ALK-rearranged non-small cell lung cancer with progression on (or intolerance to) crizotinib, due to evidence of significant and durable treatment responses [69]. Neurologic adverse events (regardless of attribution to study drug) in phase I clinical trial data included headache (15%), dizziness (11%), muscle spasms (8%), dysphonia (7%), tremor (7%), and convulsion (6%) [70].

MET Inhibitors

Cabozantinib

Cabozantinib is an inhibitor of MET, VEGFR2, and RET that is FDA approved for the treatment of metastatic medullary thyroid cancer. It is associated with significant toxicity, requiring dose reduction in 79% of patients in the phase III trial.

With regard to neurologic toxicity, side effects noted in 10% or more of patients included dysphonia, back pain, headache, and dizziness. RPLS was reported in one patient, and other VEGF inhibitor-associated complications were seen, including hemorrhage, venous thrombosis, and arterial thrombosis [71].

Crizotinib

Crizotinib, a small molecule inhibitor of ALK, MET and ROS1 tyrosine kinases, is FDA approved for the treatment of ALK-rearranged non-small cell lung cancer. Neurologic complications associated with this agent are discussed in greater detail earlier in this chapter.

BCR-ABL Inhibitors

Imatinib Mesylate

Imatinib is a potent inhibitor of BCR-ABL, PDGFRα, PDGFRβ, c-Fms, and c-Kit tyrosine kinases. Initially pioneered in the treatment of Philadelphia chromosome-positive chronic myelogenous leukemia (CML), it is also FDA approved for the treatment of Philadelphia chromosome-positive acute lymphoblastic leukemia (ALL), chronic eosinophilic leukemia, dermatofibrosarcoma protuberans, gastrointestinal stromal tumor, myelodysplastic/myeloproliferative neoplasms, and systemic mastocytosis. Neurologic adverse effects include headache, which may be severe, and muscle spasms, which are generally mild and respond to treatment with quinine, calcium or magnesium [72–74]. In a phase I/II study of imatinib for the treatment of recurrent malignant gliomas, central nervous system hemorrhage was observed at a rate higher than the expected spontaneous hemorrhage rate in these patients [75]. Subdural hemorrhage in association with imatinib use also has been described [74, 76].

Nilotinib

The second-generation BCR-ABL tyrosine kinase inhibitor nilotinib has a higher selectivity and binding affinity than imatinib, and is FDA approved for the treatment of newly diagnosed and previously treated patients with CML [77]. Headaches (grade 3 or 4 in some cases, at higher incidence than with imatinib) and less commonly muscle spasm have been associated with nilotinib therapy. Rare cases of CNS hemorrhage have been described [72, 73].

Dasatinib

Dasatinib is a second-generation oral BCL-ABL inhibitor that also has activity against the SRC family kinases Lyn and Src. It is used in the treatment of Philadelphia chromosome-positive ALL and Philadelphia chromosome-positive CML. [78]. Headache, generally mild, is reported in 12–27% of patients [72, 79]. There have been several reported cases of spontaneous subdural hemorrhage

in patients on dasatinib treatment, including one case in the absence of thrombocytopenia; dasatinib-induced platelet dysfunction has been implicated as the putative mechanism [80, 81].

Bosutinib

Bosutinib is an oral, dual SRC/ABL1 tyrosine kinase inhibitor that is FDA approved for the treatment of patients with Philadelphia chromosome-positive CML, resistant to or intolerant of prior therapy. In long-term follow-up of the Bosutinib Efficacy and Safety in Newly Diagnosed CML trial (BELA trial), neurologic side effects included headache in 13% of bosutinib-treated patients (vs. 11% with imatinib) and muscle spasms in 4% of bosutinib-treated patients (vs. 22% of those treated with imatinib) [82].

Ponatinib

Ponatinib is an oral multi-target tyrosine kinase inhibitor designed as a pan-BCR-ABL inhibitor but also effective against VEGFR, PDGFR, FGFR, ephrin receptor, Src family kinases, c-Kit, RET, TIE2, and FLT-3 [30]. It is used in the treatment of patients with chronic myeloid leukemia (CML) or Philadelphia chromosome-positive acute lymphoblastic leukemia. Neurologic complications of this agent are described in greater detail earlier in this chapter.

Bruton's Tyrosine Kinase (BTK) Inhibitors

Ibrutinib

Ibrutinib is an irreversible non-receptor tyrosine kinase inhibitor that targets Bruton's tyrosine kinase, a B-cell receptor signaling component which plays a role in the pathogenesis of chronic lymphocytic leukemia [83]. It is FDA approved for use in the treatment of chronic lymphocytic leukemia, mantle cell lymphoma, and Waldenström's macroglobulinemia. In long-term follow-up of a phase II trial of 111 mantle cell lymphoma patients treated with single-agent ibrutinib, bleeding (including bruising) occurred in 50% of patients during the total study period, the majority of which were not neurologic. Subdural hematomas were reported in four patients, all of which were associated with head trauma and/or falls, and all four patients had received anti-platelet (aspirin) or anticoagulant (warfarin) agents in close proximity to the event. Other neurologic adverse events included confusional state in 3% of patients, and back pain [84].

Janus Kinase (JAK) Inhibitors

Ruxolitinib

The potent and selective JAK 1 and 2 inhibitor ruxolitinib is FDA approved for the treatment of polycythemia vera and for the treatment of intermediate and high-risk myelofibrosis. It is well tolerated from the neurologic standpoint. Although headache, dizziness, and muscle spasms have been described with its use, the phase III trial examining ruxolitinib in comparison with standard therapy in polycythemia vera found that 49% of patients treated with ruxolitinib had an at least 50% reduction in their Myeloproliferative Neoplasm Symptom Assessment Form (MPN-SAF), with decrease in hyperviscosity-related neurologic symptoms including vision problems, dizziness, concentration problems, headache, numbness or tingling in the hands or feet, and tinnitus [85, 86].

Serine/Threonine Kinase Inhibitors

BRAF Inhibitors

Vemurafenib

40–60% of cutaneous melanomas have activating mutations in BRAF at codon 600; 80–90% of these are the V600E valine to glutamic acid substitution. These mutations result in constitutive activation of the MAPK pathway and are thought to be a driver of melanoma proliferation [87, 88]. Vemurafenib is a potent BRAF inhibitor, and is FDA approved for the treatment of unresectable or metastatic melanoma with the BRAF V600E mutation. In the randomized trial which led to its approval, 675 previously untreated patients with BRAF V600E mutation positive metastatic or unresectable melanoma were randomized to treatment with vemurafenib versus dacarbazine. Headaches were common in the vemurafenib group (23.2% vs. 10.4% in the dacarbazine group). Otherwise, neurologic side effects were uncommon [89]. Rarely, there have been cases of facial palsy attributed to vemurafenib therapy [90]. There is an isolated case report of acute inflammatory demyelinating polyneuropathy (AIDP) in the setting of vemurafenib treatment, in a patient previously treated with nivolumab [91].

Dabrafenib

Dabrafenib is a reversible, competitive inhibitor of BRAF with selective inhibition of the BRAF V600E kinase. It is FDA approved alone or in conjunction with trametinib for the treatment of unresectable or metastatic melanoma with the BRAF V600E or V600 K mutation. There are no serious neurologic complications; in the phase III trial comparing dabrafenib with dacarbazine in melanoma patients, headache was noted in 5% of dabrafenib patients (vs. 0% with dacarbazine) but it was otherwise well tolerated from the neurologic standpoint [88].

Sorafenib

Sorafenib is a multikinase inhibitor active against numerous targets, including VEGFR-2 and -3, a PDGFR, Raf kinase, KIT and FLT-3, and is used in the treatment of renal cell carcinoma, hepatocellular carcinoma, and radioactive iodine-refractory thyroid cancer. Neurologic complications associated with this agent are described in detail earlier in this chapter.

Mitogen-Activated Protein Kinase Kinase (MEK) Inhibitors

Trametinib

Trametinib is a MEK inhibitor that is FDA approved for use in the treatment of patients with unresectable or metastatic melanoma with a BRAF V600E or V600K mutation. Ocular toxicities have been noted with trametinib administration, including blurred vision and chorioretinopathy. Neurologic side effects are uncommon [92].

Cyclin-Dependent Kinase (CDK) Inhibitors

Palbociclib

CDK4 and CDK6 signaling play a critical role in the G1 to S transition in the cell cycle; CDK inhibitors have been developed in an attempt to disrupt tumor cell growth and division. Palbociclib is FDA approved for the treatment of estrogen receptor-positive (ER+) metastatic breast cancer in postmenopausal women, in conjunction with letrozole, an aromatase inhibitor. In a phase II trial evaluating letrozole versus letrozole plus palbociclib, neurologic complications were relatively infrequent and mild (grades 1–2 only); headache was reported in 14% of patients in the combined therapy group (vs. 10% with letrozole alone), dizziness in 10% (vs. 4% with letrozole alone), and peripheral neuropathy in 10% of patients in the combined therapy group (vs. 5% with letrozole alone) [93].

Lipid Kinase Inhibitors

Phosphoinositide-3-Kinase (PI3K) Inhibitors

Idelalisib

PI3K delta plays a critical role in the growth and survival of malignant B lymphocytes [94]. Idelalisib is a selective PI3K delta inhibitor approved for the treatment of chronic lymphocytic leukemia (CLL) in conjunction with rituximab, as well as for the treatment of recurrent follicular B-cell non-Hodgkin lymphoma and small lymphocytic lymphoma.

In a phase II trial of 125 patients with indolent non-Hodgkin lymphoma treated with this agent, neurologic side effects were uncommon; headache was reported by 10% of patients receiving idelalisib [94]. Other PI3K inhibitors including buparlisib (BKM120), which produces reversible anxiety and irritability, are being tested in clinical trials, but have yet to receive FDA approval.

Histone Deacetylase (HDAC) Inhibitors

Vorinostat

Histone deacetylase inhibitors are thought to work in cancer treatment by interfering with epigenetic regulation of gene expression in tumor cells [95]. Vorinostat is a histone deacetylase (HDAC) inhibitor that is FDA approved for the treatment of cutaneous manifestations of cutaneous T-cell lymphoma, and its use is under investigation in other cancers including B-cell lymphoma, leukemia, non-small cell lung cancer, and multiple myeloma. There were no serious neurologic complications in the trial leading to its approval; muscle spasms were reported in 19.8% of patients and headaches in 11.6% of patients [95].

Belinostat

The second-generation, pan-HDAC inhibitor belinostat was granted accelerated FDA approval in July 2014 for the treatment of relapsed or refractory peripheral T-cell lymphoma. Belinostat has anti-angiogenic and antitumor effects. In the open-label phase II trial in which 53 patients were treated with this agent, neurologic side effects included dizziness in 20.8%, and headache in 13.2%. One patient experienced grade 3 apraxia felt to be related to the drug [96].

Romidepsin

Romidepsin is an HDAC inhibitor used in the treatment of cutaneous T-cell lymphoma. Other than headache (reported in 14% of patients in one study and 15% in another study (11% felt to be drug-related), all grades 1–2), there are no notable neurologic side effects attributed to this agent [97, 98].

Panobinostat

Panobinostat is a pan-HDAC inhibitor approved by the FDA in February 2015 for the treatment of multiple myeloma, in combination with bortezomib and dexamethasone. In a phase III randomized, placebo-controlled trial of 768 relapsed or refractory multiple myeloma patients treated with panobinostat versus placebo in combination with bortezomib and dexamethasone, neurologic complications seen at increased frequency in the patients treated with panobinostat

in comparison with those treated with placebo included headache (14% vs. 11%), dizziness (19% vs. 16%), and back pain (13% vs. 12%). Peripheral neuropathy was reported in 61% of patients; this was slightly less frequent than in the placebo group (61% vs. 67%), although there was a slightly higher incidence of grades 3–4 neuropathy in panobinostat-treated patients (18% vs. 15%) [99].

Mammalian Target of Rapamycin (MTOR) Inhibitors

Everolimus

The mTOR signaling pathway is dysregulated in many types of cancers, and mTOR inhibitors are designed to interfere with this aberrant signaling. Everolimus is an mTOR inhibitor that is FDA approved for use in the treatment of advanced hormone receptor-positive, HER2 negative breast cancer, progressive pancreatic cancer, advanced renal cell carcinoma, and subependymal giant cell astrocytoma in tuberous sclerosis patients. There are few neurologic side effects other than headache; everolimus-treated tuberous sclerosis patients have a high incidence of convulsions, but at a rate that is not increased in comparison with placebo [100, 101].

Sirolimus

Sirolimus is an mTOR inhibitor used as an immunosuppressant in solid organ transplant patients and recently approved for the treatment of lymphangioleiomyomatosis. There are studies suggesting no significant neurologic complications with sirolimus use in heart, kidney, liver, and combined multi-organ transplants, but cases of possibly associated PRES have been described [102].

Temsirolimus

Temsirolimus is an mTOR inhibitor indicated for the treatment of advanced renal cell carcinoma. It is generally well tolerated from the neurologic standpoint; however, there is an increased risk of CNS hemorrhage in patients with primary or metastatic brain tumors and/or patients on anticoagulation [103].

Smoothened (SMO) Inhibitors

Vismodegib

Alterations in the hedgehog signaling pathway are a driver of basal cell carcinoma pathogenesis, with about 10% incidence of activating mutations in SMO, leading to constitutive activation of the hedgehog pathway. Vismodegib is an SMO inhibitor approved for the treatment of metastatic or recurrent locally advanced basal cell carcinoma. There are no associated serious neurologic complications. Muscle spasms are common, reported in 64% of patients in a large safety analysis [104].

Sonidegib

Sonidegib is an oral, selective SMO inhibitor that is FDA approved for the treatment of locally advanced basal cell carcinoma in patients not suitable for surgery or radiation therapy, or those whose disease has recurred after surgery or radiation therapy. In the randomized, double-blind phase II trial leading to its approval, the recommended 200 mg dose was associated with muscle spasms in 49% of patients (3% grade 3–4) and headache in 15% of patients [105].

Poly (ADP-Ribose) Polymerase (PARP) Inhibitors

Olaparib

The first-in-class FDA approved PARP inhibitor olaparib is indicated for the treatment of progressive BRCA mutant ovarian cancer. By interfering with the poly (ADP-ribose) polymerase enzyme, PARP inhibitors interfere with tumor cells' ability to repair DNA damage caused by other chemotherapeutic agents. Significant neurologic complications are few. In an ovarian cancer trial of olaparib plus paclitaxel and carboplatin followed by olaparib maintenance monotherapy versus paclitaxel and carboplatin alone (with no maintenance therapy), headache during combination therapy was reported in 33% of patients in the olaparib group versus 9% in the chemotherapy only group, and during the maintenance therapy phase, headache was reported in 12% of the olaparib group, versus 2% in the group receiving no maintenance treatment. Peripheral neuropathy was reported in 31% of patients in the olaparib group during combination therapy (vs. 19% in the chemo alone group) but only 2% in the olaparib group during maintenance treatment (vs. 7% in the no treatment group) [106]. Another trial looking at olaparib maintenance therapy versus placebo in platinum-responsive ovarian cancer reported headaches in 21% of olaparib-treated patients (vs. 13% of placebo-treated patients). One patient in this trial experienced a grade 5 hemorrhagic stroke [107].

Antibodies and Antibody–Drug Conjugates

Monoclonal antibodies have become an important component of treatment for many different cancer types. They may be of murine, chimeric (65% human), humanized (95% human) or human (100% human) forms, and are designed to bind to specific target antigens on cancer cells. Once bound

to their target, they may disrupt necessary cancer cell functions by binding to ligands or receptors, or may recruit the immune system of the host to fight against the tumor [2]. Monoclonal antibodies are most commonly naked (unconjugated) but more recently, there has been growing interest in the development of conjugated monoclonal antibodies, in which a monoclonal antibody is combined with a cytotoxic agent to form an antibody–drug conjugate, or combined with a radioactive particle, in an attempt to deliver cytotoxic therapies or radiation directly to cells targeted by the monoclonal antibody [108]. A new class of drugs known as bi-specific T-cell engagers (BiTE®, Amgen, Thousand Oaks, CA, USA) has emerged, and is discussed in greater detail later in this chapter. Neurologic complications associated with antibodies and antibody–drug conjugates are summarized in Table 16.3.

Naked Monoclonal Antibodies

Anti-CD20 Antibodies

Rituximab

Rituximab is a chimeric monoclonal antibody against CD20 on the surface of B cells. It is FDA approved for the treatment of B-cell non-Hodgkin lymphoma and chronic lymphocytic leukemia (CLL) but there is also growing use of rituximab in the treatment of a variety of autoimmune diseases. Neurologic side effects of rituximab include mild to moderate headache, dizziness, and paresthesias [109]. Rituximab, like other monoclonal antibodies, has been associated with increased risk for the development of progressive multifocal leukoencephalopathy (PML). PML is a rare demyelinating disease associated with reactivation of latent JC polyoma virus, seen in immunocompromised patients including patients with HIV/AIDS and lymphoproliferative disorders. Patients may present with a variety of neurologic signs and symptoms, and brain MRI typically shows multiple non-enhancing lesions which may be symmetric or asymmetric and are often seen in subcortical and periventricular white matter. The only proven effective treatment is reconstitution of the host's immune system, and the condition is usually fatal [110, 111].

Ofatumumab

The fully human anti-CD20 monoclonal antibody ofatumumab is FDA approved for the treatment of previously treated chronic lymphocytic leukemia, and also approved in combination with chlorambucil for previously untreated chronic lymphocytic leukemia. It is generally well tolerated from the neurologic standpoint. However, as with other anti-CD20 monoclonal antibodies, rare cases of PML have been reported [112].

Table 16.3 Neurological complications of antibodies and antibody–drug conjugates

Agent	Therapeutic target(s)/ mechanism of action	Use(s) in cancer treatment	Common neurologic toxicities (≥ 10% of patients)	Rare neurologic toxicities (<10%)
Naked monoclonal antibodies				
Rituximab	CD20	B-cell NHL, CLL	Headache	Dizziness, paresthesias, PML
Ofatumumab	CD20	CLL	–	PML
Obinutuzumab	CD20	CLL	–	Headache, stroke
Cetuximab	EGFR	Colorectal cancer, head and neck cancer	Headache	Aseptic meningitis, RPLS
Panitumumab	EGFR	Colorectal cancer	None	–
Ipilimumab	CTLA-4	Melanoma	Hypophysitis	RPLS, Myasthenia gravis-like syndrome, Guillain–Barre Syndrome, temporal arteritis, transverse myelitis, CIDP, aseptic meningitis, inflammatory myopathy, meningo-radiculo-neuritis, encephalopathy
Pembrolizumab	PD-1	Melanoma	–	Dizziness, headache, muscle spasm, hypoesthesia, lethargy, peripheral neuropathy, paresthesias, encephalopathy/confusion, hypophysitis
Nivolumab	PD-1	Squamous NSCLC, melanoma	–	Headache, paresthesias, vertigo, hypophysitis
Trastuzumab	HER2	HER2 positive breast cancer, HER2 positive gastric or GE junction adenocarcinoma	Headache	RPLS
Pertuzumab	HER2	HER2 positive breast cancer	Headache, muscle spasms	Peripheral neuropathy
Alemtuzumab	CD52	B-cell CLL, cutaneous T-cell lymphoma	–	PML, HHV-6 encephalitis, polyneuropathy, myelitis, extrapyramidal symptoms, guillain–barre syndrome
Siltuximab	IL-6	Multicentric castleman disease	–	Headache
Denosumab	RANKL	Giant cell tumor of bone, osteoporosis, bone metastasis, patients with high fracture risk, e.g., due to hormone deprivation therapy	Headache	–
Dinutuximab	Ganglioside GD2	Pediatric high-risk neuroblastoma	Neuropathic pain	–
Bi-specific monoclonal antibodies				
Blinatumomab	Anti-CD19/anti-CD3 BiTE® (Amgen, Thousand Oaks, CA, USA) antibody construct	B-cell ALL	Headache, tremor, dizziness, confusion/encephalopathy	Ataxia, psychosis, convulsions, aphasia, dysarthria, dysesthesia, bradyphrenia, hemiparesis
Antibody–drug conjugates				
Ado-trastuzumab emtansine	Anti-HER2 mAb + cytotoxic agent	HER2 positive breast cancer	Headache, peripheral neuropathy	Subarachnoid hemorrhage
Brentuximab vedotin	Anti-CD30 mAb + cytotoxic agent	Hodgkin lymphoma, anaplastic large cell lymphoma	Peripheral neuropathy (sensory > motor)	PML
Radiolabeled antibodies				
^{90}Y-Ibritumomab tiuxetan	Anti-CD20 mAb + radionuclide	B-cell NHL	Headache, dizziness	PML

ALL acute lymphoblastic leukemia, *BiTE®* Bi-specific T-cell Engager, *CIDP* chronic inflammatory demyelinating polyneuropathy, *CLL* chronic lymphocytic leukemia, CTLA-4 cytotoxic T-lymphocyte-associated antigen-4, *EGFR* epidermal growth factor receptor, *GE junction* gastroesophageal junction, *HER* human epidermal growth factor receptor, IL-6 interleukin-6, *mAb* monoclonal antibody, *NHL* non-Hodgkin lymphoma, *NSCLC* non-small cell lung cancer, *PD-1* programmed cell death 1 receptor, *PML* progressive multifocal leukoencephalopathy, *RANKL* receptor activator of nuclear factor-kappa B ligand

Obinutuzumab

Obinutuzumab is a glycoengineered, humanized type II anti-CD20 antibody FDA approved for use in conjunction with chlorambucil in the treatment of previously untreated chronic lymphocytic leukemia (CLL). The drug was approved based on the results of an open-label, three-group study of patients with CD20-positive CLL in which patients were assigned to treatment with chlorambucil alone, chlorambucil plus obinutuzumab, or chlorambucil plus rituximab. There were no neurologic complications unique to obinutuzumab therapy. Headache was reported in 6–7% of all patients, across the three groups. Stroke/cerebrovascular accident was an extremely rare complication, reported in none of the chlorambucil-only patients and in <1% of both the obinutuzumab and rituximab arms [113].

Anti-epidermal Growth Factor Receptor (EGFR) Antibodies

Cetuximab

Cetuximab is a recombinant chimeric monoclonal antibody targeting the epidermal growth factor receptor (EGFR). It is FDA approved for the treatment of colorectal cancer and head and neck cancer. Other than headaches, neurologic complications are uncommon [114]. Cetuximab rarely has been associated with aseptic meningitis occurring after the first cetuximab dose, which may recur with drug rechallenge, even at a decreased dose [115]. PRES has also been described in association with cetuximab use [116].

Panitumumab

Panitumumab is a fully human monoclonal antibody against the epidermal growth factor receptor (EGFR), FDA approved for the treatment of patients with EGFR-expressing, metastatic colorectal cancer with disease progression on or following fluoropyrimidine-, oxaliplatin-, and irinotecan-containing chemotherapy regimens. Its approval was based on a phase III study of panitumumab plus best supportive care versus best supportive care alone in patients with chemotherapy-refractory metastatic colorectal cancer. In this study, no significant neurologic side effects were reported [117].

Anti-human Epidermal Growth Factor Receptor 2 (HER2) Antibodies

Trastuzumab

Trastuzumab is a monoclonal antibody against human epidermal growth factor receptor 2 (HER2) that is FDA approved for the treatment of HER2-overexpressing metastatic gastric or gastroesophageal junction adenocarcinoma, and the treatment of HER2-overexpressing breast cancer.

Neurologic complications are few, likely because trastuzumab is thought to have limited blood–brain barrier penetration, although data surrounding this are conflicting [118]. Headaches have been described in 10% of patients on trastuzumab monotherapy [119]. An isolated case of RPLS has been reported, possibly related to trastuzumab's antiangiogenic properties [120].

Pertuzumab

The anti-HER2 humanized monoclonal antibody pertuzumab is approved for use in combination with trastuzumab and docetaxel for neoadjuvant treatment of HER2-positive breast cancer, and in combination with trastuzumab and docetaxel to treat HER 2-positive metastatic breast cancer. In a randomized, double-blind, placebo-controlled, phase III trial comparing pertuzumab, trastuzumab, and docetaxel versus placebo, trastuzumab and docetaxel, neurologic complications noted with increased incidence in the pertuzumab-containing regimen included headache (25.7% vs. 19.2%) and muscle spasms (10.3% vs. 5.1%). Grade 3 or higher peripheral neuropathy was noted in 2.7% of pertuzumab treated patients versus 1.8% in the placebo group [121].

Immune Checkpoint Inhibitors

Immunotherapy is a rapidly growing area of research in cancer treatment, and immune checkpoint inhibitors, a relatively new class of drugs, have shown significant promise in the treatment of numerous cancer types. Immune checkpoint inhibitors are designed to interfere with T-cell inhibitory signals, thereby facilitating T-cell antitumor activity [122]. Neurologic complications associated with the three FDA approved immune checkpoint inhibitors, ipilimumab, pembrolizumab and nivolumab, will be discussed briefly in the following section. These agents are discussed in greater detail in Chap. 17.

Ipilimumab

Ipilimumab is a monoclonal antibody directed against cytotoxic T-lymphocyte-associated antigen-4 (CTLA-4), and is approved for the treatment of unresectable or metastatic melanoma. Overall, serious neurologic complications are rare, but cases of myasthenia gravis-like syndrome, Guillain–Barre syndrome, temporal arteritis, transverse myelitis, chronic inflammatory demyelinating polyneuropathy (CIDP), aseptic meningitis, inflammatory myopathy, RPLS and meningo-radiculo-neuritis have been described [123, 124]. A case of ipilimumab-induced encephalopathy with a reversible splenial lesion has also been reported [125]. Ipilimumab has also been associated with the development of hypophysitis, seen in 11% of patients in one retrospective series, and associated with pituitary enlargement on brain imaging and clinical hypopituitarism [126]. Ipilimumab is discussed in greater detail in Chap. 17.

Pembrolizumab

Pembrolizumab is a monoclonal antibody against the programmed cell death 1 (PD-1) receptor, and is FDA approved for the treatment of unresectable or metastatic melanoma with disease progression following ipilimumab and, if BRAF V600 mutation positive, a BRAF inhibitor. Drug-related neurologic complications in the trial leading to its approval were very rare, including grades 1–2 dizziness (1.2%), headache (4%), muscle spasms (2.3%), hypoesthesia (1.7%), lethargy (2.3%), peripheral neuropathy (1.7%) and paresthesias (1.2%); only lethargy was deemed immune-related. Rare grades 3–4 toxicity included encephalopathy, confusion, and peripheral motor neuropathy, each in <1% of patients. Hypophysitis was noted in 1.2% of patients [127]. Pembrolizumab is discussed in greater detail in Chap. 17.

Nivolumab

The PD-1 inhibitor nivolumab is approved for the treatment of progressive metastatic squamous non-small cell lung cancer, and nonoperative or metastatic melanoma. Neurologic complications are very uncommon. In a phase III study comparing nivolumab with dacarbazine in previously untreated melanoma, neurologic side effects were quite rare, with headache in 4.4%, paresthesia in 1% and vertigo in 1%. Hypophysitis was noted in 0.5% of patients [128]. Nivolumab is discussed in greater detail in Chap. 17.

Other Naked Monoclonal Antibodies

Alemtuzumab

Alemtuzumab is an anti-CD52 humanized monoclonal antibody approved for the treatment of B-cell chronic lymphocytic leukemia as well as other hematologic malignancies, including cutaneous T-cell lymphomas. It binds to CD52 on the surface of B and T lymphocytes, natural killer cells, monocytes and macrophages, and some granulocytes [129]. It is also used for immunosuppression in solid organ transplantation. Neurologic adverse effects are rare. However, one series of patients undergoing alemtuzumab-based reduced intensity allogeneic transplantation reported a variety of severe neurologic complications in the first year after transplant, including progressive peripheral sensorimotor polyneuropathy, HHV-7 related transverse myelitis, extrapyramidal symptoms with enhancing basal ganglia lesions, Guillain–Barre Syndrome, axonal polyneuropathy with sensory ataxia, and myelitis plus optic neuritis

following varicella zoster virus infection. Viral infections appeared to be a risk factor for the development of neurologic complications, with immune dysfunction caused by T-cell depletion secondary to alemtuzumab as a possible contributing factor [130]. Other neurologic adverse events associated with alemtuzumab use have included cases of PML and human herpes virus-6 (HHV-6) encephalitis [131, 132].

Siltuximab

Siltuximab is a chimeric murine-human monoclonal antibody against IL-6, approved by the FDA for the treatment of multicentric Castleman disease in HIV-negative, HHV8-negative patients. In clinical trials, grade 1–2 headache was reported in 8% of patients receiving siltuximab, in comparison with 4% of patients receiving placebo. There have been no serious neurologic complications associated with this medication [133].

Denosumab

Denosumab is a fully human monoclonal antibody against the receptor activator of nuclear factor-kappa B ligand (RANKL). It is FDA approved for the treatment of unresectable giant cell tumor of bone, high-risk osteoporosis in postmenopausal women, skeletal-related events in patients with bone metastases in solid tumors, and to increase bone mass in patients with high fracture risk (including those receiving androgen deprivation therapy for nonmetastatic prostate cancer or adjuvant aromatase inhibitor therapy for breast cancer). In the interim safety and efficacy analysis of a phase II open-label study of 281 patients with giant cell tumor of bone receiving this drug, headache was common, reported in 18% of patients, but generally mild, with grade 3 or 4 headache reported in only 2 patients (1%) [134].

Dinutuximab

Dinutuximab is a chimeric murine/human monoclonal antibody against ganglioside GD2, a tumor cell surface glycolipid overexpressed in neuroblastoma, malignant melanoma, osteosarcoma, and small cell carcinoma of the lung. It was FDA approved in March 2015 for the treatment of pediatric high-risk neuroblastoma. A phase III study of dinutuximab in combination with granulocyte-macrophage colony-stimulating factor (GM-CSF), interleukin-2 (IL-2), and isotretinoin was associated with a high incidence of grades 3 and 4 neuropathic pain (52% vs. 6% in isotretinoin-only arm), for which premedication with analgesics, including intravenous opioids, is recommended before, during and for 2 hours after dinutuximab administration [135, 136].

Bi-Specific Monoclonal Antibodies

Blinatumomab

Blinatumomab is an anti-CD19/anti-CD3 bi-specific T-cell engager (BiTE®) antibody construct, which is FDA approved for the treatment of recurrent or refractory Philadelphia chromosome negative B-cell acute lymphoblastic leukemia (ALL). Blinatumomab simultaneously binds CD3-positive cytotoxic T-cells that are part of the patient's endogenous immune system and CD19-positive B cells, in an attempt to recruit the patient's own immune system in the fight against CD19 positive B-precursor ALL blasts. In a multicenter, single-arm, phase II, open-label study in which 189 patients were treated with blinatumomab, headaches were frequently reported, experienced by 34% of patients. Overall, neurologic complications were very common in this study, reported in 52% of patients, and were generally mild (grade 1–2 in severity), including most commonly tremor (17% of patients), dizziness (14%), and confusion or encephalopathy (12%); less common neurologic side effects included ataxia, aphasia, dysarthria, convulsion, dysesthesia, bradyphrenia, and hemiparesis. Neurologic complications were at times severe, with grade 3 neurologic complications in 11% of patients and grade 4 complications in 2% of patients. Most common among these were encephalopathy or confusional state, ataxia, and unspecified "nervous system disorder." There were no fatal neurologic events [137]. An earlier phase II study of 36 blinatumomab-treated patients reported six patients with significant nervous system and/or psychiatric adverse events leading to treatment interruption or discontinuation, including encephalopathy, psychosis and convulsions [138].

Antibody–Drug Conjugates

Ado-Trastuzumab Emtansine

Ado-trastuzumab emtansine is an antibody–drug conjugate linking the HER2-targeted agent trastuzumab with the cytotoxic, anti-microtubule agent DM1 (derivative of maytansine) [139]. In a randomized controlled trial comparing trastuzumab emtansine (T-DM1) versus lapatinib plus capecitabine (LC) in patients with advanced HER2 positive breast cancer, headache was common, reported in 28.2% of T-DM1 treated patients, in comparison with 14.5% in the LC arm. Peripheral neuropathy was also common but rarely severe; grade 3–4 peripheral neuropathy occurred in 2.2% of T-DM1 treated patients, in comparison with 0.2% in the LC arm, and resolved in all but one of the affected T-DM1 treated patients [139, 140]. In a phase III trial comparing trastuzumab emtansine with treatment of physician's choice in patients with pretreated HER2-positive advanced breast cancer, there was one grade 5 subarachnoid hemorrhage;

however, this occurred in a patient with grade 4 thrombocytopenia on concurrent anticoagulation [141].

Brentuximab Vedotin

Brentuximab vedotin is an antibody–drug conjugate composed of an anti-CD30 monoclonal antibody linked to monomethyl auristatin E, a cytotoxic agent; this drug design is intended to facilitate delivery of a cytotoxic agent directly into tumor cells in patients with CD30-positive lymphomas [142]. It is FDA approved for the treatment of recurrent Hodgkin lymphoma after autologous stem cell transplant, and the treatment of systemic anaplastic large cell lymphoma after multi-agent chemotherapy failure [143]. Brentuximab vedotin therapy is associated with a high rate of neuropathy; in a phase II study in which the drug was given to 102 patients with relapsed or refractory Hodgkin's lymphoma, peripheral sensory neuropathy was experienced by 42% of patients and peripheral motor neuropathy in 11% of patients; neuropathy was also the most common reason for treatment discontinuation or dose reduction, and the second most common cause of dose delays. 80% of patients affected by neuropathy did have either resolution or some improvement (of one or more grades), with median time to improvement or resolution of 13.2 weeks. The high incidence of neuropathy was not unexpected, as the cytotoxic component of the drug has potent anti-microtubule effects [142]. Brentuximab is also associated with an increased risk of PML, leading the FDA to issue a Boxed Warning on brentuximab vedotin in January 2012 [143].

Radiolabeled Antibodies

Ibritumomab Tiuxetan (^{90}Y-Ibritumomab Tiuxetan)

^{90}Y-Ibritumomab tiuxetan is a radioimmunotherapy agent combining an anti-CD20 murine IgG1 monoclonal antibody with the chelator tiuxetan, which provides a high-affinity site for binding of a radionuclide (indium-111 or yttrium-90). This allows for the combination of radiation, which is effective in treating lymphoma cells, with B-cell directed immunotherapy. It is FDA approved for use in patients with relapsed B-cell non-Hodgkin lymphoma. In a randomized controlled trial of yttrium-90–labeled ibritumomab tiuxetan versus rituximab in patients with relapsed or refractory low-grade, follicular, or transformed B-cell non-Hodgkin's lymphoma, ^{90}Y-Ibritumomab tiuxetan (which is given after pretreatment with two rituximab doses) was fairly well tolerated from the neurologic standpoint, with grade 1 or 2 headache in 16% of patients (in comparison with 23% in the rituximab group) and dizziness in 15% of patients (in comparison with 7% in the rituximab group). There were no grades 3 or 4 neurologic toxicities reported [144]. There is a case report of a patient with follicular lymphoma who developed PML one year after treatment with bendamustine, rituximab, and ibritumomab tiuxetan [111].

Summary

Advances in our molecular understanding of cancer have led to the approval by the FDA of an increasing number of targeted molecular therapies. Neurotoxicities are relatively uncommon, in part because most of these agents do not pass through the blood–brain barrier to any significant extent. VEGF and VEGFR inhibitors are associated with the highest incidence of CNS toxicity, including a slightly increased risk of bleeding, stroke and RPLS. Neuropathies are common with the first-generation proteasome inhibitor bortezomib and with thalidomide, but uncommon with most targeted agents. Experience with many of the newer agents is relatively short and it is possible that with time, more neurologic complications will be identified.

References

1. Aggarwal S. Targeted cancer therapies. Nat Rev Drug Discov. 2010;9(6):427–8.
2. Gerber DE. Targeted therapies: a new generation of cancer treatments. Am Fam Physician. 2008;77(3):311–9.
3. Weidner N, Folkman J, Pozza F, Bevilacqua P, Allred EN, Moore DH, Meli S, Gasparini G. Tumor angiogenesis: a new significant and independent prognostic indicator in early-stage breast carcinoma. J Natl Cancer Inst. 1992;84(24):1875–87.
4. Hanahan D, Weinberg RA. The hallmarks of cancer. Cell. 2000;100(1):57–70.
5. Folkman J. Tumor angiogenesis: therapeutic implications. N Engl J Med. 1971;285(21):1182–6.
6. Kerbel RS. Tumor angiogenesis: past, present and the near future. Carcinogenesis. 2000;21(3):505–15.
7. Genentech USA, Inc. Avastin [Internet] 2015 [cited 2015 June 3]. Available from: http://www.avastin.com/patient.
8. Khasraw M, Holodny A, Goldlust SA, DeAngelis LM. Intracranial hemorrhage in patients with cancer treated with bevacizumab: the Memorial Sloan-Kettering experience. Ann Oncol. 2012;23(2):458–63.
9. Hapani S, Sher A, Chu D, Wu S. Increased risk of serious hemorrhage with bevacizumab in cancer patients: a meta-analysis. Oncology. 2010;79(1–2):27–38.
10. Besse B, Lasserre SF, Compton P, Huang J, Augustus S, Rohr UP. Bevacizumab safety in patients with central nervous system metastases. Clin Cancer Res. 2010;16(1):269–78.
11. Friedman HS, Prados MD, Wen PY, Mikkelsen T, Schiff D, Abrey LE, Yung WK, Paleologos N, Nicholas MK, Jensen R, Vredenburgh J, Huang J, Zheng M, Cloughesy T. Bevacizumab alone and in combination with irinotecan in recurrent glioblastoma. J Clin Oncol. 2009;27(28):4733–40.
12. Scappaticci FA, Skillings JR, Holden SN, Gerber HP, Miller K, Kabbinavar F, Bergsland E, Ngai J, Holmgren E, Wang J, Hurwitz H. Arterial thromboembolic events in patients with metastatic carcinoma treated with chemotherapy and bevacizumab. J Natl Cancer Inst. 2007;99(16):1232–9.
13. Fraum TJ, Kreisl TN, Sul J, Fine HA, Iwamoto FM. Ischemic stroke and intracranial hemorrhage in glioma patients on antiangiogenic therapy. J Neurooncol. 2011;105(2):281–9.
14. Tlemsani C, Mir O, Boudou-Rouquette P, Huillard O, Maley K, Ropert S, Coriat R, Goldwasser F. Posterior reversible encephalopathy syndrome induced by anti-VEGF agents. Target Oncol. 2011;6(4):253–8.
15. Fugate JE, Rabinstein AA. Posterior reversible encephalopathy syndrome: clinical and radiological manifestations, pathophysiology, and outstanding questions. Lancet Neurol. 2015;14(9):914–25.
16. Sherman JH, Aregawi DG, Lai A, Fathallah-Shaykh HM, Bierman PJ, Linsky K, Larner JM, Newman SA, Schiff D. Optic neuropathy in patients with glioblastoma receiving bevacizumab. Neurology. 2009;73(22):1924–6.
17. Kelly PJ, Dinkin MJ, Drappatz J, O'Regan KN, Weiss SE. Unexpected late radiation neurotoxicity following bevacizumab use: a case series. J Neurooncol. 2011;102(3):485–90.
18. Eli Lilly and Company. CYRAMZA Prescribing Information [Internet]. 2015 [updated 2015 April; cited 2015 June 4]. Available from: http://pi.lilly.com/us/cyramza-pi.pdf.
19. National Cancer Institute at the National Institutes of Health. FDA Approval for Ziv-Aflibercept [Internet]. 2013 [Updated 2013 July 3; cited 2015 Jun3 6]. Available from: http://www.cancer.gov/about-cancer/treatment/drugs/fda-ziv-aflibercept.
20. Schlumberger M, Tahara M, Wirth LJ, Robinson B, Brose MS, Elisei R, Habra MA, Newbold K, Shah MH, Hoff AO, Gianoukakis AG, Kiyota N, Taylor MH, Kim SB, Krzyzanowska MK, Dutcus CE, de las Heras B, Zhu J, Sherman SI. Lenvatinib versus placebo in radioiodine-refractory thyroid cancer. N Engl J Med. 2015;372(7):621–30.
21. Choueiri TK1, Schutz FA, Je Y, Rosenberg JE, Bellmunt J. Risk of arterial thromboembolic events with sunitinib and sorafenib: a systematic review and meta-analysis of clinical trials. J Clin Oncol. 2010;28(13):2280–5.
22. van der Veldt AA, van den Eertwegh AJ, Hoekman K, Barkhof F, Boven E. Reversible cognitive disorders after sunitinib for advanced renal cell cancer in patients with preexisting arteriosclerotic leukoencephalopathy. Ann Oncol. 2007;18 (10):1747–50.
23. Martín G, Bellido L, Cruz JJ. Reversible posterior leukoencephalopathy syndrome induced by sunitinib. J Clin Oncol. 2007;25(23):3559.
24. Sternberg CN, Davis ID, Mardiak J, Szczylik C, Lee E, Wagstaff J, Barrios CH, Salman P, Gladkov OA, Kavina A, Zarbá JJ, Chen M, McCann L, Pandite L, Roychowdhury DF, Hawkins RE. Pazopanib in locally advanced or metastatic renal cell carcinoma: results of a randomized phase III trial. J Clin Oncol. 2010;28(6):1061–8.
25. Motzer RJ, Hutson TE, Cella D, Reeves J, Hawkins R, Guo J, Nathan P, Staehler M, de Souza P, Merchan JR, Boleti E, Fife K, Jin J, Jones R, Uemura H, De Giorgi U, Harmenberg U, Wang J, Sternberg CN, Deen K, McCann L, Hackshaw MD, Crescenzo R, Pandite LN, Choueiri TK. Pazopanib versus sunitinib in metastatic renal-cell carcinoma. N Engl J Med. 2013;369 (8):722–31.
26. GlaxoSmithKline Inc. Votrient® Product Monograph [Internet]. 2015 [updated 2015 January 20; cited 2015 June 6]. Available from: http://www.gsk.ca/english/docs-pdf/product-monographs/Votrient.pdf.
27. Foerster R, Welzel T, Debus J, Gruellich C, Jaeger D, Potthoff K. Posterior reversible leukoencephalopathy syndrome associated with pazopanib. Case Rep Oncol. 2013;6(1):204–8.

28. Asaithambi G, Peters BR, Hurliman E, Moran BP, Khan AS, Taylor RA. Posterior reversible encephalopathy syndrome induced by pazopanib for renal cell carcinoma. J Clin Pharm Ther. 2013;38(2):175–6.

29. Chelis L, Souftas V, Amarantidis K, Xenidis N, Chamalidou E, Dimopoulos P, Michailidis P, Christakidis E, Prassopoulos P, Kakolyris S. Reversible posterior leukoencephalopathy syndrome induced by pazopanib. BMC Cancer. 2012;22(12):489.

30. Price KE, Saleem N, Lee G, Steinberg M. Potential of ponatinib to treat chronic myeloid leukemia and acute lymphoblastic leukemia. Onco Targets Ther. 2013;20(6):1111–8.

31. Cortes JE, Kim DW, Pinilla-Ibarz J, le Coutre P, Paquette R, Chuah C, Nicolini FE, Apperley JF, Khoury HJ, Talpaz M, DiPersio J, DeAngelo DJ, Abruzzese E, Rea D, Baccarani M, Müller MC, Gambacorti-Passerini C, Wong S, Lustgarten S, Rivera VM, Clackson T, Turner CD, Haluska FG, Guilhot F, Deininger MW, Hochhaus A, Hughes T, Goldman JM, Shah NP, Kantarjian H; PACE Investigators. A phase 2 trial of ponatinib in Philadelphia chromosome-positive leukemias. N Engl J Med. 2013;369(19):1783–96.

32. U.S. Food and Drug Administration. FDA Drug Safety Communication: FDA asks manufacturer of the leukemia drug Iclusig (ponatinib) to suspend marketing and sales [Internet]. 2013 November 5 [cited 2015 June 6]. Available from: http://www.fda.gov/Drugs/DrugSafety/ucm373040.htm#safety.

33. ARIAD Pharmaceuticals, Inc. Iclusig® Highlights of Prescribing Information [Internet]. 2012 [updated 2014 September; cite 2015 August 19]. Available from: http://iclusig.com/hcp/wp-content/uploads/2014/10/October-2014-Iclusig-Prescribing-Information.pdf.

34. Grothey A, Van Cutsem E, Sobrero A, Siena S, Falcone A, Ychou M, Humblet Y, Bouché O, Mineur L, Barone C, Adenis A, Tabernero J, Yoshino T, Lenz HJ, Goldberg RM, Sargent DJ, Cihon F, Cupit L, Wagner A, Laurent D; CORRECT Study Group. Regorafenib monotherapy for previously treated metastatic colorectal cancer (CORRECT): an international, multicentre, randomised, placebo-controlled, phase 3 trial. Lancet. 2013;381(9863):303–12.

35. Myint ZW, Sen JM, Watts NL, Druzgal TJ, Nathan BR, Ward MD, Boyer JE, Fracasso PM. Reversible posterior leukoencephalopathy syndrome during regorafenib treatment: a case report and literature review of reversible posterior leukoencephalopathy syndrome associated with multikinase inhibitors. Clin Colorectal Cancer. 2014;13(2):127–30.

36. Tian S, Nissenblatt M, Goyal S. Regorafenib-induced transverse myelopathy after stereotactic body radiation therapy. J Gastrointest Oncol. 2014;5(6):E128–31.

37. Hutson TE, Lesovoy V, Al-Shukri S, Stus VP, Lipatov ON, Bair AH, Rosbrook B, Chen C, Kim S, Vogelzang NJ. Axitinib versus sorafenib as first-line therapy in patients with metastatic renal-cell carcinoma: a randomised open-label phase 3 trial. Lancet Oncol. 2013;14(13):1287–94.

38. U.S. Food and Drug Administration. Axitinib [Internet]. 2012 [updated 2012 January 27; cited 2015 June 7]. Available from: http://www.fda.gov/Drugs/InformationOnDrugs/ApprovedDrugs/ucm289439.htm.

39. Andhavarapu S, Roy V. Immunomodulatory drugs in multiple myeloma. Expert Rev Hematol. 2013;6(1):69–82.

40. Singhal S, Mehta J, Desikan R, Ayers D, Roberson P, Eddlemon P, Munshi N, Anaissie E, Wilson C, Dhodapkar M, Zeddis J, Barlogie B. Antitumor activity of thalidomide in refractory multiple myeloma. N Engl J Med. 1999;341(21):1565–71.

41. Delforge M, Bladé J, Dimopoulos MA, Facon T, Kropff M, Ludwig H, Palumbo A, Van Damme P, San-Miguel JF, Sonneveld P. Treatment-related peripheral neuropathy in multiple myeloma: the challenge continues. Lancet Oncol. 2010;11(11):1086–95.

42. Patel UH, Mir MA, Sivik JK, Raheja D, Pandey MK, Talamo G. Central neurotoxicity of immunomodulatory drugs in multiple myeloma. Hematol Rep. 2015;7(1):5704.

43. Crystal SC, Leonidas J, Jakubowski A, Di Rocco A. Thalidomide induced acute worsening of Parkinson's disease. Mov Disord. 2009;24(12):1863–4.

44. Richardson PG, Siegel DS, Vij R, Hofmeister CC, Baz R, Jagannath S, Chen C, Lonial S, Jakubowiak A, Bahlis N, Song K, Belch A, Raje N, Shustik C, Lentzsch S, Lacy M, Mikhael J, Matous J, Vesole D, Chen M, Zaki MH, Jacques C, Yu Z, Anderson KC. Pomalidomide alone or in combination with low-dose dexamethasone in relapsed and refractory multiple myeloma: a randomized phase 2 study. Blood. 2014;123(12):1826–32.

45. Stenger M. Pomalidomide in previously treated multiple myeloma. The ASCO Post [Internet]. 2013 March 15 [cited 2015 June 7]. Available from: http://www.ascopost.com/issues/march-15,-2013/pomalidomide-in-previously-treated-multiple-myeloma.aspx.

46. Hoelder S, Clarke PA, Workman P. Discovery of small molecule cancer drugs: successes, challenges and opportunities. Mol Oncol. 2012;6(2):155–76.

47. Richardson PG, Delforge M, Beksac M, Wen P, Jongen JL, Sezer O, Terpos E, Munshi N, Palumbo A, Rajkumar SV, Harousseau JL, Moreau P, Avet-Loiseau H, Lee JH, Cavo M, Merlini G, Voorhees P, Chng WJ, Mazumder A, Usmani S, Einsele H, Comenzo R, Orlowski R, Vesole D, Lahuerta JJ, Niesvizky R, Siegel D, Mateos MV, Dimopoulos M, Lonial S, Jagannath S, Bladé J, Miguel JS, Morgan G, Anderson KC, Durie BG, Sonneveld P. Management of treatment-emergent peripheral neuropathy in multiple myeloma. Leukemia. 2012;26(4):595–608.

48. Richardson PG. Towards a better understanding of treatment-related peripheral neuropathy in multiple myeloma. Lancet Oncol. 2010;11(11):1014–6.

49. Argyriou AA, Kyritsis AP, Makatsoris T, Kalofonos HP. Chemotherapy-induced peripheral neuropathy in adults: a comprehensive update of the literature. Cancer Manag Res. 2014;19(6):135–47.

50. Richardson PG, Xie W, Mitsiades C, Chanan-Khan AA, Lonial S, Hassoun H, Avigan DE, Oaklander AL, Kuter DJ, Wen PY, Kesari S, Briemberg HR, Schlossman RL, Munshi NC, Heffner LT, Doss D, Esseltine D-L, Weller E, Anderson KC, Amato AA. Single-agent bortezomib in previously untreated multiple myeloma: efficacy, characterization of peripheral neuropathy, and molecular correlates of response and neuropathy. J Clin Oncol. 2009;27(21):3518–25.

51. Ho CH, Lo CP, Tu MC. Bortezomib-induced posterior reversible encephalopathy syndrome: clinical and imaging features. Intern Med. 2014;53(16):1853–7.

52. Kelly K, Kalachand R, Murphy P. Bortezomib-induced reversible posterior leucoencephalopathy syndrome. Br J Haematol. 2008;141(5):566.

53. Martin TG. Peripheral neuropathy experience in patients with relapsed and/or refractory multiple myeloma treated with carfilzomib. Oncology (Williston Park). 2013;27(Suppl 3):4–10.

54. Siegel D, Martin T, Nooka A, Harvey RD, Vij R, Niesvizky R, Badros AZ, Jagannath S, McCulloch L, Rajangam K, Lonial S. Integrated safety profile of single-agent carfilzomib: experience from 526 patients enrolled in 4 phase II clinical studies. Haematologica. 2013;98(11):1753–61.

55. Cohen MH, Johnson JR, Chen YF, Sridhara R, Pazdur R. FDA drug approval summary: erlotinib (Tarceva) tablets. Oncologist. 2005;10(7):461–6.

56. Moore MJ, Goldstein D, Hamm J, Figer A, Hecht JR, Gallinger S, Au HJ, Murawa P, Walde D, Wolff RA, Campos D, Lim R, Ding K, Clark G, Voskoglou-Nomikos T, Ptasynski M, Parulekar W; National Cancer Institute of Canada Clinical Trials Group. Erlotinib plus gemcitabine compared with gemcitabine alone in patients with advanced pancreatic cancer: a phase III trial of the National Cancer Institute of Canada Clinical Trials Group. J Clin Oncol. 2007;25(15):1960–6.

57. National Cancer Institute at the National Institutes of Health. FDA Approval for Gefitinib [Internet]. 2011 January 18 [cited 2015 June 16]. Available from: http://www.cancer.gov/about-cancer/treatment/drugs/fda-gefitinib.

58. U.S. Food and Drug Administration. FDA approves targeted therapy for first-line treatment of patients with a type of metastatic lung cancer [Internet]. 2015 July 13 [Updated 2015 July 14; cited 2015 August 19]. Available from: http://www.fda.gov/NewsEvents/Newsroom/PressAnnouncements/ucm454678.htm#.

59. Goodman A. IMPRESS trial: lung cancer progression on first-line tyrosine kinase inhibitor indicates the drug should be stopped. The ASCO Post [Internet]. 2014 November 15 [cited 2015 June 16]. Available from: http://www.ascopost.com/issues/november-15,-2014/impress-trial-lung-cancer-progression-on-first-line-tyrosine-kinase-inhibitor-indicates-the-drug-should-be-stopped.aspx.

60. U.S. Food and Drug Administration. Iressa label [Internet]. 2004 April 7 [cited 2015 June 16]. Available from: http://www.accessdata.fda.gov/drugsatfda_docs/label/2005/021399s008lbl.pdf.

61. Sequist LV, Yang JC, Yamamoto N, O'Byrne K, Hirsh V, Mok T, Geater SL, Orlov S, Tsai CM, Boyer M, Su WC, Bennouna J, Kato T, Gorbunova V, Lee KH, Shah R, Massey D, Zazulina V, Shahidi M, Schuler M. Phase III study of afatinib or cisplatin plus pemetrexed in patients with metastatic lung adenocarcinoma with EGFR mutations. J Clin Oncol. 2013;31(27):3327–34.

62. Yang JC, Wu YL, Schuler M, Sebastian M, Popat S, Yamamoto N, Zhou C, Hu CP, O'Byrne K, Feng J, Lu S, Huang Y, Geater SL, Lee KY, Tsai CM, Gorbunova V, Hirsh V, Bennouna J, Orlov S, Mok T, Boyer M, Su WC, Lee KH, Kato T, Massey D25, Shahidi M, Zazulina V, Sequist LV. Afatinib versus cisplatin-based chemotherapy for EGFR mutation-positive lung adenocarcinoma (LUX-Lung 3 and LUX-Lung 6): analysis of overall survival data from two randomised, phase 3 trials. Lancet Oncol. 2015;16(2):141-51.

63. Geyer CE, Forster J, Lindquist D, Chan S, Romieu CG, Pienkowski T, Jagiello-Gruszfeld A, Crown J, Chan A, Kaufman B, Skarlos D, Campone M, Davidson N, Berger M, Oliva C, Rubin SD, Stein S, Cameron D. Lapatinib plus capecitabine for HER2-positive advanced breast cancer. N Engl J Med. 2006;355 (26):2733–43.

64. Goss PE, Smith IE, O'Shaughnessy J, Ejlertsen B, Kaufmann M, Boyle F, Buzdar AU, Fumoleau P, Gradishar W, Martin M, Moy B, Piccart-Gebhart M, Pritchard KI, Lindquist D, Chavarri-Guerra Y, Aktan G, Rappold E, Williams LS, Finkelstein DM; TEACH investigators. Adjuvant lapatinib for women with early-stage HER2-positive breast cancer: a randomised, controlled, phase 3 trial. Lancet Oncol. 2013 Jan;14(1):88–96.

65. Wells SA Jr, Robinson BG, Gagel RF, Dralle H, Fagin JA, Santoro M, Baudin E, Elisei R, Jarzab B, Vasselli JR, Read J, Langmuir P, Ryan AJ, Schlumberger MJ. Vandetanib in patients with locally advanced or metastatic medullary thyroid cancer: a randomized, double-blind phase III trial. J Clin Oncol. 2012;30 (2):134–41.

66. Thornton K, Kim G, Maher VE, Chattopadhyay S, Tang S, Moon YJ, Song P, Marathe A, Balakrishnan S, Zhu H, Garnett C, Liu Q, Booth B, Gehrke B, Dorsam R, Verbois L, Ghosh D,

Wilson W, Duan J, Sarker H, Miksinski SP, Skarupa L, Ibrahim A, Justice R, Murgo A, Pazdur R. Vandetanib for the treatment of symptomatic or progressive medullary thyroid cancer in patients with unresectable locally advanced or metastatic disease: U.S. food and drug administration drug approval summary. Clin Cancer Res. 2012;18(14):3722–30.

67. Shaw AT, Kim DW, Nakagawa K, Seto T, Crinó L, Ahn MJ, De Pas T, Besse B, Solomon BJ, Blackhall F, Wu YL, Thomas M, O'Byrne KJ, Moro-Sibilot D, Camidge DR, Mok T, Hirsh V, Riely GJ, Iyer S, Tassell V, Polli A, Wilner KD, Jänne PA. Crizotinib versus chemotherapy in advanced ALK-positive lung cancer. N Engl J Med. 2013;368(25):2385–94.

68. Camidge DR, Bang YJ, Kwak EL, Iafrate AJ, Varella-Garcia M, Fox SB, Riely GJ, Solomon B, Ou SH, Kim DW, Salgia R, Fidias P, Engelman JA, Gandhi L, Jänne PA, Costa DB, Shapiro GI, Lorusso P, Ruffner K, Stephenson P, Tang Y, Wilner K, Clark JW, Shaw AT. Activity and safety of crizotinib in patients with ALK-positive non-small-cell lung cancer: updated results from a phase 1 study. Lancet Oncol. 2012;13 (10):1011–9.

69. National Cancer Institute at the National Institutes of Health. FDA Approval for Ceritinib [Internet]. 2014 May 14 [cited 2015 June 16]. Available from: http://www.cancer.gov/about-cancer/treatment/drugs/fda-ceritinib.

70. Shaw AT, Kim DW, Mehra R, Tan DS, Felip E, Chow LQ, Camidge DR, Vansteenkiste J, Sharma S, De Pas T, Riely GJ, Solomon BJ, Wolf J, Thomas M, Schuler M, Liu G, Santoro A, Lau YY, Goldwasser M, Boral AL, Engelman JA. Ceritinib in ALK-rearranged non-small-cell lung cancer. N Engl J Med. 2014;370(13):1189–97.

71. Elisei R, Schlumberger MJ, Müller SP, Schöffski P, Brose MS, Shah MH, Licitra L, Jarzab B, Medvedev V, Kreissl MC, Niederle B, Cohen EE, Wirth LJ, Ali H, Hessel C, Yaron Y, Ball D, Nelkin B, Sherman SI. Cabozantinib in progressive medullary thyroid cancer. J Clin Oncol. 2013;31(29):3639–46.

72. Wei G, Rafiyath S, Liu D. First-line treatment for chronic myeloid leukemia: dasatinib, nilotinib, or imatinib. J Hematol Oncol. 2010;26(3):47.

73. Kantarjian HM, Hochhaus A, Saglio G, De Souza C, Flinn IW, Stenke L, Goh YT, Rosti G, Nakamae H, Gallagher NJ, Hoenekopp A, Blakesley RE, Larson RA, Hughes TP. Nilotinib versus imatinib for the treatment of patients with newly diagnosed chronic phase, Philadelphia chromosome-positive, chronic myeloid leukaemia: 24-month minimum follow-up of the phase 3 randomised ENESTnd trial. Lancet Oncol. 2011;12 (9):841–51.

74. Schiff D, Wen PY, van den Bent MJ. Neurological adverse effects caused by cytotoxic and targeted therapies. Nat Rev Clin Oncol. 2009;6(10):596–603.

75. Wen PY, Yung WK, Lamborn KR, Dahia PL, Wang Y, Peng B, Abrey LE, Raizer J, Cloughesy TF, Fink K, Gilbert M, Chang S, Junck L, Schiff D, Lieberman F, Fine HA, Mehta M, Robins HI, DeAngelis LM, Groves MD, Puduvalli VK, Levin V, Conrad C, Maher EA, Aldape K, Hayes M, Letvak L, Egorin MJ, Capdeville R, Kaplan R, Murgo AJ, Stiles C, Prados MD. Phase I/II study of imatinib mesylate for recurrent malignant gliomas: North American Brain Tumor Consortium Study 99-08. Clin Cancer Res. 2006;12(16):4899–907.

76. Song KW, Rifkind J, Al-Beirouti B, Yee K, McCrae J, Messner HA, Keating A, Lipton JH. Subdural hematomas during CML therapy with imatinib mesylate. Leuk Lymphoma. 2004;45 (8):1633–6.

77. Kantarjian H, Giles F, Wunderle L, Bhalla K, O'Brien S, Wassmann B, Tanaka C, Manley P, Rae P, Mietlowski W, Bochinski K, Hochhaus A, Griffin JD, Hoelzer D, Albitar M,

Dugan M, Cortes J, Alland L, Ottmann OG. Nilotinib in imatinib-resistant CML and Philadelphia chromosome-positive ALL. N Engl J Med. 2006;354(24):2542–51.

78. Abbott BL. Dasatinib: from treatment of imatinib-resistant or -intolerant patients with chronic myeloid leukemia to treatment of patients with newly diagnosed chronic phase chronic myeloid leukemia. Clin Ther. 2012;34(2):272–81.

79. Kantarjian H, Cortes J, Kim DW, Dorlhiac-Llacer P, Pasquini R, DiPersio J, Müller MC, Radich JP, Khoury HJ, Khoroshko N, Bradley-Garelik MB, Zhu C, Tallman MS. Phase 3 study of dasatinib 140 mg once daily versus 70 mg twice daily in patients with chronic myeloid leukemia in accelerated phase resistant or intolerant to imatinib: 15-month median follow-up. Blood. 2009;113(25):6322–9.

80. Mustafa Ali MK, Sabha MM, Al-Rabi KH. Spontaneous subdural hematoma in a patient with Philadelphia chromosome-positive acute lymphoblastic leukemia with normal platelet count after dasatinib treatment. Platelets. 2015;26(5):491–4.

81. Yhim HY, Kim HS, Lee NR, Song EK, Kwak JY, Yim CY. Bilateral subdural hemorrhage as a serious adverse event of dasatinib in a patient with Philadelphia chromosome-positive acute lymphoblastic leukemia. Int J Hematol. 2012;95(5):585–7.

82. Brümmendorf TH, Cortes JE, de Souza CA, Guilhot F, Duvillié L, Pavlov D, Gogat K, Countouriotis AM, Gambacorti-Passerini C. Bosutinib versus imatinib in newly diagnosed chronic-phase chronic myeloid leukaemia: results from the 24-month follow-up of the BELA trial. Br J Haematol. 2015;168(1):69–81.

83. Wu P, Nielsen TE, Clausen MH. FDA-approved small-molecule kinase inhibitors. Trends Pharmacol Sci. 2015;36(7):422–39.

84. Wang ML, Blum KA, Martin P, Goy A, Auer R, Kahl BS, Jurczak W, Advani RH, Romaguera JE, Williams ME, Barrientos JC, Chmielowska E, Radford J, Stilgenbauer S, Dreyling M, Jedrzejczak WW, Johnson P, Spurgeon SE, Zhang L, Baher L, Cheng M, Lee D, Beaupre DM, Rule S. Long-term follow-up of MCL patients treated with single-agent ibrutinib: updated safety and efficacy results. Blood. 2015;126(6):739–45.

85. Vannucchi AM, Kiladjian JJ, Griesshammer M, Masszi T, Durrant S, Passamonti F, Harrison CN, Pane F, Zachee P, Mesa R, He S, Jones MM, Garrett W, Li J, Pirron U, Habr D, Verstovsek S. Ruxolitinib versus standard therapy for the treatment of polycythemia vera. N Engl J Med. 2015;372 (5):426–35.

86. Harrison C, Kiladjian JJ, Al-Ali HK, Gisslinger H, Waltzman R, Stalbovskaya V, McQuitty M, Hunter DS, Levy R, Knoops L, Cervantes F, Vannucchi AM, Barbui T, Barosi G. JAK inhibition with ruxolitinib versus best available therapy for myelofibrosis. N Engl J Med. 2012;366(9):787–98.

87. Chapman PB, Hauschild A, Robert C, Haanen JB, Ascierto P, Larkin J, Dummer R, Garbe C, Testori A, Maio M, Hogg D, Lorigan P, Lebbe C, Jouary T, Schadendorf D, Ribas A, O'Day SJ, Sosman JA, Kirkwood JM, Eggermont AM, Dreno B, Nolop K, Li J, Nelson B, Hou J, Lee RJ, Flaherty KT, McArthur GA; BRIM-3 Study Group. Improved survival with vemurafenib in melanoma with BRAF V600E mutation. N Engl J Med. 2011;364(26):2507-16.

88. Hauschild A, Grob JJ, Demidov LV, Jouary T, Gutzmer R, Millward M, Rutkowski P, Blank CU, Miller WH Jr, Kaempgen E, Martín-Algarra S, Karaszewska B, Mauch C, Chiarion-Sileni V, Martin AM, Swann S, Haney P, Mirakhur B, Guckert ME, Goodman V, Chapman PB. Dabrafenib in BRAF-mutated metastatic melanoma: a multicentre, open-label, phase 3 randomised controlled trial. Lancet. 2012;380(9839):358–65.

89. Kim G, McKee AE, Ning YM, Hazarika M, Theoret M, Johnson JR, Xu QC, Tang S, Sridhara R, Jiang X, He K, Roscoe D, McGuinn WD, Helms WS, Russell AM, Miksinski SP, Zirkelbach JF, Earp J, Liu Q, Ibrahim A, Justice R, Pazdur R. FDA approval summary: vemurafenib for treatment of unresectable or metastatic melanoma with the BRAFV600E mutation. Clin Cancer Res. 2014;20(19):4994–5000.

90. Klein O, Ribas A, Chmielowski B, Walker G, Clements A, Long GV, Kefford RF. Facial palsy as a side effect of vemurafenib treatment in patients with metastatic melanoma. J Clin Oncol. 2013;31(12):e215–7.

91. Johnson DB, Wallender EK, Cohen DN, Likhari SS, Zwerner JP, Powers JG, Shinn L, Kelley MC, Joseph RW, Sosman JA. Severe cutaneous and neurologic toxicity in melanoma patients during vemurafenib administration following anti-PD-1 therapy. Cancer Immunol Res. 2013;1(6):373–7.

92. Flaherty KT, Robert C, Hersey P, Nathan P, Garbe C, Milhem M, Demidov LV, Hassel JC, Rutkowski P, Mohr P, Dummer R, Trefzer U, Larkin JM, Utikal J, Dreno B, Nyakas M, Middleton MR, Becker JC, Casey M, Sherman LJ, Wu FS, Ouellet D, Martin AM, Patel K. Schadendorf D; METRIC Study Group. Improved survival with MEK inhibition in BRAF-mutated melanoma. N Engl J Med. 2012;367(2):107–14.

93. Finn RS, Crown JP, Lang I, Boer K, Bondarenko IM, Kulyk SO, Ettl J, Patel R, Pinter T, Schmidt M, Shparyk Y, Thummala AR, Voytko NL, Fowst C, Huang X, Kim ST, Randolph S, Slamon DJ. The cyclin-dependent kinase 4/6 inhibitor palbociclib in combination with letrozole versus letrozole alone as first-line treatment of oestrogen receptor-positive, HER2-negative, advanced breast cancer (PALOMA-1/TRIO-18): a randomised phase 2 study. Lancet Oncol. 2015;16(1):25–35.

94. Gopal AK, Kahl BS, de Vos S, Wagner-Johnston ND, Schuster SJ, Jurczak WJ, Flinn IW, Flowers CR, Martin P, Viardot A, Blum KA, Goy AH, Davies AJ, Zinzani PL, Dreyling M, Johnson D, Miller LL, Holes L, Li D, Dansey RD, Godfrey WR, Salles GA. PI3 Kδ inhibition by idelalisib in patients with relapsed indolent lymphoma. N Engl J Med. 2014;370(11): 1008–18.

95. Mann BS, Johnson JR, Cohen MH, Justice R, Pazdur R. FDA approval summary: vorinostat for treatment of advanced primary cutaneous T-cell lymphoma. Oncologist. 2007;12(10):1247–52.

96. Foss F, Advani R, Duvic M, Hymes KB, Intragumtornchai T, Lekhakula A, Shpilberg O, Lerner A, Belt RJ, Jacobsen ED, Laurent G, Ben-Yehuda D, Beylot-Barry M, Hillen U, Knoblauch P, Bhat G, Chawla S, Allen LF, Pohlman B. A phase II trial of belinostat (PXD101) in patients with relapsed or refractory peripheral or cutaneous T-cell lymphoma. Br J Haematol. 2015;168(6):811–9.

97. Whittaker SJ, Demierre MF, Kim EJ, Rook AH, Lerner A, Duvic M, Scarisbrick J, Reddy S, Robak T, Becker JC, Samtsov A, McCulloch W, Kim YH. Final results from a multicenter, international, pivotal study of romidepsin in refractory cutaneous T-cell lymphoma. J Clin Oncol. 2010;28 (29):4485–91.

98. Coiffier B, Pro B, Prince HM, Foss F, Sokol L, Greenwood M, Caballero D, Borchmann P, Morschhauser F, Wilhelm M, Pinter-Brown L, Padmanabhan S, Shustov A, Nichols J, Carroll S, Balser J, Balser B, Horwitz S. Results from a pivotal, open-label, phase II study of romidepsin in relapsed or refractory peripheral T-cell lymphoma after prior systemic therapy. J Clin Oncol. 2012;30(6):631–6.

99. San-Miguel JF, Hungria VT, Yoon SS, Beksac M, Dimopoulos MA, Elghandour A, Jedrzejczak WW, Günther A, Nakorn TN, Siritanaratkul N, Corradini P, Chuncharunee S, Lee JJ, Schlossman RL, Shelekhova T, Yong K, Tan D, Numbenjapon T, Cavenagh JD, Hou J, LeBlanc R, Nahi H, Qiu L, Salwender H, Pulini S, Moreau P, Warzocha K, White D,

Bladé J, Chen W, de la Rubia J, Gimsing P, Lonial S, Kaufman JL, Ocio EM, Veskovski L, Sohn SK, Wang MC, Lee JH, Einsele H, Sopala M, Corrado C, Bengoudifa BR, Binlich F, Richardson PG. Panobinostat plus bortezomib and dexamethasone versus placebo plus bortezomib and dexamethasone in patients with relapsed or relapsed and refractory multiple myeloma: a multicentre, randomised, double-blind phase 3 trial. Lancet Oncol. 2014;15(11):1195–206.

100. Bissler JJ, Kingswood JC, Radzikowska E, Zonnenberg BA, Frost M, Belousova E, Sauter M, Nonomura N, Brakemeier S, de Vries PJ, Whittemore VH, Chen D, Sahmoud T, Shah G, Lincy J, Lebwohl D, Budde K. Everolimus for angiomyolipoma associated with tuberous sclerosis complex or sporadic lymphangioleiomyomatosis (EXIST-2): a multicentre, randomised, double-blind, placebo-controlled trial. Lancet. 2013;381 (9869):817–24.

101. Franz DN, Belousova E, Sparagana S, Bebin EM, Frost M, Kuperman R, Witt O, Kohrman MH, Flamini JR, Wu JY, Curatolo P, de Vries PJ, Berkowitz N, Anak O, Niolat J, Jozwiak S. Everolimus for subependymal giant cell astrocytoma in patients with tuberous sclerosis complex: 2-year open-label extension of the randomised EXIST-1 study. Lancet Oncol. 2014;15(13):1513–20.

102. van de Beek D, Kremers WK, Kushwaha SS, McGregor CG, Wijdicks EF. No major neurologic complications with sirolimus use in heart transplant recipients. Mayo Clin Proc. 2009;84 (4):330–2.

103. U.S. Food and Drug Administration. TORISEL™ highlights of prescribing information [Internet]. 2007 [updated 2007 May; cited 2015 June 12]. Available from: http://www.accessdata.fda. gov/drugsatfda_docs/label/2007/022088lbl.pdf.

104. Basset-Seguin N, Hauschild A, Grob JJ, Kunstfeld R, Dréno B, Mortier L, Ascierto PA, Licitra L, Dutriaux C, Thomas L, Jouary T, Meyer N, Guillot B, Dummer R, Fife K, Ernst DS, Williams S, Fittipaldo A, Xynos I, Hansson J. Vismodegib in patients with advanced basal cell carcinoma (STEVIE): a pre-planned interim analysis of an international, open-label trial. Lancet Oncol. 2015;16(6):729–36.

105. Migden MR, Guminski A, Gutzmer R, Dirix L, Lewis KD, Combemale P, Herd RM, Kudchadkar R, Trefzer U, Gogov S, Pallaud C, Yi T, Mone M, Kaatz M, Loquai C, Stratigos AJ, Schulze HJ, Plummer R, Chang AL, Cornélis F, Lear JT, Sellami D, Dummer R. Treatment with two different doses of sonidegib in patients with locally advanced or metastatic basal cell carcinoma (BOLT): a multicentre, randomised, double-blind phase 2 trial. Lancet Oncol. 2015;16(6):716–28.

106. Oza AM, Cibula D, Benzaquen AO, Poole C, Mathijssen RH, Sonke GS, Colombo N, Špaček J, Vuylsteke P, Hirte H, Mahner S, Plante M, Schmalfeldt B, Mackay H, Rowbottom J, Lowe ES, Dougherty B, Barrett JC, Friedlander M. Olaparib combined with chemotherapy for recurrent platinum-sensitive ovarian cancer: a randomised phase 2 trial. Lancet Oncol. 2015;16(1):87–97.

107. Ledermann J, Harter P, Gourley C, Friedlander M, Vergote I, Rustin G, Scott CL, Meier W, Shapira-Frommer R, Safra T, Matei D, Fielding A, Spencer S, Dougherty B, Orr M, Hodgson D, Barrett JC, Matulonis U. Olaparib maintenance therapy in patients with platinum-sensitive relapsed serous ovarian cancer: a preplanned retrospective analysis of outcomes by BRCA status in a randomised phase 2 trial. Lancet Oncol. 2014;15(8):852–61.

108. American Cancer Society. Monoclonal antibodies to treat cancer [Internet]. 2014 [Updated 2014 December 8; cited 2015 June 10]. Available from: http://www.cancer.org/treatment/treatment sandsideeffects/treatmenttypes/immunotherapy/immunotherapy-monoclonal-antibodies.

109. Foran JM, Rohatiner AZ, Cunningham D, Popescu RA, Solal-Celigny P, Ghielmini M, Coiffier B, Johnson PW, Gisselbrecht C, Reyes F, Radford JA, Bessell EM, Souleau B, Benzohra A, Lister TA. European phase II study of rituximab (chimeric anti-CD20 monoclonal antibody) for patients with newly diagnosed mantle-cell lymphoma and previously treated mantle-cell lymphoma, immunocytoma, and small B-cell lymphocytic lymphoma. J Clin Oncol. 2000;18(2):317–24.

110. Al-Tawfiq JA, Banda RW, Daabil RA, Dawamneh MF. Progressive multifocal leukoencephalopathy (PML) in a patient with lymphoma treated with rituximab: A case report and literature review. J Infect Public Health. 2015;8(5):493–7.

111. Lane MA, Renga V, Pachner AR, Cohen JA. Late occurrence of PML in a patient treated for lymphoma with immunomodulatory chemotherapies, bendamustine, rituximab, and ibritumomab tiuxetan. Case Rep Neurol Med. 2015;2015:892047.

112. Moreno C, Montillo M, Panayiotidis P, Dimou M, Bloor A, Dupuis J, Schuh A, Norin S, Geisler C, Hillmen P, Doubek M, Trněný M, Obrtlikova P, Laurenti L, Stilgenbauer S, Smolej L, Ghia P, Cymbalista F, Jaeger U, Stamatopoulos K, Stavroyianni N, Carrington P, Zouabi H, Leblond V, Gomez-Garcia JC, Rubio M, Marasca R, Musuraca G, Rigacci L, Farina L, Paolini R, Pospisilova S, Kimby E, Bradley C, Montserrat E. Ofatumumab in poor-prognosis chronic lymphocytic leukemia: a phase IV, non-interventional, observational study from the European Research Initiative on Chronic Lymphocytic Leukemia. Haematologica. 2015;100(4):511–6.

113. Goede V, Fischer K, Busch R, Engelke A, Eichhorst B, Wendtner CM, Chagorova T, de la Serna J, Dilhuydy MS, Illmer T, Opat S, Owen CJ, Samoylova O, Kreuzer KA, Stilgenbauer S, Döhner H, Langerak AW, Ritgen M, Kneba M, Asikanius E, Humphrey K, Wenger M, Hallek M. Obinutuzumab plus chlorambucil in patients with CLL and coexisting conditions. N Engl J Med. 2014;370(12):1101–10.

114. Wierzbicki R, Jonker DJ, Moore MJ, Berry SR, Loehrer PJ, Youssoufian H, Rowinsky EK. A phase II, multicenter study of cetuximab monotherapy in patients with refractory, metastatic colorectal carcinoma with absent epidermal growth factor receptor immunostaining. Invest New Drugs. 2011;29(1):167–74.

115. Ulrich A, Weiler S, Weller M, Rordorf T, Tarnutzer AA. Cetuximab induced aseptic meningitis. J Clin Neurosci. 2015;22 (6):1061–3.

116. Palma JA, Gomez-Ibañez A, Martin B, Urrestarazu E, Gil-Bazo I, Pastor MA. Nonconvulsive status epilepticus related to posterior reversible leukoencephalopathy syndrome induced by cetuximab. Neurologist. 2011;17(5):273–5.

117. Van Cutsem E, Peeters M, Siena S, Humblet Y, Hendlisz A, Neyns B, Canon JL, Van Laethem JL, Maurel J, Richardson G, Wolf M, Amado RG. Open-label phase III trial of panitumumab plus best supportive care compared with best supportive care alone in patients with chemotherapy-refractory metastatic colorectal cancer. J Clin Oncol. 2007;25(13):1658–64.

118. Pieńkowski T, Zielinski CC. Trastuzumab treatment in patients with breast cancer and metastatic CNS disease. Ann Oncol. 2010;21(5):917–24.

119. Baselga J, Carbonell X, Castañeda-Soto NJ, Clemens M, Green M, Harvey V, Morales S, Barton C, Ghahramani P. Phase II study of efficacy, safety, and pharmacokinetics of trastuzumab monotherapy administered on a 3-weekly schedule. J Clin Oncol. 2005;23(10):2162–71.

120. Kaneda H, Okamoto I, Satoh T, Nakagawa K. Reversible posterior leukoencephalopathy syndrome and trastuzumab. Invest New Drugs. 2012;30(4):1766–7.

121. Swain SM, Baselga J, Kim SB, Ro J, Semiglazov V, Campone M, Ciruelos E, Ferrero JM, Schneeweiss A, Heeson S, Clark E, Ross G,

Benyunes MC, Cortés J; CLEOPATRA Study Group. Pertuzumab, trastuzumab, and docetaxel in HER2-positive metastatic breast cancer. N Engl J Med. 2015;372(8):724–34.

122. Sharma P, Allison JP. The future of immune checkpoint therapy. Science. 2015;348(6230):56–61.

123. Tarhini A. Immune-mediated adverse events associated with ipilimumab ctla-4 blockade therapy: the underlying mechanisms and clinical management. Scientifica (Cairo). 2013;2013:857519.

124. Liao B, Shroff S, Kamiya-Matsuoka C, Tummala S. Atypical neurological complications of ipilimumab therapy in patients with metastatic melanoma. Neuro Oncol. 2014;16(4):589–93.

125. Conry RM, Sullivan JC, Nabors LB 3rd. Ipilimumab-induced encephalopathy with a reversible splenial lesion. Cancer Immunol Res. 2015;3(6):598–601.

126. Faje AT, Sullivan R, Lawrence D, Tritos NA, Fadden R, Klibanski A, Nachtigall L. Ipilimumab-induced hypophysitis: a detailed longitudinal analysis in a large cohort of patients with metastatic melanoma. J Clin Endocrinol Metab. 2014;99 (11):4078–85.

127. Robert C, Ribas A, Wolchok JD, Hodi FS, Hamid O, Kefford R, Weber JS, Joshua AM, Hwu WJ, Gangadhar TC, Patnaik A, Dronca R, Zarour H, Joseph RW, Boasberg P, Chmielowski B, Mateus C, Postow MA, Gergich K, Elassaiss-Schaap J, Li XN, Iannone R, Ebbinghaus SW, Kang SP, Daud A. Anti-programmed-death-receptor-1 treatment with pembrolizumab in ipilimumab-refractory advanced melanoma: a randomised dose-comparison cohort of a phase 1 trial. Lancet. 2014;384(9948):1109–17.

128. Robert C, Long GV, Brady B, Dutriaux C, Maio M, Mortier L, Hassel JC, Rutkowski P, McNeil C, Kalinka-Warzocha E, Savage KJ, Hernberg MM, Lebbé C, Charles J, Mihalcioiu C, Chiarion-Sileni V, Mauch C, Cognetti F, Arance A, Schmidt H, Schadendorf D, Gogas H, Lundgren-Eriksson L, Horak C, Sharkey B, Waxman IM, Atkinson V, Ascierto PA. Nivolumab in previously untreated melanoma without BRAF mutation. N Engl J Med. 2015;372(4):320–30.

129. Genzyme Corporation. About Campath [Internet]. 2009 [Cited 11 June 2015]. Available from: http://www.campath.com/hcp/AboutCampath.html.

130. Avivi I, Chakrabarti S, Kottaridis P, Kyriaku C, Dogan A, Milligan DW, Linch D, Goldstone AH, Mackinnon S. Neurological complications following alemtuzumab-based reduced-intensity allogeneic transplantation. Bone Marrow Transplant. 2004;34(2):137–42.

131. Isidoro L, Pires P, Rito L, Cordeiro G. Progressive multifocal leukoencephalopathy in a patient with chronic lymphocytic leukaemia treated with alemtuzumab. BMJ Case Rep. 2014;2014 (2014):1–3.

132. Vu T, Carrum G, Hutton G, Heslop HE, Brenner MK, Kamble R. Human herpesvirus-6 encephalitis following allogeneic hematopoietic stem cell transplantation. Bone Marrow Transplant. 2007;39(11):705–9.

133. Deisseroth A, Ko CW, Nie L, Zirkelbach JF, Zhao L, Bullock J, Mehrotra N, Del Valle P, Saber H, Sheth C, Gehrke B, Justice R, Farrell A, Pazdur R. FDA approval: siltuximab for the treatment of patients with multicentric Castleman disease. Clin Cancer Res. 2015;21(5):950–4.

134. Chawla S, Henshaw R, Seeger L, Choy E, Blay JY, Ferrari S, Kroep J, Grimer R, Reichardt P, Rutkowski P, Schuetze S, Skubitz K, Staddon A, Thomas D, Qian Y, Jacobs I. Safety and efficacy of denosumab for adults and skeletally mature adolescents with giant cell tumour of bone: interim analysis of an open-label, parallel-group, phase 2 study. Lancet Oncol. 2013;14(9):901–8.

135. Dhillon S. Dinutuximab: first global approval. Drugs. 2015;75 (8):923–7.

136. Yu AL, Gilman AL, Ozkaynak MF, London WB, Kreissman SG, Chen HX, Smith M, Anderson B, Villablanca JG, Matthay KK, Shimada H, Grupp SA, Seeger R, Reynolds CP, Buxton A, Reisfeld RA, Gillies SD, Cohn SL, Maris JM, Sondel PM; Children's Oncology Group. Anti-GD2 antibody with GM-CSF, interleukin-2, and isotretinoin for neuroblastoma. N Engl J Med. 2010;363(14):1324-34.

137. Topp MS, Gökbuget N, Stein AS, Zugmaier G, O'Brien S, Bargou RC, Dombret H, Fielding AK, Heffner L, Larson RA, Neumann S, Foà R, Litzow M, Ribera JM, Rambaldi A, Schiller G, Brüggemann M, Horst HA, Holland C, Jia C, Maniar T, Huber B, Nagorsen D, Forman SJ, Kantarjian HM. Safety and activity of blinatumomab for adult patients with relapsed or refractory B-precursor acute lymphoblastic leukaemia: a multicentre, single-arm, phase 2 study. Lancet Oncol. 2015;16(1):57–66.

138. Topp MS, Gökbuget N, Zugmaier G, Klappers P, Stelljes M, Neumann S, Viardot A, Marks R, Diedrich H, Faul C, Reichle A, Horst HA, Brüggemann M, Wessiepe D, Holland C, Alekar S, Mergen N, Einsele H, Hoelzer D, Bargou RC. Phase II trial of the anti-CD19 bispecific T cell-engager blinatumomab shows hematologic and molecular remissions in patients with relapsed or refractory B-precursor acute lymphoblastic leukemia. J Clin Oncol. 2014;32(36):4134–40.

139. Verma S, Miles D, Gianni L, Krop IE, Welslau M, Baselga J, Pegram M, Oh DY, Diéras V, Guardino E, Fang L, Lu MW, Olsen S, Blackwell K; EMILIA Study Group. Trastuzumab emtansine for HER2-positive advanced breast cancer. N Engl J Med. 2012;367(19):1783-91.

140. Amiri-Kordestani L, Blumenthal GM, Xu QC, Zhang L, Tang SW, Ha L, Weinberg WC, Chi B, Candau-Chacon R, Hughes P, Russell AM, Miksinski SP, Chen XH, McGuinn WD, Palmby T, Schrieber SJ, Liu Q, Wang J, Song P, Mehrotra N, Skarupa L, Clouse K, Al-Hakim A, Sridhara R, Ibrahim A, Justice R, Pazdur R, Cortazar P. FDA approval: ado-trastuzumab emtansine for the treatment of patients with HER2-positive metastatic breast cancer. Clin Cancer Res. 2014;20(17):4436–41.

141. Krop IE, Kim SB, González-Martín A, LoRusso PM, Ferrero JM, Smitt M, Yu R, Leung AC, Wildiers H; TH3RESA study collaborators. Trastuzumab emtansine versus treatment of physician's choice for pretreated HER2-positive advanced breast cancer (TH3RESA): a randomised, open-label, phase 3 trial. Lancet Oncol. 2014;15(7):689–99.

142. Younes A, Gopal AK, Smith SE, Ansell SM, Rosenblatt JD, Savage KJ, Ramchandren R, Bartlett NL, Cheson BD, de Vos S, Forero-Torres A, Moskowitz CH, Connors JM, Engert A, Larsen EK, Kennedy DA, Sievers EL, Chen R. Results of a pivotal phase II study of brentuximab vedotin for patients with relapsed or refractory Hodgkin's lymphoma. J Clin Oncol. 2012;30(18):2183–9.

143. National Cancer Institute at the National Institutes of Health. FDA Approval for Brentuximab Vedotin [Internet]. 2013 [updated 2013 July 1; cited 2015 June 10]. Available from: http://www.cancer.gov/about-cancer/treatment/drugs/fda-brentuximabvedotin#Anchor-Drug.

144. Witzig TE, Gordon LI, Cabanillas F, Czuczman MS, Emmanouilides C, Joyce R, Pohlman BL, Bartlett NL, Wiseman GA, Padre N, Grillo-López AJ, Multani P, White CA. Randomized controlled trial of yttrium-90-labeled ibritumomab tiuxetan radioimmunotherapy versus rituximab immunotherapy for patients with relapsed or refractory low-grade, follicular, or transformed B-cell non-Hodgkin's lymphoma. J Clin Oncol. 2002;20(10):2453–63.

Neurological Complications of Immune-Based Therapies

Martha R. Neagu, Russell W. Jenkins, and David Reardon

Introduction

FDA approval of the Sipuleucel-T (APC8015) prostate cancer vaccine, and the immune checkpoint inhibitors ipilimumab, pembrolizumab, and nivolumab for treatment of melanoma and non-small cell lung cancer (NSCLC), as well as success in treating refractory leukemias with engineered chimeric antigen receptor (CAR) autologous T cells have completely changed the landscape of cancer treatment [1–4], leading to an ever-growing number of FDA-approved immune-based cancer therapies. Immune-based therapies encompass active therapies consisting of anti-tumor vaccines and cellular-based therapies including CAR T cells as well as passive therapies in the form of monoclonal antibodies blocking immune checkpoints. While they are generally more easily tolerated than cytotoxic or targeted therapies, they carry their own unique toxicities. It will become increasingly important for oncologists and neurooncologists to become familiar with the toxicity profiles of these agents, especially with approaches combining immunotherapy with targeted agents, cytotoxic chemotherapies, and/or radiotherapy on the horizon. Immune therapies are generally well tolerated from the neurologic standpoint, and serious neurological sequelae are rare. This chapter highlights the neurologic complications described with the use of cancer vaccines, cytokines, and immune-active antibodies including checkpoint blockade.

M.R. Neagu · R.W. Jenkins
Department of Medical Oncology, Dana Farber Cancer Institute, 450 Brookline Avenue, Boston, MA 02215, USA
e-mail: mneagu@partners.org

R.W. Jenkins
e-mail: rwjenkins@partners.org

D. Reardon (✉)
Center for Neuro-Oncology, Dana-Farber Cancer Institute, 450 Brookline Avenue, Suite D2134, Boston, MA 02215, USA
e-mail: david_reardon@dfci.harvard.edu

© Springer International Publishing AG 2018
D. Schiff et al. (eds.), *Cancer Neurology in Clinical Practice*,
DOI 10.1007/978-3-319-57901-6_17

Tumor Vaccines

Vaccines direct multiple branches of the immune system against target antigens, thereby providing both specificity and durability of anti-tumor responses through immunological editing and memory. The FDA approval of the Sipuleucel-T (APC8015, Provenge®, Dendreon Corp, Seattle, WA, USA) prostate cancer vaccine heralds the potential for using vaccines in cancer eradication [3]. Vaccines are a form of active immunotherapy since they activate and educate an immune response, with repeated exposures leading to a refinement in both quality and speed of the response that is in general associated with a favorable safety and low side effect profile.

Therapeutic Tumor Vaccines

Sipuleucel-T (Provenge®)

Sipuleucel-T is a cell-based prostate cancer vaccine that received FDA approved for the treatment of metastatic castration-resistant prostate cancer [3] after showing a four-month improved survival in a phase III trial. The vaccine consists of patient's autologous peripheral blood mononuclear cells (including dendritic and other antigen-presenting cells) activated ex vivo with a recombinant fusion protein (PA2024) of the tumor-specific antigen prostatic acid phosphatase fused to granulocyte–macrophage colony-stimulating factor (GM-CSF), an immune cell activator [3]. Overall, the vaccine was well tolerated and the most common complication reported was an acute, but mild, infusion reaction. Common adverse events included chills, fever, and fatigue in 20% of patients with few grade III or IV adverse events reported [3, 5]. Neurological complications were rare and when present generally mild (Grade 1 and 2), with headache reported in 18% of Provenge-treated patients compared to 6.6% in the control patients. Asthenia and tremor were reported by 10.8 and 5% of patients, respectively, in the treatment group compared to 6.6 and 3%, respectively, in the control group [3, 5]. Other neuromuscular events such as paresthesias and muscle cramps were comparable between Sipuleucel-T-treated and control-treated patients, while depression rates were higher in patients receiving control treatment [3, 5]. In the initial randomized phase III trial, cerebrovascular events were observed in 2.4% of patients in the Provenge group compared with 1.8% of patients in controls, which was neither statistically significant ($P = 1.00$, Fisher's exact test) nor clearly temporally related. Given multiple preexisting stroke risk factors in both groups, a causal relationship is unlikely [3, 5].

Talimogene Laherparepvec (T-VEC, Imlygic°, Amgen, Thousand Oaks, CA, USA)

In October 2015, the FDA approved the first oncolytic virus therapy, talimogene laherparepvec (T-VEC, or Imlygic®), for the treatment of unresectable stage IIIb to IV metastatic melanoma [6, 7]. It went on to approval in Europe by the European Medicines Association (EMA) in January of 2016 [8]. This global approval was based on significant improvement in durable response rate and improvement in overall survival combined with a favorable safety profile [6, 7]. Imlygic consists of a live-attenuated herpes simplex virus 1 strain genetically modified to express GM-CSF [7], and is injected directly into unresectable cutaneous, subcutaneous, or nodal melanoma lesions. T-VEC is engineered to promote replication and lysis of infected cancer cells (but not healthy cells) at the injection site. Infected cells then produce GM-CSF, allowing recruited dendritic cells to activate cytotoxic T lymphocytes that in turn induce an anti-tumor immune response in distant lesions, reminiscent of tumor vaccine function [7]. Imlygic safety was evaluated among 419 patients and compared to 127 patients receiving GM-CSF control only in a phase III trial [6, 7]. Overall, it was very well tolerated, with the most common adverse events related to injection site reaction and quickly resolving fever, chills, and flu-like symptoms [7]. Neurological side effects were limited to headache (18.8% of Imlygic-treated patients compared to 9.5% of patients treated with GM-CSF alone) and dizziness (9.6% of Imlygic-treated patients compared to 3.2% of controls) [6, 7]. The EMA also lists occasional confusional state, anxiety, depression, dizziness, and insomnia [8] as potential side effects.

Bacillus Calmette-Guerin (BCG)

BCG is an attenuated strain of mycobacterium tuberculosis that was used in pioneering immunotherapy experiments to show that a vaccine could inhibit tumor growth in experimental animals [9]. Marketed as TheraCysR® (Sanofi-Pasteur, Swiftwater, PA USA), intravesical BCG was FDA approved in 1990 [10, 11] after having proven to significantly reduce the recurrence of non-muscle invasive bladder cancer (NMIBC); it remains a cornerstone in treatment of NMIBC [11–13]. The majority of patients report local side effects including cystitis and some report systemic side effects including BCG infection and generalized BCG reaction. Neurological side effects are negligible, limited to grade 1–2 headache and dizziness in 1.8 and 0.9% of patients treated with intravesical BCG, respectively, compared to 3.8 and 0.8% in the control arm treated with intravesical doxorubicin [10, 11]. Subsequent studies focused on side effect improvement with dose or schedule alterations do not mention neurological side effects [12, 14].

Prophylactic Tumor Vaccines

Human Papillomavirus Quadrivalent (Types 6, 11, 16, 18) Vaccine, Recombinant (Gardasil°, Merck, Kenilworth, NJ, USA, Silgard°, Merck, Kenilworth, NJ, USA)

The cervical cancer vaccine, Gardasil®, FDA approved in 2006 as a cancer prevention vaccine, offers protection from those HPV strains accounting for approximately 90% of all cases of cervical cancer [15–19]. Despite remarkable results with prevalence reduction in cancer-causing HPV serotypes from 11.5 to 4.3% among women aged 14–19 years and from 18.5 to 12.1% among 20–24-year-olds when comparing the pre-vaccine era (2003–2006) to 4 years of the vaccine era (2009–2012) [16], Gardasil® has been highly politicized. The FDA analyzed its safety data across 7 clinical trials (18,983 individuals), and aside from minor injection site reactions, the vaccine has been found to have an excellent safety profile. The most common reported side effect in both Gardasil (28.2%) and control/placebo (28.4%) was headache in females aged 9–26 years. In males aged 9–26, the same held true although headaches were only reported in 12.3% in the Gardasil group and 11.2% in the control/placebo group [15]. There were a small number of autoimmune events including two multiple sclerosis (MS) cases in 10,706 women in the Gardasil group and four MS cases reported in the 9412 control/placebo group [15]. A thorough summary of published, post-licensure safety data spanning 9 years failed to find any increase in incidence of serious adverse events including Guillain–Barre Syndrome, MS, or stroke and showed an excellent safety profile for Gardasil® [19].

Cytokines

With the notable exception of melanoma and renal cell carcinoma (RCC) treatment, cytokine cancer immunotherapy has met with little success due to systemic toxicity, difficulty in obtaining sufficient intratumoral cytokine concentrations, and the ability of tumors to suppress the transient immune activation induced by cytokines therapy [20, 21]. Falling into the category of interleukins, interferons, and colony-stimulating factors (used as immune adjuvants for vaccines), cytokines are the main modulators and messengers of the immune system. Thus, they have a rich, albeit somewhat disappointing, history in cancer immunotherapy [20, 21].

Interleukin 2 (IL-2)

Interleukin-2 (IL-2) is a potent activator of cellular immunity, acting as a growth factor and activator of natural killer (NK) and T cells. IL-2 is FDA approved for the treatment of metastatic melanoma and RCC; it induces a clinical response in up to 20 and 25% of patients for melanoma and RCC, respectively, with durable responses in less than 7% of treated patients [22–24]. Due to its potent systemic activity, IL-2 is poorly tolerated potentially causing extensive systemic toxicity including vascular leak syndrome as well as immune exhaustion at high doses through preferential activation of T regs and subsequent elimination of T cell effectors, limiting its use [21, 22]. Treatment with IL-2 commonly causes dose-dependent neuropsychiatric complications in 30–50% of patients [23, 24], which usually resolve upon treatment cessation. IL-2 can cause mental status changes ranging from cognitive impairment, depression, confusion, disorientation, delusions, and visual hallucinations to coma in very rare instances (two patients in 270 treated melanoma patients, 1% [25]) [23, 24]. While combination of IL-2 with other chemotherapies seems to result in less confusion than high-dose monotherapy [26], combination of IL-2 with the immunologically active GM-CSF resulted in one report of fatal intracranial hemorrhage secondary to multifocal venous sinus thrombosis [27], although a causal relationship remains unclear [28, 29]. Additional case reports highlight brachial plexopathy [30], myositis [31], myasthenia gravis [32], and one case of fatal acute leukoencephalopathy [33].

Tumor Necrosis Factor Alpha (TNF-α)

The acute phase reactant and pro-inflammatory cytokine, TNF-α, is a central player in inflammation-induced carcinogenesis and tumor control. Through complex mechanisms, it effects changes in vascular permeability, activating natural killer and cytotoxic T cells, and controls apoptotic and growth pathways in multiple cell types [34, 35]. Despite its biological importance in cancer, TNF-α use is limited due to systemic toxicity [36] including encephalopathy, transient focal neurological symptoms, headaches, and aphasia [36].

TNF-α is used in isolated limb perfusion for soft tissue sarcoma or melanoma patients. Here, it is instilled in closed systems with limited systemic or central nervous system diffusion, limiting neurological complications to a mild, mainly sensory peripheral neuropathy within two weeks after treatment that resolved by 8 weeks [37].

Interferon Alpha (IFN-α)

Produced largely by antigen-presenting cells, IFN-α has diverse immunomodulatory effects and an extensive track record in cancer treatment [20, 21]. IFN-α has direct anti-tumor effects, inhibiting tumor proliferation and augmenting immune recognition through activation of resident antigen-presenting cells [20, 21] and in 1986 was the first immunotherapeutic approved by the US FDA. Initially utilized for hairy cell leukemia, it has since found use in multiple cancers including melanoma, chronic myelogenous leukemia, advanced renal cell cancer, Kaposi's sarcoma, and other hematologic cancers (e.g., non-Hodgkin lymphoma, low-grade lymphoma) [38–40] as well as cervical intraepithelial neoplasia [20].

Unfortunately, IFN-α has a broad toxicity profile that is in general dose-dependent. The extensive experience with its use in cancer therapy has resulted in established guidelines for diagnosis and treatment of complications. More than 80% of patients will suffer constitutional symptoms such as fever, fatigue, headaches, gastrointestinal symptoms, and myalgias as well as increased liver enzymes with high-dose therapy. Cytopenias are also common and managed with dose reduction [41, 42].

Neuropsychiatric symptoms are dose related and common, especially during high-dose administration. They include depression (45% patients), confusion (10%), and mania (<1%) [43]. Depression develops over weeks to months and resolves within weeks of IFN-α discontinuation; it responds well to selective serotonin reuptake inhibitors, although rare cases of suicide while on IFN-α have been reported [43, 44]. Confusion ranges from reports of cognitive and memory dysfunction, encephalopathy, and lethargy. While once again generally reversible with discontinuation of IFN-α [43], reports of permanent dementia as well as persistent vegetative states exist [45]. Hallucinations and seizures have also been observed [46]. The most common neurotoxicity with lower doses is tremor (22%) [43]. Other more rare reported neurological complications fall in the autoimmune spectrum and include oculomotor palsy [43], neuropathy [47], myasthenia gravis [48], brachial plexopathy, and polyradiculopathy [43].

Due to the extensive experience with IFN-α in cancer treatment, many neurological and neurobehavioral symptoms have been noted that differ only slightly between the two preparations (IFN-α 2a and 2b) in clinical use and span irritability (15%), dizziness (21%) and vertigo (19%), insomnia (14%), mental status changes (12%) as well as somnolence, lethargy, cognitive complications, and confusion, and rare motor weakness with high-dose IFN-α 2a [49]. Similarly, IFN-α 2b treatment has been associated with emotional and mood symptoms (irritability, emotional liability, anxiety, depression) (4–40%), insomnia (1–12%), somnolence (1–33%), confusion (1–12%), decreased concentration (1–14%), dizziness (7–23%) and vertigo (8%) paresthesias (1–21%), and hypertonia (5%), although neuropsychiatric effects may be more prominent with IFN-α 2b [50, 51].

For the special case of intrathecal administration of IFN-α, which was occasionally used for neoplastic meningitis associated with melanoma [52], acute headache, nausea, vomiting, and dizziness can develop within hours of administration as is common for intrathecal administration of many agents with symptoms typically resolving 12–24 h thereafter. Patients can also develop severe, dose-dependent encephalopathy days after treatment, particularly in the setting of prior CNS radiotherapy [53].

Immune-Active Antibodies

Monoclonal antibodies are used in the treatment of various different cancer types. In addition to binding specific growth or survival-related target antigens on cancer cells, they can be also designed to bind antigens on cancer, immune, or endothelial cells; once bound to their target, these antibodies modulate the tumor immune environment [54]. Monoclonal antibodies are most commonly naked (unconjugated), but increasingly sophisticated modifications have led to new cancer therapies including bispecific T cell engagers (BiTE®, Amgen, Thousand Oaks, CA, USA) with the ability to specifically target cytotoxic T cells to cancer cells [55].

Naked Monoclonal and Bispecifc Antibodies

Bevacizumab (Avastin®, Genentech, South San Francisco, CA, USA)

Bevacizumab, a recombinant, humanized monoclonal antibody against vascular endothelial growth factor A (VEGF-A) is emerging as an interesting molecule in immunotherapy as it seems to be a highly immune-active anti-angiogenic drug [56]. In addition to effects on tumor vascularization, VEGF signaling is profoundly immunosuppressive [56]. With oxygen starvation, tumor-elaborated VEGF-A effects on the tumor immune environment range from restriction of activated T cell migration through tumor vasculature, to enhancement of regulatory T cell activity and

preferential recruitment into the tumor, inhibition of dendritic cell maturation, and induction of apoptosis in CD8 cells [56–58]. Since VEGF signaling is an inhibitory immune modulator, VEGF blockade can enhance anti-tumor immune responses [57] and trials combining bevacizumab with checkpoint blockade are underway for multiple cancers [59].

Neurological complications of bevacizumab are discussed in detail in Chap. 16. Like most antibodies, bevacizumab is well tolerated. Its vascular effects, however, can promote both increased hemorrhage and increased thrombosis, reflected neurologically in an increased rate of intracranial hemorrhage and stroke. Incidence of intracranial hemorrhage with bevacizumab treatment was increased both in patients with CNS cancer (primary or metastatic) (0.8–3.3%) and those with systemic cancers and no CNS involvement (0.3–0.7%) [60–63]. The risk of serious thromboembolic events such as ischemic stroke is also increased with bevacizumab treatment [64] with the incidence of ischemic stroke at 1.9% in one study [65]. Microvascular dysfunction can also occur, and <0.1% of patients develop posterior reversible encephalopathy syndrome (PRES). While the etiology of this syndrome is unknown, it is characterized by pathognomonic findings on MRI and presents with headache, confusion, visual symptoms, and seizures. With supportive treatment, PRES resolves [66]. Optic neuropathy was a complication described in 1.2% of bevacizumab-treated glioblastoma patients [67].

Blinatumomab (Blincyt, BiTE®)

The first of its kind, blinatumomab, a bispecific T cell engager antibody construct (BiTE®) designed to target the CD19 antigen on B cell leukemia and the CD3 antigen on T cells, was FDA approved in 2014 for the treatment of recurrent or refractory Philadelphia chromosome-negative B cell acute lymphoblastic leukemia [68]. BiTE®s recruit the patient's own polyclonal cytotoxic T cells to antigen targeting cells (including tumor cells) both providing specificity and activating the T cells to kill tumor cells [68]. Adverse neurological events were reported in >50% of 189 blinatumomab-treated patients in a multicenter phase II study [69]. While the majority were mild and included headaches (34%), tremor (17%), dizziness (14%), and confusion (12%), there were grade 3 and 4 neurological complications including encephalopathy and ataxia in 11 and 2% of patients, respectively [69]. This study slightly modified blinatumomab administration based on a previous phase II study, where six (17%) of 36 treated patients discontinued the drug following significant neurological complications including encephalopathy, psychosis, and convulsions [70]. Symptom resolution occurred in all six patients, and they were subsequently re-exposed to blinatumomab. Patients who had developed seizures were well controlled on AEDs, but two encephalopathy patients had to discontinue the medication for symptom recurrence on re-exposure [70]. The modular nature of bispecific engagers makes them excellent T cell activation platforms for multiple targets. As bispecific engagers with other specificity are under development, it will be interesting to determine whether neurologic complications are related to tumor antigen target or are a T cell activation specific phenomenon [68].

Checkpoint Inhibitors

Immune checkpoint inhibitors neutralize inhibitory T cell signaling, thereby enabling recognition and destruction of tumor cells by the immune system [71]. These immunomodulatory monoclonal antibodies have transformed the treatment of melanoma in recent years, and are now demonstrating activity in several other cancers [72]. Cytotoxic T-lymphocyte antigen-4 (CTLA-4) and programmed cell death receptor-1 (PD-1) are immune checkpoints that have been successfully targeted with monoclonal antibodies, and now represent first-line treatment options in metastatic melanoma. In melanoma, these agents have response rates that range from 20 to 40% as single agents, and response rates as high as 60% when given in combination [73, 74]. Durable responses have been reported in many patients, presumably from induction of immunologic memory, providing promise of long-term disease control making these very attractive options for treatment [75]. While these are powerful and promising therapeutic agents, their use can be limited by unique inflammatory and autoimmune toxicities, known as immune-related adverse events (irAEs), which can involve the skin, colon, liver, thyroid, kidney, and other organ systems [76]. These side effects are distinct from chemotherapy-related toxicities and while only rarely life-threatening, can be challenging to manage and result in significant morbidity. There is now a growing body of literature devoted to the management of side effects of immune checkpoint inhibitors [76–78]. Immune-related neurological adverse events (irNAEs) are rare events, but can be particularly devastating and can necessitate permanent discontinuation of the inciting immunotherapy.

Ipilimumab

The CTLA-4 monoclonal antibody ipilimumab (Yervoy®, Bristol-Myers Squibb, New York, NY, USA) was the first immune checkpoint inhibitor approved for melanoma in 2011, based on overall survival benefit [2, 79]. Ipilimumab has a response rate ranging from 10 to 20% as a single agent, with many of the responders having durable disease control [75]. Neurological toxicities associated with ipilimumab occur in <1% of patients and may have non-specific early manifestations including headaches, dizziness, lethargy, and fatigue [80, 81]. The varied diagnoses and syndromes described in patients treated with ipilimumab include encephalopathy [82], posterior reversible encephalopathy syndrome [83], aseptic meningitis [81], late-onset paraplegia [84], enteric neuropathy [85], transverse myelitis [86], Guillain-Barre syndrome [87], chronic inflammatory demyelinating polyneuropathy [86], myasthenia gravis [88], neurosarcoidosis [89], granulomatous inflammation of the CNS [81], Tolosa–Hunt syndrome [81], in addition to well-described neuroendocrine side effects, such as hypophysitis (Fig. 17.1a, b) [90, 91] and neuroophthalmologic and ocular side effects including uveitis [92], optic neuropathy [93], and orbital inflammation [94–96]. Many of these syndromes and conditions appear autoimmune in nature. Neuropsychiatric disturbances in response to cytokine treatments are well-described, and while psychological side effects (e.g., depression and anxiety) have been reported in patients treated with ipilimumab, these appear to be less common that in patients treated with interferon [97]. The median time to onset of irAEs from ipilimumab is ∼6 weeks (i.e., after 2 doses of ipilimumab), with some events occurring as early as 2 weeks, and the majority occurring within the 12-week induction period [98, 99]. In general, side effects were more common with the higher dose of ipilimumab (10 mg/kg), but many of the above side effects were noted at the standard (3 mg/kg) dose. Management of irAEs/irNAEs involves discontinuation of the immune checkpoint agent and if moderate to severe (grade 3 or 4), temporary administration of immunosuppressive steroids, typically high-dose intravenous corticosteroids. In the event of steroid-refractory irAEs/irNAEs, tumor necrosis factor alpha (TNF-α) antagonists, mycophenolate mofetil, and other agents may have a role. For serious, life-threatening neurological complications such as Guillain–Barre syndrome, plasmapheresis and intravenous immune globulin have been utilized, although their effectiveness remains unclear [80, 86, 87]. Many of these side effects are reversible with discontinuation, and improvement in symptoms may be seen as early as 1–2 weeks with complete resolution 1–2 months after onset [98, 99]. However, permanent organ damage and dysfunction is possible and specific irNAEs such as Guillain–Barre can potentially be fatal. With severe (grade 3–4) toxicity, the offending agent should be permanently discontinued.

Pembrolizumab and Nivolumab

PD1 monoclonal antibodies, pembrolizumab (Keytruda®, Merck, Kenilworth, NJ, USA), and nivolumab (Opdivo®, Bristol-Myers Squibb, New York, NY, USA) are now approved for metastatic melanoma, with superior response rates and lower adverse event rates compared to ipilimumab [73, 74]. As a consequence, PD1 inhibitors may supplant

(a)   **(b)**

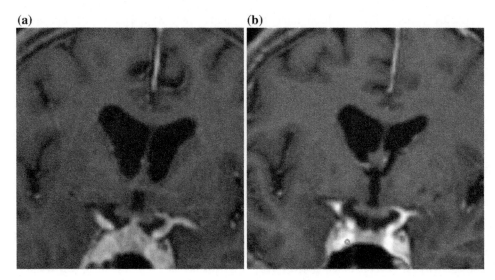

Fig. 17.1 Ipilimumab-related hypophysitis. MRI of the brain in a 77-year-old woman with metastatic melanoma. After the fourth cycle of ipilimumab, she developed profound weakness, fatigue, and confusion, with significant endocrine and electrolyte abnormalities relating to pituitary hypophysitis attributed to ipilimumab treatment. On T1-weighted, contrast-enhanced imaging, her MRI **a** shows an enhancing pituitary and stalk. The lesion abuts the optic chiasm. **b** shows the region prior to ipilimumab treatment, where no enhancement or enlargement is noted (Image courtesy of Sashank Prasad, M.D., Brigham and Women's Hospital)

CTLA-4 inhibitors as monotherapy for first-line treatment for metastatic melanoma. Indeed, responses rates (30–35% vs. 12%), progression-free survival, and overall survival favored pembrolizumab over ipilimumab, when compared head-to-head in a randomized phase III trial, using two different schedules of pembrolizumab compared to ipilimumab (given at standard dose and schedule of 3 mg/kg every 3 weeks for 4 doses) (Keynote-006) [74]. The toxicity profile of pembrolizumab was also favorable compared to ipilimumab with nearly half the number of grade 3–5 adverse events (10–13% vs. 19.2%). In a phase 3 study comparing nivolumab with dacarbazine in previously untreated melanoma, for instance, rare neurologic complications included headache (4.4%), paresthesias (1%), vertigo (1%), and hypophysitis (0.5%) [74]. Case reports highlight rare irNAEs including vasculitis [100], and encephalitis [101].

Notwithstanding the somewhat more favorable irAE profile, response rates to monotherapy with either PD-1 or CTLA-4 inhibitors remain <50%, prompting evaluation of dual immune checkpoint blockade and several combined approaches with targeted therapies, radiation, and chemotherapy. Two recent studies evaluating concurrent immunotherapy with CTLA-4 and PD1 inhibition reported improved response rates compared to monotherapy with either ipilimumab or nivolumab [73, 102]. While overall survival data are not yet available, the rate of severe (grade 3 or 4) adverse events was >50% leading to a 30–40% discontinuation rate in the combination setting, although irNAEs were not addressed. Future studies will address the issue of whether sequential immune checkpoint inhibition is comparable to concurrent therapy, but these studies underscore the importance of evaluation of adverse event monitoring with single-agent immunotherapies, combinations of immune checkpoint inhibitors, and the emerging combinations of immune checkpoint inhibitors with targeted agents or traditional chemotherapy. The adverse event rate in patients treated with nivolumab following prior treatment with ipilimumab was 18–33%, which is lower than seen with combined therapy but higher than reported rates of irAEs with nivolumab in the first line [103, 104]. There is a paucity of data regarding the side effect profile of patients receiving ipilimumab following progression on nivolumab or pembrolizumab, although there are some recent reports of early and severe toxicities following sequential immune checkpoint inhibition [105].

Immune Therapy Under Development

Chimeric Antigen Receptor (CAR) T Cells

An innovative approach to potent and specific cancer immunotherapy is the generation of engineered chimeric antigen receptor (CAR) autologous T cells [106]. Based on recent impressive results, these agents are likely to be FDA approved in the near future for acute B lineage leukemias. CARs are cytotoxic T cells that have the MHC-restricted T cell receptor replaced with an engineered chimeric receptor targeting the desired tumor cell-specific surface antigen. CARs improve on bispecific engagers by delivering tumor-specific cytotoxic T cells, activated through engineered chimeric receptors, which are able to bypass certain aspects of tumor-elaborated immune inhibition. Bispecific engagers, in contrast, rely on the recruitment of patient's endogenous polyclonal T cells, and can be suppressed by tumor-elaborated factors, leading to immune evasion of tumors. The first CAR T cell in clinical trials targets CD19 (CD19 CAR) and has been tested in patients with relapsed ALL and refractory diffuse large B cell lymphoma (DLBCL) [1, 107]. Five adult patients with relapsed B cell acute lymphoblastic leukemia (B-ALL) were treated with CD19 CAR transfer. Amazingly, all patients had a complete response; there were no comments on neurological toxicity [108]. Among 15 patients with advanced B cell malignancies including DLBCL receiving with CD19 CAR in a phase 1/2a clinical trial, the majority showed complete remission with a 92% objective response rate [106]. Interestingly, in this study (much like in studies with bispecific engagers), neurological toxicity was prominent with common confusion and obtundation. Three of 15 patients also developed aphasia with various associated neurological symptoms ranging from myoclonus, to confusion, hemifacial spasm, facial hemiparesis, apraxia, and gait disturbance [106]. All patients improved between 11 and 20 days after administration, and one patient had lymphocytosis in the CSF that consisted 97% of T cells (32.9% CD19 CAR), despite lack of CD19 expression in the CNS (confirmed with serial brain biopsies and reported by multiple investigators) [106].

Summary

Advances in our understanding of cancer immunology are leading to rapid FDA approval of novel cancer treatments, harnessing the power of the immune system to fight cancer. While most of these immune therapies are well tolerated due to the exquisite self-regulation of the immune system, immune-related adverse events, including neurological side effects, can occur. Of the agents discussed here, vaccines cause the least neurologic complications, since they are both the most specific and allow for immune self-regulation. With global activation of the immune system, such as using IL-2 or checkpoint inhibition, rare autoimmune neurological complications can be seen such as myasthenia gravis, neuropathies, plexopathies, cranial nerve involvement, to name but a few. While irNAEs are rare with checkpoint inhibitors, they can cause neuroendocrine complications in the form of autoimmune hypophysitis, and rare but dangerous conditions such as Guillain–Barre syndrome (GBS). Cytokines such as IL-2 and especially IFN cross the blood–brain barrier and have CNS effects including neuropsychiatric changes ranging from depression to confusion. Some immunotherapies

such as the anti-angiogenic and immune-active bevacizumab (Avastin) have neurotoxicities directly related to their mechanism of action, such that bevacizumab presents with increased risk of bleeding (intracranial hemorrhage), clotting (stroke), as well as complications related to microvascular dysfunction (PRES). CD19 targeting methods such as BiTEs or CD19 CAR T cells are the most neurologically active and can cause confusion, ataxia, encephalitis, aphasia, and neuropsychiatric complications; some neurotoxicities can be severe enough to force medication discontinuation. Many in the field are looking toward combination therapies either combining multiple immunotherapies, or combining immunotherapy with targeted, biological, or cytotoxic treatments with the hope of increased responses and durability. These trials have just begun, and it will be important to see how this changes the landscape of neurotoxicity in cancer treatment.

References

1. Grupp SA, et al. Chimeric antigen receptor-modified T cells for acute lymphoid leukemia. N Engl J Med. 2013;368(16):1509–18.
2. Hodi FS, et al. Improved survival with ipilimumab in patients with metastatic melanoma. N Engl J Med. 2010;363(8):711–23.
3. Kantoff PW, et al. Sipuleucel-T immunotherapy for castration-resistant prostate cancer. N Engl J Med. 2010;363 (5):411–22.
4. Robert C, et al. Nivolumab in previously untreated melanoma without BRAF mutation. N Engl J Med. 2015;372(4):320–30.
5. Administration, U.S.F.A.D. Provenge [Internet]. 2010. Available from: http://www.fda.gov/downloads/BiologicsBloodVaccines/CellularGeneTherapyProducts/ApprovedProducts/UCM210031.pdf.
6. Administration, U.S.F.A.D. Imlygic [Internet]. 2015. Available from: http://www.fda.gov/BiologicsBloodVaccines/CellularGeneTherapyProducts/ApprovedProducts/ucm469411.htm.
7. Andtbacka RH, et al. Talimogene laherparepvec improves durable response rate in patients with advanced melanoma. J Clin Oncol. 2015;33(25):2780–8.
8. Agency EM. Talimogene laherparepvec [Internet]. 2015. Available from: http://www.ema.europa.eu/docs/en_GB/document_library/EPAR_-_Product_Information/human/002771/WC500201079.pdf.
9. Old LJ, et al. Effect of prior splenectomy on the growth of sarcoma 180 in normal and bacillus Calmette-Guerin infected mice. Experientia. 1962;18:335–6.
10. Administration, U.S.F.A.D. TheraCys [Internet]. 1990. Available from:http://www.fda.gov/downloads/BiologicsBloodVaccines/CellularGeneTherapyProducts/ApprovedProducts/UCM310364.pdf.
11. Lamm DL, et al. A randomized trial of intravesical doxorubicin and immunotherapy with bacille Calmette-Guerin for transitional-cell carcinoma of the bladder. N Engl J Med. 1991;325(17):1205–9.
12. Lamm DL, et al. Maintenance bacillus Calmette-Guerin immunotherapy for recurrent TA, T1 and carcinoma in situ transitional cell carcinoma of the bladder: a randomized Southwest oncology group study. J Urol. 2000;163(4):1124–9.
13. Morales A, Eidinger D, Bruce AW. Intracavitary bacillus Calmette-Guerin in the treatment of superficial bladder tumors. J Urol. 1976;116(2):180–3.

14. Brausi M, et al. Side effects of bacillus Calmette-Guerin (BCG) in the treatment of intermediate- and high-risk Ta, T1 papillary carcinoma of the bladder: results of the EORTC genito-urinary cancers group randomised phase 3 study comparing one-third dose with full dose and 1 year with 3 years of maintenance BCG. Eur Urol. 2014;65(1):69–76.

15. Administration, U.S.F.A.D. Gardasil [Internet]. 2006. Available fhttp://www.fda.gov/downloads/BiologicsBloodVaccines/Vaccines/ApprovedProducts/UCM111263.pdf.

16. Markowitz LE, et al. Reduction in human papillomavirus (HPV) prevalence among young women following HPV vaccine introduction in the United States, National health and nutrition examination surveys, 2003–2010. J Infect Dis. 2013;208(3):385–93.

17. Reisinger KS, et al. Safety and persistent immunogenicity of a quadrivalent human papillomavirus types 6, 11, 16, 18 L1 virus-like particle vaccine in preadolescents and adolescents: a randomized controlled trial. Pediatr Infect Dis J. 2007;26(3):201–9.

18. Thaxton L, Waxman AG. Cervical cancer prevention: immunization and screening 2015. Med Clin N Am. 2015;99(3):469–77.

19. Vichnin M, et al. An overview of quadrivalent human papillomavirus vaccine safety: 2006 to 2015. Pediatr Infect Dis J. 2015;34(9):983–91.

20. Muller D. Antibody fusions with immunomodulatory proteins for cancer therapy. Pharmacol Ther. 2015;154:57–66.

21. Patel MA, et al. The future of glioblastoma therapy: synergism of standard of care and immunotherapy. Cancers (Basel). 2014;6(4):1953–85.

22. Liao W, Lin JX, Leonard WJ. Interleukin-2 at the crossroads of effector responses, tolerance, and immunotherapy. Immunity. 2013;38(1):13–25.

23. Denicoff KD, et al. The neuropsychiatric effects of treatment with interleukin-2 and lymphokine-activated killer cells. Ann Intern Med. 1987;107(3):293–300.

24. Petrella T, et al. Single-agent interleukin-2 in the treatment of metastatic melanoma: a systematic review. Cancer Treat Rev. 2007;33(5):484–96.

25. Atkins MB, et al. High-dose recombinant interleukin 2 therapy for patients with metastatic melanoma: analysis of 270 patients treated between 1985 and 1993. J Clin Oncol. 1999;17(7):2105–16.

26. Buzaid AC, Atkins M. Practical guidelines for the management of biochemotherapy-related toxicity in melanoma. Clin Cancer Res. 2001;7(9):2611–9.

27. Hotton KM, et al. A phase Ib/II trial of granulocyte-macrophage-colony stimulating factor and interleukin-2 for renal cell carcinoma patients with pulmonary metastases: a case of fatal central nervous system thrombosis. Cancer. 2000;88(8):1892–901.

28. Correale P, et al. Recruitment of dendritic cells and enhanced antigen-specific immune reactivity in cancer patients treated with hr-GM-CSF (Molgramostim) and hr-IL-2. results from a phase Ib clinical trial. Eur J Cancer. 2001;37(7):892–902.

29. Westermann J, et al. Granulocyte/macrophage-colony-stimulating-factor plus interleukin-2 plus interferon alpha in the treatment of metastatic renal cell carcinoma: a pilot study. Cancer Immunol Immunother. 2001;49(11):613–20.

30. Loh FL, et al. Brachial plexopathy associated with interleukin-2 therapy. Neurology. 1992;42(2):462–3.

31. Esteva-Lorenzo FJ, et al. Myositis associated with interleukin-2 therapy in a patient with metastatic renal cell carcinoma. Cancer. 1995;76(7):1219–23.

32. Freeman HJ. Colitis associated with biological agents. World J Gastroenterol. 2012;18(16):1871–4.

33. Vecht CJ, et al. Acute fatal leukoencephalopathy after interleukin-2 therapy. N Engl J Med. 1990;323(16):1146–7.

34. Kashii Y, et al. Constitutive expression and role of the TNF family ligands in apoptotic killing of tumor cells by human NK cells. J Immunol. 1999;163(10):5358–66.

35. Waters JP, Pober JS, Bradley JR. Tumour necrosis factor and cancer. J Pathol. 2013;230(3):241–8.

36. Balkwill F. Tumour necrosis factor and cancer. Nat Rev Cancer. 2009;9(5):361–71.

37. Drory VE, et al. Neurotoxicity of isolated limb perfusion with tumor necrosis factor. J Neurol Sci. 1998;158(1):1–4.

38. Golomb HM, et al. Alpha-2 interferon therapy of hairy-cell leukemia: a multicenter study of 64 patients. J Clin Oncol. 1986;4(6):900–5.

39. Kirkwood JM, et al. A pooled analysis of eastern cooperative oncology group and intergroup trials of adjuvant high-dose interferon for melanoma. Clin Cancer Res. 2004;10(5):1670–7.

40. Quesada JR, Gutterman JU. Alpha interferons in B-cell neoplasms. Br J Haematol. 1986;64(4):639–46.

41. Hauschild A, et al. Practical guidelines for the management of interferon-alpha-2b side effects in patients receiving adjuvant treatment for melanoma: expert opinion. Cancer. 2008;112(5):982–94.

42. Jonasch E, Haluska FG. Interferon in oncological practice: review of interferon biology, clinical applications, and toxicities. Oncologist. 2001;6(1):34–55.

43. Caraceni A, et al. Neurotoxicity of interferon-alpha in melanoma therapy: results from a randomized controlled trial. Cancer. 1998;83(3):482–9.

44. Musselman DL, et al. Paroxetine for the prevention of depression induced by high-dose interferon alfa. N Engl J Med. 2001;344(13):961–6.

45. Meyers CA, Scheibel RS, Forman AD. Persistent neurotoxicity of systemically administered interferon-alpha. Neurology. 1991;41(5):672–6.

46. Rohatiner AZ, et al. Central nervous system toxicity of interferon. Br J Cancer. 1983;47(3):419–22.

47. Rutkove SB. An unusual axonal polyneuropathy induced by low-dose interferon alfa-2a. Arch Neurol. 1997;54(7):907–8.

48. Bora I, et al. Myasthenia gravis following IFN-alpha-2a treatment. Eur Neurol. 1997;38(1):68.

49. Lipton JH, et al. Phase II, randomized, multicenter, comparative study of peginterferon-alpha-2a (40 kD) (Pegasys) versus interferon alpha-2a (Roferon-A) in patients with treatment-naive, chronic-phase chronic myelogenous leukemia. Leuk Lymphoma. 2007;48(3):497–505.

50. Hensley ML, et al. Risk factors for severe neuropsychiatric toxicity in patients receiving interferon alfa-2b and low-dose cytarabine for chronic myelogenous leukemia: analysis of cancer and leukemia group B 9013. J Clin Oncol. 2000;18(6):1301–8.

51. Michallet M, et al. Pegylated recombinant interferon alpha-2b vs recombinant interferon alpha-2b for the initial treatment of chronic-phase chronic myelogenous leukemia: a phase III study. Leukemia. 2004;18(2):309–15.

52. Dorval T, et al. Malignant melanoma: treatment of metastatic meningitis with intrathecal interferon alpha-2b. Eur J Cancer. 1992;28(1):244–5.

53. Meyers CA, et al. Neurotoxicity of intraventricularly administered alpha-interferon for leptomeningeal disease. Cancer. 1991;68(1):88–92.

54. Mahoney KM, Rennert PD, Freeman GJ. Combination cancer immunotherapy and new immunomodulatory targets. Nat Rev Drug Discov. 2015;14(8):561–84.

55. Klinger M, et al. Harnessing T cells to fight cancer with BiTE ((R)) antibody constructs—past developments and future directions. Immunol Rev. 2016;270(1):193–208.

56. Terme M, et al. Modulation of immunity by antiangiogenic molecules in cancer. Clin Dev Immunol. 2012;2012:492920.
57. Reardon DA, et al. Immunotherapy advances for glioblastoma. Neuro Oncol. 2014;16(11):1441–58.
58. Neagu MR, Reardon DA. An update on the role of immunotherapy and vaccine strategies for primary brain tumors. Curr Treat Options Oncol. 2015;16(11):54.
59. Hodi FS, et al. Bevacizumab plus ipilimumab in patients with metastatic melanoma. Cancer Immunol Res. 2014;2(7):632–42.
60. Besse B, et al. Bevacizumab safety in patients with central nervous system metastases. Clin Cancer Res. 2010;16(1):269–78.
61. Khasraw M, et al. Intracranial hemorrhage in patients with cancer treated with bevacizumab: the memorial Sloan-Kettering experience. Ann Oncol. 2012;23(2):458–63.
62. Friedman HS, et al. Bevacizumab alone and in combination with irinotecan in recurrent glioblastoma. J Clin Oncol. 2009;27 (28):4733–40.
63. Hapani S, et al. Increased risk of serious hemorrhage with bevacizumab in cancer patients: a meta-analysis. Oncology. 2010;79(1–2):27–38.
64. Scappaticci FA, et al. Arterial thromboembolic events in patients with metastatic carcinoma treated with chemotherapy and bevacizumab. J Natl Cancer Inst. 2007;99(16):1232–9.
65. Fraum TJ, et al. Ischemic stroke and intracranial hemorrhage in glioma patients on antiangiogenic therapy. J Neurooncol. 2011;105(2):281–9.
66. Tlemsani C, et al. Posterior reversible encephalopathy syndrome induced by anti-VEGF agents. Target Oncol. 2011;6(4):253–8.
67. Sherman JH, et al. Optic neuropathy in patients with glioblastoma receiving bevacizumab. Neurology. 2009;73(22):1924–6.
68. Stieglmaier J, Benjamin J, Nagorsen D. Utilizing the BiTE (bispecific T-cell engager) platform for immunotherapy of cancer. Expert Opin Biol Ther. 2015;15(8):1093–9.
69. Topp MS, et al. Safety and activity of blinatumomab for adult patients with relapsed or refractory B-precursor acute lymphoblastic leukaemia: a multicentre, single-arm, phase 2 study. Lancet Oncol. 2015;16(1):57–66.
70. Topp MS, et al. Phase II trial of the anti-CD19 bispecific T cell-engager blinatumomab shows hematologic and molecular remissions in patients with relapsed or refractory B-precursor acute lymphoblastic leukemia. J Clin Oncol. 2014;32(36):4134–40.
71. Pardoll DM. The blockade of immune checkpoints in cancer immunotherapy. Nat Rev Cancer. 2012;12(4):252–64.
72. Pennock GK, Chow LQ. The evolving role of immune checkpoint inhibitors in cancer treatment. Oncologist. 2015;20(7):812–22.
73. Larkin J, et al. Combined nivolumab and ipilimumab or monotherapy in untreated melanoma. N Engl J Med. 2015;373 (13):1270–1.
74. Robert C, et al. Pembrolizumab versus ipilimumab in advanced melanoma. N Engl J Med. 2015;372(26):2521–32.
75. Ugurel S, et al. Survival of patients with advanced metastatic melanoma: the impact of novel therapies. Eur J Cancer. 2016;53:125–34.
76. Weber JS, et al. Toxicities of immunotherapy for the practitioner. J Clin Oncol. 2015;33(18):2092–9.
77. Postow MA. Managing immune checkpoint-blocking antibody side effects. American Society of Clinical Oncology educational book/ASCO. American Society of Clinical Oncology. Meeting 2015;35: 76–83.
78. Teply BA, Lipson EJ. Identification and management of toxicities from immune checkpoint-blocking drugs. Oncology. 2014;28 (Suppl 3):30–8.
79. Robert C, et al. Ipilimumab plus dacarbazine for previously untreated metastatic melanoma. N Engl J Med. 2011;364 (26):2517–26.
80. Bot I, et al. Neurological immune-related adverse events of ipilimumab. Pract Neurol. 2013;13(4):278–80.
81. Voskens CJ, et al. The price of tumor control: an analysis of rare side effects of anti-CTLA-4 therapy in metastatic melanoma from the ipilimumab network. PLoS ONE. 2013;8(1):e53745.
82. Conry RM, Sullivan JC, Nabors LB 3rd. Ipilimumab-induced encephalopathy with a reversible splenial lesion. Cancer Immunol Res. 2015;3(6):598–601.
83. Maur M, et al. Posterior reversible encephalopathy syndrome during ipilimumab therapy for malignant melanoma. J Clin Oncol. 2012;30(6):e76–8.
84. O'Kane GM, et al. Late-onset paraplegia after complete response to two cycles of ipilimumab for metastatic melanoma. Oncol Res Treat. 2014;37(12):757–60.
85. Bhatia S, et al. Inflammatory enteric neuropathy with severe constipation after ipilimumab treatment for melanoma: a case report. J Immunother. 2009;32(2):203–5.
86. Liao B, et al. Atypical neurological complications of ipilimumab therapy in patients with metastatic melanoma. Neuro-Oncology. 2014;16(4):589–93.
87. Wilgenhof S, Neyns B. Anti-CTLA-4 antibody-induced Guillain-Barre syndrome in a melanoma patient. Ann Oncol. 2011;22(4):991–3.
88. Johnson DB, et al. Myasthenia gravis induced by ipilimumab in patients with metastatic melanoma. J Clin Oncol. 2015;33(33): e122–4.
89. Murphy KP, et al. New-onset mediastinal and central nervous system sarcoidosis in a patient with metastatic melanoma undergoing CTLA4 monoclonal antibody treatment. Oncol Res Treat. 2014;37(6):351–3.
90. Lam T, et al. Ipilimumab-induced hypophysitis in melanoma patients: an Australian case series. Int Med J. 2015;45(10):1066–73.
91. Mahzari M, et al. Immune checkpoint inhibitor therapy associated hypophysitis. Clin Med Insights Endocrinol Diab. 2015;8:21–8.
92. Miserocchi E, et al. New-onset uveitis during CTLA-4 blockade therapy with ipilimumab in metastatic melanoma patient. Can J Ophthalmol J Can Ophtalmol 2015; 50(1): e2–4.
93. Yeh OL, Francis CE. Ipilimumab-associated bilateral optic neuropathy. J Neuro-Ophthalmol. 2015;35(2):144–7.
94. Sheldon CA, Kharlip J, Tamhankar MA. Inflammatory orbitopathy associated with ipilimumab. Ophthalmic Plast Reconstr Surg. 2015 [Epub ahead of print].
95. Papavasileiou E, et al. Ipilimumab-induced ocular and orbital inflammation—a case series and review of the literature. Ocular Immunol Inflamm. 2015; 1–7.
96. Henderson AD, Thomas DA. A case report of orbital inflammatory syndrome secondary to ipilimumab. Ophthalmic Plast Reconstr Surg. 2015;31(3):e68–70.
97. Kovacs P, et al. Psychological changes in melanoma patients during ipilimumab treatment compared to low-dose interferon alpha therapy—a follow-up study of first experiences. Pathol Oncol Res. 2014;20(4):939–44.
98. Patel SP, Woodman SE. Profile of ipilimumab and its role in the treatment of metastatic melanoma. Drug Des Dev Ther. 2011;5:489–95.
99. Andrews S, Holden R. Characteristics and management of immunerelated adverse effects associated with ipilimumab, a new immunotherapy for metastatic melanoma. Cancer Manage Res. 2012;4:299–307.
100. Khoja L, et al. Eosinophilic fasciitis and acute encephalopathy toxicity from pembrolizumab treatment of a patient with metastatic melanoma. Cancer Immunol Res. 2016;4(3):175–8.

101. Salam S, Lavin T, Turan A. Limbic encephalitis following immunotherapy against metastatic malignant melanoma. BMJ Case Rep. 2016;. doi:10.1136/bcr-2016-215012.

102. Postow MA, et al. Nivolumab and ipilimumab versus ipilimumab in untreated melanoma. N Engl J Med. 2015;372(21):2006–17.

103. Weber JS, et al. Safety, efficacy, and biomarkers of nivolumab with vaccine in ipilimumab-refractory or -naive melanoma. J Clin Oncol. 2013;31(34):4311–8.

104. Wolchok JD, et al. Nivolumab plus ipilimumab in advanced melanoma. N Engl J Med. 2013;369(2):122–33.

105. Danlos FX, et al. Atypical severe immune-related adverse effects resulting from sequenced immunotherapy in melanoma. Melanoma Res. 2015;25(2):178–9.

106. Kochenderfer JN, et al. Chemotherapy-refractory diffuse large B-cell lymphoma and indolent B-cell malignancies can be effectively treated with autologous T cells expressing an anti-CD19 chimeric antigen receptor. J Clin Oncol. 2015;33 (6):540–9.

107. Kochenderfer JN, et al. B-cell depletion and remissions of malignancy along with cytokine-associated toxicity in a clinical trial of anti-CD19 chimeric-antigen-receptor-transduced T cells. Blood. 2012;119(12):2709–20.

108. Brentjens RJ, et al. CD19-targeted T cells rapidly induce molecular remissions in adults with chemotherapy-refractory acute lymphoblastic leukemia. Sci Transl Med. 2013; 5(177): 177ra38.

Neurologic Complications of Hematopoietic Stem Cell Transplantation

Eudocia Q. Lee and Patrick Y. Wen

Introduction

Hematopoietic stem cell transplantation (HSCT) is the transfer of hematopoietic stem cells to re-establish bone marrow function destroyed by the conditioning regimen (i.e., the chemotherapy and/or radiation regimen given to eradicate neoplastic or disease-causing cells) [1]. The vast majority of transplants are used to treat hematologic and lymphoid cancers, although HSCT has been used to treat other cancers and neurologic disorders [2]. An estimated 18,250 bone marrow or umbilical cord blood transplants were performed in the USA in 2013, and the number of transplant recipients continues to increase annually [3], with multiple myeloma and lymphoma accounting for 57% of all HSCT in 2012 [3].

The hematopoietic progenitor cells may be obtained from the patient (i.e., autologous transplant), an allogeneic donor who is not immunological identical (i.e., allogeneic transplant), or a syngeneic donor who is immunologically identical to the recipient, such as a twin sibling. Many of the complications described in this chapter can occur in autologous, allogeneic, and syngeneic transplants. However, unlike patients undergoing autologous or syngeneic transplantation, patients undergoing allogeneic transplantation are at risk of graft-versus-host disease (GVHD) due to mismatched histocompatibility antigens and may require chronic immunosuppressants to prevent graft rejection. This places this population at higher risk of infections and GVHD-related complications.

Hematopoietic stem cells (HSC) can be harvested from bone marrow, peripheral blood, or umbilical cord blood. Bone marrow contains a high concentration of HSCs and can be collected from the posterior or anterior iliac crests. Peripheral blood normally contains HSCs at very low concentrations although these concentrations can increase with administration of granulocyte-colony-stimulating factor (G-CSF) or granulocyte-macrophage colony-stimulating factor (GM-CSF), or during recovery from intensive chemotherapy. Peripheral blood stem cells result in more rapid hematopoietic recovery than autologous marrow. With umbilical cord blood, engraftment is slower leading to a longer period during which patients are susceptible to infections, but patients are less likely to develop GVHD. As the amount of cord blood is small, cord blood transplants are usually more suitable for pediatric populations.

Prior to transplantation, the patient receives a preparative or conditioning regimen that kills cancer cells and suppresses the immune system to prevent rejection of donor cells. This stage is known as conditioning, and the regimen used depends on the underlying disease. Regimens may include busulfan, cyclophosphamide, melphalan, thiotepa, carmustine, etoposide, and/or total body irradiation. HSCs are then infused, and the cells hone to the bone marrow. Engraftment is first evident with recovery of peripheral counts. The time to engraftment depends on the source of the stem cells, whether growth factors are used following transplant, and which GVHD prophylaxis is administered, if any.

Despite significant advances since the first human bone marrow transplant in the 1950s [4], HSCT is still associated with significant morbidity and mortality. Neurologic complications can adversely affect survival in HSCT patients [5–8], and between 10 and 40% of patients undergoing HSCT will develop a clinically significant neurologic complication [9, 10]. Encephalopathy with or without seizures, central nervous system (CNS) infections, and cerebrovascular disorders are the most commonly reported neurologic complications in clinical series [8]. The causes of neurologic complications in HSCT patients are numerous, including chemoradiotoxicity, medication toxicity, metabolic abnormalities, organ failure, GVHD, infection, pancytopenia, and

E.Q. Lee (✉) · P.Y. Wen
Center for Neuro-Oncology, Dana-Farber/Brigham and Women's Cancer Center, 450 Brookline Avenue, Boston, MA 02215, USA
e-mail: eqlee@partners.org

P.Y. Wen
e-mail: pywen@partners.org

© Springer International Publishing AG 2018
D. Schiff et al. (eds.), *Cancer Neurology in Clinical Practice*,
DOI 10.1007/978-3-319-57901-6_18

Table 18.1 Timeline of common neurologic complications

Time point	Complication
Stem cell harvest	Intracranial hypotension due to entry into subarachnoid space during bone marrow aspiration
	Worsening neurologic manifestations of underlying autoimmune syndrome, possibly related to G-CSF
Conditioning	Chemoradiation toxicity (see Table 18.2)
Infusion	Encephalopathy due to DMSO
	Ischemic stroke, possibly related to DMSO or debris across a PFO
	Transient global amnesia
Prior to engraftment and marrow reconstitution	Cerebrovascular accidents related to aspergillus or infectious emboli
	CNS infections including Aspergillus and CMV
	Coagulopathies resulting in SDH
	Drug toxicities including tacrolimus and cyclosporine for GVHD causing PRES as well as antimicrobials causing seizures
	Idiopathic hyperammonemia
	Metabolic abnormalities
	Neuromuscular complications including steroid myopathy, pressure related peroneal nerve palsies, GBS
	Systemic organ failure
Chronic complications (after bone marrow reconstitution)	CNS infections including toxoplasmosis, herpes viruses, and nocardia
	CNS manifestations of chronic GVHD including neuromuscular complications and CNS angiitis
	Drug toxicities including tacrolimus and cyclosporine for GVHD

CNS central nervous system; *DMSO* dimethyl sulfoxide; *PRES* posterior reversible encephalopathy

platelet dysfunction. Risk factors associated with developing neurologic complications include allogeneic HSCT, unrelated donors, and high-grade GVHD [10]. Patients are more susceptible to certain pathologies depending on the timing since transplant (Table 18.1). This chapter will focus on the main etiologies and manifestations.

Encephalopathy

Encephalopathy is the most common neurologic complication encountered in HSCT patients [8]. In a retrospective study of 116 adult HSCT patients, a depressed level of consciousness was a principal reason for admission to intensive care units and conferred a poor prognosis [11]. Similarly, in a study of pediatric HSCT patients, encephalopathy was associated with a poor prognosis [12]. A wide array of neurotoxic insults can cause encephalopathy and/or seizures including chemotherapy, electrolyte imbalance, infections, acid–base disorders, increased intracranial pressure, antimicrobials, organ failure, immunosuppressants, and vitamin deficiencies. Encephalopathy related to chemotherapy, organ failure, antimicrobials, and posterior reversible leukoencephalopathy (PRES) are discussed in more detail below.

Although signs and symptoms may differ depending on the etiology and severity, the hallmark of encephalopathy is an altered mental status manifesting as personality changes, inattentiveness, lack of concentration, lethargy, cognitive dysfunction, and/or depressed consciousness. Other findings that may accompany an acute confusional state include autonomic changes (fever, tachycardia, diaphoresis) and abnormal movements (tremor, asterixis, myoclonus).

Diagnosis is based on clinical history and examination. Fever suggests an infectious etiology such as meningitis or sepsis. Common etiologies that can be easily evaluated through blood or urine studies include electrolyte abnormalities, endocrine disorders, nutritional deficiencies, acid–base disorders, and alcohol/drug intoxication. Patients with an unexplained encephalopathy or with focal neurologic deficits should undergo imaging. Brain MRI with contrast is generally recommended over a head CT unless a neurologic emergency such as hemorrhage or hydrocephalus is suspected or the patient is too unstable to tolerate an MRI. Lumbar puncture is indicated if there is concern for infection, an inflammatory disorder, or neoplastic meningitis. Electroencephalogram (EEG) is useful to evaluate for nonconvulsive status epiletpicus or subclinical seizures.

Prognosis depends on the underlying etiology. Encephalopathy without focal neurologic deficits is often reversible with conservative management and removal of the offending agent or cause. However, certain types of encephalopathy can occasionally result in permanent structural changes, brain damage, and even death.

Chemotherapy-Induced Encephalopathy

Chemotherapy can cause encephalopathy in a dose-dependent fashion. Onset can be acute or delayed. Table 18.2 provides a list of chemotherapies commonly used in HSCT associated with encephalopathy. Acute encephalopathy may present within days of receiving chemotherapy. Pyramidine analogues 5-FU (fluorouracil) and cytarabine (cytosine arabinoside, Ara-C) are associated with a dose-dependent acute encephalopathy that can resolve over several weeks. For example, high-dose cytarabine (HIDAC) may cause an acute cerebellar syndrome occurring after 3–8 days and (less commonly) acute onset generalized encephalopathy characterized

by somnolence, disorientation, headache, and psychosis [13]. Delayed encephalopathy, occurring months after undergoing HSCT, can occur with purine analogues such as fludarabine, which are often used in preparative regimens [14, 15]. Imaging may demonstrate white matter changes similar to posterior reversible encephalopathy syndrome (discussed further below) or toxic leukoencephalopathy. In one series, the incidence of severe CNS toxicity associated with fludarabine conditioning was 2.4%, with cases presenting approximately 2 months after starting fludarabine and evolving over 1 month. Common presenting symptoms included confusion, generalized seizure, severe headache, and blurred vision.

Antimicrobial-Induced Encephalopathy

Because of the increased risk of infection, especially prior to engraftment, many patients will require prophylaxis and/or treatment with antimicrobial agents. The Centers for Disease

Table 18.2 Neurologic complications associated with chemotherapeutic agents commonly used in preparative regimens for hematopoietic stem cell transplantation

Agent	Central nervous system	Peripheral nervous system
Busulfan	• Seizures are common but preventable by seizure prophylaxis with antiepileptics • Headaches	
Carmustine (BCNU)	• Delayed onset encephalopathy (25–47 days after treatment) with lesions in basis pontis, corpus callosum, spinal cord, cerebral hemispheres reported with high-dose BCNU	
Cyclophosphamide	• Impaired cognition reported in breast cancer patients receiving high-dose therapy • Transient dizziness after intravenous push doses	• Guillain–Barre syndrome reported
Cytarabine (cytosine arabinoside, Ara-C, Cytosar)	CNS effects are not common with standard doses of cytarabine, but CNS toxicity may be associated with high-dose therapy: • Acute cerebellar syndrome characterized by dysarthria, dysmetria, and ataxia occurring 3–8 days after initiation of treatment • Acute encephalopathy (with or without cerebellar toxicity) • Seizures	• Motor and sensory neuropathies reported with high-dose therapy.
Etoposide (VP-16)	• Rarely, cerebral edema with capillary leak syndrome • Acute dystonia • Neuropathy	• Neuropathy rarely reported with high-dose therapy
Fludarabine	• CNS toxicity infrequent with conventional doses (≤ 125 mg/m^2 per course of treatment) • High doses can cause delayed, severe encephalopathy characterized by cortical blindness, confusion, and coma • Progressive multifocal leukoencephalopathy reported • Headaches	• Paresthesias reported
Melphalan	• Seizures and encephalopathy in patients with renal failure receiving high-dose melphalan	

Data from Micromedex

Table 18.3 Drugs used in HSCT that can cause encephalopathy ± seizures

Antineoplastic agents
Cytarabine (Ara-C)
Busulfan
Methotrexate
BCNU
Mechlorethamine
Ifosfamide
Cisplatin
Immunosuppressive agents
Cyclosporin
Tacrolimus
Muromonab-CD3
Antibiotics
Aminoglycosides (gentamicin, streptomycin, amikacin, tobramycin, neomycin, kanamycin)
Penicillin
Cephalosporins (cefazolin, cefoselis, ceftazidime, cefoperazone, cefepime)
Carbapenems (imipenem, meropenem, ertapenem)
Vancomycin
Isoniazid
Metronidazole
Trimethoprim/sulfamethoxazole (TMP-SMX)
Antiviral agents
Acyclovir
Ganciclovir
Foscarnet
Antifungal agents
Amphotericin B

Control (CDC) recommends preventing cytomegalovirus (CMV) disease with prophylactic or preemptive gancyclovir, herpes simplex virus (HSV) disease with prophylactic acyclovir, candidiasis with fluconazole, and *Pneumocystis jirovecii* pneumonia (PJP) with trimethoprim–sulfamethoxazole. While an infection is more likely to be the underlying cause of encephalopathy, some antimicrobial agents may directly cause encephalopathy with or without seizures (Table 18.3) [16, 17]. Acyclovir can cause acute neurotoxicity in rare patients, particularly in older patients with renal dysfunction [18]. Symptoms may include confusion, tremor, hallucinations, coma, ataxia, and seizures. Cases of acyclovir-associated neurotoxicity have been reported even after standard oral doses. CSF is typically normal. Complete neurologic recovery after stopping acyclovir is observed in most cases.

Encephalopathy Related to Organ Failure

Encephalopathy may rise in the setting of liver, lung, or kidney dysfunction. Hepatic veno-occlusive disease (VOD), also known as sinusoidal obstruction syndrome (SOS), is characterized by tender hepatomegaly, fluid retention, weight gain, and hyperbilirubinemia following high-dose myeloablative conditioning therapy [19]. VOD occurs in approximately 14% of patients undergoing HSCT (in modern series), typically within the first month after HSCT, and is associated with cyclophosphamide-based conditioning regimens either with total body irradiation or with busulfan [20]. CNS dysfunction may also be an early manifestation of multiple organ dysfunction syndromes (MODS) associated with severe forms of VOD. HSCT patients presenting with either pulmonary or CNS dysfunction are up to 18 times more likely to die from MODS than patients without pulmonary of CNS dysfunction [21]. Treatment is required for severe VOD and includes rigorous fluid management, pharmaceutics such as defibrotide, coagulolytic agents, or methylprednisolone, and liver transplantation [20].

Calcineurin Inhibitor Neurotoxicity and Posterior Reversible Encephalopathy Syndrome

Posterior reversible encephalopathy syndrome (PRES) in the HSCT population has been associated with chemotherapies such as fludarabine [22], hypertension, renal disease (Fig. 18.1a, b), fluid weight gain, hypomagnesemia, and calcineurin inhibitors such as cyclosporine and tacrolimus [23]. The calcineurin inhibitors are often used to prevent GVHD following allogeneic transplants. Most cases occur in the early post-transplantation period [24, 25] with the median time to onset of tacrolimus-associated PRES onset 61–85 days post-transplant [23]. Patients may present with headache, seizures, visual changes, and encephalopathy. MRI may demonstrate vasogenic cerebral edema, predominantly involving the white matter but can also involve the gray matter. PRES is often reversible with supportive care and removal of the offending agent. While stopping a calcineurin inhibitor may help reverse PRES, some patients may need to remain on a calcineurin inhibitor or switch to another immunosuppressant to prevent or manage GVHD.

Seizures

The incidence of seizures (generalized, partial, or status epilepticus) in HSCT patients ranges from 2 to 15% depending on the clinical series [26]. Potential causes of

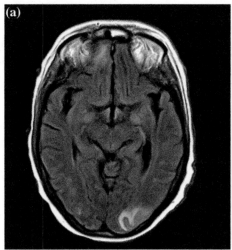 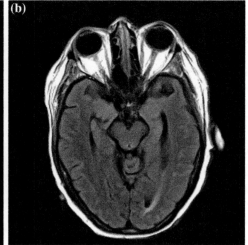

Fig. 18.1 PRES. A 69-year-old woman with a history of CNS lymphoma who presented 4 months after autologous HSCT with seizures, confusion, and acute renal failure from thrombotic thrombocytopenic purpura–hemolytic uremic syndrome. MRI shows increased T2 signal in the subcortical white matter throughout the brain consistent with PRES (**a**). Imaging findings resolved on repeat imaging 6 months later (**b**)

seizures are numerous. CNS imaging may be normal or abnormal depending on the underlying etiology. CNS infections, strokes, hemorrhages, and leukoencephalopathies often produce imaging findings, whereas electrolyte disturbances and acid–base abnormalities are typically associated with normal CNS imaging.

Busulfan, an agent used in preparative regimens, is associated with generalized seizures in up to 10% in adults treated with this agent [27]. Seizures typically occur on the third or fourth day of busulfan administration. The mechanism of toxicity is unknown but may relate to busulfan kinetics in the cerebrospinal fluid [28]. Several agents have been used for seizure prophylaxis. Phenytoin can be easily loaded intravenously but does induce cytochrome P450 enzymes and increases clearance of oral busulfan. Benzodiazepines, such as clonazepam and lorazepam, do not induce cytochrome P450 enzymes but can be sedating. Although case series suggest that newer nonenzyme-inducing antiepileptics such as levetiracetam can be used for seizure prophylaxis with busulfan administration [29], this has not been well studied. With the use of seizure prophylaxis, the incidence of seizures in children receiving a busulfan-containing regimen is low (1.3%) [30].

CNS Infections

CNS Infections occur in 3–8% of patients after allogeneic, syngeneic, or autologous HSCT [31]. Even though they are less common than systemic infections, CNS infections are potentially fatal [32]. A discussion of atypical/opportunistic pathogens seen in the HSCT population is as follows.

The post-transplantation risk of infection is based on the status of immune recovery [33]. Prior to engraftment (0–30 days post-transplantation), patients are neutropenic with weakened mucosal barriers. The most common pathogens are bacteria, *Candida,* and herpes simplex virus (HSV) reactivation. If the neutropenic period is prolonged, the risk of *Aspergillus* increases. Patients undergoing autologous transplantation are primarily at risk during this phase. In the early post-engraftment period (30–100 days post-transplantation), allogeneic HSCT patients have deficient cellular immunity caused by acute GVHD and immunosuppressant medications. In this setting, fungal (*Aspergillus* and *Pneumocystis jirovecii*), cytomegalovirus (CMV), and gram-positive bacterial infections are seen. In the late post-engraftment period (>100 post-transplantation), autologous transplant patients recover immune function more rapidly and have a lower risk of opportunistic infections than allogeneic transplant patients. Because of cell-mediated and humoral immunity defects and impaired functioning of the reticuloendothelial system, allogeneic transplant patients with chronic GVHD and recipients of allogeneic transplant with matched unrelated, cord blood, or mismatched family-related donors are at risk of infections with CMV, VZV, EBV-related post-transplantation lymphoproliferative disease, community-acquired respiratory virus infection, and infections with encapsulated bacteria such as *Haemophilus influenzae* and *Streptococcus pneumoniae* [34].

Aspergillus

Aspergillus fumigatus and *Aspergillus flavum* are the most common fungal CNS infections in HSCT patients [35]. The lungs are the most common site of involvement. Retrospective studies of CNS involvement in allogeneic SCT patients with invasive aspergillosis report rates as high as 40% [36] and as low as 3% [37]. Infection usually occurs following engraftment and typically occurs through inhalation of excessive Aspergillus spores in contaminated air. Following hematogenous dissemination, invasion of cerebral arteries eventually leads to occlusion by hyphal elements, infarction, and frequently secondary hemorrhagic conversion. These lesions may be localized in the subcortical areas of the cerebral hemispheres, the cerebellum [38], or the basal ganglia [39]. Rarely, patients may develop fungal vasculitis or mycotic aneurysms with resultant subarachnoid hemorrhage. Involvement of the meninges in the inflammatory process is distinctly uncommon.

Clinical and laboratory diagnosis of aspergillosis is difficult. Presenting symptoms are nonspecific and may include hemiparesis, unilateral cranial nerve palsies, intention tremor, seizures, headaches, or dysmetria [38, 39]. Fever and nuchal rigidity may be absent. There is a relative paucity of CSF abnormalities. Pleocytosis (usually a mix of polymorphonuclear and mononuclear cells) is usually less than 100/mm^3; CSF protein content is only mildly elevated; and glucose level is normal or mildly decreased. CSF cultures for Aspergillus are rarely positive [39]. Serologic testing in immunocompromised patients yields inconclusive results. Several MRI patterns have been described: (a) nonenhancing lesions located in the basal ganglia and thalami representing small infarctions of the lenticulostriate and thalamoperforator arteries and (b) large cerebral artery infarctions with early intravascular and meningeal enhancement [39]. Most cases do not demonstrate contrast enhancement, but ring or nodular enhancement has been described in patients who survived [40].

Early diagnosis and treatment is important since mortality is almost 100% in most series with only a few case reports of HSCT patients surviving CNS aspergillosis [38–42]. Survival is usually only 2 days to 3 weeks after onset of neurologic symptoms [40]. Therefore, a positive test for galactomannan antigen or clinical signs and symptoms compatible with invasive aspergillosis should trigger further workup [43]. Patients with pulmonary aspergillosis and neurologic deficits should be treated as CNS aspergillosis. Diagnosis of CNS aspergillosis in a patient with characteristic neuroimaging may be established by direct detection of mold from the lungs, but occasionally biopsy of a cerebral lesion may be necessary to document CNS infection [41, 42].

Prevention of aspergillosis is very important and includes clear air supply by high-efficiency particulate air filters on the hospital ward, prevention of CMV infection (which seems to predispose to invasive aspergillosis), and preemptive antifungal therapy once colonization of airways with Aspergillus species is found. Treatment consists of intravenous amphotericin B or intravenous voriconazole [43]. Duration of treatment is unknown, but treatment should probably be continued for two to three months after the MRI scan has normalized.

Candida

Candidiasis is a common systemic infection in HSCT patients but rarely leads to CNS involvement [35]. The risk of candidal infection is high during the pre-engraftment period due to neutropenia and severe mucositis, which facilitates *Candida* colonization and subsequent invasion [44, 45]. In granulocytopenic HSCT patients, candidiasis is often disseminated, involving the liver, spleen, kidney, heart, gastrointestinal tract, lungs, skin, and brain [46]. Mortality rates with disseminated Candida may be as high as 90% and is almost always fatal when brain parenchyma is involved [32]. *Candida* can lead to meningitis, meningoencephalitis, vascular complications such as mycotic aneurysms, or cerebral abscesses. One retrospective series of 58 HSCT patients identified 19 patients with Candida abscesses (15 *Candida albicans*, 2 *Candida tropicalis*, 2 unknown species) [47]. Only one patient survived but ultimately died from congestive heart failure. Twelve of these 19 patients had positive blood cultures. Another study by Maschke and collaborators reported one patient with *Candida* encephalitis occurring 24 days after HSCT [31]. Brain MRI demonstrated multiple lesions in the basal ganglia and cerebellum that were hypointense on T1-weighted images, intermediate signal on T2-weighted images, and ring-enhancing after gadolinium administration. The patient died after 19 days from respiratory failure. All allogeneic recipients and select autologous recipients should receive fluconazole prophylaxis (400 mg per day) during neutropenia to prevent invasive disease [48]. In patients who develop candidiasis, early treatment with antifungal therapy such as amphotericin B and reversal of underlying host defects are critical to good outcomes [45].

Toxoplasma

Toxoplasmosis is caused by *Toxoplasma gondii*, an obligate intracellular protozoan parasite, and most often affects immunocompromised patients or pregnant women. Transmission may occur transplacentally, via ingestion of raw or undercooked meat containing T. gondii cysts, or by exposure to oocytes from cat feces. The incidence of toxoplasmosis following allogeneic stem cell transplantation varies between 0.1 and 6.0% depending on the series [49].

Clinical disease usually results from reactivation of latent disease during immunosuppression, particularly with concurrent GVHD. Rarely, it occurs as a primary infection acquired from the allograft into the seronegative recipient [50]. Following a mononucleosis-like prodromal stage, toxoplasmosis disseminates to the lungs, liver, bone marrow, and brain. Encephalitis is the most common CNS presentation. Symptoms and signs include headaches, low-grade fever, lethargy, focal seizures without or with secondary generalization, and focal neurologic deficits depending on the location of the lesions. Clinical onset usually occurs between the second and sixth months following transplant, but may occur as early as nine days. Most patients present within three months of transplant [51–55].

Definitive diagnosis may be difficult to achieve. Polymerase chain reaction (PCR) testing for T. gondii DNA is the main method of diagnosing toxoplasmosis in HSCT patients [56] although a negative blood PCR should not rule out disease [57]. Serological tests measuring IgG antibodies against T.gondii in blood are of limited value given the prevalence of latent infection. Increased IgM levels may indicate recent activation of infection, but false-positive and false-negative cases have been reported [50, 53, 58, 59]. Routine CSF parameters such as cell count and protein level are either normal or mildly elevated due to the immunosuppressed state of the patient. PCR assay in CSF may be a useful diagnostic tool in the early detection of T. gondii [60, 61]. However, even PCR assay in CSF may be negative, at least early in the infection [52]. Proof of CNS toxoplasmosis relies upon histologic demonstration of tachyzoites of T. gondii from brain biopsy [53, 54, 60].

Multiple lesions in the basal ganglia and at the corticomedullary junction are usually present [54] (Fig. 18.2a–d). Enhancement after gadolinium administration may or may not be present, depending on the ability of the patient's immune system to muster a meaningful inflammatory response [54]. Unlike the HIV population, toxoplasmic lesions in the HSCT population may be initially hemorrhagic [62]. Differential diagnosis based on MRI characteristics would include other opportunistic infections such as aspergillosis, mucormycosis, as well as progressive multifocal leukoencephalopathy and post-transplant lymphoproliferative disorders/primary CNS lymphoma.

The CDC recommends prophylaxis for seropositive allogeneic recipients with active GVHD or a prior history of toxoplasmic chorioretinitis [33]. Trimethoprim–sulfamethoxazole (TMP/SMX) 80/400 mg once per day or 160/800 mg three times per week should be started after engraftment and be administered for as long as the patient remains on immunosuppressive therapy (which is generally for six months following HSCT). It should be noted that this prophylactic regimen may not be sufficient for a seronegative recipient with a seropositive donor who then also develops severe GVHD.

Treatment should consist of pyrimethamine and a sulfonamide. Since some patients cannot tolerate sulfonamides (due to allergic reactions or gastrointestinal symptoms), alternative options include clindamycin, atovaquone, azithromycin, or clarithromycin. Despite effective therapy, the prognosis of HSCT patients with toxoplasmosis is poor with mortality rates 60–90% [49]. Patients who receive adequate therapy and those who develop late infection (>63 days after HSCT) are less likely to die from toxoplasmosis [63].

Human Herpesvirus-6

Human herpesvirus-6 (HHV-6) is a herpes virus with a predilection for the central nervous system [64]. The HHV-6B variant is more frequently associated with disease than variant A [65]. The virus is generally acquired during childhood, presenting as exanthema subitum (roseola infantum) and febrile illness in the case of HHV-6B, and establishes latency in lymphocytes and monocytes. HHV-6 infections in the HSCT population generally represent reactivation, as opposed to primary infection, and have been documented in 38–60% of patients following HSCT [66]. In the CNS, HHV-6 reactivation causes encephalitis and most cases occur within 12 weeks of transplantation [67]. While the incidence of HHV-6 reactivation is high in the HSCT population, the incidence of HHV-6 encephalitis is low with the reported incidence in allogeneic HSCT patients ranging from 1 to 12% [68].

The most common clinical manifestations are mental changes, seizures, memory disturbance, headaches, and speech disturbance. Focal neurologic symptoms and fever are less common. Brain MRI demonstrates T2 hyperintensities involving one or both hippocampi with variable involvement of adjacent medial temporal lobe structures of the limbic system, including amygdalae and parahippocampal gyri [69, 70] (Fig. 18.3a, b). These findings are similar to other infectious etiologies of limbic encephalitis including HSV, VZV, and neurosyphilis. HHV-6 encephalitis is typically diagnosed by CSF PCR although HHV-6 DNA has occasionally been found in CSF from asymptomatic patients [71]. CSF may also be remarkable for elevated protein levels and pleocytosis. Antibody tests are not useful in adults due to the high prevalence of seropositivity in the general population. Antiviral prophylaxis is generally not recommended to prevent HHV-6 encephalitis

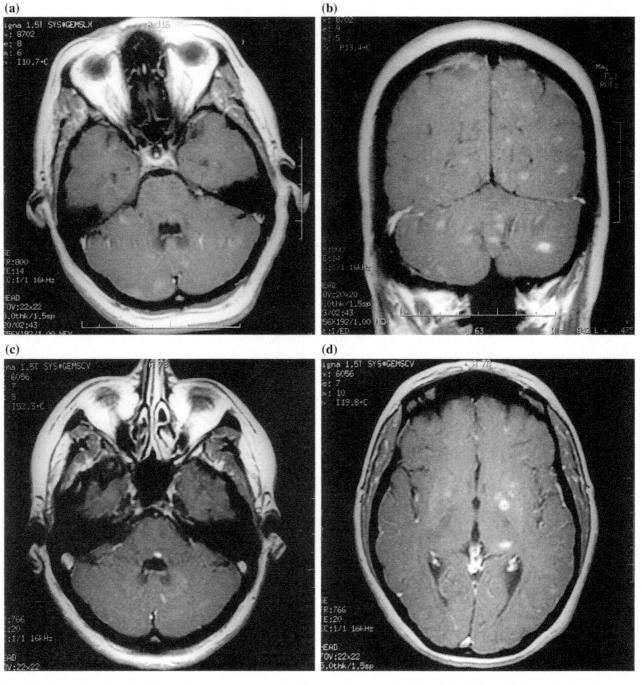

Fig. 18.2 Toxoplasmosis. A 46-year-old woman presented with dizziness, ataxia, nystagmus, and diplopia 8 months after allogeneic HSCT for chronic myelogenous leukemia. MRI demonstrates multiple lesions in both cerebral and cerebellar hemispheres (**a** and **b**). CSF analyses including toxoplasmosis IgG and IgM were normal, but serum toxoplasmoses including IgG, IgM, and IgG quantitative index were elevated. After >4 months of treatment with pyrimethamine, sulfadiazine, and leucovorin, the patient improved clinically but imaging findings did not resolve completely (**c** and **d**)

[65]. Because neurologic symptoms progress rapidly, patients should be started on antiviral therapy with gancyclovir or foscarnet as soon as possible [64, 68]. Despite treatment, mortality in HSCT patients remains high at 25% and many who survive are left with permanent cognitive deficits [68].

JC Virus

Progressive multifocal leukoencephalopathy (PML) is another rare complication following HSCT associated with chronic immunosuppression and impaired cellular response. PML is a demyelinating disorder caused by John

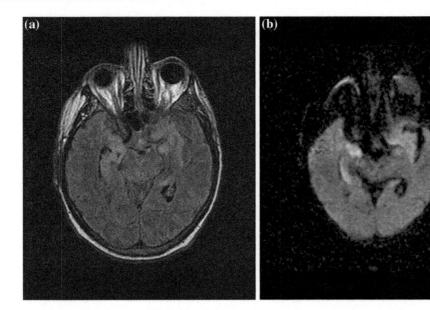

Fig. 18.3 a, b HHV-6 encephalitis. A 61-year-old man 16 days after myeloablative double-cord transplant for myeloproliferative disorder presented with mental status changes (disorientation, agitation, paranoia, and visual hallucinations). Imaging revealed T2 hyperintense lesions in bilateral temporal lobes extending to the orbital frontal cortex and associated with subtle restricted diffusion. HHV-6 PCR was positive from the CCF. His mental status and renal dysfunction declined rapidly over the next several days. Despite broad-spectrum antimicrobials including foscarnet, patient died

Cunningham (JC) virus, a neurotropic polyomavirus of the Papovaviridae family. JC virus is endemic in humans, with seroconversion up to 60% in young adults and up to 80% in the elderly [72]. Primary infection with JC virus occurs during childhood and is often asymptomatic. With viral reactivation (typically in the setting of immune suppression), patients may develop personality changes, confusion, dementia, aphasia, apraxia, hemiparesis, cerebellar dysfunction, or visual processing abnormalities. MRI is the imaging modality of choice, usually demonstrating multifocal hyperintensities on T2-weighted and FLAIR images. The lesions typically do not enhance. Changes are mostly located in the white matter but may extend into the gray matter. Diagnosis is based on demonstration of JC virus in CSF by means of PCR assay, in situ hybridization, or immunohistochemistry. However, PCR is negative in approximately 25% of PML cases [73]. No effective treatment exists for PML in HIV-negative patients. Most cases are fatal with a median survival of less than six months. There are rare reports of HSCT patients who survived more than one year after developing PML [73, 74]. In these cases, a relatively prominent inflammatory response in the biopsied brain tissue was found.

Cerebrovascular Disorders

Cerebrovascular accidents including ischemic strokes, intraparenchymal hemorrhages (IPH), subarachnoid hemorrhages (SAH), and subdural hemorrhages (SDH) occur in approximately 3% of HSCT patients [75]. In a retrospective series examining all cerebrovascular events occurring within months of HSCT, the most common mechanisms were noninfectious intracranial hemorrhage (secondary to thrombocytopenia), infectious infarction (predominantly fungal), and noninfectious infarction [75]. Table 18.4 describes risk factors and causes of cerebrovascular complications less common in the general population but found in the HSCT population.

The clinical presentation depends on the location and extent of the lesion. Ischemic strokes usually present with focal neurologic deficits, although patients who develop multiple bilateral strokes from an embolic shower present with confusion. Hemorrhages may present with variety of symptoms including altered consciousness, headaches, focal deficits, and seizures [76].

Although hemorrhages are typically diagnosed on imaging, some clinical features may suggest one type of hemorrhage over another. SAH and SDH typically occur within 60 days of allogeneic HSCT [76, 77], while ICH occurs later [76, 77]. Intraparenchymal and subarachnoid hemorrhages have also been described in the setting of PRES (previously discussed in this chapter) [78]. In patients following allogeneic transplant, PRES-related hemorrhage was associated with severe hypertension.

Ischemic strokes can occur early following HSCT (i.e., *Aspergillus*) or as a delayed complication (i.e., cerebral angiitis). In addition to well-established risk factors for stroke in the general population (such as smoking, hypertension, diabetes, and dyslipidemia), treatments may

Table 18.4 Risk factors and causes of cerebrovascular complications that are less common in the general population but found in the HSCT population

Cerebrovascular complication	Risk factors and/or causes
Ischemic strokes	Hypercoagulable states (e.g., protein C deficiency) Paradoxical emboli during infusions Medication toxicity Infectious vasculitis (e.g., Aspergillus) Endocarditis (infectious and noninfectious) GVHD vasculitis/cerebral angiitis Post-transplantation thrombotic microangiopathy
Intraparenchymal hemorrhage [76]	Thrombocytopenia or platelet refractoriness Coagulopathies Infectious vasculitis Hypertension Acute GVHD VOD Radiation therapy PRES
Subarachnoid hemorrhage	Mycotic aneurysms Relapsing leukemia PRES
Subdural hemorrhage [81, 85]	Thrombocytopenia or platelet refractoriness Coagulopathy Lumbar puncture and intrathecal treatment Leukemia meningeal infiltration and hyperleukocytosis

predispose HSCT patients to premature cardiovascular disease [79]. Endothelial damage can be induced by conditioning regimens with or without total body irradiation as well as by GVHD. The relative risk of an arterial event is higher following allogeneic transplants than autologous transplants. In one retrospective study, the cumulative incidence of arterial events (including cerebrovascular disease, coronary artery disease, and peripheral arterial disease) at 15 years was 7.5% after allogeneic HSCT versus 2.3% after autologous HSCT [80].

Any signs or symptoms concerning for stroke or hemorrhage should prompt an emergency referral to a hospital. Imaging is often required for diagnosis. For hemorrhagic lesions, a head CT scan is the usual modality of choice. For acute ischemic strokes, a brain MRI is recommended. Further workup and management of cerebrovascular events in HSCT patients should generally follow the same recommendations as the general population with special consideration of etiologies specific to HSCT patients.

Immediate correction of any underlying cause (e.g., platelet transfusions for patients with severe thrombocytopenia or antifungals for patients with *Aspergillus*) is recommended. Patients with hemorrhage may require monitoring in an intensive care unit with strict blood pressure control and other supportive measures. Surgical options may be limited due to severity of the hemorrhage and transfusion-refractory thrombocytopenia. SDH can generally

be managed conservatively with good outcomes; surgical intervention is typically reserved for patients with neurologic deterioration [81].

Outcomes from cerebrovascular events are generally worse in the HSCT population compared to the general population [75]. The 5-year overall survival rate in HSCT patients following ICH is 17.9% compared to 55.8% in HSCT patients without ICH [76]. Prognosis also depends on the type of hemorrhage and underlying etiology. For example, many patients with IPH die soon after the event, but death from SAH or SDH is much less common [76, 77].

Neurologic Complications Associated with GVHD

GVHD occurs when donor allogeneic T cells attack the transplant recipient's organs or tissues. Chronic GVHD, historically defined as occurring after the first 100 days post-transplant, resembles autoimmune vascular diseases and occurs in 30–65% of allogeneic HSCT patients [82]. Established risk factors associated with chronic GVHD include previous acute GVHD, HLA disparities, recipient's and donor's age, peripheral blood stem cells, T-cell replete graft, cord blood stem cells, viral infection, and conditioning regimens used [83]. Neurologic complications directly associated with GVHD primarily affect the peripheral nervous system and include polymyositis, myasthenia gravis, acute inflammatory demyelinating polyneuropathy (AIDP), and chronic inflammatory demyelinating polyneuropathy (CIDP) [1]. GVHD-associated CNS toxicity is rare although demyelinating events such as acute demyelinating encephalomyelitis (ADEM) have been reported [84].

Conclusions

Neurologic complications following HSCT have long been recognized. The causes are numerous, including chemoradiotoxicity, medication toxicity, metabolic abnormalities, organ failure, GVHD, infection, pancytopenia, and platelet dysfunction. As the number of transplants performed annually increases, clinicians must be aware of the potential neurologic complications seen in this patient population.

References

1. Saiz A, Graus F. Neurologic complications of hematopoietic cell transplantation. Semin Neurol. 2010;30(3):287–95.
2. Copelan EA. Hematopoietic stem-cell transplantation. N Engl J Med. 2006;354(17):1813–26.
3. Pasquini MC, Zhu X. Current uses and outcomes of hematopoietic stem cell transplantation: 2014 CIBMTR Summary Slides 2014 [June 29, 2015]. Available from: http://www.cibmtr.org/referencecenter/slidesreports/summaryslides/pages/index.aspx.
4. Little M-T, Storb R. History of haematopoietic stem-cell transplantation. Nat Rev Cancer. 2002;2(3):231–8.
5. Antonini G, Ceschin V, Morino S, Fiorelli M, Gragnani F, Mengarelli A, et al. Early neurologic complications following allogeneic bone marrow transplant for leukemia: a prospective study. Neurology. 1998;50(5):1441–5.
6. Bleggi-Torres LF, de Medeiros BC, Werner B, Neto JZ, Loddo G, Pasquini R, et al. Neuropathological findings after bone marrow transplantation: an autopsy study of 180 cases. Bone Marrow Transplant. 2000;25(3):301–7.
7. Gordon B, Lyden E, Lynch J, Tarantolo S, Pavletic ZS, Bishop M, et al. Central nervous system dysfunction as the first manifestation of multiple organ dysfunction syndrome in stem cell transplant patients. Bone Marrow Transplant. 2000;25(1):79–83.
8. Bhatt VR, Balasetti V, Abduall JJ, Giri S, Armitage JO, Loberiza FR Jr, et al. Central nervous system complications and outcomes after allogeneic hematopoietic stem cell transplantation. Clin Lymphoma Myeloma Leuk. 2015;15(10):606–11.
9. Rosenfeld MR, Pruitt A. Neurologic complications of bone marrow, stem cell, and organ transplantation in patients with cancer. Semin Oncol. 2006;33(3):352–61.
10. Kang JM, Kim YJ, Kim JY, Cho EJ, Lee JH, Lee MH, et al. Neurologic complications after allogeneic hematopoietic stem cell transplantation in children: analysis of prognostic factors. Biol Blood Marrow Transplant J Am Soc Blood Marrow Transplant. 2015;21(6):1091–8.
11. Jackson SR, Tweeddale MG, Barnett MJ, Spinelli JJ, Sutherland HJ, Reece DE, et al. Admission of bone marrow transplant recipients to the intensive care unit: outcome, survival and prognostic factors. Bone Marrow Transplant. 1998;21(7):697–704.
12. Woodard P, Helton K, McDaniel H, Khan RB, Thompson S, Hale G, et al. Encephalopathy in pediatric patients after allogeneic hematopoietic stem cell transplantation is associated with a poor prognosis. Bone Marrow Transplant. 2004;33(11):1151–7.
13. Baker WJ, Royer GL Jr, Weiss RB. Cytarabine and neurologic toxicity. J Clin Oncol. 1991;9(4):679–93.
14. Cheson BD, Vena DA, Foss FM, Sorensen JM. Neurotoxicity of purine analogs: a review. J Clin Oncol. 1994;12(10):2216–28.
15. Beitinjaneh AM, McKinney AM, Cao Q, Weisdorf DJ. Toxic Leukoencephalopathy following Fludarabine-associated hematopoietic cell transplantation. Biol Blood Marrow Transplant. 2011;17(3):300–8.
16. Snavely SR, Hodges GR. The neurotoxicity of antibacterial agents. Ann Intern Med. 1984;101(1):92–104.
17. Grill MF, Maganti RK. Neurotoxic effects associated with antibiotic use: management considerations. Br J Clin Pharmacol. 2011;72(3):381–93.
18. Berry L, Venkatesan P. Aciclovir-induced neurotoxicity: utility of CSF and serum CMMG levels in diagnosis. J Clin Virol. 2014;61 (4):608–10.
19. McDonald GB. Hepatobiliary complications of hematopoietic cell transplantation, 40 years on. Hepatology. 2010;51(4):1450–60.
20. Fan CQ, Crawford JM. Sinusoidal obstruction syndrome (hepatic veno-occlusive disease). J Clin Exp Hepatol. 2014;4(4):332–46.
21. Haire WD. Multiple organ dysfunction syndrome in hematopoietic stem cell transplantation. Crit Care Med. 2002;30(5 Suppl): S257–62.
22. Beitinjaneh A, McKinney AM, Cao Q, Weisdorf DJ. Toxic leukoencephalopathy following fludarabine-associated hematopoietic cell transplantation. Biol Blood Marrow Transplant J Am Soc Blood Marrow Transplant. 2011;17(3):300–8.
23. Hammerstrom AE, Howell J, Gulbis A, Rondon G, Champlin RE, Popat U. Tacrolimus-associated posterior reversible encephalopathy syndrome in hematopoietic allogeneic stem cell transplantation. Am J Hematol. 2013;88(4):301–5.
24. Memon M, deMagalhaes-Silverman M, Bloom EJ, Lister J, Myers DJ, Pincus SM, et al. Reversible cyclosporine-induced cortical blindness in allogeneic bone marrow transplant recipients. Bone Marrow Transplant. 1995;15(2):283–6.
25. Steg RE, Kessinger A, Wszolek ZK. Cortical blindness and seizures in a patient receiving FK506 after bone marrow transplantation. Bone Marrow Transplant. 1999;23(9):959–62.
26. Zhang XH, Xu LP, Liu DH, Chen H, Han W, Chen YH, et al. Epileptic seizures in patients following allogeneic hematopoietic stem cell transplantation: a retrospective analysis of incidence, risk factors, and survival rates. Clin Transplant. 2013;27(1):80–9.
27. Ciurea SO, Andersson BS. Busulfan in hematopoietic stem cell transplantation. Biol Blood Marrow Transplant. 2009;15(5):523–36.
28. Busulfan. In: DRUGDEX System [Internet database] Greenwood Village, CO: Thomas Reuters (Healthcare) Inc. Updated periodically.
29. Soni S, Skeens M, Termuhlen AM, Bajwa RP, Gross TG, Pai V. Levetiracetam for busulfan-induced seizure prophylaxis in children undergoing hematopoietic stem cell transplantation. Pediatr Blood Cancer. 2012;59(4):762–4.
30. Caselli D, Rosati A, Faraci M, Podda M, Ripaldi M, Longoni D, et al. Risk of seizures in children receiving busulphan-containing regimens for stem cell transplantation. Biol Blood Marrow Transplant J Am Soc Blood Marrow Transplant. 2014;20 (2):282–5.
31. Maschke M, Dietrich U, Prumbaum M, Kastrup O, Turowski B, Schaefer UW, et al. Opportunistic CNS infection after bone marrow transplantation. Bone Marrow Transplant. 1999;23 (11):1167–76.

32. de Medeiros BC, de Medeiros CR, Werner B, Neto JZ, Loddo G, Pasquini R, et al. Central nervous system infections following bone marrow transplantation: an autopsy report of 27 cases. J Hematother Stem Cell Res. 2000;9(4):535–40.

33. Guidelines for preventing opportunistic infections among hematopoietic stem cell transplant recipients. MMWR Recomm Rep. 2000;49(RR-10):1–125, CE1-7.

34. Dykewicz CA. Centers for Disease C, Prevention, Infectious Diseases Society of A, American Society of B, Marrow T. Summary of the Guidelines for Preventing Opportunistic Infections among Hematopoietic Stem Cell Transplant Recipients. Clin Infect Dis. 2001;33(2):139–44.

35. Quant EC, Wen PY. Neurological complications of hematopoietic stem cell transplantation. In: Schiff D, Kesari S, Wen PY, editors. Cancer Neurology in Clinical Practice. 2nd ed. Totowa, New Jersey: Humana Press; 2008. p. 327–52.

36. Saugier-Veber P, Devergie A, Sulahian A, Ribaud P, Traore F, Bourdeau-Esperou H, et al. Epidemiology and diagnosis of invasive pulmonary aspergillosis in bone marrow transplant patients: results of a 5 year retrospective study. Bone Marrow Transplant. 1993;12(2):121–4.

37. Jantunen E, Volin L, Salonen O, Piilonen A, Parkkali T, Anttila VJ, et al. Central nervous system aspergillosis in allogeneic stem cell transplant recipients. Bone Marrow Transplant. 2003;31(3):191–6.

38. Walsh TJ, Hier DB, Caplan LR. Aspergillosis of the central nervous system: clinicopathological analysis of 17 patients. Ann Neurol. 1985;18(5):574–82.

39. Miaux Y, Ribaud P, Williams M, Guermazi A, Gluckman E, Brocheriou C, et al. MR of cerebral aspergillosis in patients who have had bone marrow transplantation. Ajnr. 1995;16(3):555–62.

40. Guermazi A, Gluckman E, Tabti B, Miaux Y. Invasive central nervous system aspergillosis in bone marrow transplantation recipients: an overview. Eur Radiol. 2003;13(2):377–88.

41. Baslar Z, Soysal T, Hanci M, Aygun G, Ferhanoglu B, Sarioglu AC, et al. Successfully treated invasive central nervous system aspergillosis in an allogeneic stem cell transplant recipient. Bone Marrow Transplant. 1998;22(4):404–5.

42. Khoury H, Adkins D, Miller G, Goodnough L, Brown R, DiPersio J. Resolution of invasive central nervous system aspergillosis in a transplant recipient. Bone Marrow Transplant. 1997;20(2):179–80.

43. Ruping MJ, Vehreschild JJ, Cornely OA. Patients at high risk of invasive fungal infections: when and how to treat. Drugs. 2008;68 (14):1941–62.

44. Marr KA, Bow E, Chiller T, Maschmeyer G, Ribaud P, Segal B, et al. Fungal infection prevention after hematopoietic cell transplantation. Bone Marrow Transplant. 2009;44(8):483–7.

45. Richardson M, Lass-Florl C. Changing epidemiology of systemic fungal infections. Clin Microbiol Infect. 2008;14(Suppl 4):5–24.

46. LaRocco MT, Burgert SJ. Infection in the bone marrow transplant recipient and role of the microbiology laboratory in clinical transplantation. Clin Microbiol Rev. 1997;10(2):277–97.

47. Hagensee ME, Bauwens JE, Kjos B, Bowden RA. Brain abscess following marrow transplantation: experience at the Fred Hutchinson Cancer Research Center, 1984–1992. Clin Infect Dis. 1994;19 (3):402–8.

48. Centers for Disease Control. Guidelines for preventing opportunistic infections among hematopoietic stem cell transplant recipients: recommendations of CDC, the Infectious Disease Society of America, and the American Society of Blood and Marrow Transplantation. MMWR. 2000;49:23,6,107.

49. Mulanovich VE, Ahmed SI, Ozturk T, Khokhar FA, Kontoyiannis DP, de Lima M. Toxoplasmosis in allo-SCT patients: risk factors and outcomes at a transplantation center with a low incidence. Bone Marrow Transplant. 2011;46(2):273–7.

50. Chandrasekar PH, Momin F. Disseminated toxoplasmosis in marrow recipients: a report of three cases and a review of the literature. Bone Marrow Transplant Team. Bone Marrow Transplant. 1997;19(7):685–9.

51. Bretagne S, Costa JM, Kuentz M, Simon D, Vidaud M, Fortel I, et al. Late toxoplasmosis evidenced by PCR in a marrow transplant recipient. Bone Marrow Transplant. 1995;15(5):809–11.

52. Brinkman K, Debast S, Sauerwein R, Ooyman F, Hiel J, Raemaekers J. Toxoplasma retinitis/encephalitis 9 months after allogeneic bone marrow transplantation. Bone Marrow Transplant. 1998;21(6):635–6.

53. Derouin F, Devergie A, Auber P, Gluckman E, Beauvais B, Garin YJ, et al. Toxoplasmosis in bone marrow-transplant recipients: report of seven cases and review. Clin Infect Dis. 1992;15(2):267–70.

54. Dietrich U, Maschke M, Dorfler A, Prumbaum M, Forsting M. MRI of intracranial toxoplasmosis after bone marrow transplantation. Neuroradiology. 2000;42(1):14–8.

55. Tefferi A, O'Neill BP, Inwards DJ. Late-onset cerebral toxoplasmosis after allogeneic bone marrow transplantation. Bone Marrow Transplant. 1998;21(12):1285–6.

56. Edvinsson B, Lundquist J, Ljungman P, Ringden O, Evengard B. A prospective study of diagnosis of Toxoplasma gondii infection after bone marrow transplantation. APMIS. 2008;116(5):345–51.

57. Cibickova L, Horacek J, Prasil P, Slovacek L, Kohout A, Cerovsky V, et al. Cerebral toxoplasmosis in an allogeneic peripheral stem cell transplant recipient: case report and review of literature. Transpl Infect Dis. 2007;9(4):332–5.

58. Lowenberg B, van Gijn J, Prins E, Polderman AM. Fatal cerebral toxoplasmosis in a bone marrow transplant recipient with leukemia. Transplantation. 1983;35(1):30–4.

59. Slavin MA, Meyers JD, Remington JS, Hackman RC. Toxoplasma gondii infection in marrow transplant recipients: a 20 year experience. Bone Marrow Transplant. 1994;13(5):549–57.

60. Khoury H, Adkins D, Brown R, Goodnough L, Gokden M, Roberts T, et al. Successful treatment of cerebral toxoplasmosis in a marrow transplant recipient: contribution of a PCR test in diagnosis and early detection. Bone Marrow Transplant. 1999; 23(4):409–11.

61. Roemer E, Blau IW, Basara N, Kiehl MG, Bischoff M, Gunzelmann S, et al. Toxoplasmosis, a severe complication in allogeneic hematopoietic stem cell transplantation: successful treatment strategies during a 5-year single-center experience. Clin Infect Dis. 2001;32(1):E1–8.

62. Mueller-Mang C, Mang TG, Kalhs P, Thurnher MM. Imaging characteristics of toxoplasmosis encephalitis after bone marrow transplantation: report of two cases and review of the literature. Neuroradiology. 2006;48(2):84–9.

63. Martino R, Maertens J, Bretagne S, Rovira M, Deconinck E, Ullmann AJ, et al. Toxoplasmosis after hematopoietic stem cell transplantation. Clin Infect Dis. 2000;31(5):1188–95.

64. Ljungman P, Singh N. Human herpesvirus-6 infection in solid organ and stem cell transplant recipients. J Clin Virol. 2006;37 (Suppl 1):S87–91.

65. Ljungman P, de la Camara R, Cordonnier C, Einsele H, Engelhard D, Reusser P, et al. Management of CMV, HHV-6, HHV-7 and Kaposi-sarcoma herpesvirus (HHV-8) infections in patients

with hematological malignancies and after SCT. Bone Marrow Transplant. 2008;42(4):227–40.

66. Bosi A, Zazzi M, Amantini A, Cellerini M, Vannucchi AM, De Milito A, et al. Fatal herpesvirus 6 encephalitis after unrelated bone marrow transplant. Bone Marrow Transplant. 1998; 22(3):285–8.

67. Singh N, Paterson DL. Encephalitis caused by human herpesvirus-6 in transplant recipients: relevance of a novel neurotropic virus. Transplantation. 2000;69(12):2474–9.

68. Ogata M, Fukuda T, Teshima T. Human herpesvirus-6 encephalitis after allogeneic hematopoietic cell transplantation: what we do and do not know. Bone Marrow Transplant. 2015;50(8):1030–6.

69. Gorniak RJ, Young GS, Wiese DE, Marty FM, Schwartz RB. MR imaging of human herpesvirus-6-associated encephalitis in 4 patients with anterograde amnesia after allogeneic hematopoietic stem-cell transplantation. AJNR Am J Neuroradiol. 2006; 27(4):887–91.

70. Wainwright MS, Martin PL, Morse RP, Lacaze M, Provenzale JM, Coleman RE, et al. Human herpesvirus 6 limbic encephalitis after stem cell transplantation. Ann Neurol. 2001;50(5):612–9.

71. Wang FZ, Linde A, Hagglund H, Testa M, Locasciulli A, Ljungman P. Human herpesvirus 6 DNA in cerebrospinal fluid specimens from allogeneic bone marrow transplant patients: does it have clinical significance? Clin Infect Dis. 1999;28(3):562–8.

72. Demeter L. JC, BK, and other polyomavirus; progressive multifocal leukoencephalopathy. In: Mandell G, Bennett J, Dolin R, editors. Principles and practice of infectious diseases. 5th edition ed. London: Churchill Livingstone; 2000:1645–51.

73. Re D, Bamborschke S, Feiden W, Schroder R, Lehrke R, Diehl V, et al. Progressive multifocal leukoencephalopathy after autologous bone marrow transplantation and alpha-interferon immunotherapy. Bone Marrow Transplant. 1999;23(3):295–8.

74. Przepiorka D, Jaeckle KA, Birdwell RR, Fuller GN, Kumar AJ, Huh YO, et al. Successful treatment of progressive multifocal leukoencephalopathy with low-dose interleukin-2. Bone Marrow Transplant. 1997;20(11):983–7.

75. Coplin WM, Cochran MS, Levine SR, Crawford SW. Stroke after bone marrow transplantation: frequency, aetiology and outcome. Brain J Neurol. 2001;124(Pt 5):1043–51.

76. Najima Y, Ohashi K, Miyazawa M, Nakano M, Kobayashi T, Yamashita T, et al. Intracranial hemorrhage following allogeneic hematopoietic stem cell transplantation. Am J Hematol. 2009; 84(5):298–301.

77. Pomeranz S, Naparstek E, Ashkenazi E, Nagler A, Lossos A, Slavin S, et al. Intracranial haematomas following bone marrow transplantation. J Neurol. 1994;241(4):252–6.

78. Hefzy HM, Bartynski WS, Boardman JF, Lacomis D. Hemorrhage in posterior reversible encephalopathy syndrome: imaging and clinical features. AJNR Am J Neuroradiol. 2009;30(7):1371–9.

79. Tichelli A, Bhatia S, Socie G. Cardiac and cardiovascular consequences after haematopoietic stem cell transplantation. Br J Haematol. 2008;142(1):11–26.

80. Tichelli A, Bucher C, Rovo A, Stussi G, Stern M, Paulussen M, et al. Premature cardiovascular disease after allogeneic hematopoietic stem-cell transplantation. Blood. 2007;110(9):3463–71.

81. Colosimo M, McCarthy N, Jayasinghe R, Morton J, Taylor K, Durrant S. Diagnosis and management of subdural haematoma complicating bone marrow transplantation. Bone Marrow Transplant. 2000;25(5):549–52.

82. Blazar BR, Murphy WJ, Abedi M. Advances in graft-versus-host disease biology and therapy. Nat Rev Immunol. 2012;12(6): 443–58.

83. Socie G, Ritz J. Current issues in chronic graft-versus-host disease. Blood. 2014;124(3):374–84.

84. Delios AM, Rosenblum M, Jakubowski AA, DeAngelis LM. Central and peripheral nervous system immune mediated demyelinating disease after allogeneic hemopoietic stem cell transplantation for hematologic disease. J Neurooncol. 2012;110(2):251–6.

85. Kannan K, Koh LP, Linn YC. Subdural hematoma in two hematopoietic stem cell transplant patients with post-dural puncture headache and initially normal CT brain scan. Ann Hematol. 2002;81(9):540–2.

Neurologic Complications of Corticosteroids in Cancer Therapy

Erin M. Dunbar, Yue Wang, and Santosh Kesari

Introduction

Corticosteroids are chemically related to the steroid hormones aldosterone and cortisol, naturally produced by the adrenal glands as a response to pituitary adrenocorticotropic hormone (ACTH). Based on their major actions, they are divided into two main groups: glucocorticoids (GCs) and mineralocorticoids. Aldosterone is a mineralocorticoid that influences salt and water balance. Cortisol is a GC that influences a variety of general cellular, nervous system, metabolic, inflammatory, stress response, and other systemic functions. Both natural (endogenous) and synthesized (exogenous) corticosteroids share a similar chemical structure whose synthesis begins with cholesterol. Because GCs inhibit many portions of the immune response, they are used in treatment of many diseases and conditions, including cancer.

Chemical modifications of the naturally occurring steroid hormones and de novo synthetic productions have resulted in the availability of numerous synthetic corticosteroids since the 1940s. GCs have been a therapeutic standard for systemic inflammatory and autoimmune conditions since their introduction for use against rheumatoid arthritis in 1949. In addition, GCs have become an essential therapeutic adjunct in the amelioration of cancer conditions and treatment of several hematologic and solid malignancies [1]. Since 1952, GCs have revolutionized the therapy of central and peripheral nervous system (CNS, PNS) conditions as well as malignancies such as primary CNS lymphoma [2].

Treatment of systemic and nervous system conditions requires steroids at supra-physiologic doses, i.e., higher than the adrenal gland would endogenously produce. However, at therapeutic doses, a wide variety of deleterious side effects frequently occur. This chapter will address common therapeutic uses of GCs in cancer chemotherapy, as well as what is known about mechanisms of action and resistance. In addition, common complications of GC therapy, particularly neurologic ones, will be discussed, including strategies to monitor, prevent, and treat them. Lastly, potential GC alternatives and ongoing investigations will be highlighted.

Mechanisms of Action

Endogenous (natural) and exogenous (synthesized) GCs have similar mechanisms of action and will therefore be discussed together. Collectively, the mechanisms of action of GCs on target tissues are characterized by a relatively slow onset and long duration of action and can be classified as genomic (a.k.a. involving DNA) and non-genomic [3] (Fig. 19.1). Genomic alterations involve effects on transcription and transduction factors via three main mechanisms [3–9]. The first mechanism is trans-activation (responsible for most of the secondary effects of steroids), in which the GCs, via their nuclear receptor, promote DNA transcription with subsequent mRNA production and protein synthesis of targets [4, 5]. The second is trans-repression (responsible for most therapeutic effects), where they can act as negative transcription factors [6–8]. The third is post-transcriptional regulation (also responsible for therapeutic effects), which manifests from interactions between transcription factors, effects on mRNA stability and chromatin remodeling [4–6, 9].

E.M. Dunbar
Piedmont Hospital, Brain Tumor Center, 2001 Piedmont Road NE, #645, Atlanta, GA 30309, USA
e-mail: erin.dunbar@piedmont.org

Y. Wang
Department of Neurology, University of Florida, HSC PO Box 100236, Gainesville, FL 32610-0236, USA
e-mail: yue.wang@neurology.ufl.edu

S. Kesari (✉)
Department of Translational Neuro-Oncology and Neurotherapeutics, John Wayne Cancer Institute at Providence Saint John's Health Center, 2200 Santa Monica Blvd, Santa Monica, CA 90404, USA
e-mail: kesaris@jwci.org; santoshkesari@gmail.com

© Springer International Publishing AG 2018
D. Schiff et al. (eds.), *Cancer Neurology in Clinical Practice*,
DOI 10.1007/978-3-319-57901-6_19

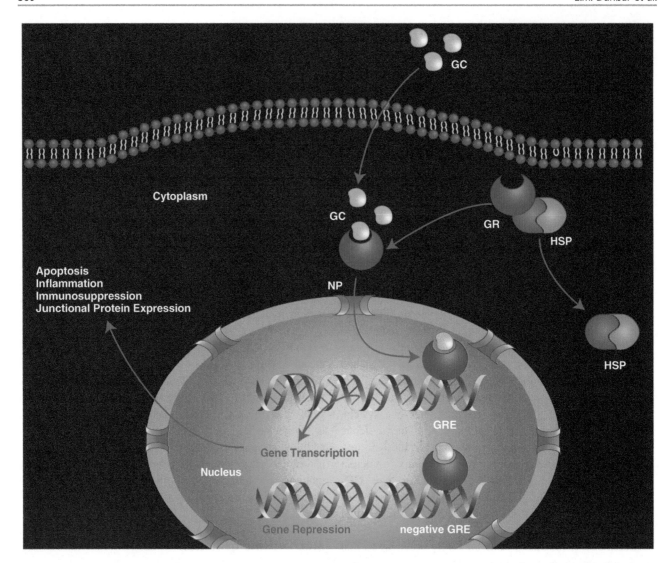

Fig. 19.1 Glucocorticoid mechanisms of action. Mechanisms of glucocorticoid (GC) action. GC crosses the cell membrane and binds to the glucocorticoid receptor (GR) in the cytoplasm. GRs are kept in an inactive state and prevented from moving into the nucleus by heat shock proteins (HSP). Upon binding of a GC to a GR, the HSP dissociates and the GC-GR complex moves to the nucleus via a nuclear pore (NP). The complex then binds to GC responsive elements (GRE) in the 5′ promoter region of DNA. Transcription is then activated. However, if the region contains a negative GRE, transcription is repressed. (*Source* Salvador et al. [3]. Open Access)

Glucocorticoid Actions on Target Tissues

In order to respond to physiologic and pathologic states, GCs affect nearly every cell of the body and modulate the expression of approximately ten percent of the body's genes. Actions of particular relevance to this chapter will be divided into effects on general cellular function, inflammation, systemic function, and nervous system function.

General cellular effects of GCs include the promotion of apoptosis and necrosis, which occur through the genomic mechanisms of gene trans-activation and trans-repression by the GR [10, 11]. The apoptotic effect of GCs is cell-type-specific, as well as time- and concentration-dependent [12]. However, the specific mechanisms of GC-induced apoptosis, their target genes, and their respective proteins remain incompletely understood [13–20]. An example of one such protein is NF-kB, whose DNA-independent repression induces apoptosis in many hematologic cell lines [15].

Anti-inflammatory effects of GCs include both the prevention and suppression of the inflammatory response. Specific actions depend on the type and dose of GCs used, the type and location of inflammation, and the type and number of immune cells involved. Anti-inflammatory actions of GCs occur via several mechanisms, including direct and indirect genomic repression. One example of such a mechanism includes the indirect repression of several mediators occurs via inhibition of transcriptional factor NF-kB. Collectively, these mechanisms minimize the proliferation, recruitment, and functional activity of

Table 19.1 Complications of pharmacologic glucocorticoid use

Complications of glucocorticoid use	
Acute	Chronic
Infectious	Infectious
Bacterial, viral, fungal	Pneumocystis pneumonia, tuberculosis
Neurologic	Neurologic
Psychosis, euphoria, anxiety, insomnia, increased appetite	Memory impairment, insomnia, depression, pseudotumor cerebri
Cutaneous	Cutaneous
Poor wound healing, acneiform eruptions	Striae, purpura, hirsutism, alopecia, non-melanoma skin cancer
Cardiovascular	Cardiovascular
Fluid retention, arrhythmia	Hypertension
Endocrine	Endocrine
Hyperglycemia, suppression of adrenal function	Suppression of adrenal function
	Musculoskeletal
	Osteoporosis, myopathy, avascular necrosis, growth retardation
	Gastrointestinal
	Peptic ulcer
	Ocular
	Cataracts

lymphocytes, neutrophils, macrophage, and monocytes by blocking the expression of endothelial and intercellular adhesion molecules, decreasing prostaglandin-mediated cell adhesion, decreasing chemokine binding to leukocytes, and inhibiting plasminogen activator synthesis [21–24]. These mechanisms also minimize the functions of pro-inflammatory mediators such as chemokines, cytokines, adhesion molecules, arachidonic acid metabolites, platelet-activating factor release, and pro-inflammatory enzymes and peptides [25]. The above mechanisms have been preferentially exploited for use in various hematologic and solid malignancies.

Systemic effects of GCs cannot be fully addressed in this chapter; however, those particularly relevant to the treatment and complications of cancer therapy will be addressed in subsequent sections and are listed in Table 19.1. GCs have a multitude of effects on a wide range of organ systems including the vascular, gastrointestinal, hematologic, dermatologic, and metabolic systems. Specific examples of these effects include regulation of blood pressure via the alteration of tissue sensitivity to catecholamine and the aldosterone-like effect on fluid retention, alterations in the number of circulating red blood cells and neutrophils, promotion of protein catabolism, gluconeogenesis, and glycogen synthesis, as well as alteration of lipid and bone metabolism. GCs also regulate protective prostaglandins and cellular integrity in the GI tract and can result in the thinning of epithelial and connective tissue throughout the body, thereby affecting skin integrity.

Nervous system effects of GCs involve both the central nervous system (CNS) and peripheral nervous system (PNS) levels. Mechanistically, acute exposure to GCs results in neuronal hyper-polarization, which is the result of alterations in intracellular calcium levels, interactions with GC protein-coupled receptors, and induction of MAP kinase cascades. Chronic exposure results in decreased quantity of neurons, induction of apoptotic cell death, impaired regenerative properties, and decreased neuronal survival [26]. Clinically, GC exposure impacts cognition (memory, mood, and personality), sleep patterns, pain perception, body temperature, muscle strength, and vasogenic edema.

Mechanisms of Resistance

Mechanisms of GC resistance remain poorly understood and vary with the genetic background of the patient, steroid type, disease type, and treatment regimen.

One mechanism of GC resistance involves apoptosis, which, amazingly, can produce seemingly dichotomous results. Such dichotomies are epitomized by the paradoxical effects that GCs have across various malignancies, as well as in response to various chemotherapy agents. One such example includes the pro-apoptotic effect of GCs on hematopoietic malignancies (discussed in the Mechanism of Action section), in contrast to the anti-apoptotic effects of GCs on many solid malignancies. For example, Zhang et al. [27] demonstrated dexamethasone and other GCs cause resistance to several cytotoxic chemotherapies and radiation in xenografted prostate cancer cells. A second mechanism of GC resistance involves inhibiting apoptosis-inducing receptors, signaling molecules, caspase enzymes, and mitochondrial membrane stabilizing proteins [28]. For example, dexamethasone has been shown to antagonize both mitochondrial and death receptor apoptotic pathways across various cancer cell lines [28], thus resulting in dexamethasone-induced apoptotic resistance in cell lines of solid malignancies, such as melanoma, neuroblastoma, gliomas, adenocarcinomas (e.g., breast), carcinomas (e.g., cervical), and bone cancers. Interestingly, many of the apoptosis genes repressed by GCs in carcinoma cell lines are the very same genes induced by GCs in hematopoietic malignancy cell lines [28, 29]. These seemingly paradoxical effects have been postulated and include cell-type specific differences in both transcriptional regulation and cell cycle progression, as well as cell-type differences in the development of mutations of GC function [28, 30–34]. A third mechanism of resistance involves perturbations of the GR gene and the GR receptor [32, 35–41]. A fourth mechanism of resistance involves activities essential to epithelial cell survival, including alterations of intercellular communication and extracellular matrix attachment, which have resulted in the chemotherapy resistance of many solid malignancies [42].

A fifth mechanism of resistance involves iatrogenic factors. For example, chronic exposure to GCs reduces both GR expression and GR protein stability [43–46]. In another example, concomitant use of medications that interact with the cytochrome P450 system can reduce the efficacy of GC metabolism and bioavailability [47–49]. In a third example, states of chronic inflammation can reduce the efficacy of GCs through the activation of both GR-dependent and GR-independent signaling pathways. Chronic inflammation can be induced by: (1) cigarette smoking, which induces an oxidative stress that affects both GR nuclear translocation and nuclear cofactors (2) inflammatory conditions such as asthma, which promote immune-mediated cytokines such as IL2 and IL-4, which diminish GR translocation and binding affinity at target cells, (3) viral infections, which reduce both GR nuclear translocation and GC functions, (4) allergen exposures, which affect both GR function and GR-binding affinity, (5) changes in the cellular micro-environment, such as during disease progression, which alter GR translocation and P-glycoprotein-mediated cellular ligand accumulation, (6) oxidative stress, which attenuates histone deacetylase-2 (HDAC2) activity and expression, thereby limiting recruitment of GC to sites of action in the genome by GR, and (7) hypoxia, which induces cellular dysfunction and impairs GR trans-activation [32].

Metabolism of Glucocorticoids

Endogenous

The adrenal cortex is responsible for the production and regulation of corticosteroids. The most peripheral of its three zones, the zona glomerulosa, produces mineralocorticoids, predominantly aldosterone, while the zona fasciculata and reticularis produce GCs and androgens, respectively. These latter two zones respond to pituitary adrenocorticotropic hormone (ACTH) that is secreted into the systemic

circulation in response to corticotropin-releasing hormone (CRH). CRH is released through the pituitary portal circulation by the hypothalamus in response to various physiologic and pathologic stressors.

Corticosteroid synthesis begins with a four-ringed cholesterol substrate, comprising three hexane rings and one pentane ring. The majority of substrate is esterified and stored in the adrenal gland, while a minority is synthesized directly from acetyl-CoA. Upon stimulation by ACTH, an esterase is activated and free cholesterol is released into the mitochondria, where it is converted to pregnenolone by a cytochrome P-450 side chain cleavage enzyme. Pregnenolone is the precursor to all other adrenal hormones, and its fate is carefully controlled by a series of feedback mechanisms. Corticosteroids are differentially synthesized by the sequential action of three hydroxylases at the C11, C17 and C21 positions. The end products include GCs (predominantly cortisol), mineralcorticoids (predominantly aldosterone), and androgens. Cortisol is secreted into the systemic circulation immediately upon production. Only 4–8% circulates in the blood in its active, unbound form. Approximately 92–96% of cortisol circulates in its inactive form, bound mainly to corticosteroid-binding globulin. Adrenal cortisol has a half-life of sixty to ninety minutes in the circulation [50].

Adrenal cortisol secretion is moderated by three main influences. The first influence comes from cortisol's direct negative feedback inhibition of both CRH and ACTH secretion on the hypothalamus and pituitary, respectively. The second influence comes from the circadian rhythm-related pulsatile release of ACTH that intensifies three to five hours after sleep initiation, peaks at the time of waking, and troughs within an hour or two after sleep initiation. The third influence comes from various physiologic and pathologic stressors, whose release of catecholamine and vasopressin cause the stimulation of hypothalamic-pituitary axis and the release of ACTH. Due to their lipophilicity, endogenous GCs readily cross the plasma membrane and interact with the GC receptor complex, as described above.

Exogenous

Synthetic steroids are manufactured from cholic acid obtained from cattle or from steroid sapogenins (diosgenin) from plants to optimize their bioavailability, plasma half-life, metabolism, and interactions with the GC receptors in target tissues [50]. The time to peak plasma level of most synthetic steroids is between 60 and 90 min, regardless of oral versus parenteral administration and co-administration with food or most other medicines. Most synthetic steroids are transported to the liver where they require metabolism into their active form [51]. Thus, as shown in Table 19.2, the

Table 19.2 Relative biologic potencies of exogenous (synthetic glucocorticoids)

Agent	Equivalency (mg)	Relative potency		Half-life	
		Anti-inflammatory	Mineralocorticoid	Plasma [32]	Biologic (h)
Short acting					
Cortisone acetate	25	0.8	0.8	30	8–12
Hydrocortisone	20	1	1	90	8–12
Intermediate acting					
Prednisone	5	4	0.8	60	12–36
Prednisolone	5	4	0.8	200	12–36
Methylprednisolone	4	5	0.5	180	12–36
Triamcinolone	4	5	0	300	12–36
Long acting					
Dexamethasone	0.75	20–30	0	200	36–72
Betamethasone	0.8	20–30	0	300	36–72

half-lives of various synthetic GCs are significantly affected by the level of overall hepatic and cytochrome p450 enzyme [52–54]. Unlike most endogenous steroids, exogenous steroids tend not to bind to the cortisol binding globulin, but instead circulate attached to either albumin or in its unbound state [55]. This binding difference does not appear to affect the serum half-life of exogenous GCs, which range from about one to four hours. Like endogenous steroids, exogenous GCs readily cross the plasma membrane and interact with steroid receptors in the nucleus. However, the resultant exogenous GC receptor complex produces a two to 11-fold greater effect than its endogenous counterpart. Lastly, as with any agent that acts by affecting nuclear receptors, the disappearance of exogenous GCs does not represent the cessation of effect [56].

The metabolism of exogenous GCs is clinically relevant in several ways. For example, the modifications that certain exogenous GCs undergo during synthesis result in differential cross-reactivity with the mineralocorticoid receptor, and thus differential complications. Also, requirement of many exogenous GCs to undergo activation in the liver results in the preferential administration of steroids not requiring liver activation, such as prednisolone, to patients with severely compromised liver function. Lastly, the requirement of many exogenous GCs to bind albumin results in higher free GC levels and more side effects in patients with low albumin [57].

Common Therapeutic Uses

General Principles

Despite decades of use in systemic and nervous system conditions, the majority of our clinical knowledge is empiric

and not evidence based. Although this has likely limited our optimal use of GCs, the impact of GCs on cancer therapy remains tremendous.

Tumor-Directed Treatment

Exogenous GCs promote death of cancer cells via a variety of mechanisms, including apoptosis. GCs have been historical mainstays in the treatment of systemic solid tumors, including breast, prostate, thymoma, and endocrine-responsive cancers [58]. GCs, with or without concomitant chemotherapy agents, have also been historical mainstays in the treatment of systemic *hematologic malignancies*, including chronic myelogenous leukemia (CML), multiple myeloma, chronic lymphocytic leukemia (CLL), and virtually all non-Hodgkin's lymphomas. For instance, GCs provide lifesaving relief to rapidly growing diffuse large B-cell lymphoma affecting the mediastinum [59].

GCs are also instrumental in the control of hematopoetic malignancies affecting the nervous system, presumably due to their previously described lympholytic mechanism, excellent penetration of the blood–brain barrier, and relatively long half-life [1, 60]. For example, dexamethasone, in combination with other chemotherapy agents, has resulted in improved CNS control of acute lymphoblastic leukemia, which has a high predilection for the CNS, and primary CNS lymphoma (PCNSL) [61, 62]. Rapid initial clinical response is a hallmark of GCs in hematologic malignancies affecting the nervous system, secondary to their ability to induce apoptosis in a p38 mitogen-activated protein kinase (MAPK)-dependent manner in B and T cells [63]. However, the effects of steroids are too transient and inefficient not to be coupled to radiotherapy and/or chemotherapy. GCs also indirectly provide anti-neoplastic effects to tumors being treated by allogeneic hematopoetic stem cell transplants by helping to prevent transplant rejection as well as prevent graft-versus-host disease [64].

Historically, there has been no clinical evidence that steroids inhibit the growth of gliomas or metastases in human patients. However, data from preclinical studies suggest that the invasiveness and proliferation of some glioma cells may be reduced by exposure to dexamethasone [65, 66]. GCs should be avoided in the initial management of patients suspected of having a hematologic malignancy of the nervous system, such as PCNSL, or infection, whenever clinically safe, as their lympholytic effects can obscure the histopathologic diagnosis. Fortunately, techniques to improve analysis yield by spinning down a CSF cytospin into a cell block, as well as the availability of other tests highly relevant to PCNSL, such as EBV, clonal heavy chain gene rearrangement, and pathologic expression of BCL2 and BCL-6 family proteins, are overcoming this historic challenge [67].

The emerging field of cancer immunotherapy is elucidating the profound complexities of the body's immune system, including the ability to harness it to fight nervous system and systemic malignancies. In brief, immunotherapy is an attempt to correct a failed or inadequate immune system, whether caused by innate, acquired, or iatrogenic immunosuppression, or by a tumor or a tumor-associated virus. Historical agents include IL-2 and interferon, and newer agents include effectors of checkpoints on T cells: PD-1, PD1-Ligand, CTLA-4, etc. Thus, understanding the interplay of GC immunomodulatory capabilities is paramount. Despite an incomplete translational understanding, several clinical trends have manifested. First, there exists the recommendation for using the "least clinically needed" GC dose during treatment with immunotherapy. Second is the use of GCs to suppress the often profound inflammatory sequela of immunotherapy. This can not only be lifesaving, but also allow for eventual resumption of treatment. A severe immune reaction necessitating prolonged GC use may require consideration of infliximab. Information about the immune-related toxicities of immunotherapy agents, which are measured by NCI's Common Toxicity Criteria [68] can be found within product inserts, FDA product safety releases, and Risk Evaluation and Management Strategies. Third, in available studies and practical experience, the judicious use of GCs with immunotherapy has not shown deleterious efficacy or overall survival. Lastly, opportunistic infection, such as *Aspergillus* pneumonia, Fournier's gangrene, *Pneumocystis jiroveci* pneumonia, cytomegalovirus colitis, and mucor mycosis, is another comorbidity of both GC use and immunotherapy that clinicians must identify and manage aggressively [69].

GCs should always be maintained at the lowest clinically needed dose, not only to minimize side effects, but also because numerous translational and clinical studies across tumor types suggest that GCs may result in chemotherapy resistance, via a variety of mechanisms [70].

Symptom-Directed Treatment

GCs serve a major role in cancer therapy by increasing the safety and tolerance of many chemotherapies, including cytotoxic drugs, monoclonal antibodies, immunotherapy, and other agents.

Anti-Emetic

One of the most important uses of GCs is the prevention or reduction in anticipatory nausea, a complex psychological–physiological phenomenon where patients experience nausea and vomiting at the mere memory trigger of the chemotherapy experience [71]. Mechanisms for these effects are not fully elucidated; however, reduced release of $5\text{-}HT_3$ from blood mononuclear cells upon administration of steroids as well as direct inhibitory effect on $5\text{-}HT_3$ receptor have been suggested as important factors [72, 73]. Furthermore, animal study data suggest a direct effect of corticosteroids in the medulla oblongata [74]. Methylprednisolone and dexamethasone have been shown to directly antagonize the serotonin receptors and GR associated decreased prostaglandin synthesis at target tissue [75].

Improve Tolerance of Treatments

GCs are used in numerous chemotherapy preparatory regimens ameliorate the symptoms associated with hypersensitivity. For example, GCs prevent various hypersensitivity reactions known to occur with certain chemotherapies and monoclonal antibodies [76]. GCs are used to reduce the hematologic toxicity associated with various chemotherapies or even the cancer itself. For example, GCs have been shown to reduce hematologic toxicity in advanced breast cancer patients receiving GCs concurrently with chemotherapy and reduce the severity of autoimmune conditions related to cancer or its treatments, including autoimmune hemolytic anemia or thrombocytopenia [58]. GCs are used to treat lethargy (fatigue), weakness, anorexia and can even induce a short-term euphoria [1]. GCs are used in the treatment of hypercalcemia associated with cancer when bisphosphonates are either contraindicated or ineffective [77]. GCs are also used to alleviate pain associated with bone metastases and their treatments, likely through the reduction in peri-neural edema and the inhibition of prostaglandin synthesis [78].

Anti-Inflammatory

GCs are frequently used to treat dyspnea, pleural effusion, ascites, pleuritis, lymphangitic carcinomatosis, and hemoptysis. This anti-inflammatory effect is caused, in part, by a reduction in the levels of eosinophils, monocytes and lymphocytes (despite a paradoxical increase in neutrophils), and an impairment of their function [79]. Similarly, GCs prevent or minimize a variety of cutaneous syndromes, including rashes, resulting from chemotherapy [80]. Lastly, GCs have been shown to ameliorate a symptomatic immune reaction in patients receiving immunotherapy for CNS and systemic malignancies, and to date, without documented diminution in their effects on tumor control and survival [69].

Anti-Edema

Since their first reported use for post-operative cerebral vasogenic edema in 1952, GCs have been mainstays in the treatment of vasogenic edema from primary and metastatic tumors throughout the nervous system [81–83]. Vasogenic edema is caused by a disrupted blood-brain barrier (BBB), resulting from breakdown of inter-endothelial tight junctions, increased endothelial pinocytosis, and increased endothelial fenestrations. Though the mechanism of BBB disruption remains unclear, VEGF release and tumor under expression of tight junction proteins likely play a role [84–86]. Steroids decrease the permeability of the blood brain barrier and limit the extravasation of fluid. This effect is mediated in part by the induction of occludin, transendothelial electrical resistance (TER) and zonula occludens (ZO)-1 expression. An increase in claudin-5 promoter activity and mRNA expression, as well as a decrease in expression of vascular endothelial-cadherin, intercellular adhesion molecule-1 (ICAM-1) and vascular cell adhesion molecule-1 (VCAM-1) , are also involved [87, 88].

The GCdexamethasone has been shown to ameliorate symptoms of vasogenic edema in over 70% of both primary and metastatic CNS cancer patients, including headache, somnolence, confusion, and to a lesser extent, seizure and focal neurologic deficits [2]. High-dose dexamathasone can also reverse life-threatening effects of vasogenic edema such as cerebral herniation or neoplastic epidural spinal cord compression (ESCC) [89, 90].

Given the desire to minimize GC side effects, dexamethasone "alternatives" continue to be explored, including corticotrophin-releasing factor, carbonic anhydrase inhibitors (e.g., acetazolamide), diuretics (e.g., furosemide, mannitol), and VEGFR-modulators (e.g., bevacizumab), and many others—discussed later in this chapter. To date, none have completely replaced GCs.

Common Therapeutic Regimens

General Principles

The determinants of GC dosing include pharmacokinetics of the different drug preparations, effects of underlying disorders on drug kinetics, and interactions of GCs with concurrently administered non-GC drugs. In addition, GCs must be individualized to specific target tissues, conditions and patient's organ function and comorbidities.

In addition, GCs cannot be titrated optimally without knowledge of how to monitor drug activity and how they impact each organ. For example, GCs significantly impact the ability for contrast dye to cross the blood-brain barrier in neuro-imaging studies. As a result, the dose and duration of GCs must be carefully taken into account when scans are interpreted [91, 92] (Fig. 19.2a–d). Furthermore, GCs cannot be titrated optimally without knowledge regarding how to safely withdraw steroids (discussed below) [93, 94].

Dexamethasone is the mainstay in primary and metastatic CNS cancers, given its minimal mineralocorticoid effects (e.g., less fluid retention, electrolyte imbalances) and long half-life, which allows for administration of a single daily dose [62]. Because of the unavoidable side effects of steroids, the "least clinically needed" dose and duration should always be attempted. Discontinuation must be gradual to prevent withdrawal symptoms.

Anti-Edema

Neurologic symptoms from cerebral vasogenic edema typically improve within 48 h and often within 12–24 h of steroid administration [95]. This is notably sooner than the improvements on MRI and CT imaging, which can take up to 48–72 h. Insufficient benefit either signifies an alternative mechanism of dysfunction or the need for additional therapies, including urgent surgical intervention, hyperosmotic mannitol [81], as well as other "dexamethasone alternatives" listed in the above section.

For patients with highly symptomatic cerebral edema, an initial dose of 16 mg/day is typically used. This dose was empirically established in the 1960s and continues to be recommended [96–99], despite a lack of prospective clinical trial evidence to support it use. In the setting of severe signs and symptoms, a loading dose of 10–20 mg of dexamethasone is often administered intravenously [100]. The bioavailability of IV and oral formulations are equivalent but GI absorption is usually 30–60 min. Maintenance doses of dexamethasone are commonly 4–24 mg daily. Importantly, given its long biologic half-life of 36–54 h, dosing more than once or twice daily is unnecessary, with administration times preferably in the morning to, the latest, early afternoon. This is particularly important for compliance and quality of life of patients after hospital discharge. For additional management principles and applications of GCs in CNS cancers, readers are directed to comprehensive reviews by Kostaras et al. [93], Ryken et al. [60], and Roth et al. [62].

Fig. 19.2 Serial MRIs of metastatic melanoma patient presenting with acute neurologic decline and showing reduction in edema and enhancement after 16 mg oral glucocorticoid administration for several days. Axial T2-weighted pre-steroids (**a**) and post-steroids (**b**). Axial T1-weighted pre-steroids (**c**) (attention to the blunting of left rostral ventricle and the effacement of the gyri) and post-steroids (**d**) (attention to the resumption of the anatomy of the ventricle and the gyri spaces)

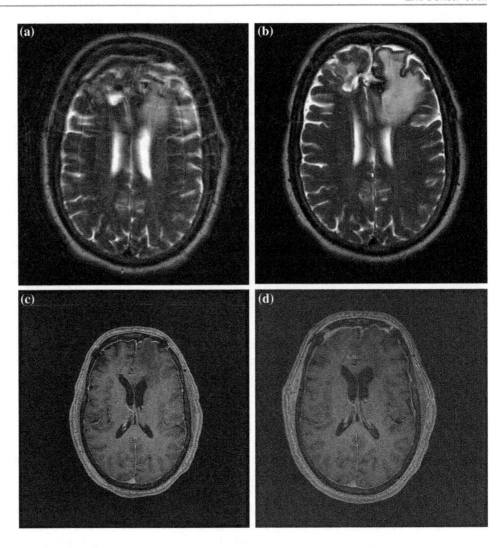

For patients with highly symptomatic spinal cord edema, such as from a tumor, immediate commencement of dexamethasone at 50–100 mg is recommended, followed by 16 mg daily [89, 90]. The onset and degree of symptomatic improvement, usually beginning within several hours, helps to determine the urgency of surgical intervention or other treatments.

Ameliorating Symptoms

GCs use to increase the safety and tolerance of many chemotherapy agents, which is highly individualized. For example, pre-medication for chemotherapy usually involves a one-time dose of 10 mg IV dexamethasone. The steroid is administered at least thirty minutes prior to the chemotherapy and is used to prevent acute transfusion reactions, anaphylaxis, or severe nausea. Patients on chemotherapy agents known to cause a more protracted cutaneous toxicity or nausea are often prescribed oral dexamethasone between 1 and 4 mg twice daily for three to five days prior to and after chemotherapy, often in combination with other supportive medications [75]. For the treatment of immunotherapy toxicity, dexamethasone is used at a dose ranging from 4 to 24 mg/day, and sometimes exchanged for once or biweekly infliximab [69]. Similar dosing can be used to treat other inflammatory conditions, including pleuritis, ascites, hemolytic anemia associated with malignancy, though prednisone is often favored over dexamethasone.

Tumor-Directed Treatment

GCs are used for their lympholytic properties in hematologic malignancies that affect the nervous system, including PCNSL and systemic lymphomas and leukemias with CNS involvement. Importantly, if the initial diagnosis of suspected lymphoma or leukemia is being investigated, dexamethasone should be withheld unless signs and symptoms are significant. This recommendation results from the disappearance of classic imaging or pathologic features that often occur after rapid and significant lympholysis. Although advances in imaging and pathology are minimizing this necessity, the general recommendation remains. Once the tumor has been diagnosed, starting doses usually range from 4 to 16 mg of dexamethasone a day. Similarly, GCs remain important components of regimens for various systemic and hematopoetic malignancies, both for their anti-neoplastic as well as symptom–amelioration roles. Across malignancies, the choice of GC, route of administration, dose and duration are highly individualized and, therefore, must be reviewed prior to prescription.

Tapering Regimens

Safe and optimal tapering involves knowledge of the dose, duration, drug activity, and status of the condition for which the GCs was used. The goal of tapering is to prevent an exacerbation of the underlying condition as well as prevent symptomatic adrenal insufficiency, a.k.a. steroid withdrawal symptoms, characterized by nausea, headache, myalgias, anorexia, and diverse nervous system symptoms [101]. Monitoring of tapering regimens predominantly involve close evaluations of signs and symptoms of withdrawl, but may include laboratory and imaging tests.

An attempt at tapering should be made in all patients and anticipation of the re-emergence of symptoms should not deter attempts [102]. Tapering of dexamethasone usually occurs over several weeks. For example, patients with brain tumors who have undergone gross or near total resections can usually be tapered down to off within a week or two after surgery and rarely need dexamethasone during radiotherapy. In contrast, brain tumor patients who have minimal or no surgical debulking usually require dexamethasone through-out radiotherapy. Spine tumor patients are generally recommended to maintain dexamethasone throughout radiotherapy and can usually be tapered down to off within two to three weeks depending on neurologic improvement. All patients should be observed for symptoms of adrenal insufficiency if dexamethasone is discontinued abruptly or used for a prolonged time, and advice from an endocrinologist should be sought if needed.

Despite the paucity of prospective, randomized trials, various tapering protocols are used, as illustrated in Table 19.3. For dexamethasone, the duration of one month at moderate dose is generally accepted as the threshold to recommend a tapering regimen. The attempted rate of tapering should be fast in the first 10 days of corticosteroid therapy (e.g., every 1–3 days) but slower after this (e.g., every 4–7 days, and even slower once physiological doses are reached). One commonly used strategy is to reduce the total daily dose by 25% each week; however, a more gradual discontinuance over 8–12 weeks may be needed for patients who have received dexamethasone for long periods of time.

If steroids have been used for more than a few weeks, then assessing for occult hypocorticolism is prudent. Baseline fasting morning (basal) cortisol levels can be tested before steroids have stopped. Patients with low cortisol levels benefit from replacement with hydrocortisone, with the first dose, (usually ~ 20 mg) given in the morning, and the second dose, (usually ~ 10 mg) at noon, to mimic the physiological secretion of the hormone [93, 103]. See additional information in the section below, entitled Management of Adverse Events Associated with Dexamethasone Therapy.

Common Non-Neurologic Clinical Toxicities

In general, GC side effects are common, correlated to dose and duration. For example, in a chart review of 88 patients with brain metastases, Sturdza et al. [97] reported that 91% of the patients receiving 16 mg or more daily and 65% of the patients receiving less than 16 mg daily experienced at least one side effect ($p = 0.006$). Hypoalbuminemia exacerbates GC side effects because such a state results in an increased percentage of unbound steroid [102].

Management of Adverse Events Associated with Dexamethasone Therapy

Drug–Drug Interactions

Exogenous GCs co-administered with other drugs (including topical and mucosal preparations) can produce drug–drug interactions as a results of disrupted globulin binding or induction/inhibition the hepatic p450 system enzymes. For example, enzyme-inducing medications such as rifampin, phenytoin, carbamazepine, and barbituates can stimulate the

Table 19.3 Suggested glucocorticoid tapering strategies

Duration	<1 month[a]	1 month—1 year[c]	>1 year[c]
Tapering strategy	Can stop immediately[a]	Reduce dose by 25% each week over four weeks[a,c]	Taper first 75% of dose over a month, and the residual over another four weeks[a,c]

[a]Beware frequent glucocorticoid courses
[b]Warn patient to report symptoms of glucocorticoid deficiency
[c]Consider formal adrenal testing when dose approaches physiologic replacement

metabolism of GCs and thus require an increased dose to achieve the desired effect [101, 104]. Alternatively, ketaconazole and many hormone-containing oral contraceptives can cause a 50% higher dose of unbound GCs concentration [105].

Glucocorticoid-Induced Adrenal Insufficiency

Prolonged exogenous GC use leads to atrophy of the zona fasciculata layer of the adrenal gland. Abrupt cessation or insufficient tapering can result in either symptomatic acute or insidious adrenal insufficiency (AI), often termed steroid withdrawal syndrome. Suppression of hypothalamic-pituitary-adrenal function by chronic administration of high doses of GCs is the most common cause. The presentation, diagnosis, and management of GC-induced AI are briefly summarized below.

The adrenal gland secretes ~ 20 mg of cortisol daily, and thus GC administration at doses greater than what is equivalent to ~ 5 mg of prednisone daily could cause suppression of the hypothalamic-pituitary-adrenal axis, a.k.a. secondary adrenal insufficiency (AI). Importantly, this can occur with any route of GC administration, including topical and inhaled. Because the adrenal gland recovers quickly from suppression, even after large doses, the use of GCs for less than a week is unlikely to cause AI with abrupt withdrawal. In contrast, patients receiving doses of ~ 20 mg of prednisone daily (or other steroid equivalent), those receiving doses in the evenings for more than a few weeks, and those with a cushingoid appearance, are recommended to undergo a tapering regimen to prevent symptomatic steroid withdrawal syndrome [106].

When evaluating a patient for suspected AI, it is important to distinguish primary AI, such as caused by a pituitary tumor, from secondary AI, such as caused by insufficient GC tapering, because the evaluation and treatment can differ. In primary AI, cortisol secretion is deficient despite the ability to secrete ACTH. In secondary AI, deficient ACTH secretion results in atrophy of the zona fasciculata and zona reticularis of the adrenal gland and impaired cortisol production and secretion. Another important difference is that secondary AI maintains nearly normal mineralocorticoid secretion because this function depends mostly on the renin-angiotensin system rather than on ACTH. Collectively, these differences form the basis of the laboratory confirmation of AI, and ultimately, their management.

The most common clinical features of secondary AI caused by GCs are listed in Table 19.1 [107], and include nausea, vomiting, abdominal pain, fever, confusion or coma, myalgia, arthralgia, and psychiatric symptoms, chronic fatigue worsened by exertion and improved with rest, generalized weakness, anorexia, weight loss, and in the case of adrenal crisis- hemodynamic shock. Patients with primary AI will also have symptoms of mineralocorticoid deficiency,

including abnormal electrolytes, hemodynamics, hyperpigmentation (because ACTH secretion is increased), and in women, androgen deficiency.

Distinguishing between primary and secondary AI requires a thorough H&P and complementary laboratory tests. A comprehensive review of laboratory tests for the evaluation of AI is beyond the scope of this chapter, but given the nuances of these laboratory tests and the variable presentations of patients, the early involvement of endocrinology is often very helpful. Notably, laboratory tests prior to urgent treatment may not always be practical, and work-up for possible causes of AI should be considered, including evaluation for infection, bleeding, or metastatic disease, which may require their own urgent empiric treatment.

Patients in adrenal crisis or those with AI and undergoing physiologic stress, such as trauma or surgery, frequently require treatment with hydrocortisone at 10–15 mg/m^2 (~ 100 mg) IV of body surface area daily (a.k.a. stress dose steroids). Equivalent doses of IV dexamethasone are favored if cortisol assays for adrenal function testing are being considered. Patients may also require aggressive hemodynamic support, intensive care monitoring, and evaluation and treatment for possible causes of AI [108]. A response is typically seen within 4–6 h of initiating treatment. Patients not presenting in crisis may be empirically treated with dexamethasone, usually 4–16 mg PO daily [109].

Infection

GC exposure can increase the risk of infection by Pneumocystis jirovecii pneumonia (PJP) (formally known as PCP), Listeria, Legionella, cryptococcus, cytomegalovirus, and many other organisms [110–113]. Furthermore, GCs can mask the features of acute infection, since symptoms such as erythema, swelling, and pain are dependent on the presence of functioning leukocytes. Lastly, they can falsely simulate true infection by the neutrophilia caused by de-margination. In this situation, the presence of more than 6% bandemia substantiates true infection [114].

There are no prospective trials or guidelines for the prevent of infection with GC use in malignancy; however, common wisdom recommends minimizing the burden of malignancy contributing to immunosuppression, using the least dose/duration of GCs clinically necessary, and having a low threshold for investigation of common and opportunistic organisms. Tests of exposure, such as for tuberculosis, and vaccinations are not routinely recommended as little is known about the patient's ability to mount a response [115]. The most evidence-based recommendation for patient with brain tumors receiving GCs for more than six weeks is the use of PJP prophylaxis with trimethoprim/sulfamethoxazole,

Table 19.4 Suggested prophylactic strategies for patients on long-term glucocorticoids

Use lowest effective steroid dose, for the shortest time possible
PJP infection prophylaxis: Trimethoprim/sulfamethoxazole, dapsone, or pentamidine
Skeletal health: Calcium 1500 mg/d, Vitamin D 800–1200 iu/d, consider bisphosphonate
Growth: Alternate-day steroid dosing
Muscle strength: Frequent exercise
Endocrine: Fasting glucose measurements every 6 months
Ophthalmology: Examination for cataract and glaucoma yearly

dapsone, or aerosolized pentamidine, as illustrated in Table 19.4 [116, 117].

Ocular

GCs can cause various acute ocular symptoms, including the sensation of dry, blurry, and fatigue-prone eyes. Chronic symptoms include increased intraocular pressure (glaucoma) and cataracts, which head & neck radiation may further exacerbate [118]. The use of saline eye drops, adequate rest, surveillance for concomitant infection, and routine eye examinations are recommended.

Cutaneous

GCs are most notoriously known for their ability to cause cushingoid features, including striae, easy bruising, purpura, hirsutism, alopecia, folliculitis, acne, and occasionally hyperpigmentation [109]. With the increasing use of chemotherapy agents that also cause various cutaneous toxicities, such as small molecule tyrosine kinase inhibitors, it may be challenging to correctly identify the causative agent. Strategies to prevent or minimize cutaneous toxicities include avoidance of harsh contacts, sunscreen, and good hygiene. Treatment strategies include minimizing the use of GCs and early intervention.

Chronic cushingoid features also include truncal obesity, buffalo hump, moon face, and weight gain [119]. In addition, chronic GCs, especially dexamethasone, impair normal wound healing through their effect on leukocytes, collagen, and fibroblasts [120]. This is a particular challenge to patients and neurosurgeons during recovery from brain and spine surgery [121].

Secondary Malignancies

Immunosuppression, regardless of whether from a genetic or acquired cause, is associated with an increased risk of secondary malignancies. Immunosuppression resulting from GC use has been associated with the development of non-melanoma skin cancer, including squamous cell and basal cell carcinoma and Kaposi's sarcoma [113]. Similarly, various lympho-proliferative disorders can occur, including PCNSL and post-transplant lympho-proliferative disorder [122, 123]. Prevention and treatment include minimizing immunosuppressive and carcinogenic contributors, close surveillance, including mucocutaneous and retinal examinations, and prompt intervention.

Vascular

Chronic GCs are associated with arterial hypertension resulting from sodium retention, volume expansion, and increased responsiveness to catecholamines [124]. Hypertension develops in roughly 20% of patients treated with steroids in a dose-dependent manner [125]. Treatment involves limiting sodium intake and the use of antihypertensive medication. Careful monitoring of electrolytes should be undertaken, especially when antihypertensives like thiazide diuretics are used concurrently with antiepileptics or other agents known to effect electrolytes. Cardiac dysrhythmias and sudden death have also been reported with the use of high-dose pulse steroids, likely related to electrolyte disturbances [126]. GC-induced fluid retention can be a particular risk for patients with underlying vascular disease and can sometimes be confused with the presentation of lower extremity thromboembolic disease. Once the latter is ruled out, elevation, compression hose, range of motion, and diuretics are used for treatment.

Thrombosis

Venous thromboembolism (VTE) is also more common in patients receiving GCs, both because of the direct thrombogenic effect of GCs, but also secondary to the comorbid conditions in patients receiving them, e.g., immobility, inflammation, cancer [127, 128]. An example of a management algorithm for symptomatic VTEs in patients with CNS cancers is reviewed elsewhere [129].

Metabolic

Hyperglycemia affects up to 72% of patients with primary brain tumors receiving dexamethasone [130]. This is often asymptomatic, mild, and reversible in patients without underlying metabolic disorders such as diabetes mellitus, but can be symptomatic, severe, and less reversible in patients with such disorders. The hyperglycemia from corticosteroid therapy usually occurs within the first 6 weeks of therapy and is believed to be secondary to insulin resistance and increased hepatic gluconeogenesis [131]. Furthermore, as many as 20–40% of patients with underlying glucose intolerance receiving GCs eventually meet the criteria of new onset diabetes mellitus [132].

Hyperglycemia has been correlated with inferior survival in many conditions, including malignant brain tumors, even when controlled for confounders [133, 134]. Treatment involves institution of a diet-limiting concentrated sweets and the judicious use of anti-hyperglycemic medications during GC therapy.

GC use is the most common form of iatrogenic osteoporosis and may occur in up to 50% of patients [135]. GCs cause a dose, duration, and age-dependent loss of 10–50% of bone mineral density leading to GC-induced osteoporosis (GIO). Although often asymptomatic, osteoporosis can lead to pain, fractures, and collapse, particularly in hips, wrists, and lumbar spine. For example, patients taking GCs for a prolonged period can have a more than fivefold increased risk of hip or vertebral fractures [136–138]. Causes are multifactorial and include direct actions on skeletal cells, reduced calcium absorption, secondary hyperparathyroidism, decreased gonadal hormones, and reduction in factors that stimulate bone growth, including insulin-like growth factor-1 and prostaglandin E2 [139]. Another cause can be concurrent medications. For example, certain antiepileptic medications, such as valproic acid or phenytoin, may further promote osteoporosis, and thus consideration for avoiding or switching these agents is warranted [140].

Treatment includes bisphosphonates, which are the most widely evaluated treatments for GIO and are generally regarded as the first line. Other treatments include parathyroid hormone peptides, daily exercise, calcium (1500 mg daily) and vitamin D (800–1200 IU daily) supplementation and use of pain medications [141–143]. Prevention includes dual-energy x-ray absorption (DEXA) and vitamin D level monitoring. Recently, a computer-based algorithm (FRAX®) was developed by the WHO to predict an absolute fracture risk score.

Lastly, avascular necrosis can occur in any patient on GCs. Special attention should be given to patients on long-term or high-dose GCs or with advanced age, underlying metabolic disorders, previous radiation, concomitant bisphosphonate use or who report musculoskeletal pain. Treatment ranges from avoidance of weight bearing to joint salvaging operations.

Gastrointestinal

GCs increase the risk of gastritis, gastro-esophageal reflux disease, ulceration, bleeding, and perforation. The risk is increased with co-administration of other agents, including anti-inflammatory drugs, certain chemotherapy agents, and alcohol [144]. As a result, the concomitant use of H2-blockers, proton-pump inhibitors, or coating agents have become standard practice. Of note, it is important to select a protective agent that does not interfere with absorption or metabolism of prescribed medications, to acknowledge the potential deficiency of absorption of agents and vitamins relying on the presence of gastrointestinal acidity, and to monitor for the development of resultant bacterial overgrowth. Chronic GC use can also cause pancreatitis, non-alcoholic fatty liver disease, or other liver dysfunction [145]. The latter forms the basis for the general recommendation to periodically monitor liver function tests, especially when co-administered with agents, including chemotherapy agents such as oxaliplatin and irinotecan, which increase this risk. Upon identification of GI toxicities, aggressive treatment is warranted.

Hematologic

GCs reduce the levels of eosinophils, monocytes, and lymphocytes, but paradoxically increase the release of neutrophils from the bone marrow, lymphatic organs, and walls of vessels causing neutrophilia without bandemia. Red blood cell number and cell volume can increase but platelets are usually less affected [146]. In the presence of GCs, hematopoietic cells appear to have reduced access to sites of inflammation and impaired function, as detailed in previous sections.

Special Patient Populations

Exposure of pregnant women to supra-physiologic exogenous GCs can result in obesity, fluid retention, hypertension, and gestational diabetes. Although clinical experience and prospective trials demonstrate that exposure of the fetus to modest doses of GCs is usually safe, potential sequelae include the development of adrenal suppression, abnormal birth-weight, potentially growth defects such as cleft lip and palate, and potentially life-threatening hypoglycemia upon delivery [147]. Dexamethasone and betamethasone cross the placenta more readily than hydrocortisone and prednisone. Careful monitoring and early intervention in the pregnant women and their fetuses are paramount. Breast feeding while taking GCs is considered generally safe, although there is some excretion of the steroids in breast milk, and thus it is generally recommended to delay for several hours after GCingestion. Children exposed to chronic GCs are at risk for various disorders, including osteoporosis, diabetes mellitus, growth retardation, and cataracts [109]. Middle aged through elderly patients exposed to chronic GCs tend to be at elevated risk for all types of GC-related side effects and therefore require special attention.

Central Nervous System Effects

GCs produce dose and duration-dependent cerebral atrophy that produces unique effects across the anatomic-functional continuum. Mechanisms underlying these effects include alterations in metabolism, electrochemical channels, and neurotransmitters. For example, memory and cognitive deficits have been shown in animal studies to be the result of structural and functional changes in dendrites and synaptic terminals, neuron loss, and inhibition of regeneration. In addition, GCs influence behavioral disorders, anxiety, depression, anger, emotional liability, euphoria, insomnia, psychosis, sun-downing, and alteration in pain and body temperature [148]. Extended dose and duration, as well as patients of advanced age and underlying mood and behavioral disorders, represent the most risk. Discrimination between symptoms of the condition for which GCs were indicated and those of GCs can be challenging. Psychiatric effects can occur in up to 60% of patients, with severe effects in $\approx$6% [149, 150]. Psychiatric effects are dose and duration-dependent. Early symptoms typically occur within 1–2 weeks (e.g., insomnia, emotional liability, hypomanic and manic episodes), whereas later symptoms typically occur after numerous weeks (e.g., depression) [151, 152]. Furthermore, GCs can also cause cognitive impairment such as memory disturbances. Like other psychiatric side effects, these also tend to be dose and duration-dependent and resolve after termination of steroids [153].

Prevention and treatment of GC-induced behavioral and psychiatric symptoms includes behavioral modification, counseling, and medications ranging from anti-psychotics to anti-depressants. For example, neuroleptic drugs (e.g., olanzapine) are known to ameliorate behavioral sequelae. In addition, maximal separation between the administration and sleep may be beneficial. Thankfully, almost all psychiatric symptoms tend to resolve with cessation of steroids.

Peripheral Nervous System Effects

Diagnosis of the PNS effects of GCs is challenging because of difficulties in discriminating them from worsening of the primary condition for which GCs were initiated. The most common and stereotypical is myopathy. Myopathy, classically presents as painless, symmetric, proximal motor weakness in both the upper and lower extremities, with preserved reflexes. Proximal muscles are most affected and muscle wasting can ensue, especially of the pelvic girdle, the proximal arm muscles, neck and respiratory muscles [141].

Myopathy has been reported in up to 20% of adults receiving a wide range of dose and durations of GCs and is usually subacute [154]. Another study reported a much higher incidence of steroid-induced myopathy in cancer patients (60%), but the sample size was much smaller [155]. Muscle atrophy occurs in approximately 10% of patients, and more frequently in the elderly and those with higher doses and durations [131].

Two distinct forms of steroid-induced myopathy are described. The first, an acute and less common form, is a generalized myopathy partially associated with rhabdomyolysis and occurs within days of steroid onset. The second, a chronic and more common form, is a myopathy characterized by proximal muscle weakness and occurs over several weeks of steroid onset [155–157].

Myopathy is especially devastating in those with pre-existing or concomitant neurologic or muscular deficits. Recovery from myopathy after dose reduction or tapering may take months, and physical therapy is recommended to attenuate the symptoms [158]. Prevention and treatment includes minimizing use, avoidance of nervous system toxins (such as vitamin deficiencies or alcohol), physical activity, and consideration of alternate-day dosing [159].

Treatment for Toxicities

Although individual GC-induced toxicities are addressed in above sections, a few general principles are worth mentioning. Any dose, duration and route of administration of GC can produce toxicity. The risk increases with extremes of age, health, duration, and dose. Although toxicities can occur without warning or reversibility, the majority can be prevented, minimized, or treated. Knowledge about GCs, communication between patients and providers, minimization of use, close surveillance and prompt therapy are successful strategies.

Future Directions and Investigations

The large number of complications associated with GCs has led to the search for alternative therapies. For example, corticotropin-releasing factor (CRF) has been shown in animals to reduce peritumoral edema by a direct effect on blood vessels through CRF 1 and 2 receptors, independent of the release of adrenal steroids [160]. In a recent phase III prospective randomized trial [a.k.a., Xerecept® (hCRF) trial (Celtic Pharma, Hamilton, Bermuda)], the administration of corticorelin acetate, a synthetic analog of human corticotropin-releasing factor, to the interventional group of malignant glioma patients, allowed for a statistically significant higher maximal reduction in the dexamethasone, as compared to the control group. Furthermore, patients in the corticorelin acetate group were less likely to experience myopathy and cushingoid appearance [161]. Prospective phase I–III clinical trials of hCRF suggest that it is relatively well tolerated and may have a future role as a GC alternative.

Given extensive preclinical studies demonstrating the important, multifaceted role VEGF plays in the pathogenesis of peritumoral edema, several agents targeted to inhibit the levels or actions of VEGF are currently being investigated. Bevacizumab (Avastin®, Genentech, South San Francisco, CA, USA), the monoclonal antibody against VEGF, is FDA approved for the treatment of glioblastoma [162]. It has been shown to reduce malignant brain tumor appearance on T1-w gadolinium-enhanced MRI, as well as peritumor vasogenic edema, and can result in improvement in neurologic symptoms—mimicking the mechanisms of GCs [163]. However, approval for this indication is lacking, and both cost and side effects preclude its widespread use. Inhibitors of VEGF receptors, such as sorafenib (Nexavar®, Bayer, Whippany, NJ, USA) and sunitinib (Sutent®, Pfizer, New York, NY, USA) are also under investigation [164] as possible steroid-sparing agents. Of note, anti-VEGF therapies have also become incorporated (often off-label) in the treatment of radiation necrosis, third space edema, malignant ascites, pleural effusions, macular neovascularization, and more recently, endolymphatic sac tumors and vestibular schwannomas [165–167].

Drugs with uncertain effects on the edema surrounding brain tumors include Boswellia serrata (an extract of Indian frankincense), cyclooxygenase (COX)-2 inhibitors, and angiotensin-II inhibitors [168, 169]. Prospective randomized trials are needed to confirm the efficacy and safety of such potential alternatives to GC therapy.

Summary

The introduction of corticosteroids over 60 years ago was a monumental advance in the treatment of cancer—both systemically and in the nervous system. GCs remain essential to the treatment of cancer and its complications. Knowledge of their metabolism and mechanisms of action and resistance form the basis for their optimal use. Knowledge of how best to prevent, surveille, and treat their potential side effects will facilitate their optimal use. Lastly, commitments for communication, patient individualization, and participation in trials exploring improved GC use and alternatives will secure improved outcomes in our patients.

References

1. Walsh D, Avashia J. Glucocorticoids in clinical oncology. Cleve Clin J Med. 1992;59(5):505–15.
2. Kaal EC, Vecht CJ. The management of brain edema in brain tumors. Curr Opin Oncol. 2004;16(6):593–600.
3. Buckingham JC. Glucocorticoids: exemplars of multi-tasking. Br J Pharmacol. 2006;147(Suppl 1):S258–68.
4. Barnes PJ. Molecular mechanisms and cellular effects of glucocorticosteroids. Immunol Allergy Clin North Am. 2005;25(3):451–68.
5. Barnes PJ. Mechanisms and resistance in glucocorticoid control of inflammation. J Steroid Biochem Mol Biol. 2010;120(2–3):76–85.
6. Piette C, Munaut C, Foidart JM, et al. Treating gliomas with glucocorticoids: from bedside to bench. Acta Neuropathol. 2006;112(6):651–64.
7. Gehring U, Segnitz B, Foellmer B, Francke U. Assignment of the human gene for the glucocorticoid receptor to chromosome 5. Proc Natl Acad Sci U S A. 1985;82(11):3751–5.
8. Turner JD, Schote AB, Macedo JA, et al. Tissue specific glucocorticoid receptor expression, a role for alternative first exon usage? Biochem Pharmacol. 2006;72(11):1529–37.
9. Janknecht R, Hunter T. Transcription. A growing coactivator network. Nature. 1996;383(6595):22–3.
10. Ramdas J, Harmon JM. Glucocorticoid-induced apoptosis and regulation of NF-{kappa}B activity in human leukemic T cells. Endocrinology. 1998;139(9):3813–21.
11. Smith LK, Cidlowski JA. Glucocorticoid-induced apoptosis of healthy and malignant lymphocytes. Prog Brain Res. 2010;182:1–30.
12. Higgins SC, Pilkington GJ. The in vitro effects of tricyclic drugs and dexamethasone on cellular respiration of malignant glioma. Anticancer Res. 2010;30(2):391–7.
13. Rogatsky I, Hittelman AB, Pearce D, Garabedian MJ. Distinct glucocorticoid receptor transcriptional regulatory surfaces mediate the cytotoxic and cytostatic effects of glucocorticoids. Mol Cell Biol. 1999;19(7):5036–49.
14. Lu NZ, Collins JB, Grissom SF, Cidlowski JA. Selective regulation of bone cell apoptosis by translational isoforms of the glucocorticoid receptor. Mol Cell Biol. 2007;20:7143–60.
15. Helmberg A, Auphan N, Caelles C, et al. Glucocorticoid-induced apoptosis of human leukemic cells is caused by the repressive function of the glucocorticoid receptor. EMBO J. 1995;14(3):452–60.

16. Wang Z, Rong YP, Malone MH, Davis MC, Zhong F, Distelhorst CW. Thioredoxin-interacting protein (txnip) is a glucocorticoid-regulated primary response gene involved in mediating glucocorticoid-induced apoptosis. Oncogene. 2006; 25(13):1903–13.

17. Schlossmacher G, Stevens A, White A. Glucocorticoid receptor-mediated apoptosis: mechanisms of resistance in cancer cells. J Endocrinol. 2011;211(1):17–25.

18. Nagao K, Iwai Y, Miyashita T. RCAN1 is an important mediator of glucocorticoid-induced apoptosis in human leukemic cells. PLoS ONE. 2012;7(11):e49926.

19. Distelhorst CW. Recent insights into the mechanism of glucocorticosteroid-induced apoptosis. Cell Death Differ. 2002;9(1):6–19.

20. Manoli I, Alesci S, Blackman MR, Su YA, Rennert OM, Chrousos GP. Mitochondria as key components of the stress response. Trends Endocrinol Metab. 2007;18(5):190–8.

21. Miyata M, Lee JY, Susuki-Miyata S, Wang WY, Xu H, Kai H, Kobayashi KS, Flavell RA, Li JD. Glucocorticoids suppress inflammation via the upregulation of negative regulator IRAK-M. Nat Commun. 2015;6:6062.

22. Caramori G, Adcock I. Anti-inflammatory mechanisms of glucocorticoids targeting granulocytes. Curr Drug Targets Inflamm Allergy. 2005;4(4):455–63.

23. Cronstein BN, Kimmel SC, Levin RI, et al. A mechanism for the antiinflammatory effects of corticosteroids: the glucocorticoid receptor regulates leukocyte adhesion to endothelial cells and expression of endothelial-leukocyte adhesion molecule 1 and intercellular adhesion molecule 1. Proc Natl Acad Sci U S A. 1992;89(21):9991–5.

24. Skubitz KM, Craddock PR, Hammerschmidt DE, et al. Corticosteroids block binding of chemotactic peptide to its receptor on granulocytes and cause disaggregation of granulocyte aggregates in vitro. J Clin Invest. 1981;68(1):13–20.

25. Ingawale DK, Satish KM, Snehal SP. An emphsis on molecular mechanisms of anti-inflammatory effects of glucocorticoid resistance. J Complement. Integr Med. 2015;12(1):1–13.

26. Sapolsky RM. Glucocorticoids and hippocampal atrophy in neuropsychiatric disorders. Arch Gen Psychiatry. 2000;57(10): 925–35.

27. Zhang C, Wenger T, Mattern J, et al. Clinical and mechanistic aspects of glucocorticoid-induced chemotherapy resistance in the majority of solid tumors. Cancer Biol Ther. 2007;6(2):278–87.

28. Herr I, Buchler MW, Mattern J. Glucocorticoid-mediated apoptosis resistance of solid tumors. Results Probl Cell Differ. 2009;49:191–218.

29. Zhang C, Beckermann B, Kallifatidis G, et al. Corticosteroids induce chemotherapy resistance in the majority of tumour cells from bone, brain, breast, cervix, melanoma and neuroblastoma. Int J Oncol. 2006;29(5):1295–301.

30. Glick RD, Medary I, Aronson DC, et al. The effects of serum depletion and dexamethasone on growth and differentiation of human neuroblastoma cell lines. J Pediatr Surg. 2000;35(3):465–72.

31. Sengupta S, Vonesch JL, Waltzinger C, et al. Negative cross-talk between p53 and the glucocorticoid receptor and its role in neuroblastoma cells. EMBO J. 2000;19(22):6051–64.

32. Gross KL, Lu NZ, Cidlowski JA. Molecular mechanisms regulating glucocorticoid sensitivity and resistance. Mol Cell Endocrinol. 2009;300(1–2):7–16.

33. Russcher H, Smit P, van den Akker EL, et al. Two polymorphisms in the glucocorticoid receptor gene directly affect glucocorticoid-regulated gene expression. J Clin Endocrinol Metab. 2005;90(10):5804–10.

34. Russcher H, van Rossum EF, de Jong FH, et al. Increased expression of the glucocorticoid receptor-A translational isoform as a result of the ER22/23EK polymorphism. Mol Endocrinol. 2005;19(7):1687–96.

35. Koper JW, Stolk RP, de Lange P, et al. Lack of association between five polymorphisms in the human glucocorticoid receptor gene and glucocorticoid resistance. Hum Genet. 1997;99(5):663–8.

36. Hillmann AG, Ramdas J, Multanen K, Norman MR, Harmon JM. Glucocorticoid receptor gene mutations in leukemic cells acquired in vitro and in vivo. Cancer Res. 2000;60(7):2056–62.

37. Irving JA, Minto L, Bailey S, Hall AG. Loss of heterozygosity and somatic mutations of the glucocorticoid receptor gene are rarely found at relapse in pediatric acute lymphoblastic leukemia but may occur in a subpopulation early in the disease course. Cancer Res. 2005;65(21):9712–8.

38. Schaaf and Cidolowski 2002 in neuroendocrinology. In: Martini L, Chorous G, Labrie F, et al. editors. Progress in brain research, vol. 181. Elsevier; 2010. p. 160.

39. Wallace and Cidlowski 2001, 7.4.1, In: Cato ACB, Schacke H, Asadullah K, editors. Recent advances in glucocorticoid receptor action. Springer Science & Business Media; 2013.

40. Haarman EG, Kaspers GJ, Pieters R, Rottier MM, Veerman AJ. Glucocorticoid receptor alpha, beta and gamma expression vs in vitro glucocorticod resistance in childhood leukemia. Leukemia. 2004;18(3):530–7.

41. Kfir S, Sionov RV, Zafrir E, Zilberman Y, Yefenof E. Staurosporine sensitizes T lymphoma cells to glucocorticoid-induced apoptosis: role of Nur77 and Bcl-2. Cell Cycle. 2007;6(24): 3086–96.

42. Sasson R, Amsterdam A. Pleiotropic anti-apoptotic activity of glucocorticoids in ovarian follicular cells. Biochem Pharmacol. 2003;66(8):1393–401.

43. Lacroix A, Bonnard GD, Lippman ME. Modulation of glucocorticoid receptors by mitogenic stimuli, glucocorticoids and retinoids in normal human cultured T cells. J Steroid Biochem. 1984;21(1):73–80.

44. Schlechte JA, Ginsberg BH, Sherman BM. Regulation of the glucocorticoid receptor in human lymphocytes. J Steroid Biochem. 1982;16(1):69–74.

45. Rosewicz S, McDonald AR, Maddux BA, et al. Mechanism ofglucocorticoid receptor down-regulation by glucocorticoids. J BiolChem. 1988;263(6):2581–4.

46. Burnstein KL, Jewell CM, Sar M, et al. Intragenic sequences of the human glucocorticoid receptor complementary DNA mediate hormone-inducible receptor messenger RNA down-regulation through multiple mechanisms. Mol Endocrinol. 1994;8(12): 1764–73.

47. Xu J, Winkler J, Derendorf H. A pharmacokinetic/pharmacodynamics approach to predict total prednisolone concentrations in human plasma. J Pharmacokinet Pharmacodyn. 2007;34(3):355–72.

48. Chalk JB, Ridgeway K, Brophy T, et al. Phenytoin impairs the bioavailability of dexamethasone in neurological and neurosurgical patients. J Neurol Neurosurg Psychiatry. 1984;47(10): 1087–90.

49. Ruegg S. Dexamethasone/phenytoin interactions: neurooncological concerns. Swiss Med Wkly. 2002;132(29–30):425–6.

50. Fotherby K. Metabolism of synthetic steroids by animals and man. Acta Endocrinol Suppl (Copenh). 1974;185:119–47.

51. Meikle AW, Weed JA, Tyler FH. Kinetics and interconversion of prednisolone and prednisone studied with new radioimmunogassays. J Clin Endocrinol Metab. 1975;41(4):717–21.

52. Bergrem H. The influence of uremia on pharmacokinetics and protein binding of prednisolone. Acta Med Scand. 1983;213 (5):333–7.

53. Schimmer BP, Parker KL. Adrenocorticotropic hormone; adrenocortical steroids and their synthetic analogs; inhibitors of the

synthesis and actions of adrenocortical hormones. In: Brunton LL, Lazo JS, Parker KL, editors. The pharmacological basis of therapeutics, 11th ed. New York: McGraw Hill; 2006. p. 1587.

54. Donohoue PA. The adrenal gland and its disorders. In: Kappy MS, Allen DB, Geffner ME, editors. Pediatric practice endocrinology. New York: McGraw-Hill; 2009.

55. Ballard PL. Delivery and transport of glucocorticoids to target cells. Monogr Endocrinol. 1979;12:25–48.

56. Axelrod L. Glucocorticoid therapy. Medicine (Baltimore). 1976;55(1):39–65.

57. Frey BM, Frey FJ. The effect of altered prednisolone kinetics in patients with the nephrotic syndrome and in women taking oral contraceptive steroids on human mixed lymphocyte cultures. J Clin Endocrinol Metab. 1985;60(2):361–9.

58. Keith BD. Systematic review of the clinical effect of glucocorticoids on nonhematologic malignancy. BMC Cancer. 2008;8:84.

59. Rowell NP, Gleeson FV. Steroids, radiotherapy, chemotherapy and stents for superior vena caval obstruction in carcinoma of the bronchus: a systematic review. Clin Oncol (R Coll Radiol). 2002;14(5):338–51.

60. Ryken TC, McDermott M, Robinson PD, et al. The role of steroids in the management of brain metastases: a systematic review and evidence-based clinical practice guideline. J Neurooncol. 2010;96(1):103–14.

61. Mitchell CD, Richards SM, Kinsey SE, et al. Benefit of dexamethasone compared with prednisolone for childhood acute lymphoblastic leukaemia: results of the UK medical research council ALL97 randomized trial. Br J Haematol. 2005;129(6):734–45.

62. Roth P, Stupp R, Eisele G, Weller M. Treatment of primary CNS lymphoma. Curr Treat Options Neurol. 2014;16(1):277.

63. Kullmann MK, Grubbauer C, Goetsch K, et al. The p27-Skp2 axis mediates glucocorticoid-induced cell cycle arrest in T-lymphoma cells. Cell Cycle. 2013;12(16):2625–35.

64. Quellmann S, Schwarzer G, Hubel K, et al. Corticosteroids in the prevention of graft-vs-host disease after allogeneic myeloablative stem cell transplantation: a systematic review and meta-analysis. Leukemia. 2008;22(9):1801–3.

65. Lin YM, Jan HJ, Lee CC, Tao HY, Shih YL, Wei HW, Lee HM. Dexamethasone reduced invasiveness of human malignant glioblastoma cells through a MAPK phosphatase-1 (MKP-1) dependent mechanism. Eur J Pharmacol. 2008;593(1–3):1–9.

66. Fan Z, Sehm T, Rauh M, Buchfelder M, Eyupoglu IY, Savaskan NE. Dexamethasone alleviates tumor-associated brain damage and angiogenesis. PLoS ONE. 2014;9(4):e93264.

67. Porter AB, Giannini C, Kaufmann T, Lucchinetti CF, Wu W, Decker PA, Atkinson JL, O'Neill BP. Primary central nervous system lymphoma can be histologically diagnosed after previous corticosteroid use: a pilot study to determine whether corticosteroids prevent the diagnosis of primary central nervous system lymphoma. Ann Neurol. 2008;63(5):662–7.

68. https://evs.nci.nih.gov/ftp1/CTCAE/CTCAE_4.03_2010-06-14_QuickReference_5x7.pdf. p. 65. Last accessed 15 July 2015.

69. Horvat TZ, Adel NG, Dang TO, et al. Immune-related adverse events, need for systemic immunosuppression, and effects on survival and time to treatment failure in patients with melanoma treated with ipilimumab at memorial sloan kettering cancer center. J Clin Oncol. 2015;33(28):3193.

70. Weller M, Schmidt C, Roth W, et al. Chemotherapy of human malignant glioma: prevention of efficacy by dexamethasone? Neurology. 1997;48(6):1704–9.

71. Markman M. Progress in preventing chemotherapy-induced nausea and vomiting. Cleve Clin J Med, 2002;69(8): 609–10, 612, 615–7.

72. Mantovani G, Macciò A, Esu S, Lai P. Evidence that cisplatin induces serotonin release from human peripheral blood mononuclear cells and that methylprednisolone inhibits this effect. Eur J Cancer. 1996;32A(11):1983–5.

73. Suzuki T, Sugimoto M, Koyama H, Mashimo T, Uchida I. Inhibitory effect of glucocorticoids on human-cloned 5-hydroxytryptamine3A receptor expressed in xenopus oocytes. Anesthesiology. 2004;101(3):660–5.

74. Ho CM, Ho ST, Wang JJ, Tsai SK, Chai CY. Dexamethasone has a central antiemetic mechanism in decerebrated cats. Anesth Analg. 2004;99(3):734–9.

75. Grunberg SM. Antiemetic activity of corticosteroids in patients receiving cancer chemotherapy: dosing, efficacy, and tolerability analysis. Ann Oncol. 2007;18(2):233–40.

76. Sehn LH, Donaldson J, Filewich A, et al. Rapid infusion rituximab in combination with corticosteroid-containing chemotherapy or as maintenance therapy is well tolerated and can safely be delivered in the community setting. Blood. 2007;109(10):4171–3.

77. Stewart AF. Clinical practice. Hypercalcemia associated with cancer. N Engl J Med. 2005;352(4):373–9.

78. Baines MJ. Cancer pain. Postgrad Med J. 1984;60(710):852–7.

79. Fauci AS, Dale DC, Balow JE. Glucocorticosteroid therapy: mechanisms of action and clinical considerations. Ann Intern Med. 1976;84(3):304–15.

80. Drake RD, Lin WM, King M, et al. Oral dexamethasone attenuates Doxil-induced palmar-plantar erythrodysesthesias in patients with recurrent gynecologic malignancies. Gynecol Oncol. 2004;94(2):320–4.

81. Miller JD, Leech P. Effects of mannitol and steroid therapy on intracranial volume-pressure relationships in patients. J Neurosurg. 1975;42(3):274–81.

82. Miller JD, Sakalas R, Ward JD, et al. Methylprednisolone treatment in patients with brain tumors. Neurosurgery. 1977;1(2):114–7.

83. Marantidou A, Levy C, Duquesne A, Ursu R, Bailon O, Coman I, Belin C, Carpentier AF. Steroid requirements during radiotherapy for malignant gliomas. J Neurooncol. 2010;100(1):89–94.

84. Heiss JD, Papavassiliou E, Merrill MJ, et al. Mechanism of dexamethasone suppression of brain tumor-associated vascular permeability in rats. Involvement of the glucocorticoid receptor and vascular permeability factor. J Clin Invest. 1996;98(6):1400–8.

85. Machein MR, Plate KH. VEGF in brain tumors. J Neurooncol. 2000;50(1–2):109–20.

86. Papadopoulos MC, Saadoun S, Binder DK, et al. Molecular mechanisms of brain tumor edema. Neuroscience. 2004;129(4):1011–20.

87. Salvador E, Shityakov S, Förster C. Glucocorticoids and endothelial cell barrier function. Cell Tissue Res. 2014;355(3):597–605.

88. Bebawy JF. Perioperative steroids for peritumoral intracranial edema: a review of mechanisms, efficacy, and side effects. J Neurosurg Anesthesiol. 2012;24(3):173–7.

89. Graham PH, Capp A, Delaney G, et al. A pilot randomised comparison of dexamethasone 96 mg vs 16 mg per day for malignant spinal-cord compression treated by radiotherapy: TROG 01.05 Superdex study. Clin Oncol (R Coll Radiol). 2006;18(1):70–6.

90. Patchell RA, Tibbs PA, Regine WF, et al. Direct decompressive surgical resection in the treatment of spinal cord compression caused by metastatic cancer: a randomised trial. Lancet. 2005;366(9486):643–8.

91. Macdonald DR, Cascino TL, Schold SC Jr, et al. Response criteria for phase II studies of supratentorial malignant glioma. J Clin Oncol. 1990;8(7):1277–80.

92. van den Bent MJ, Vogelbaum MA, Wen PY, et al. End point assessment in gliomas: novel treatments limit usefulness of classical Macdonald's Criteria. J Clin Oncol. 2009;27(18): 2905–8.

93. Kostaras X, Cusano F, Kline GA, et al. Use of dexamethasone in patients with high-grade gliomas: a clinical practice guideline. Curr Oncol. 2014;21:e493–503.

94. NCCN clinical practice guidelines in oncology: central nervous system tumours. Ver. 2.2013. Fort Washington, PA; 2013. Current version available online at: http://www.nccn.org/professionals/physician_gls/pdf/cns.pdf (free registration required); cited 3 Apr 2013.

95. Bell BA, Smith MA, Kean DM, et al. Brain water measured by magnetic resonance imaging. Correlation with direct estimation and changes after mannitol and dexamethasone. Lancet. 1987;1 (8524):66–9.

96. Wissinger JP, French LA, Gillingham FJ. The use of dexamethasone in the control of cerebral edema. J Neurol Neurosurg Psychiatry. 1967;30:588.

97. Sturdza A, Millar BA, Bana N, Laperriere N, Pond G, Wong RK, Bezjak A. The use and toxicity of steroids in the management of patients with brain metastases. Support Care Cancer. 2008;16:1041–8.

98. Pruitt AA. Medical management of patients with brain tumors. Curr Treat Options Neurol. 2011;13:413–26.

99. Ryan R, Booth S, Price S. Corticosteroid-use in primary and secondary brain tumour patients: a review. J Neurooncol. 2012;106:449–59.

100. Vecht CJ, Hovestadt A, Verbiest HB, et al. Dose-effect relationship of dexamethasone on Karnofsky performance in metastatic brain tumors: a randomized study of doses of 4, 8, and 16 mg per day. Neurology. 1994;44(4):675–80.

101. Zaccara G, Perucca E. Interactions between antiepileptic drugs, and between antiepileptic drugs and other drugs. Epileptic Disord. 2014;16(4):409–31.

102. Weissman DE, Dufer D, Vogel V, Abeloff MD. Corticosteroid toxicity in neuro-oncology patients. J Neurooncol. 1987;5:125–8.

103. Oki K, Yamane K. Therapies for adrenal insufficiency. Expert Opin Pharmacother. 2007;8(9):1283–91.

104. Bergrem H, Refvem OK. Altered prednisolone pharmacokinetics in patients treated with rifampicin. Acta Med Scand. 1983;213 (5):339–43.

105. Zurcher RM, Frey BM, Frey FJ. Impact of ketoconazole on the metabolism of prednisolone. Clin Pharmacol Ther. 1989;45(4): 366–72.

106. Lester RS, Knowles SR, Shear NH. The risks of systemic corticosteroid use. Dermatol Clin. 1998;16(2):277–88.

107. Burke CW. Adrenocortical insufficiency. Clin Endocrinol Metab. 1985;14(4):947–76.

108. Todd GR, Acerini CL, Buck JJ, et al. Acute adrenal crisis in asthmatics treated with high-dose fluticasone propionate. Eur Respir J. 2002;19(6):1207–9.

109. Truhan AP, Ahmed AR. Corticosteroids: a review with emphasis on complications of prolonged systemic therapy. Ann Allergy. 1989;62(5):375–91.

110. Stuck AE, Minder CE, Frey FJ. Risk of infectious complications in patients taking glucocorticosteroids. Rev Infect Dis. 1989;11 (6):954–63.

111. Hughes MA, Parisi M, Grossman S, et al. Primary brain tumors treated with steroids and radiotherapy: low CD4 counts and risk of infection. Int J Radiat Oncol Biol Phys. 2005;62(5):1423–6.

112. Choi JD, Powers CJ, Vredenburgh JJ, et al. Cryptococcal meningitis in patients with glioma: a report of two cases. J Neurooncol. 2008;89(1):51–3.

113. Ganiere V, Christen G, Bally F, et al. Listeria brain abscess, Pneumocystis pneumonia and Kaposi's sarcoma after temozolomide. Nat Clin Pract Oncol. 2006;3(6): 339–43; quiz following 343.

114. Segal BH, Sneller MC. Infectious complications of immunosuppressive therapy in patients with rheumatic diseases. Rheum Dis Clin North Am. 1997;23(2):219–37.

115. Recommended adult immunization schedule. United States, 2010. Ann Intern Med. 2010;152(1):36–9.

116. Henson JW, Jalaj JK, Walker RW, et al. Pneumocystis carinii pneumonia in patients with primary brain tumors. Arch Neurol. 1991;48(4):406–9.

117. Slivka A, Wen PY, Shea WM, et al. Pneumocystis carinii pneumonia during steroid taper in patients with primary brain tumors. Am J Med. 1993;94(2):216–9.

118. Black RL, Oglesby RB, Von Sallmann L, et al. Posterior subcapsular cataracts induced by corticosteroids in patients with rheumatoid arthritis. JAMA. 1960;174:166–71.

119. Shubin H. Long term (five or more years) administration of corticosteroids in pulmonary diseases. Dis Chest. 1965;48(3): 287–90.

120. Talas DU, Nayci A, Polat G, et al. The effects of dexamethasone on lipid peroxidation and nitric oxide levels on the healing of tracheal anastomoses: an experimental study in rats. Pharmacol Res. 2002;46(3):265–71.

121. Weiner HL, Rezai AR, Cooper PR. Sigmoid diverticular perforation in neurosurgical patients receiving high-dose corticosteroids. Neurosurgery. 1993;33(1):40–3.

122. Kleinschmidt-DeMasters BK, Damek DM, Lillehei KO, et al. Epstein Barr virus-associated primary CNS lymphomas in elderly patients on immunosuppressive medications. J Neuropathol Exp Neurol. 2008;67(11):1103–11.

123. Parker A, Bowles K, Bradley JA, et al. Diagnosis of post-transplant lymphoproliferative disorder in solid organ transplant recipients—BCSH and BTS Guidelines. Br J Haematol. 2010;149(5):675–92.

124. Krakoff LR. Glucocorticoid excess syndromes causing hypertension. Cardiol Clin. 1988;6(4):537–45.

125. Grossman E, Messerli FH. Drug-induced hypertension: an unappreciated cause of secondary hypertension. Am J Med. 2012;125(1):14–22.

126. Bonnotte B, Chauffert B, Martin F, et al. Side-effects of high-dose intravenous (pulse) methylprednisolone therapy cured by potassium infusion. Br J Rheumatol. 1998;37(1):109.

127. Huerta C, Johansson S, Wallander MA, et al. Risk factors and short-term mortality of venous thromboembolism diagnosed in the primary care setting in the United Kingdom. Arch Intern Med. 2007;167(9):935–43.

128. Johannesdottir SA, Horvath-Puho E, Dekkers OM, et al. Use of glucocorticoids and risk of venous thromboembolism: a nationwide population-based case-control study. JAMA Intern Med. 2013;173(9):743–52.

129. Gerber DE, Grossman SA, Streiff MB. Management of venous thromboembolism in patients with primary and metastatic brain tumors. J Clin Oncol. 2006;24(8):1310–8.

130. Hempen C, Weiss E, Hess CF. Dexamethasone treatment in patients with brain metastases and primary brain tumors: do the benefits outweigh the side-effects? Support Care Cancer. 2002;10:322–8.

131. Wen PY, Schiff D, Kesari S, Drappatz J, Gigas DC, Doherty L. Medical management of patients with brain tumors. J Neurooncol. 2006;80:313–32.

132. Gurwitz JH, Bohn RL, Glynn RJ, et al. Glucocorticoids and the risk for initiation of hypoglycemic therapy. Arch Intern Med. 1994;154(1):97–101.

133. Nesbitt LT Jr. Minimizing complications from systemic glucocorticosteroid use. Dermatol Clin. 1995;13:925–39.

134. McGirt MJ, Chaichana KL, Gathinji M, et al. Persistent outpatient hyperglycemia is independently associated with decreased survival after primary resection of malignant brain astrocytomas. Neurosurgery. 2008;63:286–91.

135. Compston J. Management of glucocorticoid-induced osteoporosis. Nat Rev Rheumatol. 2010;6(2):82–8.

136. Steinbuch M, Youket TE, Cohen S. Oral glucocorticoid use is associated with an increased risk of fracture. Osteoporos Int. 2004;15(4):323–8.

137. Kanis JA, Johansson H, Oden A, et al. A meta-analysis of prior corticosteroid use and fracture risk. J Bone Miner Res. 2004;19(6):893–9.

138. Lester RS, Knowles SR, Shear NH. The risks of systemic corticosteroid use. Dermatol Clin. 1998;16:277–88.

139. Gulko PS, Mulloy AL. Glucocorticoid-induced osteoporosis: pathogenesis, prevention and treatment. Clin Exp Rheumatol. 1996;14(2):199–206.

140. Shen C, Chen F, Zhang Y, et al. Association between use of antiepileptic drugs and fracture risk: a systematic review and meta-analysis. Bone. 2014;64:246–53.

141. Maricic M. Update on glucocorticoid-induced osteoporosis. Rheum Dis Clin North Am. 2011;37(3):415–31.

142. Lane NE. An update on glucocorticoid-induced osteoporosis. Rheum Dis Clin North Am. 2001;27(1):235–53.

143. Reid DM, Hughes RA, Laan RF, et al. Efficacy and safety of daily risedronate in the treatment of corticosteroid-induced osteoporosis in men and women: a randomized trial. European corticosteroid-induced osteoporosis treatment study. J Bone Miner Res. 2000;15(6):1006–13.

144. Piper JM, Ray WA, Daugherty JR, et al. Corticosteroid use and peptic ulcer disease: role of nonsteroidal anti-inflammatory drugs. Ann Intern Med. 1991;114(9):735–40.

145. Chun YS, Laurent A, Maru D, et al. Management of chemotherapy-associated hepatotoxicity in colorectal liver metastases. Lancet Oncol. 2009;10(3):278–86.

146. Golde DW, Bersch N, Cline MJ. Polycythemia vera: hormonal modulation of erythropoiesis in vitro. Blood. 1977;49(3):399–405.

147. Park-Wyllie L, Mazzotta P, Pastuszak A, et al. Birth defects after maternal exposure to corticosteroids: prospective cohort study and meta-analysis of epidemiological studies. Teratology. 2000;62(6):385–92.

148. Hall RC, Popkin MK, Stickney SK, et al. Presentation of the steroid psychoses. J Nerv Ment Dis. 1979;167(4):229–36.

149. Lewis DA, Smith RE. Steroid-induced psychiatric syndromes. A report of 14 cases and a review of the literature. J Affect Disord. 1983;5(4):319–32.

150. Bolanos SH, Khan DA, Hanczyc M, et al. Assessment of mood states in patients receiving long-term corticosteroid therapy and in controls with patient-rated and clinician-rated scales. Ann Allergy Asthma Immunol. 2004;92(5):500–5.

151. Brown ES, Suppes T, Khan DA, et al. Mood changes during prednisone bursts in outpatients with asthma. J Clin Psychopharmacol. 2002; 22(1): 55–61. 69.

152. Sonino N, Fava GA, Raffi AR, et al. Clinical correlates of major depression in Cushing's disease. Psychopathology. 1998;31(6):302–6.

153. Poetker DM, Reh DD. A comprehensive review of the adverse effects of systemic corticosteroids. Otolaryngol Clin North Am. 2010;43:753–68.

154. Batchelor TT, Byrne TN. Supportive care of brain tumor patients. Hematol Oncol Clin North Am. 2006;20:1337–61.

155. Dropcho EJ, Soong SJ. Steroid-induced weakness in patients with primary brain tumors. Neurology. 1991;41(8):1235–9.

156. Batchelor TT, Taylor LP, Thaler HT, Posner JB, DeAngelis LM. Steroid myopathy in cancer patients. Neurology. 1997;48(5):1234–8.

157. Pereira RM, Freire de Carvalho J. Glucocorticoid-induced myopathy. Joint Bone Spine. 2011;78(1):41–4.

158. Levin OS, Polunina AG, Demyanova MA, et al. Steroid myopathy in patients with chronic respiratory diseases. J Neurol Sci. 2014;338(1–2):96–101.

159. Frieze DA. Musculoskeletal pain associated with corticosteroid therapy in cancer. Curr Pain Headache Rep. 2010;14:256–60.

160. Villalona-Calero MA, Eckardt J, Burris H, et al. A phase I trial of human corticotropin-releasing factor (hCRF) in patients with peritumoral brain edema. Ann Oncol. 1998;9(1):71–7.

161. Recht L, Mechtler LL, Wong ET, O'Connor PC, Rodda BE. Steroid-sparing effect of corticorelin acetate in peritumoral cerebral edema is associated with improvement in steroid-induced myopathy. J Clin Oncol. 2013;31(9):1182–7.

162. Cohen MH, Shen YL, Keegan P, et al. FDA drug approval summary: bevacizumab (Avastin) as treatment of recurrent glioblastoma multiforme. Oncologist. 2009;14(11):1131–8.

163. Gerstner ER, Duda DG, di Tomaso E, et al. VEGF inhibitors in the treatment of cerebral edema in patients with brain cancer. Nat Rev Clin Oncol. 2009;6(4):229–36.

164. Hill KL Jr, Lipson AC, Sheehan JM. Brain magnetic resonance imaging changes after sorafenib and sunitinib chemotherapy in patients with advanced renal cell and breast carcinoma. J Neurosurg. 2009;111(3):497–503.

165. Bressler SB. Introduction: Understanding the role of angiogenesis and antiangiogenic agents in age-related macular degeneration. Ophthalmology. 2009;116(Suppl 10):S1–7.

166. Kobold S, Hegewisch-Becker S, Oechsle K, et al. Intraperitoneal VEGF inhibition using bevacizumab: a potential approach for the symptomatic treatment of malignant ascites? Oncologist. 2009;14(12):1242–51.

167. Wong HK, Lahdenranta J, Kamoun WS, et al. Anti-vascular endothelial growth factor therapies as a novel therapeutic approach to treating neurofibromatosis-related tumors. Cancer Res. 2010;70(9):3483–93.

168. Roth P, Regli L, Tonder M, et al. Tumor-associated edema in brain cancer patients: pathogenesis and management. Expert Rev Anticancer Ther. 2013;11:1319–25.

169. Kirste S, Treier M, Wehrle SJ, Becker G, Abdel-Tawab M, Gerbeth K, Hug MJ, Lubrich B, Grosu AL, Momm F. Boswellia serrata acts on cerebral edema in patients irradiated for brain tumors: a prospective, randomized, placebo-controlled, double-blind pilot trial. Cancer. 2011;117(16):3788–95.

Amy A. Pruitt

Introduction

Central nervous system (CNS) infections in patients receiving immunosuppressive therapy for cancer or other systemic conditions complicate treatment and result in prolonged hospitalizations, additional diagnostic procedures, and high mortality [1]. CNS infections present complex diagnostic challenges for a clinician whose goal is timely diagnosis that will ensure meaningful survival without devastating neurologic sequelae.

These challenges, many of which occur simultaneously for any given patient, include:

1. Classic signs of infection such as fever, headache, and meningismus may be absent or atypical in heavily immunosuppressed patients, particularly those receiving corticosteroids. Conversely, as the host's immune system reconstitutes after effective treatment, the resultant inflammatory response can mimic recurrent infection.
2. Multiple infections may be present concurrently.
3. The list of potential pathogens may include organisms of low pathogenicity in the immunocompetent host. In addition, infections such as West Nile Virus often are especially virulent in patients with impaired immunity [2]. With increasing global travel and climate change, a range of infections not seen often by North American consultants such as Dengue and Chikungunya must be considered [3].
4. Alternate causes of fever and nonspecific encephalopathy may include many noninfectious causes such as drug toxicity, venous thromboembolism, CNS vasculitis, nonbacterial thrombotic endocarditis (NBTE), and, in transplantation recipients, engraftment syndrome, graft-versus-host disease (GVHD), and post-transplantation lymphoproliferative disorder (PTLD).

5. Laboratory studies may be nonspecific. In a series from Memorial Sloan-Kettering Cancer Center, cerebrospinal fluid (CSF) cell counts, glucose, and protein were normal in one-third of neutropenic patients with bacterial or fungal meningitis [4].
6. Neuroimaging may be nonspecific or may mimic treatment-related abnormalities such as radiation necrosis, drug-induced leukoencephalopathy, vascular pathology such as stroke or arteritis, or disease recurrence.
7. The ever-changing landscape of new drug combinations and toxicities and changes in invasive procedures, infection risk factors, drug resistance patterns, and pathogen spectrum continues to challenge diagnostic acumen. Just a few are mentioned in this paragraph. The clinician must consider possible zoonotic exposures (rabies, anthrax), travel (Chikungunya, Chagas, Dengue), and vaccination status and efficacy. Methicillin-resistant *Staphylococcus aureus* (*MRSA*) infection acquired both nosocomially and in the community has emerged as a major infection associated at times with an often poorly recognized necrotizing fasciitis [5]. Appreciation for newly recognized parainfectious complications such as the triggering of brain autoimmunity has emerged with the description of N-methyl-D-aspartate receptor (NMDAR) encephalitis after herpesvirus encephalitis and the finding of anti-Yo (Purkinje cell) autoantibody in a patient with *Bornavirus* encephalitis [6, 7].

The Three-Step Diagnostic Approach

Step One: Epidemiology

Most CNS infections occur in a relatively small subset of cancer patients, and epidemiologic clues help the consultant to restrict the range of possible diagnoses. Patients with HCT are a particularly high-risk group, while patients with

A.A. Pruitt (✉)
Department of Neurology, Perelman School of Medicine, University of Pennsylvania, 3400 Spruce St, Philadelphia, PA 19104, USA
e-mail: pruitt@mail.med.upenn.edu

© Springer International Publishing AG 2018
D. Schiff et al. (eds.), *Cancer Neurology in Clinical Practice*,
DOI 10.1007/978-3-319-57901-6_20

leukemia or lymphoma represent more than a quarter of those with CNS infections. Another 16% of patient with CNS infections have primary CNS tumors [8]. The at-risk groups can be categorized by four types of immune deficits, though more than one may coexist at a given time in some patients:

- *Barrier Disruption*: Shunts, monitoring devices, ventricular reservoirs, cranial surgery and irradiation, central lines or ports, gastrointestinal surgery, urinary catheters, and loss of cutaneous or mucosal integrity predispose to infection by skin or gut-derived organisms. These include bacteria such as *Staphylococcus aureus* or *epidermidis, Enterobacter, Escherichia coli, Klebsiella, Streptococcus bovis, Propionibacterium acnes, Listeria monocytogenes,* and *Acinetobacter*) and fungi (*Aspergillus fumigatus, Candida albicans*). Another gastrointestinal pathogen that can cause gram-negative bacillary meningitis is the nematode *Strongyloides stercoralis*.
- *Neutropenia*: Patients with neutropenia due to bone marrow failure from a primary myelodysplastic condition or from drug-induced depletion (for hematopoietic cell transplantation), and radiation therapy are primarily at risk of the bacterial pathogens *Staphylococcus aureus, Streptococcus pneumoniae, Pseudomonas aeruginosa,* and *Escherichia coli*. Fungal pathogens include *Aspergillus fumigatus, Candida albicans,* and *Mucoraceae*. Viruses that thrive in the neutropenic host include cytomegalovirus (CMV), herpes simplex type I (HSV), human herpesviruses (HHV) 6 and 7, blood transfusion-associated infections such as adenoviruses, and West Nile Virus (WNV).
- *B Lymphocyte/Immunoglobulin Depletion*: Patients with chronic lymphocytic leukemia, multiple myeloma, splenectomy, lymphoplasmacytic lymphoma, and therapy with the CD20 monoclonal antibody rituximab are at special risk of bacterial infections with *S. pneumoniae, Haemophilus influenzae, Klebsiella,* and *Pseudomonas*. Viruses such as measles and enteroviruses will have particularly virulent courses in such patients who are also at risk of progressive multifocal leukoencephalopathy (PML) from the John Cunningham virus (JCV).
- *T Lymphocyte/Macrophage Deficiency*: The growing group of patients with heavily treated lymphomas, hematopoietic cell transplants and immunosuppressive therapies with corticosteroids, calcineurin inhibitors (cyclosporine, tacrolimus) bortezomib, alemtuzumab, mycophenolate, fludarabine, and cladribine are at risk of various viral infections including CMV, HSV, Varicella zoster virus (VZV), JCV, Epstein–Barr virus (EBV), HHV 6,7, and Adenovirus. Fungi such as *Cryptococcus neoformans, Aspergillus, Candida, Mucoraceae,* and *Pseudoallescheria boydii* affect this population as do the parasites *Strongyloides* and *Toxoplasma gondii*. Bacteria particularly likely to infect this group include *Listeria monocytogenes, Nocardia asteroides, Mycobacterium tuberculosis,* and *Treponema pallidum* (in HIV patients).

Step Two: Clinical Syndromes

While many patients with CNS infections will present with diffuse signs and symptoms such as headache and altered sensorium without localizing features, the presence of specific focal signs may suggest specific tropisms that offer important etiologic clues. Figure 20.1 offers an algorithm for differential diagnosis based on clinical syndromes and imaging studies. Meningeal signs without focal findings are typical of most infections due to bacteria, *Candida*, or *Cryptococcus*. Abscesses causing focal deficits are more likely to be caused by *Nocardia* or *Aspergillus*, whereas subdural or extradural empyemas are usually of bacterial etiology. Ischemic or hemorrhagic infarctions raise the specter of VZV, infective endocarditis, *Aspergillus,* or *Mucoraceae*. Other processes target the brainstem, spinal cord, or temporal lobes ("limbic encephalitis"). Thus, the clinician moves quickly to confirm initial impression with neuroimaging and CSF examination as indicated.

Given the inherent variability in CNS infection presentations, it is hazardous to place too much emphasis on the specific tropisms of pathogens, most of which can infect multiple sites simultaneously or sequentially. However, the presence of an exclusively brainstem, cerebellar, or spinal cord syndrome at times helps to narrow infectious possibilities.

Brainstem

Infectious conditions that preferentially affect the brainstem include *Listeria* (rhombencephalitis) and JCV-associated PML. However, noninfectious brainstem disorders including osmotic demyelination, Wernicke encephalopathy, lymphoma, and chronic lymphocytic inflammation with peripontine enhancement responsive to steroids (CLIPPERS) enter into the differential as well.

Cerebellum

Infectious pathogens that frequently or preferentially affect the cerebellum include *Listeria*, VZV, JCV and Creutzfeldt–Jakob disease. All but the last on this list are of relevance to potentially infected cancer patients. Acute postinfectious cerebellitis, more common in children and young adults, follows infections with EBV, influenza A and B, VZV, and other viruses, but is not a problem particular to the cancer population considered here. Some fungi such as *Aspergillus*

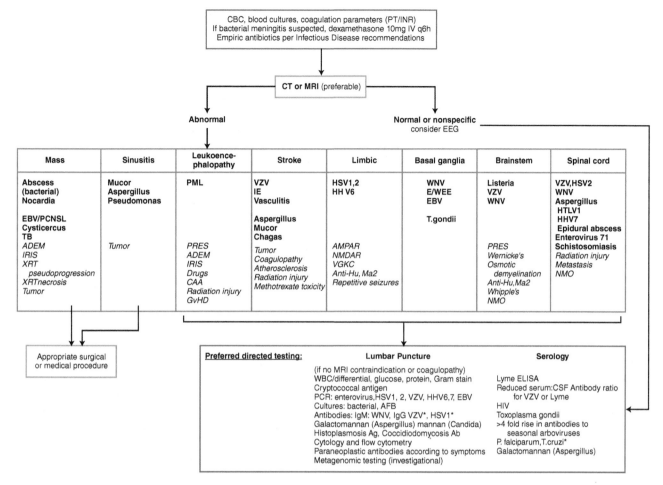

Fig. 20.1 A general approach to suspected CNS infection in a patient immunocompromised by cancer and its therapies involves basic blood tests and an urgent imaging procedure, preferably MRI, before directed testing with lumbar puncture and additional serologies. For patients with normal MRI scans but impaired level of alertness, continuous EEG is advised

have a tropism for the posterior circulation [9]. In JCV-associated granule cell neuronopathy, the affected cerebellar neurons produce a pure cerebellar syndrome of ataxia, tremor, and nystagmus [10].

Spinal Cord Infections

Infectious processes with a predilection for spinal cord involvement can be divided into those that produce a compressive myelopathy versus those that have root or parenchymal involvement that may occur in the course of a meningoencephalitis [11]; epidural cord compression is usually bacterial or occasionally fungal. The herpes family including herpes simplex virus types 1 and 2, Varicella zoster virus, cytomegalovirus, and human herpesvirus 7 causes spinal cord dysfunction both by direct infiltration after reactivation in the dorsal root ganglia with detectable CSF viral DNA and by inciting a vigorous, damaging inflammatory response. Enteroviruses (EV), most recently EV 71 and EV D68, generally produce a self-limited illness

in noncompromised hosts but can produce paralytic disease whose severity is worse in immunocompromised patients. West Nile Virus with an ascending acute poliomyelitis or ventral root infection can present as acute flaccid paralysis, and such infection is usually more severe in immunocompromised patients. Human T cell leukemia virus-1 (HTLV1)-associated myelopathy transmitted after living donor liver transplant has been described [12]. JCV-associated PML isolated to the spinal cord has been reported [13] as has paraneoplastic-isolated myelopathy resulting in some instances in a lateral spinothalamic tract "tractopathy" [14].

Noninfectious processes that produce a longitudinally extensive transverse myelitis include PRES and paraneoplastic disorders such as neuromyelitis optica (NMO), occasionally reported as a paraneoplastic phenomenon in patients with metastatic cancer. Underlying neoplasms have included metastatic carcinoid and lung cancer [15]. Paraneoplastic NMO usually occurs at an older age than does the idiopathic variety (55 years vs. 39 years) [16].

Extra-CNS Sites

General physical examination may disclose abnormalities outside the CNS that can help with diagnosis. This discussion is necessarily incomplete, but examination of eyes, skin, and lungs should be the main focus of consultants' attention. Ocular examination can be useful in diagnosing Varicella zoster and *Aspergillus*. Skin examination may disclose a rash or other lesion that when biopsied could confirm the presence of Cryptococcosis, Aspergillosis, VZV, or HSV. Since the lungs are the portal of entry for many fungal and bacterial pathogens, chest X-ray or chest computed tomography is additional valuable modalities.

Step Three: Investigations

Because of the numerous possibilities for mass lesions and frequent paucity of specific signs and symptoms, all immunocompromised patients should have at least a screening head CT before lumbar puncture and many will benefit from MRI investigation [17, 18].

Neuroimaging

As indicated in Fig. 20.1, an initial triage strategy begins with neuroimaging, preferably MRI scanning, and then considers possible pathogens by sites, recognize that there are *always* exceptions. While MRI is an invaluable addition to the diagnostic process, there are many pitfalls:

1. The use of corticosteroids reduces contrast enhancement on both CT and MRI.
2. Renal insufficiency or contrast allergy may preclude contrast use.
3. Diffuse dural or meningeal enhancement can be seen after repetitive seizures as can parenchymal signal abnormalities on fluid-attenuated inversion recovery (FLAIR) sequences in affected areas. Additionally, a recent lumbar puncture with low intracranial pressure can cause dural enhancement as can neoplastic or chemical meningitis.
4. Increased fluid-attenuated inversion recovery (FLAIR) signal intensity in the subarachnoid space could suggest proteinaceous fluid such as blood or pus, but is also frequently seen in patients ventilated with high partial pressure of oxygen.
5. Ring-enhancing lesions are nonspecific and can represent abscesses or tumor recurrence, or pseudoprogression in patients treated with radiation and concurrent temozolomide [19]. They can also be seen days to weeks after a hemorrhage or can represent demyelinating lesions in the appropriate situation.
6. Because gadolinium-enhanced sequences may be nonspecific, diffusion-weighted imaging (DWI) has been invoked to improve distinction between infections and other processes, though increased cellularity as seen with CNS lymphoma also can produce significant diffusion restriction. Restricted water diffusion is seen in fungal and bacterial abscesses, and purulent ventricular fluid is similarly hyperintense (Fig. 20.2a–f). Magnetic resonance angiography (MRA) would be most useful in evaluating potential aneurysms in suspected *Aspergillus*, arteritis associated with VZV or Mucormycosis.

Electroencephalography

Seizures are very common during CNS infections, so EEG may be useful in explaining altered mental status and long-term monitoring should be encouraged in any unresponsive patient with CNS infection. In one study, seizures or paroxysmal epileptic discharges occurred in nearly half of patients and were independently associated with poor prognoses. Half of the patients with seizures had no obvious clinical correlation on bedside examination [20].

Cerebrospinal Fluid

If there is no intracerebral lesion that contraindicates lumbar puncture and if clotting factor or platelet support is provided for cytopenic patients, this procedure can be useful when employed properly. Absolute CSF white blood cell count and differential are less useful than in the noncancer population. Not only can bacterial processes evoke very little inflammation in the heavily immunosuppressed cytopenic patient, but lymphocytic pleocytosis can have many noninfectious etiologies including drug reactions to nonsteroidal anti-inflammatory drugs, valacyclovir, azathioprine, isoniazid, intravenous immunoglobulin (IVIG) intrathecal chemotherapy, and lamotrigine. Disease states that can evoke a CSF pleocytosis include prolonged status epilepticus, arachnoiditis, and neoplastic meningitis.

Expeditious discovery of an infectious etiology for meningoencephalitis in this population can be challenging. Polymerase chain reaction (PCR) testing is expensive and time-consuming, and cultures may require prolonged incubation. Metagenomic deep sequencing (MDS) approaches, still investigational and not readily clinically available, are beginning to yield specific etiologies as this powerful diagnostic tool demonstrates potential for rapid and unbiased pathogen identification [21, 22].

Appropriate Use of Polymerase Chain (PCR) Reaction Testing

It is important to note that the confirmation of a viral infection by PCR can be done when the patient is seen early in the course of an infection due to a herpesvirus or other pathogen, but that if the patient is seen more than 7–10 days after onset of symptoms, the better test is a comparison of intrathecal pathogen-specific antibody level with concurrent serum antibody. This is particularly true for herpesvirus infections

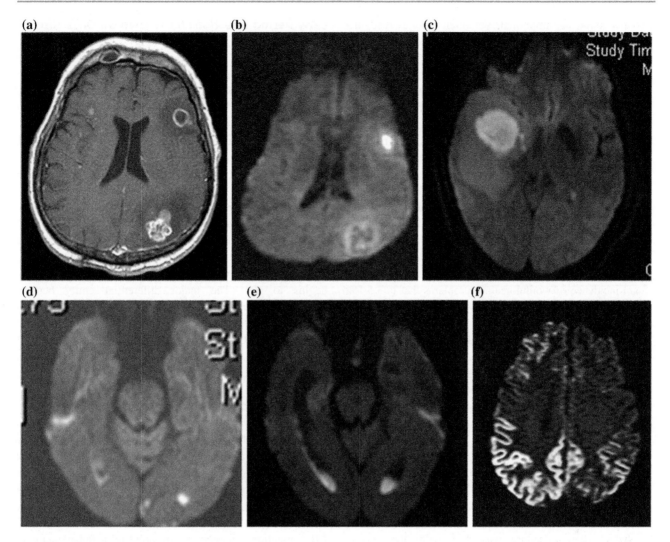

Fig. 20.2 MRI diffusion-weighted (*DWI*) imaging sequences are most frequently used in stroke evaluation, but DWI is useful for diverse infections as well. **a** shows gadolinium-enhanced T1 sequence of two mass lesions that were found to be *Nocardia asteroides*. These infections are hyperintense on DWI (**b**), as is the large right temporal abscess in a patient with colon cancer whose operation was complicated by endocarditis with *E. coli* (**c**). The possibility of VZV-related stroke was raised by the MRI sequence in **d** and led to appropriate testing for VZV vasculopathy. **e** shows diffusion positive CSF in a patient with *S. aureus* meningitis, and **f** shows the characteristic cortical hyperintensity of a prion disease, Creutzfeldt–Jakob disease

in which a negative PCR could lead to discontinuation of acyclovir in the presence of an active infection [23].

Brain or Leptomeningeal Biopsy

This procedure ideally should be reserved for situations in which an invasive procedure might lead to both specific antimicrobial diagnosis and therapeutic advantage such as debridement of a suspected fungal sinus infection or brain or spinal abscess drainage. As a procedure of last resort, sampling of an area of meningeal or parenchymal enhancement is likely of higher yield than targeting areas without contrast enhancement. Subcubic centimeter stereotactically biopsied lesions have a lower yield than larger lesions for which diagnostic yield exceeds 90%, though the former still succeeds in providing a diagnosis in 76.2% of procedures [24].

High-Risk Patient Groups

Neurosurgery-Related Infections

Patients with primary and secondary brain tumors account for up to one-quarter of CNS infections that occur among cancer patients. Bacterial meningitis due to a combination of barrier disruption, T cell immunity deficits due to corticosteroids, and poor wound healing after radiation therapy or multiple craniotomies predispose to this serious infection. Bacterial abscesses with or without subdural empyema usually occur within one month of craniotomy, but indolent skin-derived organisms can produce symptomatic infection many months to years after the surgery [25].

Three clinically important, yet often hard to recognize syndromes should be recognized among patients with brain tumors:

1. Tumor cavity-implantable carmustine-containing wafers are approved for treatment of high-grade astrocytic tumors both at initial diagnosis and at recurrence. These induce a significant cerebritis with accompanying vasogenic edema. A characteristic "Swiss cheese-like" appearance in addition to a more typical ring-enhancing abscess has been described [26].
2. Radiation therapy exacerbates wound-healing problems, a risk further compounded with the advent of bevacizumab, and other vascular endothelial growth factor (VEGF) inhibitors. These agents should not be used within one month before or after surgery as they lead to an incidence of wound-healing problems that is 3.5-fold greater than that seen without VEGF therapies [27].
3. Radiation therapy with or without concomitant chemotherapy with temozolomide can predispose patients to reactivation of herpes simplex virus or, less commonly cytomegalovirus (CMV) with resultant encephalitis. HSV reactivation also has been related to anti-epileptic hypersensitivity reactions [28, 29].

Hematopoietic Cell Transplantation (HCT)

Approach to the diagnosis of potential CNS infections in transplantation patients involves consideration of the disease for which the procedure was performed, the specific pre-transplant conditioning regimen or other therapies, and, most importantly, the interval from the transplant to the presenting clinical syndrome. In one large retrospective study of allogeneic HCT, almost 70% of clinically significant neurologic complications and 86% of all episodes of posterior reversible encephalopathy syndrome (PRES) occurred within the first 100 days after the procedure [30]. Table 20.1 presents a summary of neurologic complications whose main point can be reduced to the fact that that transplantation patients present a remarkable array of diagnostic possibilities and that, while the specific complications vary with indication for and type of procedure, many infections and their mimics are common to all types of transplantation and associated medications and it is the time out from transplantation that helps to weight diagnostic priorities [31, 32]. Here the focus will be on infections associated with commonly used immunosuppressive regimens, including corticosteroids, mycophenolate, cyclosporine, tacrolimus, rituximab, and alemtuzumab. Other complications of HCT are covered in Chap. 18.

Early Period Infections (Less Than 30 Days After Transplantation)

During this period of neutropenia, major concerns are bacterial, viral or fungal infections, donor or nosocomially acquired infections, and reactivation of preexisting infections (such as neurocysticercosis or toxoplasmosis). Emerging viruses and new patterns of infections that should be considered include donor-derived West Nile Virus, lymphocytic choriomeningitis virus, HTLV 1-associated myelitis, and rabies [33, 34]. This last pathogen usually surfaces within a month of transplantation, but recently it has been recognized that rabies can strike the recipient many months after infection by donor tissue [35–37].

A clinical problem specific to HCT is engraftment syndrome characterized by rash, fever, and headache 2–4 weeks following transplantation as the absolute neutrophil count begins to rise. The major differential entity here is post-transplant acute limbic encephalitis (PALE) caused by human herpesvirus 6 (HHV6) and accompanied by amnesia, hyponatremia, CSF pleocytosis, and abnormal EEG [38]. HHV6 is discussed in greater detail in the specific pathogens section of this chapter.

Middle Period Infections (1–6 Months After Transplantation)

Patients more than one month post-HCT remain at risk of invasive fungal infections. *Toxoplasma gondii* may resurface as encephalitis or as multiple ring-enhancing lesions, often deep in corona radiata and basal ganglia. VZV may emerge during this period despite valacyclovir prophylaxis, and PML begins to become a risk several months after HCT. EBV infection can occur at any point post-transplantation.

Late Period (>6 Months Post-transplantation)

Late complications of transplantation include secondary neoplasms such as melanoma and lymphomas as well as astrocytoma or meningioma in patients who have received cranial irradiation as part of their conditioning regimen. VZV, PTLD, and PML remain possibilities. The CNS is rarely the site of graft-versus-host disease (GVHD), but when this question arises biopsy is necessary and in the few patients so investigated there have been mature lymphohistiocytic inflammatory infiltrates with perivascular cuffing and without viral cytopathic changes [39].

Hematologic Malignancies Treated Intensively but Without Transplant

As intensive chemotherapy regimens for hematologic malignancies have produced long-term survivors of hematologic malignancies, the risk of CNS infection has risen in

Table 20.1 Time course of neurologic complications of hematopoietic cell transplantation

Time from transplant	Infectious conditions	Noninfectious conditions
Conditioning and infusion		Drug-related encephalopathy (busulfan, etoposide, ifosfamide, methotrexate, cytosine arabinoside), DMSO-related stroke, PRES, seizures, intracranial hypotension post-LP
<1 month, neutropenic period	CMV HHV-6 Aspergillus Toxoplasmosis Infections acquired from donor tissue: LCMV, WNV, rabies, adenovirus, Coxsackie B4 From IV lines: Candida	Engraftment syndrome Delirium due to organ failure Seizures: cefepime, imipenem PRES: cyclosporine, tacrolimus > sirolimus Parkinsonism: Amphotericin B, valproate SDH or SAH due to coagulopathy Intraparenchymal brain hemorrhage
1–6 months	Aspergillus HHV-6 HSV PML PTLD Toxoplasmosis VZV	ADEM Osmotic demyelination syndrome IRIS GVHD
>6 months	VZV CMV PML EBV-associated PTLD Aspergillus Mucoraceae	Autoimmune: graves, sarcoidosis, demyelinating IRIS GVHD (polymyositis, myasthenia, CIDP) Secondary malignancy Disease relapse

ADEM acute disseminated encephalomyelitis, *CIDP* chronic inflammatory demyelinating polyneuropathy, *CMV* cytomegalovirus, *EBV* Epstein–Barr virus, *GVHD* graft-versus-host disease, *HHV* human herpesvirus 5, *IRIS* immune reconstitution inflammatory syndrome, *LCMV* lymphocytic choriomeningitis virus, *PRES* posterior reversible encephalopathy syndrome, *PTLD* post-transplant lymphoproliferative disorder, *SAH* subarachnoid hemorrhage, *SDH* subdural hematoma, *WNV* West Nile Virus

patients who do not undergo transplantation. Such patients are often in hospital for extended periods and are at risk of sepsis from intravenous lines and *Candida* bacteremia. Necessary transfusion support for chemotherapy-induced cytopenias carries attendant risk of transfusion-transmitted disease caused by protozoa, prions, hepatitis virus, HIV CMV, EBV, HHV8, *Cryptococcus*, and *Trypanosoma cruzi* (Chagas disease) [40].

Several drugs used in these situations such as fludarabine, cyclophosphamide, methotrexate, mycophenolate, alemtuzumab, and rituximab carry defined increased risk of specific infections. Fludarabine and mycophenolate are particularly associated with PML because they deplete T lymphocytes. Rituximab-associated infectious complications are discussed elsewhere in this chapter. Alemtuzumab, recently approved for therapy of multiple sclerosis, has long been used as induction therapy for solid organ and HCT, for treatment of rejection after HCT, and for chronic lymphocytic leukemia. Patients receiving the drug for rejection as opposed to as induction therapy have increased risk of developing an opportunistic infection including invasive fungal infections, HHV6, Listeria meningitis, CMV viremia, and Guillain Barre syndrome or myelitis due to VZV or HHV7 [41, 42].

Clinical Manifestations and Management of Specific Infections

In this section, common clinical variants and therapeutic strategies for several commonly encountered infections are summarized. Specific antibiotic recommendations are not offered as institutional variability in antibiotic resistance, and nosocomial trends must be respected. Neurologic consultants should work with their own institutional infectious disease departments to assure appropriate coverage for pathogens based on institutional antibiotic resistance and nosocomial trends.

General Medical Management Issues

Two major medical management issues present opportunities for effective neurologic consultative advice:

1. Corticosteroid supplementation may be necessary, as many cancer patients may have been treated with large doses of corticosteroids as part of their cytotoxic regimens in the recent past. When stressed with an acute infection, some will have insufficient adrenal reserve that

can present as hypotension unresponsive to volume repletion requiring urgent intravenous hydrocortisone [43, 44].

2. Seizures complicate treatment of many patients with meningoencephalitis or infectious mass lesions. Some may be isolated events due to toxic drug reactions (Table 20.2), metabolic or electrolyte abnormalities, or posterior reversible encephalopathy syndrome (PRES) and therefore will not require long-term anti-seizure medicine. However, other pathologies in the cancer population such as bland or hemorrhagic cerebrovascular disease, venous sinus thrombosis, or abscess may carry longer-term seizure risks. Choice of anti-epileptic drug (AED) should weigh interactions between seizure treatment and ongoing cancer or transplant immunosuppressive therapy [45]. Phenytoin, fosphenytoin, carbamazepine, oxcarbazepine, and phenobarbital are potent hepatic enzyme inducers that can reduce blood levels of many chemotherapeutic agents, including corticosteroids and immunosuppressives such as tacrolimus and cyclosporine. Phenytoin and valproate are heavily protein-bound and so in patients with low serum albumin levels, free level drug measurements are indicated. Levetiracetam, available orally and parenterally, has the advantage of rapid onset of activity and absence of significant protein-binding or hepatic enzyme induction. However, up to 5% of levetiracetam-treated patients may experience adverse neuropsychiatric effects including psychosis that can mimic behaviors associated more commonly with corticosteroid-induced psychiatric problems. Lacosamide shares similar advantages with levetiracetam over the older AEDs and does not carry the psychiatric adverse effect risk. Renal failure may reduce clearance of both of these AEDs, and, as hemodialysis removes small nonprotein-bound drugs, dosing must be adjusted for renal failure and supplementation after dialysis should conform to manufacturers' recommendations.

Bacterial Meningitis

Streptococcus pneumoniae (*S. pneumo*) meningitis remains the most common community-acquired meningitis, and a quarter of such patients have an immunocompromising condition [46]. Nosocomially acquired meningitis includes a larger percentage of patients with gram-negative and MRSA

Table 20.2 Neurologic toxicities of antimicrobial and immunosuppressive agents

Neurologic problem	Potential causative agents[a]
Seizures	Penicillin G, imipenem, aztreonam, gentamicin ciprofloxacin, ofloxacin, **cefepime, ceftazidime** metronidazole, amphotericin B, acyclovir, foscarnet, meropenem, praziquantel, tacrolimus, cyclosporine
Potentiation of neuromuscular junction transmission blockade	**Aminoglycosides, cephalosporins**
Pseudotumor cerebri	Minocycline, tetracycline, tacrolimus
Ototoxicity/vestibular toxicity	**Vancomycin, aminoglycosides**, erythromycin, tacrolimus
Delirium	**Cefepime, ceftazidime**, ciprofloxacin, ofloxacin, metronidazole, foscarnet, praziquantel, amphotericin B
Visual hallucinations	Voriconazole
Extrapyramidal signs	Amphotericin B
Headache	Ciprofloxacin, ofloxacin, fluconazole, itraconazole, foscarnet, praziquantel, trimethoprim/sulfamethoxazole
Dizziness/Cerebellar signs	Metronidazole[b], **aminoglycosides,** minocycline, isoniazid, fluconazole, itraconazole, varicella vaccine
Lymphocytic meningitis	Trimethoprim/sulfamethoxazole, cephalosporins, IV immunoglobulin, valacyclovir
Optic neuropathy	**Ethambutol**, linezolid
PRES	Linezolid, roxithromycin, tacrolimus, cyclosporine
Serotonin syndrome	Linezolid (with selective serotonin reuptake inhibitors or serotonin–norepinephrine reuptake inhibitors)
Tremor	**Acyclovir, cephalosporins, tacrolimus, cyclosporine**

[a]Agents in bold have particularly strong association
[b]Dentate nucleus abnormal, usually reversible
Data updated and modified from Pruitt [17]

infections [47]. Patients with active cancer have a several fold increased risk of bacterial meningitis compared to patients without cancer and may have lower peripheral blood and CSF leukocyte cell counts. Coverage of immunocompromised patients with bacterial meningitis must include *Listeria*, and, for patients recently in the hospital, gram-negative aerobic organisms. Based on Dutch studies demonstrating decreased mortality for gram-positive meningitis patients receiving corticosteroids, current recommendations for dexamethasone use prior the first dose antibiotics (10 mg every 6 h for 4 days) [48].

Although the overall incidence of neurosurgical infections appears to be decreasing in most centers, cancer patients undergo the procedures most likely to be complicated by infections. Patients having spinal tumor biopsy or CSF shunting remain a group at highest risk of infection. In one series, half of all infections were associated with shunt or Ommaya reservoir placement [49]. In these situations, removal of drains and intrathecal instillation of antibiotics can be considered in addition to recommended antibiotics appropriate to institutional resistance patterns.

Other Nosocomial Bacterial Infections

Brain Abscess

Risk factors for postoperative bacterial brain abscess are similar to those associated with meningitis: postoperative bone infections, septicemia, dental caries, and ear and pharyngeal infections. *S. aureus* is the most common postoperative pathogen, but other organisms more likely in cancer patients than in the general neurosurgical population require consideration: These include *T. gondii, Taenia solium, Aspergillus, Mucoraceae, Histoplasma capsulatum,* and *Nocardia asteroides*. Surgical intervention may be necessary for diagnosis or therapy in abscesses greater than 2 cm in maximal diameter. Some critical care specialists use steroids for short-term vasogenic edema management. Most consultants agree that no AEDs need be given prophylactically.

Infective Endocarditis

Twenty-five percent of patients with infective endocarditis (IE) have had recent health care contact. *S. aureus*, the most common causative organism, is associated with the highest mortality among bacterial endocarditis pathogens and is also associated with the highest risk of stroke. In-hospital mortality from all-cause IE is 14–20% [50].

Invasive Fungal Infections

Invasive fungal infections are among the most feared complications of chronic immunosuppression. The most common infections are Aspergillosis, Cryptococcosis, Mucormycosis, and Candidiasis. Prophylactic, empiric, and targeted strategies remain incompletely successful often because of delayed diagnosis. Invasive fungal infections can present with abscess or infarction due to hematogenous dissemination from extracranial, particularly pulmonary, sites. Extension from adjacent sinuses can produce an optic neuropathy sometimes mistaken for steroid-responsive giant cell arteritis [51].

Fungal infection can be suspected based on clinical presentation. An important and common syndromic constellation is persistent headache, visual changes, and cranial neuropathies in neutropenic patients with sinus disease. All neurologic consultants should recognize and pursue such symptoms vigorously with MRI, MRA, CSF sampling, and, when necessary, sinus debridement for diagnosis.

Neuroimaging of fungal infections provides valuable clues. Hyperintensity on FLAIR sequences in the basal cisterns and subarachnoid space, sometimes with contrast enhancement, suggests infection. High viscosity and cellularity of fungal pus lead to early reduced diffusion that can precede enhancement [52]. Aspergillosis, an angioinvasive organism, can produce hemorrhagic infarction (Fig. 20.3a–f). Cryptococcosis tends to produce pseudocysts in the basal ganglia. Mucormycosis, like Aspergillosis, can spread from the sinuses, producing frontal lobe abscesses and infarction. Candidiasis more often produces multiple microabscesses.

Aspergillosis

Cancer patients at most risk of rapidly fatal *Aspergillus*-related infections are those with acute myeloid leukemia, myelodysplastic syndromes, allogeneic HCT recipients [especially those with active graft-versus-host disease (GVHD)], patients with longstanding intravenous lines, and those receiving long-term corticosteroids or conditioning regimens that include fludarabine or alemtuzumab [53]. Neutropenia lasting longer than 10 days with a neutrophil count less than 500/µL is the most important risk factor. High-risk patients should be monitored with daily serum galactomannan antigen that can be detected in serum up to a week before abnormal chest radiographic or clinical symptoms. *Aspergillus* species invade the internal elastic lamina of arteries leading to focal microhemorrhage or mycotic aneurysm formation. Fungal components also can occlude vessels leading to infarction with hemorrhagic transformation with a predilection for small perforating arteries of the basal ganglia, thalamus, and corpus callosum. Since infarction of the corpus callosum is rarely seen in noninfectious thromboembolic infarction or pyogenic infection, its presence should suggest Aspergillosis [54]. In a series of 14 cases from a single institution with an additional 123 literature-based cases, lung was the primary focus with paranasal sinuses nearly as common. Mortality with medial

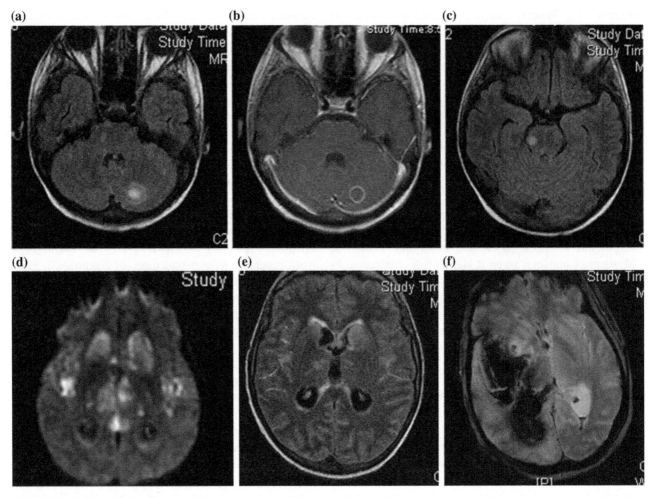

Fig. 20.3 *Aspergillus fumigatus.* MRI findings can be nonspecific, though often in the posterior circulation as seen in the fluid-attenuated inversion recovery (*FLAIR*) (**a**, **c**) and gadolinium-enhanced T1-weighted sequences (**b**). Diffusion-weighted imaging (**d**) suggestive of infarction by this angiotropic fungus and FLAIR images show increased signal in the subarachnoid space consistent with infection or blood (**e**). **f** shows a catastrophic hemorrhage form an infectious aneurysm due to *Aspergillus*

treatment alone was 60–100%, whereas those able to have surgical procedures that ranged from orbital exenteration to dural biopsies and abscess drainage had about a 25% mortality. Selection bias in favor of healthier patients undergoing surgery was a confounding factor in this retrospective study [55]. The treatment of choice is voriconazole [56].

Cryptococcus Neoformans

Cryptococcus is the most frequent cause of lymphocyte-predominant meningitis in HIV patients. In patients immunocompromised by cancer or its treatment, particularly when corticosteroids are used, meningitis can be either acute or quite indolent. Markedly elevated intracranial pressure or direct optic nerve invasion can lead to visual compromise. Gradually developing hydrocephalus, at times requiring repetitive lumbar punctures or ultimately ventriculoperitoneal shunting, occurs frequently. Cell counts may be misleading in significantly immunocompromised patients, whereas cryptococcal polysaccharide antigen in CSF is a sensitive and specific diagnostic modality. Treatment requires both acute combination therapy (amphotericin B and flucytosine) and lifelong prophylaxis in immunocompromised patients. Immune reconstitution-related exacerbation of symptoms has been observed after successful cryptococcal treatment.

Viral Infections

Table 20.3 summarizes many viruses and associated clinical parameters to be considered by clinicians consulting on oncology or transplantation services. The most important of these is Varicella zoster virus (VZV) whose diversity of clinical manifestations makes diagnosis difficult.

Table 20.3 Overview of viral infections in cancer patients

Virus	Disease and/or therapy-related risk group	Clinical manifestations	Diagnostic tests
Varicella zoster (VZV)	Glucocorticoids, calcineurin inhibitors, TNF-alpha inhibitors bortezomib HCT/SOT	Dermatomal or disseminated skin rash Zoster sine herpete Strokes Cranial neuritis (V, VII, III, IX, X) Transverse myelitis Cerebellar ataxia Necrotizing retinitis Delayed ischemic optic neuropathy Postherpetic neuralgia	Biopsy skin lesions CSF: PCF or IgG antibody reduced serum to CSF anti-VZV IgG ratio
Herpes simplex type I	Cranial irradiation HCT/SOT	Seizures, limbic features Unmasking of NMDA receptor encephalitis	Characteristic MRI may be less common in immunocompromised CSF PCR 24 h to 10 days; IgM antibody after 10 days
Cytomegalovirus (CMV)	Alemtuzumab, rituximab, cyclosporine, anti-thymocyte globulin, HIV, HCT/SOT	Retinitis Cauda equina polyradiculitis or myelitis Encephalitis, Increased risk of Listeria and EBV Hepatitis B and C reactivation	CSF: PCR
Human herpes virus type 6	HCT, alemtuzumab, anti-thymocyte globulin Hypersensitivity reaction to phenytoin or carbamazepine	Limbic encephalitis Hyponatremia Seizures, Cytomegalovirus reactivation Thrombocytopenia	CSF PCR Attention to possible chromosomal integration (see text)
Human herpes virus type 7	HCT	Optic neuritis Transverse myelitis Cytomegalovirus reactivation	CSF: PCR
JC virus	Fludarabine, Rituximab Methotrexate, Mycophenolate, Corticosteroids	PML Granule cell neuronopathy Encephalitis PML/IRIS	CSF: PCR, brain biopsy
Epstein–Barr virus (EBV)	Graft-versus-host disease HCT/SOT Anti-thymocyte globulin Azathioprine	Meningoencephalitis Post-transplant lymphoproliferative disorder Primary CNS lymphoma Parkinsonism Transverse myelitis	Quantitative serum PCR CSF: PCR

EBV Epstein–Barr virus, *HCT* hematopoietic cell transplantation, *PCR* polymerase chain reaction, *PML* progressive multifocal leukoencephalopathy, *SOT* solid organ transplantation

Varicella Zoster Virus (VZV)

VZV is an exclusively human neurotropic herpesvirus causing chicken pox in primary infection and later becoming latent in cranial and spinal sensory ganglia. Patients on long-term corticosteroids, a group that includes many primary brain tumor patients, are the largest at-risk group. The diverse spectrum of VZV-associated neurologic disorders includes the most common syndrome of dermatomal VZV with its associated risk of postherpetic neuralgia. Other complications comprise infratentorial and supratentorial stroke, retinal necrosis, pontine myelitis, cerebellar ataxia, cranial and spinal neuropathies, and spinal cord infarction [57]. Up to 35% of patients with VZV vasculopathy have no rash, and many have no CSF pleocytosis [58]. Diagnosis is based on either biopsy of skin lesions, CSF PCR, or measurement of anti-VZV IgG antibody in the CSF compared to that of serum with serum to CSF IgG ratio of less than 20 indicative of intrathecal infection.

Recent clinico-virologic studies of temporal artery biopsies from patients with clinically suspect giant cell arteritis but pathologically negative biopsies revealed infection with VZV [59]. Antiviral treatment may confer additional benefit to such patients, and while the issue of VZV temporal arteritis in immunocompromised patients has not been specifically investigated, it is important to consider this diagnosis and advocate for biopsy in patients presenting with symptoms of fever, night sweats, weight loss, fatigue, elevated ESR, and C-reactive protein, symptoms that might be attributed erroneously to the known underlying cancer [60].

VZV vaccine is a live attenuated vaccine that reduces incidence of postherpetic neuralgia in patients of all ages, though preventive efficacy decreases with age [61, 62]. The current vaccine is contraindicated in patients with impaired cellular immunity, a group that unfortunately includes those at highest risk of herpes zoster and for postherpetic neuralgia [63]. The results of a phase 3 trial of herpes zoster subunit vaccine consisting of a single VZV glycoprotein (HZ/su vaccine) have been published for immunocompetent patients over age 50. Though associated with a 17% risk of grade 3 symptoms, the vaccine had an impressive 97.2% efficacy [64]. This vaccine contains only a single virus protein and cannot replicate, so it likely will be safer in the immunocompromised patient population. A phase 1–2 trial of the vaccine involving HCT patients demonstrated induced VZV-specific CD4+ T cells lasting up to one year [65].

Human Herpes 6 Virus (HHV6)

Primary infection with HHV-6 occurs in early childhood. Similar to other herpesviruses, HHV-6 can remain latent in brain, kidneys, salivary glands, and T lymphocytes. About 1–2% of the population has viral DNA sequences integrated into chromosomes and such patients have very high viral loads in whole blood and serum, a situation that can complicate accurate attribution of pathogenicity of an acute infectious syndrome to the organism [66, 67]. Viral reactivation occurs primarily in HCT and less commonly in SOT and HIV/AIDS. Clinical manifestations include altered mental status and headache. Some patients can be characterized as specifically having amnesia, and seizures are seen in about 50% of patients. MRI may show hyperintensity in limbic areas, but this finding may be delayed. CSF can be acellular. Therefore, a high degree of suspicion is necessary to request PCR testing for early diagnosis. HHV6 lacks thymidine kinase and for this reason is not sensitive to acyclovir. While treatment with prolonged ganciclovir, valganciclovir, and foscarnet improves survival rates, these drugs can cause bone marrow suppression and renal toxicity

that in turn contribute to delayed engraftment and/or graft failure. Mortality is roughly doubled among allogeneic HCT recipients with HHV6 infection compared to those without HHV 6 infection [68]. The natural history of the disease with respect to relapse or secondary relapse prophylaxis is unknown.

Herpes Simplex Viruses (HSV)

Herpes simplex type 1 encephalitis (HSE) is the most common cause of sporadic viral encephalitis in the developed world. In the thirty years since the introduction of acyclovir, the mortality has been reduced, but resistance to acyclovir can emerge in immunocompromised hosts. Only 15–38% of such patients return to normal function. Although not generally considered an opportunistic infection, HSE in immunocompromised patients may have atypical presentations and worse outcome. In one recent series, fewer immune impaired patients had both fewer prodromal symptoms and fewer focal deficits, possibly delaying diagnosis. Three of 14 immunocompromised patients had normal CSF profiles [69]. In this series, MRI showed more widespread (extrahippocampal) cortical, brainstem, or cerebellar involvement, and mortality rate was six times higher in the immunocompromised patients. Recurrence of herpes encephalitis may occur because the available antiviral drugs prevent viral replication and the host's immune system is required to eliminate replicating virus or to reduce it to a latent state. Search for HSV IgM antibody in CSF may be critical to expeditious diagnosis, as the viral copy number may be below detection in patients with cancer [70]. Recently, the emergence of N-methyl-D-aspartate (NMDA) receptor antibody has been described in patients who appear to relapse after HSV 1 encephalitis [71]. The uncovering or induction of autoimmunity by infectious processes is just beginning to be characterized. NMDA antibody should be tested in both serum and CSF.

A specific situation in which HSE should be suspected is in the instance of reactivation of latent virus in the dorsal root ganglia and/or brain by cranial irradiation, which presumably results in breakdown of local immune surveillance [72] (Fig. 20.4a–c).

HSV 2, usually associated with lumbar radicular or urinary symptoms, can cause encephalitis in elderly immunocompromised patients. Imaging studies can resemble those of HSV 1 encephalitis, and, like that organism, HSV 2 can be seen in the context of apparent reactivation after neurosurgical procedures. Thus, immunocompromised cancer patients who have encephalitis clinically consistent with HSV-1 but in whom HSV 1 is not detected, should also be tested for HSV 2 [73].

Epstein–Barr Virus (EBV)

Post-transplant lymphoproliferative disorders (PTLD) are a variable group of proliferations occurring after solid or organ

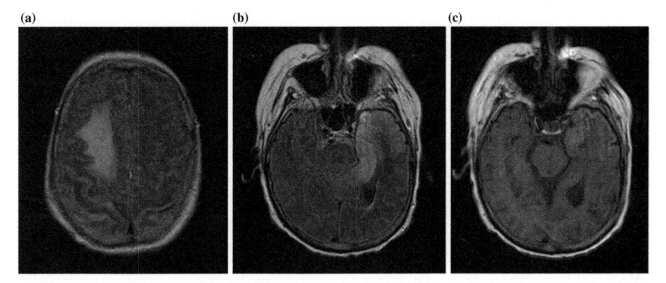

Fig. 20.4 A patient with right frontal primary CNS lymphoma refractory to methotrexate and rituximab-based chemotherapy became confused at the end of her radiation therapy (**a**), New FLAIR abnormality was seen in the left temporal lobe (**b**), and the patient was found to be seizing from Herpes simplex encephalitis that left her with laminar necrosis in the affected lobe (**c**)

or HCT whose spectrum ranges from a polyclonal B cell hyperplasia to monoclonal malignancies such as primary central nervous system lymphoma (PCNSL). CNS involvement is seen in only 10–15% of PTLD patients, and the majority of these exclusively involved the CNS. Up to 70% of PTLDs are EBV positive, whereas EBV-negative PTLDs usually occur many years after organ transplantation [74]. Treatment in the immunosuppressed patient requires balancing decreased immunosuppression with adequate immunosuppression to preserve the solid or HCT transplanted tissue or organ. Methotrexate and rituximab are used [75–77]. MRI appearance is both variable and nonspecific. Ring-enhancing lesions are the most common. A subacute Parkinsonian-like state with progression to akinetic mutism was recently reported with an MRI that showed striatal hyperintensity. EBV antibodies cross-react with alpha synuclein, effectively producing a postencephalitic Parkinsonism [78]. While CSF sampling may reveal a significant EBV viral load and confirm diagnosis, a stereotactic biopsy often is required (Fig. 20.5a–e).

Progressive Multifocal Leukoencephalopathy (PML)

PML is an often fatal demyelinating disease caused by the human neurotropic polyoma virus known as the John Cunningham or JC virus (JCV). Definitive diagnosis requires neuropathologic demonstration of demyelination, unusual astrocytes, and enlarged oligodendroglial nuclei with JC virus identified in brain by electron microscopy, immunohistochemical techniques, or PCR in brain or CSF [79]. A wide variety of neuroimaging characteristics with variable degrees of enhancement makes suspicion of the process imperative in the differential diagnosis of many clinically and radiographically disparate presentations [80, 81] (Fig. 20.6a–g). Visual symptoms are present in up to one half of all PML patients due to involvement of visual pathways rather than to direct involvement of the optic nerve itself [82].

Defining the molecular nature of persistence, reactivation of the virus, and viral avoidance of antibody-driven control has been difficult. It appears that some patients are unable to neutralize the most common PML-associated viral coat protein (VP1)-associated mutations. This raises the possibility that either active vaccination or passive transfer of antibodies could be a potential treatment [83]. Unfortunately, the only currently available therapeutic strategy is to reduce the degree of immunosuppression [84].

Clinicians have encountered an ever-broader spectrum of predisposing disease states and drug regimens. Drugs reported to increase the risk of PML include adalimumab, alemtuzumab, azathioprine, brentuximab, cyclophosphamide, cyclosporine, dimethyl fumarate, efalizumab, fingolimod, fludarabine, ibritumomab, infliximab, methotrexate, mycophenolate, natalizumab, rituximab, and tacrolimus. More recently, ruxolitinib, an inhibitor of Janus kinases 1 and 2 approved for treatment of myelofibrosis, has been tentatively linked to PML as early as 10 weeks after institution of treatment. Rituximab is the drug best studied as a factor predisposing to the development of PML. Approved by the United States Food and Drug Administration in 1997, this anti-CD20 monoclonal antibody produces prolonged B cell depletion for many months, though immunoglobulin levels are largely stable. Reactivation of hepatitis B, PML, and CMV and increased severity of enterovirus meningitis, WNV,

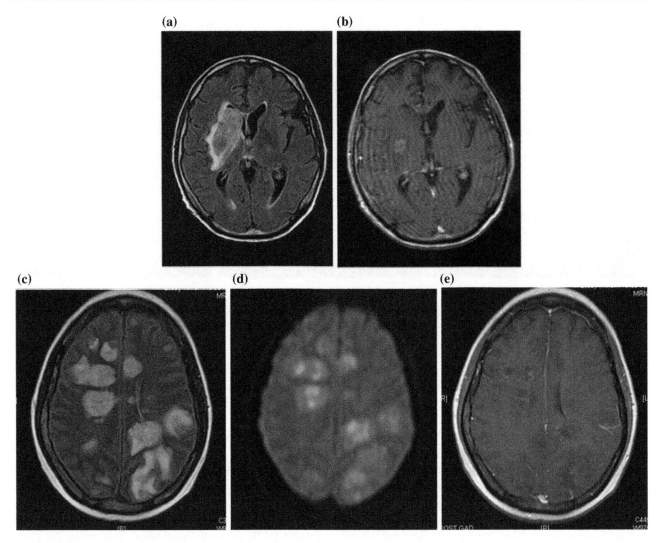

Fig. 20.5 MRI of Epstein–Barr virus (*EBV*)-associated lymphoproliferative disorders is variable as is the syndrome that can range from an indolent solitary enhancing mass evolving over several months in a patient 16 months after cardiac transplant in **a** and **b** to fulminant multifocal DWI positive and gadolinium-enhancing lesions seen in a patient 2 months after allogeneic HCT at a time of profound pancytopenia (**c–e**)

Babesiosis, and Pneumocystis jiroveci all have been reported [85–90]. For HCT and solid organ recipients, the risk of PML exists throughout the post-transplantation period. Bone marrow recipients tend to have symptoms earlier than solid organ recipients (11 vs. 27 months after transplantation in one study) [91].

After discontinuation of the potentially offending medicine, worsening neurologic signs may raise the possibility of immune reconstitution inflammatory syndrome (IRIS) [92]. The beneficial role of steroids in improving the acute symptoms of IRIS has been counterbalanced by impairment of JCV-specific T cell response [93]. Management of PML remains disappointing, and there is no evidence base for the use of cytarabine or mefloquine [94]. When immune suppression can be reduced, survival in HIV-negative patients is approximately the same as in HIV-positive patients (59 and 52%, respectively) [95].

Noninfectious Conditions Mimicking or Coexisting with CNS Infections

It is important to consider noninfectious entities in the differential diagnosis of infection in often complicated and critically ill cancer patients on multiple medications. At times, careful thought to noninfectious and non-neoplastic conditions will spare patients invasive procedures such as brain or meningeal biopsy. Some of these conditions have been emerged as diagnostic considerations in earlier sections of this chapter, but are presented here in greater detail.

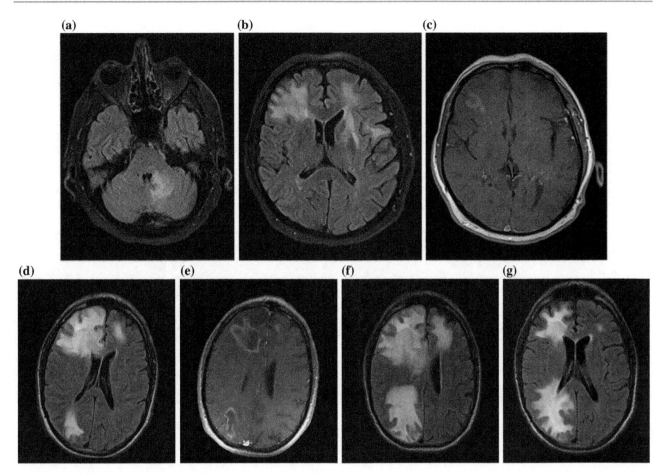

Fig. 20.6 Spectrum of progressive multifocal leukoencephalopathy (*PML*) and PML immune reconstitution (*PML/IRIS*) is presented here. **a** shows a typical posterior fossa MRI FLAIR abnormality without mass effect or enhancement (not shown). **a** and **b** show larger bifrontal areas of FLAIR abnormality with partial ring enhancement in a right cortical-based lesion but little or no enhancement elsewhere in the areas that are abnormal on FLAIR. **c–g** show a patient with PML at presentation (**c, d**) with cognitive changes. There is ring enhancement of most of the FLAIR areas of abnormality. When immunosuppression was reduced and scan repeated one month later (**e**) patient experienced worsening of symptoms along with increased FLAIR abnormality consistent with IRIS. When steroids were instituted, follow-up MRI showed diminished area of FLAIR abnormality and absence of enhancement (not shown)

Posterior Reversible Encephalopathy Syndrome (PRES)

First described twenty years ago, this form of vasogenic edema resulting from endothelial dysfunction has been reported in numerous clinical situations, the common denominators of which are failure of autoregulation such as hypertensive encephalopathy or pre-eclampsia or endothelial toxicity from various medications. There are often bilateral supratentorial, subcortical areas of white matter edema. Vasoconstriction, restricted diffusion, contrast enhancement, and hemorrhage all appear variably [96] (Fig. 20.7a–h). Atypical findings are hydrocephalus and exclusively brainstem, basal ganglia, thalamic or spinal cord signal abnormalities. The syndrome is not always completely reversible, and persistent seizures can be an uncommon sequel to the process [97]. PRES is recurrent in up to 10% of cases.

Immune Reconstitution Inflammatory Syndrome (IRIS)

IRIS, initially described in HIV patients, connotes a vigorous, often dysfunctional host inflammatory response to recent systemic or CNS infections in the setting of rapid host immune system recovery. The shift in dominant T helper (Th) response from one that constrains inflammation (Th2) to a pro-inflammatory pattern (Th1) produces a brain parenchymal or meningeal reaction, often granulomatous, that can mimic infection or sarcoidosis. IRIS is a diagnosis of exclusion to be considered in patients with previously diagnosed invasive fungal infections, tuberculosis, toxoplasmosis, CMV or PML when (a) there is new or worsening clinical and radiographic evidence of inflammation, (b) symptoms occur during receipt of appropriate antimicrobial therapy, and (c) culture results are negative. Dramatic

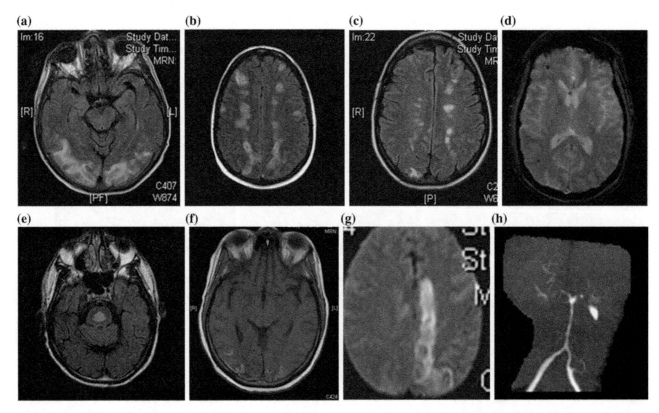

Fig. 20.7 Posterior reversible encephalopathy syndrome (*PRES*) has many radiographic appearances. All patients in **a–h** have received chemotherapy known to be associated with PRES, and some were hypertensive at the time of symptoms. **a** is the most typical with posterior predominance of FLAIR abnormality, whereas **b**, a different patient, shows more widespread cortical and subcortical frontal and posterior abnormalities. **c** and **d** are from a third patient with lesions that look demyelinating and microhemorrhages on diffusion-weighted sequences. The FLAIR image in **e** resembles osmotic demyelination, and PRES abnormalities were confined to the brainstem. Complications of the usually reversible PRES physiology are illustrated in the final three patients and include laminar necrosis in a patient who has had persistent seizures (**f**), stroke illustrated in the DWI sequence in **g** and MRA showing vasculopathy with severe vasoconstriction in the basilar artery in a different patient (**h**)

elevation in CSF pressure and pleocytosis with enhancement of affected areas can occur. In the population of HCT recipients, IRIS can occur both during engraftment and up to several months after reduction of immunosuppression. In the non-HIV population IRIS has been associated with crypto-coccal immune reconstitution following alemtuzumab for lymphoma, chronic disseminated candidiasis after neutrophil recovery in acute leukemia, and a relapsing-remitting MS-like illness involving the brain and spine [98]. Other infections demonstrating IRIS-like physiology include toxoplasmosis, PML, and CMV [99] (Fig. 20.7a–h).

Inflammatory Pseudotumor and Other Autoimmune Reactions

Unusual immune inflammatory reactions continue to be reported in the setting of manipulation of the immune system, altered T cell repertoire, and immune recovery. Some of these mimic infection and others appear more granulomatous leading to a differential diagnosis that includes tuberculosis and sarcoidosis. Acute disseminated encephalomyelitis (ADEM) can take the form of multifocal demyelination or may be a unifocal inflammatory pseudotumor that mimics neoplasm or infection [100, 101].

Novel cases of CNS sarcoidosis in patients undergoing treatment with the anti-cytotoxic T lymphocyte-associated antigen-4 (CTLA-4) agent ipilimumab have been reported. Immune-mediated adverse events should not be misinterpreted as tumor progression [102, 103]. However, when hilar adenopathy and abnormal enhancing tissue in such areas as the sella turcica and pituitary infundibulum are discovered, malignancy must be differentiated from pulmonary and neurologic sarcoidosis. Autoimmune hypophysitis occurs in up to 5% of patients treated with ipilimumab [104]. Additional adverse effects include uveitis and a chronic inflammatory demyelinating polyneuropathy responsive to steroids and intravenous immunoglobulin [105].

Neurologic Complications of Drug Regimens: Antibiotics and Immunosuppressives

Table 20.2 summarizes the major antibiotic and immunosuppressive toxicities whose contribution must be considered in the differential diagnosis of virtually any type of neurologic complication in cancer patients. A particularly versatile repertoire of toxicities is seen with tacrolimus, the most commonly employed calcineurin inhibitor. Tacrolimus, a heterocyclic macrolide, blocks production of interleukin-2, thereby inhibiting proliferation of antigen specific T lymphocytes. It has been associated with all of the following symptoms, some occurring simultaneously and not all associated with elevated tacrolimus levels. These symptoms include tremor, PRES, seizures, leukoencephalopathy, tumefactive MS, pseudotumor cerebri, chronic inflammatory demyelinating polyneuropathy (CIDP), brachial plexopathy, akinetic mutism, central pontine myelinolysis, hearing loss, and optic neuropathy [106]. Bioavailability of the drug is variable because of active secretion into the intestinal lumen by P-glycoprotein (PGP). The excretory mechanism is impaired by diarrhea, particularly *Clostridium difficile* whose destruction of colonic epithelial cells results in elevated trough tacrolimus levels [107]. Nonhepatic enzyme-inducing AEDs should be used to avoid reduction of tacrolimus levels and caution should be exercised when new oral anticoagulants are required, as they interfere with P-glycoprotein-mediated excretion leading to increased tacrolimus levels.

Among the many antibiotics associated with adverse neurologic effects, cefepime perhaps ranks first in severity and potential misleading clinical signs. This cephalosporin antibiotic increasingly is recognized as a cause of encephalopathy in intensive care units with a clinical picture characterized by impaired consciousness, jaw and other body site myoclonus, and at times nonconvulsive status epilepticus [108]. As this antibiotic complication could be misconstrued as postanoxic myoclonic status epilepticus, it is important to consider this reversible condition, particularly in patients with chronic kidney disease, though the complication can occur even when renal dosing adjustments are made [109].

Conclusion

The diagnosis and management of CNS infections remain evolving and persistently challenging areas of clinical care. Despite better epidemiologic understanding of at-risk populations, recognition of variable clinical syndromes, and timely diagnostic studies, morbidity and mortality from CNS infections remain high in the cancer population. The effective neurologic consultant, working with infectious disease colleagues, will consider emerging infections, transfusion safety issues, changing microbial susceptibilities, synergistic infections, and evolving novel cancer therapies that impact the CNS in novel ways.

References

1. Tan K, Patel S, Gandhi N, et al. Burden of neuroinfectious diseases on the neurology service in a tertiary care center. Neurology. 2008;71(15):1160–6.
2. Kleinschmidt-DeMasters BK, Marder BA, Levi ME, et al. West Nile virus encephalomyelitis in transplant recipients. Arch Neurol. 2004;61:1210–20.
3. Tyler KT. Emerging viral infections of the central nervous system: Part 1. Arch Neurol. 2009;66(8):940–8. Part 2 66(9):1065–74.
4. Safdieh JE, Mead PA, Sepkowitz KA, et al. Bacterial and fungal meningitis in patients with cancer. Neurology. 2008;70(12):943–7.
5. King MD, Humphrey BJ, Wang YF, et al. Emergence of community-acquired methicillin-resistant Staphylococcus aureus USA 300 clone as the predominant cause of skin and soft-tissue infections. Ann Intern Med. 2006;144:309–17.
6. Armangue T, Leypoldt F, Malaga I, et al. Herpes simplex virus encephalitis is a trigger of brain autoimmunity. Ann Neurol. 2014;75L:317–23.
7. Hoffmann B, Tappe D, Höper D, et al. A variegated squirrel bornavirus associated with fatal human encephalitis. N Engl J Med. 2015;373:154–62.
8. Pruitt AA. Central nervous system infections in cancer patients. Semin Neurol. 2010;30(3):296–310.
9. Pruitt AA. Infections of the cerebellum. Neurol Clin. 2014;32:1117–31.
10. Henry C, Jouan F, DeBroucker T. JC virus granule cell neuronopathy a cause of infectious cerebellar degeneration. J Neurol Sci 2015;354(1–2):86–90.
11. Richie MB, Pruitt AA. Spinal cord infections. Neurol Clin. 2013;31:19–53.
12. Soyama A, Eguchi S, Takatsuki M, et al. Human T-cell leukemia virus type 1-associated myelopathy following living donor liver transplant. Liver Transp. 2008;14(6):647–50.
13. Murayi R, Schmitt J, Woo JH, Berger JR. Spinal cord progressive multifocal leukoencephalopathy detected premortem by MRI. J Neurovirol. 2015;21(6):688–90.
14. Flanagan EP, McKeon A, Lennon VA, et al. Paraneoplastic isolated myelopathy: clinical course and neuroimaging clues. Neurology. 2011;76(24):2089–95.
15. Figueroa M, Guo Y, Tselis A, et al. Paraneoplastic neuromyelitis optica spectrum disorder associated with metastatic carcinoid expressing aquaporin-4. JAMA Neurol. 2014;71(4):495–8.
16. Quek AM, McKeon A, Lennon VA, et al. Effects of age and sex on aquaporin-4 autoimmunity. Arch Neurol. 2012;69(8):1039–43.
17. Pruitt AA. CNS infections in patients with cancer. Continuum Lifelong Learn Neurol. 2012;18(2):384–405.
18. Hasbun R, Abrahams J, Jekel J, et al. Computed tomography of the head before lumbar puncture in adults with suspected meningitis. N Engl J Med. 2001;345(24):1727–33.
19. Fink J, Born DK, Chamberlain MC. Pseudoprogression: relevance with respect to treatment of high-grade gliomas. Curr Treat Options Oncol. 2011;12(3):240–52.
20. Carrera E, Claassen J, Oddo M, et al. Continuous electroencephalographic monitoring in critically ill patients with central nervous system infections. Arch Neurol. 2008;65(12):1612–8.

21. Wilson MR, Shanbhag NM, Reid MJ, et al. Diagnosing *Balamuthia mandrillaris* encephalitis with metagenomic deep sequencing. Ann Neurol. 2015;78:722–30.

22. Wilson MR, Naccache SN, Samayoa E, et al. Actionable diagnosis of neuroleptospirosis by next-generation sequencing. N Engl J Med. 2014;370:2408–17.

23. Greenlee JE, Carroll KC. Cerebrospinal fluid in central nervous system infections. In: Scheld WM, Whitley RJ, Marra CM, editors. Infections of the central nervous system. 3rd ed. Philadelphia, PA: Lippincoctt Williams and Wilkins; 2004. p. 6–30.

24. Waters JD, Gonda DD, Reddy H, et al. Diagnostic yield of stereotactic needle biopsies of sub-cubic centimeter intracranial lesions. Surg Neurol Int. 2013;4:176–81.

25. Kranick SM, Vinnard C, Kolson DL. Propionibacterium acnes brain abscess appearing 10 years after neurosurgery. Arch Neurol. 2009;66(6):793–5.

26. Rogers LR, Gutierrez J, Scarpace L, et al. Morphologic magnetic resonance imaging features of therapy-induced cerebral necrosis. J Neurooncol. 2011;10(1):25–32.

27. Clark AJ, Butowski NA, Chang SM, et al. Impact of bevacizumab chemotherapy on craniotomy wound healing. J Neurosurg. 2011;114(6):1609–16.

28. Suzuki HI, Hangaishi A, Hosoya N, et al. Herpes simplex encephalitis and subsequent cytomegalovirus encephalitis after chemoradiotherapy for central nervous system lymphoma: a case report and literature review. Int J Hematol. 2008;87(5):538–41.

29. Kocher M, Kunze S, Eich HT, et al. Efficacy and toxicity of temozolomide radiochemotherapy in malignant glioma. Strahlenter Onkol. 2005;181(3):157–63.

30. Siegel D, Keller A, Xu W, et al. Central nervous system complications after allogeneic hematopoietic stem cell transplantation: incidence, manifestations, and clinical significance. Biol Blood Marrow Transplant 2007;13(11):1369–79.

31. Pruitt AA, Graus F, Rosenfeld MR. Neurological complications of hematopoietic cell transplantation. Neurohospitalist. 2013;3(1):24–38.

32. Pruitt AA, Graus F, Rosenfeld MR. Neurological complications of solid organ transplantation. Neurohospitalist. 2013;3(3):152–66.

33. Fischer SA, Graham MB, Kuehnert MJ, et al. Transmission of lymphocytic choriomeningitis virus by organ transplantation. N Engl J Med. 2006;354(21):2235–49.

34. Shaz BH. Transfusion transmitted diseases. In: Hilyer CD, Shaz BH, Zimring JG, Abshire TC, editors. Transfusion medicine and hemostasis: clinical and laboratory aspects. New York, NY: Elsevier; 2009. p. 361–71.

35. Srinivasen A, Burton EC, Kuehnert MJ, et al. Transmission of rabies virus from an organ donor to four transplant recipients. N Engl J Med. 2005;352(11):1103–11.

36. Burton EC, Burns DK, Opatowsky MJ, et al. Rabies encephalomyelitis: clinical, neuroradiological, and pathological findings in 4 transplant recipients. Arch Neurol. 2005;62(6):8783–882.

37. Vora NM, Basavaraju SV, Feldman KA, et al. Raccoon rabies virus variant transmission through solid organ transplantation. JAMA. 2013;310:398–407.

38. Seeley WW, Marth FM, Holmes TM, et al. Post-transplant acute limbic encephalitis: clinical features and relationship to HH6. Neurology. 2007;69(2):156–65.

39. Kamble RT, Chang CC, Sanchez S, et al. Central nervous system graft-versus-host disease: report of two cases and literature review. Bone Marrow Transplant. 2007;39(1):49–52.

40. Sun HY, Wagener MM, Singh N. Cryptococcosis in solid-organ, hematopoietic stem cell, and tissue transplant recipients: evidence-based evolving trends. Clin Infect Dis. 2009;48(11):1566–76.

41. Safdar N, Smith J, Knasisnski V, et al. Infections after the use of alemtuzumab in SOT recipients: a comparative study. Diagn Microbiol Infect Dis. 2010;66(1):7–15.

42. Peleg AY, Husain S, Kwak EJ, et al. Opportunistic infections in 547 organ transplant recipients receiving alemtuzumab, a humanized monoclonal CD-52 antibody. Clin Infect Dis. 2007;44(2):212–94.

43. Coursin D, Wood K. Corticosteroid supplementation for adrenal insufficiency. JAMA. 2002;287:236–40.

44. Neary N, Nieman L. Adrenal insufficiency: etiology, diagnosis and treatment. Curr Opin Endocrinol Diabetes Obes. 2010;17(3):217–33.

45. Yap KY, Chui WK, Chan A. Drug interactions between chemotherapeutic regimens and antiepileptics. Clin Ther. 2009;30(8):1385–407.

46. Thigpen MC, Whitney CG, Messonnier NE, et al. Bacterial meningitis in the United States, 1998–2007. N Engl J Med. 2011;364(21):2016–25.

47. Van de Beek D, Drake JM, Tunkel AR. Nosocomial bacterial meningitis. N Engl J Med. 2010;362(2):146–54.

48. Brouwer MC, McIntyre P, de Gans J, et al. Corticosteroids for acute bacterial meningitis. Cochrane Database Syst Rev. 2010;9: CD004405.

49. McClelland S, Hall WA. Postoperative central nervous system infection: incidence and associated factors in 2111 neurosurgical procedures. Clin Infect Dis. 2007;45(1):55–9.

50. Murdoch DR, Corey GR, Hoen BK, et al. Clinical presentation, etiology, and outcome of infective endocarditis in the 21st century: the International Collaboration on Endocarditis-Prospective Cohort Study. Arch Int Med. 2009;169(5):463–73.

51. Seton M, Pless M, Fishman JA, et al. Case records of the Massachusetts General Hospital. Case 18-2008. A 68-year old-man with headache and visual changes after liver transplantation. N Engl J Med. 2008;358(24):2619–28.

52. Starkey J, Moritani T, Kirby P. MRI of CNS fungal infections: review of aspergillosis to histoplasmosis and everything in between. Clin Neuroradiol. 2014;24:217–30.

53. Labbe AC, Su SH, Laverdiere M, et al. High incidence of invasive aspergillosis associated with intestinal graft-versus-host disease following nonmyeloablative transplantation. Boil Bone Marrow Transplant. 2007;13(10):1192–200.

54. DeLone DR, Goldstein RA, Petermann G, et al. Disseminated aspergillosis involving the brain: distribution and imaging characteristics. AJNR Am J Neuroradiol. 1999;20(9):1597–604.

55. Kourkoumpetis TK, Desalermos A, Muhammed M, Mylonakis E. Central nervous system aspergillosis. Medicine. 2012;91:328–36.

56. Schwartz S, Ruhnke M, Ribaud P, et al. Improved outcome in central nervous system aspergillosis, using voriconazole treatment. Blood. 2005;106:2641–5.

57. Nagel MA, Gilden DH. The protean neurologic manifestations of varicella-zoster virus infection. Cleve Clin J Med. 2007;74(7):489–94.

58. Gilden D, Cohrs RJ, Mahalingam R, et al. Varicella zoster virus vasculopathies: diverse clinical manifestations, laboratory features, pathogenesis, and treatment. Lancet Neurol. 2009;8(8):731–40.

59. Nagel MA, White T, Khmeleva N, et al. Analysis of varicella-zoster virus in temporal arteries biopsy positive and negative for giant cell arteritis. JAMA Neurol. 2015;72(11):L1281–7.

60. Gilden D, White T, Khmeleva N, et al. Prevalence and distribution of VZV in temporal arteries of patients with giant cell arteritis. Neurology. 2015;84:1948–55.

61. Morrison VA, Johnson GR, Schmader KE, et al. Long-term persistence of zoster vaccine efficacy. Clin Infect Dis. 2015;60:900–9.

62. Johnson RW, Rice ASC. Postherpetic neuralgia. N Engl J Med. 2014;371(16):1526–33.
63. Cohen JI. Herpes zoster. N Engl J Med. 2013;369(3):L255–63.
64. Lal H, Cunningham AL, Godeaux O, et al. Efficacy of an adjuvanted herpes zoster subunit vaccine in older adults. N Engl J Med. 2015;372:2087–96.
65. Stadtmauer EA, Sullivan KM, Marty FM, et al. A phase 1/2 study of an adjuvanted varicella-zoster virus subunit vaccine in autologous hematopoietic cell transplant recipients. Blood. 2014;124:29291-2929.
66. Ogata M. Human herpesvirus 6 in hematological malignancies. J ClinExp Hematop. 2009;49:57–67.
67. Morissette G, Flamand L. Herpesviruses and chromosomal integration. J Virol. 2010;84(23):12100–9.
68. Bhanushali MJ, Kranick SM, Freeman AF, et al. Human herpes 6 virus encephalitis complicating allogeneic hematopoietic stem cell transplantation. Neurology. 2013;80:1494–500.
69. Tan IL, McArthur JC, Venkatesan A, Nath A. Atypical manifestations and poor outcome of herpes simplex encephalitis in the immunocompromised. Neurology. 2012;79:2125–32.
70. Graber JJ, Rosenblum MK, DeAngelis LM. Herpes simplex encephalitis in patients with cancer. J Neurooncol. 2011;105: 415–21.
71. Titulaer M, Leypoldt F, Dalmau J. Antibodies to NMDA and other synaptic receptors in choreoathetosis and relapsing symptoms post herpes simplex encephalitis. Mov Disord. 2014;29(1): 3–6.
72. Koudriavtseva T, Onesti E, Tonachella R, et al. Fatal herpetic encephalitis during brain radiotherapy in a cerebral metastasized breast cancer patient. J Neurooncol. 2010;100:137–40.
73. Mateen FJ, Miller SA, Aksamit AJ. Herpes simplex virus 2 encephalitis in adults. Mayo Clin Proc. 2014;89(2):274–6.
74. Evens AM, Roy R, Sterrenberg D, et al. Post-transplantation lymphoproliferative disorders: diagnosis, prognosis and current approaches to therapy. Curr Oncol Rep. 2010;12(6):383–94.
75. Evens AM, Choquet S, Kroll-Desrosiers AR, et al. Primary CNS posttransplant lymphoproliferative disease (PTLD): an international report of 84 cases in the modern era. Am J Transplant. 2013;13(6):1512–22.
76. Kempf C, Tinguely M, Rushing EJ. Posttransplant lymphoproliferative disorder of the CNS. Pathobiology. 2013;80(6): 310–8.
77. Singavi AK, Harrington AM, Fenske TS. Post-transplant lymphoproliferative disorders. Cancer Treat Res. 2015;165: 305–27.
78. Espay AJ, Henderson KK. Postencephalitic parkinsonism and basal ganglia necrosis due to Epstein-Barr virus infection. Neurology. 2011;76(17):1529–30.
79. Berger JR, Aksamit AJ, Clifford DB, et al. PML diagnostic criteria: Consensus statement from the AAN Neuroinfectious Disease Section. Neurology. 2013;80:1430–8.
80. Horger M, Beschorner R, Beck R, et al. Common and uncommon imaging findings in progressive multifocal leukoencephalopathy (PML), with differential diagnostic considerations. Clin Neurol Neurosurg. 2012;114(8):1123–230.
81. Tan CS, Koralnik IIM. Progressive multifocal leukoencephalopathy and other disorders caused by JC virus: clinical features and pathogenesis. Lancet Neurol. 2010;9(4):425–37.
82. Sudhakar P, Bachman DM, Mark AS, et al. Progressive multifocal leukoencephalopathy: recent advances and a neuro-ophthalmological review. J Neuro-Ophthal. 2015;35(3): 296–305.
83. Ray U, Cinque P, Gerevini S, et al. JC polyomavirus mutants escape antibody-mediated neutralization. Sci Transl Med. 2015;7 (306):306ra151.
84. Wollebo HS, White MK, Gordon J, et al. Persistence and pathogenesis of the neurotropic polyomavirus JC. Ann Neurol. 2015;77:560–70.
85. Carson KR, Focosi D Major EO, et al. Monoclonal antibody-associated progressive multifocal leukoencephalopathy inpatients treated with rituximab, natalizumab and efalizumab: a review from the research on adverse drug events and reports (RADAR) project. Lancet Oncol. 2009;10:816–24.
86. Gea-Banacloche JC. Rituximab-associated infections. Semin Hematol. 2010;47(2):187–98.
87. Ganjoo KN, Raman R, Ra Sobel, et al. Opportunistic enteroviral meningoencephalitis: an unusual treatable complication of rituximab therapy. Leuk Lymphoma. 2009;50(4):673–5.
88. Aksamit AJ. Progressive multifocal leukoencephalopathy. Continuum Lifelong Learn Neurol. 2012;18(6):1374–91.
89. Levi ME, Quan D, Ho JT, et al. Impact of rituximab-associated B-cell defects on West Nile virus meningoencephalitis in solid organ transplant recipients. Clin Transplant. 2009;24(2):223–8.
90. Tuccori Mk, Focosi D, Balndizzii C, et al. Inclusion of rituximab in treatment protocols for non-Hodgkin's lymphoma and risk for progressive multifocal leukoencephalopathy. The Oncolgoist. 2010;15:1214–9.
91. Mateen FJ, Muralidharan RN, Carone M, et al. Progressive multifocal leukoencephalopathy in transplant recipients. Ann Neurol. 2011;70:305–22.
92. Moule S, Milojkovic D. PML associated with ruxolitinib. N Engl J Med. 2013;369(2):197(2):197–8.
93. Antoniol C, Jilek S, Schluep M, et al. Impairment of JC-specific T-cell response by corticotherapy: effect on PML-IRIS management? Neurology. 2012;79(23):2258–64.
94. Berger JR. Progressive multifocal leukoencephalopathy. Handb Clin Neurol. 2014;123:357–76.
95. Marzocchetti A, Tompkins T, Clifford DB, et al. Determinants of survival in progressive multifocal leukoencephalopathy. Neurology. 2009;73(19):1551–8.
96. Fugate JE, Rabinstein AA. Posterior reversible encephalopathy syndrome: clinical and radiological manifestations, pathophysiology, and outstanding questions. Lancet Neurol. 2015;14: 914–25.
97. Datar S, Rabinstein A, Fugate JE, et al. Long-term risk of seizures and epilepsy in patients with posterior reversible encephalopathy syndrome. Epilepsia. 2015;56:564–8.
98. Delios AM, Rosenblum M, Jakubowski AA, DeAngelis LM. Central and peripheral nervous system immune mediated demyelinating disease after allogeneic hematopoietic stem cell transplantation for hematologic disease. J Neurooncol. 2012;110 (2):251–6.
99. Airas L, Paivarinta M, Roytta M, et al. Central nervous system immune reconstitution inflammatory syndrome (IRIS) after hematopoietic SCT. Bone Marrow Transplant. 2010;45(3):593–6.
100. Young NP, Weinshenker BG, Lucchinetti CF. Acute disseminated encephalomyelitis: current understanding and controversies. Semin Neurol. 2008;28(1):84–94.
101. Brandao E, Mel-Pires M, Veria C. Relapsing-remitting tumefactive demyelination. JAMA Neurol. 2014;71(3):366–7.
102. Murphy KP, Kennedy MP, Barry JE, et al. New-onset mediastinal and central nervous system sarcoidosis in a patient with metastatic melanoma undergoing CTLA4 monoclonal antibody treatment. Oncol Res Treat. 2014;37:351–3.
103. Vogel WV, Guislai A, Kvistborg P, et al. Ipilimumab-induced sarcoidosis in a patient with metastatic melanoma undergoing a compete remission. J Clin Oncol. 2012;30:e7–10.
104. Eckert A, Schoeffler A, Dalle S, et al. Anti-CTLA4 monoclonal antibody induced sarcoidosis in a metastatic melanoma patient. Dermatology. 2009;218:699–700.

105. Manousakis G, Koch J, Sommerville RB, et al. Multifocal radiculoneuropathy during ipilimumab treatment of melanoma. Muscle Nerve. 2013;48(3):440–4.

106. Balu R, Pruitt AA. Neurologic complications of immunosuppressive drugs. In: Quant E, Wen PY, editors. Neurological complications of cancer therapy. New York: Demos; 2012. p. 107–24.

107. Lemahieu W, Maes B, Verbeke IK, et al. Cytochrome P450 3A4 and P-glycoprotein activity and assimilation of tacrolimus in transplant patients with persistent diarrhea. Am J Transplant. 2005;5(6):961–72.

108. Fugate JE, Kalimullah EA, Hocker SE, et al. Cefepime neurotoxicity in the intensive care unit: a cause of severe underappreciated encephalopathy. Crit Care. 2013;17:R264.

109. Hocker S, Rabinstein AA. Cefepime neurotoxicity can mimic postanoxic coma with myoclonic status epilepticus. Neurol Clin Pract. 2011;1:73–4.

Part VI

Neurological Complications of Specific Malignancies

Neurological Complications of Primary Brain Tumors

Justin T. Jordan, Thomas N. Byrne, and Tracy Batchelor

Introduction

The supportive care of brain tumor patients includes the treatment of brain edema, seizures, and cognitive dysfunction. Each of these complications may occur in patients with either primary or metastatic brain tumors. The development of any of these complications significantly increases the morbidity and mortality associated with brain tumors. However, effective treatment is usually possible and can result in an improved quality of life for these patients.

Clinical Manifestations of Primary Brain Tumors

Primary brain tumors typically present with progressive focal and/or diffuse clinical manifestations or seizures. If the lesion is in an eloquent area of brain, the initial clinical manifestation may be dysfunction attributable to that brain locus such as paresis, aphasia, or visual loss. Alternatively, patients may present with large space-occupying lesions arising in other locations such as the frontal or temporal lobes causing diffuse cerebral symptoms. Additionally, masses of posterior fossa, leading to obstructive hydrocephalus, may initially present with diffuse symptoms and signs. Common examples of diffuse dysfunction include cognitive or behavioral disturbance, headache, and gait disorder without focal symptoms.

J.T. Jordan (✉) · T. Batchelor
Department of Neurology, Massachusetts General Hospital, 55 Fruit Street Yawkey 9E, Boston, MA 02114, USA
e-mail: jtjordan@mgh.harvard.edu

T. Batchelor
e-mail: tbatchelor@mgh.harvard.edu

T.N. Byrne
Massachusetts General Hospital, Neurology, 55 Fruit St. WACC 7, Boston, MA 02114, USA
e-mail: tnbyrne@mgh.harvard.edu

The headache of primary brain tumors arises from compression of innervated large intracranial blood vessels and meninges. While the classical brain tumor headache is more severe after recumbency when intracranial venous pressure is increased leading to worsening of cerebral edema (see edema section below), the most common headache type to herald a primary brain tumor is one that is of insidious onset and is progressive.

The location of the primary brain tumor determines the focal neurological manifestations that occur. Frontal lobe lesions may exhibit inattention, depression, and lack of motivation. Some patients may be considered to have a psychiatric disease since there are few, if any, focal neurological signs to alert the clinician to a neurological etiology. In some such cases imaging reveals an extensive glioma crossing the corpus callosum without involving motor pathways.

Tumors in the temporal lobes also often present with neuropsychiatric manifestations such as memory impairment, hypergraphia, mood disturbance, and *déjà vu*. Lesions located in the right temporal-parietal region may lead to a sensation of being outside one's body. Dominant temporal lobe lesions may cause aphasia. A homonymous superior quadrantanopia may be seen on visual field testing since the visual pathways may be interrupted.

Parietal lobe tumors may exhibit contralateral motor and sensory disturbances and homonymous hemianopia. Dominant parietal lobe tumors may cause dysphasia. Non-dominant lesions may cause geographic agnosia, dressing apraxia, and rarely denial of the contralateral side, anosognosia.

Occipital lobe tumors may cause a contralateral homonymous hemianopia. The corpus callosum is often eventually involved by invasion of tumor along white matter tracts, which leads to invasion of the contralateral occipital lobe. This may lead to the inability to read and inability to name objects presented in the non-dominant visual field or cortical blindness.

© Springer International Publishing AG 2018
D. Schiff et al. (eds.), *Cancer Neurology in Clinical Practice*,
DOI 10.1007/978-3-319-57901-6_21

Fig. 21.1 A right frontal non-enhancing glioma with increased T2 (*left*) and FLAIR (*right*) signal abnormality. It can be difficult to distinguish vasogenic edema from infiltrative tumor in a case such as this

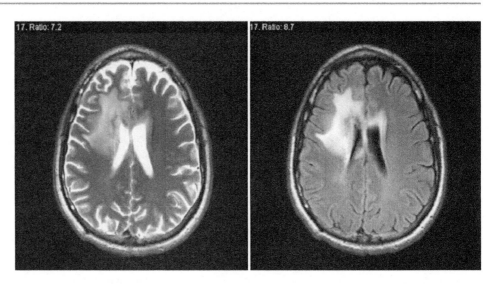

There are some clinical brain tumor syndromes that warrant special mention. Midline tumors resulting in ventricular obstruction may cause the "3 M" syndrome, namely maximal disability, minimal signs, and midline lesion. Common clinical manifestations include diffuse headache, cognitive or behavioral changes, and gait/truncal ataxia without lateralizing findings. Tumors of the fourth ventricle are common causes of the "3 M" syndrome. Another manifestation of a posterior fossa mass causing obstructive hydrocephalus is projectile vomiting which is more common in children than adults. Posterior fossa medulloblastomas, ependymomas, and astrocytomas may all present in this manner. A rare presentation of primary brain tumors that may cause focal symptoms, but not focal signs, can be seen with gliomas of the insula or floor of the posterior fossa irritating the area postrema. The authors have observed patients with non-specific symptoms such as nausea and vomiting who had extensive gastrointestinal workups including CT and endoscopy only to have a glioma of the insula or ependymoma/subependymoma of the fourth ventricle discovered after some years. Resection of the gliomas aborted the gastrointestinal complaints.

Seizures are a common manifestation of gliomas. A seizure in a middle-aged person without a history of head trauma or toxic-metabolic cause should raise the suspicion of an underlying primary brain tumor and prompt imaging of the brain, preferably contrast-enhanced MRI.

Brain Edema

Classification

Primary brain tumor blood vessels are abnormal both anatomically and functionally [1]. The consequences of this are multiple and include cerebral edema, impairment of drug delivery and regions of hypoxia [2]. The most common type of edema related to brain tumors is vasogenic edema, both within and surrounding the tumor (Fig. 21.1) [3–5]. Vasogenic edema, which is an increase in brain volume from increased water and sodium content, generally with the characteristics of plasma exudate [6, 7], may lead to focal or generalized brain dysfunction [8]. In cases with marked peritumoral edema, patients may additionally be at risk of plateau waves, which are sudden transient increases in intracranial pressure that may increase transtentorial herniation and lead to temporary increase in neurological symptoms.

Blood–Brain Barrier and Edemagenesis

The pathogenesis of vasogenic brain edema involves disruption of the blood–brain barrier. This physiologic barrier separates the systemic circulation from the central nervous system (CNS) and consists of the specialized endothelium of blood vessels supplying the CNS surrounded by pericytes. This barrier normally impedes the entry of most water-soluble but not lipid-soluble agents [8, 9]. The anatomic features essential for the normal function of the blood–brain barrier are highlighted in Fig. 21.2 [10].

Disruption of the blood–brain barrier by a brain tumor results in increased entry of water-soluble substances and macromolecules such as plasma protein into the tumor and surrounding brain. Because there is no lymphatic system in the CNS, these substances are not easily eliminated, and are driven into surrounding brain tissue by increased hydrostatic pressure within the tumor, resulting in vasogenic brain edema. The edema tends to extend along white matter tracts rather than in the more closely packed gray matter [11].

The mechanisms of blood–brain barrier disruption and formation of brain edema are incompletely understood, and

Fig. 21.2 Normal blood–brain barrier demonstrating tight junctions between endothelial cells; a normal basement membrane and adjacent astrocyte foot processes (used with permission of Cambridge University Press from Francis et al. [10])

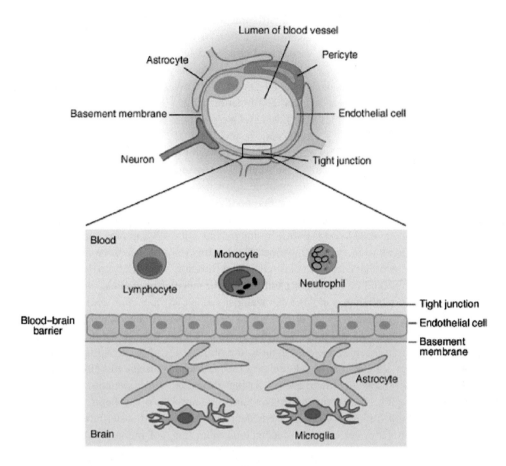

multiple factors are involved. When brain tumors grow to a size greater than 1–2 mm, they promote formation of new blood vessels that lack a normal blood–brain barrier. This tumor-associated vascular endothelium is characterized by an increased number of intercellular junctions, discontinuous tight junctions, membranous fenestrations, non-contiguous basement membranes, and active micropinocytosis. This results in increased permeability of these new blood vessels to macromolecules, ions, and proteins, with the formation of vasogenic edema. All of these microvascular abnormalities are most common in the central portion of the tumor and least common at the interface between brain and tumor [12–16]. Vascular endothelial growth factor (VEGF), secreted by tumor cells, may be responsible for the disruption of the blood–brain barrier in the tumor as well as the peritumoral region [17]. There is also evidence that arachidonic acid and its leukotriene metabolites promote vasogenic edema formation by selectively increasing capillary permeability within the tumor. Arachidonic acid is a normal constituent of membrane phospholipids in the CNS but may be released into the extracellular space under certain pathologic conditions [18–21]. Finally, immunologic mechanisms may be important, as tumor growth is associated with macrophage infiltration in and around the tumor. These inflammatory cells are capable of elaborating a variety of secretory factors that are associated with increased vascular permeability [6]. One study demonstrated that the amount of tumor-associated edema visible on CT scans correlated with the extent of macrophage infiltration found on pathologic study [22]. The relative contribution of each of these mechanisms to edemagenesis is unknown.

Blood–brain barrier disruption and the subsequent development of vasogenic edema lead to increased intracranial pressure (ICP). Because the process is caused by a focal brain lesion, the increased intracranial pressure is distributed unevenly within the intracranial compartment and may result in brain herniation and compromise of local blood supply [23]. These events contribute to the neurological symptoms and signs observed in patients with increased ICP secondary to brain tumors.

Steroid Therapy

Glucocorticoids are the mainstay of treatment for vasogenic brain edema. Kofman and colleagues [24] were the first to demonstrate the responsiveness of brain tumor edema to corticosteroids, and Galicich and French [25] introduced dexamethasone therapy as the standard treatment for tumor-associated edema. The mechanism of action of corticosteroids in the treatment of vasogenic brain edema is incompletely understood [26]. A mechanism commonly thought to account for the beneficial effects of corticosteroids is a direct action on endothelial cell function which restores normal vascular permeability [27, 28]. One possible mechanism by which corticosteroids may restore normal permeability involves the ability of corticosteroids to inhibit the release of arachidonic acid, a substance known to increase vascular permeability and promote formation of brain edema [29–31]. It has been shown that corticosteroids can have both direct and indirect effects on endothelial cells and may inhibit increased permeability by interfering with the ability of the cell to interact with permeability factors [8, 31]. It is also known that corticosteroids reduce the filtration of plasma-derived fluid across tumor capillaries and reduce the movement of albumin through the extracellular space by solvent drag [32]. Finally, there is indirect evidence that dexamethasone causes cerebral vasoconstriction [33]. Likely, all of these mechanisms contribute to the ability of corticosteroids to stabilize the blood–brain barrier and lead to reduction of vasogenic brain edema. Using diffusion tensor MR imaging, Sinha and colleagues have demonstrated that administration of corticosteroids decreases peritumoral extracellular water content in edematous brain but does not affect the water content of contralateral normal brain [34]. This finding was seen in cerebral metastases, gliomas, and extra-axial tumors.

The optimal dose of corticosteroids for vasogenic brain edema has not been established. Dexamethasone is commonly used in clinical practice and is probably the best steroid for the treatment of brain tumors [8]. The advantages of dexamethasone include the absence of mineralocorticoid effect, which makes salt retention and systemic edema less likely. There is also evidence that of all the corticosteroids, dexamethasone is less likely to be associated with infection and cognitive impairment [30, 35]. Nevertheless, like other fluorinated corticosteroids, dexamethasone is more likely to cause myopathy [36].

Since corticosteroids cause adverse side effects and induce metabolism of other drugs, the benefits of corticosteroids in patients with asymptomatic brain edema are generally outweighed by these side effects. Alternatively, patients with symptomatic brain edema typically respond and, therefore, usually benefit from the use of corticosteroids. The patient should be maintained on the lowest dose that controls neurological symptoms in order to avoid the development of adverse effects. The drug is absorbed from the gastrointestinal tract, but first-pass hepatic metabolism may decrease effectiveness, especially in patients also receiving phenytoin [37, 38]. Dexamethasone can be given twice daily because of the longer half-life of this steroid,

although clinicians sometimes prescribe it 4 times daily [39]. A commonly used starting schedule is a 10-mg oral dose followed by 4 mg 4 times a day, which is 20 times the rate of endogenous cortisol production; however, the dosage should be tailored to the individual patient's clinical and imaging characteristics [30]. There is evidence that doses lower than 16 mg daily may be just as effective with the same degree of clinical improvement after 1 week of treatment [39]. Approximately 70–80% of patients with brain tumors will experience improvement of symptoms with dexamethasone [8, 40]. A rapid clinical response to steroid administration indicates that the symptoms may be primarily due to the tumor-associated edema rather than actual tumor mass [30]. Symptoms and signs of generalized brain dysfunction such as headache and lethargy respond more rapidly and dramatically to corticosteroids than focal neurological signs. If the standard dose fails to achieve a clinical response in 48 h, then the dose can be doubled every 48 h until response occurs. Rarely, up to 100 mg of dexamethasone over 24 h may be required in occasional patients; however, the advent of bevacizumab has led to an alternative to corticosteroids as discussed below [41, 42].

In patients with brain tumors, symptomatic improvement usually begins within hours of an intravenous injection of corticosteroids. Positron emission tomography (PET) scans of humans with brain tumors demonstrate an effect on the blood–brain barrier as soon as 6 h after the intravenous bolus [43]. Maximal clinical improvement usually occurs within 24–72 h. It has been shown that the first change is a decrease in plateau waves followed by a gradual decline of increased intracranial pressure over a period of 48–70 h [44]. Improvement on CT and MR imaging studies may lag behind clinical improvement, although early scans may show decreased contrast enhancement within the tumor, suggesting partial restoration of the blood–brain barrier [27, 45, 46].

In order to avoid the deleterious effects of corticosteroids, the patient should be treated with the smallest effective dose for the shortest time possible [47]. The patient should be tapered from corticosteroids during or after more definitive treatment such as surgery, radiation therapy, or chemotherapy. The taper should generally start 3–4 days after surgery and during the second week of radiation therapy. In general, patients with malignant brain tumors should receive standard dose corticosteroids for 48–72 h prior to starting brain irradiation to reduce intracranial pressure and minimize acute radiation toxicity. For patients on a standard dose of 16 mg of dexamethasone per day, decreasing the dose by 2–4 mg every fifth day is reasonable. If symptoms of steroid withdrawal or increased brain edema occur, the drug should be increased to the immediately preceding level for 4–8 days before starting the taper again. If symptoms of brain edema recur after discontinuation, the dexamethasone may need to be resumed to control symptoms if alternative strategies are not available [8]. A more rapid taper may be used safely to minimize steroid toxicity, decreasing the dose from 16 mg/d for 4 days to 8 mg/d for 4 days followed by 4 mg/d until completion of radiation therapy [48]. In patients on corticosteroids for many months who fail the usual taper schedule or in patients with a large amount of residual tumor, the drug is tapered more slowly (e.g., 1–2 mg/wk) to the lowest dose possible. Patients on large doses of corticosteroids (e.g., 100 mg of dexamethasone per day) who have stabilized and are receiving definitive treatment can have the dose halved every 4–5 days depending on the clinical condition [8]. As discussed below, the advent of bevacizumab has provided an alternative to corticosteroid therapy.

Deleterious Steroid Effects

The classic features of excessive corticosteroids, including weight gain, moon facies, acne, hirsutism, and abdominal striae, are easily recognized by most clinicians but rarely produce significant morbidity. Adverse effects that are potentially more serious include myopathy, cognitive impairment, gastrointestinal dysfunction, and opportunistic infection [8, 11].

There are conflicting reports on the frequency of steroid toxicity in patients with brain tumors [42, 49–51]. Duration of treatment appears to be an important variable with prolonged treatment (>3 weeks) associated with greater toxicity [47]. Hypoalbuminemia also appears to confer greater risk of steroid toxicity as the percentage of unbound steroid increases, especially with serum albumin levels less than 2.5 g/dL [47, 52, 53]. Because patients with brain tumors are often debilitated, they may be particularly susceptible to the deleterious effects of corticosteroids.

Most patients treated with conventional doses of corticosteroids (e.g., 16 mg of dexamethasone per day) for more than 2–3 weeks will develop some degree of myopathy. In one study, 15 cancer patients being treated with dexamethasone were followed for the development of myopathy. Within 15 days, nine patients had developed myopathy, which, in most, was sufficient to interfere with activities of daily living. The cumulative dose ranged from 186 to 1846 mg. The development of myopathy correlated with the total dose rather than the duration or daily dose of dexamethasone [54]. In steroid-induced myopathy, muscle biopsy shows atrophy of type II fibers, the fibers characterized by high glycolytic and low oxidative capacity [55]. Serum muscle enzymes are not elevated. Steroid myopathy is characterized clinically by proximal muscle weakness and eventual muscle wasting, especially in the pelvic girdle. One

of the most common complaints is an inability to arise from the seated position. The myopathy may progress to involve the proximal arms and neck. Evaluation of neck and hip flexor strength usually provides the most sensitive clinical assessment for steroid myopathy [56]. It has also been recognized that respiratory muscle may be affected, and this can result in symptomatic dyspnea in severely myopathic patients [57]. Treatment includes reduction or discontinuation of corticosteroids, if possible. Since fluorinated corticosteroids (dexamethasone, triamcinolone) are associated with more type IIb fiber atrophy than non-fluorinated corticosteroids (prednisolone, methylprednisolone) avoidance of the former may lower the risk of steroid myopathy, although this has not been studied systematically. Preclinical experimental observations have suggested that alternate-day dosing of methylprednisolone reduces the severity of myopathy compared to continuous daily dosing of the same drug [58]. Exercise, physiotherapy, and a high-protein diet during steroid treatment may attenuate the disorder [59]. One study reported a decreased frequency of myopathy in brain tumor patients treated with corticosteroids who also received phenytoin, potentially due to increased catabolism of the steroid after induction of the hepatic microsomal system by phenytoin [37].

Psychiatric complications may develop in as many as 5% of patients receiving exogenous corticosteroids. The majority of these are either affective or psychotic reactions, but other complications include delirium and neuropsychological impairment with selective involvement of attention, concentration, and memory [60, 61]. A prior history of an adverse psychiatric reaction to corticosteroids does not predict such future complication, and corticosteroids should not be withheld if medically indicated in such patients. Most patients with psychiatric complications make a full recovery, but symptomatic treatment may be necessary. Steroid reduction and neuroleptic administration are usually effective for psychotic symptoms [60]. One report suggests that lithium prophylaxis lessens the likelihood of a psychotic reaction to corticosteroids, although it is not routinely recommended [62]. Steroid withdrawal can also lead to depressive symptoms [63].

The major gastrointestinal effects of corticosteroids are ulceration and perforation [64, 65], although upper gastrointestinal bleeding is rare in patients taking corticosteroids with no previous history of such bleeding. The incidence is much higher with simultaneous use of anticoagulants or in patients with a prior history of upper gastrointestinal bleeding, although the overall risk in one study was less than 1% for such patients if treated with corticosteroids for less than 1 month [66]. In a study of nearly 46,000 patients using corticosteroids, Nielsen and colleagues found the relative risk of hospitalizations due to gastrointestinal bleeding was 4.9 compared to expected. The relative risk fell to 2.9 among patients using corticosteroids alone, without the use of other drugs known to cause gastrointestinal bleeding (e.g., aspirin) [67]. Whether or not patients on corticosteroids benefit from receiving gastrointestinal prophylaxis with antacids, H2-blockers, proton pump inhibitors, or other anti-ulcer agents remains controversial [8, 68]. Bowel perforation is a serious complication in steroid-treated patients and is associated with high mortality. It usually occurs in patients treated with high doses of corticosteroids who have been constipated as a result of medication, immobility, or neurological dysfunction. The perforation usually affects the sigmoid colon and may not be accompanied by the usual abdominal symptoms and signs due to the masking effects of corticosteroids or comorbid neurological disease. This usually delays diagnosis and may account for the high mortality rate in this group of patients [69, 70]. Plain radiographs usually are diagnostic, and surgical repair remains the definitive treatment. The goal, however, should be prevention of this complication with careful attention and treatment of constipation, including adequate bulk in the diet, hydration, stool softeners, and laxatives as necessary.

Steroids are immunosuppressive drugs. In one study, 24% of primary brain tumor patients receiving concurrent corticosteroids and radiation experienced a reduction in their CD4+ cell count to <200 cells/mm^3 [71, 72]. Opportunistic infections secondary to immunosuppression from corticosteroids include *Candida* mucositis and esophagitis as well as *Pneumocystis jiroveci* pneumonia (PJP). The rate of PJP in patients with brain tumors is increasing, and studies have demonstrated incidence rates of 1–6% for this group of patients. Most of these patients were also receiving corticosteroids for prolonged periods, and infection was most likely to occur during the steroid taper [73–76]. Trimethoprim–sulfamethoxazole given as a single double-strength tablet either daily or thrice weekly during steroid administration and for 1 additional month afterward reduces the incidence of PJP by approximately 85% and should be considered in patients with brain tumors who are likely to require prolonged steroid treatment [73, 77].

Osteoporosis is a common complication of prolonged steroid use. While most patients with brain tumors do not live long enough for this to lead to fractures, it is important to recognize that steroid-induced osteoporosis can be prevented and treatments instituted, as appropriate, to the individual patient [78, 79]. Calcium in combination with vitamin D may prevent bone loss [80]. There are several recent studies that demonstrate the efficacy of biphosphonates, such as alendronate or risedronate, in the prevention of osteoporosis in patients taking chronic corticosteroids [81–83].

Another bone complication of steroid use is avascular necrosis of the hip or other bones which may develop following prolonged use of corticosteroids or may occur after only a few weeks of therapy [84–86].

Lipomatosis is the result of chronic steroid use, which stimulates redistribution of fat. Deposition of fat may occur in the epidural space and result in spinal cord compression. MR imaging is usually diagnostic, and surgical treatment may be necessary [87–89].

Visual problems consist mainly of blurring, which is a common complaint and is probably due to a change in refraction caused by corticosteroids. This usually improves with reduction or discontinuation of the corticosteroids. Longer-term steroid use may result in glaucoma or cataract formation [8].

Other possible side effects include hyperglycemia, which occurred in 19% of neuro-oncology patients receiving corticosteroids in one survey [47]. The majority of such patients required insulin or modification of the steroid dose to control hyperglycemia in another study [50]. Transient anogenital burning or tingling may occur with intravenous administration of dexamethasone and can be distressing if the patient is not warned of such a possibility [90]. Hiccups, nocturia, and diminished sense of smell and taste have also been reported as complications of corticosteroids [8, 91, 92].

Another potential hazard of steroid use is the development of a withdrawal syndrome during the steroid taper. Steroid pseudorheumatism is the most common withdrawal syndrome and is heralded by the onset of diffuse arthralgias and myalgias mimicking rheumatoid arthritis. These symptoms may be debilitating, but there are usually few physical findings. Either reintroduction of low-dose corticosteroids followed by a slower taper or treatment with aspirin or other nonsteroidal anti-inflammatory agents may result in improvement [11]. Amatruda and colleagues [93] described a steroid withdrawal syndrome which may include lethargy, headache, dizziness, anorexia, and nausea. These symptoms may confuse the clinician by suggesting worsening of the underlying brain tumor [11].

Due to the fact that dexamethasone results in the potent induction of specific cytochrome P450 (CYP450) isozymes (CYP3A4; CYP2C8; CYP2C9), there is a potential for significant drug interactions with other agents metabolized by this system.

Bevacizumab Therapy

Bevacizumab is a recombinant humanized monoclonal antibody that binds all isoforms of vascular endothelial growth factor (VEGF) [94], a protein which is central to vascular proliferation and permeability. While the precise mechanism is not yet known, competing theories on the action of bevacizumab include either direct suppression of angiogenesis or normaliziation of dysmorphic vessels within tumors [95].

With bevacizumab therapy, MR imaging is often rapidly and dramatically changed, and interpretation thereof may be challenging. Whereas anti-angiogenic therapy targets the vasculature, the blood–brain barrier is altered, as well as gadolinium and fluid extravasation. As such, contrast enhancement and peritumoral FLAIR hyperintensity decrease on MRI, yet tumors may still progress in a non-enhancing fashion [96].

While bevacizumab received an accelerated approval for recurrent glioblastoma in 2009 [97] based on two positive phase II trials [98], subsequent large phase III studies of bevacizumab in newly diagnosed glioblastoma failed to demonstrate overall survival advantage over standard therapy alone [99, 100]. Nonetheless, many clinicians still use bevacizumab for glioblastoma, not only for the benefit of progression-free survival (which was borne out in the aforementioned trials), but also for the purpose of reducing tumor-associated edema. While the latter has not been studied directly in trials, a surrogate marker of edema reduction was reported in several clinical trials where average dose of corticosteroids was decreased in bevacizumab-treated patients. In general practice, many neuro-oncologists use bevacizumab for the reduction of neurological symptoms from brain tumors and brain tumor-associated edema.

On the whole, bevacizumab is felt to have a reduced side effect profile when compared to corticosteroids, though still may cause adverse events, some life-threatening. Potential adverse events include both intra- and extracrial hemorrhage, thromboembolic events, hypertension, proteinuria, wound dehiscence, and others. For a more complete discussion of bevacizumab adverse events, refer to the chapter on complications of targeted agents, Chap. 16.

Emergency Therapy of Brain Edema and Increased Intracranial Pressure

Hyperventilation

Immediate treatment of brain edema and increased intracranial pressure (ICP) may occasionally be necessary to prevent death or cerebral herniation. The methods available for such treatment are outlined in Table 21.1.

Hyperventilation is the most rapidly effective technique available for decreasing ICP. Hyperventilation decreases the partial pressure of carbon dioxide (pCO_2) which causes cerebral vasoconstriction in undamaged areas of the brain and a consequent decrease in cerebral blood volume and ICP. Intracranial pressure decreases within 30 s of lowering pCO_2 and remains low for 15–20 min but usually returns to the original level by 1 h [101]. Usually, the patient is intubated and is ventilated to decrease the pCO_2 to 25–30 mm Hg. The patient must be monitored carefully, as mechanical ventilation may occasionally increase ICP and patients with brain lesions are especially susceptible to this effect [102].

Osmotherapy

The mechanism by which hyperosmolar agents lower ICP remains a matter of dispute [103, 104]. At least part of the explanation is the ability of these agents to create an osmotic gradient between the blood and that part of the brain with an intact blood–brain barrier driving the movement of water from the extracellular space to the site of the higher osmolarity in the blood. The agent most commonly used for osmotherapy is mannitol, which is usually given as 20–25% solution in a 0.5- to 2.0-g/kg intravenous bolus over 10–20 min. Mannitol is effective within minutes, and the effect is sustained for several hours [105–107]. If there is clinical worsening after initial improvement, smaller intravenous boluses of mannitol may be administered, but repeated doses of mannitol may cause a rebound increase in ICP, especially in patients with vasogenic brain edema [30]. There is also some evidence to suggest that the combination of mannitol and a loop diuretic such as furosemide produces a more significant and sustained decline in ICP, although furosemide has no role in the chronic management of tumor-related edema [108]. Varying concentrations of intravenous sodium chloride (e.g. hypertonic saline) are also used to reduce intracranial pressure through osmotic gradient formation.

High-Dose Steroid Therapy

In patients with cerebral herniation, plateau waves, or signs of increased ICP, an intravenous bolus of dexamethasone (e.g., 40–100 mg) followed by doses of 40–100 mg/d may

Table 21.1 Emergency treatment of cerebral herniation

Therapy	Dosage or procedure	Onset (duration) of action
Hyperventilation (minutes)	Lower $pCO2$ to 25–30 mm Hg	Seconds
Osmotherapy	Mannitol, 0.5–2.0 g/kg (IV) over 15 min followed by 25-g booster doses (IV) as needed	Minutes (hours)
Corticosteroids	Dexamethasone 100 mg IV push followed by 40–100 mg every 24 h depending on symptoms	Hours (days)

Used with permission of Oxford University Press from Posner [8: 51]

be effective in reversing brain herniation [8]. The addition of furosemide (40–120 mg intravenously) to the steroid dose may be better than corticosteroids alone [109]. Similarly, bevacizumab may be used to reduce cerebral edema causing raised intracranial pressure. Other available methods of lowering ICP such as barbiturate anesthesia and hypothermia are reviewed in detail elsewhere [106]. With the above-mentioned emergency therapies, most patients herniating from the effects of a brain tumor stabilize and improve.

Seizures

Epidemiology and Pathogenesis

Seizures are common in patients with primary brain tumors. The frequency of epilepsy varies with the tumor type. Vertosick and colleagues reported that >80% of patients with low-grade gliomas have epilepsy [110], whereas the reported prevalence of epilepsy in glioblastoma ranges from 30 to 50% [111], Lieu and colleagues reported epilepsy in 40% of meningiomas [112], and Hochberg and colleagues reported epilepsy in 20% of patients with primary CNS lymphoma [113].

In a series of patients receiving chemotherapy for supratentorial tumors (nearly all gliomas), Hildebrand and colleagues found that 78% of 234 patients had epilepsy [114]. In 86% of the patients with epilepsy, the epilepsy was an early manifestation of the disease and usually the presenting manifestation. In only 14% did the epilepsy begin with malignant transformation of the glioma. Seizures were clinically characterized as focal, focal with secondary generalization and generalized. Focal seizures alone were more common late in the course of the disease.

The cause for this high rate of seizures in brain tumor patients may be related to neoplastic astrocytes. While normal astrocytes take up extracellular glutamate, glioma cells have been reported to release excitotoxic levels of glutamate [115, 116], which has been hypothesized as a mechanism for tissue invasion and genesis of seizures [117, 118]. Furthermore, this report indicates that the anticonvulsants valproate, phenytoin, and gabapentin decreased the calcium-mediated glutamate release by astrocytes and decreased seizures as well. Whether glutamate antagonists could have a clinical anti-neoplastic role as demonstrated in animal models by Takano and coworkers [117], or serve as an antiepileptic for patients with brain tumors, is unknown.

Since seizures are associated with increased CNS blood flow, they may significantly increase ICP and potentially lead to a herniation syndrome. Furthermore, seizures in patients with primary brain tumors are more likely to result in a post-ictal neurological deficit (Todd's paralysis) [8, 119, 120]. Status epilepticus is rare in patients with brain tumors but can occur and has an associated mortality of 6–35% [8, 121].

Symptomatic Treatment

Since patients with brain tumors and seizures have a high risk of recurrence of seizures, treatment of these patients with AEDs is warranted. The selection of a particular anticonvulsant requires consideration of individual patient and drug factors as well as the other types of therapy the patient is receiving. Many of the older anticonvulsants either induce cytochrome P450 (CYP450) enzymes (phenytoin, carbamazepine, oxcarbamazepine, phenobarbital) or inhibit CYP450 enzymes (valproic acid). Thus, there is a potential for significant drug interactions or altered metabolism in brain tumor patients who are receiving anti-neoplastic drugs metabolized by the same enzymes. In fact, changes in the plasma levels of chemotherapeutic drugs that could be clinically significant have been observed (Table 21.2)

Table 21.2 Influence of enzyme-inducing anti-seizure drugs on the total body clearance of intravenously administered chemotherapeutic agents in cancer patients

Anticancer agent	Infusion time (h)	Dose (mg/m^2)		Total body clearance^a (l/h/m^2)		Difference (%)	Ref.
		−EIASD	+EIASD	−EIASD	+EIASD		
Etoposide	6.0	320–500	320–500	0.80	1.42	76.9	110
Irinotecan	1.5	112–125	411	18.8	29.7	58.0	111
Paclitaxel	3.0	240	240	4.76	9.75	104.8	112
Teniposide	4.0	200	200	0.78	1.92	146.2	113
Topotecan	0.5	2.0	2.0	20.8	30.6	47.1	112
Vincristine^b	0.25	2.0	2.0	34.1	55.5	62.6	114

^{a}Mean or median values
^{b}Dose and clearance values are not normalized to body surface area
Adapted with permission from Mrugala MM, Batchelor TT, Supko JG. Delivering anticancer drugs to brain tumors. In: Chabner BA, Longo DL, eds. Cancer Chemotherapy and Biotherapy, 4th ed. Philadelphia: Lippincott–Raven; 2005: 484–501

[122–126]. When available, blood levels of AEDs should be monitored, as many patients with brain tumors are also receiving other medications such as dexamethasone which may cause AED levels to fluctuate.

Since many of the newer AEDs (gabapentin, lacosamide, lamotrigine, levetiracetam, pregabalin, tiagibine, topiramate, zonisamide) do not induce the CYP450 system, these drugs are attractive options for brain tumor patients. To date, few studies have been performed to evaluate the efficacy and safety of these newer agents in patients with brain tumors. Levetiracetam is the most studied with three prospective, non-randomized studies demonstrating efficacy and acceptable safety, with the most notable adverse events of cognitive and psychiatric effects [127–129]. Further, Lim and colleagues randomized 29 patients treated with phenytoin to either continue phenytoin or switch to levetiracetam after craniotomy, and found that switching to levetiracetam was safer and resulted in fewer (but not significantly) seizures [130]. Only one randomized trial of non-enzyme-inducing seizure medications has been performed to date by Rossetti and colleagues, evaluating the use of either levetiracetam or pregabalin for the treatment of brain tumor-related epilepsy [131]. In this non-comparative, open-label study, the authors found that both levetiracetam and pregabalin were efficacious and safe for brain tumor-related epilepsy.

One controversial line of retrospective study is also worth mentioning: There may be a potential survival advantage of brain tumor patients whose seizures are treated with various AEDs. Weller and colleagues performed a subgroup analysis of the phase III European Organization for Research and Treatment of Cancer (EORTC) study of temozolomide for glioblastoma and reported an overall survival advantage with the use of valproic acid. However, this was an unplanned and underpowered subgroup analysis [132]. A retrospective analysis of subjects in the Nort Central Cancer Treatment Group suggested that treatment with enzyme-inducing seizure medications correlated with prolonged survival [133]. Additional prospective work is needed to better understand the interaction between AEDs and survival of brain tumor patients.

Treatment of gliomas with anti-neoplastic therapy can reduce the incidence of seizures. In an EORTC trial of early versus delayed radiotherapy in the management of low-grade gliomas, 25% of patients who had received early radiotherapy had seizures at one year versus 41% for those who did not receive early radiotherapy ($p = 0.03$); the prevalence of seizures was the same at diagnosis [134]. Hildebrand and coworkers reported that 56% were on monotherapy, 28% were on a combination of two AEDs, and 12% were on three AEDs. Additionally, there has been a report of a patient with an oligodendroglioma-induced epilepsy that was refractory to 14 anticonvulsants but responded to temozolomide [135].

Prophylactic Treatment

Although as noted above, many patients with primary brain tumors have seizures, the question often arises as to whether primary brain tumor patients without seizures should be placed on prophylactic AEDs. A meta-analysis of four randomized trials of seizure prophylaxis revealed no evidence of reduction in the frequency of first seizures in patients receiving prophylactic anticonvulsants [136]. As such, the potential benefit of prophylactic AED therapy with the studied drugs may not outweigh the risk of side effects in these patients, which include those commonly seen in any seizure patient, as well as some unique or far more common and serious in primary brain tumor patients. On the whole, available data suggest that brain tumor patients experience a higher frequency of AED complications (20–40% of patients) compared to the general population [136]. In six studies reporting AED side effects, 24% (5–38%) of brain tumor patients experienced adverse effects severe enough to warrant discontinuation of the drug. Complications included rash (14%); nausea or vomiting (5%); encephalopathy (5%); myelosuppression (3%); ataxia, increased liver enzymes or gum pain (5%) [136, 137]. A side effect worthy of special mention in patients with brain tumors is the Stevens–Johnson syndrome, which has been reported in patients on phenytoin and, less frequently, carbamazepine who are also receiving cranial radiation while on a decreasing dose of corticosteroids [6]. An additional consideration against prophylactic AED therapy is the interaction of certain AEDs with the CYP450 system and metabolism of chemotherapeutic agents, as discussed above. Finally, Klein and coworkers reported that AEDs were associated with six times the risk of reduced psychomotor speed and attention/executive dysfunction in patients who had undergone focal radiotherapy [138].

Based on the overall analysis of insufficient first-seizure reduction compared to potential side effects, the American Academy of Neurology (AAN) published a practice parameter in 2000 advising against the use of prophylactic AEDs. However, many clinicians still report treating brain tumor patients with prophylactic AEDs. In a survey of physicians in one state, 55% of the neurologists and 81% of the neurosurgeons prescribed prophylactic AEDs to brain tumor patients [139]. Since more clinically tolerable AEDs with less drug interaction have come into practice, no subsequent survey has been performed.

Perioperative seizure prophylaxis following craniotomy for tumor resection is generally considered as a separate category from long-term seizure prophylaxis in brain tumor patients. A prospective, randomized trial evaluated the risk of perioperative seizure either with or without prophylactic phenytoin therapy. Whereas the risk of seizures was quite low in both groups, the authors suggested that prophylactic phenytoin may not be necessary [140]. Further, two retrospective studies compared the reported incidence of perioperative seizures on levetiracetam prophylaxis versus the expected incidence without prophylactic AED, finding that perioperative levetiracetam prophylaxis was safe and effective [141, 142]. Finally, in a head-to-head comparison, Iuchi and colleagues prospectively randomized patients to either levetiracetam or phenytoin and found that levetiracetam lowered the incidence of postoperative seizures significantly more so than phenytoin [143]. In addition, the AAN has also issued a guideline that it is appropriate to taper and discontinue anticonvulsants after the first postoperative week in brain tumor patients who have not had a seizure, who are medically stable, and who are experiencing anticonvulsant-related side effects [136].

Non-convulsive Status Epilepticus

It is well established that brain tumors can cause seizures and non-convulsive status epilepticus. A single-institution review identified that, of 259 patients with an ICD-9 brain tumor diagnosis who underwent electroencephalogram (EEG), 2% were diagnosed with non-convulsive status epilepticus [144]. Treatment resolved the non-convulsive status epilepticus in 92% of those individuals, with accompanying clinical improvement in 75% of patients. Notably, the EEG may not always be helpful in establishing a definitive diagnosis of non-convulsive status epilepticus, which can only be made at times if the patient awakens following the administration of AEDs [145]. Interestingly, it has also been shown that non-convulsive status epilepticus can cause transient abnormal contrast-enhancing cortical lesions that could be confused with a brain tumor [146]. This information reinforces the fact that clinicians should maintain a high suspicion for non-convulsive status epilepticus in brain tumor patients with altered mental status, as this may represent a reversible cause.

Cognitive Effects of Brain Tumors

One of the hallmarks of brain tumors is cognitive dysfunction, which may be either acute and temporary or chronic and progressive. Cognitive dysfunction may result from the tumor itself, tumor-directed therapy, delirium, non-convulsive status epilepticus, medications, depression, or fatigue. Interestingly, in addition to location-specific dysfunction of a primary brain tumor and its therapies, the biology of the tumor itself may play a role in cognitive decline. A recent study revealed glioma grade to be an independent predictor of cognitive performance for certain locations of tumor, without regard to therapies delivered [147].

The potential neurotoxicity and cognitive effect of anti-tumor therapy is of great consideration when treating patients. This is especially true in patients with low-grade gliomas, who have a relatively longer prognosis. Reports are mixed on the cognitive effects of surgery, mostly based on small and observational studies. While some reports have demonstrated decline in short-term perioperative cognitive function, including domains such as memory, attention, and naming after surgery in eloquently located gliomas [148], others have suggested no such hazard [149]. Longer-term follow-up after surgical resection in eloquent areas is clearer, though, and overall suggests improvement in verbal memory after surgery for low-grade gliomas [150, 151].

Data are also sparse for the cognitive effects of chemotherapy for primary brain tumors. Prabhu et al. [152] evaluated the cognitive effects of adding procarbazine, lomustine, and vincristine chemotherapy to radiotherapy in a large, randomized trial among patients with low-grade gliomas. Performing the Mini-Mental State Examination (MMSE) at various intervals until five years post-therapy, they found no significant difference between patients receiving radiation alone or radiation followed by chemotherapy. Further, both groups had a significant improvement in MMSE over time. Among glioblastoma patients treated with temozolomide both concurrent and adjuvant to cranial irradiation, cognitive performance was stable after six months of therapy for those with stable tumors [153]. For treatment with bevacizumab, data are mixed. In the two large, phase III randomized trials evaluating the addition of bevacizumab to up-front glioblastoma therapy, neurocognitive findings were contradictory between trials [99, 100], with greater deterioration reported in patients treated with bevacizumab in RTOG 0825 than in AVAglio. Laboratory research has shown that bevacizumab may reduce the synaptic plasticity in hippocampi, elucidating a potential mechanism of cognitive decline with this drug [154]. Consensus guidelines now exist for further research on cognitive impairment related to chemotherapy for patients with all cancers [155].

Information about cognitive function and radiation therapy is clearer and more robust; cognitive deficits are one of the most common delayed-onset adverse effect of radiation [156]. Patients receiving brain radiotherapy commonly complain of fatigue in the hours following each treatment. Brain edema commonly develops subacutely following brain radiotherapy, especially in the case of stereotactic radiosurgery [157]. Later, patients suffer with various neurocognitive deficits at a far greater rate than similar patients without radiotherapy [158, 159]. These may occur reversibly weeks to months after radiation, or irreversibly and progressively months to years after radiation. In adults who receive radiotherapy, the most common domains to be affected include executive function, information processing speed, novel problem solving, verbal and spatial memory, and attention [159–161]. In survivors of childhood brain tumors who receive radiation, the greatest concern is long-term intelligence quotient impairment and impaired learning [162]. Notably, recent studies of proton therapy for the treatment of childhood brain tumors, in lieu of more common photon therapy, showed no evidence for cognitive decline [163, 164]. Further research on this radiation source is under way.

While the mechanisms underlying radiation-induced neurotoxicity are incompletely understood, recent studies have suggested that a critical event is injury to neural precursor cells. In both animal and human studies, hippocampal injury has been reported to be a major cause of cognitive dysfunction [165, 166]. Furthermore, neurogenesis, which is known to occur in the hippocampus of the adult [167], can be inhibited by both irradiation [168] and corticosteroids [169]. The vulnerability of these proliferating neural precursor cells may account for the deleterious cognitive effects of radiation [170–172]. Preliminary studies of hippocampal-sparing radiation have demonstrated early, promising findings with regard to preserved cognition without deleterious effect on prognosis or local tumor control [173–176]. There may be other methods to prevent radiation-induced injury to hippocampal neurogenesis as well. There is increasing evidence that radiation-induced inhibition of neurogenesis may relate, in part, to hippocampal inflammation [177, 178]. Monje et al. [177] observed that the concurrent administration of indomethacin with radiation reduced the inhibition of neurogenesis in animal models. Similarly, study of PPAR alpha and gamma antagonists, as well as RAS blockers, has demonstrated reduction of radiation-induced inflammation and improvement in cognitive status and neurogenesis [179].

Pharmacologic therapies have been tried to prevent or reverse cognitive decline related to brain tumor therapy. A placebo-controlled, phase III trial of the acetylcholinesterase inhibitor donepezil in 198 patients ≥ 6 months after partial or whole brain irradiation demonstrated no significant improvement in the primary composite cognitive score outcome after 24 weeks of therapy, but did show significant improvement in several cognitive subscores including memory, motor speed, and dexterity [180]. Notably, individuals with worse pretreatment impairment received the most benefit from this therapy. Another placebo-controlled trial studied the glutamate receptor inhibitor memantine concurrently with whole brain radiation and continued treatment for 24 weeks [181]. Similar to the prior study, the relative improvement (less post-radiation decline) seen in the treatment group lacked statistical significance, though improvement in secondary outcomes was noted including time to cognitive decline as well as function in several cognitive domains. Finally, the effects of alpha tocopherol (vitamin E) on neuroprotection were studied in a small, non-randomized, open-label, phase II study of individuals with unilateral or bilateral temporal lobe radiation necrosis [182]. While this study showed significant improvement in the treatment arm in global cognitive ability and memory after one year of treatment, it was not powered for such comparison and thus further study is necessary.

Outside of treatment-related effects, delirium (also referred to as encephalopathy in neurology literature) is a common cause of acute and reversible cognitive decline in brain tumor patients. Delirum in elderly patients has been associated with an increased risk of death after hospitalization and an increased risk of institutionalization [183]. In a meta-analysis of over 16,000 critically ill patients, delirium was associated with a significantly increased risk of in-hospital mortality [184]. Studies in cancer patients have shown brain tumors to be a major contributor to delirium (21–42%) [185–187]. While identification and treatment of any concurrent cause of delirium (e.g., infection, metabolic disturbance) is performed, antipsychotics are the most commonly used therapy to treat the agitation, sleep-wake cycle disturbance, and hallucinations of delirium, and to hasten recovery [188].

Medications may also cause altered mental status. While corticosteroids are a well-known cause of confusion and occasional psychosis, these drugs may also cause acute memory impairment, possibly through inhibition of blood flow to the medial temporal lobe [189]. Healthy subjects were injected with stress doses of hydrocortisone (25 mg) and underwent declarative memory testing and blood flow measurements using cranial PET studies. The cortisone induced a significant reduction in blood flow to the right posterior medial temporal lobe, a region associated with successful verbal retrieval. The cortisone also significantly impaired word recall in these subjects. The authors concluded that the impaired recall could be due to the impaired blood flow. This study is of interest to physicians and patients with brain tumors because of the widespread use of corticosteroids in such patients to control cerebral edema.

Depression is a major concern in patients with brain tumors, and may contribute to cognitive decline. One prospective cohort study of 155 glioma patients diagnosed 20% of patients with depression within the first 8 months after diagnosis, with the highest risk in those with severe functional impairment or with a past history of depression [175]. Another study identified that asking depression symptom inventory questions of healthcare proxies yielded increased information and reliability, emphasizing the importance of collateral information in caring for individuals with brain tumors [176]. In another, longitudinal study of 598 malignant glioma patients, physicians diagnosed depression using DSM-IV criteria in 15% of the study subjects in the early postoperative period. However, 93% of these patients reported symptoms of depression during this period. At follow-up intervals of 3 months and 6 months, physicians reported depression in 22% of patients while 90% of patients reported symptoms of depression [137]. These observations suggest that depression may be underdiagnosed and, hence, undertreated, in the brain tumor patient population. Of significant concern is that in this study, subjects who were depressed had a shorter survival compared to those patients who did not report symptoms of depression. Even when physicians diagnose depression in brain tumor patients, there is a reluctance to treat. Only 29.7% of newly diagnosed and 60% of follow-up brain tumor patients who were *diagnosed* as depressed by their physicians were prescribed antidepressant medications. Remarkably, only 15% of brain tumor patients who reported depressive symptoms were prescribed antidepressant medications by their healthcare providers [137]. This underscores the importance of a thorough psychiatric history in all brain tumor patients, early referral to a psychiatrist or to a support group as appropriate, and the use of antidepressant medications when indicated.

Finally, fatigue from brain tumors and their therapy may also play an important role in cognitive dysfunction and is one of the most highly reported symptoms among brain tumor patients [190, 191]. As such, several groups have studied the effects of stimulants in this setting. Methylphenidate has been studied in cancer patients with evidence of benefit [192–194], as well as in brain tumor patients specifically, with preliminary evidence pointing toward improvement in cognition and functional status, though definitive studies have not yet been performed [195]. Modafinil was also studied in a randomized, placebo-controlled, crossover study for primary brain tumor patients and found no significant difference between the treatment and placebo arms. This study had slow accrual and poor subject retention due to medication side effects [196]. Similarly, a phase II, double-blind, placebo-controlled trial of armodafinil was performed, enrolling 54 patients, and finding no significant difference in fatigue between groups [197]. Notably, those with greater fatigue at enrollment realized the most improvement in fatigue and quality of life in the armodafinil arm. Finally, a randomized trial of modafinil versus methylphenidate in 24 patients treated for four weeks found evidence of improvement in processing speed and executive function with either treatment, but inconsistent and non-significant results between groups [198]. To date, the data remain inconclusive with regard to stimulant medications and their effect on fatigue or cognitive dysfunction. While use of these medications may be reasonable on a patient-by-patient basis, it should be noted that modafinil and armodafinil are metabolized by the P450 system and therefore may affect chemotherapeutic

Conclusion

Brain edema, seizures, and cognitive dysfunction are frequently encountered complications of brain tumors that result in increased morbidity and mortality. Medical management of these processes can result in symptomatic improvement and lead to a better quality of life in these patients.

Steroids are the mainstay of therapy for brain edema associated with brain tumors and lead to symptomatic improvement in 70–80% of patients. Due to the significant deleterious effects associated with corticosteroids, however, they should be used in the smallest effective dose for the shortest time possible. Bevacizumab, a VEGF-targeted therapy, may be used in conjunction with corticosteroids to reduce tumor-associated edema, or even with the intention of weaning corticosteroids altogether.

Seizures will occur in a large proportion of patients with brain tumors and are usually simple partial or complex partial in variety. AEDs should be administered after a first seizure, but are not routinely prescribed for brain tumor patients without a history of seizures. Whereas older AEDs may have deleterious effects that may increase morbidity and the potential for clinically significant drug interactions in patients with brain tumors, this is not the case with newer AEDs. As such, when an AED is required, newer agents associated with less adverse events and no effect on the CYP450 system should be considered.

Cognitive side effects of treatment or the underlying tumor are prevalent and have a major deleterious impact on quality of life. The use of corticosteroids at the lowest dose necessary and for the shortest time possible may lower the frequency of steroid-induced cognitive impairment. Depression is underdiagnosed and undertreated in the primary brain tumor patient population. A thorough psychiatric history and early referral for appropriate patients to mental health professionals are critical elements in the overall management of brain tumor patients. Data remain inconclusive for improvement of treatment-associated cognitive decline with acetylcholinesterase inhibitors, glutamate receptor antagonists, or stimulant medications. Improved understanding of the biological basis of radiation-induced and chemotherapy-induced neurotoxicity may allow opportunities to study novel methods of prevention.

References

1. Jain RK, di Tomaso E, Duda DG, Loeffler JS, Sorensen AG, Batchelor TT. Angiogenesis in brain tumours. Nat Rev Neurosci. 2007;8(8):610–22.

2. Batchelor TT, Sorensen AG, di Tomaso E, Zhang WT, Duda DG, Cohen KS, et al. AZD2171, a pan-VEGF receptor tyrosine kinase inhibitor, normalizes tumor vasculature and alleviates edema in glioblastoma patients. Cancer Cell. 2007;11(1):83–95.

3. Reichman HR, Farrell CL, Del Maestro RF. Effects of steroids and nonsteroid anti-inflammatory agents on vascular permeability in a rat glioma model. J Neurosurg. 1986;65(2):233–7.

4. Shivers RR, Edmonds CL, Del Maestro RF. Microvascular permeability in induced astrocytomas and peritumor neuropil of rat brain. A high-voltage electron microscope-protein tracer study. Acta Neuropathol. 1984;64(3):192–202.

5. Yamada KUY, Hayakawa T, et al. Effects of methylprednisolone on peritumoral brain edema. A quantitative autoradiographic study. J Neurosurg. 1983;59:612–9.

6. Del Maestro RF, Megyesi JF, Farrell CL. Mechanisms of tumor-associated edema: a review. Can J Neurol Sci. 1990;17(2):177–83.

7. Klatzo I. Presidental address. Neuropathological aspects of brain edema. J Neuropathol Exp Neurol. 1967;26(1):1–14.

8. Posner J. Neurologic complications of cancer. Contemporary Neurology series. Philadelphia: FA Davis; 1995.

9. Rosenblum WI. Biology of disease. Aspects of endothelial Malfunction and function in cerebral microvessels. Lab Invest. 1986;55:252–68.

10. Francis K, Van Beek J, Canova C, Neal JW, Gasque P. Innate immunity and brain inflammation: the key role of complement. Expert Rev Mol Med. 2003;2003:1–19.

11. Weissman DE. Glucocorticoid treatment for brain metastases and epidural spinal cord compression: a review. J Clin Oncol. 1988;(6):543–51.

12. Costello P, Del Maestro R. Human cerebral endothelium: isolation and characterization of cells derived from microvessels of non-neoplastic and malignant glial tissue. J Neurooncol. 1990;8(3):231–43.

13. Criscuolo GR, Merrill MJ, Oldfield EH. Further characterization of malignant glioma-derived vascular permeability factor. J Neurosurg. 1988;69(2):254–62.

14. Long DM. Capillary ultrastructure in human metastatic brain tumors. J Neurosurg. 1979;51:53–8.

15. Silbergeld DL, Ali-Osman F. Isolation and characterization of microvessels from normal brain and brain tumors. J Neurooncol. 1991;11(1):49–55.

16. Zhang RD, Price JE, Fujimaki T, Bucana CD, Fidler IJ. Differential permeability of the blood-brain barrier in experimental brain metastases produced by human neoplasms implanted into nude mice. Am J Pathol. 1992;141(5):1115–24.

17. Machelen MRPK. VEGF in brain tumors. J Neurooncol. 2000;50:109–20.

18. Baba T, Chio CC, Black KL. The effect of 5-lipoxygenase inhibition on blood-brain barrier permeability in experimental brain tumors. J Neurosurg. 1992;77(3):403–6.

19. Black KLHJ, McGillicuddy JE, et al. Increased leukotriene C4 and vasogenic edema surronding brain tumors in humans. Ann Neurol. 1986;19:592–5.

20. Chio CC, Baba T, Black KL. Selective blood-tumor barrier disruption by leukotrienes. J Neurosurg. 1992;77(3):407–10.

21. Ohnishi T, Posner JB, Shapiro WR. Vasogenic brain edema induced by arachidonic acid: role of extracellular arachidonic acid in blood-brain barrier dysfunction. Neurosurgery. 1992;30(4):545–51.

22. Shinonaga M, Chang CC, Suzuki N, Sato M, Kuwabara T. Immunohistological evaluation of macrophage infiltrates in brain tumors. Correlation with peritumoral edema. J Neurosurg. 1988;68(2):259–65.

23. Weaver DD, Winn HR, Jane JA. Differential intracranial pressure in patients with unilateral mass lesions. J Neurosurg. 1982;56(5):660–5.

24. Kofman S, Garvin JS, Nagamani D, Taylor SG 3rd. Treatment of cerebral metastases from breast carcinoma with prednisolone. J Am Med Assoc. 1957;163(16):1473–6.

25. Galicich JH, French LA. Use of dexamethasone in the treatment of cerebral edema resulting from brain tumors and brain surgery. Am Pract Dig Treat. 1961;12:169–74.

26. Heiss JD, Papavassiliou E, Merrill MJ, Nieman L, Knightly JJ, Walbridge S, et al. Mechanism of dexamethasone suppression of brain tumor-associated vascular permeability in rats. Involvement of the glucocorticoid receptor and vascular permeability factor. J Clin Invest. 1996;98(6):1400–8.

27. Andersen C, Astrup J, Gyldensted C. Quantitative MR analysis of glucocorticoid effects on peritumoral edema associated with intracranial meningiomas and metastases. J Comput Assist Tomogr. 1994;18(4):509–18.

28. Hedley-Whyte ET, Hsu DW. Effect of dexamethasone on blood-brain barrier in the normal mouse. Ann Neurol. 1986;19(4):373–7.

29. Chan PH, Fishman RA. The role of arachidonic acid in vasogenic brain edema. Fed Proc. 1984;43(2):210–3.

30. Fishman RA. Cerebrospinal Fluid in Diseases of the Nervous system, ed 2. Philadelphia: Saunders; 1992.

31. Weissman DE, Stewart C. Experimental drug therapy of peritumoral brain edema. J Neurooncol. 1988;6(4):339–42.

32. Nakagawa H, Groothuis DR, Owens ES, Fenstermacher JD, Patlak CS, Blasberg RG. Dexamethasone effects on [125I] albumin distribution in experimental RG-2 gliomas and adjacent brain. J Cereb Blood Flow Metab. 1987;7(6):687–701.

33. Leenders KL, Beaney RP, Brooks DJ, Lammertsma AA, Heather JD, McKenzie CG. Dexamethasone treatment of brain tumor patients: effects on regional cerebral blood flow, blood volume, and oxygen utilization. Neurology. 1985;35(11):1610–6.

34. Sinha S, Bastin ME, Wardlaw JM, Armitage PA, Whittle IR. Effects of dexamethasone on peritumoural oedematous brain: a DT-MRI study. J Neurol Neurosurg Psychiatry. 2004;75(11):1632–5.

35. Peters WP, Holland JF, Senn H, Rhomberg W, Banerjee T. Corticosteroid administration and localized leukocyte mobilization in man. N Engl J Med. 1972;286(7):342–5.

36. van Balkom RH, van der Heijden HF, van Herwaarden CL, Dekhuijzen PN. Corticosteroid-induced myopathy of the respiratory muscles. Neth J Med. 1994;45(3):114–22.

37. Dropcho EJ, Soong SJ. Steroid-induced weakness in patients with primary brain tumors. Neurology. 1991;41(8):1235–9.

38. Lackner TE. Interaction of dexamethasone with phenytoin. Pharmacotherapy. 1991;11(4):344–7.

39. Vecht CJ, Hovestadt A, Verbiest HB, van Vliet JJ, van Putten WL. Dose-effect relationship of dexamethasone on Karnofsky performance in metastatic brain tumors: a randomized study of doses of 4, 8, and 16 mg per day. Neurology. 1994;44(4):675–80.

40. Ruderman NB, Hall TC. Use of glucocorticoids in the palliative treatment of metastatic brain tumors. Cancer. 1965;18:298–306.

41. Lieberman A, LeBrun Y, Glass P, Goodgold A, Lux W, Wise A, et al. Use of high dose corticosteroids in patients with inoperable brain tumours. J Neurol Neurosurg Psychiatry. 1977;40(7):678–82.

42. Renaudin J, Fewer D, Wilson CB, Boldrey EB, Calogero J, Enot KJ. Dose dependency of decadron in patients with partially excised brain tumors. J Neurosurg. 1973;39(3):302–5.

43. Jarden JO, Dhawan V, Moeller JR, Strother SC, Rottenberg DA. The time course of steroid action on blood-to-brain and blood-to-tumor transport of 82Rb: a positron emission tomographic study. Ann Neurol. 1989;25(3):239–45.

44. Alberti E, Hartmann A, Schutz HJ, Schreckenberger F. The effect of large doses of dexamethasone on the cerebrospinal fluid pressure in patients with supratentorial tumors. J Neurol. 1978;217(3):173–81.

45. Crocker EF, Zimmerman RA, Phelps ME, Kuhl DE. The effect of steroids on the extravascular distribution of radiographic contrast material and technetium pertechnetate in brain tumors as determined by computed tomography. Radiology. 1976;119 (2):471–4.

46. Yeung WT, Lee TY, Del Maestro RF, Kozak R, Bennett J, Brown T. Effect of steroids on iopamidol blood-brain transfer constant and plasma volume in brain tumors measured with X-ray computed tomography. J Neurooncol. 1994;18(1):53–60.

47. Weissman DE, Dufer D, Vogel V, Abeloff MD. Corticosteroid toxicity in neuro-oncology patients. J Neurooncol. 1987;5(2): 125–8.

48. Weissman DE, Janjan NA, Erickson B, Wilson FJ, Greenberg M, Ritch PS, et al. Twice-daily tapering dexamethasone treatment during cranial radiation for newly diagnosed brain metastases. J Neurooncol. 1991;11(3):235–9.

49. Green D, Lee MY, Lim AC, Chmiel JS, Vetter M, Pang T, et al. Prevention of thromboembolism after spinal cord injury using low-molecular-weight heparin. Ann Intern Med. 1990;113(8): 571–4.

50. Marshall LF, King J, Langfitt TW. The complications of high-dose corticosteroid therapy in neurosurgical patients: a prospective study. Ann Neurol. 1977;1(2):201–3.

51. Martenson JA Jr, Evans RG, Lie MR, Ilstrup DM, Dinapoli RP, Ebersold MJ, et al. Treatment outcome and complications in patients treated for malignant epidural spinal cord compression (SCC). J Neurooncol. 1985;3(1):77–84.

52. Boston Collaborative Drug Surveillance Program. Acute adverse reactions to prednisone in relation to dosage. Clin Pharmacol Ther. 1972;13:694–8.

53. Lewis GP, Jusko WJ, Graves L, Burke CW. Prednisone side-effects and serum-protein levels. A collaborative study. Lancet. 1971;2(7728):778–80.

54. Batchelor TT, Taylor LP, Thaler HT, Posner JB, DeAngelis LM. Steroid myopathy in cancer patients. Neurology. 1997;48(5): 1234–8.

55. Sieb JP, Gillessen T. Iatrogenic and toxic myopathies. Muscle Nerve. 2003;27(2):142–56.

56. Taylor LPPJ. Steroid myopathy in cancer patients trated with dexamethasone [abstract PP78]. Neurology. 1989; 39(suppl 1):129.

57. Gallagher CG. Respiratory steroid myopathy. Am J Respir Crit Care Med. 1994;150(1):4–6.

58. van Balkom RH, van der Heijden HF, van Moerkerk HT, Veerkamp JH, Fransen JA, Ginsel LA, et al. Effects of different treatment regimens of methylprednisolone on rat diaphragm contractility, immunohistochemistry and biochemistry. Eur Respir J. 1996;9(6):1217–23.

59. Bowyer SL, LaMothe MP, Hollister JR. Steroid myopathy: incidence and detection in a population with asthma. J Allergy Clin Immunol. 1985;76(2 Pt 1):234–42.

60. Lewis DA, Smith RE. Steroid-induced psychiatric syndromes. A report of 14 cases and a review of the literature. J Affect Disord. 1983;5(4):319–32.

61. Wolkowitz DWRV, Weingartner H, et al. Cognitive effects of corticosteroids Am J Psychiatry. 1990;147:1297–303.

62. Falk WE, Mahnke MW, Poskanzer DC. Lithium prophylaxis of corticotropin-induced psychosis. JAMA. 1979;241(10):1011–2.

63. Patten SB, Neutel CI. Corticosteroid-induced adverse psychiatric effects: incidence, diagnosis and management. Drug Saf. 2000; 22(2):111–22.

64. Conn HO, Blitzer BL. Nonassociation of adrenocorticosteroid therapy and peptic ulcer. N Engl J Med. 1976;294(9):473–9.

65. Messer J, Reitman D, Sacks HS, Smith H Jr, Chalmers TC. Association of adrenocorticosteroid therapy and peptic-ulcer disease. N Engl J Med. 1983;309(1):21–4.

66. Carson JL, Strom BL, Schinnar R, Duff A, Sim E. The low risk of upper gastrointestinal bleeding in patients dispensed corticosteroids. Am J Med. 1991;91(3):223–8.

67. Nielsen GL, Sorensen HT, Mellemkjoer L, Blot WJ, McLaughlin JK, Tage-Jensen U, et al. Risk of hospitalization resulting from upper gastrointestinal bleeding among patients taking corticosteroids: a register-based cohort study. Am J Med. 2001;111(7):541–5.

68. Tryba M. Side effects of stress bleeding prophylaxis. Am J Med. 1989;86(6A):85–93.

69. Fadul CE, Lemann W, Thaler HT, Posner JB. Perforation of the gastrointestinal tract in patients receiving steroids for neurologic disease. Neurology. 1988;38(3):348–52.

70. ReMine SG, McIlrath DC. Bowel perforation in steroid-treated patients. Ann Surg. 1980;192(4):581–6.

71. Ambrus JL, Ambrus CM, Mink IB, Pickren JW. Causes of death in cancer patients. J Med. 1975;6(1):61–4.

72. Hughes MA, Parisi M, Grossman S, Kleinberg L. Primary brain tumors treated with steroids and radiotherapy: low CD4 counts and risk of infection. Int J Radiat Oncol Biol Phys. 2005;62(5): 1423–6.

73. Henson JW, Jalaj JK, Walker RW, Stover DE, Fels AO. Pneumocystis carinii pneumonia in patients with primary brain tumors. Arch Neurol. 1991;48(4):406–9.

74. Sepkowitz KA, Brown AE, Telzak EE, Gottlieb S, Armstrong D. Pneumocystis carinii pneumonia among patients without AIDS at a cancer hospital. JAMA. 1992;267(6):832–7.

75. Slivka AWP, Shea WM, et al. Pneumocystis carini pneumonia during steroid taper in patients with primary brain tumors. Am J Med. 1983;94:216–9.

76. Schiff D. Pneumocystis pneumonia in brain tumor patients: risk factors and clinical features. J Neurooncol. 1996;27(3):235–40.

77. Stern A, Green H, Paul M, Vidal L, Leibovici L. Prophylaxis for Pneumocystis pneumonia (PCP) in non-HIV immunocompromised patients. Cochrane Database Syst Rev. 2014;10:CD005590.

78. Sambrook PN. How to prevent steroid induced osteoporosis. Ann Rheum Dis. 2005;64(2):176–8.

79. Dougherty JA. Risedronate for the prevention and treatment of corticosteroid-induced osteoporosis. Ann Pharmacother. 2002; 36(3):512–6.

80. Buckley LM, Leib ES, Cartularo KS, Vacek PM, Cooper SM. Calcium and vitamin D3 supplementation prevents bone loss in the spine secondary to low-dose corticosteroids in patients with rheumatoid arthritis. A randomized, double-blind, placebo-controlled trial. Ann Intern Med. 1996;125(12):961–8.

81. Saag KG, Emkey R, Schnitzer TJ, Brown JP, Hawkins F, Goemaere S, et al. Alendronate for the prevention and treatment of glucocorticoid-induced osteoporosis. Glucocorticoid-induced osteoporosis intervention study group. N Engl J Med. 1998; 339(5):292–9.

82. Wallach S, Cohen S, Reid DM, Hughes RA, Hosking DJ, Laan RF, et al. Effects of risedronate treatment on bone density and vertebral fracture in patients on corticosteroid therapy. Calcif Tissue Int. 2000;67(4):277–85.

83. Warriner AH, Saag KG. Prevention and treatment of bone changes associated with exposure to glucocorticoids. Curr Osteoporos reports. 2013;11(4):341–7.

84. Fast A, Alon M, Weiss S, Zer-Aviv FR. Avascular necrosis of bone following short-term dexamethasone therapy for brain edema. Case report. J Neurosurg. 1984;61(5):983–5.

85. Lukert BP, Raisz LG. Glucocorticoid-induced osteoporosis: pathogenesis and management. Ann Intern Med. 1990;112(5): 352–64.

86. Assouline-Dayan Y, Chang C, Greenspan A, Shoenfeld Y, Gershwin ME. Pathogenesis and natural history of osteonecrosis. Semin Arthritis Rheum. 2002;32(2):94–124.

87. Haddad SF, Hitchon PW, Godersky JC. Idiopathic and glucocorticoid-induced spinal epidural lipomatosis. J Neurosurg. 1991;74(1):38–42.

88. Kaneda A, Yamaura I, Kamikozuru M, et al. Paraplegia as a complication of corticosteroid therapy. J Bone Joint Surg Br. 1985;26:1–14.

89. Russell NA, Belanger G, Benoit BG, Latter DN, Finestone DL, Armstrong GW. Spinal epidural lipomatosis: a complication of glucocorticoid therapy. Can J Neurol Sci. 1984;11(3):383–6.

90. Baharav E, Harpaz D, Mittelman M, Lewinski UH. Dexamethasone-induced perineal irritation. N Engl J Med. 1986;314(8):515–6.

91. Baethge BA, Lidsky MD. Intractable hiccups associated with high-dose intravenous methylprednisolone therapy. Ann Intern Med. 1986;104(1):58–9.

92. LeWitt PA, Barton NW, Posner JB. Hiccup with dexamethasone therapy. Ann Neurol. 1982;12(4):405–6.

93. Amatruda TT Jr, Hurst MM, D'Esopo ND. Certain endocrine and metabolic facets of the steroid withdrawal syndrome. J Clin Endocrinol Metab. 1965;25(9):1207–17.

94. Ferrara N, Hillan KJ, Gerber HP, Novotny W. Discovery and development of bevacizumab, an anti-VEGF antibody for treating cancer. Nat Rev Drug Discovery. 2004;3(5):391–400.

95. Field KM, Jordan JT, Wen PY, Rosenthal MA, Reardon DA. Bevacizumab and glioblastoma: scientific review, newly reported updates, and ongoing controversies. Cancer. 2015;121(7): 997–1007.

96. Taylor J, Gerstner ER. Anti-angiogenic therapy in high-grade glioma (treatment and toxicity). Curr Treat Options Neurol. 2013;15(3):328–37.

97. Cohen MH, Shen YL, Keegan P, Pazdur R. FDA drug approval summary: bevacizumab (Avastin) as treatment of recurrent glioblastoma multiforme. Oncologist. 2009;14(11):1131–8.

98. Jordan JT, Wen PY. Novel chemotherapeutic approaches in adult high-grade gliomas. Cancer Treat Res. 2015;163:117–42.

99. Gilbert MR, Dignam JJ, Armstrong TS, Wefel JS, Blumenthal DT, Vogelbaum MA, et al. A randomized trial of bevacizumab for newly diagnosed glioblastoma. N Engl J Med. 2014;370(8):699–708.

100. Chinot OL, Wick W, Mason W, Henriksson R, Saran F, Nishikawa R, et al. Bevacizumab plus radiotherapy-temozolomide for newly diagnosed glioblastoma. N Engl J Med. 2014;370(8):709–22.

101. Ropper A. Raised intracranial pressure in neurologic disease. Semin Neurol. 1984;4:397–407.

102. Colice G. How to ventilate patients when IC_P elevation is a risk: Monitor pressure, consider hyperventilation therapy. J Crit Illness. 1993;8:1003–20.

103. Donato T, Shapira Y, Artru A, Powers K. Effect of mannitol on cerebrospinal fluid dynamics and brain tissue edema. Anesth Analg. 1994;78(1):58–66.

104. Hartwell RC, Sutton LN. Mannitol, intracranial pressure, and vasogenic edema. Neurosurgery. 1993;32(3):444–50; discussion 50.

105. Ravussin P, Abou-Madi M, Archer D, Chiolero R, Freeman J, Trop D, et al. Changes in CSF pressure after mannitol in patients with and without elevated CSF pressure. J Neurosurg. 1988; 69(6):869–76.

106. Ropper A. Neurological and neurosurgical intensive care. 3rd ed. New York, Raven; 1993.

107. Wise BL, Chater N. The value of hypertonic mannitol solution in decreasing brain mass and lowering cerebro-spinal-fluid pressure. J Neurosurg. 1962;19:1038–43.

108. Pollay M, Fullenwider C, Roberts PA, Stevens FA. Effect of mannitol and furosemide on blood-brain osmotic gradient and intracranial pressure. J Neurosurg. 1983;59(6):945–50.

109. Rottenberg DA, Hurwitz BJ, Posner JB. The effect of oral glycerol on intraventricular pressure in man. Neurology. 1977; 27(7):600–8.

110. Vertosick FT Jr, Selker RG, Arena VC. Survival of patients with well-differentiated astrocytomas diagnosed in the era of computed tomography. Neurosurgery. 1991;28(4):496–501.

111. van Breemen MS, Wilms EB, Vecht CJ. Epilepsy in patients with brain tumours: epidemiology, mechanisms, and management. Lancet Neurol. 2007;6(5):421–30.

112. Lieu AS, Howng SL. Intracranial meningiomas and epilepsy: incidence, prognosis and influencing factors. Epilepsy Res. 2000;38(1):45–52.

113. Hochberg FH, Miller DC. Primary central nervous system lymphoma. J Neurosurg. 1988;68(6):835–53.

114. Hildebrand J, Lecaille C, Perennes J, Delattre JY. Epileptic seizures during follow-up of patients treated for primary brain tumors. Neurology. 2005;65(2):212–5.

115. Ye ZC, Sontheimer H. Glioma cells release excitotoxic concentrations of glutamate. Can Res. 1999;59(17):4383–91.

116. Behrens PF, Langemann H, Strohschein R, Draeger J, Hennig J. Extracellular glutamate and other metabolites in and around RG2 rat glioma: an intracerebral microdialysis study. J Neurooncol. 2000;47(1):11–22.

117. Takano T, Lin JH, Arcuino G, Gao Q, Yang J, Nedergaard M. Glutamate release promotes growth of malignant gliomas. Nat Med. 2001;7(9):1010–5.

118. Tian GF, Azmi H, Takano T, Xu Q, Peng W, Lin J, et al. An astrocytic basis of epilepsy. Nat Med. 2005;11(9):973–81.

119. Jacobs M, Phuphanich S. Seizures in brain metastasis and meningeal carcinomatosis [abstract 373]. In Proceedings of the American Society of clinical oncology, Houston, TX; 1990. p. 96.

120. Weaver S, Forsyth P, Fulton D, et al. A prospective, randomized study of prophylactic anticonvulsants inpatients with primary brain tumors or metastatic brain tumors and without prior seizures. A preliminary analysis of 67 patients [abstract 371P]. Neurology. 1995;45((suppl 4)A):263.

121. Engel J. Seizures and epilepsy. Philadelphia: FA Davis; 1989.

122. Rodman JH, Murry DJ, Madden T, Santana VM. Altered etoposide pharmacokinetics and time to engraftment in pediatric patients undergoing autologous bone marrow transplantation. J Clin Oncol. 1994;12(11):2390–7.

123. Gilbert MR, Supko JG, Batchelor T, Lesser G, Fisher JD, Piantadosi S, et al. Phase I clinical and pharmacokinetic study of irinotecan in adults with recurrent malignant glioma. Clin Cancer Res. 2003;9(8):2940–9.

124. Zamboni WC, Gajjar AJ, Heideman RL, Beijnen JH, Rosing H, Houghton PJ, et al. Phenytoin alters the disposition of topotecan and N-desmethyl topotecan in a patient with medulloblastoma. Clin Cancer Res. 1998;4(3):783–9.

125. Baker DK, Relling MV, Pui CH, Christensen ML, Evans WE, Rodman JH. Increased teniposide clearance with concomitant anticonvulsant therapy. J Clin Oncol. 1992;10(2):311–5.

126. Villikka K, Kivisto KT, Maenpaa H, Joensuu H, Neuvonen PJ. Cytochrome P450-inducing antiepileptics increase the clearance of vincristine in patients with brain tumors. Clin Pharmacol Ther. 1999;66(6):589–93.

127. Maschio M, Dinapoli L, Sperati F, Pace A, Fabi A, Vidiri A, et al. Levetiracetam monotherapy in patients with brain tumor-related epilepsy: seizure control, safety, and quality of life. J Neurooncol. 2011;104(1):205–14.

128. Rosati A, Buttolo L, Stefini R, Todeschini A, Cenzato M, Padovani A. Efficacy and safety of levetiracetam in patients with glioma: a clinical prospective study. Arch Neurol. 2010;67(3): 343–6.

129. Usery JB, Michael LM 2nd, Sills AK, Finch CK. A prospective evaluation and literature review of levetiracetam use in patients with brain tumors and seizures. J Neurooncol. 2010;99(2): 251–60.

130. Lim DA, Tarapore P, Chang E, Burt M, Chakalian L, Barbaro N, et al. Safety and feasibility of switching from phenytoin to levetiracetam monotherapy for glioma-related seizure control following craniotomy: a randomized phase II pilot study. J Neurooncol. 2009;93(3):349–54.

131. Rossetti AO, Jeckelmann S, Novy J, Roth P, Weller M, Stupp R. Levetiracetam and pregabalin for antiepileptic monotherapy in patients with primary brain tumors. A phase II randomized study. Neuro-Oncol. 2014;16(4):584–8.

132. Weller M, Gorlia T, Cairncross JG, van den Bent MJ, Mason W, Belanger K, et al. Prolonged survival with valproic acid use in the EORTC/NCIC temozolomide trial for glioblastoma. Neurology. 2011;77(12):1156–64.

133. Jaeckle KA, Ballman K, Furth A, Buckner JC. Correlation of enzyme-inducing anticonvulsant use with outcome of patients with glioblastoma. Neurology. 2009;73(15):1207–13.

134. van den Bent MJ, Afra D, de Witte O, Ben Hassel M, Schraub S, Hoang-Xuan K, et al. Long-term efficacy of early versus delayed radiotherapy for low-grade astrocytoma and oligodendroglioma in adults: the EORTC 22845 randomised trial. Lancet. 2005;366 (9490):985–90.

135. Ngo L, Nei M, Glass J. Temozolomide treatment of refractory epilepsy in a patient with an oligodendroglioma. Epilepsia. 2006;47(7):1237–8.

136. Glantz MJ, Cole BF, Forsyth PA, Recht LD, Wen PY, Chamberlain MC, et al. Practice parameter: anticonvulsant prophylaxis in patients with newly diagnosed brain tumors. Report of the Quality Standards Subcommittee of the American Academy of Neurology. Neurology. 2000;54(10):1886–93.

137. Chang SM, Parney IF, Huang W, Anderson FA Jr, Asher AL, Bernstein M, et al. Patterns of care for adults with newly diagnosed malignant glioma. JAMA. 2005;293(5):557–64.

138. Klein M, Heimans JJ, Aaronson NK, van der Ploeg HM, Grit J, Muller M, et al. Effect of radiotherapy and other treatment-related factors on mid-term to long-term cognitive sequelae in low-grade gliomas: a comparative study. Lancet. 2002;360(9343):1361–8.

139. Glantz MJ, Cole BF, Friedberg MH, Lathi E, Choy H, Furie K, et al. A randomized, blinded, placebo-controlled trial of divalproex sodium prophylaxis in adults with newly diagnosed brain tumors. Neurology. 1996;46(4):985–91.

140. Wu AS, Trinh VT, Suki D, Graham S, Forman A, Weinberg JS, et al. A prospective randomized trial of perioperative seizure prophylaxis in patients with intraparenchymal brain tumors. J Neurosurg. 2013;118(4):873–83.

141. Zachenhofer I, Donat M, Oberndorfer S, Roessler K. Perioperative levetiracetam for prevention of seizures in supratentorial brain tumor surgery. J Neurooncol. 2011;101(1):101–6.

142. Gokhale S, Khan SA, Agrawal A, Friedman AH, McDonagh DL. Levetiracetam seizure prophylaxis in craniotomy patients at high risk for postoperative seizures. Asian J Neurosurg. 2013;8 (4):169–73.

143. Iuchi T, Kuwabara K, Matsumoto M, Kawasaki K, Hasegawa Y, Sakaida T. Levetiracetam versus phenytoin for seizure prophylaxis during and early after craniotomy for brain tumours: a phase II prospective, randomised study. J Neurol Neurosurg Psychiatry. 2015;86(10):1158–62.

144. Marcuse LV, Lancman G, Demopoulos A, Fields M. Nonconvulsive status epilepticus in patients with brain tumors. Seizure. 2014;23(7):542–7.

145. El Kamar FG, Posner JB. Brain metastases. Semin Neurol. 2004;24(4):347–62.

146. Hormigo A, Liberato B, Lis E, DeAngelis LM. Nonconvulsive status epilepticus in patients with cancer: imaging abnormalities. Arch Neurol. 2004;61(3):362–5.

147. Noll KR, Sullaway C, Ziu M, Weinberg JS, Wefel JS. Relationships between tumor grade and neurocognitive functioning in patients with glioma of the left temporal lobe prior to surgical resection. Neuro-oncology. 2015;17(4):580–7.

148. Santini B, Talacchi A, Squintani G, Casagrande F, Capasso R, Miceli G. Cognitive outcome after awake surgery for tumors in language areas. J Neurooncol. 2012;108(2):319–26.

149. Habets EJ, Kloet A, Walchenbach R, Vecht CJ, Klein M, Taphoorn MJ. Tumour and surgery effects on cognitive functioning in high-grade glioma patients. Acta Neurochir. 2014; 156(8):1451–9.

150. Satoer D, Visch-Brink E, Smits M, Kloet A, Looman C, Dirven C, et al. Long-term evaluation of cognition after glioma surgery in eloquent areas. J Neurooncol. 2014;116(1):153–60.

151. Teixidor P, Gatignol P, Leroy M, Masuet-Aumatell C, Capelle L, Duffau H. Assessment of verbal working memory before and after surgery for low-grade glioma. J Neurooncol. 2007;81(3): 305–13.

152. Prabhu RS, Won M, Shaw EG, Hu C, Brachman DG, Buckner JC, et al. Effect of the addition of chemotherapy to radiotherapy on cognitive function in patients with low-grade glioma: secondary analysis of RTOG 98-02. J Clin Oncol. 2014;32(6):535–41.

153. Hilverda K, Bosma I, Heimans JJ, Postma TJ, Peter Vandertop W, Slotman BJ, et al. Cognitive functioning in glioblastoma patients during radiotherapy and temozolomide treatment: initial findings. J Neurooncol. 2010;97(1):89–94.

154. Fathpour P, Obad N, Espedal H, Stieber D, Keunen O, Sakariassen PO, et al. Bevacizumab treatment for human glioblastoma. Can it induce cognitive impairment? Neuro-oncology. 2014;16 (5):754–6.

155. Tannock IF, Ahles TA, Ganz PA, Van Dam FS. Cognitive impairment associated with chemotherapy for cancer: report of a workshop. J Clin Oncol. 2004;22(11):2233–9.

156. Crossen JR, Garwood D, Glatstein E, Neuwelt EA. Neurobehavioral sequelae of cranial irradiation in adults: a review of radiation-induced encephalopathy. J Clin Oncol. 1994;12(3): 627–42.

157. El Shehaby A, Ganz JC, Reda WA, Hafez A. Temporary symptomatic swelling of meningiomas following gamma knife surgery. Report of two cases. J Neurosurg. 2005;102(Suppl): 293–6.

158. Surma-aho O, Niemela M, Vilkki J, Kouri M, Brander A, Salonen O, et al. Adverse long-term effects of brain radiotherapy in adult low-grade glioma patients. Neurology. 2001;56 (10):1285–90.

159. Douw L, Klein M, Fagel SS, van den Heuvel J, Taphoorn MJ, Aaronson NK, et al. Cognitive and radiological effects of radiotherapy in patients with low-grade glioma: long-term follow-up. Lancet Neurol. 2009;8(9):810–8.

160. Hochberg FH, Slotnick B. Neuropsychologic impairment in astrocytoma survivors. Neurology. 1980;30(2):172–7.
161. Laukkanen E, Klonoff H, Allan B, Graeb D, Murray N. The role of prophylactic brain irradiation in limited stage small cell lung cancer: clinical, neuropsychologic, and CT sequelae. Int J Radiat Oncol Biol Phys. 1988;14(6):1109–17.
162. Mulhern RK, Merchant TE, Gajjar A, Reddick WE, Kun LE. Late neurocognitive sequelae in survivors of brain tumours in childhood. Lancet Oncol. 2004;5(7):399–408.
163. Shih HA, Sherman JC, Nachtigall LB, Colvin MK, Fullerton BC, Daartz J, et al. Proton therapy for low-grade gliomas: Results from a prospective trial. Cancer. 2015;121(10):1712–9.
164. Pulsifer MB, Sethi RV, Kuhlthau KA, MacDonald SM, Tarbell NJ, Yock TI. Early cognitive outcomes following proton radiation in pediatric patients with brain and central nervous system tumors. Int J Radiat Oncol Biol Phys. 2015;93(2):400–7.
165. Sarkissian V. The sequelae of cranial irradiation on human cognition. Neurosci Lett. 2005;382(1–2):118–23.
166. Armstrong CL, Gyato K, Awadalla AW, Lustig R, Tochner ZA. A critical review of the clinical effects of therapeutic irradiation damage to the brain: the roots of controversy. Neuropsychol Rev. 2004;14(1):65–86.
167. Eriksson PS, Perfilieva E, Bjork-Eriksson T, Alborn AM, Nordborg C, Peterson DA, et al. Neurogenesis in the adult human hippocampus. Nat Med. 1998;4(11):1313–7.
168. Raber J, Rola R, LeFevour A, Morhardt D, Curley J, Mizumatsu S, et al. Radiation-induced cognitive impairments are associated with changes in indicators of hippocampal neurogenesis. Radiat Res. 2004;162(1):39–47.
169. Garcia A, Steiner B, Kronenberg G, Bick-Sander A, Kempermann G. Age-dependent expression of glucocorticoid- and mineralocorticoid receptors on neural precursor cell populations in the adult murine hippocampus. Aging Cell. 2004;3(6):363–71.
170. Monje ML, Palmer T. Radiation injury and neurogenesis. Curr Opin Neurol. 2003;16(2):129–34.
171. Kempermann G, Wiskott L, Gage FH. Functional significance of adult neurogenesis. Curr Opin Neurobiol. 2004;14(2):186–91.
172. Redmond KJ, Mahone EM, Terezakis S, Ishaq O, Ford E, McNutt T, et al. Association between radiation dose to neuronal progenitor cell niches and temporal lobes and performance on neuropsychological testing in children: a prospective study. Neuro-oncology. 2013;15(3):360–9.
173. Kim KH, Cho BC, Lee CG, Kim HR, Suh YG, Kim JW, et al. Hippocampus-sparing whole-brain radiotherapy and simultaneous integrated boost for multiple brain metastases from lung adenocarcinoma: early response and dosimetric evaluation. Technol Cancer Res Treat. 2016;15(1):122–9.
174. Lin SY, Yang CC, Wu YM, Tseng CK, Wei KC, Chu YC, et al. Evaluating the impact of hippocampal sparing during whole brain radiotherapy on neurocognitive functions: a preliminary report of a prospective phase II study. Biomed J. 2015;38(5):439–49.
175. Rooney AG, Brown PD, Reijneveld JC, Grant R. Depression in glioma: a primer for clinicians and researchers. J Neurol Neurosurg Psychiatry. 2014;85(2):230–5.
176. Rooney AG, McNamara S, Mackinnon M, Fraser M, Rampling R, Carson A, et al. Screening for major depressive disorder in adults with glioma using the PHQ-9: a comparison of patient versus proxy reports. J Neurooncol. 2013;113(1):49–55.
177. Monje ML, Toda H, Palmer TD. Inflammatory blockade restores adult hippocampal neurogenesis. Science. 2003;302(5651):1760–5.
178. Schnegg CI, Greene-Schloesser D, Kooshki M, Payne VS, Hsu FC, Robbins ME. The PPARdelta agonist GW0742 inhibits neuroinflammation, but does not restore neurogenesis or prevent early delayed hippocampal-dependent cognitive impairment after whole-brain irradiation. Free Radic Biol Med. 2013;61:1–9.
179. Greene-Schloesser D, Moore E, Robbins ME. Molecular pathways: radiation-induced cognitive impairment. Clin Cancer Res. 2013;19(9):2294–300.
180. Rapp SR, Case LD, Peiffer A, Naughton MM, Chan MD, Stieber VW, et al. Donepezil for irradiated brain tumor survivors: a phase iii randomized placebo-controlled clinical trial. J Clin Oncol. 2015;33(15):1653–9.
181. Brown PD, Pugh S, Laack NN, Wefel JS, Khuntia D, Meyers C, et al. Memantine for the prevention of cognitive dysfunction in patients receiving whole-brain radiotherapy: a randomized, double-blind, placebo-controlled trial. Neuro-oncology. 2013;15(10):1429–37.
182. Chan AS, Cheung MC, Law SC, Chan JH. Phase II study of alpha-tocopherol in improving the cognitive function of patients with temporal lobe radionecrosis. Cancer. 2004;100(2):398–404.
183. Witlox J, Eurelings LS, de Jonghe JF, Kalisvaart KJ, Eikelenboom P, van Gool WA. Delirium in elderly patients and the risk of postdischarge mortality, institutionalization, and dementia: a meta-analysis. JAMA. 2010;304(4):443–51.
184. Salluh JI, Wang H, Schneider EB, Nagaraja N, Yenokyan G, Damluji A, et al. Outcome of delirium in critically ill patients: systematic review and meta-analysis. BMJ. 2015;350:h2538.
185. Tuma R, DeAngelis LM. Altered mental status in patients with cancer. Arch Neurol. 2000;57(12):1727–31.
186. McCusker J, Cole M, Abrahamowicz M, Han L, Podoba JE, Ramman-Haddad L. Environmental risk factors for delirium in hospitalized older people. J Am Geriatr Soc. 2001;49(10):1327–34.
187. Sarhill N, Walsh D, Nelson KA, LeGrand S, Davis MP. Assessment of delirium in advanced cancer: the use of the bedside confusion scale. Am J Hosp Palliat Care. 2001;18(5):335–41.
188. Thekdi SM, Trinidad A, Roth A. Psychopharmacology in cancer. Curr psychiatry Rep. 2015;17(1):529.
189. de Quervain DJ, Henke K, Aerni A, Treyer V, McGaugh JL, Berthold T, et al. Glucocorticoid-induced impairment of declarative memory retrieval is associated with reduced blood flow in the medial temporal lobe. Eur J Neurosci. 2003;17(6):1296–302.
190. Osoba D, Aaronson NK, Muller M, Sneeuw K, Hsu MA, Yung WK, et al. Effect of neurological dysfunction on health-related quality of life in patients with high-grade glioma. J Neurooncol. 1997;34(3):263–78.
191. Osoba D, Brada M, Prados MD, Yung WK. Effect of disease burden on health-related quality of life in patients with malignant gliomas. Neuro-oncology. 2000;2(4):221–8.
192. Bruera E, Driver L, Barnes EA, Willey J, Shen L, Palmer JL, et al. Patient-controlled methylphenidate for the management of fatigue in patients with advanced cancer: a preliminary report. J Clin Oncol. 2003;21(23):4439–43.
193. Hanna A, Sledge G, Mayer ML, Hanna N, Einhorn L, Monahan P, et al. A phase II study of methylphenidate for the treatment of fatigue. Support Care Cancer. 2006;14(3):210–5.
194. Sugawara Y, Akechi T, Shima Y, Okuyama T, Akizuki N, Nakano T, et al. Efficacy of methylphenidate for fatigue in advanced cancer patients: a preliminary study. Palliat Med. 2002;16(3):261–3.
195. Meyers CA, Weitzner MA, Valentine AD, Levin VA. Methylphenidate therapy improves cognition, mood, and function of brain tumor patients. J Clin Oncol. 1998;16(7):2522–7.
196. Boele FW, Douw L, de Groot M, van Thuijl HF, Cleijne W, Heimans JJ, et al. The effect of modafinil on fatigue, cognitive functioning, and mood in primary brain tumor patients: a

multicenter randomized controlled trial. Neuro-oncology. 2013;15(10):1420–8.

197. Page BR, Shaw EG, Lu L, Bryant D, Grisell D, Lesser GJ, et al. Phase II double-blind placebo-controlled randomized study of armodafinil for brain radiation-induced fatigue. Neuro-oncology. 2015;17(10):1393–401.

198. Gehring K, Patwardhan SY, Collins R, Groves MD, Etzel CJ, Meyers CA, et al. A randomized trial on the efficacy of methylphenidate and modafinil for improving cognitive functioning and symptoms in patients with a primary brain tumor. J Neurooncol. 2012;107(1):165–74.

Ming Chi and Manmeet S. Ahluwalia

Introduction

Lung cancer is the leading cause of cancer-related mortality in the USA. An estimated 159,260 Americans were projected to die from lung cancer in 2014, accounting for approximately 27% of all cancer deaths [1]. The number of deaths due to lung cancer has increased approximately 3.5% between 1999 and 2012 from 152,156 to 157,499. Whereas the number of deaths among men has reached a plateau, the number is still rising among women, with 86,740 deaths in men and 70,759 in women in 2012. The incidence of lung cancer over the past 37 years has dropped for men (28% decrease), while it has risen for women (98% increase). The rate of new cases for women has peaked in 1998 and now started to decline [2]. This difference is likely due to the lag of 20 years in the prevalence of smoking among women compared to men. African Americans are more likely to develop and die from lung cancer than a person of any other racial or ethnic group.

Approximately 402,326 Americans living today have ever been diagnosed with lung cancer and 82% were 60 years of age or older [2]. Smoking, a main cause of lung cancer, contributes to 80 and 90% of lung cancer deaths in women and men, respectively [3]. Between 2005 and 2010, an average of 130,659 Americans (74,300 men and 56,359 women) died of smoking-attributable lung cancer each year. Exposure to secondhand smoke causes approximately 7330 lung cancer deaths among non-smokers every year [4].

The two major clinicopathologic subtypes of lung cancer include non-small cell lung cancers (NSCLC) and small cell lung carcinoma (SCLC), which account for 85 and 15% of total cases, respectively [5, 6]. Non-small cell lung cancer is further subdivided histologically into squamous cell carcinoma, adenocarcinoma, and large cell carcinoma, although they can coexist in a single tumor. Squamous cell carcinoma and SCLC are strongly associated with cigarette smoking.

Non-small cell lung cancer is staged by the TNM (tumor node metastasis) system and approximately two-thirds of patients with NSCLC have locally advanced or metastatic disease (stage IV) at initial diagnosis. Small cell lung carcinoma is staged either as limited stage or extensive stage based on whether all tumor(s) can be encompassed by a single radiation therapy port or not. About two-thirds of the SCLC cases are extensive-stage disease at the time of diagnosis. Management of SCLC is dependent on stage and incorporates surgery, radiation therapy, chemotherapy, and targeted therapy. The overall 5-year survival is approximately 15% for patients with NSCLC and only about 2% for patients with SCLC [7]. Lung cancer is a frequent cause of neurological complication in these patients most commonly as a result of direct metastases or leptomeningeal disease or indirect paraneoplastic effect of the cancer.

Parenchymal Brain Metastases

Incidence

Parenchymal brain metastases are common in patients with lung cancer and represent the most common neurologic complication of lung cancer. Lung cancer is the most common source cause of brain metastases in adults, accounting for 40–50% of all cases, followed by breast cancer, and melanoma [8–10].

In patients with SCLC, the incidence of brain metastases at diagnosis is 10% (Fig. 22.1a–e) and increases to 20% during therapy, with the cumulative risk at 2 years post-diagnosis of approximately 50% for limited-stage disease and 70% for extensive-stage disease [11–13]. In two

M. Chi (✉)
Atlanta Cancer Care, Northside Hospital, 5670 Peachtree Dunwoody Road, Suite 1100, Atlanta, GA 30342, USA
e-mail: mchi@atlantacancercare.com

M.S. Ahluwalia
9500 Euclid Ave, S73, Cleveland, OH 44195, USA
e-mail: ahluwam@ccf.org

© Springer International Publishing AG 2018
D. Schiff et al. (eds.), *Cancer Neurology in Clinical Practice*,
DOI 10.1007/978-3-319-57901-6_22

large series of patients with SCLC, the lifetime incidence of symptomatic brain metastases was 25 and 40% compared to 3.6 and 5.6% for spinal epidural metastases, 2.2 and 8.6% for leptomeningeal metastases [14, 15]. In one-third of these patients, brain was the only metastatic site, and up to half of these patients are asymptomatic at the time of detection of brain metastases [16].

In patients with NSCLC and brain metastases, half of the cases are discovered/developed upon initial diagnosis whereas half are developed subsequently [17]. With overall improvement of systemic treatment, there has been an increase in the incidence of brain metastases as brain as serve as a sanctuary site. In most series to date, both young age at diagnosis and adenocarcinoma have been recognized as risk factors for developing brain metastases [7].

Treatment

Treatment options for patients with parenchymal brain metastases include surgical resection, whole brain radiotherapy (WBRT), stereotactic radiosurgery, chemotherapy, molecular targeted agents, immunotherapy and supportive measures that include anticonvulsants and corticosteroids. Selection of single or multiple modalities of treatment should be individualized in every patient and is dependent

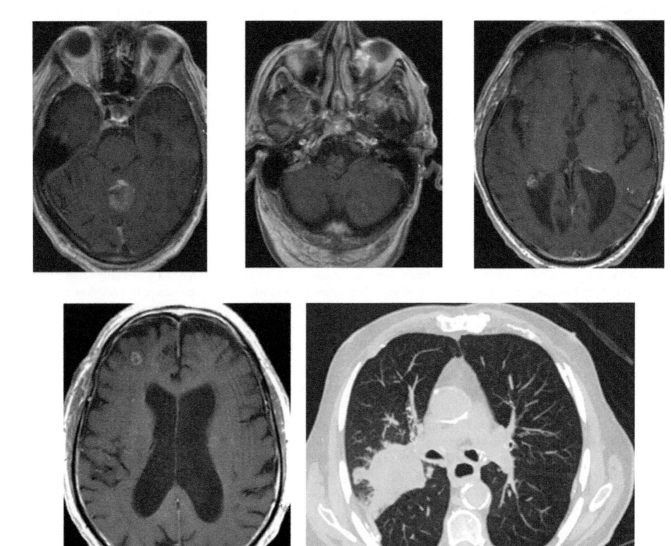

Fig. 22.1 a–d Brain MRI with contrast obtained in an 86-year-old former smoker with a 2-week history of gait unsteadiness revealing multiple peripherally enhancing supratentorial and infratentorial metastases. **e** Subsequent chest CT revealed numerous lung lesions. One dominant spiculated mass in the *right upper lobe* measuring up to 6 cm was biopsied and was consistent with small cell lung cancer

on several factors that include patient characteristics (co-morbidities, age, neurological status), primary tumor characteristics (histology, extent of primary cancer and whether it is controlled), and the brain metastases (size, location, number, prior treatment). Overall survival for lung cancer patients with brain metastases is usually influenced by systemic disease control rather than intracranial process.

Whole Brain Radiation Therapy (WBRT)

WBRT is a common treatment modality for patients with brain metastases, especially those with multiple lesions and is utilized either alone or in combination with other modalities such as stereotactic radiosurgery (SRS), surgery or medical therapies. It is usually delivered as 30–40 Gy over 10–15 fractions [18]. Studies have shown that altered fractionation, extra boost dose to tumor bed, or addition of radiosensitizing agents offered no additional benefits [19]. Neither the use of lower dose nor higher dose over variable time periods resulted in any significant improvement in survival in these patients [20, 21].

Overall, approximately 60% of patients respond to radiotherapy with improvement or stabilization of their symptoms [22]. At least 75% of patients with SCLC show a partial or complete radiographic response compared to about 50% patients with NSCLC [23]. There is time delay for treatment response, with about 50–60% of these patients having a partial response (i.e., at least 50% shrinkage in the tumor) at 6 weeks post-treatment. Usually, small metastases respond better than large lesions and are more likely to regress. The median overall survival after treatment with WBRT is usually 3–9 months [17, 24–26], and patients more often are likely to die of progressive systemic disease than intracranial process.

Surgical Resection

Surgery is usually reserved for patients with NSCLC and with single brain metastases or oligometastases when one single lesion is the cause of impending neurological deficit. Unlike in infiltrative glioma, brain metastases are well demarcated from surrounding tissues and more amenable for resection. A randomized study demonstrated that surgical resection followed by WBRT improves time to recurrence of brain metastases, functional independence, and lower risk of death from neurological complications, compared to WBRT alone [20, 27]. The combination of surgery and WBRT is also superior to surgery alone, in terms of controlling intracranial disease locally and distantly [28]. Favorable prognostic factors for surgical intervention include stable systemic disease, good performance status, and adenocarcinoma among other histology [27, 29]. In contrast, in patients with brain metastases from SCLC, the benefit of resecting solitary lesion is less clear, due to the greater radiosensitivity of SCLC than NSCLC.

With the advent of SRS, it has been shown that combination of SRS and WBRT is equivalent to surgery and WBRT for solitary metastasis. Nevertheless, surgery does offer the advantage of immediate debulking and relief of mass effect and the ability of managing large tumors, whereas the role of SRS has not been well defined for large metastasis (more than 3 cm in size) or a lesion causing midline shift (>1 cm). Surgical resection to remove more than one lesion either during single or staged procedure is less preferred these days, especially with the advancement of SRS [18].

Stereotactic Radiosurgery (SRS)

SRS has been increasingly employed in the management of brain metastases from lung cancer and is indicated in several clinical settings: (1) as primary treatment of single metastasis in addition to surgical resection, (2) as the sole modality of treatment for newly diagnosed solitary or multiple brain metastases (up to three brain metastases), (3) in combination with WBRT for newly diagnosed metastases (up to four brain metastases), (4) and as treatment for recurrent brain metastases [30]. It is delivered in a highly focused single dose to a circumscribed target (maximal diameter 3–3.5 cm) while avoiding the surrounding tissues. Stereotactic radiosurgery is well-suited treatment for metastases due to their circumscribed, round margin. It can also be delivered "hypofractionated," i.e., 30–40 Gy in 3–5 fractions [31]. RTOG 9005 showed that prescription doses of 15, 18, and 24 Gy to the tumor margin were the maximal safe doses for lesions with diameters of 3.1–4.0, 2.1–3.0, and 2.0 cm or less, respectively [32]. The optimal SRS dose for lung cancer patients and lesion sizes is not determined [33, 34].

Compared to surgery, SRS can be used for multiple lesions in single or several sessions, carries lower risk of complications, and is more cost-effective due to its outpatient setting. Studies have shown that it produces equivalent local tumor control when compared to surgery [35], with 12-month local control rates of approximately 90% [36–39]. The disease control rates are better in smaller metastases (<2.0 cm) as compared to larger metastases (>2.0 cm) [34, 38]. In addition, treatment outcomes are also influenced by the total volume of brain metastases rather than simply the number of these lesions [40].

Studies have also evaluated the combination of SRS and other modalities, such as surgery and WBRT. One approach for treatment of single brain metastases is to surgically resect the lesion followed by SRS to the margin of resected cavity. This results in a local control rate of 70–90% [41, 42].

Radiation Therapy Oncology Group (RTOG) 9508 evaluated the combination of WBRT followed by SRS boost compared to WBRT alone for patients with one to three brain metastases [43]. Sixty-four percent of patients had primary lung cancer, and patients were stratified on the number of brain metastases and a brain metastasis prognostic index [recursive partitioning analysis (RPA)]. This study did not demonstrate any survival benefit for all patients treated with combination of SRS and WBRT (median survival time [MST] 6.5 months compared to those treated with WBRT alone (MST of 5.7 months [$p = 0.14$]). However, planned subgroup analysis revealed that patients with solitary brain metastases derived benefit from the combined approach of WBRT and SRS (MST 6.5 vs. 4.9 months, $p = 0.04$). An independent secondary analysis was also reported [44]. This report utilized a disease-specific prognostic index, graded prognostic assessment (GPA), and 84% of patients in this study had a diagnosis of lung cancer. Again, no survival benefit was seen in patients with one to three brain metastases treated with a combinatorial approach of WBRT and SRS. However, patients with GPA score of 3.5–4.0 derived benefit from the addition of SRS to WBRT compared to WBRT alone with MST of 21.0 months versus 10.4 months ($p = 0.05$), and this benefit was independent of the number of brain metastases.

The addition of WBRT to initial local therapy (SRS or surgery) is an area of active ongoing research. The rationale of addition of upfront WBRT is to improve local control and prevent distant intracranial metastases; however, the concern over this strategy lies in long-term, adverse effects on neurocognitive function (NCF) [18]. Two large retrospective studies [45, 46] showed that upfront WBRT after SRS indeed improved local control and reduced distant intracranial metastases, but offered no survival benefit. Five prospective studies have tried to address this question and randomized patients to upfront WBRT versus observation after initial local therapy (radiosurgery or surgery), and more than 50% of the patients on these studies had the diagnosis of lung cancer [47–51]. The addition of upfront WBRT was associated with improved local control and reduced the distant intracranial metastases in all five studies, as well as reduced neurological-related death in two studies [47, 50]. However, no survival benefit was observed across five studies. The Japanese study evaluated NCF using Mini-Mental State Examination (MMSE) and revealed that controlling intracranial disease outweighed neurotoxicity from WBRT in stabilizing NCF [52]. In contrast, one of other studies that used Hopkins Verbal Learning Test (HVLT) at 4-month post-treatment was closed prematurely because an interim analysis revealed NCF at 4 month was significantly worse with the combination of SRS and WBRT compared to the use of SRS alone (median posterior probability decline of 52% vs. 24%) [49]. Similarly, a cooperative group study recently reported worsening cognitive function with the addition of WBRT to SRS, specifically immediate recall and memory and verbal fluency [51].

Whether WBRT can be postponed until disease progression remains to be determined, and individualized treatment decisions are needed based on patients' age, comorbidities, disease status, and overall prognosis. However, based on the emerging evidence, there is decreased use of upfront WBRT in treatment of patients with 1–3 brain metastases and SRS is often the preferred treatment alone.

SRS is also a commonly used therapeutic modality for treatment of brain metastases that have progressed or recurred after WBRT, and the RTOG 9005 trial has established the dose levels for tumors <4 cm and demonstrated good local control [32]. Prognostic factors affecting overall survival with salvage SRS include tumor volume, time between initial diagnosis of primary tumor and development of brain metastasis, performance status and dose of SRS delivered [53–55].

Chemotherapy

In the past, the role of cytotoxic chemotherapy has been limited in the treatment of brain metastases from lung cancer for several reasons: (1) inherent chemoresistance of lung cancer, especially NSCLC; (2) prior exposure to chemotherapy that renders further disease progression and/or metastases less sensitive to chemotherapy, either systemic or intracranial, and (3) limited penetration of water-soluble or large molecular weight compounds through the blood–brain barrier (BBB). There is controversy regarding the impact of BBB on the drug delivery to the brain metastases [18]. When brain metastases reach a certain size, they become associated with BBB disruption, peritumoral edema, and neongiogenesis. This is reflected on brain imaging studies in enhancement of tumor tissue with intravenous contrast [56]. Hence, there is at least a partial breakdown of the BBB.

The brain response rate (RR) to platinum-based regimen for NSCLC patients with brain metastases was 20–50% in those who were treatment naïve compared to 10% in those who had received prior treatment. For SCLC, the brain RR is relatively higher due to its chemosensitivity, 60–85% if previously untreated versus 20–50% if treated [57, 58]. A MST of 4–9 months has been reported in this patient population. In addition, single agent temozolomide, with relevant permeability through BBB, has been extensively studied in patients with brain metastases despite its minimal systemic activity against lung cancer. Response rates of 0–20% have been reported, and therefore, temozolomide is not routinely used in this patient population [59–61].

Optimal sequencing of chemotherapy and radiotherapy for patients with asymptomatic multiple brain metastases remains uncertain. It has been well recognized that administering chemotherapy and radiation concurrently carries higher risks of brain toxicity, especially adverse neurocognitive deficits [62]. As a result, sequential treatments with chemotherapy and radiotherapy are offered for most eligible patients. Until recently medical therapies had only limited role in management of lung cancer brain metastases, and hence, most patients received some form of radiation prior to being managed with medical therapies. One pilot study [63] randomized 48 neurologically asymptomatic patients with synchronous brain metastases into primary chemotherapy (vinorelbine/gemcitabine) followed by RT versus WBRT followed by chemotherapy. It demonstrated close correlation between intracranial and extracranial tumor response and statistically nonsignificant intracranial response rates (28.0% vs. 39.1%). There was no difference in survival between the two arms (9.1 months vs. 9.9 months). However, in the WBRT arm, more patients developed neutropenia and delayed or deferred chemotherapy due to deteriorating performance status. Hence, the authors concluded that use of upfront chemotherapy was a preferred option. Another phase III randomized study of 176 patients [64] evaluated the use of delayed versus upfront concurrent WBRT with chemotherapy (cisplatin/vinorelbine) and showed equivalent response rate and survival benefits. Hence, in select group of patients it is reasonable to pursue primary chemotherapy for patients with asymptomatic brain metastases, reserving WBRT for disease recurrence/progression. This approach has been endorsed by the European Society of Medical Oncology clinical practice guidelines (II, B).

Molecular Targeted Agents

In the past two decades, increasing recognition of specific driver mutations has shifted the treatment strategies for advanced NSCLC from standard chemotherapy toward development of targeted therapies in selected patients. Activating mutations in the epidermal growth factor receptor (EGFR) occur in about 10–15% of NSCLC. A number of studies have investigated gefitinib and erlotinib, tyrosine kinase inhibitors (TKIs) that target EGFR in patients with EGFR-mutation positive NSCLC with brain metastases [65–68]. Response rates of 70–90%, MST of 15–20 months, and intracranial PFS of 6–12 months have been observed in these studies. Erlotinib may have higher intracranial efficacy compared to gefitinib [69], likely due to its higher concentration in cerebrospinal fluid (CSF) [70, 71]. In addition, high-dose pulsatile weekly erlotinib has been used and noted to result in increased CSF concentration and improved intracranial response after treatment failure with standard dose [72–74].

The combination of TKIs with radiotherapy was evaluated in a phase III trial with 126 NSCLC patients where patients were treated either with a combination of WBRT and SRS with erlotinib or temozolomide or placebo [75]. No survival benefit was observed by addition of either TKI or temozolomide to WBRT and SRS. However, the patients were not stratified according to EGFR mutational status in this study. The combination of WBRT and erlotinib was shown to be safe in a phase II study of 40 NSCLC patients with brain metastases, and increase in neurotoxicity was seen [76]. The MST of 11.8 months for the whole cohort was reported in the study. However, the mutant EGFR patients derived more benefit and OS of 19.1 months seen in that group compared to OS of 9.3 months in the wild-type EGFR patients [76].

Limited data exist for anaplastic lymphoma kinase (ALK)-inhibitors for patients with ALK + NSCLC and brain metastases. Brain metastases have been exceptionally frequent in patients with ALK + NSCLC despite their good systemic control, with 35% (120/357) prevalence being reported in a large phase III study [77]. The underlying mechanism is yet to be defined, due to either low CSF concentration [78] or secondary resistance, and there is a study describing an intracranial response to high-dose crizotinib after treatment failure with standard dose [79]. Improved pharmacokinetics with greater CSF concentrations and improved CNS activity has been noted in second-generation ALK inhibitors in several early-phase clinical trials. AP26113 showed intracranial response in four of five ALK+ patients, including one crizotinib-resistant patient [80], and responses in brain metastases have been reported with both LDK378 [81] and CH5424802 [82].

Bevacizumab is a humanized monoclonal antibody that targets the vascular endothelial growth factor (VEGF) and inhibits tumor angiogenesis, and has been used with the combination of chemotherapy for non-squamous NSCLC without hemoptysis, based on two large phase III studies (E4599 [83] and Avail [84]). However, initially there was concern over the use of bevacizumab in the patients with brain metastases due to the risk of development of intracranial hemorrhage (ICH) in these patients. Several retrospective studies tried to address this issue [85–88]. Srivastava and colleagues showed that the rate of spontaneous ICH was higher in patients with brain metastases than those who did not have brain metastases when treated with bevacizumab [85]. However, the rates of symptomatic ICH were not statistically different between the two groups [85]. Several other retrospective studies have shown that bevacizumab did not further increase risk of ICH even for patients with brain metastases [86–88].

Furthermore, prospective studies have evaluated the safety of bevacizumab in patients with brain metastases. The PASSPORT study of 115 patients with treated brain metastases employed a combination of either bevacizumab and chemotherapy as first-line therapy or bevacizumab and erlotinib as second-line therapy [89]. This study confirmed the safety of bevacizumab in this patient population, and no reported grade 2 or higher ICH was seen in the study. Another prospective study showed similar results and confirmed the findings of the PASSPORT study [90]. Bevacizumab has been shown to be safe for patients with symptomatic or active brain metastases in other retrospective reports [91, 92].

Bevacizumab has also been evaluated to treat cerebral radiation necrosis (RN) due to its ability to target VEGF. Cerebral RN is a difficult to treat complication of SRS or WBRT that can lead to continuing neurological decline, and until recently steroids were the main therapy used despite its side effects and limited efficacy in select group of patients. In a study of six NSCLC and five breast cancer patients with brain metastases and RN, use of bevacizumab resulted in reduced steroid dosage in all patients and improved or stabilized RN symptoms in all but one patient [93].

Prophylactic cranial radiation (PCI) is considered standard of care for patients with limited SCLC who achieve complete remission after concurrent chemoradiation in order to prevent brain metastases. This is due to the high prevalence of brain metastases after completion of systemic treatment and the sensitivity of SCLC to RT [94]. This practice is based on several well-conducted randomized studies and meta-analysis that demonstrated significantly reduced cumulative incidence of brain metastases (from 50–60% to 25–30%) and improvement in overall survival (5% survival advantage at 3-year follow-up) [95–97].

Moreover, PCI is advocated in select patients with extensive-stage SCLC patients who have had a response to chemotherapy, based on a randomized phase III study by Slotman et al. [98]. This study showed that PCI lowers risk of symptomatic brain metastases by 73% ($p < 0.001$), with one-year cumulative risk of brain metastases dropped from 40.4 to 14.6% ($p < 0.001$). PCI was associated with improved PFS from 12.0 to 14.7 weeks ($p = 0.02$) and improved OS from 5.4 to 6.7 months ($p = 0.003$).

Studies that evaluated the use of PCI in select patients with NSCLC who has responded well to initial systemic therapy showed that PCI reduced overall incidence of brain metastases in patients with stage III NSCLC, but this did not translate into survival benefit [99, 100]. Therefore, PCI is currently not standard of care for such patient population.

Leptomeningeal Metastases

Incidence

Leptomeningeal metastasis (LM) affects approximately 5% of cancer patients [101–103]. LM occurs in approximately 10% of lung cancer patients, based on autopsy series [104–106] and is an important cause of morbidity and mortality for this population. LM is usually accompanied by extensive and/or progressive systemic disease and presence of metastases in other parts of CNS or usually extensive extracranial disease burden [102, 107].

In SCLC patients, the overall prevalence of LM is 2% and the cumulative incidence 10% at 2 years [15, 107]. These numbers are likely underestimates of the actual rates, since only symptomatic patients undergo investigations to diagnose LM. In NSCLC, LM is more commonly seen in adenocarcinoma than other NSCLC histologies [108].

Clinical Features

The multifocal nature of LM means that there may be signs and symptoms at multiple levels of the neuraxis, and combination of mental status changes, cranial nerve, and spinal nerve root signs is often seen in these patients [109, 110]. About half of patients present with headache, vomiting, lethargy, and/or altered mental status at diagnosis, and up to 25% of patients have hydrocephalus and increased intracranial pressure. Cognitive dysfunction occurs in 25–33% of patients, while focal or generalized seizures are present in 3–12%. Signs of parenchymal brain dysfunction, e.g., aphasia, hemipharesis, and hemisensory loss, are uncommon and, when present, are suggestive of coexisting cerebral metastases or significant invasion of tumor cells into brain along Virchow-Robin spaces [111]. Mental status changes are seen in about 50% of patients.

Cranial nerve involvement is seen in approximately 20% of SCLC patients with LM [112]. Such patients report a loss of visual acuity, diplopia, dysarthria, dysphagia, hoarseness, hearing loss, tinnitus, facial numbness, or pain. Cranial nerve signs noted during examination can be mild and involve paresis of extraocular muscles, decreased facial sensation, facial paresis, and hearing loss [110, 111].

Spinal cord and nerve root symptoms occur in more than 50% of patients with LM [7] (Fig. 22.2). Radicular pattern of involvement, such as cauda equina syndrome, involves lower extremities more common than upper extremities and can manifest as multifocal radicular pain, sensory loss, weakness, fasciculations, reflex asymmetry, and autonomic failure with sexual dysfunction and sphincter disturbances. In comparison, tumor infiltration of the parenchyma of the spinal cord may present predominantly with upper motor neuron type, such as weakness, spasticity, hyperreflexia, and Babinski signs.

Treatment

The goal of treatment in patients with LM from lung cancer is generally to provide palliation, relieve pain, and improve or maintain neurologic function. RT has been commonly used in this setting [113]. In general, focal RT with a dose of 30 Gy is delivered to area (s) causing rapidly progressive symptoms (usually of cranial nerve or cauda equine origin), areas causing CSF compartmental blockage, and/or sites of "bulky" disease on MR scans. WBRT is used in patients with seizures or other signs of brain parenchymal involvement. The use of craniospinal axis RT is uncommon due to significant side effects such as mucositis and myelosuppression with no

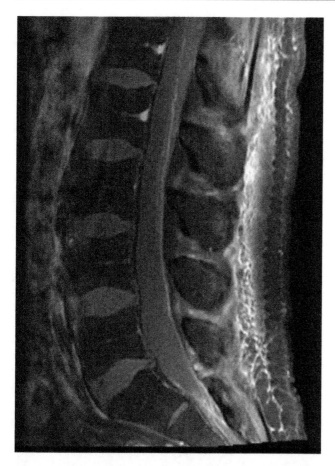

Fig. 22.2 Diffuse abnormal leptomeningeal enhancement along the conus medullaris and cauda equina nerve roots consistent with leptomeningeal metastases in a patient with NSCLC

additional clinical or survival benefit seen with the use of such an approach. PCI, which prevents brain parenchymal metastases, is not effective in preventing LM in SCLC [111].

Intrathecal or intraventricular chemotherapy is employed in select patients, if clinically indicated, after any CSF flow blockage has been relieved surgically or by focal RT [113]. Historically, methotrexate (MTX), cytarabine, and liposomal cytarabine are the most common agents used to treat LM caused by any primary cancer including lung cancer, despite their lack of activity against lung cancer [114]. A retrospective study also evaluated the combination of intrathecal MTX and cytarabine in 30 patients with LM from solid tumors, including five lung cancer patients, and showed that it was relatively tolerable, with six patients experiencing grade III toxicity including two patients with meningitis [115]. Most systemic chemotherapy agents used to treat lung cancer are not used in LM due to their poor CNS penetration. However, there are reports of good response to EGFR TKI erlotinib or gefitinib in patients with LM from NSCLC [71, 72, 116]. Lee et al. retrospectively reviewed 25 patients with LM from NSCLC who all received intrathecal chemotherapy and also received either gefinitib (11 patients)

or erlotinib (14 patients); use of erlotinib resulted in higher cytologic conversion rate of LM than gefinitib (64.3% [9/14] vs. 9.1% [1/11]) [71].

The average survival time in patients with LM from lung cancer is 6–12 weeks [102, 108, 117]. Several studies have identified poor performance status and/or neurological function, high protein levels, and high WBC counts in initial CSF and bulky CNS disease as adverse prognostic factors whereas EGFR TKI use, VP shunt operation as favorable prognostic factors in this patient population [116, 118]

Epidural Spinal Cord Compression

Epidural spinal cord compression (ESCC) is a frequent and often devastating complication of lung cancer. In a large series of patients with ESCC due to cancer, lung, breast, and prostate were the most common primary cancers, with each comprising 20–25% of the total cases [18]. The cumulative incidence of symptomatic ESCC is approximately 3–6% for patients with lung cancer [15].

Fractionated radiation is the most common definitive treatment for epidural spinal metastases, generally given in 30–40 Gy over 10–15 days, and centered on the site of ESCC and incorporating one or two vertebral bodies above and below the full extent of the epidural lesion(s). Intensity-modulated RT (IMRT) and SRS have been used in the past primarily for recurrence in previously irradiated field of lung or spinal metastases [119, 120] and have been increasingly used as the primary treatment of spinal metastases [121, 122]. The theoretical advantages of such focused RT techniques are higher capacity of delivering high-dose radiation to the targeted lesion and sparing the surrounding tissues as compared to standard fractionated RT.

Surgical decompression should be considered for diagnostic and/or therapeutic purposes in patients with ESCC with no known cancer, in patients with otherwise limited or indolent systemic disease, or cases of RT failure or patients with spinal instability. A systemic literature review of 33 non-randomized studies (2495 patients from 1970 to 2007, including 416 patients with lung cancer) showed that more patients with ESCC regained their ability to ambulate after aggressive surgery with or without RT compared to RT alone (64% vs. 29%, p < 0.001) [123]. In a recent randomized trial that compared surgery followed by RT versus RT alone in 101 patients with ESCC (including 26% of patients with lung carcinoma), patients treated with surgery and RT had a significantly higher rate of regaining ambulation than RT alone (42/50, 84% vs. 29/51, 57%; p = 0.001) for longer duration (median 122 days vs. 13 days; p = 0.003) and significantly reduced use of corticosteroids and analgesics [124].

The best result from treatment are seen with pain control, with 70–80% of patients with ESCC experiencing durable improvement of pain, and improved motor function is observed in approximately one-third of patients [125]. Improvement in ambulation largely depends on pre-treatment functional status, and studies have shown that approximately 80% of patients who are fully ambulatory before treatment maintaining ambulation compared to 20–30% of those with paraparesis and fewer than 10% of paraplegic patients are able to ambulate after treatment [126, 127]. Favorable prognostic factors include tumor histology (lung cancer is an unfavorable histology), good performance status, complete surgical resection of epidural metastasis, cervical location, and single epidural lesion [128–130]. Among different lung cancer histologies, a trend to worse outcome is observed with squamous cell carcinoma while patients with SCLC having the best outcome [131]. For a complete discussion on malignant ESCC, please refer to Chap. 6.

Intramedullary Spinal Cord Metastases

Incidence

Intramedullary spinal cord metastases (ISCMs) are unusual complication of solid tumors and believed to arise from hematogenous spread. Lung cancer accounts for more than 50% of ISCM cases (Fig. 22.3), followed by breast cancer, melanoma, and renal cell cancer; ISCM is more commonly seen in SCLC compared to NSCLC [132–134].

Treatment

Commonly patients with ISCM are treated with standard fractionated RT that leads to partial improvement or stabilization of neurologic function [132], and results seen in SCLC patients are more favorable compared to NSCLC patients. In highly selected patients with NSCLC and solitary ISCM with no leptomeningeal disease, partial or complete resection of ISCM may be performed [134]. However, regardless of treatment modality, patients with ISCM have a poor prognosis with median overall survival of 4 months [135]. Early diagnosis and initiation of appropriate treatment are important to preserve neurological function in such patients.

Brachial Plexus and Peripheral Nerve Metastases

Brachial Plexus Metastases

Apical lung cancer, also termed as Pancoast tumor, arises in about 5% of NSCLC cases and 1% of SCLC. Lung cancer can spread to the nearby C8 and T1 nerve roots or into the

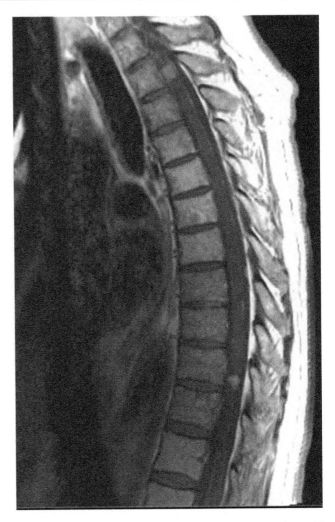

Fig. 22.3 Intramedullary spinal cord metastasis in a patient with NSCLC

brachial plexus, especially the inferior trunk and medial cord [136]. Pain is the most common initial symptom, and rapidly progresses from a dull, throbbing sensation in the upper back or lateral shoulder to the medial portion of upper arm, elbow, and forearm. Dysesthesias can also occur in the C8-T1 nerve distributed area, followed by weakness and atrophy of the intrinsic hand muscles. Continued tumor spread can involve the rest of the plexus, including the medial and radial nerve, and result in weakness in the flexors and extensors of the hand and wrist and extensors of the elbow. When tumor involves the sympathetic trunk, it can result in partial Horner's syndrome with ptosis and anhydrosis. The tumor invades the adjacent vertebrae and extends into the epidural space in approximately 30% of patients. Lung cancer metastases to the axillary or supraclavicular lymph nodes can also involve the brachial plexus [137].

Brachial plexus metastases need to be distinguished from radiation plexopathy in patients with history of prior chest RT [18]. Most important, distinguishing clinical features include Horner's syndrome, which almost always indicates lung metastasis, and early onset, severe pain, which is more commonly seen with plexus metastases than radiation-related injury. MRI of the brachial plexus is generally highly sensitive in detecting brachial plexus metastases. FDG-PET can be helpful in select patients who may not have clearly visible tumor mass or in cases where MRI changes in radiation plexopathy are difficult to distinguish from nerve infiltration by the tumor.

The goal of treatment is to improve symptoms including pain and to stabilize or improve motor function. Analgesics including opioids and drugs such as gabapentin or pregabalin are commonly used to help with neuropathic pain. Radiation is the standard treatment and results in significant pain relief in majority of patients; however, less than one-third of patients report major improvement in their motor and/or sensory deficits. In cases when the conservative measures and RT do not result in pain control, rhizotomy, or cordotomy, and in the setting of a reflex sympathetic disorder, stellate ganglion block are alternatives [7].

Peripheral Nerve Metastases

Lung cancer metastases can compress the recurrent laryngeal nerve, a distal branch of the vagal nerve that innervates the muscles of the larynx, and cause weak cough, hoarseness, and/or dysphagia, and increased risk of aspiration secondary to paralyzed vocal cord. Treatment of lung cancer with chemotherapy and radiation can occasionally improve these symptoms, and laryngoplasty of the paralyzed vocal cord is performed to decrease the risk of aspiration. Atypical facial pain has also been described in patients with lung cancer, as constant aching around the ear, always ipsilateral to the thoracic tumor and is likely due to the intrathoracic vagus nerve compression by the metastatic deposits [7]. Local intervention with surgery or radiation usually alleviates the pain.

Paraneoplastic Disorders

Overview

Small cell lung cancer (SCLC) is the most common cancer that is associated with neurologic paraneoplastic disorders in adults [138]. One to four percent of SCLC patients develop Lambert–Eaton myasthenic syndrome [15, 139] and other neurologic paraneoplastic disorders seen in 1% in SCLC. Any paraneoplastic disorder can occur in NSCLC, though at much lower frequency compared to SCLC. The etiology of most neurologic paraneoplastic disorders is believed to be an autoimmune response against shared tumor neuronal antigens, and the higher incidence of these disorders in SCLC is likely due to neuroendocrine origin seen in SCLC. Patients with neurologic paraneoplastic disorders usually have limited-stage SCLC, due to either early detection or the anti-tumor immune response [139–141]. In the past two decades, numerous tumor neuronal antibodies in serum or CSF have been identified, among which anti-Hu and anti-CV2 are more associated with SCLC and NSCLC [138, 142, 143]. The identification of such antibodies may help in diagnosis of the primary tumor in patients with a suspected paraneoplastic neurologic disorder but no known cancer diagnosis. Sometimes the detection of such antibodies can precede radiologic detection of primary tumor for months to years, posing a challenge for clinical diagnosis.

Clinical Syndromes

Multifocal Encephalomyelitis

Paraneoplastic encephalomyelitis is most commonly seen in SCLC [138, 144–146] and less commonly in NSCLC patients. It is characterized pathologically by patchy, multifocal involvement of any or multiple areas of the central nervous system, seen as neuronal loss and variable degree of infiltration by mononuclear cells, lymphocytes, and plasma cells. Clinically, patients commonly present with subacute sensory neuronopathy and cerebellar degeneration. However, some exhibit focal cortical encephalitis, limbic encephalitis, extrapyramidal movement disorder [147], and brainstem encephalitis [148]. In addition, patients may have peripheral nerve involvement, including sensorimotor polyneuropathy, mononeuritis multiplex, or Lambert–Eaton syndrome. Most patients have circulating antibodies, especially anti-Hu antibodies against a group of RNA-binding proteins [144–146] or anti-CV2 (CRMP-5) antibodies directed against a group of proteins expressed by neurons and oligodendrocytes [149].

Most patients with paraneoplastic encephalomyelitis usually deteriorate over weeks to months, and then stabilize at a level of severe neurologic disability, regardless of treatment. In patients with incomplete response to lung cancer-targeted treatment, subsequent neurological decline is common [140].

Limbic Encephalitis

Approximately one-half of patients with paraneoplastic limbic encephalitis have SCLC [150–152]; this is less commonly seen in NSCLC. The diagnostic criteria for paraneoplastic limbic encephalitis include subacute onset of memory loss, seizures, and psychiatric symptoms, neuropathologic, neuroimaging, or EEG evidence for involvement of the limbic system and a cancer diagnosis within a few years of onset of the neurologic syndrome [151, 153]. Paraneoplastic limbic encephalitis generally evolves over days to weeks and manifests as amnestic syndrome (short-term antegrade and retrograde) or psychiatric disorder or both. Denial of deficits and confabulation are common. The psychiatric disorders seen include depression, anxiety, emotional lability, personality change, hallucinations, or paranoid delusions. Other features include obsessive-compulsive behavior, disinhibited behavior, hyperphagia, and hypersexuality. Generalized or partial complex seizures occur in most patients, may be the initial neurologic feature, and can be medically intractable. MRI shows abnormal T2-weighted or FLAIR signal in the mesial temporal lobe and amygdala bilaterally and less commonly in the hypothalamus and basal frontal cortex [151, 152]. In many patients the MRI lesions subsequently resolve and may not correspond with clinical improvement. Temporal lobe biopsy shows extensive neuronal loss, gliosis, and microglial nodules in the hippocampus and amygdale [151]. Most patients with paraneoplastic limbic encephalitis and SCLC have multifocal encephalomyelitis. Most patients have circulating tumor neural autoantibodies [150, 154], with anti-Hu and anti-CV2 being most prevalent.

Cerebellar Degeneration

Ninety percent of patients with paraneoplastic cerebellar degeneration have SCLC, Hodgkin lymphoma, or carcinoma of the breast or ovary, with SCLC being the most common primary tumor [18]. The most striking and consistent neuropathologic finding is severe, diffuse loss of Purkinje cells throughout the cerebellar cortex [155, 156]. The clinical onset can be abrupt [157], and signs and symptoms reflect diffuse dysfunction of the cerebellum, including truncal ataxia, dysarthria, nystagmus, vertigo, diplopia, and oscillopsia. Many patients may also develop multifocal encephalomyelitis, paraneoplastic peripheral neuropathy, or Lambert–Eaton myasthenic syndrome [158, 159]. After a period of subacute progression, the disease usually stabilizes, leaving the typical patient severely disabled [157]. Anti-Hu antibodies are the most common onconeural antibodies seen in this patient population [157, 158], while others may have anti-CV2 antibodies [143] or anti-Zic4 antibodies [160]. Anti-Yo antibodies that are strongly associated with breast or ovarian cancer, and anti-Tr that is associated with Hodgkin lymphoma, are rarely associated with lung carcinoma.

Opsoclonus-Myoclonus

Opsoclonus is characterized as chaotic, continuous multidirectional rapid eye movements (saccadic oscillations) without an intersaccadic interval, less common in adults and most often associated with SCLC or breast carcinoma, occasionally with NSCLC [161, 162]. The specific pathophysiology is unclear; postmortem cases implicate injury to cerebellar neurons and/or to brainstem ocular motor nuclei in opsoclonus may play a role. Anti-Hu, anti-Ri (ANNA-2), anti-CV2, or antiamphiphysin antibodies are present in select patients [162].

Extrapyramidal Syndrome

Extrapyramidal syndrome is manifested as chorea, athetosis, dystonia, or parkinsonism, occurring most often in SCLC and rarely in NSCLC [163]. MRI shows focal lesions in the basal ganglia. Anti-Hu and anti-CV2 are the most commonly associated antibodies.

Brainstem Encephalitis

Paraneoplastic brainstem encephalitis manifests as a variety of gaze palsies or other ocular motor disturbance, possibly along with dysarthria, dysphagia, central respiratory failure, or other signs and symptoms referable to the brainstem [148]. It most commonly occurs in the setting of paraneoplastic multifocal encephalomyelitis in SCLC and is associated with anti-Hu antibodies. The neurologic prognosis is generally poor, and the brainstem dysfunction can be fatal in some patients.

Carcinoma-Associated Retinopathy

More than 75% of patients with carcinoma-associated paraneoplastic retinopathy have SCLC [164, 165]. The visual symptoms usually precede tumor detection by months to years and include painless bilateral blurry vision, night blindness, episodic obscurations, distortions, or photosensitivity. Examination shows severely impaired visual acuity and diffuse dysfunction of both rod and cone photoreceptor cells. The clinical course is subacute and worsens over weeks to months to severe impairment. A great majority of patients have circulating autoantibodies against recoverin, a 23-kd calcium-binding protein, and some have antibodies against other retinal proteins [18].

Stiff Person Syndrome

Stiff person syndrome refers to a presentation of muscle rigidity and spasms that are associated with SCLC and other neoplasms. Rigidity is likely the result of injury to the spinal cord and/or brainstem. Patients develop progressive aching and rigidity of the axial and proximal muscles, sometimes with painful, violent spasms that can occur spontaneously or triggered by voluntary or passive movement. Patients may eventually develop fixed flexion of the limbs or even opisthotonus and respiratory difficulty. Autoantibodies against the synaptic vesicle-associated protein amphiphysin can be detected in some patients [166, 167].

Motor Neuron Disease

Paraneoplastic lower motor neuron dysfunction occurs in up to 25% of patients with SCLC and multifocal encephalomyelitis [145] and generally does not improve with treatment. However, several well-described patients with a lower motor neuron syndrome or combined upper and lower motor neuron syndrome experienced significant neurologic improvement after resection of lung cancer.

Subacute Sensory Neuronopathy

This syndrome is the most common manifestation of paraneoplastic encephalomyelitis with more than 90% of patients having SCLC and a minority having NSCLC [144–146]. Pathologically, there is inflammation of the dorsal root ganglion with loss of neuronal cell bodies [111, 155]. Early symptoms include patchy or asymmetric numbness and burning dysesthesias that involve the legs and progressively involve the arms and the face over days to weeks. Examination reveals severe sensory ataxia that mimics cerebellar dysfunction and hypoactive or absent muscle stretch reflexes, whereas normal muscle strength is preserved. Both small and large neurons are affected, which is different from the large fiber neuropathy seen with cisplatin. Characteristic EEG/NCS studies show normal motor nerve findings but severely reduced or absent sensory potentials [168, 169]. Most patients will have subacute deterioration over weeks to months, and then stabilize at a severely debilitated level regardless of treatment, while others may have subsequent stepwise or gradual neurologic decline. Rarely patients have minimal CNS manifestations and an indolent course of sensory neuropathy, independent of treatment modalities [170].

Neuromyotonia

Patients with SCLC may develop paraneoplastic peripheral nerve hyperexcitability as the "cramp-fasciculation syndrome" or as a syndrome of diffuse muscle stiffness similar to neuromyotonia or continuous muscle fiber activity (Isaacs' syndrome) [171]. Needle EMG shows repetitive bursts of rapidly firing motor unit discharges and/or very high-frequency trains of discharges. Occasionally, autoantibodies against proteins in the voltage-gated potassium channel complex can be detected, including contacting-associated protein-2 (Caspr2) [172, 173].

Other Neuropathies

A minority of patients with SCLC as well as anti-Hu and/or anti-CV2 antibodies have a mixed sensorimotor polyneuropathy with a mixed axonal-demyelinating electrophysiologic pattern [143, 174]. Mononeuritis multiplex with biopsy-proven nerve vasculitis can occur in SCLC or NSCLC, with or without anti-Hu antibodies [175].

Autonomic Insufficiency

Paraneoplastic autonomic dysfunction most commonly occurs as part of encephalomyelitis in patients with SCLC, rarely in NSCLC. These patients may present with severe and progressive gastrointestinal dysmotility up to several months prior to detection of the cancer [176–178]. Other symptoms include sympathetic and/or parasympathetic dysfunction, such as orthostatic hypotension, dry mouth, and urinary retention. Neurologic outcome is usually poor, and patients are at risk for sudden death.

Lambert–Eaton Myasthenic Syndrome

Lambert–Eaton myasthenic syndrome (LEMS) is a disorder of the neuromuscular junction, and antibodies to voltage-gated calcium channels at the presynaptic terminal are pathogenic. Approximately one-half of patients LEMS have an associated neoplasm, among whom 90% have SCLC [141, 179–181]. On the other hand, LEMS is the most frequently described paraneoplastic syndrome associated with SCLC. Paraneoplastic LEMS precedes the detection of tumor in more than 75% of patients by months to years. Clinical course is often insidious with gradual onset of weakness and fatigue. The initial symmetric weakness predominantly involving the proximal leg muscles and sometimes shoulder girdle muscles over time can progress to involve distal muscles. Weakness can involve respiratory muscles as well. In contrast to myasthenia gravis, in LEMS the oculobulbar muscles are usually spared and the strength increases with initial effort before the weakness returns. Muscle stretch reflexes are characteristically diminished or absent. Over time, 90% of patients eventually develop other cholinergic disturbances such as dry mouth, constipation, and impotence. The characteristic electrophysiologic profile of LEMS includes a decrement of the compound muscle action potential (CMAP) at slow rates of stimulation but an increment at faster rates [169]. This is different from normal musculature that has a similar size CMAP at slow or fast rates, and from myasthenia gravis, which has a decremental response to both [111]. Before the identification of primary tumor, it can be challenging to differentiate paraneoplastic LEMS from non-paraneoplastic LEMS based on their neuromuscular symptoms, EMG abnormalities, or the presence of anti-calcium channel antibodies. Antibodies against the SOX1 transcription factor are present in nearly two-thirds of patients with LEMS associated with SCLC but only in 5% of patients with non-paraneoplastic LEMS [182, 183]. Anti-SOX antibodies are also present in 40% of patients with SCLC who do not develop neurological symptoms. Although anti-SOX antibodies are not known to be directly involved in the pathogenesis of LEMS, they may well serve as a valuable serologic marker for SCLC [18].

Myopathies

Both dermatomyositis (DM) and polymyositis (PM) are inflammatory myopathies of autoimmune origin and are rarely associated with underlying malignancies, among which lung cancer is a frequent cause. Dermatomyositis is more likely than PM to be associated with cancer [184–186]. Laboratory findings include autoantibodies such as anti-Jo and increased serum creatine kinase level, and EMG often confirms the presence of a myopathy. Some patients improve after tumor resection and/or immunosuppressant, while others can become severely disabled or die as a result of bulbar and respiratory weakness.

Treatment

The neurologic outcomes in patients with paraneoplastic neurologic disorders vary widely following tumor treatment, depending on the specific paraneoplastic syndrome, the time interval between onset of symptoms and clinical intervention and tumor response to treatment. Increasing evidence demonstrates that successful tumor treatment is a major factor in determining neurologic outcome, and that immunosuppressive therapy is more likely to be effective when the tumor is treated successfully [145, 146].

Most patients with paraneoplastic LEMS have neurological improvement after successful treatment of the associated SCLC [141]. Pyridostigmine is of benefit but is less effective than for myasthenia gravis. The potassium channel antagonist 3,4-diaminopyridine prolongs the action potential at motor nerve terminals, increases the time available for calcium entry into the cell, enhances acetylcholine release, and therefore improves strength in nearly all patients with LEMS [181]. Immunosuppressive therapy is usually reserved for patients with severe weakness or in those where tumor treatment is not an option. Prednisone and/or azathioprine is commonly used, followed by cyclosporin as second line of therapy. Plasma exchange or intravenous immunoglobulin can produce improvement in most patients and lasts for 2–3 months. There are case reports of response to rituximab as well [187].

In several other syndromes including neuromyotonia and stiff person syndrome, successful tumor treatment and/or immunosuppressive therapy often results in significant neurologic improvement. It has been postulated that onconeural antibodies cause neuronal or peripheral nerve dysfunction but not neuronal cell death, allowing for recovery if the autoimmune response can be suppressed [18]. Most patients with paraneoplastic retinal degeneration and antirecoverin antibodies treated with prednisone show mild to moderate vision improvement, while some patients can have a fluctuating steroid-dependent course or deteriorate after an initial partial response. There are no definite reports of visual improvement following tumor treatment without concomitant corticosteroid therapy. Intravenous immunoglobulin may also be beneficial in select patients.

In patients with paraneoplastic opsoclonus-myoclonus, symptoms may improve spontaneously [162], with successful treatment of the tumor [161], or with immunosuppressive therapy [162], while others show little neurological improvement with treatment. In patients with paraneoplastic limbic encephalitis, the neurological course is variable, partly due to the type of associated autoantibody. Overall, 30–50% of patients with limbic encephalitis and SCLC improve after tumor treatment, with or without immunosuppressive therapy [144, 150, 151].

The poorest neurologic outcomes are seen in patients with paraneoplastic cerebellar degeneration [157, 188], encephalomyelitis, or other syndrome associated with anti-Hu antibodies [140, 146]. Fewer than 10% of these patients show significant neurologic improvement despite successful tumor treatment and aggressive immunosuppressive therapy. It is likely that patients have already suffered neuronal death or irreversible injury by the time of diagnosis being made. Therefore, the decision to treat with use of immunosuppressive therapies must be based on the particular syndrome and be individualized.

Conclusion

As improved systemic treatment allows patients with lung cancer to live longer, relapse and the involvement of central nervous system is more frequently observed in these patients. The treatment of neurological complications from lung cancer is also rapidly evolving, and the role of radiation has been further refined in lung cancer patients with brain metastases and radiosurgery been increasingly used. In the past, chemotherapy had limited role in the management of these patients due to poor BBB penetration and chemoresistance of the relapsed tumor. However, newer targeted agents have better CNS penetration and can be effective in select group of patients. Continued advancements in these areas will further improve the survival and quality of life of these patients.

References

1. American Cancer Society. Cancer facts and figures; 2014.
2. U.S. National Institutes of Health. National Cancer Institute. SEER cancer statistics review; 1975–2011.
3. U.S. Department of Health and Human Services. The health consequences of smoking: a report of the U.S. surgeon general; 2004.
4. U.S. Department of Health and Human Services. The health consequences of smoking—50 years of progress: a report of the surgeon general; 2014.

5. Goldstraw P, Ball D, Jett JR, Le Chevalier T, Lim E, Nicholson AG, et al. Non-small-cell lung cancer. Lancet. 2011;378 (9804):1727–40.
6. van Meerbeeck JP, Fennell DA, De Ruysscher DK. Small-cell lung cancer. Lancet. 2011;378(9804):1741–55.
7. Jeyapalan SA, Mahadevan A. Neurologic complications of lung cancer. In: Schiff D, Kesari S, Wen PY, editors. Current clinical oncology: cancer neurology in clinical practice. second ed.: Humana Press; 2008. p. 397–398–421.
8. Sperduto PW, Chao ST, Sneed PK, Luo X, Suh J, Roberge D, et al. Diagnosis-specific prognostic factors, indexes, and treatment outcomes for patients with newly diagnosed brain metastases: a multi-institutional analysis of 4259 patients. Int J Radiat Oncol Biol Phys. 2010;77(3):655–61.
9. Giordana MT, Cordera S, Boghi A. Cerebral metastases as first symptom of cancer: a clinico-pathologic study. J Neurooncol. 2000;50(3):265–73.
10. Mavrakis AN, Halpern EF, Barker FG, Gonzalez RG, Henson JW. Diagnostic evaluation of patients with a brain mass as the presenting manifestation of cancer. Neurology 2005;65 (6):908–911.
11. Postmus PE, Haaxma-Reiche H, Smit EF, Groen HJ, Karnicka H, Lewinski T, et al. Treatment of brain metastases of small-cell lung cancer: comparing teniposide and teniposide with whole-brain radiotherapy–a phase III study of the european organization for the research and treatment of cancer lung cancer cooperative group. J Clin Oncol. 2000;18(19):3400–8.
12. Glantz MJ, Choy H, Yee L. Prophylactic cranial irradiation in small cell lung cancer: rationale, results, and recommendations. Semin Oncol. 1997;24(4):477–83.
13. van Oosterhout AG, van de Pol M, ten Velde GP, Twijnstra A. Neurologic disorders in 203 consecutive patients with small cell lung cancer. Results of a longitudinal study. Cancer. 1996;77 (8):1434–41.
14. Sculier JP, Feld R, Evans WK, DeBoer G, Shepherd FA, Payne DG, et al. Neurologic disorders in patients with small cell lung cancer. Cancer. 1987;60(9):2275–83.
15. Seute T, Leffers P, ten Velde GP, Twijnstra A. Neurologic disorders in 432 consecutive patients with small cell lung carcinoma. Cancer. 2004;100(4):801–6.
16. Seute T, Leffers P, ten Velde GP, Twijnstra A. Detection of brain metastases from small cell lung cancer: consequences of changing imaging techniques (CT versus MRI). Cancer. 2008;112 (8):1827–34.
17. Rodrigus P, de Brouwer P, Raaymakers E. Brain metastases and non-small cell lung cancer. Prognostic factors and correlation with survival after irradiation. Lung Cancer 2001;32(2):129–136.
18. Dropcho EJ. Neurologic complications of lung cancer. In: Billler J, Ferro JM, editors. Handbook of clinical neurology, vol. 119. Neurologic aspects of systemic disease part I, third series ed.; 2014. p. 335–336–361.
19. Tsao MN, Lloyd N, Wong R, Chow E, Rakovitch E, Laperriere N. Whole brain radiotherapy for the treatment of multiple brain metastases. Cochrane Database Syst Rev. 2006;3 (3):CD003869.
20. Gaspar LE, Mehta MP, Patchell RA, Burri SH, Robinson PD, Morris RE, et al. The role of whole brain radiation therapy in the management of newly diagnosed brain metastases: a systematic review and evidence-based clinical practice guideline. J Neurooncol. 2010;96(1):17–32.
21. Wen PY, Loeffler JS. Management of brain metastases. Oncology (Williston Park) 1999;13 (7):941–54, 957–61; discussion 961–2, 9.
22. Postmus PE, Haaxma-Reiche H, Gregor A, Groen HJ, Lewinski T, Scolard T, et al. Brain-only metastases of small cell lung cancer; efficacy of whole brain radiotherapy. An EORTC phase II study. Radiother Oncol. 1998;46(1):29–32.

23. Nieder C, Berberich W, Schnabel K. Tumor-related prognostic factors for remission of brain metastases after radiotherapy. Int J Radiat Oncol Biol Phys. 1997;39(1):25–30.
24. Lagerwaard FJ, Levendag PC, Nowak PJ, Eijkenboom WM, Hanssens PE, Schmitz PI. Identification of prognostic factors in patients with brain metastases: a review of 1292 patients. Int J Radiat Oncol Biol Phys. 1999;43(4):795–803.
25. Videtic GM, Adelstein DJ, Mekhail TM, Rice TW, Stevens GH, Lee SY, et al. Validation of the RTOG recursive partitioning analysis (RPA) classification for small-cell lung cancer-only brain metastases. Int J Radiat Oncol Biol Phys. 2007;67(1):240–3.
26. Videtic GM, Reddy CA, Chao ST, Rice TW, Adelstein DJ, Barnett GH, et al. Gender, race, and survival: a study in non-small-cell lung cancer brain metastases patients utilizing the radiation therapy oncology group recursive partitioning analysis classification. Int J Radiat Oncol Biol Phys. 2009;75(4):1141–7.
27. Patchell RA, Tibbs PA, Walsh JW, Dempsey RJ, Maruyama Y, Kryscio RJ, et al. A randomized trial of surgery in the treatment of single metastases to the brain. N Engl J Med. 1990;322 (8):494–500.
28. Kalkanis SN, Kondziolka D, Gaspar LE, Burri SH, Asher AL, Cobbs CS, et al. The role of surgical resection in the management of newly diagnosed brain metastases: a systematic review and evidence-based clinical practice guideline. J Neurooncol. 2010;96 (1):33–43.
29. Nakagawa H, Miyawaki Y, Fujita T, Kubo S, Tokiyoshi K, Tsuruzono K, et al. Surgical treatment of brain metastases of lung cancer: retrospective analysis of 89 cases. J Neurol Neurosurg Psychiatry. 1994;57(8):950–6.
30. Linskey ME, Andrews DW, Asher AL, Burri SH, Kondziolka D, Robinson PD, et al. The role of stereotactic radiosurgery in the management of patients with newly diagnosed brain metastases: a systematic review and evidence-based clinical practice guideline. J Neurooncol. 2010;96(1):45–68.
31. Kwon AK, Dibiase SJ, Wang B, Hughes SL, Milcarek B, Zhu Y. Hypofractionated stereotactic radiotherapy for the treatment of brain metastases. Cancer. 2009;115(4):890–8.
32. Shaw E, Scott C, Souhami L, Dinapoli R, Kline R, Loeffler J, et al. Single dose radiosurgical treatment of recurrent previously irradiated primary brain tumors and brain metastases: final report of RTOG protocol 90-05. Int J Radiat Oncol Biol Phys. 2000;47 (2):291–8.
33. Shehata MK, Young B, Reid B, Patchell RA, St Clair W, Sims J, et al. Stereotatic radiosurgery of 468 brain metastases < or = 2 cm: implications for SRS dose and whole brain radiation therapy. Int J Radiat Oncol Biol Phys. 2004;59(1):87–93.
34. Vogelbaum MA, Angelov L, Lee SY, Li L, Barnett GH, Suh JH. Local control of brain metastases by stereotactic radiosurgery in relation to dose to the tumor margin. J Neurosurg. 2006;104 (6):907–12.
35. O'Neill BP, Iturria NJ, Link MJ, Pollock BE, Ballman KV, O'Fallon JR. A comparison of surgical resection and stereotactic radiosurgery in the treatment of solitary brain metastases. Int J Radiat Oncol Biol Phys. 2003;55(5):1169–76.
36. Serizawa T, Ono J, Iichi T, Matsuda S, Sato M, Odaki M, et al. Gamma knife radiosurgery for metastatic brain tumors from lung cancer: a comparison between small cell and non-small cell carcinoma. J Neurosurg. 2002;97(5 Suppl):484–8.
37. Gerosa M, Nicolato A, Foroni R, Tomazzoli L, Bricolo A. Analysis of long-term outcomes and prognostic factors in patients with non-small cell lung cancer brain metastases treated by gamma knife radiosurgery. J Neurosurg. 2005;102(Suppl):75–80.
38. Pan HC, Sheehan J, Stroila M, Steiner M, Steiner L. Gamma knife surgery for brain metastases from lung cancer. J Neurosurg. 2005;102(Suppl):128–33.

39. Wegner RE, Olson AC, Kondziolka D, Niranjan A, Lundsford LD, Flickinger JC. Stereotactic radiosurgery for patients with brain metastases from small cell lung cancer. Int J Radiat Oncol Biol Phys. 2011;81(3):e21–7.

40. Bhatnagar AK, Flickinger JC, Kondziolka D, Lunsford LD. Stereotactic radiosurgery for four or more intracranial metastases. Int J Radiat Oncol Biol Phys. 2006;64(3):898–903.

41. Jagannathan J, Yen CP, Ray DK, Schlesinger D, Oskouian RJ, Pouratian N, et al. Gamma Knife radiosurgery to the surgical cavity following resection of brain metastases. J Neurosurg. 2009;111(3):431–8.

42. Prabhu R, Shu HK, Hadjipanayis C, Dhabaan A, Hall W, Raore B, et al. Current dosing paradigm for stereotactic radiosurgery alone after surgical resection of brain metastases needs to be optimized for improved local control. Int J Radiat Oncol Biol Phys. 2012;83(1):e61–6.

43. Andrews DW, Scott CB, Sperduto PW, Flanders AE, Gaspar LE, Schell MC, et al. Whole brain radiation therapy with or without stereotactic radiosurgery boost for patients with one to three brain metastases: phase III results of the RTOG 9508 randomised trial. Lancet. 2004;363(9422):1665–72.

44. Sperduto PW, Shanley R, Luo X, Andrews D, Werner-Wasik M, Valicenti R, et al. Secondary analysis of RTOG 9508, a phase 3 randomized trial of whole-brain radiation therapy versus WBRT plus stereotactic radiosurgery in patients with 1–3 brain metastases; poststratified by the graded prognostic assessment (GPA). Int J Radiat Oncol Biol Phys. 2014;90(3):526–31.

45. Sneed PK, Suh JH, Goetsch SJ, Sanghavi SN, Chappell R, Buatti JM, et al. A multi-institutional review of radiosurgery alone vs. radiosurgery with whole brain radiotherapy as the initial management of brain metastases. Int J Radiat Oncol Biol Phys. 2002;53(3):519–26.

46. Varlotto JM, Flickinger JC, Niranjan A, Bhatnagar A, Kondziolka D, Lunsford LD. The impact of whole-brain radiation therapy on the long-term control and morbidity of patients surviving more than one year after gamma knife radiosurgery for brain metastases. Int J Radiat Oncol Biol Phys. 2005;62(1):1125–32.

47. Patchell RA, Tibbs PA, Regine WF, Dempsey RJ, Mohiuddin M, Kryscio RJ, et al. Postoperative radiotherapy in the treatment of single metastases to the brain: a randomized trial. JAMA. 1998;280(17):1485–9.

48. Aoyama H, Shirato H, Tago M, Nakagawa K, Toyoda T, Hatano K, et al. Stereotactic radiosurgery plus whole-brain radiation therapy vs stereotactic radiosurgery alone for treatment of brain metastases: a randomized controlled trial. JAMA. 2006;295(21):2483–91.

49. Chang EL, Wefel JS, Hess KR, Allen PK, Lang FF, Kornguth DG, et al. Neurocognition in patients with brain metastases treated with radiosurgery or radiosurgery plus whole-brain irradiation: a randomised controlled trial. Lancet Oncol. 2009;10(11):1037–44.

50. Kocher M, Soffietti R, Abacioglu U, Villa S, Fauchon F, Baumert BG, et al. Adjuvant whole-brain radiotherapy versus observation after radiosurgery or surgical resection of one to three cerebral metastases: results of the EORTC 22952-26001 study. J Clin Oncol. 2011;29(2):134–41.

51. Brown PD, Asher AL, Ballman KV, Farace E, Cerhan JH, Anderson SK, et al. NCCTG N0574 (Alliance): a phase III randomized trial of whole brain radiation therapy (WBRT) in addition to radiosurgery (SRS) in patients with 1–3 brain metastases. J Clin Oncol. 2015;33 (suppl; abstr LBA4).

52. Aoyama H, Tago M, Kato N, Toyoda T, Kenjyo M, Hirota S, et al. Neurocognitive function of patients with brain metastasis who received either whole brain radiotherapy plus stereotactic radiosurgery or radiosurgery alone. Int J Radiat Oncol Biol Phys. 2007;68(5):1388–95.

53. Chao ST, Barnett GH, Vogelbaum MA, Angelov L, Weil RJ, Neyman G, et al. Salvage stereotactic radiosurgery effectively treats recurrences from whole-brain radiation therapy. Cancer. 2008;113(8):2198–204.

54. Karlsson B, Hanssens P, Wolff R, Soderman M, Lindquist C, Beute G. Thirty years' experience with Gamma Knife surgery for metastases to the brain. J Neurosurg. 2009;111(3):449–57.

55. Caballero JA, Sneed PK, Lamborn KR, Ma L, Denduluri S, Nakamura JL, et al. Prognostic factors for survival in patients treated with stereotactic radiosurgery for recurrent brain metastases after prior whole brain radiotherapy. Int J Radiat Oncol Biol Phys. 2012;83(1):303–9.

56. Gerstner ER, Fine RL. Increased permeability of the blood-brain barrier to chemotherapy in metastatic brain tumors: establishing a treatment paradigm. J Clin Oncol. 2007;25(16):2306–12.

57. Walbert T, Gilbert MR. The role of chemotherapy in the treatment of patients with brain metastases from solid tumors. Int J Clin Oncol. 2009;14(4):299–306.

58. Zimmermann S, Dziadziuszko R, Peters S. Indications and limitations of chemotherapy and targeted agents in non-small cell lung cancer brain metastases. Cancer Treat Rev. 2014;40(6):716–22.

59. Kouroussis C, Vamvakas L, Vardakis N, Kotsakis A, Kalykaki A, Kalbakis K, et al. Continuous administration of daily low-dose temozolomide in pretreated patients with advanced non-small cell lung cancer: a phase II study. Oncology. 2009;76(2):112–7.

60. Siena S, Crino L, Danova M, Del Prete S, Cascinu S, Salvagni S, et al. Dose-dense temozolomide regimen for the treatment of brain metastases from melanoma, breast cancer, or lung cancer not amenable to surgery or radiosurgery: a multicenter phase II study. Ann Oncol. 2010;21(3):655–61.

61. Pietanza MC, Kadota K, Huberman K, Sima CS, Fiore JJ, Sumner DK, et al. Phase II trial of temozolomide in patients with relapsed sensitive or refractory small cell lung cancer, with assessment of methylguanine-DNA methyltransferase as a potential biomarker. Clin Cancer Res. 2012;18(4):1138–45.

62. Soussain C, Ricard D, Fike JR, Mazeron JJ, Psimaras D, Delattre JY. CNS complications of radiotherapy and chemotherapy. Lancet. 2009;374(9701):1639–51.

63. Lee DH, Han JY, Kim HT, Yoon SJ, Pyo HR, Cho KH, et al. Primary chemotherapy for newly diagnosed nonsmall cell lung cancer patients with synchronous brain metastases compared with whole-brain radiotherapy administered first: result of a randomized pilot study. Cancer. 2008;113(1):143–9.

64. Robinet G, Thomas P, Breton JL, Lena H, Gouva S, Dabouis G, et al. Results of a phase III study of early versus delayed whole brain radiotherapy with concurrent cisplatin and vinorelbine combination in inoperable brain metastasis of non-small-cell lung cancer: Groupe Francais de Pneumo-Cancerologie (GFPC) Protocol 95-1. Ann Oncol. 2001;12(1):59–67.

65. Kim JE, Lee DH, Choi Y, Yoon DH, Kim SW, Suh C, et al. Epidermal growth factor receptor tyrosine kinase inhibitors as a first-line therapy for never-smokers with adenocarcinoma of the lung having asymptomatic synchronous brain metastasis. Lung Cancer. 2009;65(3):351–4.

66. Porta R, Sanchez-Torres JM, Paz-Ares L, Massuti B, Reguart N, Mayo C, et al. Brain metastases from lung cancer responding to erlotinib: the importance of EGFR mutation. Eur Respir J. 2011;37(3):624–31.

67. Park SJ, Kim HT, Lee DH, Kim KP, Kim SW, Suh C, et al. Efficacy of epidermal growth factor receptor tyrosine kinase inhibitors for brain metastasis in non-small cell lung cancer

patients harboring either exon 19 or 21 mutation. Lung Cancer. 2012;77(3):556–60.

68. Li Z, Lu J, Zhao Y, Guo H. The retrospective analysis of the frequency of EGFR mutations and the efficacy of gefitinib in NSCLC patients with brain metastasis. J Clin Oncol. 2011;29 (suppl; abstr e18065).

69. Katayama T, Shimizu J, Suda K, Onozato R, Fukui T, Ito S, et al. Efficacy of erlotinib for brain and leptomeningeal metastases in patients with lung adenocarcinoma who showed initial good response to gefitinib. J Thorac Oncol. 2009;4 (11):1415–9.

70. Togashi Y, Masago K, Masuda S, Mizuno T, Fukudo M, Ikemi Y, et al. Cerebrospinal fluid concentration of gefitinib and erlotinib in patients with non-small cell lung cancer. Cancer Chemother Pharmacol. 2012;70(3):399–405.

71. Lee E, Keam B, Kim DW, Kim TM, Lee SH, Chung DH, et al. Erlotinib versus gefitinib for control of leptomeningeal carcinomatosis in non-small-cell lung cancer. J Thorac Oncol. 2013;8 (8):1069–74.

72. Clarke JL, Pao W, Wu N, Miller VA, Lassman AB. High dose weekly erlotinib achieves therapeutic concentrations in CSF and is effective in leptomeningeal metastases from epidermal growth factor receptor mutant lung cancer. J Neurooncol. 2010;99 (2):283–6.

73. Grommes C, Oxnard GR, Kris MG, Miller VA, Pao W, Holodny AI, et al. "Pulsatile" high-dose weekly erlotinib for CNS metastases from EGFR mutant non-small cell lung cancer. Neuro Oncol. 2011;13(12):1364–9.

74. Togashi Y, Masago K, Fukudo M, Tsuchido Y, Okuda C, Kim YH, et al. Efficacy of increased-dose erlotinib for central nervous system metastases in non-small cell lung cancer patients with epidermal growth factor receptor mutation. Cancer Chemother Pharmacol. 2011;68(4):1089–92.

75. Sperduto PW, Wang M, Robins HI, Schell MC, Werner-Wasik M, Komaki R, et al. A phase 3 trial of whole brain radiation therapy and stereotactic radiosurgery alone versus WBRT and SRS with temozolomide or erlotinib for non-small cell lung cancer and 1–3 brain metastases: Radiation Therapy Oncology Group 0320. Int J Radiat Oncol Biol Phys. 2013;85(5):1312–8.

76. Welsh JW, Komaki R, Amini A, Munsell MF, Unger W, Allen PK, et al. Phase II trial of erlotinib plus concurrent whole-brain radiation therapy for patients with brain metastases from non-small-cell lung cancer. J Clin Oncol. 2013;31(7):895–902.

77. Shaw AT, Kim DW, Nakagawa K, Seto T, Crino L, Ahn MJ, et al. Crizotinib versus chemotherapy in advanced ALK-positive lung cancer. N Engl J Med. 2013;368(25):2385–94.

78. Kim YH, Nagai H, Ozasa H, Sakamori Y, Mishima M. Therapeutic strategy for non-small-cell lung cancer patients with brain metastases (Review). Biomed Rep. 2013;1(5):691–6.

79. Takeda M, Okamoto I, Nakagawa K. Clinical impact of continued crizotinib administration after isolated central nervous system progression in patients with lung cancer positive for ALK rearrangement. J Thorac Oncol. 2013;8(5):654–7.

80. Camidge R. First-in-human dose-finding study of the ALK/EGFR inhibitor AP26113 in patients with advanced malignancies: updated results. J Clin Oncol. 2013;31 (Suppl)([abstr.8031]).

81. Shaw A. Clinical activity of the ALK inhibitor LDK378 in advanced, ALK-positive NSCLC. J Clin Oncol 2013;31 (suppl) ([abstr.8010]).

82. Nakagawa K. A phase I/II study with a highly selective ALK inhibitor CH5424802 in ALK-positive non-small cell lung cancer (NSCLC) patients: updated safety and efficacy results from AF-001JP. J Clin Oncol 2913;31 (Suppl.)([abstr.8033]).

83. Sandler A, Gray R, Perry MC, Brahmer J, Schiller JH, Dowlati A, et al. Paclitaxel-carboplatin alone or with bevacizumab for

non-small-cell lung cancer. N Engl J Med. 2006;355(24):2542–50.

84. Reck M, von Pawel J, Zatloukal P, Ramlau R, Gorbounova V, Hirsh V, et al. Overall survival with cisplatin-gemcitabine and bevacizumab or placebo as first-line therapy for nonsquamous non-small-cell lung cancer: results from a randomised phase III trial (AVAiL). Ann Oncol. 2010;21(9):1804–9.

85. Srivastava G, Rana V, Wallace S, Taylor S, Debnam M, Feng L, et al. Risk of intracranial hemorrhage and cerebrovascular accidents in non-small cell lung cancer brain metastasis patients. J Thorac Oncol. 2009;4(3):333–7.

86. Besse B, Lasserre SF, Compton P, Huang J, Augustus S, Rohr UP. Bevacizumab safety in patients with central nervous system metastases. Clin Cancer Res. 2010;16(1):269–78.

87. Carden CP, Larkin JM, Rosenthal MA. What is the risk of intracranial bleeding during anti-VEGF therapy? Neuro Oncol. 2008;10(4):624–30.

88. Khasraw M, Holodny A, Goldlust SA, DeAngelis LM. Intracranial hemorrhage in patients with cancer treated with bevacizumab: the Memorial Sloan-Kettering experience. Ann Oncol. 2012;23(2):458–63.

89. Socinski MA, Langer CJ, Huang JE, Kolb MM, Compton P, Wang L, et al. Safety of bevacizumab in patients with non-small-cell lung cancer and brain metastases. J Clin Oncol. 2009;27(31):5255–61.

90. Besse B, Moulec SL, Senellart H, Mazieres J, Barlesi F, Dansin E, et al. Phase II study of bevacizumab in combination with first-line chemotherapy or second-line erlotinib in non-squamous NSCLC patients with asymptomatic untreated brain metastases (ML21823). Ann Oncol. 2012;23(ix426):2012.

91. De Braganca KC, Janjigian YY, Azzoli CG, Kris MG, Pietanza MC, Nolan CP, et al. Efficacy and safety of bevacizumab in active brain metastases from non-small cell lung cancer. J Neurooncol. 2010;100(3):443–7.

92. Yamamoto D, Iwase S, Tsubota Y, Sueoka N, Yamamoto C, Kitamura K, et al. Bevacizumab in the treatment of five patients with breast cancer and brain metastases: Japan breast cancer research network-07 trial. Onco Targets Ther. 2012;5:185–9.

93. Boothe D, Young R, Yamada Y, Prager A, Chan T, Beal K. Bevacizumab as a treatment for radiation necrosis of brain metastases post stereotactic radiosurgery. Neuro Oncol. 2013;15 (9):1257–63.

94. Blanchard P, Le Pechoux C. Prophylactic cranial irradiation in lung cancer. Curr Opin Oncol. 2010;22(2):94–101.

95. Gregor A, Cull A, Stephens RJ, Kirkpatrick JA, Yarnold JR, Girling DJ, et al. Prophylactic cranial irradiation is indicated following complete response to induction therapy in small cell lung cancer: results of a multicentre randomised trial. United Kingdom Coordinating Committee for Cancer Research (UKCCCR) and the European Organization for Research and Treatment of Cancer (EORTC). Eur J Cancer. 1997;33(11):1752–8.

96. Auperin A, Arriagada R, Pignon JP, Le Pechoux C, Gregor A, Stephens RJ, et al. Prophylactic cranial irradiation for patients with small-cell lung cancer in complete remission. Prophylactic cranial irradiation overview collaborative group. N Engl J Med. 1999;341(7):476–84.

97. Arriagada R, Le Chevalier T, Riviere A, Chomy P, Monnet I, Bardet E, et al. Patterns of failure after prophylactic cranial irradiation in small-cell lung cancer: analysis of 505 randomized patients. Ann Oncol. 2002;13(5):748–54.

98. Slotman B, Faivre-Finn C, Kramer G, Rankin E, Snee M, Hatton M, et al. Prophylactic cranial irradiation in extensive small-cell lung cancer. N Engl J Med. 2007;357(7):664–72.

99. Pottgen C, Eberhardt W, Grannass A, Korfee S, Stuben G, Teschler H, et al. Prophylactic cranial irradiation in operable

stage IIIA non small-cell lung cancer treated with neoadjuvant chemoradiotherapy: results from a German multicenter randomized trial. J Clin Oncol. 2007;25(31):4987–92.

100. Gore EM, Bae K, Wong SJ, Sun A, Bonner JA, Schild SE, et al. Phase III comparison of prophylactic cranial irradiation versus observation in patients with locally advanced non-small-cell lung cancer: primary analysis of radiation therapy oncology group study RTOG 0214. J Clin Oncol. 2011;29(3):272–8.

101. Balm M, Hammack J. Leptomeningeal carcinomatosis. Presenting features and prognostic factors. Arch Neurol. 1996;53 (7):626–32.

102. Herrlinger U, Forschler H, Kuker W, Meyermann R, Bamberg M, Dichgans J, et al. Leptomeningeal metastasis: survival and prognostic factors in 155 patients. J Neurol Sci. 2004;223 (2):167–78.

103. Clarke JL, Perez HR, Jacks LM, Panageas KS, Deangelis LM. Leptomeningeal metastases in the MRI era. Neurology. 2010;74 (18):1449–54.

104. Elliott JA, Osterlind K, Hirsch FR, Hansen HH. Metastatic patterns in small-cell lung cancer: correlation of autopsy findings with clinical parameters in 537 patients. J Clin Oncol. 1987;5 (2):246–54.

105. Stenbygaard LE, Sorensen JB, Olsen JE. Metastatic pattern at autopsy in non-resectable adenocarcinoma of the lung—a study from a cohort of 259 consecutive patients treated with chemotherapy. Acta Oncol. 1997;36(3):301–6.

106. Balducci L, Little DD, Khansur T, Steinberg MH. Carcinomatous meningitis in small cell lung cancer. Am J Med Sci 1984;287 (1):31–33.

107. Seute T, Leffers P, ten Velde GP, Twijnstra A. Leptomeningeal metastases from small cell lung carcinoma. Cancer. 2005;104 (8):1700–5.

108. Chamberlain MC, Kormanik P. Carcinoma meningitis secondary to non-small cell lung cancer: combined modality therapy. Arch Neurol. 1998;55(4):506–12.

109. Zachariah B, Zachariah SB, Varghese R, Balducci L. Carcinomatous meningitis: clinical manifestations and management. Int J Clin Pharmacol Ther. 1995;33(1):7–12.

110. Chamberlain MC. Leptomeningeal metastases: a review of evaluation and treatment. J Neurooncol. 1998;37(3):271–84.

111. Posner J. Neurologic complications of cancer. Philadelphia: F.A. Davis; 1995.

112. Rosen ST, Aisner J, Makuch RW, Matthews MJ, Ihde DC, Whitacre M, et al. Carcinomatous leptomeningitis in small cell lung cancer: a clinicopathologic review of the National Cancer Institute experience. Medicine (Baltimore). 1982;61(1):45–53.

113. Gleissner B, Chamberlain MC. Neoplastic meningitis. Lancet Neurol. 2006;5(5):443–52.

114. Groves MD, Glantz MJ, Chamberlain MC, Baumgartner KE, Conrad CA, Hsu S, et al. A multicenter phase II trial of intrathecal topotecan in patients with meningeal malignancies. Neuro Oncol. 2008;10(2):208–15.

115. Scott BJ, van Vugt VA, Rush T, Brown T, Chen CC, Carter BS, et al. Concurrent intrathecal methotrexate and liposomal cytarabine for leptomeningeal metastasis from solid tumors: a retrospective cohort study. J Neurooncol. 2014;119(2):361–8.

116. Kwon J, Chie EK, Kim K, Kim HJ, Wu HG, Kim IH, et al. Impact of multimodality approach for patients with leptomeningeal metastases from solid tumors. J Korean Med Sci. 2014;29(8):1094–101.

117. Waki F, Ando M, Takashima A, Yonemori K, Nokihara H, Miyake M, et al. Prognostic factors and clinical outcomes in patients with leptomeningeal metastasis from solid tumors. J Neurooncol. 2009;93(2):205–12.

118. Lee SJ, Lee JI, Nam DH, Ahn YC, Han JH, Sun JM, et al. Leptomeningeal carcinomatosis in non-small-cell lung cancer patients: impact on survival and correlated prognostic factors. J Thorac Oncol. 2013;8(2):185–91.

119. Yamada Y, Bilsky MH, Lovelock DM, Venkatraman ES, Toner S, Johnson J, et al. High-dose, single-fraction image-guided intensity-modulated radiotherapy for metastatic spinal lesions. Int J Radiat Oncol Biol Phys. 2008;71 (2):484–90.

120. Gagnon GJ, Nasr NM, Liao JJ, Molzahn I, Marsh D, McRae D, et al. Treatment of spinal tumors using cyberknife fractionated stereotactic radiosurgery: pain and quality-of-life assessment after treatment in 200 patients. Neurosurgery 200964(2):297–306; discussion 306–7.

121. Yamada Y, Lovelock DM, Bilsky MH. A review of image-guided intensity-modulated radiotherapy for spinal tumors. Neurosurgery 2007;61(2):226–35; discussion 235.

122. Sahgal A, Larson DA, Chang EL. Stereotactic body radiosurgery for spinal metastases: a critical review. Int J Radiat Oncol Biol Phys. 2008;71(3):652–65.

123. Kim JM, Losina E, Bono CM, Schoenfeld AJ, Collins JE, Katz JN, et al. Clinical outcome of metastatic spinal cord compression treated with surgical excision ± radiation versus radiation therapy alone: a systematic review of literature. Spine (Phila Pa 1976) 2012 Jan 1;37(1):78–84.

124. Patchell RA, Tibbs PA, Regine WF, Payne R, Saris S, Kryscio RJ, et al. Direct decompressive surgical resection in the treatment of spinal cord compression caused by metastatic cancer: a randomised trial. Lancet 2005;366(9486):643–648.

125. Rades D, Veninga T, Stalpers LJ, Basic H, Rudat V, Karstens JH, et al. Outcome after radiotherapy alone for metastatic spinal cord compression in patients with oligometastases. J Clin Oncol. 2007;25(1):50–6.

126. Helweg-Larsen S, Sorensen PS, Kreiner S. Prognostic factors in metastatic spinal cord compression: a prospective study using multivariate analysis of variables influencing survival and gait function in 153 patients. Int J Radiat Oncol Biol Phys. 2000;46 (5):1163–9.

127. Zaidat OO, Ruff RL. Treatment of spinal epidural metastasis improves patient survival and functional state. Neurology. 2002;58(9):1360–6.

128. Bauer HC. Posterior decompression and stabilization for spinal metastases. Analysis of sixty-seven consecutive patients. J Bone Joint Surg Am. 1997;79(4):514–22.

129. Klekamp J, Samii H. Surgical results for spinal metastases. Acta Neurochir (Wien). 1998;140(9):957–67.

130. Schiff D, O'Neill BP, Wang CH, O'Fallon JR. Neuroimaging and treatment implications of patients with multiple epidural spinal metastases. Cancer. 1998;83(8):1593–601.

131. Bach F, Agerlin N, Sorensen JB, Rasmussen TB, Dombernowsky P, Sorensen PS, et al. Metastatic spinal cord compression secondary to lung cancer. J Clin Oncol. 1992;10(11):1781–7.

132. Schiff D, O'Neill BP. Intramedullary spinal cord metastases: clinical features and treatment outcome. Neurology. 1996;47 (4):906–12.

133. Kalayci M, Cagavi F, Gul S, Yenidunya S, Acikgoz B. Intramedullary spinal cord metastases: diagnosis and treatment —an illustrated review. Acta Neurochir (Wien) 2004;146 (12):1347–54; discussion 1354.

134. Dam-Hieu P, Seizeur R, Mineo JF, Metges JP, Meriot P, Simon H. Retrospective study of 19 patients with intramedullary spinal cord metastasis. Clin Neurol Neurosurg. 2009;111(1):10–7.

135. Sung WS, Sung MJ, Chan JH, Manion B, Song J, Dubey A, et al. Intramedullary spinal cord metastases: a 20-year institutional

experience with a comprehensive literature review. World Neurosurg 2013;79(3–4):576–584.

136. Arcasoy SM, Jett JR. Superior pulmonary sulcus tumors and Pancoast's syndrome. N Engl J Med. 1997;337(19):1370–6.

137. Jaeckle KA. Neurologic manifestations of neoplastic and radiation-induced plexopathies. Semin Neurol. 2010;30(3):254–62.

138. Giometto B, Grisold W, Vitaliani R, Graus F, Honnorat J, Bertolini G, et al. Paraneoplastic neurologic syndrome in the PNS Euronetwork database: a European study from 20 centers. Arch Neurol. 2010;67(3):330–5.

139. Maddison P, Lang B. Paraneoplastic neurological autoimmunity and survival in small-cell lung cancer. J Neuroimmunol. 2008;15 (201–202):159–62.

140. Keime-Guibert F, Graus F, Broet P, Rene R, Molinuevo JL, Ascaso C, et al. Clinical outcome of patients with anti-Hu-associated encephalomyelitis after treatment of the tumor. Neurology. 1999;53(8):1719–23.

141. Titulaer MJ, Lang B, Verschuuren JJ. Lambert-Eaton myasthenic syndrome: from clinical characteristics to therapeutic strategies. Lancet Neurol. 2011;10(12):1098–107.

142. Pittock SJ, Kryzer TJ, Lennon VA. Paraneoplastic antibodies coexist and predict cancer, not neurological syndrome. Ann Neurol. 2004;56(5):715–9.

143. Hoffmann LA, Jarius S, Pellkofer HL, Schueller M, Krumbholz M, Koenig F, et al. Anti-Ma and anti-Ta associated paraneoplastic neurological syndromes: 22 newly diagnosed patients and review of previous cases. J Neurol Neurosurg Psychiatry. 2008;79(7):767–73.

144. Dalmau J, Graus F, Rosenblum MK, Posner JB. Anti-Hu–associated paraneoplastic encephalomyelitis/sensory neuronopathy. A clinical study of 71 patients. Medicine (Baltimore). 1992;71(2):59–72.

145. Graus F, Keime-Guibert F, Rene R, Benyahia B, Ribalta T, Ascaso C, et al. Anti-Hu-associated paraneoplastic encephalomyelitis: analysis of 200 patients. Brain. 2001;124(Pt 6):1138–48.

146. Sillevis Smitt P, Grefkens J, de Leeuw B, van den Bent M, van Putten W, Hooijkaas H, et al. Survival and outcome in 73 anti-Hu positive patients with paraneoplastic encephalomyelitis/sensory neuronopathy. J Neurol 2002;249(6):745–753.

147. Vernino S, Tuite P, Adler CH, Meschia JF, Boeve BF, Boasberg P, et al. Paraneoplastic chorea associated with CRMP-5 neuronal antibody and lung carcinoma. Ann Neurol. 2002;51(5):625–30.

148. Saiz A, Bruna J, Stourac P, Vigliani MC, Giometto B, Grisold W, et al. Anti-Hu-associated brainstem encephalitis. J Neurol Neurosurg Psychiatry. 2009;80(4):404–7.

149. Yu Z, Kryzer TJ, Griesmann GE, Kim K, Benarroch EE, Lennon VA. CRMP-5 neuronal autoantibody: marker of lung cancer and thymoma-related autoimmunity. Ann Neurol. 2001;49 (2):146–54.

150. Alamowitch S, Graus F, Uchuya M, Rene R, Bescansa E, Delattre JY. Limbic encephalitis and small cell lung cancer. Clinical and immunological features. Brain 1997;120 (Pt 6)(Pt 6):923–928.

151. Gultekin SH, Rosenfeld MR, Voltz R, Eichen J, Posner JB, Dalmau J. Paraneoplastic limbic encephalitis: neurological symptoms, immunological findings and tumour association in 50 patients. Brain 2000;123 (Pt 7)(Pt 7):1481–1494.

152. Lawn ND, Westmoreland BF, Kiely MJ, Lennon VA, Vernino S. Clinical, magnetic resonance imaging, and electroencephalographic findings in paraneoplastic limbic encephalitis. Mayo Clin Proc. 2003;78(11):1363–8.

153. Graus F, Delattre JY, Antoine JC, Dalmau J, Giometto B, Grisold W, et al. Recommended diagnostic criteria for paraneoplastic neurological syndromes. J Neurol Neurosurg Psychiatry. 2004;75(8):1135–40.

154. Bataller L, Kleopa KA, Wu GF, Rossi JE, Rosenfeld MR, Dalmau J. Autoimmune limbic encephalitis in 39 patients: immunophenotypes and outcomes. J Neurol Neurosurg Psychiatry. 2007;78(4):381–5.

155. Newsom-Davis J. Paraneoplastic neurological disorders. J R Coll Physicians Lond 1999;33(3):225–227.

156. Greenlee JE. Cytotoxic T cells in paraneoplastic cerebellar degeneration. Ann Neurol. 2000;47(1):4–5.

157. Shams'ili S, Grefkens J, de Leeuw B, van den Bent M, Hooijkaas H, van der Holt B, et al. Paraneoplastic cerebellar degeneration associated with antineuronal antibodies: analysis of 50 patients. Brain. 2003;126(Pt 6):1409–18.

158. Mason WP, Graus F, Lang B, Honnorat J, Delattre JY, Valldeoriola F, et al. Small-cell lung cancer, paraneoplastic cerebellar degeneration and the Lambert-Eaton myasthenic syndrome. Brain. 1997;120 (Pt 8)(Pt 8):1279–1300.

159. Fukuda T, Motomura M, Nakao Y, Shiraishi H, Yoshimura T, Iwanaga K, et al. Reduction of P/Q-type calcium channels in the postmortem cerebellum of paraneoplastic cerebellar degeneration with Lambert–Eaton myasthenic syndrome. Ann Neurol. 2003;53 (1):21–8.

160. Bataller L, Wade DF, Graus F, Stacey HD, Rosenfeld MR, Dalmau J. Antibodies to Zic4 in paraneoplastic neurologic disorders and small-cell lung cancer. Neurology. 2004;62 (5):778–82.

161. Bataller L, Graus F, Saiz A, Vilchez JJ. Spanish opsoclonus-myoclonus study group. Clinical outcome in adult onset idiopathic or paraneoplastic opsoclonus-myoclonus. Brain. 2001;124(Pt 2):437–43.

162. Pittock SJ, Lucchinetti CF, Lennon VA. Anti-neuronal nuclear autoantibody type 2: paraneoplastic accompaniments. Ann Neurol. 2003;53(5):580–7.

163. Vigliani MC, Honnorat J, Antoine JC, Vitaliani R, Giometto B, Psimaras D, et al. Chorea and related movement disorders of paraneoplastic origin: the PNS EuroNetwork experience. J Neurol. 2011;258(11):2058–68.

164. Adamus G, Ren G, Weleber RG. Autoantibodies against retinal proteins in paraneoplastic and autoimmune retinopathy. BMC Ophthalmol. 2004;4(4):5.

165. Ohguro H, Yokoi Y, Ohguro I, Mamiya K, Ishikawa F, Yamazaki H, et al. Clinical and immunologic aspects of cancer-associated retinopathy. Am J Ophthalmol. 2004;137 (6):1117–9.

166. Dropcho EJ. Antiamphiphysin antibodies with small-cell lung carcinoma and paraneoplastic encephalomyelitis. Ann Neurol. 1996;39(5):659–67.

167. Pittock SJ, Lucchinetti CF, Parisi JE, Benarroch EE, Mokri B, Stephan CL, et al. Amphiphysin autoimmunity: paraneoplastic accompaniments. Ann Neurol. 2005;58(1):96–107.

168. Camdessanche JP, Antoine JC, Honnorat J, Vial C, Petiot P, Convers P, et al. Paraneoplastic peripheral neuropathy associated with anti-Hu antibodies. A clinical and electrophysiological study of 20 patients. Brain. 2002;125(Pt 1):166–75.

169. Oh SJ, Kurokawa K, Claussen GC, Ryan HF Jr. Electrophysiological diagnostic criteria of Lambert–Eaton myasthenic syndrome. Muscle Nerve. 2005;32(4):515–20.

170. Graus F, Bonaventura I, Uchuya M, Valls-Sole J, Rene R, Leger JM, et al. Indolent anti-Hu-associated paraneoplastic sensory neuropathy. Neurology. 1994;44(12):2258–61.

171. Hart IK, Maddison P, Newsom-Davis J, Vincent A, Mills KR. Phenotypic variants of autoimmune peripheral nerve hyperexcitability. Brain. 2002;125(Pt 8):1887–95.

172. Irani SR, Bera K, Waters P, Zuliani L, Maxwell S, Zandi MS, et al. *N*-methyl-D-aspartate antibody encephalitis: temporal progression of clinical and paraclinical observations in a predominantly non-paraneoplastic disorder of both sexes. Brain. 2010;133(Pt 6):1655–67.

173. Irani SR, Pettingill P, Kleopa KA, Schiza N, Waters P, Mazia C, et al. Morvan syndrome: clinical and serological observations in 29 cases. Ann Neurol. 2012;72(2):241–55.

174. Antoine JC, Honnorat J, Camdessanche JP, Magistris M, Absi L, Mosnier JF, et al. Paraneoplastic anti-CV2 antibodies react with peripheral nerve and are associated with a mixed axonal and demyelinating peripheral neuropathy. Ann Neurol. 2001;49 (2):214–21.

175. Oh SJ. Paraneoplastic vasculitis of the peripheral nervous system. Neurol Clin. 1997;15(4):849–63.

176. Condom E, Vidal A, Rota R, Graus F, Dalmau J, Ferrer I. Paraneoplastic intestinal pseudo-obstruction associated with high titres of Hu autoantibodies. Virchows Arch A Pathol Anat Histopathol. 1993;423(6):507–11.

177. Lee HR, Lennon VA, Camilleri M, Prather CM. Paraneoplastic gastrointestinal motor dysfunction: clinical and laboratory characteristics. Am J Gastroenterol. 2001;96(2):373–9.

178. McKeon A, Lennon VA, Lachance DH, Fealey RD, Pittock SJ. Ganglionic acetylcholine receptor autoantibody: oncological, neurological, and serological accompaniments. Arch Neurol. 2009;66(6):735–41.

179. O'Neill JH, Murray NM, Newsom-Davis J. The Lambert–Eaton myasthenic syndrome. A review of 50 cases. Brain. 1988;111 (Pt 3)(Pt 3):577–596.

180. Chalk CH, Murray NM, Newsom-Davis J, O'Neill JH, Spiro SG. Response of the Lambert-Eaton myasthenic syndrome to treatment of associated small-cell lung carcinoma. Neurology. 1990;40(10):1552–6.

181. Sanders DB. Lambert-eaton myasthenic syndrome: diagnosis and treatment. Ann N Y Acad Sci. 2003;998:500–8.

182. Sabater L, Titulaer M, Saiz A, Verschuuren J, Gure AO, Graus F. SOX1 antibodies are markers of paraneoplastic Lambert-Eaton myasthenic syndrome. Neurology. 2008;70(12):924–8.

183. Titulaer MJ, Klooster R, Potman M, Sabater L, Graus F, Hegeman IM, et al. SOX antibodies in small-cell lung cancer and Lambert-Eaton myasthenic syndrome: frequency and relation with survival. J Clin Oncol. 2009;27(26):4260–7.

184. Buchbinder R, Forbes A, Hall S, Dennett X, Giles G. Incidence of malignant disease in biopsy-proven inflammatory myopathy. A population-based cohort study. Ann Intern Med. 2001;134 (12):1087–95.

185. Hill CL, Zhang Y, Sigurgeirsson B, Pukkala E, Mellemkjaer L, Airio A, et al. Frequency of specific cancer types in dermatomyositis and polymyositis: a population-based study. Lancet. 2001;357(9250):96–100.

186. Fardet L, Dupuy A, Gain M, Kettaneh A, Cherin P, Bachelez H, et al. Factors associated with underlying malignancy in a retrospective cohort of 121 patients with dermatomyositis. Medicine (Baltimore). 2009;88(2):91–7.

187. Maddison P, McConville J, Farrugia ME, Davies N, Rose M, Norwood F, et al. The use of rituximab in myasthenia gravis and Lambert-Eaton myasthenic syndrome. J Neurol Neurosurg Psychiatry. 2011;82(6):671–3.

188. Keime-Guibert F, Graus F, Fleury A, Rene R, Honnorat J, Broet P, et al. Treatment of paraneoplastic neurological syndromes with antineuronal antibodies (Anti-Hu, anti-Yo) with a combination of immunoglobulins, cyclophosphamide, and methylprednisolone. J Neurol Neurosurg Psychiatry. 2000;68 (4):479–82.

Neurological Complications of Breast Cancer and Its Treatment

Emilie Le Rhun, Sophie Taillibert, and Marc C. Chamberlain

List of Abbreviations	
AED	Antiepileptic drugs
AMPAR	Amino-3-hydroxy-5-methyl-4-isoxazolepropionic acid receptor
APOE	Apolipoprotein E
ASIA	American Spinal Injury Association
BC	Breast cancer
BM	Brain metastases
BCRA	BReast CAncer
CIPN	Chemotherapy-induced peripheral neuropathy
CMF	Cyclophosphamide, methotrexate, and 5-fluorouracil
CNS	Central nervous system
COMT	Catechol-O-methyltransferase
COWA	Controlled Oral Word Association
CVD	Cerebrovascular disease
CSF	Cerebrospinal fluid
CT	Computed tomography
DTI	Diffusion tensor imaging
DNA	Desoxyribose nucleic acid
ECOG	Eastern Cooperative Oncology Group
EIAED	Enzyme-inducing antiepileptic drugs
EORTC	European Organization for Research and Treatment of Cancer
EpCAM	Epithelial cell adhesion molecule
ER	Estrogen receptors
ESCC	Epidural spinal cord compression

E. Le Rhun (✉)
Department of Neurosurgery and Neuro-oncology,
University Hospital, 59037 Lille Cedex, France
e-mail: emilie.lerhun@chru-lille.fr

E. Le Rhun
Breast unit, Department of Medical Oncology,
Oscar Lambert Center, 59020 Lille Cedex, France

E. Le Rhun
PRISM Inserm U1192, Villeneuve d'Ascq, France

S. Taillibert
Department of Neurology, Pitié-Salpétrière Hospital,
UPMC-Paris VI University, 47 Boulevard de l'Hôpital,
75013 Paris, France
e-mail: sophie.taillibert@pal.aphp.frsophie.taillibert@gmail.com

S. Taillibert
Department of Radiation Oncology, Pitié-Salpétrière Hospital,
UPMC-Paris VI University, 47 Boulevard de l'Hôpital,
75013 Paris, France

M.C. Chamberlain
Department of Neurology and Neurological Surgery,
Seattle Cancer Care Alliance, University of Washington,
835 Eastlake Ave East, Seattle, WA 98109, USA
e-mail: chambemc@uw.edu

© Springer International Publishing AG 2018
D. Schiff et al. (eds.), *Cancer Neurology in Clinical Practice*,
DOI 10.1007/978-3-319-57901-6_23

FLAIR	Fluid-attenuated inversion recovery
18FDG-PET	[(18)F] 2-fluoro-2-deoxyglucose–positron emission tomography
fMRI	Functional MRI
5-FU	5 fluorouracil
GPA	Graded prognostic assessment
Gy	Gray
HA-WBRT	Hippocampal avoidance whole-brain radiotherapy
HER2	Human epidermal growth factor receptor 2
HRQOL	Health-related quality of life
HLVT-R DR	Hopkins Verbal Learning Test-Revised Delayed Recall
HVLT-R	Hopkins Verbal Learning Test-Revised
ICCTF	International Cognition and Cancer Task Force
ICH	Intracranial hemorrhage
ISCM	Intramedullary spinal cord metastasis
KPS	Karnofsky performance status
LM	Leptomeningeal metastases
LMWH	Low molecular weight heparin
MBP	Myelin basic protein
MMSE	Mini-mental status examination
MRI	Magnetic resonance imaging
mTOR	*Mammalian target of rapamycin*
NCCN	National Comprehensive Cancer Network
NF2	Neurofibromatosis 2
NGF	Nerve growth factor
NMDA	*N*-methyl-D-aspartate
OS	Overall survival
PARP	*Poly (ADP-ribose) polymerase*
PET	Positron emission tomography
PI3K	Phosphoinositide 3-kinase
PNS	Paraneoplastic neurological syndromes
PR	Progesterone receptors
PFS	Progression-free survival
PRES	Posterior reversible encephalopathy
PS	Performance status
QoL	Quality of life
RECIST	Response Evaluation Criteria In Solid Tumors
RIBP	Radiation-induced brachial plexopathy
RT	Radiotherapy
RTOG	Radiation Treatment Oncology group
SEER	Surveillance epidemiology and end results
SMART	Stroke-like migraine attacks after radiation therapy
SRS	Stereotactic surgery
SRT	Stereotactic radiotherapy (stereotactic hypofractionated radiotherapy)
STIR	Short TI inversion recovery
tPA	Tissue-type plasminogen activator
TMT	Trail Making Test
uPA	Urokinase plasminogen activator
US	USA
VEGF	Vascular endothelial growth factor
VTE	Venous thromboembolism
WBRT	Whole-brain radiotherapy
WHO	World Health Organization

Introduction

Breast cancer (BC) is one of the most common cancers in women with approximately 1 in 8 developing BC. Neurological complications of BC can result from metastases, treatment, and other causes. Neurological signs and symptoms may involve both the central (CNS) nervous system and the peripheral (PNS) nervous system. CNS metastases portend a poor outcome in patients with BC, and in all cases, the neurological complications of BC have a significant impact on the functional status and quality of life (QoL) of the patient. An outline of the chapter is illustrated in Table 23.1.

Metastatic Complications

Central Nervous System Metastases

Parenchymal Brain Metastases (Fig. 23.1)

Breast cancer (BC) is one the most frequent systemic cancers resulting in brain metastases (BM). Between 10 and 30% of BC patients will develop BM [1]. BM often have a significant clinical impact by reducing the QoL and compromising survival [2].

Table 23.1 Neurological complications of breast cancer: outline

Metastatic complications of breast cancer	Central nervous system
	Cranial
	Parenchymal brain metastases
	Skull base metastases
	Dural metastases
	Spinal
	Intramedullary spinal cord metastases
	Spinal epidural metastases
	Leptomeningeal metastases
	Peripheral nervous system
	Peripheral nervous system metastases
	Neoplastic plexopathy
Non-metastatic, non-treatment-related complications	Paraneoplastic syndromes
	Meningiomas
Treatment related complications	Central nervous system
	Encephalopathy
	Cognitive injury
	Radionecrosis
	Cardiovascular complications
	Meningitic syndromes
	Myelopathy
	Peripheral nervous system
	Plexopathy
	Radiculopathy
	Neuropathy
	Peripheral neuropathy
	Myopathy

BM in BC most often are metachronous in presentation and seen in patients with known cancer (80%), but can also be the first manifestation of cancer (5–10%) [3] or discovered concomitantly with systemic disease. BM are solitary in 20 to 30% of patients and are oligometastatic (2 or 3 lesions) in the same proportion [2, 3]. Signs and symptoms of BM are related to the anatomic localization of the metastases. Approximately 50% of patients present with headache, and 30% present with focal neurological signs, mostly seizures [4]. Cranial computed tomography (CT) scan is able to detect BM; however, the sensitivity and specificity of magnetic resonance imaging (MRI) are considerably higher [5]. Contrast MRI permits a more precise evaluation of the number and location of BM. BM are located in the cerebral hemispheres (80% overall) and less frequently in the cerebellum (15%) or brainstem (5%). Once developed, the neurological symptoms/signs do not always resolve, even in patients responding to treatment. Early diagnosis and serial follow-up after BM are diagnosed as important to minimize emergence of CNS disease that may compromise QoL and survival. In the CEREBEL study of human epidermal growth factor receptor 2 (HER2)-positive metastatic BC, nearly 20% of the patients had asymptomatic BM. Considering the high proportion of BM in BC and the increasing treatment options in the HER2-positive population, serial brain MRI appears clinically appropriate [3].

The incidence of and the time to presentation of BM vary according to the subtype of BC (categorized as luminal A: ER/PR positive, HER2 negative; luminal B: triple positive; HER2: HER2 positive, ER/PR negative; and basal: triple negative). In a cohort of 383 BC patients treated for BM, both the median time between BC and BM diagnoses and the median overall survival (OS) following discovery of BM were significantly different among the different BC subtypes [6]. The shortest interval between BC diagnosis and BM diagnosis was observed in the basal/triple negative and the HER2 subtypes (Table 23.2) [7, 8]. The overexpression of HER2 is associated with a higher risk of BM; between 30 and 50% of HER2-positive patients will develop BM [9–12]. Several risk factors for BM have been identified in BC patients, including overexpression of HER2, estrogen receptor negativity, triple negative status, young age, nodal involvement, high-grade tumors, and larger tumor size [7, 8, 13–15].

In a Japanese retrospective cohort of 1256 BC patients with BM, the median OS was 8.7 months [16]. Shortest OS was observed in the non-HER2-positive subtypes in the cohort of Sperduto et al. [7, 8, 15]. No significant difference in OS was observed among HER2-positive tumors in a large cohort of 423 HER2-positive BC patients with BM [17]. In this cohort, BM patients treated with trastuzumab and lapatinib had a significantly longer survival as compared to patients treated with trastuzumab alone, lapatinib alone, or

Fig. 23.1 Brain metastases. Brain MRI, T1 W gadolinium-enhanced axial images

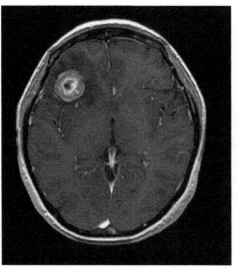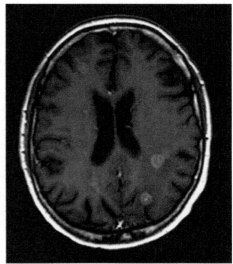

no HER2-targeting agent. The subtype of BC appears to not only influence prognosis but cause death as well. Half of all patients with HER2-positive BM die of CNS disease progression, whereas patients with triple negative BC die most commonly of systemic disease [9, 18].

The Breast Graded Prognostic Assessment (Breast-GPA) instrument developed by the RTOG (Radiation Treatment Oncology Group) can assist in determining the prognosis of BC patients with BM and guide treatment. For BC, the GPA instrument used a single prognostic factor, the Karnofsky Performance Status (KPS) [19]. In another RTOG cohort of newly diagnosed BC patients, significant prognostic factors included the KPS, the HER2, ER/PR status, and the interaction between ER/PR and HER2 [6]. The initial Breast-GPA was revised based on a larger cohort of BC patients with BM and now includes, KPS, BC subtype, and age (Table 23.3). The median OS was estimated at 3.4 months for patients with a Breast-GPA score $\geq$1 and at 25.3 months for patients with a BC-GPA score between 3.5 and 4.0 [6]. Notably, the number of BM was not integrated in the revised Breast-GPA; however, a recent analysis of another large cohort of patients with BC and BM suggested that the number of BM (>3 vs. $\leq$ 3) has a significant impact on survival [20]. In the aforementioned Japanese cohort, multivariate analyses found increased survival in patients diagnosed with BM within 6 months of metastatic BC diagnoses, with asymptomatic BM, or with HER2-positive/ estrogen receptor-positive tumors [16]. In another retrospective cohort of 215 BC patients, non-luminal subtype, presence of extracranial disease, time to CNS metastases <15 months, the presence of >3 BM, and a low Breast-GPA were associated with a shorter survival [21].

Relatively few trials have been prospectively studied in BC patients with BM. Indeed, in the majority of BM trials, lung cancer patients represent the largest population. As BC and lung cancer share a better radiosensitivity relative to melanoma [22], the management of BC BM can be in part extrapolated from the results of these trials. Initial treatment for newly diagnosed BC-related BM includes surgery, whole-brain radiotherapy (WBRT), stereotactic radiotherapy (stereotactic radiosurgery [SRS] and stereotactic radiotherapy [SRT]), systemic therapy, clinical trials, and palliative care. The choice of treatment depends on the number, localization, and volume of BM, the neurological and overall status of the patient, and the control of the systemic disease [23, 24]. The intent of BM-directed treatment in BC can be curative or palliative. Additionally, supportive care is important following BM diagnosis. The lowest effective dose of steroids is recommended for the management of vasogenic edema to avoid steroid-related toxicity that may further compromise QoL. According to the American Academy of Neurology and European guidelines, prophylactic antiseizure treatment is not recommended in patients with BM [25, 26]. In a patient with seizures and BM in whom an antiepileptic drug is indicated, the use of non enzyme-inducing agents is recommended to minimize interactions with systemic anticancer treatments.

Surgical resection is considered for patients with accessible and limited BM. In a cohort of 42 BC patients with BM, the median OS after surgery was 16 months [27]. In this case series, age was the only factor significantly correlated in multivariate analyses with OS. In another cohort of 116 BC patients with BM, the median OS was 11.5 months [28]. Surgical resection is performed in patients with a solitary BM in non-eloquent brain regions and in patients with well-controlled systemic disease. Surgical resections of all lesions in patients with up to 3 BM may improve survival as well [29, 30]. Indications are less clear in patients with multiple BM or uncontrolled extracranial disease, but in some cases, surgery can provide rapid relief of symptoms

Table 23.2 Incidence, median delay between breast cancer (BC) diagnosis and brain metastases (BM) diagnosis, and median overall survival after BM diagnosis

	Incidence of the different BC subtypes in BM (%)	Median delay between BC diagnosis and BM diagnosis (months)	Median survival after BM diagnosis (months)	References
Luminal A	20 14	54.4 30	10.0 9.3 7.4 5	Sperduto [6] Niikuara [16] Aversa [15] Bachmann [8]
Luminal B	25.5 35	47.4 96 33.5	22.9 16.5 19.2 16.5	Sperduto [6] Niikuara [16] Aversa [15] Hayashi [17]
HER2	31 49	35.8 36 33.5	17.9 11.5 7 11.5	Sperduto [6] Niikuara [16] Aversa [15] Hayashi [17]
Basal /triple negative	23.5 22	27.5 35	7.2 7.3 4.9 4.9 5	Dawood [399] Sperduto [6] Niikuara [16] Aversa [15] Bachmann [8]

Abbreviations: *BC* breast cancer, *BM* brain metastases

Table 23.3 Revised breast cancer graded prognostic assessment

Factor	0.0	0.5	1.0	1.5	2.0
KPS	≤ 50	60	70–80	90–100	–
Genetic subtype	Basal	–	Luminal A	HER2	Luminal B
Age	≥ 60	<60	–	–	–

Group	Breast-GPA	MST (months) (95% CI)	1 year OS (95% CI)	2 year OS (95% CI)	3 year OS (95% CI)
Group 1	0.0–1.0	3.4 (2.4–4.9)	15 (4–33)	0	0
Group 2	1.5–2.0	7.7 (4.8–9.7)	32 (23–41)	13 (6–20)	6 (2–13)
Group 3	2.5–3.0	15.1 (10.8–17.9)	55 (46–63)	29 (21–37)	19 (11–27)
Group 4	3.5–4.0	25.3 (20.4–30.4)	77 (69–84)	53 (43–61)	31 (22–40)

Abbreviations: *KPS* Karnofsky performance score, *MST* Median survival time, *OS* Overall survival
Used with permission of Springer Science from Sperduto et al. [6]

due to intracranial hypertension and obstructive hydrocephalus, particularly in patients with a large symptomatic lesion [31]. In summary, resective surgery is indicated for (1) therapeutic indications including a large symptomatic or asymptomatic lesion; (2) diagnostic indications including the absence of known primary tumor, doubt regarding the metastatic origin of the lesion, uncertainty between radionecrosis, and progression after brain irradiation; and (3) histological and molecular biological documentation. Advances in surgery include functional MRI (fMRI) with fiber tract mapping, transcranial stimulation, and intra-operative MRI. Piecemeal resection should be avoided as the recurrence rate is 1.7 times higher than tumors removed *en bloc*, particularly for lesions in the posterior fossa and in contact with CSF pathways [32, 33]. When feasible, a microscopic total resection with a 5-mm margin

of normal-appearing tissue may lead to a reduced incidence of local recurrence [34]. When surgery is performed, histological and molecular biomarkers should be re-examined to verify the concordance between the primary BC and the BM and to identify potential druggable targets.

The indications for stereotactic radiosurgery (SRS) or stereotactic RT (SRT) include BM in patients with surgically inaccessible metastases, post-surgical treatment of the operative cavity, and progressive BM in patients previously treated with WBRT (re-irradiation). SRT is used in patients with a limited number of BM, limited lesional volume, and controlled systemic disease. SRS is often used for patients with less than 5 BM. However, large retrospective cohorts with up to 15 lesions have reported similar outcomes to those with 1–4 BM [35–38]. The total volume of tumor has been suggested to be more important than total number of lesions [39]. Local control rates observed after SRS range from 64 to 94% [31]. SRS alone may be as effective as surgery and SRS of the resection cavity [40–42]. In a cohort of 136 BC patients presenting with 1–3 BM and treated with SRS, local failure rate was 10% at 12 months and the median OS was 17.6 months. On multivariate analyses, patients with >1 lesion, triple negative BC, and poorly controlled extracranial disease had a shorter OS [43]. In another cohort of 131 BC patients with BM treated by SRS, the median OS varied significantly according to the type of BC, ranging from 7 months in triple negative patients, to 16 months in ER-positive HER2-negative patients, 23 months in ER-negative HER2-positive patients, and 26 months in ER-positive HER2-positive patients [44]. The dose of SRS varies according to the volume of the lesion and the potential risk of radionecrosis. In a small study, the dose of SRS in BC patients with 1–3 BM was evaluated by comparing 20 patients treated with 20 Gy versus 10 patients treated with 16–18.5 Gy [45]. The local control rates were 94% after 20 Gy and 48% after 16–18.5 Gy.

WBRT has long been the standard treatment for BM, though its role has changed with the advent of SRS/SRT, new methods of WBRT, such as hippocampal avoidance, and improved knowledge of outcome based upon BC subtype. Notably, however, WBRT decreases local and distant failures after either surgery or SRS/SRT [46]. Addition of WBRT results in a clinically significant benefit in 64–83% of patients with BM and is associated with an increase of 2–6 months in overall survival [47]. BC, as well as non-small cell lung cancer (NSCLC), are more likely to respond to WBRT compared to other histologies [48]. Response rates to WBRT in BC patients with BM vary from 65 to 82% [48–50]. The combination of WBRT and systemic agents constitutes another potential treatment for BC BM. The addition of temozolomide to WBRT in BC patients did not improve local control or survival in a phase II randomized trial (NCT 00875355) [51]. The addition of veliparib, an oral PARP inhibitor, to WBRT was well tolerated and showed encouraging preliminary efficacy data in a cohort with 31% of BC patients [52].

A phase III European Organization for Research and Treatment of Cancer trial (EORTC 22952-26001) assessed the impact of WBRT after surgery or SRS on the preservation of functional independence in patients with 1–3 BM (>90% with a solitary BM) from solid tumors (excluding small cell lung cancer) with stable extracranial disease and a 0–2 WHO performance status (PS) [53]. In this study, 199 patients underwent SRS and 160 underwent surgery. The median time to a deterioration of WHO PS by more than 2 points was 10.0 months after observation and 9.5 months after WBRT. OS was not significantly different between the 2 arms (10.9 months after WBRT and 10.7 after observation). The 2-year relapse rate at both the initial treated site

and at new sites of disease was significantly reduced after WBRT, although BC represented only 12% of all tumors in this trial. The role of WBRT added to SRS in BC patients with 1–3 BM has been reported in a retrospective cohort of 30 patients treated by SRS alone and 28 treated by SRS plus WBRT [54]. The addition of WBRT to SRS resulted in significantly longer survival without new BM but no difference was observed in survival between the 2 groups. In the EORTC trial, a significantly better health-related quality of life (HRQOL) was observed in the observation arm compared to the WBRT arm during the first year after treatment [55]. The authors conclude that WBRT was detrimental to several elements of the HRQOL. This study also reported that frequent monitoring for BM recurrence did not have a negative impact on HRQOL. The impact of WBRT on cognition was assessed in a small randomized controlled study (NCT 00548756). In this trial, patients with 1–3 newly diagnosed BM were randomly assigned to SRS plus WBRT or SRS alone. The primary endpoint was cognition measured by Hopkins Verbal Learning Test-Revised (HVLT-R) total recall at 4 months. The study was stopped in accordance with trial stoppage guideline, after determination of a 96% probability that patients in the SRS + WBRT group were significantly more likely to have cognitive decline as compared to patients treated by SRS alone [56]. In the Alliance trial (NCT00377156), 213 patients with 1–3 BM, each <3 cm were randomized between SRS alone or SRS plus WBRT [57]. The primary objective was to evaluate cognitive decline. After SRS alone, intracranial tumor control with SRS was 66.1% at 6 months and 50.5% at 12 months. After SRS plus WBRT, intracranial tumor control was 88.3% at 6 months and 84.9% at 12 months. Median OS was 10.7 months after SRS alone and 7.5 months after SRS plus WBRT. Moreover, despite better local control after WBRT without improvement of OS, the cognitive decline was higher after SRS plus WBRT.

The incidence of radiation-induced white matter injury has been assessed in a retrospective cohort of 35 BC patients treated by SRS plus WBRT and 30 patients treated by SRS alone. A higher incidence of white matter hyperintensities by brain MRI was observed after combined treatment. At one year, 71.5% of the patients treated with both SRS and WBRT demonstrated white matter lesions (limited periventricular hyperintensity in 42.9%, diffuse white matter hyperintensity in 28.6%), whereas only one patient treated with SRS developed white matter lesions [58].

The use of WBRT is increasingly deferred, given evidence that WBRT negatively impacts QoL and cognition, and because BC patients, especially those with HER2 positive tumors, are living longer. Initial treatment with SRS and close radiographic monitoring is thus preferred in patients with a limited number of BM. The indications for WBRT include multiple and disseminated BM, and failure of stereotactic radiotherapy [31]. The incidence of cognitive decline as assessed by a decline in the Mini-Mental Status Examination (MMSE) was determined in a prospective randomized trial comparing WBRT plus SRS versus SRS alone in 110 patients with 1–4 BM [59]. Deterioration in the MMSE was seen in 39% of patients in the WBRT plus SRS group and 26% of patients in the SRS only group. On average deterioration occurred at 13.6 months in the WBRT plus SRS group and at 6.8 months in the SRS group. Recognizing the limitations of the MMSE as an instrument to assess cognition, these data suggested that cognitive impairment in patients with treated BM may result from radiation-related toxicity as well as recurrence of BM. Thus the control of brain disease is of particular importance for preservation of cognition.

Several approaches have been evaluated to minimize RT-associated cognitive decline. Memantine, a N-methyl-D-aspartate (NMDA) receptor agonist, was assessed in a randomized double-blind placebo controlled trial in patients treated with WBRT [60]. Memantine was well tolerated but the difference in delayed recall, the primary endpoint, was not significant between treatment arms. Nonetheless significantly longer time to cognitive deterioration, reduction in the rate of decline in delayed recognition, executive function and processing speed was observed with memantine. Perihippocampal stem cells injury as a consequence of WBRT may contribute to RT associated cognitive decline, and thus shielding the hippocampal neural stem cell compartment was evaluated in a phase II study utilizing hippocampal avoidance WBRT (HA-WBRT) in patients with BM (RTOG 0933) [61]. In this study, the median OS was 6.8 months. The mean relative decline in Hopkins Verbal Learning Test-Revised Delayed Recall (HLVT-R DR) at 4 months (primary endpoint) was 7.0%, significantly lower than historical controls.

The efficacy of liposomal doxorubicin in combination with cyclophosphamide was evaluated in a retrospective study of 29 BC patients. The objective response rate in brain was 41.4% after 3 cycles (50% in the absence of prior brain RT). The median OS from brain diagnosis was 23 months [62]. BM responses have also been reported with anthracycline-based regimens, CMF (cyclophosphamide, methotrexate and 5-fluorouracil), and high-dose methotrexate [23]. Temozolomide as single agent in metastatic BC and BM has little activity based upon two small phase II studies in which the objective response rate was <6% and transient [63, 64]. Similarly gefitinib has no activity, based on a single phase II trial [65]. Interim analyses of the phase II did not meet the efficacy point [23]. TPI-287, a microtubule-stabilizing agent, designed to bypass the MDR-1 drug efflux resistance mechanism is undergoing study [23]. Other new agents under development include cabazitaxel (NCT01913067), ANG1005 (NCT01480583), TPI-287

(NCT01332630) and 2B3-101 a glutathione-pegylated doxorubicin (NCT01386580).

Targeted therapies are highly efficacious in BC. Genomic and epigenomic profiling of metastases may provide a basis for future therapeutic strategies [66, 67]. Endocrine therapies represent the oldest targeted therapies in BC, and responses of BM to tamoxifen, aromatase inhibitors and megestrol acetate have been reported in small case reports [3]. However, loss of hormonal receptor positivity is frequent in BM (when compared to the matched primary tumor) often obviating the use of hormonal agents [68]. In a cohort of 36 paired samples of the primary BC and BM, the discordance rates were 28% for ER and 20% for PR [69]. Additionally the majority ER-positive BC is endocrine-refractory when BM is diagnosed [23].

Anti-HER2 targeted agents play an important role in the management of BM in HER2 positive breast cancer. In the cohort of 36 paired tumors mentioned above, the discordant rate was only 3% only for HER2 status [69]. Improved OS has been reported in several retrospective studies in HER2 positive BC patients with BM when treated with trastuzumab [12, 70, 71]. Approximately one third of metastatic BC patients receiving trastuzumab develop BM [12, 72]. In 50%, BM are diagnosed when systemic disease is controlled. BM has been shown to develop later in patients treated with trastuzumab [70]. Furthermore, a survival benefit has been reported with continuation of trastuzumab-based therapies after development of BM [70, 73–77]. However, the impact on OS may relate more to control of extracranial disease.

The efficacy and the safety of lapatinib alone was first evaluated in 39 patients with HER2 positive progressive BM all previously treated by trastuzumab and by WBRT in 37 cases [78]. The objective response rate was low (2.6%). The median time to progression was 3.0 months suggesting very limited activity as a single agent. In a phase II study, 242 HER2 positive BC patients with progressive BM previously treated with trastuzumab and cranial RT were treated with lapatinib alone [79]. The objective response rate was 6%; 21% had a volumetric response of 20% or more. Of the 50 patients enrolled in the extension phase of the study that added capecitabine to lapatinib, a CNS objective response was observed in 20% (according to RECIST criteria) and 40% (based on volumetric response of 20% or more). Importantly, the effect of capecitabine alone cannot be excluded in the extension phase, although lapatinib may have had an additive effect. The modest activity of lapatinib in the CNS replicates that seen in systemic disease as well [80]. The efficacy of the combination of lapatinib and capecitabine was confirmed in a cohort of 22 evaluable HER2 positive BC patients with previously treated BM [81]. Partial responses were observed in 7 patients and stabilization was observed in 6 patients. The median brain PFS was 5.6 months and the median OS was 27.9 months, significantly longer than in patients treated with trastuzumab-based therapies after CNS progression (16.7 months). The response rates observed with lapatinib and capecitabine were replicated in several expanded access programs [18% response reported by Boccardo and 21% reported by Sutherland] [82, 83]. In combination with capecitabine, CNS response rates vary from 18 to 38% [78, 79, 81–84].

Excess toxicity and lack of efficacy was observed in a study comparing the combination of lapatinib plus topotecan versus lapatinib plus capecitabine [84]. The efficacy of the combination of lapatinib and capecitabine was studied in the LANDSCAPE phase II trial (NCT00967031) in untreated asymptomatic BM with HER2 positive BC [85]. A high partial response rate of 66% was seen. The median time to progression was 5.5 months. This approach constitutes an option for patients with HER2 positive tumors that are low volume and paucisymptomatic. The CEREBEL trial, designed to demonstrate that the combination of lapatinib plus capecitabine could reduce the incidence of BM compared to trastuzumab plus capecitabine, was closed early due to a low incidence of BM (3% in the lapatinib plus capecitabine group and 4% in the trastuzumab plus capecitabine group) [86].

In a retrospective study, Bartsch evaluated the impact of trastuzumab and lapatinib on 80 HER2 positive BC patients with BM [71]. Median OS was 13 months in patients treated with trastuzumab after diagnosis of BM, 9 months in patients treated with chemotherapy and 3 months in patients treated with RT only. Addition of lapatinib to trastuzumab, either sequentially or concomitantly, prolonged OS compared to trastuzumab alone. Thus, the combination of lapatinib and trastuzumab may be an option for BC BM.

The combination of trastuzumab and WBRT resulted in a response rate of 74% suggesting possible radiosensitization [87]. The potential radiosensitizing impact of lapatinib in combination with WBRT was evaluated in a phase I trial in which a response rate of 79% was observed [88]. Further studies are ongoing. New anti-HER2 therapies (pertuzumab, TDM-1) have been approved recently; however, their impact on BM is not yet well defined. Regimens containing afatinib, an irreversible HER2 and EGFR inhibitor, failed to improve PFS in a phase III trial, compared to either trastuzumab or lapatinib [89]. Only a few responses were observed with neratinib in a phase II study enrolling 40 BC patients with progressive BM previously treated (NCT01494662) [90]. The association of neratinib and capecitabine is also under investigation [91]. Other new anti-HER2s, including ARRY-380, a HER2-selective tyrosine kinase inhibitor, are in development [24, 91].

A CNS response of 63% was observed on prespecified volumetric criteria in a phase II trial evaluating the combination of carboplatin and bevacizumab in BC BM patients [92]. By RECIST criteria, the response rate was 45%. In another phase II trial, the objective CNS response rate according to RECIST criteria was 77% for the combination of bevacizumab, etoposide and cisplatin [93]. The median CNS PFS and OS were 7.3 and 10.5 months, respectively.

mTOR, PI3 K and dual mTOR/PI3 K inhibitors are currently being explored in breast cancer. Everolimus, a rapamycin analogue that inhibits mTOR signalling, is being evaluated in a phase II trial in combination with trastuzumab and vinorelbine in HER2 positive BC with BM. BKM20, an oral pan-PI3 K inhibitor, is also being studied in HER2 positive BC patients with BM (NCT01132664). PARP inhibitors, which disrupt DNA repair, such as ABT-888, are also being investigated in BM patients (NCT00649207). Iniparib, initially developed as a PARP inhibitor but subsequently shown not to have any PARP inhibitor activity, showed a modest activity in BM [24]. Immune-based approaches including ipilimumab and anti-PD-1 therapies may also be new promising approaches if activity is confirmed in BC.

Skull Base Metastases

Skull base metastases occur in approximately 4% of cancer patients [94], and are found in 22% of autopsy cases [95]. BC is one of the most common causes of skull base metastases, accounting for 20.5–40% of all cases [94–96]. Skull base metastases are most often diagnosed in patients with disseminated disease, particularly to other skeletal elements [96]. Direct hematogenous spread is the primary route of dissemination to the skull base. Rarely, retrograde seeding through the valveless venous plexus of Batson has been proposed [97, 98]. Progressive ipsilateral involvement of cranial nerves is the main presentation of skull base metastases. The clinical manifestations depend on the size, location and growth rate of the metastases. The etiology of signs and symptoms is multifactorial and includes stretching of the dura, compression of cranial nerves, irritation of adjacent brain and occlusion of dural venous sinuses [99]. Five main clinical syndromes have been defined based on anatomic site of disease (Table 23.4) [96].

Contrast MRI is the technique of choice for the diagnosis of skull base metastases. Fat suppression techniques are particularly useful. Bone metastases are characterized by a hypointense lesion on non-enhanced T1-weighted MRI sequence [100]. Contrast enhancement is variable on T1 weighted sequences with fat suppression. MRI further permits determination of invasion of the cavernous sinus, the dura or cranial nerves. Orbital CT may help by demonstrating bone anatomy and associated erosion. Importantly, a normal imaging study does not exclude the diagnosis [94]. Radionuclide bone scan can reveal skull base metastases, but sensitivity is poor particularly for osteolytic lesions [101]. FDG-PET has a similar accuracy to that of bone scintigraphy

Table 23.4 Main clinical syndromes associated with skull base metastases

Clinical syndrome	Clinical description
Sellar and parasellar syndrome (29%)	*Sellar* Characterized by co-occurring pituitary metastases Most often silent as near complete destruction of the adenohypophysis is necessary to produce clinical manifestations Posterior metastases: diabetes insipidus Anterior metastases: hypopituitarism and visual loss Lateral extension: cranial neuropathies affecting oculomotor and trigeminal nerves *Parasellar* Oculomotor and trigeminal nerve palsies Frontal headache, facial paresthesia or pain, and periorbital swelling are also reported
Occipital condyle syndrome (16%)	Unilateral severe and constant pain in the occipital region followed by ipsilateral 12th cranial nerve palsy leading to dysarthria and dysphagia, atrophy of the ipsilateral tongue with associated fasciculations Meningismus is frequent Radiation of pain to the forehead Isolated hypoglossal nerve palsy
Orbital syndrome (12.5–15%)	Progressive frontal headaches particularly over the ipsilateral affected eye with associated blurred vision and diplopia Sensory loss of the forehead due to trigeminal sensory involvement Proptosis and ophthalmoplegia of the involved eye Local signs such as periorbital swelling
Middle fossa syndrome, or Gasserian ganglion syndrome (6%)	Facial paresthesias, numbness, and pain of the face sparing the forehead Headache uncommon Sensory loss of the second and third divisions of the trigeminal nerve and more rarely the first division Motor deficits of the trigeminal nerve or of the abducens nerve common
Jugular foramen syndrome (3.5%)	Hoarseness, dysphagia, and unilateral dull pain in the occipital and pharyngeal areas Paralysis with involvement of cranial nerves 9th–11th observed Glossopharyngeal neuralgia-associated syndrome with syncope or papilledema
Numb chin syndrome	Numbness of the chin usually unilateral
Hemibasis syndrome	Progressive ipsilateral paralysis of at least seven cranial nerves

Data from: Laigle-Donadey [94], Boldt and Nerad [400], Johnston [401]

[102]. Rarely, biopsies are needed to establish the diagnosis. The role of a cerebrospinal fluid (CSF) analysis is to exclude co-associated leptomeningeal metastases (LM).

Skull base metastases are most often a late event in the course of cancer [94].The overall prognosis depends of the type of cancer, remaining therapeutic options, and the site and extent of the skull base metastases. In the cohort of Laigle Donadey, BC had the longest survival, with a median survival of 60 months [94]. Cranial nerve palsies are associated with a poorer OS [94].

Asymptomatic skull base metastases can be followed [100] and symptomatic patients treated with supportive therapy including steroids, analgesics, and bisphosphonates, as needed. Radiotherapy, alone or in combination with chemotherapy or surgery, is the most frequently used therapy (in >70%) [94]. Excellent pain relief and regression of cranial nerve dysfunction may occur and improved neurological function is seen if treatment commences early [93, 103]. SRS may be an alternative therapy, in particular for previously irradiated areas and for small metastases [94, 100, 104]. Lastly, surgery may be used in selected patients [94, 105]. Chemotherapy and endocrine therapies may be an option for patients with chemoresponsive disease [94].

Dural Metastases

Dural metastases are localized to dural and surrounding space (epidural and subdural) [106] and are most frequently associated with breast, prostate, lung, head and neck, and hematologic malignancies. Overall, BC is the primary cancer most often associated with dural metastases, occurring in

16.5–34% of cases [106–108]. Intracranial dural metastases occur in up to 10% of BC patients in autopsy series [106, 107]. Four mechanisms of dural seeding have been proposed: direct extension from skull metastases, hematogenous dissemination, seeding through Batson's plexus, and spread from the lymphatic circulation [107]. Those derived from direct extension of skull metastases account for 60% and dural metastases from hematogenous spread for 36% [106, 108]. In most patients with BC and dural metastases, recurrent/progressive systemic disease (>80%) is found [106].

In a retrospective cohort of 122 patients with intracranial dural metastases, the most frequent symptoms include headache (due to increased intracranial pressure) and cranial nerve palsy (due skull base location), followed by visual disorders, alterations in mental status, and seizures [106]. Signs and symptoms are related to the location and the extent of the dural metastases. Between 11 and 20% of patients are asymptomatic and diagnosed incidentally by brain imaging [106, 107]. Non-traumatic subdural hematoma, also called "pachymeningitis interna hemorrhagica," can be observed in 15–40% of cases and generally are asymptomatic [106–108]. Cerebral venous thromboses have been described secondary to infiltration of the cerebral venous sinuses [106]. In one study, 56% of the patients had a single dural metastasis and 25% demonstrated diffuse dural enhancement. The most common sites of dural metastases were parietal (36%) or frontal (32%). Infratentorial lesions were observed in 11%. Dural metastases can appear as a localized thickening of the dura or as nodules, usually biconvex or lenticular in shape [106, 108]. A combination of diffuse dural enhancement and dural nodules can be observed as well. Homogeneous intense post-contrast enhancement is most often seen. MRI findings include a dural tail (44%), vasogenic edema (53%), and brain invasion (34%), most commonly by direct extension from skull [106]. Skull metastases are observed in 70% of cases [106]. Other findings may include venous sinuses involvement and subdural hematoma or effusions. Meningioma is the main differential diagnosis [106, 108]. Infections or inflammatory lesions may be considered as well in appropriate context.

Treatment is not standardized. Surgery should be considered as the first option in patients with a resectable solitary lesion, controlled extracerebral disease, and acceptable surgical risk [106–108]. In the cohort of Nayak, 25% of the patients underwent surgical resection, consisting of complete resection in 63% of the cases. Focal radiotherapy, SRS/SRT, and WBRT are also options, alone or in combination with surgery. In the cohort of Nayak, 52% of patients received RT of whom 47% received WBRT and 53% focal RT or SRS. Systemic treatment may be an option in some cases as these lesions are outside the blood–brain barrier [106]. Best supportive care, including corticosteroids, may be indicated in some patients.

In a literature review, the median OS was 6 months varying whether surgery was performed, to control extracranial disease and the primary tumor type [108]. In this review, dural metastases from BC were associated with a more favorable outcome compared to other tumor types, with a median OS of 9 months. In the cohort of Nayak, the median PFS was 3.7 months and the median OS was 9.5 months. The initial site of progression was intracranial in 30% of the patients and both intracranial and systemic in 21%. The intracranial progression was local in the dura in 86% of patients, distant in the dura in 37%, intraparenchymal in 41%, and leptomeningeal in 6% [106]. In this study, surgical resection was shown to improve PFS and OS. Chemotherapy prolonged PFS, but not OS. An impaired PS was associated with a worse outcome.

Intramedullary Spinal Cord Metastases

BC is the second most common solid tumor responsible for intramedullary spinal cord metastasis (ISCM), after lung cancer. In a meta-analysis of 96 autopsy-proven cases with ISCM, lung cancer (49%) and BC (14%) were the most common primary cancers [109]. Treatment options include best supportive care, surgery, RT, and systemic therapy. Treatment depends on the number, volume, and location of the metastases, the extent of systemic disease, the general and neurological status of the patient, and life expectancy [110]. In all cases, the treatment is urgent so as to forestall paraplegia. Symptomatic treatment with corticosteroids can be a useful adjunct. After supportive care only, clinical deterioration is observed in 89% of the cases [111].

In highly selected patients with solitary metastases, with a reasonable life expectancy, and without leptomeningeal, brain, or widespread metastases, the prognosis may be improved by surgery [111–114]. A gross total resection can sometimes be achieved in these otherwise well-circumscribed metastases [114]. After surgery, improvement in clinical symptoms can be observed in 58% of the cases, no change in 31%, and clinical deterioration in 11%. Adjuvant RT following surgery should be administered [112].

As BC is radiosensitive, RT may be effective and is the most commonly used treatment for the majority of patients. After RT, transient stabilization of neurological disease progression and a reduction in pain is often achieved [109, 111]. The schedule of RT should be shortened so as to account for the poor OS [115]. Stereotactic radiotherapy is also an option. After SRT treatment, clinical improvement is noted in 21% of the cases, no change in 63%, and clinical deterioration in 11% [110]. BC is chemosensitive as well, and systemic agents may be effective depending on the neurological status, the volume of the metastases, available systemic treatment options, and the extent of the systemic disease. Nevertheless, no clear impact on survival has been shown [110].

For a more complete review of ISCM please refer to Chap. 6 of this text.

Spinal Epidural Metastases (Fig. 23.2)

Metastatic epidural spinal cord compression (ESCC) is seen in 5–10% of all patients with BC [114, 116–120], usually in the context of known metastatic disease [114] and often (25%) with concurrent CNS metastases [121]. Median survival of patients with ESCC may be longer for patients with

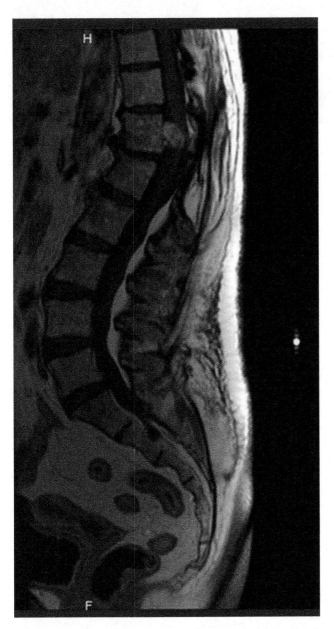

Fig. 23.2 Epidural spinal cord compression. Spinal MRI, T1 W gadolinium-enhanced sagittal image

breast cancer in comparison to other tumor types. While the median overall survival for all patients with ESCC has been reported to range between 4 and 14 months [121], survival in BC patients with ESCC was the longest (21.5 months) in a study of 81 patients that included 23.6% BC patients [119].

For a complete review of spinal epidural metastases and ESCC, including presenting symptoms, treatment, and prognostic factors, please refer to Chap. 6.

Leptomeningeal Metastases (Fig. 23.3 a, b)

Leptomeningeal metastasis (LM) or neoplastic/carcinomatous meningitis is diagnosed in 1–8% of patients with solid tumors during the course of the cancer; however, it is diagnosed at autopsy in 19% of patients with premorbid neurological signs and symptoms [122–126]. BC, in addition to lung cancer and melanoma, is one of the most common primary cancers responsible for LM. Risk factors of LM in BC include an infiltrating lobular carcinoma and cancers negative for estrogen and progesterone receptors [18, 127–130]. Triple negative status in BC has been reported as being a risk factor of LM [129, 131, 132]. In contrast, LM is observed in only 3–5% of HER2-positive BC; thus, HER2-positive status is not considered a risk factor for LM [18]. Other risk factors have been identified and include piecemeal resection instead of *en bloc* resection [33], surgical resection of parenchymal cerebellar metastases [133–135], surgical resection of supraventricular BM that violates the ventricular system [136–138], deferring WBRT after BM resection [139], and improved survival due to more effective systemic therapy often associated with poor CNS penetration [124].

The median OS of untreated patients with LM is limited to 4–6 weeks [123–125]. Despite aggressive treatment, survival is limited to a few months. Compared to patients with LM disease from other solid tumors, BC patients have a better prognosis [123–125, 140, 141]. The median OS in BC patients is estimated at 3.3–5 months [123, 124, 130, 140–153]. One-year survival varies from 7–24% [154]. Prognostic factors enumerated by the NCCN CNS guidelines include a poor risk group defined by a KPS below 60, multiple neurologic deficits, extensive systemic disease with few treatment options, bulky CNS disease, and the presence of a LM-related encephalopathy [155]. On multivariate analyses, an association has been observed between OS and the PS, age at LM diagnosis and treatment (number of prior chemotherapy regimens, receipt of combined treatment modality, coadministration of systemic chemotherapy, and intra-CSF chemotherapy) [140, 141, 156]. Other prognostic factors in BC patients include histological characteristics (histological grade and hormone receptor status), number of prior chemotherapy regimens, status of systemic disease, initial response to treatment, cytologic response to treatment, and in one study, the concentration of cyfra 21-1 (a fragment

Fig. 23.3 **a**, **b** Leptomeningeal metastases. **a** Brain MRI, T1 W gadolinium-enhanced axial images. **b** Spinal MRI, T1 W gadolinium-enhanced sagittal image

(a)

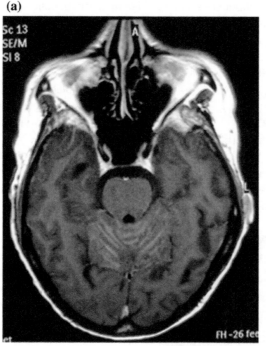

(b)

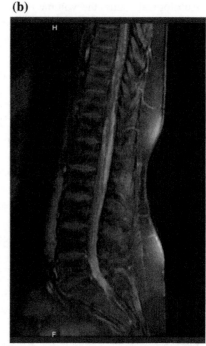

of cytokeratin 19 thought to represent a tumor marker) in the CSF [130, 143–146].

Treatment of LM should ideally be initiated as early as possible before the appearance of disabling neurologic deficits [124]. In the majority of patients, progressive extracranial disease coexists and must be taken into account in the management of LM. Only one randomized trial, prematurely closed for low accrual (n = 35), was performed in LM BC patients comparing systemic therapy and RT with or without intra-CSF methotrexate [157]. No significant difference between groups was observed in clinical response (neurologic improvement: 41 vs. 39%; disease stabilization: 18 vs. 28%) or median survival (18.3 vs. 30.3 week). However, treatment-related complications were higher in patients treated with intra-CSF chemotherapy compared to the no intra-CSF chemotherapy arm (47 vs. 6%). Further studies are needed to define the role of intra-CSF therapy in the treatment of BC LM. Combined treatment (both systemic chemotherapy and intra-CSF chemotherapy) is preferred when possible in patients considered for LM treatment due to an improvement in survival.

Chemotherapy allows simultaneous treatment of the entire neuraxis and can be administered systematically or intra-CSF. The choice of agent is based on the chemosensitivity profile of the primary tumor and the ability of drug to penetrate into the CSF compartment [124, 125]. Paclitaxel and docetaxel are effective in metastatic BC, but have poor penetration into the CNS [158].

Capecitabine in case reports has produced responses and disease stabilization in BC LM [159–163]. As in BC BM,

temozolomide for the treatment of LM was disappointing [164]. The efficacy of new agents such as eribulin has not been yet demonstrated. High-dose methotrexate or cytarabine is not often administered due to significant systemic toxicity and the requirement for hospitalization. Efficacy of endocrine therapies has been demonstrated in case reports, but acquired resistance is often present at this stage of the disease. Bevacizumab, a monoclonal antibody targeting the vascular endothelial growth factor (VEGF) ligand, has shown prolonged responses in case reports with LM [165–168]. Prospective trials are ongoing to confirm the role of bevacizumab in LM (NCT NCT00924820). A response to trastuzumab emtansine has been reported [169]. The efficacy of other anti-HER2 therapies such as lapatinib and pertuzumab has not been demonstrated. A glutathione-pegylated liposomal formulation of doxorubicin and anthracycline is under investigation in BC LM (NCT01818713).

Intra-CSF treatment, in combination with systemic therapy, is often used for the treatment of LM notwithstanding its superiority relative to systemic therapy only has never been established in a randomized trial [123, 124]. The goal of intra-CSF treatment is to bypass the blood–CSF barrier which is only partially disrupted in LM and increase drug exposure in the CSF compartment while mitigating systemic toxicity [124, 125]. Three main intra-CSF chemotherapy agents are used: cytarabine (free or liposomal), methotrexate (standard and high-dose regimens), and thiotepa with differing doses and schedules (Table 23.5). The optimal dose and schedule, particularly concerning maintenance therapy,

Table 23.5 Intra-CSF chemotherapy dose and schedule

Drug	Description of the drug	CSF half-life	Description of the regimen
Liposomal cytarabine	Pyrimidine nucleoside analogue, cell cycle specific	14–21 days	50 mg every 2 weeks (total, 8 wks) then 50 mg once every 4 weeks
Methotrexate	Folate antimetabolite, cell cycle-specific drug	4, 5–8 h	*Standard regimen* 10–15 mg twice weekly (total, 4 wks), then 10–15 mg once weekly (total, 4 wks) then 10–15 mg once monthly *Low-dose regimen* 2 mg/d (d1–d5) every other week *High-dose regimen* 15 mg/d (d1–d5) every other wk
Thiotepa	Alkylating ethyleneimine compound, cell cycle non-specific drug	3–4 min	10 mg twice weekly (total, 4 wks) then 10 mg once weekly (total, 4 wks) then 10 mg once a month

Abbreviations: *CSF* cerebrospinal fluid, *mg* milligrams, *d* day, *wk* week

are not well defined [125, 154, 170]. Many studies have reported no differences in efficacy among these agents, including in patients with BC-related LM [130, 143–150]. Liposomal cytarabine, which resulted in a significant longer survival as compared to methotrexate in one randomized trial, requires less frequent clinic visits and may have less impact on QoL [171]. Combination (multi-agent) intra-CSF chemotherapy has not demonstrated improved results and is not recommended for the treatment of BC-related LM. Intra-CSF etoposide has shown modest efficacy [172]. Prolonged responses have been reported after intra-CSF trastuzumab in case studies [173–176]. Two studies are currently ongoing to define the safety and efficacy profile of intra-CSF trastuzumab in HER2-positive BC patients (NCT01325207 and NCT01373710).

For a complete review of LM, please refer to Chap. 5.

Peripheral Nervous System Metastases

Neoplastic Plexopathy

Neoplastic plexopathy typically occurs at the time of local or regional progression of cancer. BC is the second (32%) most common cause of neoplastic brachial plexopathy after lung cancer, and the third (11%) leading cause of lumbosacral neoplastic plexopathy after lung cancer and soft tissue sarcoma [177, 178]. Neoplastic plexopathy manifests as severe pain, followed by motor weakness and sensory disturbances in the distribution of plexus involvement [177, 178]. When the brachial plexus is involved, the lower trunk is most frequently affected. Pain is observed in 75–83% of the patients and is usually located in the shoulder and axilla [177, 179]. Radicular pain is common and radiates into the arm with extension into the fourth and fifth digits. Motor weakness and loss of reflexes are seen in 75% of cases, mostly in the lower plexus distribution. More widespread

signs of whole plexus involvement are occasionally noted. A Horner's syndrome occurs in 23% of the patients with a neoplastic brachial plexopathy [177]. In lymphedema-associated plexopathy, patients present with neuropathic extremity pain (90%), followed by weakness (86%), sensory loss (73%), reflex loss (64%), and limb edema (47%) [177]. Tumor spread to the plexus most commonly occurs by direct invasion of the plexus or hematogenous spread from distant metastases. Adjacent structures, such as infiltrated lymph nodes or soft tissues, can also result in direct compression of the plexus [177, 179, 180].

Contrast MRI is more sensitive than CT in the identification of neoplastic plexopathy [177, 179]. Increased T2/FLAIR MRI intensity in nerve trunks with or without contrast enhancement is commonly observed. If no lesion is observed, a repeat MRI examination within a 4- to 6-week interval commonly reveals tumor not previously appreciated on initial examination [177]. The presence of tumor recurrence, especially in the area of plexus, in combination with a supportive examination, is presumptive for a diagnosis of metastatic plexopathy. The sensitivity and specificity of PET are not clear, but PET can be helpful in instances of negative MRI. Electromyography demonstrates a unilateral lesion often with more extensive denervation than clinically predicted [177]. Lower medial trunk/cord lesions or whole plexus lesions are more frequent than upper trunk lateral cord lesions [179].

The main differential diagnosis is radiation-induced plexopathy (Table 23.6). The pattern of distribution of weakness and the results of nerve conduction studies may help to distinguish between neoplastic and radiation-induced brachial plexopathy [181]. A more complete discussion on this topic is featured later in this chapter. Other differential diagnosis include LM, ESCC, paraneoplastic plexopathy, complications of regional intra-arterial chemotherapy, post-infectious plexopathy, and primary plexus tumors

Table 23.6 Differential diagnosis: Neoplastic brachial plexopathy and radiation-induced brachial plexopathy

Presentation	Neoplastic plexopathy	Radiation associated plexopathy
Clinical presentation	Severe and early pain, occasional edema, involvement of the lower brachial plexus, Horner's syndrome common, No tissue necrosis	Paresthesia and weakness, pain late during the course of the disease, edema common, impairment of the whole plexus, Horner's syndrome unusual, local tissue necrosis common
Electromyography	Myokymia unusual	Myokymia usually present
MRI	Nerve contrast enhancement	Usually no nerve contrast enhancement
PET scan	High SUV max	Low SUV max

Abbreviations: *MRI* magnetic resonance imaging, *PET* positron emission tomography, *SUV* standardized uptake value
Used with permission of Thieme from Jaeckle [177]

Table 23.7 Autoantibodies and common paraneoplastic syndromes (PNS) associated with breast cancer

Autoantibodies	Common paraneoplastic syndrome
Amphiphysin	Stiff person syndrome, myelopathy and myoclonus, encephalomyelitis, sensory neuronopathy
Ri (ANNA2)	Brainstem encephalitis, opsoclonus myoclonus
Yo (PCA1)	Paraneoplastic cerebellar degeneration
AMPAR	Limbic encephalitis
CAR	Retinopathy

[177]. Radiotherapy of the involved area is the most commonly used treatment and often results in durable responses. Chemotherapy and endocrine therapy may be used with some utility in chemosensitive cancer [180]. Pain should be treated according to the WHO guidelines. Physical therapy may help to augment and preserve neurologic function.

Non-metastatic, Non-treatment-related Complications

Paraneoplastic Syndromes

Paraneoplastic neurological syndromes (PNS) affect less than 1% of patients with BC [182]. BC is most often associated with the following PNS: cerebellar degeneration, sensory neuropathy, encephalomyelitis, opsoclonus myoclonus, stiff person syndrome, myelopathy, and brainstem encephalitis (Table 23.7) [183, 184]. Subacute cerebellar degeneration is the most common PNS seen with BC [185]. Other paraneoplastic syndromes, such as retinopathy, have been reported in BC (Table 23.8). Associated systemic symptoms including weight loss, anorexia, fever, and fatigue may be observed [186].

The best characterized onconeural antibodies associated with BC and PNS are amphiphysin associated with the stiff person syndrome, myelopathy, myoclonus, encephalomyelitis, and sensory neuronopathy; Ri (ANNA2) associated with brainstem encephalitis and opsoclonus myoclonus; and Yo (PCA1) associated with paraneoplastic cerebellar degeneration [184]; AMPAR (amino-3-hydroxy-5-methyl-4-isoxazolepropionic acid receptor) associated with limbic encephalitis; and anti-Ma2 (anti-Ta) associated with limbic encephalitis, brainstem encephalitis, and cerebellar degeneration [184, 187, 188].

PNS precedes the diagnosis of cancer in more than 80% of the cases by several months to years [183, 189]. In most cases, an underlying cancer is identified within 5 months after the diagnosis of PNS. The risk of a coexistent cancer decreases after 2 years and is considered as highly unlikely after 4 years [183]. When BC is considered in a patient with a PNS, a cancer screen should include a clinical examination and mammography followed by breast MRI and body FDG-PET in cases with negative initial screening [184, 188]. When the initial screen is negative, repeat assessments should be performed every 6 months for at least 2 years [188].

For a complete review of PNS, please refer to Chap. 13.

Meningiomas (Fig. 23.4)

Meningioma is one of the most common primary tumors of the CNS in adults and accounts for 13–26% of all intracranial tumors [190–192]. The only well-established risk factors are prior ionizing brain RT and some rare hereditary diseases such as neurofibromatosis [190–195]. Mutation in the NF2 gene and genetic variants in genes involved in DNA repair pathway are often identified in meningioma [196]. Several observations suggest a link between a patient's hormonal status and meningioma. In intracranial meningioma, the female: male ratio is 2–3.5, which is even higher

Table 23.8 Most frequent paraneoplastic syndromes (PNS) in breast cancer

Name of the PNS	Description of the paraneoplastic syndrome
Subacute cerebellar degeneration	Development in <12 weeks of a severe pancerebellar syndrome without cerebellar atrophy on MRI other than age expected Initial gait ataxia followed by appendicular ataxia Initial symptoms may also include dizziness, visual problems (diplopia, blurry vision, oscillopsia), nausea/vomiting, or dysarthria These rapidly progressive symptoms stabilize after culminating in a severe pancerebellar syndrome Other neurological symptoms and signs that may be seen include cognitive impairment, lethargy, bulbar palsy, or limb weakness Other PNS (paraneoplastic peripheral neuropathy or Lambert–Eaton myasthenic syndrome) sometimes associated Cerebellar atrophy on MRI in the late stages of the disease often associated with anti-Yo antibodies
Sensory neuronopathy	Subacute and asymmetric numbness, paresthesia, pain, cramps, proprioceptive loss of upper and lower extremities and abolition of deep-tendon reflexes Radicular symptoms and signs sometimes associated Involvement of the sensory fibers on electroneurography
Encephalomyelitis	Involvement of multiple parts of the CNS such as the hippocampus, brainstem, spinal cord, or dorsal root ganglia Manifests as limbic encephalopathy, brainstem encephalitis, dysautonomia, myelitis, and sensory neuronopathy
Opsoclonus myoclonus syndrome	Spontaneous large amplitude saccades occurring in all directions of gaze Myoclonus of the trunk and limbs Encephalopathy sometimes associated Often associated with Ri antibodies
Stiff person syndrome	Slowly progressive stiffness and rigidity of axial musculature Followed by proximal muscle rigidity Leads to difficulties in walking and fixed deformities. Associated with superimposed muscle spasms that are increased by sensory stimuli Variant form with an onset of stiffness in upper limbs Antibodies against amphiphysin Continuous motor activity at rest on electroneurography
Subacute progressive myelopathy	Progressive symptoms and signs of myelopathy Symmetric MRI T2 abnormalities and gadolinium enhancement that involves the spinal gray matter in usually >3 segments Antibodies against amphiphysin
Brainstem encephalitis	Rapidly progressive symptoms and signs of brainstem dysfunction. Antibodies against Ri (ANNA2)

Data from: Gatti et al. [182], Honnorat and Antoine [183], Graus and Dalmau [184], Graus and Delattre [185]

in spinal meningioma (4:1 ratio) [194, 197, 198]. Progesterone receptors are detected in 70–98% of meningiomas; estrogen and androgen receptors are seen in 20–40% of meningiomas [193, 195, 199, 200]. Increased meningioma growth rate is reported during pregnancy [193, 194]. An association between BC and meningioma has been demonstrated [193, 195, 201]. In addition, a link between use of exogenous hormones and meningioma has been reported [194], as well as a positive association with endometriosis or uterine fibrosis [196]. A non-significant association has been shown between age at menarche, age at menopause, menopausal status, parity, age at first birth, and meningioma [193, 194, 202–204]. A protective role of breastfeeding has also been observed [204–207]. The evidence that use of oral contraceptives and hormone replacement therapy increase

the risk of meningioma remains controversial; however, in most studies [194, 204], no association was found [193–195, 203–206, 208–213].

An association between BC and meningioma has been postulated. In a large Swedish cohort, an increased risk of meningioma was observed after BC with a relative risk of meningioma estimated at 1.6 [214]. In another US population-based retrospective cohort analysis, the risk of BC in patients previously diagnosed with a meningioma was 1.54, and the risk of meningioma in BC patients was 1.40 [211]. In a five-state US cancer registry, the incidence of meningioma was 2.6 cases per 100,000 women and the incidence of BC was 61 cases per 100,000 women. The association between the two cancers was higher than expected [201]. The pathophysiology of this association is

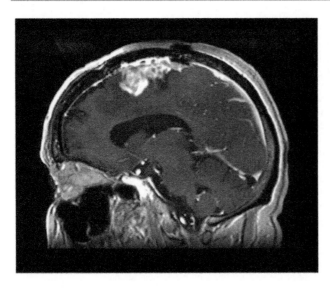

Fig. 23.4 Meningioma. Brain MRI, T1 W gadolinium-enhanced sagittal image

not well understood. BRCA1 and BRCA2 mutations do not seem to contribute to the development of meningioma [215]. In a large US SEER registry, associations between BC and meningioma were reported [216]. BC preceded meningioma by >2 months in 48% of the women, and tumors were synchronous (within 2 months) in 20%. Hormone receptor status of BC was not different between BC only and BC plus meningioma groups. BC disease stage was more advanced in the BC plus meningioma group than in the BC only group. Contrary to this study, in a large retrospective study of BC patients, the 10-year cumulative incidence of meningioma was only 0.37%, suggesting no increased risk [217]. Use of aromatase inhibitors confers a non-significant increased risk of meningioma in patients with BC [217], whereas tamoxifen use may be protective. The risk of meningioma has been shown to be lower in patients treated with tamoxifen compared to those not treated with this agent [192].

Complications of Breast Cancer Treatment

Central Nervous System Complications

Encephalopathy

Any anticancer drug given at conventional dose can be responsible for causing a toxic encephalopathy [218]. Toxic chemotherapy-related encephalopathy may manifest as a confusional state, posterior reversible leukoencephalopathy, seizures, a cerebellar syndrome, myelopathy, or cerebrovascular complications [219, 220]. The signs and symptoms can vary from mild and transient to severe and chronic [219, 221]. 5-FU (5-fluorouracil) and capecitabine represent the most frequent chemotherapy agents responsible

for CNS toxicity in BC. The symptoms can originate within days to months after the initial administration of the drug. Most toxic encephalopathies are transient, last only days, and are associated with complete neurologic recovery [222–225]. MRI changes seen with toxic encephalopathies resolve more slowly than clinical manifestations. The pathophysiology of toxic encephalopathy is not clearly understood. Direct endothelial cell injury has been proposed with associated vasogenic edema [222, 226]. Most occurrences of encephalopathy are believed to be idiosyncratic and with a low risk of recurrence [219, 220, 227].

Several antineoplastic agents used in BC may induce an encephalopathy (Table 23.9). Methotrexate results in encephalopathy in less than 2% of patients [219, 228]. Administration of methotrexate and brain RT further increases the risk of CNS neurotoxicity [221]. Acute encephalopathies have been described after the administration of paclitaxel or very rarely docetaxel, vinorelbine, and pegylated liposomal doxorubicin in BC patients, notwithstanding limited penetration of the CNS with these agents [229–233]. Anti-VEGF agents such as bevacizumab are rarely the cause of posterior reversible encephalopathy or PRES [234, 235]. Leukoencephalopathy and encephalopathy were observed in 2.5 and 5% of patients with LM following lumbar injection and 7.5 and 5% after ventricular injection of liposomal cytarabine in a large cohort of patients treated for LM [236]. In a smaller cohort of patients treated with intraventricular methotrexate, leukoencephalopathy was observed in 64% of patients [237]. Leukoencephalopathy can be delayed, developing 3–15 months after intra-CSF methotrexate [237]. Patients may manifest with personality changes, cognitive deficits, and apathy followed by hemiparesia or quadriparesia and coma. Lesions predominate in the periventricular white matter, and histological examination demonstrates demyelination, axonal degeneration, astrocytosis, and necrosis [238]. An elevation in MBP (myelin basic protein) can be observed in the CSF. Risk factors include high cumulative doses of intra-CSF methotrexate and concomitant systemic methotrexate plus WBRT [237]. An accidental overdose of intra-CSF methotrexate can lead to death. An acute transient mild encephalopathy with fever may be observed after intra-CSF methotrexate and which likely represents expansion of a treatment-related chemical meningitis discussed below [237].

Other potential causes of encephalopathy must be excluded including CNS metastases (e.g., BM or LM), other toxic agents (e.g., antiepileptics, opioids, benzodiazepines), metabolic encephalopathies (such as hyper or hypoglycemia, azotemia, hepatic failure, electrolyte disorders), stroke, and infectious etiologies [222]. Cessation of the offending drug is indicated until resolution of symptoms. Neurological manifestations usually clear within a few days after discontinuing the chemotherapy [218, 222–224]. Nonetheless, in some patients, persistent neurological deficits are reported after discontinuation of the offending agent [223]. Steroids are of questionable benefit [223–225]. Dihydropyrimidine dehydrogenase deficiency, a genetic risk factor for MTX neurotoxicity, should be excluded [224]. In the absence of alternative chemotherapy, careful re-introduction of the drug at reduced dose and under close supervision is usually safe and associated with a low risk of recurrence [224].

Cognitive Impact of Endocrine Therapy and Chemotherapy

Cognitive impairment associated with chemotherapy is referred to as *chemobrain* or *chemofog* [239]. There are no established criteria that define the syndrome, related in part to methodological inconsistencies observed between studies discussed below. In BC, post-chemotherapy cognitive deficits have been observed in 17–75% of patients, as compared with 4–11% in healthy controls in retrospective cross-sectional studies [240–251]. Most longitudinal studies have confirmed a negative cognitive effect of chemotherapy in 15–25% of patients [244, 252–254]. In several prospective cohorts of BC patients, objective cognitive impairments have been observed in 20–35% at baseline before any systemic therapy without clear explanation as to cause [239, 241, 244, 255, 256]. Cognitive impairment due to chemotherapy emerges months to years after completion of treatment [257]. In prospective cohorts, cognitive decline was observed within the first 6 months after initiation of chemotherapy [246]. The duration of cognitive impairment is poorly defined. In longitudinal studies, cognitive impact appears to resolve over time, and stable or improved cognition has been observed 12–18 months following completion of chemotherapy [245, 252, 258]. Improvements in cognition may be delayed, and there exist a small subset of patients with refractory and intractable cognitive complaints after completion of chemotherapy [258–260].

Cognitive changes observed during *chemobrain* are often mild to moderate in severity and differ clinically from encephalopathy observed after chemotherapy [261]. The most common cognitive deficits include difficulties in attention and concentration, working memory, and executive and psychomotor functions [251, 258]. Deficits in verbal learning, nonverbal and visuospatial memory, psychomotor processing speed, mental flexibility, memory retrieval, confrontational naming, complex visuoconstruction, and fine motor dexterity have been reported as well [246, 250, 258, 262]. Patients report an inability to concentrate, organize their daily activities, or multitask. They also endorse memory loss, confusion, slow thinking, and fatigue [258]. The impact of these cognitive deficits in day-to-day activities varies and may be related to the patient's pre-illness level of function, type of work or lifestyle, ability to manage, coping style, premorbid cognitive reserve, age, and other comorbidities such as mood or personality disorders, fatigue, and psychosocial issues [234, 239, 258, 261, 263–265]. Different studies have demonstrated that cognitive complaints are better correlated with emotional distress, coping skills, and cancer-related fatigue than with objective neuropsychological testing [239, 243, 261, 262, 266, 267].

The role of chemotherapy dose is not clear. One study demonstrated a greater deficit among women treated with high-dose chemotherapy compared to women treated with standard doses of chemotherapy [268]. In another longitudinal study, progressive cognitive decline was observed at each subsequent time point. This suggests a dose–response relationship with linear worsening following each cycle of chemotherapy [269]. Patients treated with combined chemotherapy and endocrine therapy have the most extensive pattern of cognitive deficits [245, 252, 260, 262]. Pretreatment cognitive impairment has been shown to be independent of fatigue or emotional distress, surgical factors, or medical comorbidities [261]. The exact mechanisms underlying the effects of chemotherapy on cognition are not clearly understood [244, 261]. Chemotherapy may have a direct neurotoxic effect and may induce oxidative stress, DNA damage, telomere shortening, damage to neural stem cells, hormonal changes, immune dysregulation, activation of pro-inflammatory cytokines, thrombosis in brain microvasculature, white matter abnormalities, metabolic abnormalities including anemia, and reduced brain functional connectivity [241, 261, 262, 270]. The role of genetic factors such as apolipoprotein E (APOE) and catechol-*O*-methyltransferase (COMT) has also been suggested [241, 244, 262, 271].

An evaluation of treatment-related cognitive disorders requires a neuropsychological assessment. In order to improve between-study comparisons, the International Cognition and Cancer Task Force (ICCTF) has developed recommendations for neuropsychological testing [242]. The Hopkins Verbal Learning Test-Revised (HVLT-R), Trail Making Test (TMT), and the Controlled Oral Word Association (COWA) of the Multilingual Aphasia Examination measuring learning and memory, processing speed, and executive function are recommended [242]. Baseline evaluation and an appropriate control group are suggested as is an evaluation of emotional functioning [261].

Volumetric brain MRI and diffusion tensor MRI (DTI) have shown widespread reduction in white matter tract integrity and gray matter volume over time in patients treated with chemotherapy and with cognitive deficits [251, 261]. A correlation has been observed between reduction in brain activation by fMRI and cognitive performance after chemotherapy in a longitudinal study [272]. Studies using fMRI have demonstrated alteration in brain activation and connectivity in BC patients after chemotherapy treatment [251, 258, 261]. Decreased activation by fMRI appears to

Table 23.9 Breast cancer chemotherapy associated with toxic encephalopathy

Agent	Clinical description	Brain MRI
5-FU (5 fluorouracil) and capecitabine	Cerebellar syndrome or multifocal leukoencephalopathy with altered mental status ranging from confusion to coma, memory deficits, ataxia, dysarthria, nystagmus, headache, seizures, trismus, slurred speech, diplopia, and paresthesias	Normal or showing diffuse white matter alterations, with T2 and FLAIR periventricular hyperintensities of both hemispheres
Methotrexate	Acute encephalopathy to severe delayed chronic encephalopathies with cognitive deficits, aphasia, and hemiparesis	Diffuse T2/FLAIR abnormalities
Bevacizumab	Headache, visual disturbances, seizures, confusion, and relative hypertension	Parieto-occipital white matter abnormalities on T2/FLAIR sequences. Less frequently involvement of anterior brain regions

Data from
5-FU (5 fluorouracil) and capecitabine: Videnovic et al. [223], Tipples et al. [224], Formica et al. [225], Niemann et al. [402], Couch et al. [403], Fantini et al. [404], Lyros et al. [222]
Methotrexate: Erbetta et al. [226]
Bevacizumab: Schiff et al. [234], Tlemsani et al. [235]

relate to impaired cognition, whereas increased activation, typically seen in the context of absent or mild cognitive deficits, is thought to represent compensatory neural activation required to be maintained. PET shows similar activation patterns as seen with fMRI [241, 258, 261, 273]. Electrophysiological studies have shown a reduction in the amplitude of the P-300 event-related brain potential and a reduction in the P-300 latency, corresponding to the timing and duration of chemotherapy. This pattern was consistent with changes in information processing capacity [241, 258].

Chemobrain is a diagnosis of exclusion wherein PNS, CNS metastases, medication toxicity (corticosteroids, antiepileptics), fatigue, sleep disorders, pain, and preexistent neurological disease need to be excluded [261, 263]. The effectiveness of donepezil, an acetylcholinesterase inhibitor, for the treatment of chemotherapy cognitive deficits is uncertain [261]. No significant positive impact of psychostimulants such as methylphenidate, dexmethylphenidate, and modafinil, has been shown for the treatment of cognitive impairment in non-CNS cancer patients [239, 261]. *Gingko biloba* administered concomitantly with chemotherapy had no effect on cognitive function [274]. New approaches are needed, and promising results in animal studies suggest agents that prevent oxidative stress (2-mercaptoethane sulfonate, *N*-acetylcysteine, or melatonin), stimulate neurogenesis (insulin-like growth factor-1, fluoxetine, or glucose), or improve chemotherapy-induced cognitive effects (dextromethorphan or memantine) may be useful [261]. Learning compensatory strategies can help to minimize the impact of chemotherapy-related cognitive deficits [265]. Cognitive rehabilitation aims to improve cognitive abilities, functional capacity, and real-world skills [261]. Several studies show a significant improvement in both subjective and objective cognitive deficits with these interventions [244, 261]. Sleep disturbances, psychological distress, and fatigue, if present,

should be addressed as treating these elements secondarily improves cognition [261]. Other medications that may affect cognition should be reduced or discontinued when possible. Physical activity has been associated with improved cognition, mostly executive function, in human and animal studies [275]. Neurofeedback and transcranial magnetic stimulation have been suggested as possibly useful interventions [261, 276].

Several studies have suggested a negative impact on cognition in BC patients treated with endocrine therapies, affecting mostly verbal memory and executive functions [277–286]. Deficits in processing speed and verbal memory were observed in postmenopausal patients compared to controls [279–281, 287]. A negative impact of tamoxifen or anastrozole on speed measures of letter fluency, complex visuomotor attention, and manual dexterity has also been reported [288]. In a separate trial, postmenopausal women with early-stage BC were treated with anastrozole or tamoxifen and the cognitive impact of each treatment was compared. A more severe impact on verbal and visual learning as well as on memory tests was observed after anastrozole [288]. Notably, no cognitive decline was reported at 6 and 24 months in the randomized IBIS II trial conducted in high-risk postmenopausal women without BC receiving anastrozole or placebo [282]. In the TEAM (tamoxifen and exemestane adjuvant multinational) study, no cognitive impact was found after exemestane treatment, but poorer performances on verbal memory and executive function were observed after tamoxifen compared to healthy controls [277]. In a phase III randomized trial, aromatase inhibitors did not appear to negatively affect verbal episodic memory during a 1-year follow-up [289]. The discordant findings in the above-mentioned studies could be explained by methodological inconsistencies such as differences in the characteristics of population studied (prior chemotherapy or not, inclusion of pre- or postmenopausal women), differences in the neurocognitive testing batteries, trial design (prospective vs. cross-sectional), timing and the duration of follow-up, and whether the evaluation of cognitive function was a primary study objective [277–281, 286, 287, 289]. Importantly, the impact of mood or fatigue on cognition is often not reported [268, 279, 290–294].

Cardiovascular Complications (Ischemic, Central Venous Thrombosis, Sinus Thrombosis)

In an autopsy cohort of cancer patients, cerebrovascular disease (CVD) was seen in 14.6%, of whom half had clinical symptoms during life [295]. In a database of the Eastern Cooperative Oncology Group (ECOG) trials for BC, the frequency of both venous thrombosis and arterial thrombosis was 5.4% among patients treated with adjuvant therapy and 1.6% in patients on observation only [296]. A higher risk of stroke in cancer patients as compared to controls without cancer was reported in a Swedish cohort [297]. In a study of hospitalized stroke patients, cancer patients represented 9.1% of all cases and BC was the second most common type of malignancy [298]. In the Norwegian Stroke Research Registry (NOR-STROKE), the prevalence of cancer was higher among patients presenting with a stroke and BC was the third most frequent cancer associated with stroke [299]. The cumulative incidence of stroke in BC is 1.5% compared to 1.1% in controls [300]. The highest risk of stroke is observed soon after diagnosis of cancer [297, 300] and is estimated at 12% [301].

Cancer is a prothrombotic state with acquired protein S or C deficiency, activated protein C resistance, antiphospholipid antibodies and the antiphospholipid syndrome, hyperfibrinogenemia, thrombocytosis, and D-dimer elevation [302, 303]. Thrombotic angiopathy has been observed in BC and was reported to be linked to cancer therapy, but was also observed after treatment when the cancer was in remission. In the ECOG cohort mentioned above, the association of chemotherapy and tamoxifen increased the risk of both venous and arterial strokes compared to chemotherapy alone in premenopausal patients [296]. In another cohort of women with BC, tamoxifen was associated with an increased risk of stroke [304]. In BC, supraclavicular and internal mammary nodal RT may accelerate atherosclerosis of the carotid artery and increase the risk of stroke [304–306]. The EORTC study NCT00002851 (Lymph Node Radiation Therapy in Patients With Stage I, Stage II, or Stage III Breast Cancer That Has Been Surgically Removed) will provide more data on the risk of stroke and RT. The management of stroke in cancer patients depends on the etiology. Patients with cancer have been for the most part excluded from trials of thrombolysis. Treatment with thrombolysis may result in a higher in-hospital mortality in patients with cancer due to medical comorbidities, but there

does not appear to be a higher risk of intracranial hemorrhage (ICH) [307].

Cancer patients also have an increased risk of venous thromboembolism (VTE), and VTE is associated with a significant risk of morbidity and mortality in cancer patients [308, 309]. In the Iowa SEER, the standardized morbidity ratio, estimated by dividing the observed number of cancers in the VTE incident cohort by expected number, was 8.4 for BC [310]. The risk of VTE has been associated with several factors including the type of cancer, the stage of the cancer, performance of surgery, administration of chemotherapy or endocrine therapy, the presence of a central venous catheter, patient age, whether non-ambulatory, and prior episode of VTE [311]. The Khorana predictive score of VTE risk in ambulatory patients includes 5 variables: the site of cancer, the prechemotherapy platelet count, the hemoglobin level, the use of erythropoietic agents, the leukocyte count, and the body mass index [312]. In this score, BC is considered at low risk of VTE.

Thromboembolic events are more frequent in women treated by chemotherapy for BC [313]. Tamoxifen, a selective estrogen receptor modulator with estrogen antagonistic effects, may also increase the risk of thromboembolic complications [314, 315]. The combination of chemotherapy and tamoxifen further increases the risk of VTE compared to tamoxifen alone in postmenopausal patients [296]. Systemic treatment may increase the risk of VTE by several mechanisms including acute and non-acute damages to vessel walls and decrease in protein C, protein S, factor VII or fibrinogen, and platelet activation [303, 308, 311].

Cerebral venous occlusion can be observed in cancer patients, either in superficial cortical veins, internal cerebral veins, or dural sinuses [302]. Systemic cancer accounts for 3.2% of all causes of cerebral venous occlusion [316]. Cerebral sinus or veins can also be affected by compression or local invasion by brain, dural, or skull metastases [317, 318]. A BC patient with VTE receiving tamoxifen in the adjuvant setting should be transitioned to an aromatase inhibitor [308]. Thrombolytic agents are contraindicated in patients with intracranial tumors [319].

For a complete review of cerebrovascular dysfunction in cancer, please refer to Chap. 10.

Meningitic Syndromes

Chemical Meningitis

Chemical meningitis is the most common side effect of intra-CSF chemotherapy and is characterized by headache, photophobia, fever, nausea and vomiting, meningismus, and confusion [320]. It occurs in 15–33.3% of patients following liposomal cytarabine administration regardless of the route of administration (lumbar vs. ventricular) [320]. The incidence of aseptic meningitis may be reduced by prophylactic oral dexamethasone initiated on the day of intra-CSF drug administration. Most symptoms of chemical meningitis occur within the first days after drug administration. Mild symptoms resolve within days; however, symptomatic treatment with intravenous corticosteroids and fluids may be required in severe cases. Subsequent intra-CSF drug administration is dose reduced and used in combination with more liberal prophylactic oral steroids [320]. Acute aseptic meningitis may also be observed after administration of any intra-CSF drug including methotrexate, cytarabine, and thiotepa [237]. The main differential diagnosis of chemical meningitis is infectious meningitis or LM disease progression and is primarily differentiated by the time course of chemical meningitis and the failure to culture bacteria from CSF [123].

Infections

Intra-CSF agents can be administered either by the intralumbar or by the ventricular route. Intraventricular injections offer several advantages compared to lumbar administration, such as the certainty of drug delivery into the CSF compartment (10% of all intrathecal injections are epi- or subdural) and a relatively pain-free procedure [321, 322]. A survival benefit has also been suggested for intraventricular administration compared to lumbar injection [321]. However, intraventricular drug administration requires placement of ventricular access device resulting in a risk of infection not unlike that seen with a vascular access device. In a prospective cohort of patients (mostly BC) with the 10% of complications seen with the use of a ventricular access device, the majority (70%) were bacterial infections [323]. The infection rate was estimated at 3.6% per patient and 0.38% per injection. This rate was similar to other series [320, 324, 325]. Bacterial meningitis is less frequent after lumbar injection (3.75% vs. 0%) [320]. In the cohort of Zairi, the ventricular access device was removed in all cases and antibiotics were administered for 2 weeks. Nevertheless, no clear recommendations exist for the management of infected ventricular access devices. Some authors propose preservation of the device and administration of combined systemic and intra-CSF organism-specific antibiotic therapy [326, 327].

Other CNS Adverse Effects

Other CNS toxicities seen after intra-CSF liposomal cytarabine administration include a communicating hydrocephalus, decreased visual acuity, and seizures [320]. Stroke-like events that rapidly resolve have been reported after intra-CSF methotrexate injection [328].

Peripheral Nervous System Complications

Plexopathy

Axillary lymph node dissection for BC is a fundamental part of treatment, but can be responsible for post-surgical injury complications including chronic pain syndromes, numbness, shoulder restriction, lymphoedema, and rarely plexopathy. Damage to the nerves traversing the axillary fat and in particular the intercostobrachial nerve prone to injury during axillary dissection can result in chronic pain.

One week after surgery, up to 78% of patients report moderate to severe pain [329]. Neuropathic pain after BC surgery is seen in 14.7–52% of patients during the first year after surgery [329–331]. Other neurological symptoms include paresthesia, dyesthesias, swelling sensation, and hypoesthesia. Number of axillary nodes dissected (more than 15 lymph nodes excised), age <40 years, African American race, diabetes, fibromyalgia, and taxane-based chemotherapy have been identified as risk factors for neuropathic pain after BC surgery [330, 331]. Sentinel lymph node biopsy has been developed for axillary staging and minimizes the morbidity of axillary lymph node dissection in patients with BC. Sentinel node dissection alone has been shown to significantly reduce the rate of paresthesia, dyesthesias, swelling sensation, or pain compared to axillary node dissection [332–334]. Pharmacological treatment of pain consists of tricyclic antidepressants, duloxetine, AEDs (carbamazepine, gabapentin, pregabalin), transdermal lidocaine, and capsaicin.

The risk of loco-regional recurrence is reduced after chest wall and axillary node RT among women with a node-positive BC [335]. Radiation-induced brachial plexopathy (RIBP) is the most frequent peripheral nervous system complication after BC irradiation [336]. The incidence is <1% with 50 in 2 Gy fractions [337]. The interval between RT and symptom onset varies from 3 months to 26 years with a median of 1.25–4.25 years [179, 337–339]. Rarely, early acute transient RIPB have been reported within 2–14 months after supraclavicular–axillary RT at 50 Gy [337]. The delay between RT and clinical deficits is partly related to the dose per fraction, total dose, and volume irradiated [340]. Signs and symptoms of RIBP include paresthesias, pain, hyporeflexia, and motor impairment with potentially flaccid paralysis of the ipsilateral arm [335, 337, 338]. RIBP usually begins with paresthesias or dyesthesias followed by hypoesthesia and anesthesia. Tinel's sign has been reported with paresthesia evoked after axillary or supraclavicular stimulation. Pain is the most common symptom and is seen in >75% of patients. Progressive motor weakness appears later and can be associated with fasciculations and amyotrophy [337]. The first motor signs are usually observed in the thenar muscles [337]. The topography varies with the level of plexus damage though typically appears distally and progressively spread to forearm and upper arm [337]. The onset is insidious, but signs and symptoms gradually increase and often lead to paralysis of the upper limb with severe impairment of useful hand function [337–339]. Rapid neurological worsening has been described after trauma related to surgery, upper limb lymphedema, or traction of the affected arm [341]. Direct neuronal and endothelial injury with associated demyelination and ischemia and compression by radiation-induced fibrosis have been suggested as potential mechanisms of RIBP [327, 338].

Pain and paresthesia can be treated with AEDs, non-opioid and opioid analgesics, tricyclic antidepressants, and benzodiazepines. Quinine may be used for cramps and carbamazepine for myokymia. The role of B vitamins, corticosteroids, or anticoagulants is controversial. A randomized phase III trial evaluating the association of pentoxifylline, tocopherol, and clodronate (PENTOCLO, NCT01291433) in radiation-induced neuropathies is currently ongoing. Physiotherapy can aid in the development of strategies to maintain and improve function. Reducing comorbid factors that may aggravate the plexopathy such as diabetes, high blood pressure, alcohol abuse, and statins is recommended. Hyperbaric oxygen has been evaluated in small case series, but currently, there is no evidence to support its use in the treatment of RIBP [342]. Surgery with nerve or muscle transfer [343–345] and neurolysis [346] have been reported to be useful in highly select patients with RIBP [342].

For a complete discussion on radiation-induced plexopathies, please refer to Chap. 14.

Radiculopathy

Isolated radiculopathy is rare in BC and may be a manifestation of ESCC, LM, or *Herpes zoster*. *Herpes zoster* infection, an opportunistic infection, may be enabled by adjuvant chemotherapy with secondary treatment-induced immunosuppression. In a large study of early-stage BC patients, 1.9% developed *zoster* [347]. In this cohort, the incidence of *Herpes zoster* infection was estimated at 55/1000 cases/year, whereas the incidence in the general population varies between 2.2 and 4.1 per 1000 patients/year. Thus, in early BC patients, the risk of infection is 13- to 25-fold higher compared to the incidence in the general population [347]. Treatment utilizes analgesics and antiviral medications such as acyclovir. Delayed late post-herpetic neuralgia, a neuropathic syndrome, may appear in a small subset and may require chronic opioid treatment.

Radiation Neuropathy

The peripheral nervous system is often characterized as radioresistant; nevertheless, radiation-induced neuropathies are reported. The signs and symptoms are heterogeneous and differ according to the affected part of the peripheral nervous system (nerve root, nerve plexus, nerve trunk). Radiation neuropathies are often progressive and irreversible and may have a considerable impact on QoL. Generally, radiation neuropathies appear years after RT [336, 337].

Peripheral Neuropathy

Chemotherapy-induced peripheral neuropathy (CIPN) is a frequent adverse consequence of BC treatment. CIPN is observed in 30–40% of patients receiving chemotherapy and varies according to the cytotoxic drug regimen, duration of treatment, cumulative dose, and neuropathy-related risk factors [348]. CIPN can be severe and have a significant impact on activities of daily living and overall QoL [349, 350]. In severe cases, chemotherapy dose delays, reductions, or discontinuation of treatment is required [348, 349, 351]. The potential impact of dose reductions or treatment delays due to CIPN on PFS CIPN is unknown [351]. The overall clinical presentation of CIPN is similar, although some differences are observed among the chemotherapy agents.

Several risk factors have been associated with CIPN. The role of older age as a risk factor for CIPN is controversial [352]. Diabetes has been shown to increase the risk and severity of CIPN related to weekly paclitaxel treatment [353]. Moreover, more frequent chemotherapy dose delays and dose reductions are observed in patients with diabetes. Treatment-related risk factors include chemotherapy dose per cycle, treatment schedule, cumulative dose, and duration of infusion [351, 354, 355]. The class of chemotherapy and the class of biochemical characteristics influence the risk of CIPN. For example, docetaxel induces less CIPN than paclitaxel (1–9% vs. 30%) [348]. Inter-individual variability in toxicity is observed, and genetic factors likely are of importance, but are difficult to determine a priori [355]. Pharmacogenomic approaches using single nucleotide polymorphisms (SNPs) have been used to correlate the risk of toxicity to specific agents. For paclitaxel, studies have focused on several candidate genes such as CYP2C8, CYP3A4, CYP3A5, and ABCB1 [350, 355, 356]. Associations have also been reported between the risk of neuropathy and FGD4, EPHA5, and FZD3 genes [350]. Higher TUBB2A gene expression may lead to a lower sensitivity to paclitaxel [357]. For docetaxel, candidates include glutathione S-transferase detoxification enzyme GSTP1 polymorphism [350, 358]. GSTP1 polymorphism has also been suggested to increase the risk of oxaliplatin and cisplatin neurotoxicity [349]. The results are not always consistent between studies, and further research is needed to confirm the relevant associations between genotype and risk of CIPN.

Taxanes, microtubule-stabilizing agents, are among the most active drugs used in BC. The most important dose-limiting toxicity is CIPN, and the incidence of all grades of CIPN after taxanes varies from 11 to 87% [354, 359]. Microtubules are critical for peripheral nerve axonal transport processes and are affected by taxanes [349]. Taxanes induce microtubule polymerization and inhibit depolymerization leading to an impairment of axonal transport [349, 351], which has been speculated to play a role in CIPN. Severe CIPN is reported in 1–18% of patients following taxane treatment. The incidence of all grades of docetaxel-induced CIPN varies from 11–64% [358, 359]. The incidence of serious (grade 3/4) sensory and motor neuropathy in patients treated with docetaxel was 1.6 and 0%, respectively [360]. Patients presenting with CIPN after initial docetaxel infusion often receive fewer cycles without dose modification as compared to patients without CIPN [361]. The incidence of all grades of CIPN with paclitaxel is higher and varies from 59 to 87% [351, 359]. Grade 3–4 CIPN is observed in 7–33% of patients treated with paclitaxel [351]. The incidence of serious (grade 3/4) sensory and motor neuropathy in patients treated with paclitaxel was 7 and 5%, respectively [362]. A dose reduction in taxanes due to a CIPN is required in 2–26% of patients [351, 354, 363–365]. One study observed a 17% dose reduction due to CIPN resulted in a decreased relative dose intensity of 73.4% [351]. The clinical manifestations of taxane CIPN are mainly sensory. Sensory symptoms include numbness, paresthesia, burning, and hyperalgesia. Loss of deep-tendon reflexes is rare in taxane-induced CIPN. Motor neuropathy occurs less frequent than sensory CIPN and may result in weakness of distal limb muscles. Myalgias and arthralgias have been associated with CIPN from paclitaxel [349]. A toxic optic neuropathy has been reported after docetaxel treatment [366].

Symptoms of acute CIPN occur within 24–72 h following taxane infusion [348, 351, 367, 368]. Symptoms may be observed after the first infusion, but are more frequent after 2 or more infusions [354]. Clinical manifestations usually disappear spontaneously after discontinuation of the drug [348]. However, axonal degeneration can sometimes be observed, especially after prolonged administration, and be responsible for permanent CIPN. Approximately 50% of the symptoms resolve within 9 months [369]. In a cohort of 69 patients treated with docetaxel, paclitaxel, or both, taxane-induced CIPN completely resolved in only 14% of the patients after cessation of treatment, and long-term neurotoxicity was observed in 60% in the docetaxel group and 70% in the paclitaxel group [353]. Long-term symptoms were, however, minor in most patients [359]. In a cohort of 1031 patients treated with adjuvant docetaxel, 23% reported grades 2–4 neuropathy, CIPN persisted for 1–3 years in 34% of patients though generally subsiding to grades 0–1. In this cohort, 15% of survivors reported a significant impact on QoL due to docetaxel CIPN at 1–3 years after cessation of treatment [370]. After paclitaxel, CIPN of all grades was observed in 41% of the 219 patients 3 years after treatment [364], while in another cohort of 50 patients, 81% of the patients still reported CIPN symptoms 6 months to 2 years after paclitaxel treatment, with up to 27% reporting severe symptoms [365].

The symptoms of neuropathy induced by taxanes appear at cumulative doses ≥ 300 mg/m^2. An increased single dose of paclitaxel is also associated with a higher risk of neurotoxicity. Shorter infusions appear to increase the risk of neurotoxicity (comparing 1–3 h(s) vs. 24 h infusions) [349]. Paclitaxel is more toxic than docetaxel and results in more frequent CIPN [348, 359]. In a phase III trial, paclitaxel versus docetaxel in patients with metastatic BC, more grade 3/4 sensory (7% vs. 4%) and motor CIPN (5% vs. 2%) was observed. In this study, more discontinuation of treatment due to CIPN was observed after docetaxel [371]. Weekly administration of paclitaxel results in more frequent CIPN than the every 3-week schedule (24% vs. 12% for grade 3 sensory CIPN and 9% vs. 5% for grade 3 CIPN) [362]. In contrast, more grade 3 CIPN has been observed after every 3-week docetaxel schedule (10% vs. 5%) [372]. New formulations of paclitaxel, such as nanoparticle albumin-bound (Nab) paclitaxel and liposomal-encapsulated paclitaxel, appear to reduce neurotoxicity [350, 362, 373].

Eribulin mesylate is a non-taxane microtubule dynamic inhibitor. Eribulin binds to microtubules and suppresses microtubule growth [374]. In trials, CIPN of any grade occurred in 14–35% after eribulin. Grade 3 CIPN was observed in 3–27% and grade 4 CIPN in less than 1% [375–377]. Drug interruption was required in 4–5% due to CIPN [375, 376, 378]. Signs and symptoms were observed after a median of 9 months of treatment and resolved after 12 months [378] of CIPN. Treatment with carboplatin may result in CIPN, but causes less CIPN as compared to cisplatin [379, 380]. Oxaliplatin and cisplatin and vinca alkaloids (vinorelbine) can cause CIPN, but are only occasionally used in BC. Vinorelbine, the most commonly used vinca alkaloids in metastatic BC, interferes with microtubule assembly [381]. Unlike with other vinca alkaloids, neuropathy is relatively infrequent with this agent. Cisplatin and carboplatin are used for the treatment of metastatic BC, in particular for triple negative BC. Cisplatin CIPN can result in a worsening of the neuropathy following discontinuation of chemotherapy, a phenomenon termed coasting [348, 370]. Additionally, cisplatin can cause progressive and irreversible hearing loss in many patients [380, 382, 383]. Bilateral sensorineural hearing loss may be observed in 19–77% of the patients treated with cisplatin, and permanent tinnitus may be seen in 19–42%. Raynaud phenomena, a localized autonomic neuropathy, may be observed with cisplatin as well [384].

A neuropathy scale exists for the cisplatin-induced neurotoxicity with elements that include CIPN, ototoxicity, and Raynaud phenomena [349, 385]. Although carboplatin is generally thought to be less frequently responsible for CIPN, a meta-analysis of platinoid chemotherapy toxicity (carboplatin vs. cisplatin) used in association with third-generation agents for advanced-stage non-small cell lung cancer demonstrated a twofold higher rate of neurotoxicity in the carboplatin group [379].

Other sensory neuropathies, such as Charcot-Marie-Tooth, diabetic neuropathy, alcoholic neuropathy, paraneoplastic neuropathy, and discogenic nerve root compression, should be excluded [221, 350, 351, 354, 355, 364, 386]. Taxanes may cause lymphedema, which can lead to a bilateral carpal tunnel syndrome mimicking or worsening signs and symptoms of CIPN [359, 387]. The onset of symptoms and their relationships with chemotherapy administration help to identify the casualty of the cytotoxic agent. Early detection and recognition of CIPN are critical so as to allow chemotherapy dose delays or dose reduction prior to the appearance of severe neurologic symptoms [349, 350]. Drug discontinuance is recommended for all high-grade neuropathies [350]. Antiepileptics (gabapentin or pregabalin) and antidepressants (tricyclics, duloxetine, or venlafaxine) are often proposed for the treatment of neuropathic pain despite relatively limited effectiveness in CIPN [348, 350, 351, 380, 388–391]. Numerous other treatments have been evaluated in preventive studies including nerve growth factor (NGF) stimulants (all-trans-retinoic acid); antioxidants or antioxidant-related agents (a-Lipoic acid, vitamin E, glutathione, glutamine, N-acetylcysteine, D-methionine, omega-3 fatty acids, amifostine); electrolytes, chelators, ion channel modulators (calcium/magnesium infusion, carbamazepine and oxcarbazepine, nimodipine), and other compounds (acetyl-L-carnitine, xaliproden [a 5-hydroxytryptamine(HT)1A agonist], venlafaxine, *goshajinkigan* [Kampo medicine composed of 10 natural ingredients], topical gel with baclofen + amitriptyline + ketamine, erythropoietin, recombinant human leukemia inhibitory factor), and none have proved effective. Dextromethorphan, a N-methyl-D-aspartate receptor antagonist, has not been evaluated in CIPN, but shows efficacy in painful diabetic neuropathy and in postoperative pain [388]. A randomized double-blind trial using dextromethorphan in CIPN is currently under recruitment (NCT02271893). Non-pharmaceutical approaches such as acupuncture have also been studied [351]. A phase II randomized trial is currently evaluating the efficacy of acupuncture in preventing dose reductions due to CIPN in patients with BC which is currently ongoing (NCT01881932). Other approaches include the non-invasive electro-analgesia device referred to as "Scrambler" therapy and manual therapy such as massage. Physiotherapy may help to improve gait impairment and assist patients by providing life-relevant adaptive strategies [349].

Myopathy

Although skeletal muscles comprise more than 50% of total body mass, skeletal muscle metastases are rare. In a cohort of 73 patients with skeletal muscle metastases, BC was identified as the primary in only 14% of the cases, preceded by lung cancer (34%) and gastrointestinal cancer (18%) [392]. Paraneoplastic necrotizing myopathy is rarely reported in BC [393, 394]. Patients present with a proximal, symmetric, and rapidly progressive myopathy. Myalgia can be absent, and deep-tendon reflexes are hypoactive. An increase in serum creatinine kinase and myoglobin is commonly observed. Electromyogram may show an incomplete interference pattern during voluntary contraction. Treatment of BC and corticosteroids may lead to an improvement in neurological deficits.

Myopathy can also be a result of treatment. Corticosteroids are frequently used in cancer patients and are a frequent cause of myopathy with clinical symptoms in up to 60% of patients [395]. Steroid myopathy is characterized by proximal muscle weakness predominantly in the lower extremities that may interfere with the activities of daily living. Symptoms may appear insidiously and can be observed within days after steroid initiation and are related in part to cumulative dose. Respiratory muscle weakness may lead to symptomatic dyspnea, sometimes in the absence of proximal muscles symptoms. Acute severe myopathy has been described after high-dose steroids [396]. Serum muscle enzymes can be normal as is electromyography [396, 397]. Muscle biopsy shows atrophy of type IIb fibers without necrosis or inflammation [397]. Steroid myopathy is reversible after reduction or discontinuation of steroids, though recovery may require weeks. Fluorinated steroids (dexamethasone, triamcinolone) are more often responsible for myopathy than non-fluorinated steroids (prednisone, hydrocortisone) [395]. Radiotherapy-induced myopathy is very rare in BC. Muscles weakness is observed, serum creatinine kinase values are normal, and electromyography shows myopathic changes [398]. Musculoskeletal symptoms and myopathy can be induced by other agents such as cytarabine, cyclophosphamide, methotrexate, and aromatase inhibitors. Other conditions such as hypercalcemia may also lead to myopathy.

References

1. Lin NU, Bellon JR, Winer EP. CNS metastases in breast cancer. J Clin Oncol. 2004;22:3608–17.
2. Barnholtz-Sloan JS, Sloan AE, Davis FG, Vigneau FD, Lai P, Sawaya RE. Incidence proportions of brain metastases in patients diagnosed (1973–2001) in the metropolitan detroit cancer surveillance system. J Clin Oncol. 2004;22:2865–72.
3. Gil-Gil MJ, Martinez-Garcia M, Sierra A, Conesa G, Del Barco S, González-Jimenez S, Villà S. Breast cancer brain

metastases: a review of the literature and a current multidisciplinary management guideline. Clin Transl Oncol Off Publ Fed
Span Oncol Soc Natl Cancer Inst Mex. 2014;16:436–46.

4. Posner JB. Neurologic complications of cancer. Philadelphia: FA
Davis; 1995.

5. Barajas RF, Cha S. Imaging diagnosis of brain metastasis. Prog
Neurol Surg. 2012;25:55–73.

6. Sperduto PW, Kased N, Roberge D, et al. The effect of tumor
subtype on the time from primary diagnosis to development of
brain metastases and survival in patients with breast cancer.
J Neurooncol. 2013;112:467–72.

7. Sperduto PW, Kased N, Roberge D, et al. Effect of tumor subtype
on survival and the graded prognostic assessment for patients
with breast cancer and brain metastases. Int J Radiat Oncol Biol
Phys. 2012;82:2111–7.

8. Bachmann C, Schmidt S, Staebler A, Fehm T, Fend F, Schittenhelm J, Wallwiener D, Grischke E. CNS metastases in breast
cancer patients: prognostic implications of tumor subtype. Med
Oncol. 2015;32:400.

9. Bendell JC, Domchek SM, Burstein HJ, Harris L, Younger J,
Kuter I, Bunnell C, Rue M, Gelman R, Winer E. Central nervous
system metastases in women who receive trastuzumab-based
therapy for metastatic breast carcinoma. Cancer. 2003;97:2972–7.

10. Clayton AJ, Danson S, Jolly S, et al. Incidence of cerebral
metastases in patients treated with trastuzumab for metastatic
breast cancer. Br J Cancer. 2004;91:639–43.

11. Stemmler HJ, Kahlert S, Siekiera W, Untch M, Heinrich B,
Heinemann V. Characteristics of patients with brain metastases
receiving trastuzumab for HER2 overexpressing metastatic breast
cancer. Breast. 2006;15:219–25.

12. Brufsky AM, Mayer M, Rugo HS, et al. Central nervous system
metastases in patients with HER2-positive metastatic breast
cancer: incidence, treatment, and survival in patients from
registHER. Clin Cancer Res. 2011;17:4834–43.

13. Kennecke H, Yerushalmi R, Woods R, Cheang MCU, Voduc D,
Speers CH, Nielsen TO, Gelmon K. Metastatic behavior of breast
cancer subtypes. J Clin Oncol. 2010;28:3271–7.

14. Lin NU, Vanderplas A, Hughes ME, Theriault RL, Edge SB,
Wong Y-N, Blayney DW, Niland JC, Winer EP, Weeks JC.
Clinicopathologic features, patterns of recurrence, and survival
among women with triple-negative breast cancer in the national
comprehensive cancer network. Cancer. 2012;118:5463–72.

15. Aversa C, Rossi V, Geuna E, Martinello R, Milani A, Redana S,
Valabrega G, Aglietta M, Montemurro F. Metastatic breast cancer
subtypes and central nervous system metastases. Breast.
2014;23:623–8.

16. Niikura N, Hayashi N, Masuda N, et al. Treatment outcomes and
prognostic factors for patients with brain metastases from breast
cancer of each subtype: a multicenter retrospective analysis.
Breast Cancer Res Treat. 2014;147:103–12.

17. Hayashi N, Niikura N, Masuda N, et al. Prognostic factors of
HER2-positive breast cancer patients who develop brain metas-
tasis: a multicenter retrospective analysis. Breast Cancer Res
Treat. 2015;149:277–84.

18. Lin NU, Claus E, Sohl J, Razzak AR, Arnaout A, Winer EP. Sites
of distant recurrence and clinical outcomes in patients with
metastatic triple-negative breast cancer: high incidence of central
nervous system metastases. Cancer. 2008;113:2638–45.

19. Sperduto PW, Chao ST, Sneed PK, et al. Diagnosis-specific
prognostic factors, indexes, and treatment outcomes for patients
with newly diagnosed brain metastases: a multi-institutional
analysis of 4259 patients. Int J Radiat Oncol Biol Phys.
2010;77:655–61.

20. Subbiah IM, Lei X, Weinberg JS, et al. Validation and
development of a modified breast graded prognostic assessment

as a tool for survival in patients with breast cancer and brain
metastases. J Clin Oncol. 2015;33:2239–45.

21. Castaneda CA, Flores R, Rojas KY, Castillo M, Dolores-Cerna
K, Flores C, Belmar-Lopez C, Milla E, Gomez H. Prognostic
factors for patients with newly diagnosed brain metastasis from
breast cancer. CNS Oncol. 2015;4:137–45.

22. Gaspar LE, Scott C, Murray K, Curran W. Validation of the RTOG
recursive partitioning analysis (RPA) classification for brain
metastases. Int J Radiat Oncol Biol Phys. 2000;47(4):1001–6.

23. Lin NU. Breast cancer brain metastases: new directions in
systemic therapy. Ecancermedicalscience. 2013;7:307.

24. Lim E, Lin NU. Updates on the management of breast cancer
brain metastases. Oncol. 2014;28:572–8.

25. Glantz MJ, Cole BF, Forsyth PA, Recht LD, Wen PY, Chamberlain MC, Grossman SA, Cairncross JG. Practice parameter:
anticonvulsant prophylaxis in patients with newly diagnosed
brain tumors. Report of the Quality Standards Subcommittee of
the American Academy of Neurology. Neurology.
2000;54:1886–93.

26. Soffietti R, Cornu P, Delattre JY, et al. EFNS Guidelines on
diagnosis and treatment of brain metastases: report of an EFNS
task force. Eur J Neurol. 2006;13:674–81.

27. Leone JP, Lee AV, Brufsky AM. Prognostic factors and survival
of patients with brain metastasis from breast cancer who
underwent craniotomy. Cancer Med. 2015;4:989–94.

28. Chong JU, Ahn SG, Lee HM, Park JT, Lee SA, Park S, Jeong J,
Kim SI. Local control of brain metastasis: treatment outcome of
focal brain treatments in relation to subtypes. J Breast Cancer.
2015;18:29–35.

29. Yaeger KA, Nair MN. Surgery for brain metastases. Surg Neurol
Int. 2013;4:S203–8.

30. Patchell RA. The management of brain metastases. Cancer Treat
Rev. 2003;29:533–40.

31. Ba JL, Jandial R, Nesbit A, Badie B, Chen M. Current and
emerging treatments for brain metastases. Oncol. 2015;29:250–7.

32. Patel TR, Knisely JPS, Chiang VLS. Management of brain
metastases: surgery, radiation, or both? Hematol Oncol Clin
North Am. 2012;26:933–47.

33. Suki D, Hatiboglu MA, Patel AJ, Weinberg JS, Groves MD,
Mahajan A, Sawaya R. Comparative risk of leptomeningeal
dissemination of cancer after surgery or stereotactic radiosurgery
for a single supratentorial solid tumor metastasis. Neurosurgery
2009;64:664–674; discussion 674–676.

34. Yoo H, Kim YZ, Nam BH, Shin SH, Yang HS, Lee JS, Zo JI,
Lee SH. Reduced local recurrence of a single brain metastasis
through microscopic total resection. J Neurosurg. 2009;110:730–
6.

35. Yamamoto M, Kawabe T, Sato Y, Higuchi Y, Nariai T,
Barfod BE, Kasuya H, Urakawa Y. A case-matched study of
stereotactic radiosurgery for patients with multiple brain metastases: comparing treatment results for 1–4 vs ≥ 5 tumors:
clinical article. J Neurosurg. 2013;118:1258–68.

36. Ojerholm E, Lee JYK, Kolker J, Lustig R, Dorsey JF,
Alonso-Basanta M. Gamma Knife radiosurgery to four or more
brain metastases in patients without prior intracranial radiation or
surgery. Cancer Med. 2014;3:565–71.

37. Jawahar A, Shaya M, Campbell P, Ampil F, Willis BK, Smith D,
Nanda A. Role of stereotactic radiosurgery as a primary treatment
option in the management of newly diagnosed multiple (3–6)
intracranial metastases. Surg Neurol. 2005;64:207–12.

38. Chang WS, Kim HY, Chang JW, Park YG, Chang JH. Analysis
of radiosurgical results in patients with brain metastases according to the number of brain lesions: is stereotactic radiosurgery
effective for multiple brain metastases? J Neurosurg. 2010;113
(Suppl):73–8.

39. Xue J, Kubicek GJ, Grimm J, LaCouture T, Chen Y, Goldman HW, Yorke E. Biological implications of whole-brain radiotherapy versus stereotactic radiosurgery of multiple brain metastases. J Neurosurg. 2014;121(Suppl):60–8.

40. Mintz AH, Kestle J, Rathbone MP, Gaspar L, Hugenholtz H, Fisher B, Duncan G, Skingley P, Foster G, Levine M. A randomized trial to assess the efficacy of surgery in addition to radiotherapy in patients with a single cerebral metastasis. Cancer. 1996;78:1470–6.

41. Paek SH, Audu PB, Sperling MR, Cho J, Andrews DW. Reevaluation of surgery for the treatment of brain metastases: review of 208 patients with single or multiple brain metastases treated at one institution with modern neurosurgical techniques. Neurosurgery 2005;56:1021–1034; discussion 1021–1034.

42. Linskey ME, Andrews DW, Asher AL, et al. The role of stereotactic radiosurgery in the management of patients with newly diagnosed brain metastases: a systematic review and evidence-based clinical practice guideline. J Neurooncol. 2010;96:45–68.

43. Yang TJ, Oh JH, Folkert MR, et al. Outcomes and prognostic factors in women with 1 to 3 breast cancer brain metastases treated with definitive stereotactic radiosurgery. Int J Radiat Oncol Biol Phys. 2014;90:518–25.

44. Cho E, Rubinstein L, Stevenson P, Gooley T, Philips M, Halasz LM, Gensheimer MF, Linden HM, Rockhill JK, Gadi VK. The use of stereotactic radiosurgery for brain metastases from breast cancer: who benefits most? Breast Cancer Res Treat. 2015;149:743–9.

45. Rades D, Huttenlocher S, Rudat V, Hornung D, Blanck O, Phuong PC, Khoa MT, Schild SE, Fischer D. Radiosurgery with 20 Gy provides better local control of 1–3 brain metastases from breast cancer than with lower doses. Anticancer Res. 2015;35:333–6.

46. Mehta MP. Brain metastases: the changing landscape. Oncol. 2015;29:257–60.

47. Gaspar L, Scott C, Rotman M, Asbell S, Phillips T, Wasserman T, McKenna WG, Byhardt R. Recursive partitioning analysis (RPA) of prognostic factors in three Radiation Therapy Oncology Group (RTOG) brain metastases trials. Int J Radiat Oncol Biol Phys. 1997;37:745–51.

48. Nieder C, Berberich W, Schnabel K. Tumor-related prognostic factors for remission of brain metastases after radiotherapy. Int J Radiat Oncol Biol Phys. 1997;39:25–30.

49. Phillips TL, Scott CB, Leibel SA, Rotman M, Weigensberg IJ. Results of a randomized comparison of radiotherapy and bromodeoxyuridine with radiotherapy alone for brain metastases: report of RTOG trial 89-05. Int J Radiat Oncol Biol Phys. 1995;33:339–48.

50. Ogura M, Mitsumori M, Okumura S, Yamauchi C, Kawamura S, Oya N, Nagata Y, Hiraoka M. Radiation therapy for brain metastases from breast cancer. Breast Cancer. 2003;10:349–55.

51. Cao KI, Lebas N, Gerber S, Levy C, Le Scodan R, Bourgier C, Pierga J-Y, Gobillion A, Savignoni A, Kirova YM. Phase II randomized study of whole-brain radiation therapy with or without concurrent temozolomide for brain metastases from breast cancer. Ann Oncol. 2015;26:89–94.

52. Mehta MP, Wang D, Wang F, et al. Veliparib in combination with whole brain radiation therapy in patients with brain metastases: results of a phase 1 study. J Neurooncol. 2015;122:409–17.

53. Kocher M, Soffietti R, Abacioglu U, et al. Adjuvant whole-brain radiotherapy versus observation after radiosurgery or surgical resection of one to three cerebral metastases: results of the EORTC 22952-26001 study. J Clin Oncol. 2011;29:134–41.

54. Rades D, Huttenlocher S, Hornung D, Blanck O, Schild SE, Fischer D. Do patients with very few brain metastases from breast cancer benefit from whole-brain radiotherapy in addition to radiosurgery? Radiat Oncol. 2014;9:267.

55. Soffietti R, Kocher M, Abacioglu UM, et al. A European organisation for research and treatment of cancer phase III trial of adjuvant whole-brain radiotherapy versus observation in patients with one to three brain metastases from solid tumors after surgical resection or radiosurgery: quality-of-life results. J Clin Oncol 31:65–72.

56. Chang EL, Wefel JS, Hess KR, et al. Neurocognition in patients with brain metastases treated with radiosurgery or radiosurgery plus whole-brain irradiation: a randomised controlled trial. Lancet Oncol. 2009;10:1037–44.

57. Brown PD et al. NCCTG N0574 (Alliance): a phase III randomized trial of whole brain radiation therapy (WBRT) in addition to radiosurgery (SRS) in patients with 1 to 3 brain metastases. J Clin Oncol. 2015;33(suppl; abstr LBA4).

58. Stokes TB, Niranjan A, Kano H, Choi PA, Kondziolka D, Dade Lunsford L, Monaco EA. White matter changes in breast cancer brain metastases patients who undergo radiosurgery alone compared to whole brain radiation therapy plus radiosurgery. J Neurooncol. 2015;121:583–90.

59. Aoyama H, Tago M, Kato N, et al. Neurocognitive function of patients with brain metastasis who received either whole brain radiotherapy plus stereotactic radiosurgery or radiosurgery alone. Int J Radiat Oncol Biol Phys. 2007;68:1388–95.

60. Brown PD, Pugh S, Laack NN, et al. Memantine for the prevention of cognitive dysfunction in patients receiving whole-brain radiotherapy: a randomized, double-blind, placebo-controlled trial. Neuro-Oncol. 2013;15:1429–37.

61. Gondi V, Pugh SL, Tome WA, et al. Preservation of memory with conformal avoidance of the hippocampal neural stem-cell compartment during whole-brain radiotherapy for brain metastases (RTOG 0933): a phase II multi-institutional trial. J Clin Oncol. 2014;32:3810–6.

62. Linot B, Campone M, Augereau P, Delva R, Abadie-Lacourtoisie S, Nebout-Mesgouez N, Capitain O. Use of liposomal doxorubicin-cyclophosphamide combination in breast cancer patients with brain metastases: a monocentric retrospective study. J Neurooncol. 2014;117:253–9.

63. Trudeau ME, Crump M, Charpentier D, Yelle L, Bordeleau L, Matthews S, Eisenhauer E. Temozolomide in metastatic breast cancer (MBC): a phase II trial of the National Cancer Institute of Canada—Clinical Trials Group (NCIC-CTG). Ann Oncol. 2006;17:952–6.

64. Siena S, Crinò L, Danova M, Del Prete S, Cascinu S, Salvagni S, Schiavetto I, Vitali M, Bajetta E. Dose-dense temozolomide regimen for the treatment of brain metastases from melanoma, breast cancer, or lung cancer not amenable to surgery or radiosurgery: a multicenter phase II study. Ann Oncol. 2010;21:655–61.

65. von Minckwitz G, Jonat W, Fasching P, et al. A multicentre phase II study on gefitinib in taxane- and anthracycline-pretreated metastatic breast cancer. Breast Cancer Res Treat. 2005;89:165–72.

66. Salhia B, Kiefer J, Ross JTD, et al. Integrated genomic and epigenomic analysis of breast cancer brain metastasis. PLoS ONE. 2014;9:e85448.

67. Bollig-Fischer A, Michelhaugh SK, Wijesinghe P, Dyson G, Kruger A, Palanisamy N, Choi L, Alosh B, Ali-Fehmi R, Mittal S. Cytogenomic profiling of breast cancer brain metastases reveals potential for repurposing targeted therapeutics. Oncotarget 2015;6:14614–14624.

68. Biernat W et al. Quantitative HER2 levels and steroid receptor expression in primary breast cancers and in matched brain metastases. J Clin Oncol 2012;30 2012 (suppl; abstr 603).

69. Shen Q, Sahin AA, Hess KR, Suki D, Aldape KD, Sawaya R, Ibrahim NK. Breast cancer with brain metastases: clinicopathologic features, survival, and paired biomarker analysis. Oncologist. 2015;20:466–73.

70. Park IH, Ro J, Lee KS, Nam BH, Kwon Y, Shin KH. Trastuzumab treatment beyond brain progression in HER2-positive metastatic breast cancer. Ann Oncol. 2009;20:56–62.

71. Bartsch R, Berghoff A, Pluschnig U, et al. Impact of anti-HER2 therapy on overall survival in HER2-overexpressing breast cancer patients with brain metastases. Br J Cancer. 2012;106:25–31.

72. Duchnowska R, Biernat W, Szostakiewicz B, et al. Correlation between quantitative HER-2 protein expression and risk for brain metastases in HER-2+ advanced breast cancer patients receiving trastuzumab-containing therapy. Oncologist. 2012;17:26–35.

73. Gori S, Rimondini S, De Angelis V, et al. Central nervous system metastases in HER-2 positive metastatic breast cancer patients treated with trastuzumab: incidence, survival, and risk factors. Oncologist. 2007;12:766–73.

74. Metro G, Sperduti I, Russillo M, Milella M, Cognetti F, Fabi A. Clinical utility of continuing trastuzumab beyond brain progression in HER-2 positive metastatic breast cancer. Oncologist 2007;12:1467–1469; author reply 1469–1471.

75. Bartsch R, Rottenfusser A, Wenzel C, et al. Trastuzumab prolongs overall survival in patients with brain metastases from Her2 positive breast cancer. J Neurooncol. 2007;85:311–7.

76. Park YH, Park MJ, Ji SH, et al. Trastuzumab treatment improves brain metastasis outcomes through control and durable prolongation of systemic extracranial disease in HER2-overexpressing breast cancer patients. Br J Cancer. 2009;100:894–900.

77. Karam I, Hamilton S, Nichol A, Woods R, Speers C, Kennecke H, Tyldesley S. Population-based outcomes after brain radiotherapy in patients with brain metastases from breast cancer in the Pre-Trastuzumab and Trastuzumab eras. Radiat Oncol. 2013;8:12.

78. Lin NU, Carey LA, Liu MC, et al. Phase II trial of lapatinib for brain metastases in patients with human epidermal growth factor receptor 2-positive breast cancer. J Clin Oncol. 2008;26:1993–9.

79. Lin NU, Diéras V, Paul D, et al. Multicenter phase II study of lapatinib in patients with brain metastases from HER2-positive breast cancer. Clin Cancer Res. 2009;15:1452–9.

80. Gomez HL, Doval DC, Chavez MA, et al. Efficacy and safety of lapatinib as first-line therapy for ErbB2-amplified locally advanced or metastatic breast cancer. J Clin Oncol. 2008;26:2999–3005.

81. Metro G, Foglietta J, Russillo M, et al. Clinical outcome of patients with brain metastases from HER2-positive breast cancer treated with lapatinib and capecitabine. Ann Oncol. 2011;22:625–30.

82. Boccardo FK, Baselga B, Dieras J, et al. Evaluation of lapatinib (Lap) plus capecitabine (Cap) in patients with brain metastases (BM) from HER2+ breast cancer (BC) enrolled in the Lapatinib Expanded Access Program (LEAP) and French Authorisation Temporaire d'Utilisation (ATU). Proc Am Soc Clin Oncol 2008;26 (suppl): abstr 1094.

83. Sutherland S, Ashley S, Miles D, et al. Treatment of HER2-positive metastatic breast cancer with lapatinib and capecitabine in the lapatinib expanded access programme, including efficacy in brain metastases–the UK experience. Br J Cancer. 2010;102:995–1002.

84. Lin NU, Eierman W, Greil R, Campone M, Kaufman B, Steplewski K, Lane SR, Zembryki D, Rubin SD,

Winer EP. Randomized phase II study of lapatinib plus capecitabine or lapatinib plus topotecan for patients with HER2-positive breast cancer brain metastases. J Neurooncol. 2011;105:613–20.

85. Bachelot T, Romieu G, Campone M, et al. Lapatinib plus capecitabine in patients with previously untreated brain metastases from HER2-positive metastatic breast cancer (LANDSCAPE): a single-group phase 2 study. Lancet Oncol. 2013;14:64–71.

86. Pivot X, Manikhas A, Żurawski B, et al. CEREBEL (EGF111438): A Phase III, Randomized, Open-Label Study of Lapatinib Plus Capecitabine Versus Trastuzumab Plus Capecitabine in patients with human epidermal growth factor receptor 2-positive metastatic breast cancer. J Clin Oncol. 2015;33:1564–73.

87. Chargari C, Idrissi HR, Pierga J-Y, Bollet MA, Diéras V, Campana F, Cottu P, Fourquet A, Kirova YM. Preliminary results of whole brain radiotherapy with concurrent trastuzumab for treatment of brain metastases in breast cancer patients. Int J Radiat Oncol Biol Phys. 2011;81:631–6.

88. Lin NU, Freedman RA, Ramakrishna N, et al. A phase I study of lapatinib with whole brain radiotherapy in patients with human epidermal growth factor receptor 2 (HER2)-positive breast cancer brain metastases. Breast Cancer Res Treat. 2013;142:405–14.

89. Cortes J, Dieras V, Ro J, et al. Randomized phase II trial of afatinib alone or with vinorelbine versus investigator's choice of treatment in patients with HER2-positive breast cancer with progressive brain metastases after trastuzumab and/or lapatinib-based therapy: LUX-Breast 3. San Antonio Breast Cancer Symposium: P5–19-07;2014.

90. Freedman RA et al. TBCRC 022: phase II trial of neratinib for patients (Pts) with human epidermal growth factor receptor 2 (HER2+) breast cancer and brain metastases (BCBM). J Clin Oncol. 2014;32:5s, (suppl; abstr 528).

91. Lin NU, Amiri-Kordestani L, Palmieri D, Liewehr DJ, Steeg PS. CNS metastases in breast cancer: old challenge, new frontiers. Clin Cancer Res. 2013;19:6404–18.

92. Lin NU, Gelman RS, Younger WJ, et al. Phase II trial of carboplatin (C) and bevacizumab (BEV) in patients (pts) with breast cancer brain metastases (BCBM). J Clin Oncol. 2013;31 (suppl; abstr 513).

93. Lu Y-S, Chen W-W, Lin C-H, et al. Bevacizumab, etoposide, and cisplatin (BEEP) in brain metastases of breast cancer progressing from radiotherapy: results of the first stage of a multicenter phase II study. J Clin Oncol. 2012;30 (suppl; abstr 1079).

94. Laigle-Donadey F, Taillibert S, Martin-Duverneuil N, Hildebrand J, Delattre J-Y. Skull-base metastases. J Neurooncol. 2005;2012(75):63–9.

95. Gloria-Cruz TI, Schachern PA, Paparella MM, Adams GL, Fulton SE. Metastases to temporal bones from primary nonsystemic malignant neoplasms. Arch Otolaryngol Head Neck Surg. 2000;126:209–14.

96. Greenberg HS, Deck MD, Vikram B, Chu FC, Posner JB. Metastasis to the base of the skull: clinical findings in 43 patients. Neurology. 1981;31:530–7.

97. Svare A, Fosså SD, Heier MS. Cranial nerve dysfunction in metastatic cancer of the prostate. Br J Urol. 1988;61:441–4.

98. Castaldo JE, Bernat JL, Meier FA, Schned AR. Intracranial metastases due to prostatic carcinoma. Cancer. 1983;52:1739–47.

99. Dmuchowska DA, Krasnicki P, Obuchowska I, Kochanowicz J, Syta-Krzyżanowska A, Mariak Z. Ophthalmic manifestation of skull base metastasis from breast cancer. Med Sci Monit Int Med J Exp Clin Res 2012;18:CS105–108.

100. Mitsuya K, Nakasu Y, Horiguchi S, Harada H, Nishimura T, Yuen S, Asakura K, Endo M. Metastatic skull tumors: MRI

features and a new conventional classification. J Neurooncol. 2011;104:239–45.

101. Haubold-Reuter BG, Duewell S, Schilcher BR, Marincek B, von Schulthess GK. The value of bone scintigraphy, bone marrow scintigraphy and fast spin-echo magnetic resonance imaging in staging of patients with malignant solid tumours: a prospective study. Eur J Nucl Med. 1993;20:1063–9.

102. Fujimoto R, Higashi T, Nakamoto Y, et al. Diagnostic accuracy of bone metastases detection in cancer patients: comparison between bone scintigraphy and whole-body FDG-PET. Ann Nucl Med. 2006;20:399–408.

103. Vikram B, Chu FC. Radiation therapy for metastases to the base of the skull. Radiology. 1979;130:465–8.

104. Kotecha R, Angelov L, Barnett GH, Reddy CA, Suh JH, Murphy ES, Neyman G, Chao ST. Calvarial and skull base metastases: expanding the clinical utility of Gamma Knife surgery. J Neurosurg. 2014;121(Suppl):91–101.

105. Michael CB, Gokaslan ZL, DeMonte F, McCutcheon IE, Sawaya R, Lang FF. Surgical resection of calvarial metastases overlying dural sinuses. Neurosurgery 20001;48:745–754; discussion 754–755.

106. Nayak L, Abrey LE, Iwamoto FM. Intracranial dural metastases. Cancer. 2009;115:1947–53.

107. Da Silva AN, Schiff D. Dural and skull base metastases. Cancer Treat Res. 2007;136:117–41.

108. Laigle-Donadey F, Taillibert S, Mokhtari K, Hildebrand J, Delattre J-Y. Dural metastases. J Neurooncol. 2005;75:57–61.

109. Lee SS, Kim MK, Sym SJ, Kim SW, Kim WK, Kim S-B, Ahn J-H. Intramedullary spinal cord metastases: a single-institution experience. J Neurooncol. 2007;84:85–9.

110. Veeravagu A, Lieberson RE, Mener A, Chen Y-R, Soltys SG, Gibbs IC, Adler JR, Tian AG, Chang SD. CyberKnife stereotactic radiosurgery for the treatment of intramedullary spinal cord metastases. J Clin Neurosci. 2012;19:1273–7.

111. Sung W-S, Sung M-J, Chan JH, Manion B, Song J, Dubey A, Erasmus A, Hunn A. Intramedullary spinal cord metastases: a 20-year institutional experience with a comprehensive literature review. World Neurosurg. 2013;79:576–84.

112. Basaran R, Tiryaki M, Yavuzer D, Efendioglu M, Balkuv E, Sav A. Spinal intramedullary metastasis of breast cancer. Case Rep Med 2014;583282.

113. Hrabalek L. Intramedullary spinal cord metastases: review of the literature. Biomed Pap Med Fac Univ Palacký Olomouc Czechoslov. 2010;154:117–22.

114. Mut M, Schiff D, Shaffrey ME. Metastasis to nervous system: spinal epidural and intramedullary metastases. J Neurooncol. 2005;75:43–56.

115. Hashii H, Mizumoto M, Kanemoto A, Harada H, Asakura H, Hashimoto T, Furutani K, Katagiri H, Nakasu Y, Nishimura T. Radiotherapy for patients with symptomatic intramedullary spinal cord metastasis. J Radiat Res (Tokyo). 2011;52:641–5.

116. Chaichana KL, Pendleton C, Wolinsky J-P, Gokaslan ZL, Sciubba DM. Vertebral compression fractures in patients presenting with metastatic epidural spinal cord compression. Neurosurgery. 2009;65:267–274; discussion 274–275.

117. Tancioni F, Navarria P, Pessina F, Attuati L, Mancosu P, Alloisio M, Scorsetti M, Santoro A, Baena RRY. Assessment of prognostic factors in patients with metastatic epidural spinal cord compression (MESCC) from solid tumor after surgery plus radiotherapy: a single institution experience. Eur Spine J Off Publ Eur Spine Soc Eur Spinal Deform Soc Eur Sect Cerv Spine Res Soc. 2012;21(Suppl 1):S146–8.

118. Cole JS, Patchell RA. Metastatic epidural spinal cord compression. Lancet Neurol. 2008;7:459–66.

119. Tancioni F, Navarria P, Lorenzetti MA, et al. Multimodal approach to the management of metastatic epidural spinal cord compression (MESCC) due to solid tumors. Int J Radiat Oncol Biol Phys. 2010;78:1467–73.

120. Giglio P, Gilbert MR. Neurologic complications of cancer and its treatment. Curr Oncol Rep. 2010;12:50–9.

121. Chamberlain MC, Kormanik PA. Epidural spinal cord compression: a single institution's retrospective experience. Neuro-Oncol. 1999;1:120–3.

122. Glass JP, Melamed M, Chernik NL, Posner JB. Malignant cells in cerebrospinal fluid (CSF): the meaning of a positive CSF cytology. Neurology. 1979;29:1369–75.

123. Chamberlain MC. Leptomeningeal metastasis. Curr Opin Oncol. 2010;22:627–35.

124. Le Rhun E, Taillibert S, Chamberlain MC. Carcinomatous meningitis: leptomeningeal metastases in solid tumors. Surg Neurol Int. 2013;4:S265–88.

125. Roth P, Weller M. Management of neoplastic meningitis. Chin Clin Oncol. 2015;4:26.

126. Lee YT. Breast carcinoma: pattern of metastasis at autopsy. J Surg Oncol. 1983;23:175–80.

127. Altundag K, Bondy ML, Mirza NQ, Kau S-W, Broglio K, Hortobagyi GN, Rivera E. Clinicopathologic characteristics and prognostic factors in 420 metastatic breast cancer patients with central nervous system metastasis. Cancer. 2007;110:2640–7.

128. Lamovec J, Bracko M. Metastatic pattern of infiltrating lobular carcinoma of the breast: an autopsy study. J Surg Oncol. 1991;48:28–33.

129. Le Rhun E, Taillibert S, Zairi F, Devos P, Pierret MF, Dubois F, Assaker R, Buisset E, Bonneterre J, Baranzelli MC. Clinicopathological features of breast cancers predict the development of leptomeningeal metastases: a case-control study. J Neurooncol. 2011;105:309–3150.

130. Gauthier H, Guilhaume MN, Bidard FC, Pierga JY, Girre V, Cottu PH, Laurence V, Livartowski A, Mignot L, Diéras V. Survival of breast cancer patients with meningeal carcinomatosis. Ann Oncol. 2010;21:2183–7.

131. Rakha EA, El-Sayed ME, Green AR, Lee AHS, Robertson JF, Ellis IO. Prognostic markers in triple-negative breast cancer. Cancer. 2007;109:25–32.

132. Niwińska A, Rudnicka H, Murawska M. Breast cancer leptomeningeal metastasis: propensity of breast cancer subtypes for leptomeninges and the analysis of factors influencing survival. Med Oncol. 2013;30:408.

133. DeAngelis LM. Current diagnosis and treatment of leptomeningeal metastasis. J Neurooncol. 1998;38:245–52.

134. Norris LK, Grossman SA, Olivi A. Neoplastic meningitis following surgical resection of isolated cerebellar metastasis: a potentially preventable complication. J Neurooncol. 1997;32:215–23.

135. Sawaya R, Hammoud M, Schoppa D, Hess KR, Wu SZ, Shi WM, Wildrick DM. Neurosurgical outcomes in a modern series of 400 craniotomies for treatment of parenchymal tumors. Neurosurgery 1998;42:1044–1055; discussion 1055–1056.

136. DeAngelis LM, Mandell LR, Thaler HT, Kimmel DW, Galicich JH, Fuks Z, Posner JB. The role of postoperative radiotherapy after resection of single brain metastases. Neurosurgery. 1989;24:798–805.

137. Ahn JH, Lee SH, Kim S, Joo J, Yoo H, Lee SH, Shin SH, Gwak H-S. Risk for leptomeningeal seeding after resection for brain metastases: implication of tumor location with mode of resection. J Neurosurg. 2012;116:984–93.

138. van der Ree TC, Dippel DW, Avezaat CJ, Sillevis Smitt PA, Vecht CJ, van den Bent MJ. Leptomeningeal metastasis after

surgical resection of brain metastases. J Neurol Neurosurg Psychiatry 1999;66:225–227.

139. Jung J-M, Kim S, Joo J, Shin KH, Gwak H-S, Lee SH. Incidence and risk factors for leptomeningeal carcinomatosis in breast cancer patients with parenchymal brain metastases. J Korean Neurosurg 2012;Soc 52:193–199.

140. Clarke JL, Perez HR, Jacks LM, Panageas KS, Deangelis LM. Leptomeningeal metastases in the MRI era. Neurology. 2010;74:1449–54.

141. Oechsle K, Lange-Brock V, Kruell A, Bokemeyer C, de Wit M. Prognostic factors and treatment options in patients with leptomeningeal metastases of different primary tumors: a retrospective analysis. J Cancer Res Clin Oncol. 2010;136:1729–35.

142. Lee S, Ahn HK, Park YH, et al. Leptomeningeal metastases from breast cancer: intrinsic subtypes may affect unique clinical manifestations. Breast Cancer Res Treat. 2011;129:809–17.

143. Le Rhun E, Taillibert S, Zairi F, et al. A retrospective case series of 103 consecutive patients with leptomeningeal metastasis and breast cancer. J Neurooncol. 2013;113:83–92.

144. de Azevedo CRAS, Cruz MRS, Chinen LTD, Peres SV, Peterlevitz MA, de Azevedo Pereira AE, Fanelli MF, Gimenes DL. Meningeal carcinomatosis in breast cancer: prognostic factors and outcome. J Neurooncol 2011;104:565–572.

145. Clatot F, Philippin-Lauridant G, Ouvrier M-J, Nakry T, Laberge-Le-Couteulx S, Guillemet C, Veyret C, Blot E. Clinical improvement and survival in breast cancer leptomeningeal metastasis correlate with the cytologic response to intrathecal chemotherapy. J Neurooncol. 2009;95:421–6.

146. Rudnicka H, Niwińska A, Murawska M. Breast cancer leptomeningeal metastasis–the role of multimodality treatment. J Neurooncol. 2007;84:57–62.

147. Regierer AC, Stroux A, Kühnhardt D, Dieing A, Lehenbauer-Dehm S, Flath B, Possinger K, Eucker J. Contrast-enhancing meningeal lesions are associated with longer survival in breast cancer-related leptomeningeal metastasis. Breast Care. 2008;3:118–23.

148. Lara-Medina F, Crismatt A, Villarreal-Garza C, Alvarado-Miranda A, Flores-Hernández L, González-Pinedo M, Gamboa-Vignolle C, Ruiz-González JDS, Arrieta O. Clinical features and prognostic factors in patients with carcinomatous meningitis secondary to breast cancer. Breast J. 2012;18:233–41.

149. Meattini I, Livi L, Saieva C, et al. Prognostic factors and clinical features in patients with leptominengeal metastases from breast cancer: a single center experience. J Chemother. 2012;24:279–84.

150. Comte A, Jdid W, Guilhaume MN, et al. Survival of breast cancer patients with meningeal carcinomatosis treated by intrathecal thiotepa. J Neurooncol. 2013;115:445–52.

151. Fusco JP, Castañón E, Carranza OE, Zubiri L, Martín P, Espinós J, Rodríguez J, Santisteban M, Aramendía JM, Gil-Bazo I. Neurological and cytological response as potential early predictors of time-to-progression and overall survival in patients with leptomeningeal carcinomatosis treated with intrathecal liposomal cytarabine: a retrospective cohort study. J Neurooncol. 2013;115:429–35.

152. Yust-Katz S, Garciarena P, Liu D, Yuan Y, Ibrahim N, Yerushalmi R, Penas-Prado M, Groves MD. Breast cancer and leptomeningeal disease (LMD): hormone receptor status influences time to development of LMD and survival from LMD diagnosis. J Neurooncol. 2013;114:229–35.

153. Kim H-J, Im S-A, Keam B, et al. Clinical outcome of central nervous system metastases from breast cancer: differences in survival depending on systemic treatment. J Neurooncol. 2012;106:303–13.

154. Le Rhun E, Taillibert S, Zairi F, Pannier D, Boulanger T, Andre C, Cazin JL, Dubois F, Bonneterre J, Chamberlain MC.

Prolonged survival of patients with breast cancer-related leptomeningeal metastases. Anticancer Res. 2013;33:2057–63.

155. National Comprehensive Cancer Network (NCCN). Clinical practice guidelines in oncology (NCCN Guidelines)—central nervous system cancers. Version I.2015. NCCN.org.

156. Herrlinger U, Förschler H, Küker W, Meyermann R, Bamberg M, Dichgans J, Weller M. Leptomeningeal metastasis: survival and prognostic factors in 155 patients. J Neurol Sci. 2004;223:167–78.

157. Boogerd W1, van den Bent MJ, Koehler PJ, Heimans JJ, van der Sande JJ, Aaronson NK, Hart AA, Benraadt J, Vecht ChJ. The relevance of intraventricular chemotherapy for leptomeningeal metastasis in breast cancer: a randomised study. Eur J Cancer. 2004;40(18):2726–33.

158. Kosmas C, Malamos NA, Tsavaris NB, Stamataki M, Stefanou S, Gregoriou A, Rokana S, Vartholomeou M, Antonopoulos MJ. Leptomeningeal carcinomatosis after major remission to taxane-based front-line therapy in patients with advanced breast cancer. J Neurooncol. 2002;56:265–73.

159. Ekenel M, Hormigo AM, Peak S, Deangelis LM, Abrey LE. Capecitabine therapy of central nervous system metastases from breast cancer. J Neurooncol. 2007;85:223–7.

160. Giglio P, Tremont-Lukats IW, Groves MD. Response of neoplastic meningitis from solid tumors to oral capecitabine. J Neurooncol. 2003;65:167–72.

161. Rogers LR, Remer SE, Tejwani S. Durable response of breast cancer leptomeningeal metastasis to capecitabine monotherapy. Neuro-Oncol. 2004;6:63–4.

162. Tham Y-L, Hinckley L, Teh BS, Elledge R. Long-term clinical response in leptomeningeal metastases from breast cancer treated with capecitabine monotherapy: a case report. Clin Breast Cancer. 2006;7:164–6.

163. Tanaka Y, Oura S, Yoshimasu T, Ohta F, Naito K, Nakamura R, Hirai Y, Ikeda M, Okamura Y. Response of meningeal carcinomatosis from breast cancer to capecitabine monotherapy: a case report. Case Rep Oncol. 2013;6:1–5.

164. Segura PP, Gil M, Balañá C, Chacón I, Langa JM, Martín M, Bruna J. Phase II trial of temozolomide for leptomeningeal metastases in patients with solid tumors. J Neurooncol. 2012;109:137–42.

165. Vincent A, Lesser G, Brown D, Vern-Gross T, Metheny-Barlow L, Lawrence J, Chan M. Prolonged regression of metastatic leptomeningeal breast cancer that has failed conventional therapy: a case report and review of the literature. J Breast Cancer. 2013;16:122–6.

166. Labidi SI, Bachelot T, Ray-Coquard I, Mosbah K, Treilleux I, Fayette J, Favier B, Galy G, Blay J-Y, Guastalla J-P. Bevacizumab and paclitaxel for breast cancer patients with central nervous system metastases: a case series. Clin Breast Cancer. 2009;9:118–21.

167. Le Rhun E, Taillibert S, Boulanger T, Zairi F, Bonneterre J, Chamberlain MC. Prolonged response and restoration of functional independence with bevacizumab plus vinorelbine as third-line treatment for breast cancer-related leptomeningeal metastases. Case Rep Oncol. 2015;8:72–7.

168. Chen I-C, Lin C-H, Jan I-S, Cheng A-L, Lu Y-S. Bevacizumab might potentiate the chemotherapeutic effect in breast cancer patients with leptomeningeal carcinomatosis. J Formos Med Assoc Taiwan Yi Zhi. 2016;115(4):243–8.

169. Torres S, Maralani P, Verma S. Activity of T-DM1 in HER-2 positive central nervous system breast cancer metastases. BMJ Case Rep. 2014 (pii: bcr2014205680).

170. Chamberlain M, Soffietti R, Raizer J, et al. Leptomeningeal metastasis: a response assessment in neuro-oncology critical review of endpoints and response criteria of published randomized clinical trials. Neuro-Oncol. 2014;16:1176–85.

171. Cole BF, Glantz MJ, Jaeckle KA, Chamberlain MC, Mackowiak JI. Quality-of-life-adjusted survival comparison of sustained-release cytosine arabinoside versus intrathecal methotrexate for treatment of solid tumor neoplastic meningitis. Cancer. 2003;97:3053–60.

172. Chamberlain MC, Tsao-Wei DD, Groshen S. Phase II trial of intracerebrospinal fluid etoposide in the treatment of neoplastic meningitis. Cancer. 2006;106:2021–7.

173. Mego M, Sycova-Mila Z, Obertova J, Rajec J, Liskova S, Palacka P, Porsok S, Mardiak J. Intrathecal administration of trastuzumab with cytarabine and methotrexate in breast cancer patients with leptomeningeal carcinomatosis. Breast. 2011;20:478–80.

174. Oliveira M, Braga S, Passos-Coelho JL, Fonseca R, Oliveira J. Complete response in HER2+ leptomeningeal carcinomatosis from breast cancer with intrathecal trastuzumab. Breast Cancer Res Treat. 2011;127:841–4.

175. Zagouri F, Sergentanis TN, Bartsch R, Berghoff AS, Chrysikos D, de Azambuja E, Dimopoulos M-A, Preusser M. Intrathecal administration of trastuzumab for the treatment of meningeal carcinomatosis in HER2-positive metastatic breast cancer: a systematic review and pooled analysis. Breast Cancer Res Treat. 2013;139:13–22.

176. Dumitrescu C, Lossignol D. Intrathecal trastuzumab treatment of the neoplastic meningitis due to breast cancer: a case report and review of the literature. Case Rep Oncol Med 2013:154674.

177. Jaeckle KA. Neurological manifestations of neoplastic and radiation-induced plexopathies. Semin Neurol. 2004;24:385–93.

178. Jaeckle KA. Neurologic manifestations of neoplastic and radiation-induced plexopathies. Semin Neurol. 2010;30:254–62.

179. Ko K, Sung DH, Kang MJ, Ko MJ, Do JG, Sunwoo H, Kwon TG, Hwang JM, Park Y. Clinical, electrophysiological findings in adult patients with non-traumatic plexopathies. Ann Rehabil Med. 2011;35:807–15.

180. Kamenova B, Braverman AS, Schwartz M, Sohn C, Lange C, Efiom-Ekaha D, Rotman M, Yoon H. Effective treatment of the brachial plexus syndrome in breast cancer patients by early detection and control of loco-regional metastases with radiation or systemic therapy. Int J Clin Oncol. 2009;14:219–24.

181. Harper CM, Thomas JE, Cascino TL, Litchy WJ. Distinction between neoplastic and radiation-induced brachial plexopathy, with emphasis on the role of EMG. Neurology. 1989;39:502–6.

182. Gatti G, Simsek S, Kurne A, Zurrida S, Naninato P, Veronesi P, Frasson A, Millen E, Rososchansky J, Luini A. Paraneoplastic neurological disorders in breast cancer. Breast. 2003;12:203–7.

183. Honnorat J, Antoine J-C. Paraneoplastic neurological syndromes. Orphanet J Rare Dis. 2007;2:22.

184. Graus F, Dalmau J. Paraneoplastic neurological syndromes. Curr Opin Neurol. 2012;795–801.

185. Graus F, Delattre JY, Antoine JC, et al. Recommended diagnostic criteria for paraneoplastic neurological syndromes. J Neurol Neurosurg Psychiatry. 2004;75:1135–40.

186. Kannoth S. Paraneoplastic neurologic syndrome: a practical approach. Ann Indian Acad Neurol. 2012;15:6–12.

187. Psimaras D, Carpentier AF, Rossi C. PNS Euronetwork. Cerebrospinal fluid study in paraneoplastic syndromes. J Neurol Neurosurg Psychiatry. 2010;81:42–5.

188. Titulaer MJ, Soffietti R, Dalmau J, et al. Screening for tumours in paraneoplastic syndromes: report of an EFNS task force. Eur J Neurol. 2011;18:19 (e3).

189. Berger B, Bischler P, Dersch R, Hottenrott T, Rauer S, Stich O. "Non-classical" paraneoplastic neurological syndromes associated with well-characterized antineuronal antibodies as compared to "classical" syndromes—More frequent than expected. J Neurol Sci. 2015;352:58–61.

190. Barnholtz-Sloan JS, Kruchko C. Meningiomas: causes and risk factors. Neurosurg Focus. 2007;23:E2.

191. Wiemels J, Wrensch M, Claus EB. Epidemiology and etiology of meningioma. J Neurooncol. 2010;99:307–14.

192. Ji J, Sundquist J, Sundquist K. Association of tamoxifen with meningioma: a population-based study in Sweden. Eur J Cancer Prev Off J Eur Cancer Prev Organ ECP. 2016;25(1):29–33.

193. Korhonen K, Raitanen J, Isola J, Haapasalo H, Salminen T, Auvinen A. Exogenous sex hormone use and risk of meningioma: a population-based case-control study in Finland. Cancer Causes Control CCC. 2010;21:2149–56.

194. Michaud DS, Gallo V, Schlehofer B, et al. Reproductive factors and exogenous hormone use in relation to risk of glioma and meningioma in a large European cohort study. Cancer Epidemiol Biomark Prev Publ Am Assoc Cancer Res Cosponsored Am Soc Prev Oncol. 2010;19:2562–9.

195. Cea-Soriano L, Blenk T, Wallander M-A, Rodríguez LAG. Hormonal therapies and meningioma: is there a link? Cancer Epidemiol. 2012;36:198–205.

196. Claus EB, Calvocoressi L, Bondy ML, Schildkraut JM, Wiemels JL, Wrensch M. Family and personal medical history and risk of meningioma. J Neurosurg. 2011;115:1072–7.

197. Klaeboe L, Lonn S, Scheie D, Auvinen A, Christensen HC, Feychting M, Johansen C, Salminen T, Tynes T. Incidence of intracranial meningiomas in Denmark, Finland, Norway and Sweden, 1968–1997. Int J Cancer J Int Cancer. 2005;117:996–1001.

198. Gottfried ON, Gluf W, Quinones-Hinojosa A, Kan P, Schmidt MH. Spinal meningiomas: surgical management and outcome. Neurosurg Focus. 2003;14:e2.

199. Schildkraut JM, Calvocoressi L, Wang F, Wrensch M, Bondy ML, Wiemels JL, Claus EB. Endogenous and exogenous hormone exposure and the risk of meningioma in men. J Neurosurg. 2014;120:820–6.

200. Fakhrjou A, Meshkini A, Shadrvan S. Status of Ki-67, estrogen and progesterone receptors in various subtypes of intracranial meningiomas. Pak J Biol Sci PJBS. 2012;15:530–5.

201. Rao G, Giordano SH, Liu J, McCutcheon IE. The association of breast cancer and meningioma in men and women. Neurosurgery 2009;65:483–489; discussion 489.

202. Lee E, Grutsch J, Persky V, Glick R, Mendes J, Davis F. Association of meningioma with reproductive factors. Int J Cancer J Int Cancer. 2006;119:1152–7.

203. Korhonen K, Auvinen A, Lyytinen H, Ylikorkala O, Pukkala E. A nationwide cohort study on the incidence of meningioma in women using postmenopausal hormone therapy in Finland. Am J Epidemiol. 2012;175:309–14.

204. Claus EB, Calvocoressi L, Bondy ML, Wrensch M, Wiemels JL, Schildkraut JM. Exogenous hormone use, reproductive factors, and risk of intracranial meningioma in females. J Neurosurg. 2013;118:649–56.

205. Custer B, Longstreth WT, Phillips LE, Koepsell TD, Van Belle G. Hormonal exposures and the risk of intracranial meningioma in women: a population-based case-control study. BMC Cancer. 2006;6:152.

206. Hatch EE, Linet MS, Zhang J, Fine HA, Shapiro WR, Selker RG, Black PM, Inskip PD. Reproductive and hormonal factors and risk of brain tumors in adult females. Int J Cancer J Int Cancer. 2005;114:797–805.

207. Wigertz A, Lönn S, Hall P, et al. Reproductive factors and risk of meningioma and glioma. Cancer Epidemiol Biomark Prev Publ Am Assoc Cancer Res Cosponsored Am Soc Prev Oncol. 2008;17:2663–70.

208. Wigertz A, Lönn S, Mathiesen T, Ahlbom A, Hall P, Feychting M. Swedish interphone study Grou. Risk of brain tumors

associated with exposure to exogenous female sex hormones. Am J Epidemiol. 2006;164:629–36.

209. Blitshteyn S, Crook JE, Jaeckle KA. Is there an association between meningioma and hormone replacement therapy? J Clin Oncol. 2008;26:279–82.

210. Andersen L, Friis S, Hallas J, Ravn P, Schrøder HD, Gaist D. Hormone replacement therapy increases the risk of cranial meningioma. Eur J Cancer. 2013;49:3303–10.

211. Custer BS, Koepsell TD, Mueller BA. The association between breast carcinoma and meningioma in women. Cancer. 2002;94:1626–35.

212. Jhawar BS, Fuchs CS, Colditz GA, Stampfer MJ. Sex steroid hormone exposures and risk for meningioma. J Neurosurg. 2003;99:848–53.

213. Benson VS, Pirie K, Green J, Casabonne D, Beral V. Million women study collaborators. Lifestyle factors and primary glioma and meningioma tumours in the Million Women Study cohort. Br J Cancer. 2008;99:185–90.

214. Malmer B, Tavelin B, Henriksson R, Grönberg H. Primary brain tumours as second primary: a novel association between meningioma and colorectal cancer. Int J Cancer J Int Cancer. 2000;85:78–81.

215. Kirsch M, Zhu JJ, Black PM. Analysis of the BRCA1 and BRCA2 genes in sporadic meningiomas. Genes Chromosomes Cancer. 1997;20:53–9.

216. Milano MT, Grossman CE. Meningioma in Breast Cancer Patients: Population-based Analysis of Clinicopathologic Characteristics. Am J Clin Oncol. 2017;40(1):11–6.

217. Criscitiello C, Disalvatore D, Santangelo M, Rotmensz N, Bazolli B, Maisonneuve P, Goldhirsch A, Curigliano G. No link between breast cancer and meningioma: results from a large monoinstitutional retrospective analysis. Cancer Epidemiol Biomark Prev Publ Am Assoc Cancer Res Cosponsored Am Soc Prev Oncol. 2014;23:215–7.

218. Hildebrand J. Neurological complications of cancer chemotherapy. Curr Opin Oncol. 2006;18:321–4.

219. Newton HB. Neurological complications of chemotherapy to the central nervous system. Handb Clin Neurol. 2012;105:903–16.

220. Soffietti R, Trevisan E, Rudà R. Neurologic complications of chemotherapy and other newer and experimental approaches. Handb Clin Neurol. 2014;121:1199–218.

221. Verstappen CCP, Heimans JJ, Hoekman K, Postma TJ. Neurotoxic complications of chemotherapy in patients with cancer: clinical signs and optimal management. Drugs. 2003;63:1549–63.

222. Lyros E, Walter S, Keller I, Papanagiotou P, Fassbender K. Subacute reversible toxic encephalopathy related to treatment with capecitabine: a case report with literature review and discussion of pathophysiology. Neurotoxicology. 2014;42:8–11.

223. Videnovic A, Semenov I, Chua-Adajar R, et al. Capecitabine-induced multifocal leukoencephalopathy: a report of five cases. Neurology 2005;65:1792–1794; discussion 1685.

224. Tipples K, Kolluri RB, Raouf S. Encephalopathy secondary to capecitabine chemotherapy: a case report and discussion. J Oncol Pharm Pract. 2009;15:237–9.

225. Formica V, Leary A, Cunningham D, Chua YJ. 5-Fluorouracil can cross brain-blood barrier and cause encephalopathy: should we expect the same from capecitabine? A case report on capecitabine-induced central neurotoxicity progressing to coma. Cancer Chemother Pharmacol. 2006;58:276–8.

226. Erbetta A, Salmaggi A, Sghirlanzoni A, Silvani A, Potepan P, Botturi A, Ciceri E, Bruzzone MG. Clinical and radiological features of brain neurotoxicity caused by antitumor and immunosuppressant treatments. Neurol Sci. 2008;29:131–7.

227. Cruz-Sanchez FF, Artigas J, Cervos-Navarro J, Rossi ML, Ferszt R. Brain lesions following combined treatment with

methotrexate and craniospinal irradiation. J Neurooncol. 1991;10:165–71.

228. Hinchey J, Chaves C, Appignani B, Breen J, Pao L, Wang A, Pessin MS, Lamy C, Mas JL, Caplan LR. A reversible posterior leukoencephalopathy syndrome. N Engl J Med. 1996;334:494–500.

229. Perry JR, Warner E. Transient encephalopathy after paclitaxel (Taxol) infusion. Neurology. 1996;46:1596–9.

230. Ziske CG, Schöttker B, Gorschlüter M, Mey U, Kleinschmidt R, Schlegel U, Sauerbruch T, Schmidt-Wolf IGH. Acute transient encephalopathy after paclitaxel infusion: report of three cases. Ann Oncol Off J Eur Soc Med Oncol ESMO. 2002;13:629–31.

231. Guglani S, Farrugia D, Elsdon M, Parmar M, Owen JR. Reversible life-threatening encephalopathy in the absence of hepatic failure following conventional doses of docetaxel. Clin Oncol R Coll Radiol G B. 2003;15:160–1.

232. Muallaoğlu S, Koçer M, Güler N. Acute transient encephalopathy after weekly paclitaxel infusion. Med Oncol. 2012;29:1297–9.

233. Baker M, Markman M, Niu J. Pegylated liposomal Doxorubicin-induced acute transient encephalopathy in a patient with breast cancer: a case report. Case Rep Oncol. 2014;7:228–32.

234. Schiff D, Wen PY, van den Bent MJ. Neurological adverse effects caused by cytotoxic and targeted therapies. Nat Rev Clin Oncol. 2009;6:596–603.

235. Tlemsani C, Mir O, Boudou-Rouquette P, Huillard O, Maley K, Ropert S, Coriat R, Goldwasser F. Posterior reversible encephalopathy syndrome induced by anti-VEGF agents. Target Oncol. 2011;6:253–8.

236. Chamberlain MC. Role for cytotoxic chemotherapy in patients with recurrent glioblastoma progressing on bevacizumab: a retrospective case series. Expert Rev Neurother. 2012;12:929–36.

237. Boogerd W, vd Sande JJ, Moffie D. Acute fever and delayed leukoencephalopathy following low dose intraventricular methotrexate. J Neurol Neurosurg Psychiatry 1988;51:1277–1283.

238. Shapiro WR, Chernik NL, Posner JB. Necrotizing encephalopathy following intraventricular instillation of methotrexate. Arch Neurol. 1973;28:96–102.

239. Moore HCF. An overview of chemotherapy-related cognitive dysfunction, or "Chemobrain". Oncol. 2014;28(9):797–804.

240. Tannock IF, Ahles TA, Ganz PA, Van Dam FS. Cognitive impairment associated with chemotherapy for cancer: report of a workshop. J Clin Oncol. 2004;22:2233–9.

241. Vardy J, Wefel JS, Ahles T, Tannock IF, Schagen SB. Cancer and cancer-therapy related cognitive dysfunction: an international perspective from the Venice cognitive workshop. Ann Oncol. 2008;19:623–9.

242. Wefel JS, Vardy J, Ahles T, Schagen SB. International cognition and cancer task force recommendations to harmonise studies of cognitive function in patients with cancer. Lancet Oncol. 2011;12:703–8.

243. Schagen SB, Muller MJ, Boogerd W, Van Dam FSAM. Cognitive dysfunction and chemotherapy: neuropsychological findings in perspective. Clin Breast Cancer. 2002;3(Suppl 3):S100–8.

244. Ahles TA, Root JC, Ryan EL. Cancer- and cancer treatment-associated cognitive change: an update on the state of the science. J Clin Oncol. 2012;30:3675–86.

245. Castellon SA, Ganz PA, Bower JE, Petersen L, Abraham L, Greendale GA. Neurocognitive performance in breast cancer survivors exposed to adjuvant chemotherapy and tamoxifen. J Clin Exp Neuropsychol. 2004;26:955–69.

246. Correa DD, Ahles TA. Neurocognitive changes in cancer survivors. Cancer J Sudbury Mass. 2008;14:396–400.

247. Brezden CB, Phillips KA, Abdolell M, Bunston T, Tannock IF. Cognitive function in breast cancer patients receiving adjuvant chemotherapy. J Clin Oncol. 2000;18:2695–701.

248. Tchen N, Juffs HG, Downie FP, et al. Cognitive function, fatigue, and menopausal symptoms in women receiving adjuvant chemotherapy for breast cancer. J Clin Oncol. 2003;21:4175–83.

249. Janelsins MC, Kohli S, Mohile SG, Usuki K, Ahles TA, Morrow GR. An update on cancer- and chemotherapy-related cognitive dysfunction: current status. Semin Oncol. 2011;38:431–8.

250. Jim HSL, Phillips KM, Chait S, Faul LA, Popa MA, Lee Y-H, Hussin MG, Jacobsen PB, Small BJ. Meta-analysis of cognitive functioning in breast cancer survivors previously treated with standard-dose chemotherapy. J Clin Oncol. 2012;30:3578–87.

251. Ahles TA. Brain vulnerability to chemotherapy toxicities. Psychooncology. 2012;21:1141–8.

252. Collins B, Mackenzie J, Stewart A, Bielajew C, Verma S. Cognitive effects of chemotherapy in post-menopausal breast cancer patients 1 year after treatment. Psychooncology. 2009;18:134–43.

253. Biglia N, Bounous VE, Malabaila A, Palmisano D, Torta DME, Alonzo MD, Sismondi P, Torta R. Objective and self-reported cognitive dysfunction in breast cancer women treated with chemotherapy: a prospective study. Eur J Cancer Care 2012; (Engl) 21:485–492.

254. Quesnel C, Savard J, Ivers H. Cognitive impairments associated with breast cancer treatments: results from a longitudinal study. Breast Cancer Res Treat. 2009;116:113–23.

255. Wefel JS, Lenzi R, Theriault R, Buzdar AU, Cruickshank S, Meyers CA. "Chemobrain" in breast carcinoma? a prologue. Cancer. 2004;101:466–75.

256. Hermelink K, Untch M, Lux MP, Kreienberg R, Beck T, Bauerfeind I, Münzel K. Cognitive function during neoadjuvant chemotherapy for breast cancer: results of a prospective, multicenter, longitudinal study. Cancer. 2007;109:1905–13.

257. Wefel JS, Saleeba AK, Buzdar AU, Meyers CA. Acute and late onset cognitive dysfunction associated with chemotherapy in women with breast cancer. Cancer. 2010;116:3348–56.

258. Taillibert S. Is systemic anti-cancer therapy neurotoxic? Does chemo brain exist? And should we rename it? Adv Exp Med Biol. 2010;678:86–95.

259. Schagen SB, Muller MJ, Boogerd W, Rosenbrand RM, van Rhijn D, Rodenhuis S, van Dam FS a. M. Late effects of adjuvant chemotherapy on cognitive function: a follow-up study in breast cancer patients. Ann Oncol 2002;13:1387–1397.

260. Bender CM. Chemotherapy may have small to moderate negative effects on cognitive functioning. Cancer Treat Rev. 2006;32:316–9.

261. Wefel JS, Kesler SR, Noll KR, Schagen SB. Clinical characteristics, pathophysiology, and management of noncentral nervous system cancer-related cognitive impairment in adults. CA Cancer J Clin. 2015;65:123–38.

262. Bower JE. Behavioral symptoms in patients with breast cancer and survivors. J Clin Oncol. 2008;26:768–77.

263. Meyers CA. Cognitive complaints after breast cancer treatments: patient report and objective evidence. J Natl Cancer Inst. 2013;105:761–2.

264. Reid-Arndt SA, Cox CR. Stress, coping and cognitive deficits in women after surgery for breast cancer. J Clin Psychol Med Settings. 2012;19:127–37.

265. Patel SK, Hurria A, Mandelblatt JS. Chemobrain: is it time to initiate guidelines for assessment and management? Oncol. 2014;28(9):809–10.

266. Ganz PA, Kwan L, Castellon SA, Oppenheim A, Bower JE, Silverman DHS, Cole SW, Irwin MR, Ancoli-Israel S, Belin TR. Cognitive complaints after breast cancer treatments: examining the relationship with neuropsychological test performance. J Natl Cancer Inst. 2013;105:791–801.

267. Shilling V, Jenkins V. Self-reported cognitive problems in women receiving adjuvant therapy for breast cancer. Eur J Oncol. 2007;11:6–15.

268. van Dam FS, Schagen SB, Muller MJ, Boogerd W, vd Wall E, Droogleever Fortuyn ME, Rodenhuis S. Impairment of cognitive function in women receiving adjuvant treatment for high-risk breast cancer: high-dose versus standard-dose chemotherapy. J Natl Cancer Inst 1998;90:210–218.

269. Collins B, MacKenzie J, Tasca GA, Scherling C, Smith A. Cognitive effects of chemotherapy in breast cancer patients: a dose-response study. Psychooncology. 2013;22:1517–27.

270. Wefel JS, Witgert ME, Meyers CA. Neuropsychological sequelae of non-central nervous system cancer and cancer therapy. Neuropsychol Rev. 2008;18:121–31.

271. Wefel JS, Schagen SB. Chemotherapy-related cognitive dysfunction. Curr Neurol Neurosci Rep. 2012;12:267–75.

272. Deprez S, Vandenbulcke M, Peeters R, Emsell L, Smeets A, Christiaens M-R, Amant F, Sunaert S. Longitudinal assessment of chemotherapy-induced alterations in brain activation during multitasking and its relation with cognitive complaints. J Clin Oncol. 2014;32:2031–8.

273. Silverman DHS, Dy CJ, Castellon SA, Lai J, Pio BS, Abraham L, Waddell K, Petersen L, Phelps ME, Ganz PA. Altered fronto-cortical, cerebellar, and basal ganglia activity in adjuvant-treated breast cancer survivors 5–10 years after chemotherapy. Breast Cancer Res Treat. 2007;103:303–11.

274. Barton DL, Burger K, Novotny PJ, et al. The use of Ginkgo biloba for the prevention of chemotherapy-related cognitive dysfunction in women receiving adjuvant treatment for breast cancer, N00C9. Support Care Cancer Off J Multinatl Assoc Support Care Cancer. 2013;21:1185–92.

275. Hötting K, Röder B. Beneficial effects of physical exercise on neuroplasticity and cognition. Neurosci Biobehav Rev. 2013;37:2243–57.

276. Alvarez J, Meyer FL, Granoff DL, Lundy A. The effect of EEG biofeedback on reducing postcancer cognitive impairment. Integr Cancer Ther. 2013;12:475–87.

277. Schilder CM, Seynaeve C, Beex LV, et al. Effects of tamoxifen and exemestane on cognitive functioning of postmenopausal patients with breast cancer: results from the neuropsychological side study of the tamoxifen and exemestane adjuvant multinational trial. J Clin Oncol. 2010;28:1294–300.

278. Bender CM, Sereika SM, Brufsky AM, Ryan CM, Vogel VG, Rastogi P, Cohen SM, Casillo FE, Berga SL. Memory impairments with adjuvant anastrozole versus tamoxifen in women with early-stage breast cancer. Menopause N Y N. 2007;14:995–8.

279. Jenkins V, Shilling V, Fallowfield L, Howell A, Hutton S. Does hormone therapy for the treatment of breast cancer have a detrimental effect on memory and cognition? A pilot study. Psychooncology. 2004;13:61–6.

280. Collins B, Mackenzie J, Stewart A, Bielajew C, Verma S. Cognitive effects of hormonal therapy in early stage breast cancer patients: a prospective study. Psychooncology. 2009;18:811–21.

281. Shilling V, Jenkins V, Fallowfield L, Howell T. The effects of hormone therapy on cognition in breast cancer. J Steroid Biochem Mol Biol. 2003;86:405–12.

282. Jenkins VA, Ambroisine LM, Atkins L, Cuzick J, Howell A, Fallowfield LJ. Effects of anastrozole on cognitive performance in postmenopausal women: a randomised, double-blind chemoprevention trial (IBIS II). Lancet Oncol. 2008;9:953–61.

283. Berga SL. Anastrozole: brain draining or sparing? Lancet Oncol. 2008;9:913–4.

284. Phillips K-A, Ribi K, Sun Z, et al. Cognitive function in postmenopausal women receiving adjuvant letrozole or

tamoxifen for breast cancer in the BIG 1-98 randomized trial. Breast. 2010;19:388–95.

285. Agrawal K, Onami S, Mortimer JE, Pal SK. Cognitive changes associated with endocrine therapy for breast cancer. Maturitas. 2010;67:209–14.

286. Ganz PA, Petersen L, Castellon SA, Bower JE, Silverman DHS, Cole SW, Irwin MR, Belin TR. Cognitive function after the initiation of adjuvant endocrine therapy in early-stage breast cancer: an observational cohort study. J Clin Oncol. 2014;32 (31):3559–67.

287. Jenkins V, Atkins L, Fallowfield L. Does endocrine therapy for the treatment and prevention of breast cancer affect memory and cognition? Eur J Cancer. 2007;43:1342–7.

288. Lejbak L, Vrbancic M, Crossley M. Endocrine therapy is associated with low performance on some estrogen-sensitive cognitive tasks in postmenopausal women with breast cancer. J Clin Exp Neuropsychol. 2010;32:836–46.

289. Le Rhun E, Delbeuck X, Lefeuvre-Plesse C, Kramar A, Skrobala E, Pasquier F, Bonneterre J. A phase III randomized multicenter trial evaluating cognition in post-menopausal breast cancer patients receiving adjuvant hormonotherapy. Breast Cancer Res Treat. 2015;152(3):569–80.

290. Gallagher J, Parle M, Cairns D. Appraisal and psychological distress six months after diagnosis of breast cancer. Br J Health Psychol. 2002;7:365–76.

291. Danhauer SC, Legault C, Bandos H, et al. Positive and negative affect, depression, and cognitive processes in the Cognition in the Study of Tamoxifen and Raloxifene (Co-STAR) Trial. Neuropsychol Dev Cogn B Aging Neuropsychol Cogn. 2013;20:532–52.

292. Paganini-Hill A, Clark LJ. Preliminary assessment of cognitive function in breast cancer patients treated with tamoxifen. Breast Cancer Res Treat. 2000;64:165–76.

293. Bender CM, Pacella ML, Sereika SM, Brufsky AM, Vogel VG, Rastogi P, Casillo FE, Richey SM, Ryan CM. What do perceived cognitive problems reflect? J Support Oncol. 2008;6:238–42.

294. Jenkins V, Shilling V, Deutsch G, et al. A 3-year prospective study of the effects of adjuvant treatments on cognition in women with early stage breast cancer. Br J Cancer. 2006;94:828–34.

295. Graus F, Rogers LR, Posner JB. Cerebrovascular complications in patients with cancer. Medicine (Baltimore). 1985;64:16–35.

296. Saphner T, Tormey DC, Gray R. Venous and arterial thrombosis in patients who received adjuvant therapy for breast cancer. J Clin Oncol. 1991;9:286–94.

297. Lee AYY, Levine MN, Baker RI, et al. Low-molecular-weight heparin versus a coumarin for the prevention of recurrent venous thromboembolism in patients with cancer. N Engl J Med. 2003;349:146–53.

298. Sanossian N, Djabiras C, Mack WJ, Ovbiagele B. Trends in cancer diagnoses among inpatients hospitalized with stroke. J Stroke Cerebrovasc Dis. 2013;22:1146–50.

299. Selvik HA, Thomassen L, Logallo N, Næss H. Prior cancer in patients with ischemic stroke: the Bergen NORSTROKE study. J Stroke Cerebrovasc Dis. 2014;23:919–25.

300. Navi BB, Singer S, Merkler AE, Cheng NT, Stone JB, Kamel H, Iadecola C, Elkind MSV, DeAngelis LM. Cryptogenic subtype predicts reduced survival among cancer patients with ischemic stroke. Stroke J Cereb Circ. 2014;45:2292–7.

301. Nilsson G, Holmberg L, Garmo H, Terent A, Blomqvist C. Increased incidence of stroke in women with breast cancer. Eur J Cancer. 2005;41:423–9.

302. Grisold W, Oberndorfer S, Struhal W. Stroke and cancer: a review. Acta Neurol Scand. 2009;119:1–16.

303. Navi BB, Reiner AS, Kamel H, Iadecola C, Elkind MSV, Panageas KS, DeAngelis LM. Association between incident cancer and subsequent stroke. Ann Neurol. 2015;77:291–300.

304. Hooning MJ, Dorresteijn LDA, Aleman BMP, Kappelle AC, Klijn JGM, Boogerd W, van Leeuwen FE. Decreased risk of stroke among 10-year survivors of breast cancer. J Clin Oncol. 2006;24:5388–94.

305. Woodward WA, Giordano SH, Duan Z, Hortobagyi GN, Buchholz TA. Supraclavicular radiation for breast cancer does not increase the 10-year risk of stroke. Cancer. 2006;106:2556–62.

306. Nilsson G, Holmberg L, Garmo H, Terent A, Blomqvist C. Radiation to supraclavicular and internal mammary lymph nodes in breast cancer increases the risk of stroke. Br J Cancer. 2009;100:811–6.

307. Masrur S, Abdullah AR, Smith EE, Hidalgo R, El-Ghandour A, Rordorf G, Schwamm LH. Risk of thrombolytic therapy for acute ischemic stroke in patients with current malignancy. J Stroke Cerebrovasc Dis. 2011;20:124–30.

308. Mandalà M, Falanga A, Roila F, ESMO guidelines working group. Management of venous thromboembolism (VTE) in cancer patients: ESMO clinical practice guidelines. Ann Oncol. 2011; 22 Suppl 6:vi85–92.

309. Hisada Y, Geddings JE, Ay C, Mackman N. Venous thrombosis and cancer: from mouse models to clinical trials. J Thromb Haemost JTH. 2015;13(8):1372–82.

310. Petterson TM, Marks RS, Ashrani AA, Bailey KR, Heit JA. Risk of site-specific cancer in incident venous thromboembolism: a population-based study. Thromb Res. 2015;135:472–8.

311. Falanga A, Zacharski L. Deep vein thrombosis in cancer: the scale of the problem and approaches to management. Ann Oncol. 2005;16:696–701.

312. Khorana AA, Kuderer NM, Culakova E, Lyman GH, Francis CW. Development and validation of a predictive model for chemotherapy-associated thrombosis. Blood. 2008;111:4902–7.

313. Rogers LR. Cerebrovascular complications in patients with cancer. Semin Neurol. 2010;30:311–9.

314. Bushnell C. The cerebrovascular risks associated with tamoxifen use. Expert Opin Drug Saf. 2005;4:501–7.

315. Kim Y, Kim OJ, Kim J. Cerebral venous thrombosis in a breast cancer patient taking tamoxifen: Report of a case. Int J Surg Case Rep. 2015;6C:77–80.

316. Ferro JM, Canhão P, Stam J, Bousser M-G, Barinagarrementeria F, ISCVT Investigators. Prognosis of cerebral vein and dural sinus thrombosis: results of the International study on cerebral vein and dural sinus thrombosis (ISCVT). Stroke J Cereb Circ 2004;35:664–6.

317. Rogers LR. Cerebrovascular complications in patients with cancer. Semin Neurol. 2004;24:453–46070.

318. Raizer JJ, DeAngelis LM. Cerebral sinus thrombosis diagnosed by MRI and MR venography in cancer patients. Neurology. 2000;54:1222–6.

319. Strowd RE, Knovich MA, Lesser GJ. The therapeutic management of bleeding and thrombotic disorders complicating CNS malignancies. Curr Treat Options Oncol. 2012;13:451–64.

320. Chamberlain MC. Neurotoxicity of intra-CSF liposomal cytarabine (DepoCyt) administered for the treatment of leptomeningeal metastases: a retrospective case series. J Neurooncol. 2012;109:143–8.

321. Glantz MJ, Van Horn A, Fisher R, Chamberlain MC. Route of intracerebrospinal fluid chemotherapy administration and efficacy of therapy in neoplastic meningitis. Cancer. 2010;116:1947–52.

322. Shapiro WR, Young DF, Mehta BM. Methotrexate: distribution in cerebrospinal fluid after intravenous, ventricular and lumbar injections. N Engl J Med. 1975;293:161–6.

323. Zairi F, Le Rhun E, Bertrand N, Boulanger T, Taillibert S, Aboukais R, Assaker R, Chamberlain MC. Complications related to the use of an intraventricular access device for the treatment of leptomeningeal metastases from solid tumor: a single centre experience in 112 patients. J Neurooncol. 2015;124(2):317–23.

324. Mead PA, Safdieh JE, Nizza P, Tuma S, Sepkowitz KA. Ommaya reservoir infections: a 16-year retrospective analysis. J Infect. 2014;68:225–30.

325. Szvalb AD, Raad II, Weinberg JS, Suki D, Mayer R, Viola GM. Ommaya reservoir-related infections: clinical manifestations and treatment outcomes. J Infect. 2014;68:216–24.

326. Lishner M, Scheinbaum R, Messner HA. Intrathecal vancomycin in the treatment of Ommaya reservoir infection by Staphylococcus epidermidis. Scand J Infect Dis. 1991;23:101–4.

327. Siegal T, Pfeffer MR, Steiner I. Antibiotic therapy for infected Ommaya reservoir systems. Neurosurgery. 1988;22:97–100.

328. Rollins N, Winick N, Bash R, Booth T. Acute methotrexate neurotoxicity: findings on diffusion-weighted imaging and correlation with clinical outcome. AJNR Am J Neuroradiol. 2004;25:1688–95.

329. Andersen KG, Aasvang EK, Kroman N, Kehlet H. Intercostobrachial nerve handling and pain after axillary lymph node dissection for breast cancer. Acta Anaesthesiol Scand. 2014;58:1240–8.

330. Wilson GC, Quillin RC, Hanseman DJ, Lewis JD, Edwards MJ, Shaughnessy EA. Incidence and predictors of neuropathic pain following breast surgery. Ann Surg Oncol. 2013;20:3330–4.

331. Alves Nogueira Fabro E, Bergmann A, do Amaral E Silva B, Padula Ribeiro AC, de Souza Abrahão K, da Costa Leite Ferreira MG, de Almeida Dias R, Santos Thuler LC. Post-mastectomy pain syndrome: incidence and risks. Breast. 2012;21:321–325.

332. Lucci A, McCall LM, Beitsch PD, et al. Surgical complications associated with sentinel lymph node dissection (SLND) plus axillary lymph node dissection compared with SLND alone in the American College of Surgeons Oncology Group Trial Z0011. J Clin Oncol. 2007;25:3657–63.

333. Helms G, Kühn T, Moser L, Remmel E, Kreienberg R. Shoulder-arm morbidity in patients with sentinel node biopsy and complete axillary dissection–data from a prospective randomised trial. Eur J Surg Oncol J Eur Soc Surg Oncol Br Assoc Surg Oncol. 2009;35:696–701.

334. Ashikaga T, Krag DN, Land SR, et al. Morbidity results from the NSABP B-32 trial comparing sentinel lymph node dissection versus axillary dissection. J Surg Oncol. 2010;102:111–8.

335. Lundstedt D, Gustafsson M, Steineck G, Alsadius D, Sundberg A, Wilderäng U, Holmberg E, Johansson K-A, Karlsson P. Long-term symptoms after radiotherapy of supraclavicular lymph nodes in breast cancer patients. Radiother Oncol J Eur Soc Ther Radiol Oncol. 2012;103:155–60.

336. Pradat P-F, Maisonobe T, Psimaras D, Lenglet T, Porcher R, Lefaix J-L, Delanian S. Radiation-induced neuropathies: collateral damage of improved cancer prognosis. Rev Neurol (Paris). 2012;168:939–50.

337. Delanian S, Lefaix J-L, Pradat P-F. Radiation-induced neuropathy in cancer survivors. Radiother Oncol J Eur Soc Ther Radiol Oncol. 2012;105:273–82.

338. Senkus-Konefka E, Jassem J. Complications of breast-cancer radiotherapy. Clin Oncol R Coll Radiol G B. 2006;18:229–35.

339. Fathers E, Thrush D, Huson SM, Norman A. Radiation-induced brachial plexopathy in women treated for carcinoma of the breast. Clin Rehabil. 2002;16:160–5.

340. Gałecki J, Hicer-Grzenkowicz J, Grudzień-Kowalska M, Michalska T, Załucki W. Radiation-induced brachial plexopathy and hypofractionated regimens in adjuvant irradiation of patients with breast cancer–a review. Acta Oncol Stockh Swed. 2006;45:280–4.

341. Pradat PF, Poisson M, Delattre JY. Radiation-induced neuropathies. Experimental and clinical data. Rev Neurol (Paris). 1994;150:664–77.

342. Pradat P-F, Delanian S. Late radiation injury to peripheral nerves. Handb Clin Neurol. 2013;115:743–58.

343. Wong M, Tang ALY, Umapathi T. Partial ulnar nerve transfer to the nerve to the biceps for the treatment of brachial plexopathy in metastatic breast carcinoma: case report. J Hand Surg. 2009;34:79–82.

344. Tung TH, Liu DZ, Mackinnon SE. Nerve transfer for elbow flexion in radiation-induced brachial plexopathy: a case report. Hand N Y N. 2009;4:123–8.

345. Gangurde BA, Doi K, Hattori Y, Sakamoto S. Free functioning muscle transfer in radiation-induced brachial plexopathy: case report. J Hand Surg. 2014;39:1967–70.

346. Lu L, Gong X, Liu Z, Wang D, Zhang Z. Diagnosis and operative treatment of radiation-induced brachial plexopathy. Chin J Traumatol Zhonghua Chuang Shang Za Zhi Chin Med Assoc. 2002;5:329–32.

347. Masci G, Magagnoli M, Gullo G, Morenghi E, Garassino I, Simonelli M, Santoro A. Herpes infections in breast cancer patients treated with adjuvant chemotherapy. Oncology. 2006;71:164–7.

348. Beijers AJM, Jongen JLM, Vreugdenhil G. Chemotherapy-induced neurotoxicity: the value of neuroprotective strategies. Neth J Med. 2012;70:18–25.

349. Park SB, Goldstein D, Krishnan AV, Lin CS-Y, Friedlander ML, Cassidy J, Koltzenburg M, Kiernan MC. Chemotherapy-induced peripheral neurotoxicity: a critical analysis. CA Cancer J Clin 2013;63:419–437.

350. Rivera E, Cianfrocca M. Overview of neuropathy associated with taxanes for the treatment of metastatic breast cancer. Cancer Chemother Pharmacol. 2015;75:659–70.

351. Bhatnagar B, Gilmore S, Goloubeva O, Pelser C, Medeiros M, Chumsri S, Tkaczuk K, Edelman M, Bao T. Chemotherapy dose reduction due to chemotherapy induced peripheral neuropathy in breast cancer patients receiving chemotherapy in the neoadjuvant or adjuvant settings: a single-center experience. SpringerPlus. 2014;3:366.

352. Schneider BP, Zhao F, Wang M, et al. Neuropathy is not associated with clinical outcomes in patients receiving adjuvant taxane-containing therapy for operable breast cancer. J Clin Oncol. 2012;30:3051–7.

353. la Morena Barrio P de, Conesa MÁV, González-Billalabeitia E, Urrego E, García-Garre E, García-Martínez E, Poves MZ, Vicente V, la Peña FA de. Delayed recovery and increased severity of Paclitaxel-induced peripheral neuropathy in patients with diabetes. J Natl Compr Cancer Netw JNCCN 2015;13:417–423.

354. Eckhoff L, Knoop AS, Jensen M-B, Ejlertsen B, Ewertz M. Risk of docetaxel-induced peripheral neuropathy among 1,725 Danish patients with early stage breast cancer. Breast Cancer Res Treat. 2013;142:109–18.

355. Postma TJ, Reijneveld JC, Heimans JJ. Prevention of chemotherapy-induced peripheral neuropathy: a matter of personalized treatment? Ann Oncol. 2013;24:1424–6.

356. Hertz DL, Roy S, Jack J, Motsinger-Reif AA, Drobish A, Clark LS, Carey LA, Dees EC, McLeod HL. Genetic heterogeneity beyond CYP2C8*3 does not explain differential sensitivity to paclitaxel-induced neuropathy. Breast Cancer Res Treat. 2014;145:245–54.

357. Leandro-García LJ, Leskelä S, Jara C, et al. Regulatory polymorphisms in β-tubulin IIa are associated with paclitaxel-induced peripheral neuropathy. Clin Cancer Res. 2012;18:4441–8.

358. Eckhoff L, Feddersen S, Knoop AS, Ewertz M, Bergmann TK. Docetaxel-induced neuropathy: a pharmacogenetic case-control

study of 150 women with early-stage breast cancer. Acta Oncol Stockh Swed. 2015;54:530–7.

359. Osmani K, Vignes S, Aissi M, Wade F, Milani P, Lévy BI, Kubis N. Taxane-induced peripheral neuropathy has good long-term prognosis: a 1- to 13-year evaluation. J Neurol. 2012;259:1936–43.

360. Harvey V, Mouridsen H, Semiglazov V, Jakobsen E, Voznyi E, Robinson BA, Groult V, Murawsky M, Cold S. Phase III trial comparing three doses of docetaxel for second-line treatment of advanced breast cancer. J Clin Oncol. 2006;24:4963–70.

361. Bakitas MA. Background noise: the experience of chemotherapy-induced peripheral neuropathy. Nurs Res. 2007;56:323–31.

362. Winer EP, Berry DA, Woolf S, et al. Failure of higher-dose paclitaxel to improve outcome in patients with metastatic breast cancer: cancer and leukemia group B trial 9342. J Clin Oncol. 2004;22:2061–8.

363. Speck RM, Sammel MD, Farrar JT, Hennessy S, Mao JJ, Stineman MG, DeMichele A. Impact of chemotherapy-induced peripheral neuropathy on treatment delivery in nonmetastatic breast cancer. J Oncol Pract. 2013;9:e234–40.

364. Tanabe Y, Hashimoto K, Shimizu C, et al. Paclitaxel-induced peripheral neuropathy in patients receiving adjuvant chemotherapy for breast cancer. Int J Clin Oncol. 2013;18:132–8.

365. Hershman DL, Weimer LH, Wang A, Kranwinkel G, Brafman L, Fuentes D, Awad D, Crew KD. Association between patient reported outcomes and quantitative sensory tests for measuring long-term neurotoxicity in breast cancer survivors treated with adjuvant paclitaxel chemotherapy. Breast Cancer Res Treat. 2011;125:767–74.

366. Moloney TP, Xu W, Rallah-Baker K, Oliveira N, Woodward N, Farrah JJ. Toxic optic neuropathy in the setting of docetaxel chemotherapy: a case report. BMC Ophthalmol. 2014;14:18.

367. Rowinsky EK, Eisenhauer EA, Chaudhry V, Arbuck SG, Donehower RC. Clinical toxicities encountered with paclitaxel (Taxol). Semin Oncol. 1993;20:1–15.

368. Argyriou AA, Koltzenburg M, Polychronopoulos P, Papapetropoulos S, Kalofonos HP. Peripheral nerve damage associated with administration of taxanes in patients with cancer. Crit Rev Oncol Hematol. 2008;66:218–28.

369. Pace A, Nisticò C, Cuppone F, et al. Peripheral neurotoxicity of weekly paclitaxel chemotherapy: a schedule or a dose issue? Clin Breast Cancer. 2007;7:550–4.

370. Eckhoff L, Knoop A, Jensen MB, Ewertz M. Persistence of docetaxel-induced neuropathy and impact on quality of life among breast cancer survivors. Eur J Cancer. 2015;1990 (51):292–300.

371. Jones SE, Erban J, Overmoyer B, et al. Randomized phase III study of docetaxel compared with paclitaxel in metastatic breast cancer. J Clin Oncol. 2005;23:5542–51.

372. Rivera E, Mejia JA, Arun BK, et al. Phase 3 study comparing the use of docetaxel on an every-3-week versus weekly schedule in the treatment of metastatic breast cancer. Cancer. 2008;112:1455–61.

373. Gradishar WJ. Taxanes for the treatment of metastatic breast cancer. Breast Cancer Basic Clin Res. 2012;6:159–71.

374. LaPointe NE, Morfini G, Brady ST, Feinstein SC, Wilson L, Jordan MA. Effects of eribulin, vincristine, paclitaxel and ixabepilone on fast axonal transport and kinesin-1 driven microtubule gliding: implications for chemotherapy-induced peripheral neuropathy. Neurotoxicology. 2013;37:231–9.

375. Cortes J, O'Shaughnessy J, Loesch D, et al. Eribulin monotherapy versus treatment of physician's choice in patients with metastatic breast cancer (EMBRACE): a phase 3 open-label randomised study. Lancet Lond Engl. 2011;377:914–23.

376. Wilks S, Puhalla S, O'Shaughnessy J, Schwartzberg L, Berrak E, Song J, Cox D, Vahdat L. Phase 2, multicenter, single-arm study of eribulin mesylate with trastuzumab as first-line therapy for locally recurrent or metastatic HER2-positive breast cancer. Clin Breast Cancer. 2014;14:405–12.

377. Cortes J, Montero AJ, Glück S. Eribulin mesylate, a novel microtubule inhibitor in the treatment of breast cancer. Cancer Treat Rev. 2012;38:143–51.

378. Vahdat LT, Garcia AA, Vogel C, Pellegrino C, Lindquist DL, Iannotti N, Gopalakrishna P, Sparano JA. Eribulin mesylate versus ixabepilone in patients with metastatic breast cancer: a randomized Phase II study comparing the incidence of peripheral neuropathy. Breast Cancer Res Treat. 2013;140:341–51.

379. de Castria TB, da Silva EMK, Gois AFT, Riera R. Cisplatin versus carboplatin in combination with third-generation drugs for advanced non-small cell lung cancer. Cochrane Database Syst Rev 2013;8:CD009256.

380. Avan A, Postma TJ, Ceresa C, Avan A, Cavaletti G, Giovannetti E, Peters GJ. Platinum-induced neurotoxicity and preventive strategies: past, present, and future. Oncologist. 2015;20:411–32.

381. Galano G, Caputo M, Tecce MF, Capasso A. Efficacy and tolerability of vinorelbine in the cancer therapy. Curr Drug Saf. 2011;6:185–93.

382. Bertolini P, Lassalle M, Mercier G, Raquin MA, Izzi G, Corradini N, Hartmann O. Platinum compound-related ototoxicity in children: long-term follow-up reveals continuous worsening of hearing loss. J Pediatr Hematol Oncol. 2004;26:649–55.

383. McHaney VA, Thibadoux G, Hayes FA, Green AA. Hearing loss in children receiving cisplatin chemotherapy. J Pediatr. 1983;102:314–7.

384. Brydøy M, Oldenburg J, Klepp O, Bremnes RM, Wist EA, Wentzel-Larsen T, Hauge ER, Dahl O, Fosså SD. Observational study of prevalence of long-term Raynaud-like phenomena and neurological side effects in testicular cancer survivors. J Natl Cancer Inst. 2009;101:1682–95.

385. Oldenburg J, Fosså SD, Dahl AA. Scale for chemotherapy-induced long-term neurotoxicity (SCIN): psychometrics, validation, and findings in a large sample of testicular cancer survivors. Qual Life Res Int J Qual Life Asp Treat Care Rehabil. 2006;15:791–800.

386. Makino H. Treatment and care of neurotoxicity from taxane anticancer agents. Breast Cancer Tokyo Jpn. 2004;11:100–4.

387. Vignes S, Lebrun-Vignes B. Sclerodermiform aspect of arm lymphoedema after treatment with docetaxel for breast cancer. J Eur Acad Dermatol Venereol JEADV. 2007;21:1131–3.

388. Martin E, Morel V, Joly D, Villatte C, Delage N, Dubray C, Pereira B, Pickering G. Rationale and design of a randomized double-blind clinical trial in breast cancer: dextromethorphan in chemotherapy-induced peripheral neuropathy. Contemp Clin Trials. 2015;41:146–51.

389. Smith EML, Pang H, Cirrincione C, et al. Effect of duloxetine on pain, function, and quality of life among patients with chemotherapy-induced painful peripheral neuropathy: a randomized clinical trial. JAMA. 2013;309:1359–67.

390. Hirayama Y, Ishitani K, Sato Y, et al. Effect of duloxetine in Japanese patients with chemotherapy-induced peripheral neuropathy: a pilot randomized trial. Int J Clin Oncol. 2015;20(5):866–71.

391. Hershman DL, Unger JM, Crew KD, et al. Randomized double-blind placebo-controlled trial of acetyl-L-carnitine for the prevention of taxane-induced neuropathy in women undergoing adjuvant breast cancer therapy. J Clin Oncol. 2013;31:2627–33.

392. Khandelwal AR, Takalkar AM, Lilien DL, Ravi A. Skeletal muscle metastases on FDG PET/CT imaging. Clin Nucl Med. 2012;37:575–9.

393. Rajabally YA, Qaddoura B, Abbott RJ. Steroid-responsive para-neoplastic demyelinating neuropathy and myelopathy associated with breast carcinoma. J Clin Neuromuscul Dis. 2008;10:65–9.

394. Silvestre J, Santos L, Batalha V, et al. Paraneoplastic necrotizing myopathy in a woman with breast cancer: a case report. J Med Case Reports. 2009;3:95.

395. Batchelor TT, Taylor LP, Thaler HT, Posner JB, DeAngelis LM. Steroid myopathy in cancer patients. Neurology. 1997;48:1234–8.

396. van Balkom RH, van der Heijden HF, van Herwaarden CL, Dekhuijzen PN. Corticosteroid-induced myopathy of the respiratory muscles. Neth J Med. 1994;45:114–22.

397. Da Silva JAP, Jacobs JWG, Kirwan JR, et al. Safety of low dose glucocorticoid treatment in rheumatoid arthritis: published evidence and prospective trial data. Ann Rheum Dis 2006;65:285–293.

398. Ghosh PS, Milone M. Clinical and laboratory findings of 21 patients with radiation-induced myopathy. J Neurol Neurosurg Psychiatry. 2015;86:152–8.

399. Dawood S, Lei X, Litton JK, Buchholz TA, Hortobagyi GN, Gonzalez-Angulo AM. Incidence of brain metastases as a first site of recurrence among women with triple receptor-negative breast cancer. Cancer. 2012;118:4652–9.

400. Boldt HC, Nerad JA. Orbital metastases from prostate carcinoma. Arch Ophthalmol Chic Ill. 1988;106:1403–8.

401. Johnston JL. Parasellar syndromes. Curr Neurol Neurosci Rep. 2002;2:423–31.

402. Niemann B, Rochlitz C, Herrmann R, Pless M. Toxic encephalopathy induced by capecitabine. Oncology. 2004;66:331–5.

403. Couch LSB, Groteluschen DL, Stewart JA, Mulkerin DL. Capecitabine-related neurotoxicity presenting as trismus. Clin Colorectal Cancer. 2003;3:121–3.

404. Fantini M, Gianni L, Tassinari D, Nicoletti S, Possenti C, Drudi F, Sintini M, Bagli L, Tamburini E. Ravaioli Toxic encephalopathy in elderly patients during treatment with capecitabine: literature review and a case report. J Oncol Pharm Pract. 2011;17:288–91.

Neurologic Complications of Gastrointestinal Cancer

Rajiv Magge and Eli L. Diamond

Introduction

Malignancies of the gastrointestinal (GI) tract are some of the most commonly presenting tumors in the USA. There were an estimated 291,150 new cases and 149,300 deaths from GI cancers in 2015 [1]. The most frequently occurring GI malignancy is colorectal cancer, which comprises 8% of all new cancer diagnoses and is the third most common malignancy in men and women.

Generally, staging takes into account the depth of invasion of the primary tumor into the wall of the viscus, the number and location of involved lymph nodes, and whether or not there are metastatic sites of disease. Treatment strategies usually favor surgical resection, when possible, followed by adjuvant chemotherapy or combined chemoradiation therapy to prevent local or distant recurrence. Neoadjuvant strategies using chemotherapy or chemoradiation therapy before surgery are sometimes necessary, especially for tumors of the pancreas, esophagus, and rectum.

Neurologic complications from GI malignancies may be direct [i.e., brain metastases (BM)] or indirect (i.e., complications related to chemotherapy). They are varied but the incidence is far less than with some other solid tumors such as breast or lung cancer. For example, gastrointestinal metastases to the central nervous system (CNS) account for approximately 4–6% of solid tumor metastatic brain lesions [2]. However, with improved therapies and survivorship, the incidence of metastatic CNS disease from GI malignancies may increase due to poor CNS penetration of most agents used for these tumors. As a rule, CNS disease is usually associated with more extensive systemic disease, especially liver and lung metastases. Intracranial metastases from gastrointestinal malignancies do not present differently from other solid tumors. CNS invasion is thought to be hematogenous via the arterial circulation or Batson's plexus, but is rarely caused by direct extension from skull or dural metastases.

We review some of the direct and indirect neurologic complications of GI malignancies. These are rare complications but need to be considered by physicians treating such patients. Symptoms from BM are based on the location of the tumor and are attributable to multiple mechanisms, including direct displacement or irritation of brain tissue, vasogenic edema, and disruption of nearby venous and arterial blood flow. The most common presenting symptoms are focal weakness, impaired cognition, and headache with or without nausea and vomiting. Imaging with contrast MRI or CT scans will identify lesions and associated edema; MRI is the modality of choice for optimal resolution of the nervous system, especially the posterior fossa.

Acute medical treatment should include corticosteroid therapy such as dexamethasone and anti-seizure medications if the patient presents or develops generalized or partial seizures. More definitive therapy is the same as for other solid tumor metastases to the brain. Patients with a solitary lesion benefit from surgical resection potentially followed by radiation therapy; patients with >4 BM in most cases should receive WBRT. Chemotherapy may be attempted for patients who fail surgery and radiation, but data on effective therapies using this approach are scarce.

Metastatic lesions to the spine, leptomeninges, and dura are rare in gastrointestinal disease and again not treated differently from other solid tumor metastases. Symptoms at presentation may sometimes be different than symptoms from brain lesions. For example, patients with epidural spinal cord compression present with focal back pain and may have weakness, sensory changes, or autonomic dysfunction such as urinary retention.

R. Magge
Weill Cornell Medicine/New York Presbyterian, Weill Cornell Brain Tumor Center, 1305 York Avenue Box 80,
New York, NY 10021, USA
e-mail: ram9116@med.cornell.edurmagge@gmail.com

E.L. Diamond (✉)
Department of Neurology, Memorial Sloan Kettering Cancer Center, 160 E. 53rd St. Second Floor Neurology, New York, NY 10022, USA
e-mail: diamone1@mskcc.org

© Springer International Publishing AG 2018
D. Schiff et al. (eds.), *Cancer Neurology in Clinical Practice*,
DOI 10.1007/978-3-319-57901-6_24

Management of these lesions from GI malignancies is not unique. In the acute setting, corticosteroids (high or low dose depending on clinical picture) should be used when the spinal cord is compromised and/or there is neurologic dysfunction or significant back pain. Treatment is radiation therapy in most cases, but surgery may be of benefit as many of the GI malignancies are radioresistant. Surgery may also be used for cases with mechanical instability, bone fragments in the spinal canal, or radiation failures.

Treatment of leptomeningeal metastases (LM) is limited to either intrathecal (IT) or systemically administered agents. The available IT agents have limited to no activity against GI malignancies, and systemically administered agents have either poor CNS penetration or limited to no activity, hence the poor outcomes for these patients. Radiation should be used to treat symptomatic sites for palliation. Dural lesions can be treated with surgery and/or radiation.

Colorectal Cancer

Colorectal cancer (CRC) is the third most common cancer and cause of cancer death in the USA [1]. About 132,700 new cases of colon cancer are estimated to be diagnosed each year, including about 93,090 colon and 39,610 rectal malignancies. More than 49,700 patients are estimated to die each year from CRC. Fortunately, both incidence and mortality have continued to decline since 1990, probably related to improved screening and treatment [3].

Several genetic disorders carry a high risk of developing colon cancer. Familial adenomatous polyposis (FAP) and Lynch Syndrome (hereditary nonpolyposis colorectal cancer (HNPCC)) account for about 5% of CRC patients [4–6]. FAP is caused by a germline mutation at the APC gene on chromosome 5 and typically presents as several colonic adenomas during childhood. Extracolonic manifestations associated with FAP include gastric/duodenal polyps, congenital hypertrophy of the retinal pigment epithelium (CHRPE), follicular or papillary thyroid, and childhood hepatoblastoma. Lynch syndrome (HNPCC) is autosomal dominant and involves defects in one of the mismatch repair genes. In addition to predominantly right-sided colorectal tumors, patients with Lynch syndrome carry increased risk for development of extracolonic tumors including endometrial, ovarian, and small bowel tumors. Turcot syndrome originally referred to the association of familial CRC with brain tumors. Both of these familial syndromes are associated with brain tumors—FAP-associated brain tumors are usually medulloblastomas, while gliomas are typically seen with Lynch syndrome [7–9]. More common risk factors for developing CRC include age, personal or family history of sporadic colorectal cancer, and inflammatory bowel disease,

as well as modifiable factors such as obesity and lack of physical activity [10].

CRC is typically diagnosed after patients present with symptoms such as occult bleeding (potentially with iron deficiency anemia), hematochezia, abdominal pain, rectal pain, weight loss, constipation, and diarrhea [11]. Patients may also present emergently with intestinal obstruction or peritonitis. Colonoscopy is the gold standard for diagnosis of CRC in the setting of suggestive symptoms.

Surgery is the only curative option for localized colorectal cancer. Chemotherapy can improve outcomes for locally advanced disease. Regimens for advanced stage CRC classically include 5-fluorouracil (5-FU), oxaliplatin, and irinotecan, but modern treatment courses have added agents such as bevacizumab, cetuximab, or panitumumab.

Brain Metastases

Metastatic disease to the brain from CRC is generally rare, especially compared to lung cancer, breast cancer, and melanoma. The incidence of brain metastases among patients with CRC has by and large ranged from 1 to 4% in prior studies [12–18]. This is much lower than more common sites of metastasis such as liver (20–30%) and lung (10–20%) [19]. Autopsy studies have shown that an additional 2–3% of patients have brain metastases at death [20]. Asian countries may have a lower incidence of colorectal brain metastasis. Brain metastases were only identified in 27/4378 (0.67%) of CRC patients diagnosed between 1995 and 2003 in Singapore, a country with one of the highest rates of CRC in the world [20, 21]. Similarly, Ko and colleagues reported brain metastases in 53/7153 CRC patients (0.74%) in their Taiwan study [17].

Patients with CRC brain metastases typically have systemic metastatic disease [22]. These seem to frequently be found concurrently with metastases to the lung (55–85%) and liver (up to 75%) [15, 20, 23]. The distal colon (sigmoid, rectosigmoid junction, and rectum) is the primary tumor site in up to 60% of patients with brain metastases [18–20, 24]. In a review of 1620 CRC patients (39 with confirmed brain metastasis), Mongan et al. [15] identified primary tumor in the left colon, long-standing pulmonary metastasis (especially with recent progression), and CXCR4 expression by tumor cells as risk factors for developing brain lesions. These tend to have a characteristic location—studies have noted cerebellar lesions in 33–55% of patients with brain metastases [16, 19].

The interval between primary diagnosis of CRC and discovery of brain metastasis likely correlates with survival [18]. This time interval appears to be longer for CRC (22.6–27.6 months) than other GI cancers and lung cancer (but shorter than breast) [20, 21, 24]. A study by Hammoud et al. [18] found the brain disease free interval (bDFI) to be longer in patients who received radiation (49 months) or chemotherapy (27 months) for extracerebral metastatic disease, compared to those who received no treatment (13 months).

As with brain metastases from other primary tumors, survival is dismal without treatment (4–6 weeks) [25]. Surgical resection, if possible, remains the best initial treatment option—Farnell and colleagues reported a median survival of 45 weeks with surgical resection alone. Although still unclear, there is suspicion that CRC brain metastases are relatively radioresistant [18, 19]. In the study by Farnell and colleagues, WBRT did not improve survival or recurrence in a statistically significant way. Radiosurgery has been found to be effective in achieving local control in retrospective studies of CRC and mixed GI cancers, including patients having undergone prior WBRT [26, 27]. In addition to the historical 5-FU-based regimens, patients with metastatic CRC often receive bevacizumab. Although it has known activity in the brain, data are still limited as to whether it is helpful with brain metastases. CEA does not appear to be helpful in predicting survival [15].

Leptomeningeal Metastases

Leptomeningeal metastasis from colorectal cancer is rare with an incidence likely under 1% [28]. Giglio and coworkers examined 5 patients with leptomeningeal disease with median survival of 5 weeks after diagnosis (range 0–14 weeks). Additional individual cases have been reported [29–31]. Treatment is palliative as outlined above.

Epidural Spinal Cord Compression (SCC)

As with brain metastases, intramedullary spinal cord metastases are uncommon with colorectal cancer. Unlike in other primary tumors, there is also decreased affinity for bone. In one review of patients with ESCC by Gilbert and coworkers, only 9 of 235 patients had a primary GI malignancy [32]. Brown and coworkers examined 34 patients with CRC and ESCC who subsequently received RT. The most common presenting symptoms were back pain (97%), weakness, sensory loss, and radiculopathy [33]. Median overall survival for the entire cohort was 4.1 months, while patients with rectal primary tumors had better survival (median 7.9 months) compared with those who had colon primary tumors (median 2.7 months). In addition, patients treated with more than 3000 cGy had a better survival (7 months) than those receiving 3000 cGy or less

(3.1 months). Although most metastases from other primary tumors are located in the thoracic spine, epidural metastases in this cohort were most frequently in the lumbar spine (55% of lesions). Most patients (88%) had systemic metastatic disease when the SCC was diagnosed.

Paraneoplastic Syndromes

Although rare, individual case reports of paraneoplastic neurologic syndromes with colorectal cancer have been reported. One patient with limbic encephalitis and paraneoplastic cerebellar degeneration (PCD) was found to have anti-Hu-like antibody. The encephalitis (but not the PCD) improved after removal of the colonic polyp [34]. Two cases note paraneoplastic retinopathy [35, 36] with colon adenocarcinoma. Paraneoplastic neuropathy has been described in another two patients [37, 38]. Although antibody analysis was negative (including anti-GAD), a clinical diagnosis of stiff person syndrome was made in a colon cancer patient [39]. Lastly, brainstem encephalitis caused by an anti-Ma1 antibody has been reported in CRC patients [28].

Esophageal Cancer (Fig. 24.1a, b)

Esophageal cancer is one of the fastest growing malignancies in the country in terms of incidence, probably related to increasing body mass index and subsequent gastroesophageal reflux disease. Almost 16,980 patients are diagnosed annually in the USA with an expected 15,590 deaths [1]. There are an estimated 482,300 new cases worldwide with the highest rates found in Southern and Eastern Africa as well as Eastern Asia [40]. Most esophageal cancers are squamous cell or adenocarcinoma, with the incidence of the latter originating from Barrett's esophagus rising significantly.

Major risk factors for squamous cell carcinoma include smoking and alcohol consumption, while Barrett's esophagus, gastroesophageal reflux disease, smoking and high body mass index increase the risk of adenocarcinoma [41–43]. Patients usually presented with progressive dysphagia (especially to solid foods) and weight loss. Many patients receive trimodality treatment with chemotherapy (including agents such as carboplatin, paclitaxel and 5-FU), radiation and surgery [44].

Brain Metastases

Brain metastases from esophageal cancer are rare, occurring in 1–5% of cases. Spread to the brain probably occurs via

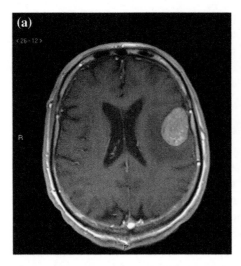

Fig. 24.1 A 73-year-old man with an 18-month history of esophageal adenocarcinoma presented in April 2013 with right hemiparesis. **a** (postcontrast T1 MRI) reveals a mass that preoperatively was felt to represent a dural metastasis. Resection confirmed this diagnosis. He then received fractionated whole brain radiotherapy. Five months later he re-presented with personality changes and weakness. **b** demonstrates a new hemorrhagic parenchymal metastasis that was subsequently resected

Batson's vertebral venous plexus which provides communication between the esophagus and the brain [20, 45]. Weinberg and coworkers identified 27 patients (1.7%) with esophageal cancer brain metastases from 1588 treated at MD Anderson Cancer Center between 1993 and 2001 [46]. Nineteen of these patients (70%) had concurrent systemic metastatic disease and 75% presented with neurologic symptoms. Median survival was 3.8 months. The only risk factor for brain metastasis was increased tumor size in association with local invasion and lymph node metastases. Ogawa and coworkers reported on 36 esophageal cancer patients with brain metastases; only 5 survived more than one year (all treated with both SRS and WBRT), but 80% of these patients had no extracranial metastatic disease, excellent KPS, and solitary brain lesions [45].

A more recent review at MD Anderson Cancer Center by Wadhwa and coworkers identified 20 patients (3.9%) with brain metastasis from a population of 518 with esophageal adenocarcinoma given trimodality treatment (chemoradiation followed by surgery) between 2000 and 2010 [47]. Twelve patients (60%) had solitary metastasis while 8 (40%) had multiple metastases; 16 (80%) had CNS symptoms at diagnosis. Extracranial metastases were documented in 9 patients (45%). Seventeen of the 20 patients received treatment (4 had surgery alone, 8 had surgery followed by WBRT, 3 had WBRT alone, and 2 had SRS); median OS for all patients was 10.5 months. Additional recent clinical reviews of patients with esophageal cancer brain metastases similarly found that the frequency of brain metastases was higher in adenocarcinoma patients compared to those with squamous cell carcinoma histology [48, 49].

Leptomeningeal Metastases

Two case series each identified seven patients with leptomeningeal disease from primary esophageal cancer [50, 51]. There was a predominance of male patients with adenocarcinoma histology. Presenting symptoms included headache, visual changes, vertigo, nausea, and vomiting. Overall survival was poor—0 to 28 weeks in the first series and 2.5–16 weeks in the second.

Paraneoplastic Syndromes

A patient with esophageal squamous cell cancer was reported to have opsoclonus–myoclonus syndrome with symptoms improving after IVIG [52]. Another patient presented with limbic encephalitis and was subsequently diagnosed with esophageal adenocarcinoma [53]. An anti-Hu antibody was identified in a woman with encephalomyelitis and esophageal small cell carcinoma [54]. Two patients with paraneoplastic cerebellar degeneration (PCD) due to anti-Yo antibody have been reported [55, 56]. Lastly, one patient with numbness and fever was found to have vasculitis on muscle biopsy with symptoms resolving after esophagectomy [57].

Gastric Cancer

Approximately 22,220 patients are diagnosed with gastric cancer annually in the USA, with an estimated 10,990 deaths [1]. Worldwide, rates of disease are highest in Eastern Asia,

Eastern Europe, and South America. Gastric ulcers, adenomatous polyps, and intestinal metaplasia are associated with increased risk of gastric cancer [58]. Additional risk factors include *H. pylori* infection, diet (nitroso compounds, high salt diet with low vegetables), smoking, and alcohol use. Gastric cancer is also associated with specific inherited cancer syndromes such as Lynch syndrome (hereditary nonpolyposis colorectal cancer), familial adenomatous polyposis (FAP), and Li–Fraumeni syndrome.

Early gastric cancer often does not have associated symptoms, but advanced disease may cause indigestion, nausea or vomiting, dysphagia, postprandial fullness, loss of appetite, and weight loss. Late complications include peritoneal or pleural effusions, obstructions, bleeding from esophageal varices, and jaundice.

Most gastric malignancies are adenocarcinoma, and diagnosis is usually made by imaging or endoscopy followed by biopsy or resection. Prognosis is good with resection of early gastric cancer. Patients with at least stage IB disease will often require postoperative chemoradiation.

Brain Metastases

Brain metastases from gastric cancer are very rare and have been reported in less than 1% of cases. York and coworkers identified only 24 brain metastasis patients (0.7%) of the 3320 gastric cancer patients treated at MD Anderson Cancer Center 1957–1997 [59]. There was a greater incidence of brain metastases from primary tumors originating in the proximal stomach, and all 24 patients had concurrent systemic metastatic disease (most commonly bone, liver, and lung). Mean interval from gastrectomy to the diagnosis of brain metastasis was 9 months. Median survival was only 2.4 months.

Kasakura et al. [60] reported brain metastasis in only 11 of 2322 (0.47%) of Japanese patients treated between 1980 and 1998. They noted median survival of 24 weeks in patients who had surgical resection, compared with 10.8 weeks with WBRT and 54 weeks for those who had both surgery and WBRT.

Leptomeningeal Metastases

Oh and colleagues reported 54 cases of cytologically confirmed leptomeningeal metastasis from gastric adenocarcinoma at four institutions in Korea from 1994 to 2007 [61]. The most common presenting symptoms were headache and nausea or vomiting. Opening pressure on lumbar puncture was elevated in 29 patients (58%), and MRI demonstrated leptomeningeal enhancement in 45 (82%). The median interval from diagnosis of the primary gastric cancer to the diagnosis of leptomeningeal disease was 6.3 months. Thirty-six patients received intrathecal chemotherapy with methotrexate alone or in combination with hydrocortisone or cytarabine. Twenty of these patients also received chemotherapy or radiation. Median overall survival was dismal at 6.7 weeks, and only conversion to negative cytology was predictive of relatively longer survival duration (14.6 weeks) on multivariate analysis. Other smaller series similarly suggest extremely poor prognosis as well as a possible modest benefit of intrathecal treatment [50, 62–66]. Leptomeningeal metastasis has also been reported as the presenting manifestation of gastric malignancy in several cases [67–71].

Paraneoplastic Syndromes

Two patients with gastric adenocarcinoma were reported to have paraneoplastic cerebellar degeneration associated with anti-Yo antibody; titers dropped in one patient after resection of the tumor [72, 73]. Another patient with paraneoplastic cerebellar degeneration due to anti-Ri antibody had a mixed tumor of neuroendocrine (reactive part of tumor) and adenocarcinoma [74]. Other cases include a sensorimotor neuropathy and encephalopathy with an antibody to alpha-enolase [75], peripheral neuropathy with arteritis of the sciatic nerve [76], and opsoclonus–myoclonus syndrome [77].

Hepatocellular Carcinoma (HCC)

The incidence of HCC continues to increase rapidly in the USA, especially in men. Approximately 20,000 patients are diagnosed with HCC each year. Worldwide, the highest incidences occur in sub-Saharan Africa and Asia. Important risk factors for the development of HCC include hepatitis B viral (HBV) infection, chronic hepatitis C virus (HCV) infection, hereditary hemochromatosis, and cirrhosis of almost any cause [78].

Patients with HCC typically present with symptoms related to chronic liver disease. There should be high suspicion for the diagnosis in patients with underlying liver disease with rising alpha-fetoprotein (AFP) levels. Most patients who develop HCC have cirrhosis and possibly thrombocytopenia, hypoalbuminemia, hyperbilirubinemia, and/or hypoprothrombinemia.

Surgery remains the only possible cure for HCC, but few patients have fully resectable disease. Additional treatment options for patients who cannot undergo resection or transplantation include radiofrequency ablation, percutaneous ethanol injection, transarterial chemoembolization, radiation therapy, and systemic chemotherapy. Studies have shown some efficacy for sorafenib in advanced HCC [79].

Brain Metastases

Earlier retrospective studies have reported an incidence of brain metastases in 0.2–2.2% of HCC patients [80–83]. However, a more recent review by Shao and colleagues identified brain metastases in 11 (7%) of 158 advanced HCC cases [84], which may be related to improved survival in the setting of new molecular targeted agents such as sorafenib. Median overall survival was poor at 4.6 months. Lim and colleagues reviewed 118 patients with HCC-brain metastases to develop an HCC-specific graded prognostic assessment (GPA) [85]. Patients with a single brain metastasis, Child–Pugh grade of A, and AFP less than 400 had the best prognosis with a median survival of 27 weeks. Sixty-five (55.1%) had associated brain hemorrhage and 101 (85.6%) had extracranial metastases. Studies suggest that treatment with surgery or radiation does improve survival [86]. Xu et al. [87] reported a median survival time of 5.0 months in 14 patients treated with gamma knife radiosurgery. However, Han et al. [88] noted better survival with surgical resection (with or without WBRT) compared to patients who received just stereotactic radiosurgery and or WBRT on analysis of 33 HCC-brain metastasis cases.

Leptomeningeal Metastases

Leptomeningeal disease with HCC is rare. One woman with HCC and headaches, hoarseness, dysphagia, and vomiting was diagnosed with leptomeningeal metastasis by CSF cytology in the setting of concomitant systemic and parenchymal brain metastases [89]. Her symptoms improved with intrathecal methotrexate and WBRT, but she passed away four months after diagnosis.

Paraneoplastic Syndromes

Several patients with demyelinating neuropathy have been reported [90–93]. In addition, there have been cases of motor neuronopathy, polymyositis, and cancer-associated retinopathy [94–97].

Gallbladder and Bile Duct (Cholangiocarcinoma) Carcinomas (Fig. 24.2)

Gallbladder cancer is rare although highly fatal. About 5000 cases are diagnosed annually in the USA [1]. Higher rates of gallbladder cancer are present in South America and East Asia. Most are adenocarcinomas, and risk factors are related to chronic gallbladder inflammation including gallstones, gallbladder polyps, and chronic infection. Patients are often asymptomatic but may present with jaundice, pain, and fever. Surgery is the only potentially curative option for gallbladder cancer, but most patients are ineligible for curative intent surgery because of local invasion and/or metastatic spread. For more advanced disease, palliation with radiation and chemotherapy is often considered.

Cholangiocarcinoma is even less common with fewer than 3000 cases a year in the USA; it is curable by surgery in less than 10% of cases. It can be difficult to treat as it is often characterized by early metastatic spread to lymph nodes and surrounding organs. The main risk factors are primary sclerosing cholangitis and choledochal cysts, but hepatobiliary flukes contribute to the high incidence in Southeast Asia. Most patients present with painless jaundice, abdominal pain, and weight loss [98]. As with gallbladder cancer,

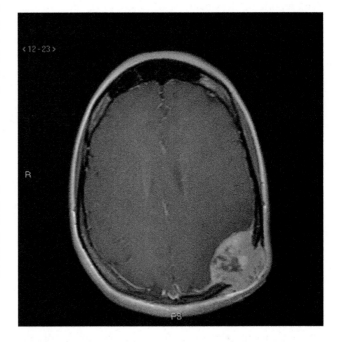

Fig. 24.2 A 39-year-old woman with no past medical history presented with 3 months of left scalp tenderness and an enlarging mass. Post-Gd T1 MRI shows an extra-axial mass invading through the calvarium. Body CT showed a large hepatic mass with satellite lesions. Resection of the calvarial mass demonstrated metastatic adenocarcinoma consistent with intrahepatic cholangiocarcinoma

radiation and chemotherapy are given for locally advanced and metastatic disease.

Brain Metastases

Large series have described the incidence of brain metastasis to be less than 0.5% of gallbladder cancer patients [99]. Few cases of brain metastasis in gallbladder cancer or cholangiocarcinoma have been reported [100–102].

Leptomeningeal Metastases

Although generally more rare than BM, several cases of leptomeningeal metastasis have been published. One patient with gallbladder cancer presented with psychosis [103], while others presented with headaches and cranial neuropathies [104, 105] and a meningitic picture [106]. Two patients with cholangiocarcinoma and LM have been described [107, 108].

Paraneoplastic Syndromes

One case of Guillain–Barré syndrome that may have been paraneoplastic has been described in association with gallbladder cancer; patients with polymyositis and opsoclonus have also been reported [109–111]. Another patient was diagnosed with an anti-Hu paraneoplastic sensory neuropathy related to small cell carcinoma of the gallbladder [112].

Pancreatic Cancer

Approximately 48,960 patients are diagnosed with exocrine pancreatic cancer (arising from the exocrine cells of the pancreas) annually, most of which are adenocarcinomas originating from the ductal epithelium [1]. Unfortunately, survival is often poor given the aggressive nature of the disease. Risk factors for the development of pancreatic cancer include obesity, cigarette smoking, chronic pancreatitis (hereditary and nonhereditary), pancreatic cysts, and potentially germline mutations in specific genes such as BRCA1, BRCA2, and STK11 [113, 114].

Patients often present late in the course of the disease with abdominal pain, jaundice, and weight loss. Surgical resection is the only potentially curative treatment, but only 15–20% of patients can get pancreatectomy. Patients who cannot undergo full resection often receive chemotherapy and radiation with limited results.

Brain Metastases

Pancreatic metastases to the brain are very rare (reported incidence of 0.33–0.57%) potentially related to poor overall survival [20, 115]. Kumar et al. [116] reported eight cases of CNS involvement with pancreatic adenocarcinoma at Johns Hopkins between 2004 and 2012. Six of the eight had other systemic metastases, and median time to diagnosis of brain metastasis was 29 months. Lemke et al. [117] retrospectively analyzed 12 patients with pancreatic cancer brain metastases reported in the literature. They identified two patients who underwent pancreatectomy with curative intent who developed solitary brain metastases (one 11 months and the other 6 years after initial diagnosis). These were surgically resected with subsequent extended survival (5 years and 4 years from diagnosis of the brain metastasis, respectively).

Leptomeningeal Metastases

As with brain metastases, leptomeningeal disease from pancreatic cancer is exceedingly rare. Several cases have been reported with poor survival [50, 118–121].

Paraneoplastic Syndromes

One patient with encephalomyelitis was found to have anti-GAD antibodies and another with small cell pancreatic cancer who presented with PCD and later polyneuropathy had anti-Hu antibodies [122, 123].

Peripheral Nervous System Complications

A rare complication of colorectal cancer is lumbosacral plexopathy. This may be a direct effect of the tumor or a secondary complication of radiation therapy. Direct compression from tumor causes back and leg pain followed by sensory changes and weakness. In a review of 85 patients with lumbosacral plexopathy, 17 had colon and 2 gastric cancer [124]. Symptoms differed slightly between colon and rectal cancers. Colon cancer produced radicular pain down the posterior aspect of the leg from lower plexus compression, while rectal cancer was associated with perineal sensory changes from coccygeal plexus involvement. Patients did poorly with a median survival of 5 months from diagnosis of plexopathy. Radiation-induced lumbosacral plexopathy is characterized by painless weakness that progresses and ultimately stabilizes with a fixed deficit. Myokymia may be seen on EMG and provide a clue that neurologic dysfunction is a complication of radiation.

Metabolic Abnormalities

Volume depletion from vomiting or diarrhea results in the secretion of antidiuretic hormone (ADH), which when coupled with free water intake may lead to hypo-osmotic hyponatremia. Low serum sodium levels can manifest symptomatically as lethargy, confusion, seizures, or even coma. Continued volume depletion can further lead to deceased renal perfusion with hypokalemia and azotemia. Severe and persistent emesis can lead to hypokalemic metabolic alkalosis. Hypokalemia and hyperkalemia can present as muscle weakness, while uremia can result in mental status changes. McKittrick–Wheelock syndrome is the constellation of dehydration, hyponatremia, hypokalemia, and azotemia that is directly associated with malignancies in the rectum, most commonly a villous adenoma, although rectal adenocarcinoma has also been implicated [125].

Treatment of volume depletion and electrolyte disorders is supportive and often can be managed with isotonic fluids. Electrolyte replacement should be done with care; it is recommended that the correction rate of serum sodium not exceed 10–12 mEq/L per day in order to prevent osmotic demyelination. Treatment for the underlying cause of the electrolyte imbalance may require surgical intervention to relieve a small bowel obstruction or resect the rectal tumor as the case of McKittrick–Wheelock syndrome. The administration of octreotide or sandostatin LAR can be very helpful in reducing the diarrhea associated with carcinoid syndrome and VIPomas.

Some of the physiologic changes that occur with gastric cancer are related to surgery [126]. One complication is a "gastric dumping" syndrome, where there is a delay in the transportation of food into the small intestine due to loss of a functional pylorus. A second complication is iron and B12 deficiency, the latter due to the loss of intrinsic factor which can cause pernicious anemia, peripheral neuropathy, and subacute combined degeneration of the spinal cord. This has a delayed onset, and patients have loss of proprioception and vibration, ataxia, and loss of deep tendon reflexes. Treatment is with parenteral vitamin B12 replacement.

Neurologic Complications of Chemotherapy

The available treatments for GI malignancy are rapidly expanding, and clinicians must be alert for neurologic complications associated with therapy. The most commonly used agents are covered here.

5-Fluorouracil (5-FU)

Intravenous fluorouracil (5-FU) can rarely be associated with acute and chronic neurotoxicities. The acute toxicities have two clinical presentations: the acute cerebellar syndrome characterized by ataxia, confusion, drowsiness, disorientation, euphoria, headache, nystagmus, and visual disturbances or an encephalopathy with the notable biochemical changes: hyperammonemia and lactic acidosis [14]. These toxicities usually develop shortly after therapy and persist for 48–72 h after therapy has stopped. Dihydropyrimidine dehydrogenase (DPD), which is necessary in clearing 5-FU, is deficient in 2.4% of cancer patients; its absence has been linked to an increase in neurotoxicity [127].

In early studies combining levamisole and 5-FU in the treatment of metastatic colorectal cancer, some patients developed a subacute multifocal leukoencephalopathy manifested as cognitive abnormalities, disturbances of consciousness, dysarthria, focal extremity weakness, and gait and limb ataxia 3–5 months post-therapy [128, 129]. Brain MRI revealed multifocal enhancing white matter lesions, which were both supra and infratentorial. Discontinuation of levamisole generally results in improvement.

Other reported side effects include ophthalmoplegia, optic neuropathy, encephalopathy, focal dystonias, and parkinsonism [28].

Bevacizumab

Bevacizumab is a monoclonal antibody against VEGF. It has been associated with reversible posterior leukoencephalopathy syndrome (RPLS), which may present with varied neurologic symptoms including headaches, seizures, lethargy, confusion, blindness, or other visual disturbances. Hypertension may precede the symptoms but is not necessary for diagnosis. Magnetic resonance imaging is used to confirm the diagnosis based on characteristic findings. The incidence is less than 0.1% [130]. Bevacizumab increases the risk of arterial thromboembolic events including stroke, transient ischemic attacks, and myocardial infarctions. Although less common than venous thrombotic disease in general, the morbidity associated with arterial events can be quite significant. The bevacizumab study AVF2107 g reported 13 (3.3%) events compared to 5 (1.3%) when treated with and without bevacizumab [131]. Similarly, AVF2192 g reported an absolute doubling of the rate of arterial thrombotic events when bevacizumab was used (10 vs. 4.8%). Of note, the study population had median age of 70 years [87]. In practice, clinicians must exercise caution in prescribing bevacizumab for patients with risk factors for or with known vascular disease. Intratumoral bleeding is another side effect that may occur in tumors; for intracranial tumors, this could be fatal.

Oxaliplatin

Oxaliplatin is a third-generation platinum compound that causes acute and chronic peripheral neuropathies. The acute neurotoxicity may occur during, shortly after, or 1–2 days postinfusion of the drug and is associated with paresthesias, hypesthesias, and dysesthesias. These usually begin in the hands or feet, but may occur around the mouth or in the throat as well. Acute side effects occur at a dose of about 130 mg/m^2 [132]. Patients may also have a sense of dyspnea or dysphagia without bronchospasm, wheezing, stridor, or laryngospasm. Patients have described an unusual sensation in the tongue, jaw spasms, eye pain, and muscle spasms or cramps, which are sometimes described as stiffness in the hands or feet or an inability to release grip. Cold temperature may exacerbate symptoms, and patients are educated to avoid cold drinks, wear gloves when handling refrigerated items, and avoid inhaling cold air. Symptoms usually last only a few days post-therapy [133].

One suggestion for the mechanism by which oxaliplatin causes an acute neurotoxicity has been coined "channelopathy." Oxaliplatin has been shown to be associated with the prolonged opening of sodium-gated channels on peripheral nerves that leads to hyperexcitability [134–136]. Whether this is a direct effect or not is unclear but may be related to the sequestration of calcium by the oxaliplatin–oxalate metabolite.

There are little published data on how to prevent and treat the acute neurotoxicity associated with oxaliplatin. Using a lower dose or increasing the infusion time has been thought to lessen the occurrence of these symptoms [137]. Administering calcium and magnesium salts like calcium gluconate and magnesium chloride has reportedly decreased the occurrence of pharyngolaryngeal dysesthesia (1.6 vs. 26%) [132, 138], although subsequent studies did not confirm this. Amifostine has also been studied as a preventative measure in reducing acute oxaliplatin-induced neuropathy. Patients receiving oxaliplatin, 5-FU, and leucovorin (a common first- or second-line therapy for metastatic colon cancer) in addition to amifostine reported less cold-induced sensitivity. However, there are significant toxicities associated with the administration of intravenous amifostine including hypotension, nausea, and vomiting that may limit its practical use; therefore, a subcutaneous preparation is recommended [139].

Symptoms associated with a more prolonged administration of oxaliplatin (total doses of $\geq$ 540–850 mg/m^2)

include paresthesia, hypesthesia, dysesthesia, and changes in proprioception that do not resolve between cycles. Proprioceptive dysfunction may present with difficulties in fine motor coordination required for writing, holding objects, picking up coins, and buttoning shirts. The chronic neuropathy is cumulative with a reported incidence of grade 3 toxicity occurring in 10% after nine cycles and in roughly 50% after 12–14 cycles (based on oxaliplatin doses of 85 mg/m^2 infused over 2 h every 14 days) [140, 141]. Lhermitte's phenomenon, an electric sensation experienced with neck flexion, has also been reported as a manifestation of chronic oxaliplatin-induced neuropathy [142]. Other central neuropathic symptoms such as urinary retention have also been reported less commonly. Symptoms usually last months with most resolving completely or to grade 1–2 toxicity within 12 months [143]. Rare symptoms include optic neuritis and visual field deficits [144].

Preventive strategies such as those outlined above (e.g., longer infusion time) have some reported efficacy in helping to prevent or at least minimize the chronic neuropathic effects of oxaliplatin. Gabapentin has also been shown to reduce the acute neuropathic toxicity but also prevents the chronic form as well.

Capecitabine

Capecitabine is a prodrug metabolized to 5-FU by thymidine phosphorylase. Neurologic toxicity is rare and limited to one case of peripheral neuropathy and several cases of encephalopathy. The latter is different from that seen with 5-FU/levamisole, as this is a reversible process with diffusion-restricted changes that do not enhance on brain MRI. This process starts earlier than that of 5-FU/levamisole [145, 146]. Capecitabine can cause an erythpalmar dysesthia that may mimic symptoms of neuropathy or give a sense that an underlying neuropathy is worsening.

Gemcitabine

Gemcitabine is a deoxycytidine analogue with minimal CNS effects. About 1% of patients complain of mild paresthesias and rare autonomic neuropathy is reported [147]. It may increase neurotoxicity when given after WBRT [148].

Cetuximab/Panitumumab

Cetuximab and panitumumab are anti-EGFR monoclonal antibodies. Neither carries significant neurologic toxicity, but both have been noted to cause headache in recent trials with metastatic colorectal cancer [149].

Conclusions

Neurologic complications from gastrointestinal cancers are relatively rare, especially compared to other solid tumors such as breast or lung cancer. However, they may occur and it is crucial that they are considered when patients with gastrointestinal cancers present with new neurologic symptoms. Although indirect neurotoxicity can occur from treatment, neurologic deficits are usually caused by metastatic disease to the CNS.

Acknowledgements The authors of this third edition chapter would like to thank the authors of this chapter in the previous (second) edition (Jeffrey Raizer, MD, and Jeffrey Cilley, MD), as this newly revised and updated chapter relies on their fine work.

References

1. Siegel RL, Miller KD, Jemal A. Cancer statistics, 2015. CA: Cancer J Clin. 2015 Jan–Feb;65(1):5–29.
2. Newton HB. Neurologic complications of systemic cancer. Am Fam Physician. 1999;59(4):878–86.
3. Jemal A, Simard EP, Dorell C, Noone AM, Markowitz LE, Kohler B, et al. Annual Report to the Nation on the Status of Cancer, 1975–2009, featuring the burden and trends in human papillomavirus(HPV)-associated cancers and HPV vaccination coverage levels. J Natl Cancer Inst. 2013;105(3):175–201.
4. Burt RW, DiSario JA, Cannon-Albright L. Genetics of colon cancer: impact of inheritance on colon cancer risk. Annu Rev Med. 1995;46:371–9.
5. Lynch HT, Smyrk TC, Watson P, Lanspa SJ, Lynch JF, Lynch PM, et al. Genetics, natural history, tumor spectrum, and pathology of hereditary nonpolyposis colorectal cancer: an updated review. Gastroenterology. 1993;104(5):1535–49.
6. Ponz de Leon M, Sassatelli R, Benatti P, Roncucci L. Identification of hereditary nonpolyposis colorectal cancer in the general population. The 6-year experience of a population-based registry. Cancer. 1993 Jun 1;71(11):3493–501.
7. Attard TM, Giglio P, Koppula S, Snyder C, Lynch HT. Brain tumors in individuals with familial adenomatous polyposis: a cancer registry experience and pooled case report analysis. Cancer. 2007;109(4):761–6.
8. Hamilton SR, Liu B, Parsons RE, Papadopoulos N, Jen J, Powell SM, et al. The molecular basis of Turcot's syndrome. New England J Med. 1995;332(13):839–47.
9. Vasen HF, Moslein G, Alonso A, Aretz S, Bernstein I, Bertario L, et al. Guidelines for the clinical management of familial adenomatous polyposis (FAP). Gut. 2008;57(5):704–13.
10. Chan AT, Giovannucci EL. Primary prevention of colorectal cancer. Gastroenterology. 2010 Jun;138(6):2029-43 e10.
11. Hamilton W, Round A, Sharp D, Peters TJ. Clinical features of colorectal cancer before diagnosis: a population-based case-control study. Br J Cancer. 2005;93(4):399–405.
12. Sundermeyer ML, Meropol NJ, Rogatko A, Wang H, Cohen SJ. Changing patterns of bone and brain metastases in patients with colorectal cancer. Clin Colorectal Cancer. 2005;5 (2):108–13.
13. Cascino TL, Leavengood JM, Kemeny N, Posner JB. Brain metastases from colon cancer. J Neurooncol. 1983;1(3):203–9.
14. Schouten LJ, Rutten J, Huveneers HA, Twijnstra A. Incidence of brain metastases in a cohort of patients with carcinoma of the breast, colon, kidney, and lung and melanoma. Cancer. 2002;94 (10):2698–705.
15. Mongan JP, Fadul CE, Cole BF, Zaki BI, Suriawinata AA, Ripple GH, et al. Brain metastases from colorectal cancer: risk factors, incidence, and the possible role of chemokines. Clin Colorectal Cancer. 2009;8(2):100–5.
16. Alden TD, Gianino JW, Saclarides TJ. Brain metastases from colorectal cancer. Dis Colon Rectum. 1996;39(5):541–5.
17. Ko FC, Liu JM, Chen WS, Chiang JK, Lin TC, Lin JK. Risk and patterns of brain metastases in colorectal cancer: 27-year experience. Dis Colon Rectum. 1999;42(11):1467–71 p.
18. Hammoud MA, McCutcheon IE, Elsouki R, Schoppa D, Patt YZ. Colorectal carcinoma and brain metastasis: distribution, treatment, and survival. Ann Surg Oncol. 1996;3(5):453–63.
19. Wronski M, Arbit E. Resection of brain metastases from colorectal carcinoma in 73 patients. Cancer. 1999;85(8):1677–85.
20. Go PH, Klaassen Z, Meadows MC, Chamberlain RS. Gastrointestinal cancer and brain metastasis: a rare and ominous sign. Cancer. 2011;117(16):3630–40.
21. Wong MT, Eu KW. Rise of colorectal cancer in Singapore: an epidemiological review. ANZ J Surg. 2007;77(6):446–9.
22. Amichetti M, Lay G, Dessi M, Orru S, Farigu R, Orru P, et al. Results of whole brain radiation therapy in patients with brain metastases from colorectal carcinoma. Tumori. 2005 Mar-Apr;91 (2):163–7.
23. Temple DF, Ledesma EJ, Mittelman A. Cerebral metastases. From adenocarcinoma of the colon and rectum. New York State J Med. 1982;82(13):1812–4.
24. Bartelt S, Momm F, Weissenberger C, Lutterbach J. Patients with brain metastases from gastrointestinal tract cancer treated with whole brain radiation therapy: prognostic factors and survival. World J Gastroenterology: WJG. 2004;10(22):3345–8.
25. Farnell GF, Buckner JC, Cascino TL, O'Connell MJ, Schomberg PJ, Suman V. Brain metastases from colorectal carcinoma. The long term survivors. Cancer. 1996;78(4):711–6.
26. Matsunaga S, Shuto T, Kawahara N, Suenaga J, Inomori S, Fujino H. Gamma Knife surgery for brain metastases from colorectal cancer. Clinical article. J Neurosurg. 2011;114(3):782–9.
27. Da Silva AN, Nagayama K, Schlesinger DJ, Sheehan JP. Gamma Knife surgery for brain metastases from gastrointestinal cancer. J Neurosurg. 2009;111(3):423–30.
28. Deangelis LM, Posner JB. Neurologic complications of cancer. New York: Oxford University Press; 2009.
29. Bresalier RS, Karlin DA. Meningeal metastasis from rectal carcinoma with elevated cerebrospinal fluid carcinoembryonic antigen. Dis Colon Rectum. 1979 May–Jun;22(4):216–7.
30. Fisher MA, Weiss RB. Carcinomatous meningitis in gastrointestinal malignancies. South Med J. 1979;72(8):930–2.
31. Kato H, Emura S, Takashima T, Ohmori K, Sunaga T. Gadolinium-enhanced magnetic resonance imaging of meningeal carcinomatosis in colon cancer. Tohoku J Exp Med. 1995;176 (2):121–6.
32. Gilbert RW, Kim JH, Posner JB. Epidural spinal cord compression from metastatic tumor: diagnosis and treatment. Ann Neurol. 1978;3(1):40–51.
33. Brown PD, Stafford SL, Schild SE, Martenson JA, Schiff D. Metastatic spinal cord compression in patients with colorectal cancer. J Neurooncol. 1999;44(2):175–80.
34. Tsukamoto T, Mochizuki R, Mochizuki H, Noguchi M, Kayama H, Hiwatashi M, et al. Paraneoplastic cerebellar degeneration and limbic encephalitis in a patient with

adenocarcinoma of the colon. J Neurol Neurosurg Psychiatry. 1993;56(6):713–6.

35. Chao D, Chen WC, Thirkill CE, Lee AG. Paraneoplastic optic neuropathy and retinopathy associated with colon adenocarcinoma. Can J Ophthalmol J Canadien d'ophtalmologie. 2013;48 (5):e116–20.

36. Jacobson DM, Adamus G. Retinal anti-bipolar cell antibodies in a patient with paraneoplastic retinopathy and colon carcinoma. Am J Ophthalmol. 2001;131(6):806–8.

37. Pantalone D, Muscas GC, Tings T, Paolucci R, Nincheri-Kunz M, Borri A, et al. Peripheral paraneoplastic neuropathy, an uncommon clinical onset of sigmoid cancer. Case report and review of the literature. Tumori. 2002 Jul–Aug;88(4):347–9.

38. Sharma BC, Ghoshal UC, Saraswat VA. Carcinoma colon presenting as paraneoplastic sensorimotor neuropathy. J Assoc Physicians India. 1998;46(2):239.

39. Badzek S, Miletic V, Prejac J, Gorsic I, Golem H, Bilic E, et al. Paraneoplastic stiff person syndrome associated with colon cancer misdiagnosed as idiopathic Parkinson's disease worsened after capecitabine therapy. World J Surg Oncol. 2013;11:224.

40. Jemal A, Bray F, Center MM, Ferlay J, Ward E, Forman D. Global cancer statistics. CA: Cancer J Clin. 2011 Mar–Apr;61 (2):69–90.

41. Engel LS, Chow WH, Vaughan TL, Gammon MD, Risch HA, Stanford JL, et al. Population attributable risks of esophageal and gastric cancers. J Natl Cancer Inst. 2003;95(18):1404–13.

42. Pandeya N, Williams G, Green AC, Webb PM, Whiteman DC, Australian Cancer S. Alcohol consumption and the risks of adenocarcinoma and squamous cell carcinoma of the esophagus. Gastroenterology. 2009 Apr;136(4):1215–24, e1–2.

43. Thun MJ, Peto R, Lopez AD, Monaco JH, Henley SJ, Heath CW Jr, et al. Alcohol consumption and mortality among middle-aged and elderly U.S. adults. New England J Med. 1997;337 (24):1705–14.

44. Sjoquist KM, Burmeister BH, Smithers BM, Zalcberg JR, Simes RJ, Barbour A, et al. Survival after neoadjuvant chemotherapy or chemoradiotherapy for resectable oesophageal carcinoma: an updated meta-analysis. Lancet Oncol. 2011;12 (7):681–92.

45. Ogawa K, Toita T, Sueyama H, Fuwa N, Kakinohana Y, Kamata M, et al. Brain metastases from esophageal carcinoma: natural history, prognostic factors, and outcome. Cancer. 2002;94 (3):759–64.

46. Weinberg JS, Suki D, Hanbali F, Cohen ZR, Lenzi R, Sawaya R. Metastasis of esophageal carcinoma to the brain. Cancer. 2003;98 (9):1925–33.

47. Wadhwa R, Taketa T, Correa AM, Sudo K, Campagna MC, Blum MA, et al. Incidence of brain metastases after trimodality therapy in patients with esophageal or gastroesophageal cancer: implications for screening and surveillance. Oncology. 2013;85 (4):204–7.

48. Smith RS, Miller RC. Incidence of brain metastasis in patients with esophageal carcinoma. World J Gastroenterology: WJG. 2011;17(19):2407–10.

49. Song Z, Lin B, Shao L, Zhang Y. Brain metastases from esophageal cancer: clinical review of 26 cases. World Neurosurg. 2014;81(1):131–5.

50. Giglio P, Weinberg JS, Forman AD, Wolff R, Groves MD. Neoplastic meningitis in patients with adenocarcinoma of the gastrointestinal tract. Cancer. 2005;103(11):2355–62.

51. Lukas RV, Mata-Machado NA, Nicholas MK, Salgia R, Antic T, Villaflor VM. Leptomeningeal carcinomatosis in esophageal cancer: a case series and systematic review of the literature. Dis Esophagus. 2015 Nov–Dec;28(8):772–81.

52. Rossor AM, Perry F, Botha A, Norwood F. Opsoclonus myoclonus syndrome due to squamous cell carcinoma of the oesophagus. BMJ Case Rep. 2014 Mar 3;2014. pii: bcr2013202849.

53. Menezes RB, de Lucena AF, Maia FM, Marinho AR. Limbic encephalitis as the presenting symptom of oesophageal adenocarcinoma: another cancer to search? BMJ Case Rep. 2013 Apr 16;2013. pii: bcr2012008201.

54. Shirafuji T, Kanda F, Sekiguchi K, Higuchi M, Yokozaki H, Tanaka K, et al. Anti-Hu-associated paraneoplastic encephalomyelitis with esophageal small cell carcinoma. Intern Med. 2012;51(17):2423–7.

55. Sutton IJ, Fursdon Davis CJ, Esiri MM, Hughes S, Amyes ER, Vincent A. Anti-Yo antibodies and cerebellar degeneration in a man with adenocarcinoma of the esophagus. Ann Neurol. 2001 Feb;49(2):253–7.

56. Xia K, Saltzman JR, Carr-Locke DL. Anti-Yo antibody-mediated paraneoplastic cerebellar degeneration in a man with esophageal adenocarcinoma. MedGenMed: Medscape General Med. 2003;5 (3):18.

57. Mita T, Nakanishi Y, Ochiai A, Shimoda T, Kato H, Yamaguchi H, et al. Paraneoplastic vasculitis associated with esophageal carcinoma. Pathol Int. 1999;49(7):643–7.

58. Correa P. A human model of gastric carcinogenesis. Can Res. 1988;48(13):3554–60.

59. York JE, Stringer J, Ajani JA, Wildrick DM, Gokaslan ZL. Gastric cancer and metastasis to the brain. Ann Surg Oncol. 1999;6(8):771–6.

60. Kasakura Y, Fujii M, Mochizuki F, Suzuki T, Takahashi T. Clinicopathological study of brain metastasis in gastric cancer patients. Surg Today. 2000;30(6):485–90.

61. Oh SY, Lee SJ, Lee J, Lee S, Kim SH, Kwon HC, et al. Gastric leptomeningeal carcinomatosis: multi-center retrospective analysis of 54 cases. World J Gastroenterology WJG. 2009;15 (40):5086–90.

62. Kim NH, Kim JH, Chin HM, Jun KH. Leptomeningeal carcinomatosis from gastric cancer: single institute retrospective analysis of 9 cases. Ann Surg Treat Res. 2014;86(1):16–21.

63. Kusumoto T, Kimura Y, Sugiyama M, Ohta M, Tsutsumi N, Sakaguchi Y, et al. Leptomeningeal carcinomatosis originating from advanced gastric cancer–a report of three cases and review of the literatures. Fukuoka igaku zasshi = Hukuoka Acta Medica. 2013;104(11):456–63.

64. Lisenko Y, Kumar AJ, Yao J, Ajani J, Ho L. Leptomeningeal carcinomatosis originating from gastric cancer: report of eight cases and review of the literature. Am J Clin Oncol. 2003;26 (2):165–70.

65. Tomita H, Yasui H, Boku N, Nakasu Y, Mitsuya K, Onozawa Y, et al. Leptomeningeal carcinomatosis associated with gastric cancer. Int J Clin Oncol. 2012;17(4):361–6.

66. Lee JL, Kang YK, Kim TW, Chang HM, Lee GW, Ryu MH, et al. Leptomeningeal carcinomatosis in gastric cancer. J Neurooncol. 2004;66(1–2):167–74.

67. Braeuninger S, Mawrin C, Malfertheiner P, Schildhaus HU, Seiler C, Dietzmann K, et al. Gastric adenocarcinoma with leptomeningeal carcinomatosis as the presenting manifestation: an autopsy case report. Eur J Gastroenterol Hepatol. 2005;17 (5):577–9.

68. Bredin C, Terris B, Sogni P, Podevin P. [Carcinomatous meningitis as a rare presentation of gastric cancer]. Presse medicale. 2005 Apr 9;34(7):509–10. Meningite carcinomateuse revelant un carcinome gastrique a cellules independantes.

69. Deeb LS, Yamout BI, Shamseddine AI, Shabb NS, Uthman SM. Meningeal carcinomatosis as the presenting manifestation of

gastric adenocarcinoma. Am J Gastroenterology. 1997;92 (2):329–31.

70. Grove A. Meningeal carcinomatosis from a clinically undiagnosed early gastric cancer. Pathology, research and practice. 1991 Mar;187(2–3):341-5; discussion 5-7.

71. Guo JW, Zhang XT, Chen XS, Zhang XC, Zheng GJ, Zhang BP, et al. Leptomeningeal carcinomatosis as the initial manifestation of gastric adenocarcinoma: a case report. World Journal of Gastroenterology: WJG. 2014;20(8):2120–6.

72. Goto A, Kusumi M, Wakutani Y, Nakaso K, Kowa H, Nakashima K. [Anti-Yo antibody associated paraneoplastic cerebellar degeneration with gastric adenocarcinoma in a male patient: a case report]. Rinsho shinkeigaku = Clin Neurol. 2006;46(2):144–7.

73. Meglic B, Graus F, Grad A. Anti-Yo-associated paraneoplastic cerebellar degeneration in a man with gastric adenocarcinoma. J Neurol Sci. 2001;185(2):135–8.

74. Kikuchi H, Yamada T, Okayama A, Hara H, Taniwaki T, Shigeto H, et al. Anti-Ri-associated paraneoplastic cerebellar degeneration without opsoclonus in a patient with a neuroendocrine carcinoma of the stomach. Fukuoka igaku zasshi = Hukuoka Acta Medica. 2000;91(4):104–9.

75. Tojo K, Tokuda T, Yazaki M, Oide T, Nakamura A, Mitsuhashi S, et al. Paraneoplastic sensorimotor neuropathy and encephalopathy associated with anti-alpha-enolase antibody in a case of gastric adenocarcinoma. Eur Neurol. 2004;51(4):231–3.

76. Naka T, Yorifuji S, Fujimura H, Takahashi M, Tarui S. [A case of paraneoplastic neuropathy with necrotizing arteritis localized in the peripheral nervous system]. Rinsho shinkeigaku = Clin Neurol. 1991;31(4):427–32.

77. Bataller L, Graus F, Saiz A, Vilchez JJ. Spanish opsoclonus-Myoclonus Study G. Clinical outcome in adult onset idiopathic or paraneoplastic opsoclonus-myoclonus. Brain J Neurol. 2001;124(Pt 2):437–43.

78. Davila JA, Morgan RO, Shaib Y, McGlynn KA, El-Serag HB. Hepatitis C infection and the increasing incidence of hepatocellular carcinoma: a population-based study. Gastroenterology. 2004;127(5):1372–80.

79. Llovet JM, Ricci S, Mazzaferro V, Hilgard P, Gane E, Blanc JF, et al. Sorafenib in advanced hepatocellular carcinoma. New Engl J Med. 2008;359(4):378–90.

80. Murakami K, Nawano S, Moriyama N, Sekiguchi R, Satake M, Fujimoto H, et al. Intracranial metastases of hepatocellular carcinoma: CT and MRI. Neuroradiology. 1996;38(Suppl 1): S31–5.

81. Kim M, Na DL, Park SH, Jeon BS, Roh JK. Nervous system involvement by metastatic hepatocellular carcinoma. J Neurooncol. 1998;36(1):85–90.

82. Chen SF, Tsai NW, Lui CC, Lu CH, Huang CR, Chuang YC, et al. Hepatocellular carcinoma presenting as nervous system involvement. European J Neurol. 2007;14(4):408–12.

83. Choi HJ, Cho BC, Sohn JH, Shin SJ, Kim SH, Kim JH, et al. Brain metastases from hepatocellular carcinoma: prognostic factors and outcome: brain metastasis from HCC. J Neurooncol. 2009;91(3):307–13.

84. Shao YY, Lu LC, Cheng AL, Hsu CH. Increasing incidence of brain metastasis in patients with advanced hepatocellular carcinoma in the era of antiangiogenic targeted therapy. Oncologist. 2011;16(1):82–6.

85. Lim S, Lee S, Lim JY, Park JS, Seong JS, Chang WS, et al. Hepatocellular carcinoma specific graded prognostic assessment can predict outcomes for patients with brain metastases from hepatocellular carcinoma. J Neurooncol. 2014;120(1):199–207.

86. Park TY, Na YC, Lee WH, Kim JH, Chang WS, Jung HH, et al. Treatment options of metastatic brain tumors from Hepatocellular

Carcinoma: Surgical Resection vs. Gamma Knife Radiosurgery vs. Whole Brain Radiation Therapy. Brain Tumor Res Treat. 2013 Oct;1(2):78–84.

87. Xu Q, Wu P, Feng Y, Ye K, Tong Y, Zhou Y. Gamma knife surgery for brain metastasis from hepatocellular carcinoma. PLoS ONE. 2014;9(2):e88317.

88. Han MS, Moon KS, Lee KH, Cho SB, Lim SH, Jang WY, et al. Brain metastasis from hepatocellular carcinoma: the role of surgery as a prognostic factor. BMC Cancer. 2013;13:567.

89. Pan Z, Yang G, Yuan T, Pang X, Wang Y, Qu L, et al. Leptomeningeal metastasis from hepatocellular carcinoma with other unusual metastases: a case report. BMC Cancer. 2014;14:399.

90. Matsui T, Hori Y, Nagano H, Eguchi H, Marubashi S, Wada H, et al. Poorly differentiated hepatocellular carcinoma accompanied by anti-Hu antibody-positive paraneoplastic peripheral neuropathy. Pathol Int. 2015;65(7):388–92.

91. Walcher J, Witter T, Rupprecht HD. Hepatocellular carcinoma presenting with paraneoplastic demyelinating polyneuropathy and PR3-antineutrophil cytoplasmic antibody. J Clin Gastroenterol. 2002;35(4):364–5.

92. Sugai F, Abe K, Fujimoto T, Nagano S, Fujimura H, Kayanoki Y, et al. Chronic inflammatory demyelinating polyneuropathy accompanied by hepatocellular carcinoma. Intern Med. 1997;36 (1):53–5.

93. Arguedas MR, McGuire BM. Hepatocellular carcinoma presenting with chronic inflammatory demyelinating polyradiculoneuropathy. Dig Dis Sci. 2000;45(12):2369–73.

94. Turgut N, Karagol H, Celik Y, Uygun K, Reyhani A. Subacute motor neuronopathy associated with hepatocellular carcinoma. J Neurooncol. 2007;83(1):95–6.

95. Chang PY, Yang CH, Yang CM. Cancer-associated retinopathy in a patient with hepatocellular carcinoma: case report and literature review. Retina. 2005;25(8):1093–6.

96. Kishore D, Khurana V, Raj A, Gambhir IS, Diwaker A. Hepatocellular carcinoma presenting as polymyositis: a paraneoplastic syndrome. Ann Saudi Med. 2011 Sep–Oct;31(5):533–5.

97. Hasegawa K, Uesugi H, Kubota K, Ugawa Y, Murayama S, Kobayashi T, et al. Polymyositis as a paraneoplastic manifestation of hepatocellular carcinoma. Hepato-gastroenterology. 2000 Sep–Oct;47(35):1425–7.

98. Blechacz B, Komuta M, Roskams T, Gores GJ. Clinical diagnosis and staging of cholangiocarcinoma. Nat Rev Gastroenterology Hepatol. 2011;8(9):512–22.

99. Takano S, Yoshii Y, Owada T, Shirai S, Nose T. Central nervous system metastasis from gallbladder carcinoma–case report. Neurol Med Chir. 1991;31(12):782–6.

100. Gudesblatt MS, Sencer W, Sacher M, Lanzieri CF, Song SK. Cholangiocarcinoma presenting as a cerebellar metastasis: case report and review of the literature. J Computed Tomogr. 1984;8 (3):191–5.

101. Kawamata T, Kawamura H, Kubo O, Sasahara A, Yamazato M, Hori T. Central nervous system metastasis from gallbladder carcinoma mimicking a meningioma. Case illustration. J Neurosurg. 1999;91(6):1059.

102. Smith WD, Sinar J, Carey M. Sagittal sinus thrombosis and occult malignancy. J Neurol Neurosurg Psychiatry. 1983;46(2):187–8.

103. Higes-Pascual F, Beroiz-Groh P, Bravo-Guillen AI, Palomo-Martinez V, Cuevas-Santos J. [Leptomeningeal carcinomatosis as presenting symptom of a gallbladder carcinoma]. Revista de neurologia. 2000 May 1–15;30(9):841–4. Carcinomatosis leptomeningea como forma de presentacion de un adenocarcinoma de vesicula biliar.

104. Gaumann A, Marx J, Bohl J, Kommoss F, Kohler H, Tews DS. Leptomeningeal carcinomatosis and cranial nerve palsy as

presenting symptoms of a clinically inapparent gallbladder carcinoma. Pathol Res Pract. 1999;195(7):495–9.

105. Tans RJ, Koudstaal J, Koehler PJ. Meningeal carcinomatosis as presenting symptom of a gallbladder carcinoma. Clin Neurol Neurosurg. 1993;95(3):253–6.

106. Miyagui T, Luchembeck L, Teixeira GH, de Azevedo KM. Meningeal carcinomatosis as the initial manifestation of a gallbladder adenocarcinoma associated with a Krukenberg tumor. Revista do Hospital das Clinicas. 2003 May–Jun;58(3):169–72.

107. William BM, Grem JL. Brain metastasis and leptomeningeal carcinomatosis in a patient with cholangiocarcinoma. Gastrointestinal Cancer Res GCR. 2011;4(4):144–5.

108. Huffman JL, Yeatman TJ, Smith JB. Leptomeningeal carcinomatosis: a sequela of cholangiocarcinoma. Am Surg. 1997;63 (4):310–3.

109. Phan TG, Hersch M, Zagami AS. Guillain-Barre syndrome and adenocarcinoma of the gall bladder: a paraneoplastic phenomenon? Muscle Nerve. 1999;22(1):141–2.

110. Corcia P, De Toffol B, Hommet C, Saudeau D, Autret A. Paraneoplastic opsoclonus associated with cancer of the gall bladder. J Neurol Neurosurg Psychiatry. 1997;62(3):293.

111. Adli B, Pakzad M, Bangash MN, Rakei S. Polymyositis as presenting manifestation of gallbladder carcinoma: a case report. Int J Surg Case Rep. 2013;4(8):665–8.

112. Uribe-Uribe NO, Jimenez-Garduno AM, Henson DE, Albores-Saavedra J. Paraneoplastic sensory neuropathy associated with small cell carcinoma of the gallbladder. Ann Diagn Pathol. 2009;13(2):124–6.

113. Iqbal J, Ragone A, Lubinski J, Lynch HT, Moller P, Ghadirian P, et al. The incidence of pancreatic cancer in BRCA1 and BRCA2 mutation carriers. Br J Cancer. 2012;107(12):2005–9.

114. Su GH, Hruban RH, Bansal RK, Bova GS, Tang DJ, Shekher MC, et al. Germline and somatic mutations of the STK11/LKB1 Peutz-Jeghers gene in pancreatic and biliary cancers. Am J Pathol. 1999;154(6):1835–40.

115. Park KS, Kim M, Park SH, Lee KW. Nervous system involvement by pancreatic cancer. J Neurooncol. 2003;63(3):313–6.

116. Kumar A, Dagar M, Herman J, Iacobuzio-Donahue C, Laheru D. CNS involvement in pancreatic adenocarcinoma: a report of eight cases from the Johns Hopkins Hospital and review of literature. J Gastrointest Cancer. 2015;46(1):5–8.

117. Lemke J, Scheele J, Kapapa T, Wirtz CR, Henne-Bruns D, Kornmann M. Brain metastasis in pancreatic cancer. Int J Mol Sci. 2013;14(2):4163–73.

118. Blows SJ, Morgan R, Dhariwal U, Petts G, Roncaroli F. Pancreatic adenocarcinoma presenting with sudden onset bilateral deafness secondary to metastatic leptomeningeal infiltration. Age Ageing. 2012;41(6):818–9.

119. Minchom A, Chan S, Melia W, Shah R. An unusual case of pancreatic cancer with leptomeningeal infiltration. J Gastrointest Cancer. 2010;41(2):107–9.

120. Rao R, Sadashiv SK, Goday S, Monga D. An extremely rare case of pancreatic cancer presenting with leptomeningeal carcinomatosis and synchronous intraparenchymal brain metastasis. Gastrointest Cancer Res: GCR. 2013;6(3):90–2.

121. Yoo IK, Lee HS, Kim CD, Chun HJ, Jeen YT, Keum B, et al. Rare case of pancreatic cancer with leptomeningeal carcinomatosis. World Journal Gastroenterol WJG. 2015;21(3):1020–3.

122. Hernandez-Echebarria L, Saiz A, Ares A, Tejada J, Garcia-Tunon L, Nieves C, et al. Paraneoplastic encephalomyelitis associated with pancreatic tumor and anti-GAD antibodies. Neurology. 2006;66(3):450–1.

123. Salmeron-Ato P, Medrano V, Morales-Ortiz A, Martinez-Garcia FA, Villaverde-Gonzalez R, Bas A, et al. [Paraneoplastic cerebellar degeneration as initial presentation of a pancreatic small-cell carcinoma]. Revista de neurologia. 2002 Dec 16–31;35 (12):1112–5. Degeneracion cerebelosa paraneoplasica como inicio de un carcinoma indiferenciado de celulas pequenas de pancreas.

124. Jaeckle KA, Young DF, Foley KM. The natural history of lumbosacral plexopathy in cancer. Neurology. 1985;35(1):8–15.

125. Lepur D, Klinar I, Mise B, Himbele J, Vranjican Z, Barsic B. McKittrick-Wheelock syndrome: a rare cause of diarrhoea. Eur J Gastroenterol Hepatol. 2006;18(5):557–9.

126. Williams JA, Hall GS, Thompson AG, Cooke WT. Neurological disease after partial gastrectomy. BMJ. 1969;3(5664):210–2.

127. Pirzada NA, Ali II, Dafer RM. Fluorouracil-induced neurotoxicity. Ann Pharmacother. 2000;34(1):35–8.

128. Chen TC, Hinton DR, Leichman L, Atkinson RD, Apuzzo ML, Couldwell WT. Multifocal inflammatory leukoencephalopathy associated with levamisole and 5-fluorouracil: case report. Neurosurgery. 1994 Dec;35(6):1138–42; discussion 42–3.

129. Hook CC, Kimmel DW, Kvols LK, Scheithauer BW, Forsyth PA, Rubin J, et al. Multifocal inflammatory leukoencephalopathy with 5-fluorouracil and levamisole. Ann Neurol. 1992;31(3):262–7.

130. Glusker P, Recht L, Lane B. Reversible posterior leukoencephalopathy syndrome and bevacizumab. New Engl J Med. 2006 Mar 2;354(9):980–2; discussion-2.

131. Johnson DH, Fehrenbacher L, Novotny WF, Herbst RS, Nemunaitis JJ, Jablons DM, et al. Randomized phase II trial comparing bevacizumab plus carboplatin and paclitaxel with carboplatin and paclitaxel alone in previously untreated locally advanced or metastatic non-small-cell lung cancer. J Clin Oncol. 2004;22 (11):2184–91.

132. Gamelin E, Gamelin L, Bossi L, Quasthoff S. Clinical aspects and molecular basis of oxaliplatin neurotoxicity: current management and development of preventive measures. Semin Oncol. 2002;29 (5 Suppl 15):21–33.

133. Cersosimo RJ. Oxaliplatin-associated neuropathy: a review. Ann Pharmacother. 2005;39(1):128–35.

134. Grolleau F, Gamelin L, Boisdron-Celle M, Lapied B, Pelhate M, Gamelin E. A possible explanation for a neurotoxic effect of the anticancer agent oxaliplatin on neuronal voltage-gated sodium channels. J Neurophysiol. 2001;85(5):2293–7.

135. Lehky TJ, Leonard GD, Wilson RH, Grem JL, Floeter MK. Oxaliplatin-induced neurotoxicity: acute hyperexcitability and chronic neuropathy. Muscle Nerve. 2004;29(3):387–92.

136. Adelsberger H, Quasthoff S, Grosskreutz J, Lepier A, Eckel F, Lersch C. The chemotherapeutic oxaliplatin alters voltage-gated Na(+) channel kinetics on rat sensory neurons. Eur J Pharmacol. 2000;406(1):25–32.

137. Screnci D, McKeage MJ. Platinum neurotoxicity: clinical profiles, experimental models and neuroprotective approaches. J Inorg Biochem. 1999;77(1–2):105–10.

138. Gamelin L, Boisdron-Celle M, Delva R, Guerin-Meyer V, Ifrah N, Morel A, et al. Prevention of oxaliplatin-related neurotoxicity by calcium and magnesium infusions: a retrospective study of 161 patients receiving oxaliplatin combined with 5-Fluorouracil and leucovorin for advanced colorectal cancer. Clin Cancer Res. 2004;10(12 Pt 1):4055–61.

139. Koukourakis MI, Simopoulos C, Minopoulos G, Patlakas G, Polychronidis A, Limberis V, et al. Amifostine before chemotherapy: improved tolerance profile of the subcutaneous over the intravenous route. Clin Cancer Res. 2003;9(9):3288–93.

140. de Gramont A, Figer A, Seymour M, Homerin M, Hmissi A, Cassidy J, et al. Leucovorin and fluorouracil with or without oxaliplatin as first-line treatment in advanced colorectal cancer. J Clin Oncol. 2000;18(16):2938–47.

141. Souglakos J, Mavroudis D, Kakolyris S, Kourousis C, Vardakis N, Androulakis N, et al. Triplet combination with irinotecan plus oxaliplatin plus continuous-infusion fluorouracil and leucovorin as first-line treatment in metastatic colorectal cancer: a multicenter phase II trial. J Clin Oncol. 2002;20 (11):2651–7.

142. Taieb S, Trillet-Lenoir V, Rambaud L, Descos L, Freyer G. Lhermitte sign and urinary retention: atypical presentation of oxaliplatin neurotoxicity in four patients. Cancer. 2002;94 (9):2434–40.

143. Andre T, Boni C, Mounedji-Boudiaf L, Navarro M, Tabernero J, Hickish T, et al. Oxaliplatin, fluorouracil, and leucovorin as adjuvant treatment for colon cancer. New Engl J Med. 2004;350 (23):2343–51.

144. Sul JK, Deangelis LM. Neurologic complications of cancer chemotherapy. Semin Oncol. 2006;33(3):324–32.

145. Videnovic A, Semenov I, Chua-Adajar R, Baddi L, Blumenthal DT, Beck AC, et al. Capecitabine-induced multifocal leukoencephalopathy: a report of five cases. Neurology. 2005 Dec 13;65(11):1792–4; discussion 685.

146. Saif MW, Wood TE, McGee PJ, Diasio RB. Peripheral neuropathy associated with capecitabine. Anticancer Drugs. 2004;15(8):767–71.

147. Dormann AJ, Grunewald T, Wigginghaus B, Huchzermeyer H. Gemcitabine-associated autonomic neuropathy. Lancet. 1998;351 (9103):644.

148. Jeter MD, Janne PA, Brooks S, Burstein HJ, Wen P, Fuchs CS, et al. Gemcitabine-induced radiation recall. Int J Radiat Oncol Biol Phys. 2002;53(2):394–400.

149. Sunakawa Y, Ichikawa W, Sasaki Y. ASPECCT: panitumumab versus cetuximab for colorectal cancer. Lancet Oncol. 2014;15 (8):e301–2.

Neurologic Complications of Genitourinary Cancer

Jennie W. Taylor

Introduction

Cancers of the genitourinary system encompass a wide variety of malignancies arising from the prostate, kidneys, bladder, and testes. Combined, an estimated 365,000 patients will be diagnosed with one of these malignancies in 2015 in the USA. Cancers of the genitourinary system comprise just over 20% of all malignancies [1]. These neoplasms affect men and women of varying ages and prognoses. Neurologic morbidity and mortality is not uncommon in this patient population with frequent metastases to the brain, spinal cord, and paraneoplastic syndromes. Neurologic sequelae may also result from systemic or localized treatments for these malignancies. Here, we will highlight the most common neurologic complications arising from malignancies of the genitourinary system.

Prostate Cancer

Prostate cancer is the third leading cause of malignancy in the USA with an estimated 220,800 new cases diagnosed in 2015 [1]. Aside from the classic TNM staging, the Gleason score is the preferred method for staging as it is more informative of prognosis [2]. Decisions about treatment are based on a combination of clinical and pathologic staging that incorporates traditional TNM staging, Gleason score, and several prognostic factors.

With the advent of screening using prostate serum antigen (PSA), many patients are diagnosed with low-risk disease, and management includes active surveillance, radiation, and radical prostatectomy [3, 4]. Patients with intermediate or high risk, but clinically localized disease, may be treated with a combination of radiation, androgen deprivation therapy (ADT) or bilateral orchiectomy, and radical prostatectomy [5]. For patients with metastatic disease, treatment is focused on ADT for castration sensitive disease [5]. However, most patients with metastatic disease eventually become castration resistant, and treatment is focused on androgen inhibition (abiraterone or enzalutamide) and chemotherapy (docetaxel, cabazitaxel, and mitoxantrone) [6].

Surgical-Related Neurologic Complications

Complications from treatment for prostate cancer result in local injury during surgery or radiation [7]. Impotence often results from injury to the neurovascular bundle during resection and is also seen in 62% of patients treated with focal radiation [8]. Advances in nerve-sparing laparoscopic surgical technique [7] and intensity-modulated radiation therapy [9] are aimed at preserving sexual function after treatment. Radical prostatectomy may also result in obturator nerve injury [10].

Brain Metastases

Intracranial involvement from prostate cancer is rare, and a marker of advanced disease with evidence of systemic metastases and average time from diagnosis of 3–4 years [11]. Autopsy studies identify brain involvement in 1–6% of patients with known diagnosis of prostate cancer [11, 12], though clinical incidence is <2% [11]. Solitary metastases are more common and location is usually supratentorial [11, 13]. Small cell histology is more likely to metastasize to the brain than the more common adenocarcinoma histology, behaving similarly to small cell malignances from other organs [11, 14]. Treatment should be considered similarly to other brain metastases with a role for surgical resection for appropriate solitary or symptomatic lesions, radiotherapy,

J.W. Taylor (✉)
Department of Neurology and Neurosurgery, University of California, 400 Parnassus Ave., Room A808, Box 0372, San Francisco, CA 94143-0372, USA
e-mail: jennie.taylor@ucsf.edu

© Springer International Publishing AG 2018
D. Schiff et al. (eds.), *Cancer Neurology in Clinical Practice*,
DOI 10.1007/978-3-319-57901-6_25

and whole-brain radiation for diffuse disease. Median survival is estimated between 3 and 9 months [11, 14].

Patients with prostate cancer may also develop metastasis to the calvarium or dura. Given prostate cancer's tendency to metastasize to bone, calvarial metastases have been reported in 2–8% of patients [15, 16]. Though often asymptomatic, calvarial metastases may exert mass effect on venous sinuses leading to increased intracranial pressure or venous infarct [17]. Metastases to the skull base may cause cranial neuropathies [18]. Radiation is often the treatment of choice, with good responses and high rates of local control, though often a marker of advanced disease with prognosis <1 year [18, 19]. Dural metastases (Fig. 25.1a, b) have also been reported in 13–21% of patients [11, 20] and may mimic meningiomas or hematomas. Treatment, again, usually includes radiation, though surgery may be needed for decompression of large lesions.

Leptomeningeal Metastases

Leptomeningeal metastasis from prostate cancer is very rare. It is a late complication of disease, and thereby often associated with hormone refractory disease and a poor prognosis [21]. As patients with prostate cancer survive longer, there may be increased incidence of relapse in the CNS, including in the leptomeninges [22]. Aside from identifying malignant cells on cytology, PSA can also be detected in the CSF [23]. Treatment is palliative with radiation as the backbone of treatment.

Epidural Spinal Cord Compression

The vertebral bodies are a common location for bone metastases in advanced prostate cancer. Prostate cancer accounts for 16% of all malignant epidural spinal cord

compression (MESCC) with 5% of patients with prostate developing MESCC [24]. Back pain in this patient population should prompt evaluation for epidural spinal cord compression, as pain often precedes neurologic symptoms by weeks or months and early intervention may prevent deficits. Patients may also present with a myelopathy and bowel/bladder dysfunction, depending on the location of the lesion. Prostate cancer rarely presents as MESCC, which is a marker of advanced metastatic disease [25]. Although the thoracic spine is the most common site of MESCC overall in cancer, the lumbar region is more often affected in prostate cancer [26].

Evaluation and treatment considerations for MESCC from prostate cancer are similar to those from other neoplasms. Importantly, the entire spine should be screened if MESCC is suspected or a lesion is identified, as it may be multifocal. The intent of treatment is palliative and focused on pain control and preservation of neurologic function. Prostate histology and ambulation prior to treatment are favorable predictors of outcome and improvement in neurologic function [27, 28]. Glucocorticoids and opioids are used acutely for pain control. Though high-level evidence is limited, surgical decompression and spinal stabilization should be considered in select patients with spinal instability who are felt to be good surgical candidates [29, 30]. This is particularly true for patients with MESCC from prostate cancer with median survival >9 months [28].

Prostate cancer is highly radiosensitive, and radiation is a cornerstone in the treatment of MESCC. Radiation, usually 30–40 Gy in 10–20 fractions, is an effective method for pain control from MESCC without spinal instability [31]. Surgery is often followed by radiation for improved rates of local control [29, 30]. Radiation is the treatment of choice for the remainder of patients who are not felt to benefit from surgery with high rates of local control and median survival of >9 months [28]. Radiation effectively preserves ambulation in nearly all patients who are ambulatory at presentation.

Fig. 25.1 MRI of 79-year-old man with a history of prostate cancer who presented with diplopia. **a** Coronal, T1 post-contrast image with arrow demonstrating dural lesion in the right anterior temporal lobe. **b** Corona, T1 post-contrast image with arrow demonstrating several dural lesions in the right frontal lobe

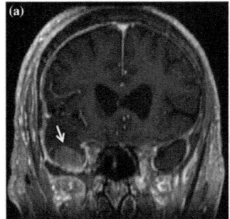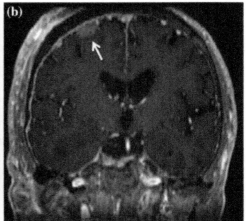

For those who are paretic at presentation, ambulation rates of 52–83% are reported after radiation, though only 20–25% of paraplegic patients will regain their ability to walk [29, 32, 33]. Though courses of hypofractionated radiation and stereotactic radiation can be considered for selected patients with short-life expectancy, protracted courses of 30–40 Gy over 10–20 fractions are recommended with evidence of improved local control rates over shorter courses [34, 35]. Patients with MESCC from prostate cancer who are hormone-naïve may also benefit from androgen deprivation in combination with radiation and/or surgery [29, 32]. Despite effect treatments, however, patients remain at risk of compression at the same site, or a new site, within two years [36].

Paraneoplastic Syndromes

Paraneoplastic syndromes have also been identified in prostate cancer. The anti-Hu antibody is associated with a subacute, distal, sensorimotor polyneuropathy found in patients with squamous cell carcinomas of the prostate [37, 38]. It has also been identified in patients with limbic encephalitis and squamous cell carcinomas of the prostate. Symptoms may respond to treatment of the underlying malignancy or immunotherapy, though overall response rates are low [39]. Anti-Hu antibodies have also been discovered in cerebellar degeneration in patients with prostate cancer [40]. Symptoms include weeks to months of progressive ataxia, dysarthria, diplopia, nystagmus, and ophthalmoplegia. Imaging reveals cerebellar atrophy late in the disease. Lambert-Eaton syndrome, a paraneoplastic disorder affecting the neuromuscular junction whereby an antibody to voltage-gated calcium channel (VGCC) impairs release of acetylcholine from nerve terminus, is rarely seen in patients with prostate carcinoma [41]. Presentation mimics that of myasthenia gravis, only the limbs are predominately weak and oculobulbar muscles are spared. Dermatomyositis has also been described in prostate cancer [42].

Renal Cell Carcinoma

There are 50,000 new cases of renal cell carcinoma diagnosed per year in the USA [43, 44]. The most common histology is clear cell adenocarcinomas, followed by papillary, chromophobe, oncocytic, and collecting duct. RCC is associated with several genetic syndromes including von Hippel-Lindau and tuberous sclerosis. Patients usually present with hematuria, abdominal pain, and palpable flank mass [45].

Localized disease is often surgically curable and, therefore, the recommended treatment in patients who are appropriate surgical candidates. Trials of adjuvant treatment with immunotherapy or anti-angiogenic-targeted therapy (sunitinib and sorafenib) have not improved disease-free or overall survival. Patients with stage I or II disease have five-year overall survival rates of 75–95%. Five-year survival rates of stage III of 59–70% with invasion of vena cava [46, 47] and urine collection system [48] associated with worse prognosis.

Treatment for advanced RCC includes immunotherapy with interleukin-2 (IL-2) and interferon alpha (INF-α). Several tyrosine kinase inhibitors such as pazopanib, sunitinib, sorafenib, and axitinib target the vascular endothelial growth factor (VEGF) pathway. Bevacizumab, the monoclonal antibody against VEGF, has also been shown to improve progression-free survival when combined with INF-α [49, 50]. Everolimus or temsirolimus target the mammalian target of rapamycin (mTOR) pathway. Treatment decisions are based on several prognostic factors, and contemporary median overall survival with stage IV disease is 28–29 months [51–53].

Brain Metastases

The incidence of metastases to the brain in RCC is estimated at 10% (Fig. 25.2a, b) [54]. Brain metastases from RCC also have increased risk of hemorrhage [26] and are more likely to present as a single lesion versus multiple [55]. Median OS is 10 months with poor KPS and increasing number of metastases at diagnoses as poor prognostic factors [56–58]. The approach to treatment is similar to brain metastases from other malignancies with consideration for resection of single metastases majority of patients succumb to systemic versus brain disease [59]. Despite its radioresistance, higher doses of radiation with stereotactic radiosurgery have demonstrated efficacy. For patients with limited number of intracranial metastases, good performance scores, and stable extracranial disease, stereotactic radiosurgery may provide rates of local control 83–95% [60–62].

The effectiveness of kinase inhibitors (KIs)—such as VEGFR inhibitors sorafenib and sunitinib and mTOR inhibitor temsirolimus—on control of brain metastases is unclear. Preclinical data suggest synergy and without significant toxicity when combining KIs with radiation [63–65]. In prospective trials of sunitinib in brain metastases from RCC, CNS toxicity was low with one instance of hemorrhage and four seizures [63]. Despite preclinical evidence that KI may be radiosensitizing, outcomes for patients with brain metastases in the KI-era are not markedly changed [56, 57]. Despite small case series suggesting efficacy of KIs as monotherapy for brain metastasis [56, 66], prospective data have failed to demonstrate efficacy [65] and local treatment with surgery and radiation is still favored. Evaluation of

Fig. 25.2 MRI of
62-year-old-man with history of
renal cell carcinoma who
presented with dizziness. **a** Axial,
T1 post-contrast image of
homogenously enhancing mass in
the right hemisphere. **b** Axial,
FLAIR image demonstrating
significant surrounding vasogenic
edema

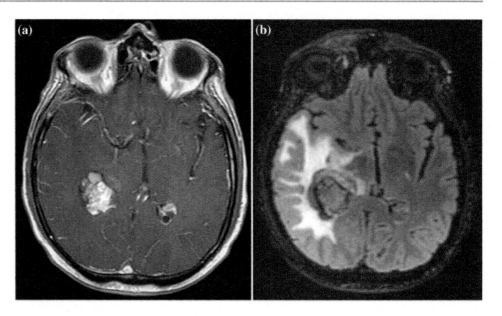

brain metastases patients in the expanded-access trials for sorafenib [67] and sunitinib [63] demonstrated response rates of at least stable disease in 74 and 64%, respectively, suggesting efficacy and need for further study [63, 67]. Prospective data have also demonstrated a decrease in incidence of brain metastases in patients treated with sorafenib versus placebo [68].

Leptomeningeal Metastases

Leptomeningeal carcinomatosis is extremely rare in RCC with only case reports in the literature. As is the case with leptomeningeal disease from other solid malignancies, it is associated with poor outcome and treatment usually includes radiation [69, 70].

Epidural Spinal Cord Compression

RCC commonly metastasizes to bone with spinal involvement in 40% of cases [71]. Spinal metastases risk metastatic epidural spinal cord compression (MESCC), which can have a marked impact on quality and duration of life [72]. Median survival of RCC metastasis to the spine is reported at 8–13 months [73–77].

Evaluation and treatment of MESCC from RCC should be similar to other neoplasms, including evaluation of the entire spine, as disease may be multifocal. The intent of treatment is palliative and focused on pain control and preservation of neurologic function. The radioresistant nature [78] of RCC and poor response to systemic therapy have set a low threshold for surgery. Prognostic factors include Fuhrman grade (a four-grade system based on nuclear size,

shape, and nucleoli appearance [79]) of the initial nephrectomy, state of systemic disease, and presurgical neurologic deficits and correlate with outcome after surgery [73]. Patients with spinal instability should also be considered for surgical decompression and stabilization.

Conventional, fractionated radiation is felt to be less effective for patients with radioresistant tumors, such as RCC [28]. However, there is increasing evidence for improved local control rates and symptomatic improvement with radiosurgery in patients with spinal metastases with stable spines [27]. Studies have also demonstrated 80% improvement in neurologic function with epidural spinal cord compression without high-grade compression [80]. Retrospective studies also report local control rates of 80% when radiosurgery doses of 18–36 Gy were used after decompression surgery [81, 82].

Intramedullary Spinal Cord Metastases

Intramedullary spinal cord metastases are rare and account for 4–9% of all CNS metastases [83]. Renal carcinoma is thought to comprise ∼4% of all cases of intramedullary metastases and is reported in small case series and case reports [84]. Patients often present first with symptoms of pain, followed by weakness and sphincter dysfunction, that is, often rapid. Patients usually have advanced metastatic disease, including other CNS metastases, though intramedullary metastases may rarely be the presenting symptom [84, 85]. Decisions regarding treatment are dependent on functional status and extent of systemic disease, with surgery reserved for those with controlled systemic disease who are good surgical candidates. Otherwise, radiation treatment is used to palliate and stabilize disease [83, 84].

Paraneoplastic Syndromes

Paraneoplastic syndromes are uncommon in RCC. There are reports of limbic encephalitis in patients with renal cell [86]. Anti-Ri antibodies have been associated with opsoclonus myoclonus syndrome in patients with RCC [87]. Patients present with spontaneous chaotic eye movements of opsoclonus, with myoclonic movements of the trunks and limbs, and cerebellar ataxia. Dermatomyositis has also been seen in RCC [88]. Presenting symptoms include progressive pain and hypertrophy of proximal muscles and violet-colored rash of the face and hands.

Bladder Cancer

Bladder cancer accounts for an estimated 4.5% of malignancies in the USA with an estimated 74,000 cases diagnosed in 2015. It is the fifth leading cause of cancer and much more common in men [1]. The most common histology is transitional cell, followed by squamous cell, adenocarcinoma, small cell carcinoma, sarcoma, rhabdmyosarcoma, and leiomyosarcoma. Spread is through local invasion and hematogenous dissemination and involves liver, lung, and bone [89, 90].

Prognosis and treatment are dependent on histology and staging based on the depth of invasion [91]. Superficial, non-muscle invasive bladder tumors may be amenable to transurethral resection and intravesical delivery of chemotherapy or immunologic agents, such as bacillus Calmette–Guerin (BCG) [91, 92]. Invasive tumors, however, often necessitate neoadjuvant systemic chemotherapy combinations followed by cystectomy. Chemotherapy regimens include MVAC (methotrexate, vinblastine, doxorubicin, and cisplatin) [93] or gemcitabine and cisplatin (or carboplatin) [94]. Overall, neurologic complications are infrequent from bladder carcinoma [95].

Brain Metastases

Brain metastases are a rare finding in bladder cancer with reports of 0–7% with longer survivors being more at risk [95, 96]. First, the use of the MVAC regimen, and more recently combination therapy with a platinum and gemcitabine, has significantly improved outcomes in patients with bladder cancer. However, these regimens have limited blood brain barrier penetration, therefore increasing the risk of late CNS relapse [97] with an estimated incidence ∼16% [98]. Multiple lesions are more common and are a marker of advanced disease [99]. Median survival is 2–7 months [97, 100, 101]. Treatment consists of surgical resection, when

appropriate, and radiation therapy—prospective studies comparing combinations of these treatments are lacking. Retrospective trials have identified the number of metastases, status of extracranial disease, and RPA status as prognostic factors [102, 103].

Leptomeningeal Metastases

Leptomeningeal carcinomatous is noted in case reports for bladder cancer. It is seen in longer survivors of pretreated patients, again indicating the propensity for relapse in the CNS when chemotherapeutics are unable to penetrate the blood–brain barrier (Fig. 25.3a, b) [104, 105]. There are also case reports of transitional cell carcinoma of the bladder presenting as leptomeningeal carcinomatosis [106].

Epidural Spinal Cord Compression

Epidural spinal cord compression from bladder cancer is rare with reports of <2% in the literature and usually presenting with pain [95]. Hematogenous dissemination to bone is the most common mechanism, though erosion from metastasis to the paraspinal lymph nodes and erosion is also reported. Treatment usually includes radiation [95].

Paraneoplastic Syndromes

Several paraneoplastic syndromes have been associated with bladder malignancies [107]. The anti-Ri [108, 109] antibody is associated with opsoclonus myoclonus syndrome in patients with transitional cell carcinoma of the bladder. Patients present with spontaneous chaotic eye movements of opsoclonus, with myoclonic movements of the trunk and limbs, and cerebellar ataxia. Polymyositis [110] and dermatomyositis [111], with progressive pain and hypertrophy of proximal muscles and violet-colored rash of the face and hands, have both been seen in bladder cancer.

Lambert-Eaton syndrome [112] is a paraneoplastic disorder affecting the neuromuscular junction where the antibody to voltage-gated calcium channel (VGCC) impairs release of acetylcholine from nerve terminus. Anti-VGCC antibodies are rarely seen in patients with bladder carcinoma. Presentation mimics that of myasthenia gravis, only the limbs are predominately weak and oculobulbar muscles are spared. Anti-Yo antibodies are associated with cerebellar degeneration in patients with bladder cancer [113]. Symptoms include weeks to months of progressive ataxia, dysarthria, diplopia, nystagmus, and ophthalmoplegia. Imaging reveals cerebellar atrophy late in the disease.

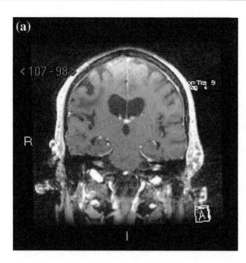

Fig. 25.3 MRIs of an 80-year-old man with bladder cancer. He had recently received carboplatin and gemcitabine with a complete systemic radiographic response but developed low back pain followed by deafness and gait ataxia. **a** Coronal T1 post-contrast images reveal patchy bilateral enhancement of VIII nerves. **b** Sagittal T1 post-contrast image demonstrates enhancement of the distal cord and cauda equina with signal abnormality involving the distal cord and conus

Other

Retroperitoneal metastases may locally invade the lumbosacral plexus causing a plexopathy. Patients commonly present with back pain and may have radiographic evidence of retroperitoneal mass on imaging. Treatment includes radiation [95].

Testicular Cancer

Although testicular cancer is the most common solid malignancy diagnosed in men between 15 and 35 years of age [105], it accounts for <1% of all newly diagnosed cancers in the USA [1]. It is among the most curable solid tumors with five-year survival rates >95% in the USA [1]. Greater than 95% are germ-cell tumors (GCT), which are broadly classified as seminomas or nonseminomatous germ-cell tumors (NSGCTs). Seminomas are more likely to present with localized disease, have a lower tendency to metastasize, and are highly radiosensitive. NSGCTs carry a worse prognosis and are more radioresistant [114]. Metastases occur most often to the chest, retroperitoneum, or neck. Early stage disease may be cured with orchiectomy. However, higher risk patients may require adjuvant chemotherapy; such as bleomycin, etoposide, and cisplatin (BEP) or etoposide plus cisplatin (EP) [115]. Though neurologic complications from testicular cancer are relatively rare, there are several syndromes of particular importance.

Brain Metastases

Brain metastases develop in 0.4–4% of men with metastatic germ-cell tumors and are associated with poor prognosis [116, 117]. Metastases to the brain are more common in nonseminomatous tumors [118]. Patients presenting with synchronous disease at the time of diagnoses are felt to have platinum-sensitive disease and have five-year survival rates of 45% [116]. However, patients who relapse in the brain either during or after chemotherapy treatment have far poorer prognosis with five-year survival rates of 12% [116, 118].

Brain metastases from testicular germ-cell tumors are felt to be sensitive to chemotherapy; first line treatment involves cisplatin and etoposide, both of which have some blood–brain barrier penetration. Surgery or focal radiation may be appropriate in certain clinical scenarios. Whole-brain radiation, however, is reserved for patients with refractory disease given the risk of delayed neurotoxicity [116, 118, 119].

Leptomeningeal Metastases

There are case reports of leptomeningeal carcinomatosis from testicular cancer in patients with seminomatous [120] and nonseminomatous [121–123] tumors. Similar to intracranial metastases, it is likely a marker of advanced disease with CNS relapse of aggressive disease after treatment with therapy that does not cross the blood–brain barrier. Treatment with radiation is usually recommended [122].

Epidural Spinal Cord Compression

Epidural spinal cord compression secondary to metastatic germ-cell tumors is rare and accounts for <1% of spinal metastases [124]. Treatment may include surgical intervention for unstable spine or rapidly deteriorating neurologic function. Radiation may be used for radiosensitive seminomas, or platinum-based therapy given the chemosensitivity of GCT [124, 125].

Paraneoplastic Syndrome

Limbic encephalitis is a constellation of symptoms in behavioral changes, sleep disruption, seizures, and memory impairment. MRI depicts non-enhancing, T2/FLAIR changes most commonly in the temporal lobes. Anti-Ma2-associated encephalitis (also known as anti-Ta) may also affect the diencephalon or brainstem and is found in patients with testicular cancer [126, 127]. Symptoms may also include ophthalmoplegia or other eye abnormalities and sleep disorders [128]. Ma2-associated encephalitis is more responsive to treatment directed against testicular cancer and immunotherapy and is associated with a better outcome than other causes of limbic encephalitis [128, 129]. Dermatomyositis has been associated with testicular cancer [130]. Presenting symptoms include progressive pain and hypertrophy of proximal muscles and violet-colored rash of the face and hands.

Chemotherapy-Related Neurologic Complications

Treatment for testicular cancer is highly dependent on platinum-based therapy. This puts patients at high risk for developing peripheral neuropathy and ototoxicity. The incidence of persistent paresthesias is estimated at 29% for testicular cancers, and neuropathy may persist for years [131]. Ototoxicity is an even more prevalent toxicity from platinum therapy with ∼20% long-term survivors reporting tinnitus and hearing loss [131, 132].

Targeted agents used to treat RCC also have associated neurologic toxicities. The VEGFR kinase inhibitors (KIs), such as sorafenib and sunitinib, have been associated with increased risk of hemorrhage and seizures [63]. This has particularly been seen in patients with brain metastases [133]. There are also several case reports in the literature of reversible posterior leukoencephalopathy syndrome (RPLS) in patients with RCC treated with sunitinib [134, 135]. Several of these neurologic toxicities are also seen with bevacizumab, including hemorrhage and RPLS, as well as the risk of intracranial ischemia [136].

Patients with prostate cancer treated with androgen deprivation therapy will frequently experience fatigue, insomnia, and cognitive changes. Though it is unclear if this is a direct medication or result of androgen withdraw, there is no clear correlation with testosterone levels [137]. Prostate cancer patients treated with taxanes, such as docetaxel or cabazitaxel, are at risk for developing a sensory neuropathy. Though less neurotoxic than paclitaxel, sensory and motor neuropathies are seen more often in cumulative doses in excess of 400 mg/m^2 for docetaxel [138]. Cabazitaxel appears less neurotoxic with peripheral neuropathy noted in <20% of patients [139, 140].

Conclusion

In conclusion, tumors of the genitourinary system are a common and heterogeneous group of malignancies affecting people of all ages with varying prognosis. Neurologic complications from these malignancies are an important cause of morbidity and mortality and can result from metastatic disease and treatment. As outcomes from patients with these malignancies improve, neurologic sequelae from delayed relapse and chronic treatment-related effects are likely to increase. Management of these neurologic complications from genitourinary cancer is an important focus for future research.

References

1. Howlader N, Noone AM, Krapcho M, Garshell J, Miller D, Altekruse SF, et al. SEER cancer statistics review, 1975–2012, National Cancer Institute. Bethesda, MD, http://seer.cancer.gov/csr/1975_2012/, based on November 2014 SEER data submission, posted to the SEER web site, April 2015. Accessed June 2015.
2. Prostate. AJCC cancer staging mannual. New York: Springer; 2010. p. 457.
3. Hoffman RM, Koyama T, Fan KH, Albertsen PC, Barry MJ, Goodman M, et al. Mortality after radical prostatectomy or external beam radiotherapy for localized prostate cancer. J Natl Cancer Inst. 2013;105(10):711–8.
4. Nepple KG, Stephenson AJ, Kallogjeri D, Michalski J, Grubb RL III, Strope SA, et al. Mortality after prostate cancer treatment with radical prostatectomy, external-beam radiation therapy, or brachytherapy in men without comorbidity. Eur Urol. 2013;64(3):372–8.
5. http://www.nccn.org/professionals/physician_gls/f_guidelines.asp NCCNNNCpgio. Accessed 21 June 2015.
6. Basch E, Loblaw DA, Oliver TK, Carducci M, Chen RC, Frame JN, et al. Systemic therapy in men with metastatic castration-resistant prostate cancer: American Society of Clinical Oncology and Cancer Care Ontario clinical practice guideline. J Clin Oncol. 2014;32(30):3436–48.
7. Talcott JA, Manola J, Clark JA, Kaplan I, Beard CJ, Mitchell SP, et al. Time course and predictors of symptoms after primary prostate cancer therapy. J Clin Oncol. 2003;21(21):3979–86.
8. Beard CJ, Lamb C, Buswell L, Schneider L, Propert KJ, Gladstone D, et al. Radiation-associated morbidity in patients

undergoing small-field external beam irradiation for prostate cancer. Int J Radiat Oncol Biol Phys. 1998;41(2):257–62.

9. Buyyounouski MK, Horwitz EM, Price RA, Hanlon AL, Uzzo RG, Pollack A. Intensity-modulated radiotherapy with MRI simulation to reduce doses received by erectile tissue during prostate cancer treatment. Int J Radiat Oncol Biol Phys. 2004;58 (3):743–9.

10. Spaliviero M, Steinberg AP, Kaouk JH, Desai MM, Hammert WC, Gill IS. Laparoscopic injury and repair of obturator nerve during radical prostatectomy. Urology. 2004;64(5):1030.

11. Tremont-Lukats IW, Bobustuc G, Lagos GK, Lolas K, Kyritsis AP, Puduvalli VK. Brain metastasis from prostate carcinoma: The M. D. Anderson Cancer Center experience. Cancer. 2003;98 (2):363–8.

12. Salvati M, Frati A, Russo N, Brogna C, Piccirilli M, D'Andrea G, et al. Brain metastasis from prostate cancer. Report of 13 cases and critical analysis of the literature. J Exp Clin Cancer Res. 2005;24(2):203–7.

13. Nussbaum ES, Djalilian HR, Cho KH, Hall WA. Brain metastases. Histology, multiplicity, surgery, and survival. Cancer. 1996;78(8):1781–8.

14. McCutcheon IE. Author reply. Cancer. 2000;89(3):707.

15. Bubendorf L, Schopfer A, Wagner U, Sauter G, Moch H, Willi N, et al. Metastatic patterns of prostate cancer: an autopsy study of 1,589 patients. Hum Pathol. 2000;31(5):578–83.

16. Long MA, Husband JE. Features of unusual metastases from prostate cancer. Br J Radiol. 1999;72(862):933–41.

17. Raizer JJ, DeAngelis LM. Cerebral sinus thrombosis diagnosed by MRI and MR venography in cancer patients. Neurology. 2000;54(6):1222–6.

18. McDermott RS, Anderson PR, Greenberg RE, Milestone BN, Hudes GR. Cranial nerve deficits in patients with metastatic prostate carcinoma: clinical features and treatment outcomes. Cancer. 2004;101(7):1639–43.

19. Seymore CH, Peeples WJ. Cranial nerve involvement with carcinoma of prostate. Urology. 1988;31(3):211–3.

20. Kleinschmidt-DeMasters BK. Dural metastases. A retrospective surgical and autopsy series. Arch Pathol Lab Med. 2001;125 (7):880–7.

21. Orphanos G, Ardavanis A. Leptomeningeal metastases from prostate cancer: an emerging clinical conundrum. Clin Exp Metastasis. 2010;27(1):19–23.

22. Lin C, Turner S, Gurney H, Peduto A. Increased detections of leptomeningeal presentations in men with hormone refractory prostate cancer: an effect of improved systemic therapy? J Med Imaging Radiat Oncol. 2008;52(4):376–81.

23. Cone LA, Koochek K, Henager HA, Fausel R, Gade-Andavolu R, Potts BE, et al. Leptomeningeal carcinomatosis in a patient with metastatic prostate cancer: case report and literature review. Surg Neurol. 2006;65(4):372–5, discussion 5–6.

24. Mak KS, Lee LK, Mak RH, Wang S, Pile-Spellman J, Abrahm JL, et al. Incidence and treatment patterns in hospitalizations for malignant spinal cord compression in the United States, 1998–2006. Int J Radiat Oncol Biol Phys. 2011;80 (3):824–31.

25. Schiff D, O'Neill BP, Suman VJ. Spinal epidural metastasis as the initial manifestation of malignancy: clinical features and diagnostic approach. Neurology. 1997;49(2):452–6.

26. Posner JB. Neurologic complications of cancer. Philadelphia: FA Davis; 1995.

27. Gerszten PC, Mendel E, Yamada Y. Radiotherapy and radiosurgery for metastatic spine disease: what are the options, indications, and outcomes? Spine (Phila Pa 1976). 2009;34(22 Suppl):S78–92.

28. Maranzano E, Latini P. Effectiveness of radiation therapy without surgery in metastatic spinal cord compression: final results from a prospective trial. Int J Radiat Oncol Biol Phys. 1995;32(4):959–67.

29. Flynn DF, Shipley WU. Management of spinal cord compression secondary to metastatic prostatic carcinoma. Urol Clin North Am. 1991;18(1):145–52.

30. Patchell RA, Tibbs PA, Regine WF, Payne R, Saris S, Kryscio RJ, et al. Direct decompressive surgical resection in the treatment of spinal cord compression caused by metastatic cancer: a randomised trial. Lancet. 2005;366(9486):643–8.

31. Zelefsky MJ, Scher HI, Krol G, Portenoy RK, Leibel SA, Fuks ZY. Spinal epidural tumor in patients with prostate cancer. Clinical and radiographic predictors of response to radiation therapy. Cancer. 1992;70(9):2319–25.

32. Tazi H, Manunta A, Rodriguez A, Patard JJ, Lobel B, Guille F. Spinal cord compression in metastatic prostate cancer. Eur Urol. 2003;44(5):527–32.

33. Smith EM, Hampel N, Ruff RL, Bodner DR, Resnick MI. Spinal cord compression secondary to prostate carcinoma: treatment and prognosis. J Urol. 1993;149(2):330–3.

34. Rades D, Lange M, Veninga T, Rudat V, Bajrovic A, Stalpers LJ, et al. Preliminary results of spinal cord compression recurrence evaluation (score-1) study comparing short-course versus long-course radiotherapy for local control of malignant epidural spinal cord compression. Int J Radiat Oncol Biol Phys. 2009;73 (1):228–34.

35. Rades D, Stalpers LJ, Veninga T, Schulte R, Hoskin PJ, Obralic N, et al. Evaluation of five radiation schedules and prognostic factors for metastatic spinal cord compression. J Clin Oncol. 2005;23(15):3366–75.

36. Huddart RA, Rajan B, Law M, Meyer L, Dearnaley DP. Spinal cord compression in prostate cancer: treatment outcome and prognostic factors. Radiother Oncol. 1997;44(3):229–36.

37. Baird AD, Cornford PA, Helliwell T, Woolfenden KA. Small cell prostate cancer with anti-Hu positive peripheral neuropathy. J Urol. 2002;168(1):192.

38. Graus F, Keime-Guibert F, Rene R, Benyahia B, Ribalta T, Ascaso C, et al. Anti-Hu-associated paraneoplastic encephalomyelitis: analysis of 200 patients. Brain. 2001;124(Pt 6):1138–48.

39. Stern RC, Hulette CM. Paraneoplastic limbic encephalitis associated with small cell carcinoma of the prostate. Mod Pathol. 1999;12(8):814–8.

40. Matschke J, Kromminga A, Erbersdobler A, Lamszus K, Anders S, Kofuncu E. Paraneoplastic cerebellar degeneration and anti-Yo antibodies in a man with prostatic adenocarcinoma. J Neurol Neurosurg Psychiatry. 2007;78(7):775–7.

41. Delahunt B, Abernethy DA, Johnson CA, Nacey JN. Prostate carcinoma and the Lambert-Eaton myasthenic syndrome. J Urol. 2003;169(1):278–9.

42. Mooney CJ, Dunphy EJ, Stone B, McNeel DG. Identification of autoantibodies elicited in a patient with prostate cancer presenting as dermatomyositis. Int J Urol. 2006;13(3):211–7.

43. Jemal A, Siegel R, Ward E, Hao Y, Xu J, Murray T, et al. Cancer statistics, 2008. CA Cancer J Clin. 2008;58(2):71–96.

44. Jemal A, Siegel R, Ward E, Murray T, Xu J, Thun MJ. Cancer statistics, 2007. CA Cancer J Clin. 2007;57(1):43–66.

45. Cairns P. Renal cell carcinoma. Cancer Biomark. 2010;9(1–6):461–73.

46. Hatcher PA, Anderson EE, Paulson DF, Carson CC, Robertson JE. Surgical management and prognosis of renal cell carcinoma invading the vena cava. J Urol. 1991;145(1):20–3; discussion 3–4.

47. Cherrie RJ, Goldman DG, Lindner A, deKernion JB. Prognostic implications of vena caval extension of renal cell carcinoma. J Urol. 1982;128(5):910–2.
48. Anderson CB, Clark PE, Morgan TM, Stratton KL, Herrell SD, Davis R, et al. Urinary collecting system invasion is a predictor for overall and disease-specific survival in locally invasive renal cell carcinoma. Urology. 2011;78(1):99–104.
49. Escudier B, Szczylik C, Hutson TE, Demkow T, Staehler M, Rolland F, et al. Randomized phase II trial of first-line treatment with sorafenib versus interferon Alfa-2a in patients with metastatic renal cell carcinoma. J Clin Oncol. 2009;27(8):1280–9.
50. Rini BI, Halabi S, Rosenberg JE, Stadler WM, Vaena DA, Ou SS, et al. Bevacizumab plus interferon alfa compared with interferon alfa monotherapy in patients with metastatic renal cell carcinoma: CALGB 90206. J Clin Oncol. 2008;26(33):5422–8.
51. Heng DY, Choueiri TK, Rini BI, Lee J, Yuasa T, Pal SK, et al. Outcomes of patients with metastatic renal cell carcinoma that do not meet eligibility criteria for clinical trials. Ann Oncol. 2014;25 (1):149–54.
52. Motzer RJ, Hutson TE, McCann L, Deen K, Choueiri TK. Overall survival in renal-cell carcinoma with pazopanib versus sunitinib. N Engl J Med. 2014;370(18):1769–70.
53. Motzer RJ, Hutson TE, Cella D, Reeves J, Hawkins R, Guo J, et al. Pazopanib versus sunitinib in metastatic renal-cell carcinoma. N Engl J Med. 2013;369(8):722–31.
54. Saitoh H. Distant metastasis of renal adenocarcinoma. Cancer. 1981;48(6):1487–91.
55. Delattre JY, Krol G, Thaler HT, Posner JB. Distribution of brain metastases. Arch Neurol. 1988;45(7):741–4.
56. Bastos DA, Molina AM, Hatzoglou V, Jia X, Velasco S, Patil S, et al. Safety and efficacy of targeted therapy for renal cell carcinoma with brain metastasis. Clin Genitourin Cancer. 2015;13(1):59–66.
57. Shuch B, La Rochelle JC, Klatte T, Riggs SB, Liu W, Kabbinavar FF, et al. Brain metastasis from renal cell carcinoma: presentation, recurrence, and survival. Cancer. 2008;113 (7):1641–8.
58. Sperduto PW, Kased N, Roberge D, Xu Z, Shanley R, Luo X, et al. Summary report on the graded prognostic assessment: an accurate and facile diagnosis-specific tool to estimate survival for patients with brain metastases. J Clin Oncol. 2012;30(4):419–25.
59. Vogl UM, Bojic M, Lamm W, Frischer JM, Pichelmayer O, Kramer G, et al. Extracerebral metastases determine the outcome of patients with brain metastases from renal cell carcinoma. BMC Cancer. 2010;10:480.
60. Muacevic A, Kreth FW, Mack A, Tonn JC, Wowra B. Stereotactic radiosurgery without radiation therapy providing high local tumor control of multiple brain metastases from renal cell carcinoma. Minim Invasive Neurosurg. 2004;47(4):203–8.
61. Shuto T, Inomori S, Fujino H, Nagano H. Gamma knife surgery for metastatic brain tumors from renal cell carcinoma. J Neurosurg. 2006;105(4):555–60.
62. Wowra B, Siebels M, Muacevic A, Kreth FW, Mack A, Hofstetter A. Repeated gamma knife surgery for multiple brain metastases from renal cell carcinoma. J Neurosurg. 2002;97 (4):785–93.
63. Gore ME, Hariharan S, Porta C, Bracarda S, Hawkins R, Bjarnason GA, et al. Sunitinib in metastatic renal cell carcinoma patients with brain metastases. Cancer. 2011;117(3):501–9.
64. Stadler WM, Figlin RA, McDermott DF, Dutcher JP, Knox JJ, Miller WH Jr, et al. Safety and efficacy results of the advanced renal cell carcinoma sorafenib expanded access program in North America. Cancer. 2010;116(5):1272–80.
65. Chevreau C, Ravaud A, Escudier B, Amela E, Delva R, Rolland F, et al. A phase II trial of sunitinib in patients with renal cell cancer and untreated brain metastases. Clin Genitourin Cancer. 2014;12(1):50–4.
66. Richey SL, Tamboli P, Ng CS, Lin E, Lim ZD, Araujo JC, et al. Phase II trial of pemetrexed plus gemcitabine in patients with locally advanced and metastatic nonclear cell renal cell carcinoma. Am J Clin Oncol. 2013;36(5):450–4.
67. Henderson CA, Bukowski RM, Stadler WM, Dutcher JP, Kindwall-Keller TL, Hotte SJ, et al. The Advanced Renal Cell Carcinoma Sorafenib (ARCCS) expanded access trial: subset analysis of patients (pts) with brain metastases (BM). J Clin Oncol. 2007;25(18S (June 20 Supplement)).
68. Massard C, Zonierek J, Gross-Goupil M, Fizazi K, Szczylik C, Escudier B. Incidence of brain metastases in renal cell carcinoma treated with sorafenib. Ann Oncol. 2010;21(5):1027–31.
69. Crino PB, Sater RA, Sperling M, Katsetos CD. Renal cell carcinomatous meningitis: pathologic and immunohistochemical features. Neurology. 1995;45(1):189–91.
70. Chilkulwar A, Pottimutyapu R, Wu F, Padooru KR, Pingali SR, Kassem M. Leptomeningeal carcinomatosis associated with papillary renal cell carcinoma. Ecancermedicalscience. 2014;8:468.
71. Zekri J, Ahmed N, Coleman RE, Hancock BW. The skeletal metastatic complications of renal cell carcinoma. Int J Oncol. 2001;19(2):379–82.
72. Hosono N, Ueda T, Tamura D, Aoki Y, Yoshikawa H. Prognostic relevance of clinical symptoms in patients with spinal metastases. Clin Orthop Relat Res. 2005;436:196–201.
73. Tatsui CE, Suki D, Rao G, Kim SS, Salaskar A, Hatiboglu MA, et al. Factors affecting survival in 267 consecutive patients undergoing surgery for spinal metastasis from renal cell carcinoma. J Neurosurg Spine. 2014;20(1):108–16.
74. Giehl JP, Kluba T. Metastatic spine disease in renal cell carcinoma–indication and results of surgery. Anticancer Res. 1999;19(2C):1619–23.
75. Jackson RJ, Loh SC, Gokaslan ZL. Metastatic renal cell carcinoma of the spine: surgical treatment and results. J Neurosurg. 2001;94(1 Suppl):18–24.
76. King GJ, Kostuik JP, McBroom RJ, Richardson W. Surgical management of metastatic renal carcinoma of the spine. Spine (Phila Pa 1976). 1991;16(3):265–71.
77. Sundaresan N, Scher H, DiGiacinto GV, Yagoda A, Whitmore W, Choi IS. Surgical treatment of spinal cord compression in kidney cancer. J Clin Oncol. 1986;4(12):1851–6.
78. Halperin EC, Harisiadis L. The role of radiation therapy in the management of metastatic renal cell carcinoma. Cancer. 1983;51 (4):614–7.
79. Fuhrman SA, Lasky LC, Limas C. Prognostic significance of morphologic parameters in renal cell carcinoma. Am J Surg Pathol. 1982;6(7):655–63.
80. Ryu S, Rock J, Jain R, Lu M, Anderson J, Jin JY, et al. Radiosurgical decompression of metastatic epidural compression. Cancer. 2010;116(9):2250–7.
81. Moulding HD, Elder JB, Lis E, Lovelock DM, Zhang Z, Yamada Y, et al. Local disease control after decompressive surgery and adjuvant high-dose single-fraction radiosurgery for spine metastases. J Neurosurg Spine. 2010;13(1):87–93.
82. Laufer I, Iorgulescu JB, Chapman T, Lis E, Shi W, Zhang Z, et al. Local disease control for spinal metastases following "separation surgery" and adjuvant hypofractionated or high-dose single-fraction stereotactic radiosurgery: outcome analysis in 186 patients. J Neurosurg Spine. 2013;18(3):207–14.
83. Sung WS, Sung MJ, Chan JH, Manion B, Song J, Dubey A, et al. Intramedullary spinal cord metastases: a 20-year institutional experience with a comprehensive literature review. World Neurosurg. 2013;79(3–4):576–84.

84. Fakih M, Schiff D, Erlich R, Logan TF. Intramedullary spinal cord metastasis (ISCM) in renal cell carcinoma: a series of six cases. Ann Oncol. 2001;12(8):1173–7.

85. Donovan DJ, Freeman JH. Solitary intramedullary spinal cord tumor presenting as the initial manifestation of metastatic renal cell carcinoma: case report. Spine (Phila Pa 1976). 2006;31(14): E460–3.

86. Bell BB, Tognoni PG, Bihrle R. Limbic encephalitis as a paraneoplastic manifestation of renal cell carcinoma. J Urol. 1998;160(3 Pt 1):828.

87. De Luca S, Terrone C, Crivellaro S, De Zan A, Polo P, Vigliani MC, et al. Opsoclonus-myoclonus syndrome as a paraneoplastic manifestation of renal cell carcinoma. a case report and review of the literature. Urol Int. 2002;68(3):206–8.

88. Schaefer O, Lohrmann C, Harder J, Veelken H, Langer M. Treatment of renal cell carcinoma-associated dermatomyositis with renal arterial embolization and percutaneous radiofrequency heat ablation. J Vasc Interv Radiol. 2004;15(1 Pt 1):97–9.

89. Kishi K, Hirota T, Matsumoto K, Kakizoe T, Murase T, Fujita J. Carcinoma of the bladder: a clinical and pathological analysis of 87 autopsy cases. J Urol. 1981;125(1):36–9.

90. Wallmeroth A, Wagner U, Moch H, Gasser TC, Sauter G, Mihatsch MJ. Patterns of metastasis in muscle-invasive bladder cancer (pT2-4): An autopsy study on 367 patients. Urol Int. 1999;62(2):69–75.

91. Babjuk M, Burger M, Zigeuner R, Shariat SF, van Rhijn BW, Comperat E, et al. EAU guidelines on non-muscle-invasive urothelial carcinoma of the bladder: update 2013. Eur Urol. 2013;64(4):639–53.

92. Hall MC, Chang SS, Dalbagni G, Pruthi RS, Seigne JD, Skinner EC, et al. Guideline for the management of nonmuscle invasive bladder cancer (stages Ta, T1, and Tis): 2007 update. J Urol. 2007;178(6):2314–30.

93. Grossman HB, Natale RB, Tangen CM, Speights VO, Vogelzang NJ, Trump DL, et al. Neoadjuvant chemotherapy plus cystectomy compared with cystectomy alone for locally advanced bladder cancer. N Engl J Med. 2003;349(9): 859–66.

94. von der Maase H, Hansen SW, Roberts JT, Dogliotti L, Oliver T, Moore MJ, et al. Gemcitabine and cisplatin versus methotrexate, vinblastine, doxorubicin, and cisplatin in advanced or metastatic bladder cancer: results of a large, randomized, multinational, multicenter, phase III study. J Clin Oncol. 2000;18(17):3068–77.

95. Anderson TS, Regine WF, Kryscio R, Patchell RA. Neurologic complications of bladder carcinoma: a review of 359 cases. Cancer. 2003;97(9):2267–72.

96. Clatterbuck RE, Sampath P, Olivi A. Transitional cell carcinoma presenting as a solitary brain lesion: a case report and review of the world literature. J Neurooncol. 1998;39(1):91–4.

97. Dhote R, Beuzeboc P, Thiounn N, Flam T, Zerbib M, Christoforov B, et al. High incidence of brain metastases in patients treated with an M-VAC regimen for advanced bladder cancer. Eur Urol. 1998;33(4):392–5.

98. Sternberg CN, Yagoda A, Scher HI, Watson RC, Herr HW, Morse MJ, et al. M-VAC (methotrexate, vinblastine, doxorubicin and cisplatin) for advanced transitional cell carcinoma of the urothelium. J Urol. 1988;139(3):461–9.

99. Bianchi M, Roghmann F, Becker A, Sukumar S, Briganti A, Menon M, et al. Age-stratified distribution of metastatic sites in bladder cancer: a population-based analysis. Can Urol Assoc J. 2014;8(3–4):E148–58.

100. Mahmoud-Ahmed AS, Suh JH, Kupelian PA, Klein EA, Peereboom DM, Dreicer R, et al. Brain metastases from bladder carcinoma: presentation, treatment and survival. J Urol. 2002;167 (6):2419–22.

101. Bloch JL, Nieh PT, Walzak MP. Brain metastases from transitional cell carcinoma. J Urol. 1987;137(1):97–9.

102. Fokas E, Henzel M, Engenhart-Cabillic R. A comparison of radiotherapy with radiotherapy plus surgery for brain metastases from urinary bladder cancer: analysis of 62 patients. Strahlenther Onkol. 2010;186(10):565–71.

103. Rades D, Meyners T, Veninga T, Stalpers LJ, Schild SE. Hypofractionated whole-brain radiotherapy for multiple brain metastases from transitional cell carcinoma of the bladder. Int J Radiat Oncol Biol Phys. 2010;78(2):404–8.

104. Eng C, Cunningham D, Quade BJ, Schwamm L, Kantoff PW, Skarin AT. Meningeal carcinomatosis from transitional cell carcinoma of the bladder. Cancer. 1993;72(2):553–7.

105. Mandell S, Wernz J, Morales P, Weinberg H, Steinfeld A. Carcinomatous meningitis from transitional cell carcinoma of bladder. Urology. 1985;25(5):520–1.

106. Bruna J, Rojas-Marcos I, Martinez-Yelamos S, Catala I, Vidaller A, Galan C, et al. Meningeal carcinomatosis as the first manifestation of a transitional cell carcinoma of the bladder. J Neurooncol. 2003;63(1):63–7.

107. Sacco E, Pinto F, Sasso F, Racioppi M, Gulino G, Volpe A, et al. Paraneoplastic syndromes in patients with urological malignancies. Urol Int. 2009;83(1):1–11.

108. Lowe BA, Mershon C, Mangalik A. Paraneoplastic neurological syndrome in transitional cell carcinoma of the bladder. J Urol. 1992;147(2):462–4.

109. Prestigiacomo CJ, Balmaceda C, Dalmau J. Anti-Ri-associated paraneoplastic opsoclonus-ataxia syndrome in a man with transitional cell carcinoma. Cancer. 2001;91(8):1423–8.

110. Hill CL, Zhang Y, Sigurgeirsson B, Pukkala E, Mellemkjaer L, Airio A, et al. Frequency of specific cancer types in dermatomyositis and polymyositis: a population-based study. Lancet. 2001;357(9250):96–100.

111. Sabio JM, Vargas-Hitos JA, Jimenez-Alonso J. Paraneoplastic dermatomyositis associated with bladder cancer. Lupus. 2006;15 (9):619–20.

112. Collins DR, Connolly S, Burns M, Offiah L, Grainger R, Walsh JB. Lambert-eaton myasthenic syndrome in association with transitional cell carcinoma: a previously unrecognized association. Urology. 1999;54(1):162.

113. Greenlee JE, Dalmau J, Lyons T, Clawson S, Smith RH, Pirch HR. Association of anti-Yo (type I) antibody with paraneoplastic cerebellar degeneration in the setting of transitional cell carcinoma of the bladder: detection of Yo antigen in tumor tissue and fall in antibody titers following tumor removal. Ann Neurol. 1999;45(6):805–9.

114. Horwich A, Shipley J, Huddart R. Testicular germ-cell cancer. Lancet. 2006;367(9512):754–65.

115. Feldman DR, Bosl GJ, Sheinfeld J, Motzer RJ. Medical treatment of advanced testicular cancer. JAMA. 2008;299(6):672–84.

116. Fossa SD, Bokemeyer C, Gerl A, Culine S, Jones WG, Mead GM, et al. Treatment outcome of patients with brain metastases from malignant germ cell tumors. Cancer. 1999;85(4):988–97.

117. Raina V, Singh SP, Kamble N, Tanwar R, Rao K, Dawar R, et al. Brain metastasis as the site of relapse in germ cell tumor of testis. Cancer. 1993;72(7):2182–5.

118. Bokemeyer C, Nowak P, Haupt A, Metzner B, Kohne H, Hartmann JT, et al. Treatment of brain metastases in patients with testicular cancer. J Clin Oncol. 1997;15(4):1449–54.

119. Spears WT, Morphis JG II, Lester SG, Williams SD, Einhorn LH. Brain metastases and testicular tumors: long-term survival. Int J Radiat Oncol Biol Phys. 1992;22(1):17–22.

120. Mackey JR, Venner P. Seminoma with isolated central nervous system relapse, and salvage with craniospinal irradiation. Urology. 1998;51(6):1043–5.

121. Miranda P, Ramos A, Ricoy JR. Images in neuro-oncology: brain metastases and leptomeningeal dissemination of nonseminomatous germ cell tumor. J Neurooncol. 2005;73(1):51–2.

122. Onesti E, Fabi A, Mingoia M, Savarese A, Anelli V, Koudriavtseva T. Leptomeningeal carcinomatosis in aggressive germ non-seminoma testicular tumor: a case report and review of literature. Clin Neurol Neurosurg. 2012;114(7):1081–5.

123. Denissen NH, van Spronsen DJ, Smilde TJ, De Mulder PH. Leptomeningeal carcinomatosis in relapsed non-seminoma testis: a 1-year complete remission with high-dose chemotherapy. Anticancer Drugs. 2005;16(8):897–9.

124. Arnold PM, Morgan CJ, Morantz RA, Eckard DA, Kepes JJ. Metastatic testicular cancer presenting as spinal cord compression: report of two cases. Surg Neurol. 2000;54(1):27–33.

125. Cooper K, Bajorin D, Shapiro W, Krol G, Sze G, Bosl GJ. Decompression of epidural metastases from germ cell tumors with chemotherapy. J Neurooncol. 1990;8(3):275–80.

126. Gultekin SH, Rosenfeld MR, Voltz R, Eichen J, Posner JB, Dalmau J. Paraneoplastic limbic encephalitis: neurological symptoms, immunological findings and tumour association in 50 patients. Brain. 2000;123(Pt 7):1481–94.

127. Voltz R, Gultekin SH, Rosenfeld MR, Gerstner E, Eichen J, Posner JB, et al. A serologic marker of paraneoplastic limbic and brain-stem encephalitis in patients with testicular cancer. N Engl J Med. 1999;340(23):1788–95.

128. Dalmau J, Graus F, Villarejo A, Posner JB, Blumenthal D, Thiessen B, et al. Clinical analysis of anti-Ma2-associated encephalitis. Brain. 2004;127(Pt 8):1831–44.

129. Hoffmann LA, Jarius S, Pellkofer HL, Schueller M, Krumbholz M, Koenig F, et al. Anti-Ma and anti-Ta associated paraneoplastic neurological syndromes: 22 newly diagnosed patients and review of previous cases. J Neurol Neurosurg Psychiatry. 2008;79(7):767–73.

130. Di Stasi SM, Poggi A, Giannantoni A, Zampa G. Dermatomyositis associated with testicular germ cell cancer. J Urol. 2000;163(1):240.

131. Brydoy M, Oldenburg J, Klepp O, Bremnes RM, Wist EA, Wentzel-Larsen T, et al. Observational study of prevalence of long-term Raynaud-like phenomena and neurological side effects in testicular cancer survivors. J Natl Cancer Inst. 2009;101 (24):1682–95.

132. Bokemeyer C, Berger CC, Hartmann JT, Kollmannsberger C, Schmoll HJ, Kuczyk MA, et al. Analysis of risk factors for cisplatin-induced ototoxicity in patients with testicular cancer. Br J Cancer. 1998;77(8):1355–62.

133. Pouessel D, Culine S. High frequency of intracerebral hemorrhage in metastatic renal carcinoma patients with brain metastases treated with tyrosine kinase inhibitors targeting the vascular endothelial growth factor receptor. Eur Urol. 2008;53(2):376–81.

134. Chen A, Agarwal N. Reversible posterior leucoencephalopathy syndrome associated with sunitinib. Int Med J. 2009;39(5):341–2.

135. Duchnowska R, Miciuk B, Bodnar L, Wasniewski L, Szczylik C. Severe neurological symptoms in a patient with advanced renal cell carcinoma treated with sunitinib. J Oncol Pharm Pract. 2013;19(2):186–9.

136. Armstrong TS, Wen PY, Gilbert MR, Schiff D. Management of treatment-associated toxicites of anti-angiogenic therapy in patients with brain tumors. Neuro Oncol. 2012;14(10):1203–14.

137. Kumar RJ, Barqawi A, Crawford ED. Adverse events associated with hormonal therapy for prostate cancer. Rev Urol. 2005;7 (Suppl 5):S37–43.

138. Grisold W, Cavaletti G, Windebank AJ. Peripheral neuropathies from chemotherapeutics and targeted agents: diagnosis, treatment, and prevention. Neuro Oncol. 2012;14 Suppl 4:iv45–54.

139. Pivot X, Koralewski P, Hidalgo JL, Chan A, Goncalves A, Schwartsmann G, et al. A multicenter phase II study of XRP6258 administered as a 1-h i.v. infusion every 3 weeks in taxane-resistant metastatic breast cancer patients. Ann Oncol. 2008;19(9):1547–52.

140. de Bono JS, Oudard S, Ozguroglu M, Hansen S, Machiels JP, Kocak I, et al. Prednisone plus cabazitaxel or mitoxantrone for metastatic castration-resistant prostate cancer progressing after docetaxel treatment: a randomised open-label trial. Lancet. 2010;376(9747):1147–54.

Neurologic Complications of Female Reproductive Tract Cancers

K. Ina Ly and Maciej M. Mrugala

Introduction

Malignancies of the female reproductive tract can cause direct and indirect complications on the central and peripheral nervous system. Direct effects include malignant cell infiltration of the brain, spinal cord, nerve roots and plexi, and peripheral nerves, as well as compression of surrounding structures by the tumor itself or regional lymph nodes. With the exception of choriocarcinoma, gynecologic cancers, however, are regarded as "neurophobic" due to their low metastatic potential to the central nervous system (CNS). The most common gynecologic tumors to cause CNS metastases are chorio-, ovarian, and endometrial carcinoma. Indirect effects of gynecologic cancers include paraneoplastic syndromes, particularly paraneoplastic cerebellar degeneration and anti-NMDA receptor encephalitis, and complications of cancer treatment, such as chemotherapy-related peripheral neuropathy, surgery-induced peripheral nerve, and radiation-induced plexopathy. This chapter reviews the epidemiology, clinical features, treatment, and prognostic data of some of the most common metastatic, paraneoplastic, and treatment-related complications of gynecologic cancers.

K.I. Ly
Stephen E and Catherine Pappas Center for Neuro-Oncology, Massachusetts General Hospital, Yawkey 9E, 55 Fruit Street, Boston, MA 02114, USA
e-mail: ily@partners.org

K.I. Ly
Center for Neuro-Oncology, Dana-Farber Cancer Institute, Boston, MA, USA

M.M. Mrugala (✉)
Department of Neurology, University of Washington Medical School, Fred Hutchinson Cancer Research Center, 1959 NE Pacific St, Box 356465Seattle, WA 98195-6097, USA
e-mail: mmrugala@uw.edu

M.M. Mrugala
Department of Neurology and Division of Medical Oncology, Mayo Clinic, 5777 East Mayo Boulevard, Phoenix, AZ 85054, USA

© Springer International Publishing AG 2018
D. Schiff et al. (eds.), *Cancer Neurology in Clinical Practice*, DOI 10.1007/978-3-319-57901-6_26

Nervous System Metastases from Gynecologic Cancers

Choriocarcinoma

Choriocarcinomas are classified under the category of gestational trophoblastic diseases (GTDs). All types of GTDs arise from placental trophoblastic tissue after normal or abnormal fertilization [1]. They are grouped into hydatidiform moles (also known as "molar pregnancy" and subclassified into complete and partial hydatidiform moles) and gestational trophoblastic neoplasia (GTN; subclassified into invasive moles, choriocarcinoma, placental site trophoblastic tumor, and epithelioid trophoblastic tumor) [2]. Choriocarcinoma is the most aggressive type of GTN, due to its propensity for early vascular invasion and widespread metastasis, and causes CNS metastases in up to 40% of patients [3]. Although most cases of choriocarcinoma are gestational (i.e., arising from a normal or abnormal pregnancy), a non-gestational form also exists, which can be of gonadal (e.g., ovarian or testicular) or extragonadal origin (e.g., the pineal body, mediastinum, and retroperitoneum) [4].

The incidence of choriocarcinoma varies greatly with geographical location. According to the National Cancer Institute, the estimated incidence in the USA is 2–7 per 100,000 pregnancies [5], similar to incidence ratios in Europe, Australia, some areas of Latin America, and the Middle East [1]. In Asia, the incidence ranges from 5 to 12 per 100,000 in Japan and 63–202 per 100,000 in Thailand, India, Indonesia, and China [1]. These wide ranges are partly attributed to differences in reporting and diagnostic criteria. The two best established risk factors for choriocarcinoma are extremes of maternal age (<20 years, >40 years) and previous molar pregnancy [1]. The latter increases the risk of a subsequent one to 1%. With two or more previous molar pregnancies, this risk further increases to 25% [1, 6]. Most choriocarcinomas occur after a molar pregnancy but they can also be preceded by a normal term pregnancy, abortion, or ectopic pregnancy [4].

Histopathologically, choriocarcinoma is characterized by highly invasive and vascular masses of cytotrophoblasts and syncytiotrophoblasts without villi surrounded by necrosis and hemorrhage [1]. Human chorionic gonadotrophin (hCG) produced by malignant cells is characteristically elevated and serves as a tumor marker for diagnosis, monitoring of treatment response, and posttreatment surveillance [1, 6].

Classically, patients present with abnormal uterine bleeding. In addition, a rapidly enlarging uterus, pelvic pain, and signs of hCG overstimulation, including hyperemesis gravidarum, pre-eclampsia, and hyperthyroidism may be elicited. The most common sites of metastases are lung (80%), vagina (30%), brain (10%), and liver (10%) [7]. Patients may come to medical attention due to symptoms related to metastatic rather than primary disease such as dyspnea, cough, vaginal bleeding or purulent discharge, neurologic symptoms, jaundice, and epigastric pain [8]. Work-up of suspected choriocarcinoma should include pelvic examination, quantitative measurement of serum hCG, pelvic ultrasound, thyroid, liver, and renal function tests, and chest X-ray due to the high risk of pulmonary metastases. Further evaluation with CT of the chest, abdomen, and pelvis and brain MRI may be necessary if the initial work-up or clinical presentation is concerning for metastatic disease [8].

Choriocarcinoma is staged according to a combined system defined by the International Federation of Gynecology and Obstetrics (FIGO) and World Health Organization (WHO). The former includes the conventional anatomic staging criteria, whereas the latter incorporates a prognostic scoring system of eight variables that predicts response to single-agent chemotherapy (CHT) with methotrexate (MTX) and actinomycin D: age, antecedent pregnancy, interval from index pregnancy, pretreatment serum hCG level, largest tumor size (including uterus), site and number of metastases, and prior CHT [8]. Patients can be stratified as "low risk" (score 0–6) or "high risk" (score $\geq$ 7), which predicts low versus high resistance to single-agent CHT, respectively, and the need for multiple chemotherapeutic agents [8].

CNS metastases typically cause symptoms of increased intracranial pressure (ICP) , including headache, vision changes, nausea, vomiting, tinnitus, and altered mental status [8–10]. Other manifestations are hemiparesis and seizures, the latter being particularly common with cortically-based lesions. In addition to the standard aforementioned work-up, brain MRI with and without contrast is the diagnostic study of choice for CNS metastases [8]. The most common presentation is intracerebral hemorrhage, due to invasion of blood vessels by chorionic villi [10]. The diagnosis of metastatic choriocarcinoma should thus be considered in any woman of reproductive age with a hemorrhagic brain lesion.

Endovascular metastases can also lead to formation of cerebral aneurysms with subsequent rupture [11–14] (Fig. 26.1a–f) as well as arterial [15] and venous infarctions [16]. Spinal and epidural metastases are very rare [17–19].

Human chorionic gonadotropin levels can vary dramatically in metastatic CNS disease, ranging from <500 to >500,000 mIU/ml [9, 10, 20]. Given the high risk (70–100%) of concurrent lung involvement with CNS metastases [9, 10, 20–22], CT chest should be routinely performed as part of the work-up [8]. The rate of concurrent renal and liver metastases is lower, ranging from 12 to 19% [10, 20, 21]. Pelvic ultrasound is helpful to detect uterine involvement and identify those who may require hysterectomy [8].

Systemic CHT forms the cornerstone of treatment of metastatic choriocarcinoma and consists of MTX- and actinomycin D-based therapies. The most widely accepted approach is EMA-CO (etoposide, MTX, and actinomycin D, alternating weekly with cyclophosphamide and vincristine) or, in those with concurrent metastatic liver disease, EMA-EP (etoposide, MTX, and actinomycin D, alternating weekly with etoposide and cisplatin). The dose of MTX is lower (1 g/m^2) than that commonly used in other types of CNS malignancy such as primary CNS lymphoma (3.5–8 g/m^2), but higher than for metastatic choriocarcinoma to other systemic sites [20]. In those with a high burden of CNS disease or significant systemic involvement at the time of CNS diagnosis, low-dose etoposide and cisplatin can be administered before definitive treatment with EMA-CO/EP [20]. The duration of therapy varies among practitioners. The Charing Cross group recommends treatment until serum hCG levels have normalized, followed by consolidation for eight additional weeks thereafter [20, 21]. Others have given shorter courses of EMA-CO/EP (as few as two cycles) and EMA only as consolidation therapy (up to six cycles) [22]. In addition, dexamethasone should be administered to reduce cerebral edema.

The routine use of surgery, radiotherapy (XRT), and intrathecal (IT) CHT is controversial. Craniotomy with surgical resection of solitary or superficial metastases can prevent hemorrhage, relieve mass effect, and improve neurologic outcome. Whole-brain radiotherapy (WBRT) at 2000–3000 cGy (in fractions of 200–300 cGy) has been used at some centers with systemic EMA-CO/EP [9, 10]. However, the benefit of WBRT plus systemic CHT over systemic CHT alone is not clearly established. Some argue that the addition of WBRT results in disease remission if CNS disease is diagnosed at the time of clinical presentation ("early" disease) but not if it develops during active treatment with CHT or after an initial complete or partial response to treatment ("late" disease) [10]. In one case series [10], three of four patients with "early" disease achieved remission after WBRT plus EMA-CO, whereas all three patients with "late" disease undergoing the same treatment

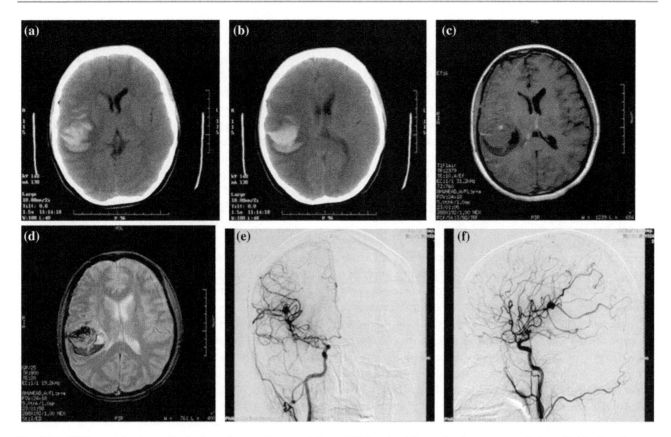

Fig. 26.1 CNS complications of choriocarcinoma. Representative images of an aneurysmal hemorrhage from choriocarcinoma. **a, b** CT head shows an intraparenchymal hemorrhage in the right temporoparietal lobe with mass effect. Axial T1 MR imaging (**c**) and T2-weighted MR imaging (**d**) reveals a heterogeneous lesion with blood products. **e, f** Cerebral angiogram demonstrates an aneurysm in the distal right middle cerebral artery. Used with permission of Elsevier from Wang et al. [11]

protocol died. This could, however, reflect the overall poor performance status and response to therapy of those with "late" disease rather than a direct effect of WBRT on survival. Given the known long-term neurotoxic sequelae of WBRT, some groups thus advocate against routine use of WBRT [20]. Instead, stereotactic radiosurgery (SRS) has assumed an increasingly important role in treating CNS metastases, particularly multiple small or unresectable lesions and after completion of systemic CHT to prevent relapse and/or treat residual disease [9, 10, 20, 21]. Lastly, IT CHT has been employed as an adjunct to systemic CHT, with the goal of achieving higher cerebrospinal fluid (CSF) drug levels. Some administer IT MTX (12.5 mg) routinely during non-EMA weeks until serum and CSF hCG levels have normalized [20, 21], whereas others [10] reserve it for patients with "late" disease. Treatment response is monitored by serial measurements of serum hCG levels, neurologic and overall clinical status, and disease burden on MRI brain.

The cure rate for metastatic choriocarcinoma is higher than that for metastatic disease from other solid tumors but reported response rates vary. The Charing Cross group observed remission in 85% of patients treated with EMA-CO/EP plus IT MTX, in the absence of WBRT [20, 21]. In another case series [9] comparing overall survival (OS) in patients treated before and after 1995, survival rates had increased from 46 to 64% but did not reach the numbers reported by the Charing Cross group. The remission rate was even lower (27%) in a cohort from the Philippines, although this was likely influenced by local confounders such as financial barriers and access to treatment [10].

The presence of neurologic symptoms at the time of presentation [9], "late" (vs. "early") disease [10], and concurrent liver metastases [21] may portend a worse outcome. Some data also suggest that a long interval from antecedent pregnancy to diagnosis of CNS metastasis is associated with poorer prognosis [23]. There is no clear established treatment protocol for those who fail to respond to EMA-CO/EP, but regimens based on etoposide and a platinum agent (e.g., cisplatin) have been used in combination with bleomycin, ifosfamide, or paclitaxel with modest success [9].

Ovarian and Fallopian Tube Cancer

Ovarian neoplasms are divided into epithelial ovarian cancer (EOC) and ovarian germ cell tumors. EOC constitutes the vast majority (95%) of ovarian malignancies and is regarded as one entity with fallopian tube and primary peritoneal cancer, given their shared embryonic origin and similarities in pathogenesis, clinical behavior, and treatment [24]. This section discusses the neurologic complications of EOC and primary fallopian tube cancer. The neurologic sequelae of ovarian germ cell tumors, specifically ovarian teratoma, are typically seen in paraneoplastic syndromes and will be discussed in a separate section of this chapter.

Ovarian cancer is the second most common gynecologic cancer after endometrial cancer and the leading cause of gynecologic cancer-related mortality [25], with a mortality rate of 7.7 per 100,000 per year [26]. The lifetime risk for a woman to develop ovarian cancer is 1.3%. The incidence is 12.1 per 100,000 [26] and highest in the developed world (Europe, USA) [24]. The most significant risk factor is family history of ovarian and breast cancer. Specifically, the presence of a genetic mutation in the *BRCA1* and *BRCA2* genes increases the risk of EOC to 39–46% and 12–20%, respectively [24]. Additional well-established risk factors are nulliparity, early menarche, late menopause, and age >50 [27]. By contrast, primary fallopian tube cancer is very rare, comprising less than 1% of all gynecologic malignancies [28]. In a Finnish study, the incidence was 5.4 per million per year [29]. Risk factors for fallopian tube cancer are less well established than for ovarian cancer, but high parity appears to be protective [29]. Most fallopian tube cancers are serous adenocarcinomas [28, 29].

Early-stage EOC often presents with nonspecific symptoms, such as anorexia, fatigue, early satiety, back pain, weight loss, nausea, vomiting, and urinary urgency and frequency. Patients rarely complain of abdominal or pelvic discomfort [24], often resulting in diagnostic delay. With disease progression, increased abdominal girth, pain, bloating, and fullness can develop [24]. About 75% of patients with EOC have stage III or IV disease at the time of diagnosis [24]. By contrast, fallopian tube cancer is rarely asymptomatic and typically presents with vaginal bleeding or spotting and abdominal pain due to tubal distension [28].

The initial step in the diagnosis of EOC is transvaginal ultrasound, which is more sensitive than CT in detecting and characterizing pelvic masses [24]. Serum CA-125 level is helpful in establishing the diagnosis as it is raised in >80% of those with advanced disease but lacks sensitivity and specificity [30]. It is also routinely used to monitor response to treatment and tumor recurrence [24, 29]. Surgical staging by exploratory laparotomy is performed in most patients and consists of total abdominal hysterectomy and bilateral salpingo-oophorectomy (TAH-BSO), examination of peritoneal surfaces, infracolic omentectomy, biopsies of pelvic and para-aortic lymph nodes, and peritoneal washings [24]. Patients with high-grade (grade 3 or higher) disease of any stage receive adjuvant CHT (a combination of a platinum agent such as carboplatin or cisplatin and a taxane such as paclitaxel or docetaxel). Individuals with stage I moderately differentiated (grade 2) cancer may also benefit from CHT [24]. The use of intraperitoneal (IP) CHT varies amongst providers due to potential problems with toxicity, drug administration, and risk of complications (e.g., intraperitoneal infections and adhesions) [24].

Local metastases involve the abdomino-pelvic-peritoneal compartment and regional lymph nodes first [24, 28]. The most common extra-abdominal metastatic sites are the pleural space (33%), liver (26%), and lung (3%) [24, 31]. Although EOC is the second most common cancer of the female reproductive tract to metastasize to the CNS, this occurrence is very rare with an incidence between <1 and 2.5% [32, 33]. Notably, these numbers may underestimate the true incidence and merely reflect symptomatic lesions, given that brain imaging is not routinely performed in ovarian cancer [33]. Given its much rarer occurrence, the incidence of CNS metastases from fallopian tube cancer is likely even lower [34].

CNS metastases can occur in isolation or in the setting of disseminated metastatic disease. Approximately, 30–44% of patients have isolated CNS relapse [32, 35, 36]. In general, CNS involvement is a manifestation of late disease that afflicts patients with prolonged survival after treatment of their systemic disease. More than 80% have stage III or IV cancer when CNS metastases are diagnosed, and most have grade III disease [35]. Figure 26.2a, b illustrates a characteristic patient with stage IIIc ovarian cancer who developed multifocal CNS involvement five years after her initial diagnosis. The median time from EOC diagnosis to CNS involvement was 21.5–46 months in different review series [32, 35], which was significantly longer than the time to development of liver and lung metastases (five and seven months, respectively) [32]. In up to two-thirds of patients, the underlying histology is of serous origin [32, 36].

In addition to parenchymal brain metastases, leptomeningeal dissemination has been described in ovarian cancer [37–39]. Although even less common than parenchymal disease, recognition and work-up of leptomeningeal involvement is important as it has significant implications for treatment and prognosis. Patients most often present with multifocal neurologic deficits, including multiple cranial nerve palsies, radiculopathy from nerve root and cauda equina infiltration, ataxia from cerebellar involvement, and signs of increased ICP secondary to hydrocephalus [40]. Contrast-enhanced MRI of the neuraxis may show

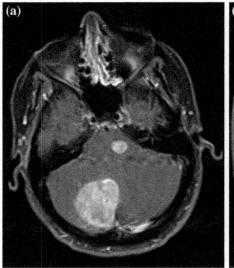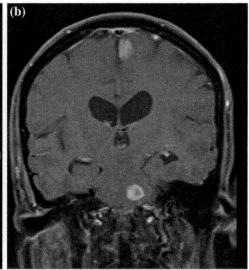

Fig. 26.2 CNS complications of ovarian cancer. Post-contrast **a** axial and **b** coronal T1-weighted MR images of a 55-year-old woman with a history of stage IIIc ovarian cancer (serous histologic subtype, *BRCA*-positive disease) who presented with headaches five years after initial diagnosis. MRI revealed parenchymal metastases in the (**a**) *right* cerebellar hemisphere, (**a**, **b**) *left upper* brainstem, and (**b**) *left frontal* lobe. CSF was positive for malignant cells. She underwent surgical resection of the right cerebellar lesion, followed by XRT to the resection cavity and residual disease. She is currently receiving IT topotecan every two months for leptomeningeal disease and is two years out from her CNS diagnosis. Courtesy of and reproduced with permission of Dr. Jose Carrillo, University of California, Irvine

enhancement in the subarachnoid space but sensitivity of imaging is low, with false negative rates ranging from 30 to 70% [40]. CSF cytology was only 71% sensitive in one study but the diagnostic yield can be increased by repeated large-volume lumbar punctures, rapid sample processing, and obtaining fluid from symptomatic sites [41]. High CSF opening pressure, pleocytosis, and elevated protein support the diagnosis of leptomeningeal carcinomatosis.

As with most parenchymal brain metastases, corticosteroids can rapidly restore neurologic function but their effects are short-lived. Median OS was two months only on corticosteroids alone [35]. In general, patients with good performance status, controlled or absent systemic disease, and a solitary and surgically accessible lesion may be good surgical candidates. In this population, prospective data have shown that surgery plus WBRT prolongs OS and reduces the rate of local relapse, compared to WBRT alone [42, 43]. Such randomized controlled data are not available for metastatic ovarian cancer specifically but a retrospective case series [44] found that resection of solitary metastases and adjuvant WBRT improved OS (23 months) compared to WBRT (5 months) or surgery alone (7 months). In an uncontrolled case series, surgery followed by either WBRT or carboplatin resulted in OS of 16 months [36]. Surgery is more difficult if multiple metastases are present. Although feasible and associated with prolonged survival (14 months vs. 3 months in those who did not undergo surgery) [45], its implementation largely depends on the anatomic location of the lesions, the patient's clinical and functional status, and expertise of the neurosurgeon.

For patients with unresectable lesions, nonsurgical candidates, or those refractory to WBRT, SRS may be an alternative option [25, 46]. SRS involves high doses of focused radiation to brain metastases, delivered either by a linear accelerator or gamma knife. The limiting factor for SRS is lesion size, and it is typically only considered for lesions <3 cm in diameter. It remains controversial whether WBRT plus SRS is superior to SRS alone [47]. Similarly, no randomized controlled trials to date have compared surgery versus SRS.

The role of systemic CHT in the management of metastatic ovarian cancer is unclear. The main disadvantage of CHT is its inability to cross the blood–brain barrier (BBB), although CNS drug penetration may partly be facilitated by a disrupted BBB as a result of metastatic disease. Systemic CHT is often administered in the presence of concurrent extracranial metastases, sometimes resulting in improved OS. Although this may merely reflect better systemic disease control rather than CNS remission, others have reported potential benefits of systemic CHT in isolated CNS disease [48, 49]. Treatment of leptomeningeal disease is largely palliative and typically consists of WBRT, IT CHT (MTX, cytarabine, thiotepa), or systemic CHT [40].

Overall prognosis for patients with parenchymal CNS metastases from ovarian and fallopian tube cancer is poor and likely significantly worse in the setting of leptomeningeal disease. Two factors appear to consistently affect OS: performance status and presence of concurrent extracranial metastases [32, 36]. For instance, median OS was nine months in those with concurrent extracranial disease versus 21 months in those with isolated CNS metastases [36]. Prolonged survival is exceptionally rare. One patient survived for 31 months after diagnosis of multiple brain metastases from stage IV EOC and successful treatment with carboplatin but ultimately succumbed to recurrent abdominal disease [48]. Micha et al. [50] reported a patient with stage IV EOC who remained in clinical remission for 7 years after surgery and WBRT. Lastly, a small number of case reports have documented prolonged OS (range of 36–82 months) in patients with advanced-stage fallopian tube cancer [34, 51].

Endometrial Cancer

The vast majority of uterine malignancies originate from the endometrium. Endometrial carcinoma is the most common gynecologic malignancy in the developed world, with an incidence of 24.6 per 100,000 women per year and a lifetime risk of 2.7% in the USA [52–54]. In developing countries, it is the second most common gynecologic malignancy after cervical cancer. More than 75% are endometrioid adenocarcinomas and most occur as a result of excess endogenous or exogenous estrogen without opposing progestin [53]. The typical presentation is abnormal uterine bleeding in post-menopausal women and intermenstrual, heavy, frequent, or prolonged uterine bleeding in pre-menopausal women [53, 55].

At the time of diagnosis, most women (80%) have grade I and II endometrioid cancer ("type I"), which is usually estrogen-responsive and portends a good prognosis [53]. The remaining 20% have grade III or non-endometrioid cancer of other histologic origin ("type II"), including papillary serous, clear cell, squamous cell, mixed, and undifferentiated subtypes [53, 56]. Prognosis in type II endometrial cancer is less favorable, partly because it responds less robustly to estrogen-based therapy. The non-endometrioid subtypes also have a higher propensity to metastasize [53], usually via the lymphatic system to pelvic lymph nodes or by local invasion [57]. Although rare, metastases can also occur via the hematogenous route to the lungs and liver [57].

Endometrial carcinoma is staged by the FIGO and "tumor, nodes, metastasis" (TNM) surgical staging system, which incorporates various risk and prognostic factors, including histologic (FIGO) and nuclear grade, depth of myometrial invasion, involvement of the uterine cervix, and presence of local or distant metastases [53]. For disease

confined to the uterus, the standard treatment is TAH-BSO with or without pelvic and para-aortic lymph node dissection [52], although conservative management may be considered in those with well-differentiated disease and lack of myometrial invasion and adnexal disease who wish to preserve fertility [56]. The use of adjuvant CHT or XRT is determined by numerous clinical and pathologic factors, including patient age and ethnicity, histologic grade, disease stage, status of peritoneal cytology, and involvement of the lower uterine segment [53]. Recurrence of disease following treatment can occur either locally or at distant sites [56].

Endometrial carcinoma is the third most common gynecologic cancer to metastasize to the brain [25, 58] but, as with ovarian and fallopian tube cancer, CNS involvement is exceedingly rare and occurs in only 0.3–0.9% of patients [59, 60]. This number increases to 3% if autopsy cases are included [61]. Tumor cells likely disseminate to the lungs first via the hematogenous route, with subsequent spread to the CNS. Factors that increase the risk of brain metastasis include certain histologic subtypes (papillary serous, clear cell, poorly differentiated tumors) and advanced surgical stage [59, 60]. Although most CNS metastases occur in the setting of widely disseminated late-stage disease, exceptions have been reported. Martinez-Manas et al. [57] treated a woman with isolated disease recurrence in the brain 1.5 years after treatment for a stage IIB papillary endometrioid adenocarcinoma. Similarly, Gien et al. [60] observed two patients with successfully treated stage IIB and IIIc endometrial carcinoma and no systemic disease who presented with multiple brain metastases two and seven months after completion of treatment, respectively. In another patient, neurologic symptoms preceded the diagnosis of an endometrioid carcinoma [60].

The reported median time between diagnosis of endometrial carcinoma and brain metastasis ranges from 0 to 52 months [58, 59, 62, 63]. Some authors have observed CNS involvement early during the disease course, especially in patients with vascular and deep myometrial invasion, thus underscoring the aggressive nature of tumors with metastatic tendency [60, 62].

Treatment recommendations for brain metastases in endometrial cancer are largely based on observational results. Similar to data from CNS metastases in ovarian cancer, surgical resection followed by WBRT is superior to surgery or XRT alone for patients with controlled extracranial disease and good performance status. In one case series of ten patients, those who underwent surgery and WBRT with or without SRS had a median OS of 15 months, compared to those who had XRT or surgery alone (median OS 2.4 and 2.7 months, respectively) [58]. Another study reported even longer OS (28 and 83 months) in two patients treated with surgery and WBRT, compared to OS of

3 months in patients receiving WBRT only [59]. For patients with multiple symptomatic brain metastases with or without uncontrolled extracranial disease, WBRT is the treatment of choice [58, 59]. The role of adjuvant CHT is less well defined but usually reserved for those with multiple brain lesions and concomitant systemic disease. One proposed regimen is four to six cycles of paclitaxel and carboplatin in addition to pelvic XRT for patients with advanced or high-risk (stage III) disease [60].

In general, prognosis is grim and median OS after diagnosis of CNS disease ranges from one to 19 months [57–60, 62, 64]. Survival may be improved in those with single compared to multiple brain lesions. For instance, two patients survived for 82 [64] and 83 [59] months, respectively, after diagnosis of a solitary brain metastasis treated with resection and WBRT.

Cervical Cancer

Cervical cancer is the third most common gynecologic cancer in the developed world, following ovarian and endometrial cancer [65]. The incidence in the USA is 7.7 per 100,000, and the estimated lifetime risk is 0.6% [66]. It has long been recognized that human papillomavirus (HPV), specifically HPV 16 and 18, is the key pathogenic driver of cervical neoplasia, being present in 99.7% of affected patients [67]. Other risk factors include early onset of sexual activity, multiple sexual partners, increasing parity, early age of first birth, low socioeconomic background, history of sexually transmitted diseases, and immunosuppression [68]. The typical clinical presentation of early disease is irregular, heavy vaginal, or post-coital bleeding, whereas pelvic or back pain can indicate advanced-stage disease [69]. Squamous cell carcinoma is by far the most common histologic subtype, followed by adenocarcinoma [68].

Most metastases from cervical cancer occur via direct local invasion or by lymphatic spread. Hematogenous spread is rare and tends to affect lungs, bone, and liver first before involving the CNS. Concurrent lung metastases have been reported in up to two-thirds of patients with CNS disease [70]. The reported incidence of metastatic CNS disease ranges from 0.4 to 1.2% [71–73]. As with ovarian and endometrial carcinoma, CNS metastases have been observed in patients of all disease stages and can occur before, during, or after completion of systemic therapy [72, 74]. Median OS with metastatic CNS disease is poor, ranging from 2.3 to 8 months [71, 72, 74, 75]. Patients undergoing surgery and adjuvant XRT tend to survive longer than those receiving either treatment modality alone [71, 72, 74, 75]. SRS alone prolonged survival to 22.5 months in one patient [72].

Paraneoplastic Diseases Associated with Gynecologic Cancers

Unlike direct malignant cell infiltration from a primary tumor, paraneoplastic syndromes (PNS) arise from an immune-mediated reaction by the host to an underlying cancer. Certain malignancies express proteins similar to those found on neuronal tissue and can trigger an immune response against these proteins, with subsequent cross-reactivity involving the nervous system. PNS can antedate the diagnosis of an underlying malignancy by months or years but also occur after a cancer has been diagnosed or during remission following cancer treatment. Of all solid tumors, small cell lung cancer (SCLC) is the leading cause of PNS, followed by breast and gynecologic malignancies [76].

The general management of PNS relies on the identification and appropriate treatment of the primary tumor (e.g., surgical resection of tumor with or without systemic CHT), immunosuppression (e.g., corticosteroids), and targeted removal of circulating onconeural antibodies (e.g., intravenous immunoglobulin (IVIG) and plasma exchange (PLEX)). Refractory cases may require treatment with a cyclophosphamide or rituximab. In some instances, long-term immunosuppression with azathioprine or mycophenolate mofetil is needed. In addition to pharmacologic treatment, physical, occupational, and speech therapy, and intensive rehabilitation should be incorporated to improve and maintain functional outcome.

Gynecologic cancers are most frequently associated with paraneoplastic cerebellar degeneration (PCD) and anti-NMDA receptor (NMDAR) encephalitis. Other PNS, including paraneoplastic peripheral neuropathies, opsoclonus myoclonus syndrome, limbic encephalitis, retinopathy, and Lambert-Eaton syndrome are rarely seen with gynecologic tumors [76, 77]. Table 26.1 provides a summary of these PNS.

Paraneoplastic Cerebellar Degeneration

Paraneoplastic cerebellar degeneration (PCD) occurs in <0.1% of gynecologic cancers [78] but is the most common paraneoplastic disease seen in reproductive tract cancers [76]. The type of underlying cancer and antibody determines the severity of symptoms, presence of other non-cerebellar features, and clinical outcome. The typical presentation is a subacute, severe, and progressive pancerebellar syndrome, with axial, appendicular, and gait ataxia, vertigo, dysarthria, and diplopia. Cognitive impairment [79] and non-cerebellar symptoms have been described. For instance, anti-Hu antibody-associated PCD can present with concomitant

Table 26.1 Paraneoplastic syndromes associated with gynecologic malignancies

Paraneoplastic syndrome	Typical onconeural antibody; gynecologic neoplasm	Treatment[a]	Prognosis
Paraneoplastic cerebellar degeneration	Anti-Yo; most commonly ovarian cancer but also fallopian tube, uterine, and cervical cancer	Corticosteroids, IVIG, PLEX Tacrolimus RTX	Poor
Anti-NMDAR encephalitis	Anti-NMDAR; ovarian teratoma	First-line: corticosteroids, IVIG, PLEX Second-line: RTX, cyclophosphamide	Good
Peripheral neuropathy	No clear antibody association; ovarian, endometrial, cervical cancer	Corticosteroids, IVIG	Variable
Opsoclonus myoclonus syndrome	Anti-Ri (weak association); ovarian and fallopian tube cancer, ovarian teratoma	Corticosteroids, IVIG Symptomatic treatment (benzodiazepines, levetiracetam, gabapentin, valproic acid, topiramate)	Variable but generally good
Limbic encephalitis, retinopathy, Lambert-Eaton syndrome	Individual cases reported with ovarian, endometrial, and cervical cancer. General treatment approach consists of corticosteroids, IVIG, PLEX, and/or immunosuppression. Guanidine and 3,4 diaminopyridine may be helpful in Lambert-Eaton syndrome. Prognosis is variable		

[a]In all cases, the underlying neoplasm should be treated

peripheral neuropathy and a brainstem/limbic encephalitis [80].

PCD is most frequently seen with ovarian, breast, and SCLC but has also been reported in association with fallopian tube, uterine, and cervical cancer [79, 81]. In most cases of PCD, the associated onconeural antibody is directed against an intracellular protein. The antibody varies depending on the underlying malignancy. In ovarian and breast cancer, there is a strong association with anti-Yo antibody (also known as Purkinje cell cytoplasmic antibody type 1 (PCA 1)) [76]. These antibodies have also been found in patients with uterine [79, 82], fallopian tube [78, 79, 82–84], cervical [76, 85], and primary peritoneal malignancy [84]. By contrast, PCD in non-gynecologic cancers is associated with anti-Hu (anti-neuronal nuclear antibody 1 or ANNA1), anti-Ri (ANNA2), and anti-Tr antibody [81]. In one case series, anti-Yo antibodies were the most frequently detected antibodies in PCD with a relative frequency of 38%, compared to lower rates of anti-Hu (32%), anti-Tr (14%), and anti-Ri (12%) antibodies [80]. Given the strong association of anti-Yo antibody with gynecologic and breast neoplasms, its presence should prompt a thorough search for underlying malignancy. Its specificity for gynecologic cancers ranges from 47 to 60% [79, 80] to >80% [76, 84, 86].

CSF studies can be normal [78] or show a lymphocyte-predominant pleocytosis, mildly elevated IgG and protein, and oligoclonal bands [79, 86, 87]. Brain MRI is usually normal in the early stages but can evolve to cerebellar or brainstem atrophy with disease progression (Fig. 26.3a, b), reflecting the histopathologic hallmark of

cerebellar cortical atrophy and loss of cerebellar Purkinje cells [79, 88]. All patients with suspected PCD should undergo comprehensive work-up for underlying malignancy, including CT of the chest, abdomen, and pelvis, mammography, pelvic ultrasound, and CA125 measurement to screen for ovarian cancer [78]. FDG-PET should be considered if CT imaging does not reveal malignancy; sensitivity and specificity of FDG-PET to detect occult malignancy in PNS can be as high as 83 and 25%, respectively [89]. If initial work-up is negative, some authors advocate for repeat mammography, pelvic examination, uterine dilatation and curettage, and eventually surgical exploration of the pelvic organs [79, 86]. When an underlying gynecologic cancer is found, it is typically high grade. In one case series, most patients with a gynecologic malignancy, a clinical syndrome consistent with PCD, and positive anti-Yo antibody titers had poorly differentiated grade III cancer [84]. Interestingly, total metastatic volume was significantly smaller compared to controls with confirmed ovarian cancer and no PCD, suggesting that the autoimmune process limits metastatic spread [84].

PCD typically follows a relentless, progressive course. Neurologic symptoms tend to stabilize at the time of diagnosis and with initiation of treatment [79, 80] but neurologic recovery is rare, even with exhaustive therapy [79, 88]. In some patients, antibody titers remain elevated despite successful treatment of the underlying primary malignancy and stabilization of neurologic disease [79]. PCD associated with gynecologic cancers and anti-Yo antibodies carries a particularly dismal prognosis. In a retrospective case series of

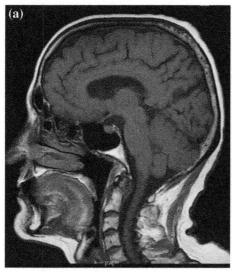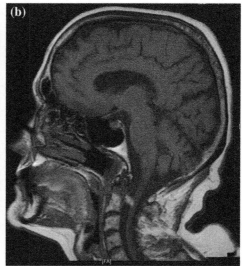

Fig. 26.3 Paraneoplastic cerebellar degeneration. Sagittal T1-weighted images of a 71-year-old woman with FIGO stage IIIc ovarian cancer (**a, b**). Following surgery, the patient was treated with carboplatin and taxol and several months into therapy started having some difficulty with balance. She underwent brain MRI (**a**) which was unremarkable. She was tested for presence of paraneoplastic antibodies and was found to have anti-Yo antibodies. She subsequently received several courses of IVIG without improvement. Her symptoms progressed gradually over the next two years and she developed severe ataxia and dysarthria. Her MRI 27 months after diagnosis of the ovarian cancer showed atrophy of the cerebellum (**b**)

fifty patients with PCD, 79% of those with anti-Yo antibodies were bedbound at the peak of disease, compared to <60% of those with anti-Tr and anti-mGluR1 antibodies and 17% of those with anti-Ri antibody [80]. The same study also showed a trend toward worse median OS in those with anti-Yo (13 months) and anti-Hu (7 months) antibodies compared to those with anti-Tr (>113 months) and anti-Ri (>69 months) antibodies [80]. In another series following patients with breast or gynecologic cancer and PCD over a median of 84 months or until death, median OS was 22 months in those with gynecologic cancers compared to 100 months in the breast cancer group [85]. Similarly, Hammack et al. [86] observed that patients with positive anti-Yo antibody survived for only 17.3 months compared to 39.9 months in those with negative antibody titers.

Given that many patients are treated with multiple agents simultaneously and the rarity of PCD, it has proven difficult to systematically study the efficacy of individual treatment modalities [81]. The general consensus is that early diagnosis of PCD is critical as unrecognized and untreated disease inevitably leads to irreversible loss of Purkinje cells. As with all PNS, treatment of PCD is based on primary tumor control and removal of circulating antibodies with immunosuppressive or -modulatory therapy with the goal to reduce antigenic burden. With ovarian cancers, this encompasses surgical resection, maximal cytoreduction, and platinum-based chemotherapy [88]. Corticosteroids are typically given as IV methylprednisolone (1 g daily) for 3–5 days, followed by oral prednisone (60–80 mg daily).

An alternative regimen is repeated courses of high-dose methylprednisolone [81].

The benefit of IVIG in anti-Yo antibody-associated PCD is controversial [81]. A typical dose is 2 g/kg over five days and 1–2 g/kg for repeated courses [81]. No improvement was seen in four patients with PCD and anti-Yo antibodies treated with one to 11 courses of IVIG [90]. A combined approach of IVIG, cyclophosphamide (600 mg/m^2 at day 1), and methylprednisolone (1 g daily from day 1 to 3) was also disappointing; it stabilized disease in one-third of patients with a modified Rankin scale (mRS) ≤ 3 (ambulatory) for up to 35 months but had no impact on disease progression in those with mRS ≥ 4 (bedridden) [91].

PCD is thought to be mediated by cellular rather than humoral immunity as supported by recent treatment results with T and B cell-targeting agents. In one trial, patients received combined tacrolimus (0.15–0.3 mg/kg daily in two divided doses) and prednisone (60 mg daily, followed by a taper over one to four weeks) [92]. Tacrolimus is a T cell inhibitor with good BBB penetration and steroids may induce apoptosis in mature T cells [93], resulting in potent induction of T cell death [92]. Thirteen patients with anti-Yo antibody and ovarian cancer were included, and significant subjective neurologic improvement was observed in eight of them. Median OS was 38 months, which is longer than in other studies [85]. In addition, there was a significant lowering of median CSF WBC count, thus substantiating the role of cellular immunity in the pathogenesis of PCD.

By contrast, rituximab (RTX) , a monoclonal antibody against CD20 used to treat B cell malignancies, has not shown convincing benefit. In a case series of nine patients (eight with anti-Hu and one with anti-Yo antibody), only one-third improved by ≥ 1 point on mRS (two with anti-Hu and one with anti-Yo antibody) [94]. The lack of improvement with RTX may support the predominant role of T cells in disease pathogenesis.

Plasma exchange (PLEX) has demonstrated variable efficacy [81]. Some studies did not show any objective improvement with PLEX [86], while others did in 50% of patients when PLEX was given with cyclophosphamide or cancer-directed treatment [95]. The trend was less favorable for those with gynecologic cancers and anti-Yo antibodies (27% with improvement) than those with other onconeural antibodies (71% with improvement) [95], again highlighting the more dismal prognosis associated with anti-Yo antibodies.

Anti-NMDA Receptor Encephalitis

Anti-NMDAR encephalitis is the most common autoimmune encephalitis after acute demyelinating encephalomyelitis [96] and, in young individuals, occurs much more frequently than any type of viral encephalitis [97]. It is thought to be the most common cause of paraneoplastic encephalitis [98].

The key mediators of anti-NMDAR encephalitis are IgG antibodies against the NR1 subunit of N-methyl D-aspartate (NMDA) receptors, which are prominently distributed on the cell membranes of GABAergic neurons [99, 100], resulting in various downstream effects, including disinhibition of excitatory pathways and concurrent release of glutamate in the extracellular space [98]. It also affects dopaminergic, noradrenergic, and cholinergic pathways, which may explain the prominent autonomic instability seen in this disease. Involvement of the brainstem respiratory center leads to central hypoventilation [98].

The typical patient is a young woman who presents with prominent psychiatric symptoms, including behavioral disturbance, psychosis, grandiose delusions, catatonia, anxiety, and paranoia [98, 101]. A history of a viral-like prodrome predating the onset of psychiatric features by a few days to two weeks may be elicited in up to 70% of patients [98]. Significant language difficulties, ranging from decreased speech output and echolalia to mutism, are often seen [98]. The psychiatric features then progress to development of memory loss and decreased level of consciousness. Movement abnormalities, including orofacial dyskinesias, choreoathetosis, dystonia, rigidity, and oculogyric crisis are common, as is autonomic dysfunction, which typically presents with hyperthermia, fluctuating blood pressure and heart rate, hypersalivation, and genitourinary dysfunction [98].

Central hypoventilation, along with impaired level of consciousness and status epilepticus, often necessitates intubation and prolonged ventilator support [98, 101]. Seizures occur early and invariably and often progress into status epilepticus [98].

The above clinical constellation, especially in a young woman, should prompt an immediate work-up for anti-NMDAR encephalitis and thorough search for an underlying malignancy as timely implementation of treatment hastens recovery and improves prognosis [101]. The associated tumor is almost always an ovarian teratoma, which expresses NMDAR [102, 103]. In some cases, no underlying tumor is found despite extensive screening; this is more common in younger (age < 12) and nonblack patients [98, 101]. Diagnostic evaluation should include CT or MRI of the chest, abdomen, and pelvis, pelvic and/or transvaginal ultrasound, contrast-enhanced brain MRI, CSF studies, and testing for paraneoplastic antibodies.

CSF studies typically show a lymphocytic pleocytosis and normal or mildly elevated protein levels. CSF oligoclonal bands are found in 60% of afflicted individuals [98]. The presence of NMDAR antibodies in CSF or serum confirms the diagnosis. CSF NMDAR antibody is more sensitive than serum NMDAR antibody (100% versus 85.6%), and higher CSF titers have been observed in those with clinical relapses, underlying teratoma, and poor outcome (defined as mRS ≥ 3). Specificity is 100% for both CSF and serum NMDAR antibodies [104].

Brain MRI and EEG are useful to exclude other causes of encephalitis and altered mental status but lack sensitivity and specificity. MRI can be normal in up to half of patients [105]. Alternatively, it may show T2/FLAIR hyperintensity in the hippocampi, cerebellar or cerebral cortex, frontobasal and insular regions, and basal ganglia, with or without associated enhancement in these areas or the meninges [98]. Brain atrophy can occur as a result of intractable seizures. EEG frequently shows nonspecific slowing, epileptiform discharges, and electrographic seizures [98].

In addition to removal of the underlying tumor, first-line treatment includes corticosteroids plus IVIG or PLEX [98]. Second-line therapy is added if patients experience little to no improvement with first-line treatment. This typically consists of combined RTX (375 mg/m^2 every week for four weeks) and cyclophosphamide (750 mg/m^2 with first dose of rituximab, then monthly thereafter) [98, 101]. Most physicians treat until a satisfactory clinical response has been achieved.

Overall prognosis is good but clinical recovery can take months to more than a year. In an observational study of 577 patients, 81% of patients had a significant clinical response to tumor removal and first-line immunotherapy at a median follow-up time of 24 months [101]. Recovery continued to occur until 18 months of follow-up. Prompt initiation of immunotherapy, tumor removal, and lower symptom severity were independent predictors of a favorable outcome [101]. In addition, patients with an underlying ovarian teratoma tend to perform better neurologically than those without [98]. In those failing first-line immunotherapy, the addition of second-line therapy led to improved clinical outcome, compared to those who did not receive second-line therapy [101]. Relapses occur more frequently in those without an underlying tumor and who do not receive immunotherapy [101]. Mortality in anti-NMDAR encephalitis is 4–7% [101, 106], and patients typically succumb to medical complications, neurologic deterioration, or tumor progression.

Paraneoplastic Peripheral Neuropathies

Paraneoplastic peripheral neuropathies (PNs) are one of the more common paraneoplastic manifestations of cancer and typically seen in SCLC, thymoma, and hematologic disease (monoclonal gammopathy of undetermined significance (MGUS), Waldenström's macroglobulinemia, and lymphoma) [107]. Their incidence in gynecologic cancers is low. They have been reported in cancer of the ovary, endometrium, and cervix [76, 108–110]. The neuropathy is usually axonal and either sensory-predominant [76], motor-predominant [108], or mixed sensorimotor [109, 110]. Concurrent involvement of the dorsal root ganglia (neuronopathy) is possible [76]. Whereas paraneoplastic PNs observed in SCLC and thymoma often associate with a specific onconeural antibody (such as anti-Hu or anti-CRMP antibody) [111], such an association is less clear for PNs in gynecologic cancers. For instance, in a series of patients with gynecologic malignancies and paraneoplastic PN, two were positive for anti-Hu antibody, one had atypical antibody, and two were negative for onconeural antibodies [76]. No clear data on response to treatment and prognosis exist. In the aforementioned case series [76], one patient with cervical cancer had progressive disease despite treatment with steroids whereas another with ovarian cancer improved with IVIG. Another case had improvement of neurologic symptoms after resection of an endometrial carcinoma [108].

Opsoclonus Mycolonus Syndrome

Opsoclonus myoclonus syndrome (OMS) is typically a disease of childhood and associated with neuroblastoma [112]. Adult-onset disease is much rarer and usually develops over a course of a few weeks. Patients present with truncal ataxia, gait problems, falls, and myoclonus. The myoclonus can affect different body segments (limbs, truncal, craniocervical) and cause dysarthria and dysphagia [113]. Opsoclonus refers to involuntary, chaotic, multidirectional, and irregular saccades, causing vision abnormalities. Patients can be afflicted by other symptoms secondary to brainstem and cerebellar involvement and present with encephalopathy [113].

OMS can be paraneoplastic, parainfectious, toxic/metabolic, autoimmune, or idiopathic in origin [113]. An underlying tumor is rarely found; if present, it is most commonly SCLC or breast cancer [113, 114]. An association with gynecologic cancers is even less common but has been reported in patients with ovarian and fallopian tube carcinoma [76, 113–115] and ovarian teratoma [116]. In a case series of 92 patients with breast or gynecologic malignancy and definitive or possible PNS, four had OMS (three breast and one ovarian carcinoma) and two had positive anti-Ri antibody [76]. A paraneoplastic antibody is only found occasionally, most commonly anti-Ri antibody [113, 117]. Brain MRI is often normal but can show T2/FLAIR hyperintensity in the dorsal pons or midbrain [118].

Based on uncontrolled observational studies, response to treatment is good. Klaas and coworkers reviewed 21 patients with OMS and found that most achieved clinical remission with immunotherapy (corticosteroids and/or IVIG) and symptomatic therapy (benzodiazepines, levetiracetam, valproic acid, and gabapentin) and remained symptom-free upon discontinuation of therapy [113]. Long-term immunosuppression, e.g., with mycophenolate mofetil, was rarely needed [113]. Prognosis is better for those without an underlying cancer and, if present, for those who undergo targeted treatment of their neoplasm [117]. A suggested treatment plan is a short course of IV methylprednisolone or IVIG for 3–5 days, followed by weekly infusions for six weeks. Patients refractory to this regimen may be considered for combination immunotherapy and PLEX [113]. Lastly, rare cases of complete response to clonazepam (8–12 mg) and topiramate have been reported [119, 120].

Hypercoagulability and Non-bacterial Thrombotic Endocarditis

Hypercoagulability of malignancy is mediated by a number of factors, including increased pro-coagulant activity and decreased fibrinolytic activity [121]. Non-bacterial thrombotic endocarditis (NBTE) is a rare manifestation of cancer-related hypercoagulability that has been described in association with gynecologic tumors, most commonly ovarian cancer, although cases of endometrial cancer have also been reported [122, 123]. Arterial thromboembolic complications include arterial strokes in multiple vascular territories and myocardial infarctions. Venous embolic events can manifest as deep venous thromboses in the lower extremities and pulmonary emboli [122]. Transthoracic or - esophageal echocardiogram reveals vegetations, typically on the mitral or aortic valve. Blood cultures are characteristically negative. The underlying gynecologic tumor can be benign [123] or malignant and of various histologic grades and stages [122, 124, 125]. Notably, NBTE has been observed more frequently in adenocarcinomas than other histologic subtypes [126]. Treatment of NBTE involves treatment of the underlying cancer and anti-coagulation, preferably low-molecular weight heparin [127].

Treatment-Related Complications of Gynecologic Cancers

Surgery-Induced Peripheral Nerve Injuries

The incidence of peripheral nerve injury after gynecologic surgery is <2%, based on prospective and retrospective data [128–130]. Injuries can occur through compression, stretch, entrapment, or transection of nerves. The risk of postoperative neuropathy and the distribution of nerve involvement depends on the type of surgery, patient positioning, and duration of surgery. For instance, the lithotomy position carries a higher risk of sciatic, femoral, and peroneal nerve injury. Deep abdominal surgery, including abdominal hysterectomy, is a common cause of femoral neuropathy due to stretch injury from hyperflexion of the thigh and compression of the femoral nerve against the pelvic wall [131]. The risk of compression injury is particularly high with self-retaining retractors [131]. The ilioinguinal and iliohypogastric nerves can be injured with transverse (e.g., Pfannenstiel) incisions, due to entrapment from sutures or neuroma formation during the healing or scarring process [132]. Other potentially affected nerves are the lateral femoral cutaneous, genitofemoral, obturator, and pudendal nerves. Bilateral nerve injury has been reported in as many as 27% of patients [128]. Patients commonly complain of sensory loss or weakness in the distribution of the affected nerve. Pain is less common but can occur with transection or ligation injuries and neuroma formation. Preventive intra-operative measures include appropriate patient positioning (avoiding excessive extension, flexion, abduction, and external rotation) [133], avoiding the lithotomy position for >2 h [134], attention to incisional technique, and positioning of retractor blades.

Treatment is typically conservative and, in most cases, symptoms resolve over weeks to months. In one study, all but one patient (91%) had complete resolution of neuropathic symptoms after a median of 31.5 days (range of 1 day–6 months) [128].

Radiation-Induced Lumbosacral Plexopathy

Patients with gynecologic cancers may receive pelvic XRT or brachytherapy, which can damage regional nerves via direct toxicity on axons, myelin, and the vasa vasorum, with resultant nerve infarction [135]. Radiation-induced lumbosacral plexopathy is a rare but potentially debilitating complication of gynecologic malignancies. It has been reported in cervical, uterine, and ovarian cancer [70, 136, 137]. Onset is typically insidious and can occur months to years after completion of treatment [138]. Toxicity of radiation is dose-dependent but has also been reported at lower doses (1700 cGy) [138]. Vaginal brachytherapy is used in the treatment of locally advanced cervical and uterine cancer to achieve better local disease control and prevent vaginal recurrence [139, 140]. Since most patients receive combined external beam radiation and brachytherapy, it is unclear whether brachytherapy alone significantly increases the risk of regional nerve damage. In a case series of 2410 patients, four cases who had received whole-pelvis XRT and intracavitary brachytherapy for cervical carcinoma developed flaccid lower extremity weakness 8–26 months after completion of radiation [136]. Pain was uncommon.

Careful differentiation of radiation-induced plexopathy from neoplastic plexopathy is important, given the different implications for treatment and prognosis. Radiation-induced plexopathy typically presents with paresthesias, flaccid weakness, and accompanying limb edema. Pain, the hallmark of neoplastic plexopathy (present in 98% of patients), is less prominent (10%) in radiation-induced injury [138]. Electromyogram (EMG) may reveal myokymia, which is generally absent in neoplastic or compressive plexopathy [138]. The imaging modality of choice is contrast-enhanced MRI of the plexus. With tumor- but not radiation-related injury, enhancement of the nerve roots is common, although radiation can produce T2-weighted hyperintense changes [141]. Most importantly, the absence of local tumor on imaging suggests a treatment-related rather than neoplastic etiology.

Management of radiation-induced plexopathy is primarily symptomatic and focuses on pain control, physical therapy, and rehabilitation. Although frequently used, there is no evidence that hyperbaric oxygen is beneficial [142, 143]. Unfortunately, most patients experience progressive functional decline [138].

Chemotherapy-Induced Peripheral Neuropathy

Platinum-based agents and taxanes are frequently used in the treatment of gynecologic cancers but are notoriously known to cause peripheral neuropathy. Cisplatin causes an axonal neuropathy of primarily large myelinated sensory fibers in up to 60% of patients receiving a cumulative dose of 225–500 mg/m² [144]. The most susceptible site is the dorsal root ganglion. Neuropathic symptoms can persist or worsen even after discontinuation of the drug [145]. The risk of peripheral neuropathy with carboplatin at conventional doses is lower than with cisplatin [144]. Paclitaxel and docetaxel can also cause a predominant sensory neuropathy. Paclitaxel appears to be more neurotoxic than doxetaxel, with an incidence of approximately 60 and 15%, respectively [146, 147]. As for platinum-based agents, the cumulative dose is the main risk factor for taxane-induced peripheral neuropathy, with a neurotoxic threshold of 1000 mg/m² for paclitaxel and 400 mg/m² for docetaxel [148].

In addition, cisplatin has been associated with dose-dependent ototoxicity, which typically manifests with bilateral and irreversible sensorineural hearing loss, ear pain, and tinnitus [149]. The underlying mechanism involves deposition of the drug and generation of reactive oxygen species in the cochlea, outer hair cells, spiral ganglia, stria vascularis, and spiral ligament. There is insufficient evidence to support use of any particular agent (such as vitamin E, sodium thiosulfate, or amifostine) to prevent cisplatin-induced ototoxicity [149].

Conclusions

Gynecologic cancers can cause a variety of neurologic complications via direct malignant cell infiltration of the nervous system, paraneoplastic phenomena, and treatment-related effects. CNS metastases from gynecologic tumors are rare except with choriocarcinoma and generally portend an unfavorable prognosis. Paraneoplastic cerebellar degeneration and anti-NMDAR encephalitis are well-characterized paraneoplastic syndromes associated with ovarian tumors and should be considered in any woman presenting with typical symptoms. Lastly, with the development of more sophisticated treatment modalities and improved survival in patients with gynecologic cancers, the incidence of long-term surgery-, chemotherapy-, and radiation-related neurologic complications will likely increase.

References

1. Altieri A, Franceschi S, Ferlay J, Smith J, La Vecchia C. Epidemiology and aetiology of gestational trophoblastic diseases. Lancet Oncol. 2003;4(11):670–8.
2. Lurain JR. Gestational trophoblastic disease I: epidemiology, pathology, clinical presentation and diagnosis of gestational trophoblastic disease, and management of hydatidiform mole. Am J Obstet Gynecol. 2010;203(6):531–9.
3. Graf AH, Buchberger W, Langmayr H, Schmid KW. Site preference of metastatic tumours of the brain. Virchows Archiv A, Pathol Anat Histopathol. 1988;412(5):493–8.
4. Guo J, Zhong C, Liu Q, Xu J, Zheng Y, Xu S, et al. Intracranial choriocarcinoma occurrence in males: two cases and a review of the literature. Oncol Lett. 2013;6(5):1329–32.
5. National Cancer Institute. General information about gestational trophoblastic disease [Internet] 2015 [updated February 2015; cited 2015 July 10]. Available from: http://www.cancer.gov/types/gestational-trophoblastic/hp/gtd-treatment-pdq#link/_380_toc.
6. Seckl MJ, Sebire NJ, Berkowitz RS. Gestational trophoblastic disease. Lancet. 2010;376(9742):717–29.
7. Berkowitz RS, Goldstein DP. Pathogenesis of gestational trophoblastic neoplasms. Pathobiol Ann. 1981;11:391–411.
8. Berkowitz RS, Goldstein DP. Current management of gestational trophoblastic diseases. Gynecol Oncol. 2009;112(3):654–62.
9. Neubauer NL, Latif N, Kalakota K, Marymont M, Small W Jr, Schink JC, et al. Brain metastasis in gestational trophoblastic neoplasia: an update. J Reprod Med. 2012;57(7–8):288–92.
10. Cagayan MS, Lu-Lasala LR. Management of gestational trophoblastic neoplasia with metastasis to the central nervous system: a 12-year review at the Philippine General Hospital. J Reprod Med. 2006;51(10):785–92.
11. Wang J, Wang R, Zhao J. Ruptured cerebral aneurysm from choriocarcinoma. J Clin Neurosci: Off J Neurosurg Soc Australas. 2013;20(9):1324–6.
12. Lefebvre G, Toledano M, Saeed Kilani M, Tempremant F, Boulanger T, Leclerc X. Brain metastatic dissemination of choriocarcinoma complicated of aneurysmal rupture. J Neuroradiol (Journal de neuroradiologie). 2013;40(1):62–4.
13. Zairi F, De Saint Denis T, Thines L, Bourgeois P, Lejeune JP. Ruptured cerebral oncotic aneurysm from choriocarcinoma: report of two cases and review of the literature. Acta Neurochirurgica. 2011;153(2):353–7.
14. Chang IB, Cho BM, Park SH, Yoon DY, Oh SM. Metastatic choriocarcinoma with multiple neoplastic intracranial microaneurysms: case report. J Neurosurg. 2008;108(5):1014–7.
15. Saad N, Tang YM, Sclavos E, Stuckey SL. Metastatic choriocarcinoma: a rare cause of stroke in the young adult. Australas Radiol. 2006;50(5):481–3.
16. May T, Rabinowe SN, Berkowitz RS, Goldstein DP. Cerebral venous sinus thrombosis presenting as cerebral metastasis in a patient with choriocarcinoma following a non-molar gestation. Gynecol Oncol. 2011;122(1):199–200.
17. Naito Y, Akeda K, Kasai Y, Matsumine A, Tabata T, Nagao K, et al. Lumbar metastasis of choriocarcinoma. Spine. 2009;34(15):E538–43.
18. Beskonakli E, Cayli S, Kulacoglu S. Metastatic choriocarcinoma in the thoracic extradural space: case report. Spinal cord. 1998;36(5):366–7.
19. Kuten A, Cohen Y, Tatcher M, Kobrin I, Robinson E. Pregnancy and delivery after successful treatment of epidural metastatic choriocarcinoma. Gynecol Oncol. 1978;6(5):464–6.
20. Savage P, Kelpanides I, Tuthill M, Short D, Seckl MJ. Brain metastases in gestational trophoblast neoplasia: an update on incidence, management and outcome. Gynecol Oncol. 2015;137(1):73–6.
21. Newlands ES, Holden L, Seckl MJ, McNeish I, Strickland S, Rustin GJ. Management of brain metastases in patients with high-risk gestational trophoblastic tumors. J Reprod Med. 2002;47(6):465–71.
22. Soper JT, Spillman M, Sampson JH, Kirkpatrick JP, Wolf JK, Clarke-Pearson DL. High-risk gestational trophoblastic neoplasia with brain metastases: individualized multidisciplinary therapy in the management of four patients. Gynecol Oncol. 2007;104(3):691–4.

23. Powles T, Young A, Sanitt A, Stebbing J, Short D, Bower M, et al. The significance of the time interval between antecedent pregnancy and diagnosis of high-risk gestational trophoblastic tumours. Br J Cancer. 2006;95(9):1145–7.

24. Hennessy BT, Coleman RL, Markman M. Ovarian cancer. Lancet. 2009;374(9698):1371–82.

25. Monaco E 3rd, Kondziolka D, Mongia S, Niranjan A, Flickinger JC, Lunsford LD. Management of brain metastases from ovarian and endometrial carcinoma with stereotactic radiosurgery. Cancer. 2008;113(9):2610–4.

26. National Cancer Institute. SEER Stat Fact Sheets: Ovary Cancer [Internet] 2015 [cited 2015 July 10]. Available from: http://seer.cancer.gov/statfacts/html/ovary.html.

27. Collaborative Group on Epidemiological Studies of Ovarian C, Beral V, Doll R, Hermon C, Peto R, Reeves G. Ovarian cancer and oral contraceptives: collaborative reanalysis of data from 45 epidemiological studies including 23,257 women with ovarian cancer and 87,303 controls. Lancet. 2008;371(9609):303–14

28. Pectasides D, Pectasides E, Economopoulos T. Fallopian tube carcinoma: a review. Oncologist. 2006;11(8):902–12.

29. Riska A, Leminen A, Pukkala E. Sociodemographic determinants of incidence of primary fallopian tube carcinoma, Finland 1953–97. Int J Cancer J (International du Cancer). 2003;104(5):643–5.

30. Bast RC Jr, Klug TL, St John E, Jenison E, Niloff JM, Lazarus H, et al. A radioimmunoassay using a monoclonal antibody to monitor the course of epithelial ovarian cancer. New Engl J Med. 1983;309(15):883–7.

31. Bonnefoi H, A'Hern RP, Fisher C, Macfarlane V, Barton D, Blake P, et al. Natural history of stage IV epithelial ovarian cancer. J Clin Oncol. 1999;17(3):767–75.

32. Kolomainen DF, Larkin JM, Badran M, A'Hern RP, King DM, Fisher C, et al. Epithelial ovarian cancer metastasizing to the brain: a late manifestation of the disease with an increasing incidence. J Clin Oncol. 2002;20(4):982–6.

33. Pietzner K, Oskay-Oezcelik G, El Khalfaoui K, Boehmer D, Lichtenegger W, Sehouli J. Brain metastases from epithelial ovarian cancer: overview and optimal management. Anticancer Res. 2009;29(7):2793–8.

34. Hidaka T, Nakamura T, Shima T, Sumiya S, Saito S. Cerebral metastasis from a primary adenocarcinoma of the fallopian tube. Gynecol Oncol. 2004;95(1):260–3.

35. Pectasides D, Pectasides M, Economopoulos T. Brain metastases from epithelial ovarian cancer: a review of the literature. Oncologist. 2006;11(3):252–60.

36. Cormio G, Maneo A, Colamaria A, Loverro G, Lissoni A, Selvaggi L. Surgical resection of solitary brain metastasis from ovarian carcinoma: an analysis of 22 cases. Gynecol Oncol. 2003;89(1):116–9.

37. Miller E, Dy I, Herzog T. Leptomeningeal carcinomatosis from ovarian cancer. Med Oncol. 2012;29(3):2010–5.

38. Li HK, Harding V, Williamson R, Blagden S, Gabra H, Agarwal R. Cerebral sinus thrombosis and leptomeningeal carcinomatosis in a patient with ovarian cancer. J Clin Oncol. 2012;30(2):e19–20.

39. Gordon AN, Kavanagh JJ Jr, Wharton JT, Rutledge FN, Obbens EA, Bodey GP Sr. Successful treatment of leptomeningeal relapse of epithelial ovarian cancer. Gynecol Oncol. 1984;18(1):119–24.

40. Chamberlain M, Soffietti R, Raizer J, Ruda R, Brandsma D, Boogerd W, et al. Leptomeningeal metastasis: a response assessment in neuro-oncology critical review of endpoints and response criteria of published randomized clinical trials. Neuro-Oncol. 2014;16(9):1176–85.

41. Glantz MJ, Cole BF, Glantz LK, Cobb J, Mills P, Lekos A, et al. Cerebrospinal fluid cytology in patients with cancer: minimizing false-negative results. Cancer. 1998;82(4):733–9.

42. Patchell RA, Tibbs PA, Walsh JW, Dempsey RJ, Maruyama Y, Kryscio RJ, et al. A randomized trial of surgery in the treatment of single metastases to the brain. New Engl J Med. 1990;322(8):494–500.

43. Vecht CJ, Haaxma-Reiche H, Noordijk EM, Padberg GW, Voormolen JH, Hoekstra FH, et al. Treatment of single brain metastasis: radiotherapy alone or combined with neurosurgery? Ann Neurol. 1993;33(6):583–90.

44. Cohen ZR, Suki D, Weinberg JS, Marmor E, Lang FF, Gershenson DM, et al. Brain metastases in patients with ovarian carcinoma: prognostic factors and outcome. J Neurooncol. 2004;66(3):313–25.

45. Bindal RK, Sawaya R, Leavens ME, Lee JJ. Surgical treatment of multiple brain metastases. J Neurosurg. 1993;79(2):210–6.

46. Corn BW, Mehta MP, Buatti JM, Wolfson AH, Greven KM, Kim RY, et al. Stereotactic irradiation: potential new treatment method for brain metastases resulting from ovarian cancer. Am J Clin Oncol. 1999;22(2):143–6.

47. Andrews DW, Scott CB, Sperduto PW, Flanders AE, Gaspar LE, Schell MC, et al. Whole brain radiation therapy with or without stereotactic radiosurgery boost for patients with one to three brain metastases: phase III results of the RTOG 9508 randomised trial. Lancet. 2004;363(9422):1665–72.

48. Cormio G, Gabriele A, Maneo A, Zanetta G, Bonazzi C, Landoni F. Complete remission of brain metastases from ovarian carcinoma with carboplatin. Eur J Obstet Gynecol Reprod Biol. 1998;78(1):91–3.

49. Watanabe A, Shimada M, Kigawa J, Iba T, Oishi T, Kanamori Y, et al. The benefit of chemotherapy in a patient with multiple brain metastases and meningitis carcinomatosa from ovarian cancer. Int J Clin Oncol. 2005;10(1):69–71.

50. Micha JP, Goldstein BH, Hunter JV, Rettenmaier MA, Brown JV. Long-term survival in an ovarian cancer patient with brain metastases. Gynecol Oncol. 2004;92(3):978–80.

51. Shimada C, Todo Y, Minobe S, Okamoto K, Kato H. Long-term disease-free survival in a patient with cerebral recurrence from adenocarcinoma of the fallopian tube. J Obstet Gynaecol Res. 2013;39(9):1425–9.

52. Arora V, Quinn MA. Endometrial cancer. Best pract & Res Clin Obstet & Gynaecol. 2012;26(3):311–24.

53. American College of O, Gynecologists. ACOG practice bulletin, clinical management guidelines for obstetrician-gynecologists, number 65, August 2005: management of endometrial cancer. Obstet Gynecol. 2005;106(2):413–25.

54. National Cancer Institute. SEER Stat Fact Sheets: Endometrial Cancer [Internet] 2015 [cited 2015 July 10]. Available from: http://seer.cancer.gov/statfacts/html/corp.html.

55. Kimura T, Kamiura S, Yamamoto T, Seino-Noda H, Ohira H, Saji F. Abnormal uterine bleeding and prognosis of endometrial cancer. Int J Gynaecol Obstet. 2004;85(2):145–50.

56. Kurra V, Krajewski KM, Jagannathan J, Giardino A, Berlin S, Ramaiya N. Typical and atypical metastatic sites of recurrent endometrial carcinoma. Cancer Imaging. 2013;13:113–22.

57. Martinez-Manas RM, Brell M, Rumia J, Ferrer E. Brain metastases in endometrial carcinoma. Gynecol Oncol. 1998;70(2):282–4.

58. Mahmoud-Ahmed AS, Suh JH, Barnett GH, Webster KD, Belinson JL, Kennedy AW. The effect of radiation therapy on brain metastases from endometrial carcinoma: a retrospective study. Gynecol Oncol. 2001;83(2):305–9.

59. Cormio G, Lissoni A, Losa G, Zanetta G, Pellegrino A, Mangioni C. Brain metastases from endometrial carcinoma. Gynecol Oncol. 1996;61(1):40–3.

60. Gien LT, Kwon JS, D'Souza DP, Radwan JS, Hammond JA, Sugimoto AK, et al. Brain metastases from endometrial carcinoma: a retrospective study. Gynecol Oncol. 2004;93(2):524–8.

61. Henriksen E. The lymphatic dissemination in endometrial carcinoma. A study of 188 necropsies. Am J Obstet Gynecol. 1975;123(6):570–6.

62. Kottke-Marchant K, Estes ML, Nunez C. Early brain metastases in endometrial carcinoma. Gynecol Oncol. 1991;41(1):67–73.

63. Wronski M, Zakowski M, Arbit E, Hoskins WJ, Galicich JH. Endometrial cancer metastasis to brain: report of two cases and a review of the literature. Surg Neurol. 1993;39(5):355–9.

64. Sawada M, Inagaki M, Ozaki M, Yamasaki M, Nakagawa H, Inoue T, et al. Long-term survival after brain metastasis from endometrial cancer. Jpn J Clin Oncol. 1990;20(3):312–5.

65. Siegel R, Ward E, Brawley O, Jemal A. Cancer statistics, 2011: the impact of eliminating socioeconomic and racial disparities on premature cancer deaths. CA Cancer J Clin. 2011;61(4):212–36.

66. National Cancer Institute. SEER Stat Fact Sheets: Cervic Uteri Cancer [Internet] 2015 [cited 2015 July 10]. Available from: http://seer.cancer.gov/statfacts/html/cervix.html.

67. Walboomers JM, Jacobs MV, Manos MM, Bosch FX, Kummer JA, Shah KV, et al. Human papillomavirus is a necessary cause of invasive cervical cancer worldwide. J Pathol. 1999;189 (1):12–9.

68. International Collaboration of Epidemiological Studies of Cervical C. Comparison of risk factors for invasive squamous cell carcinoma and adenocarcinoma of the cervix: collaborative reanalysis of individual data on 8,097 women with squamous cell carcinoma and 1,374 women with adenocarcinoma from 12 epidemiological studies. Int J Cancer (Journal International du Cancer). 2007;120(4):885–91.

69. DiSaia PJ, Creasman WT. Invasive cervical cancer. Clinical Gynecologic Oncology. 7th ed. Philadelphia: Mosby Elsevier; 2007:55.

70. Saphner T, Gallion HH, Van Nagell JR, Kryscio R, Patchell RA. Neurologic complications of cervical cancer. A review of 2261 cases. Cancer. 1989;64(5):1147–51.

71. Cormio G, Pellegrino A, Landoni F, Regallo M, Zanetta G, Colombo A, et al. Brain metastases from cervical carcinoma. Tumori. 1996;82(4):394–6.

72. Mahmoud-Ahmed AS, Suh JH, Barnett GH, Webster KD, Kennedy AW. Tumor distribution and survival in six patients with brain metastases from cervical carcinoma. Gynecol Oncol. 2001;81(2):196–200.

73. Kumar L, Tanwar RK, Singh SP. Intracranial metastases from carcinoma cervix and review of literature. Gynecol Oncol. 1992;46(3):391–2.

74. Ikeda S, Yamada T, Katsumata N, Hida K, Tanemura K, Tsunematu R, et al. Cerebral metastasis in patients with uterine cervical cancer. Jpn J Clin Oncol. 1998;28(1):27–9.

75. Chura JC, Shukla K, Argenta PA. Brain metastasis from cervical carcinoma. Int J Gynecol Cancer. 2007;17(1):141–6.

76. Rojas-Marcos I, Rousseau A, Keime-Guibert F, Rene R, Cartalat-Carel S, Delattre JY, et al. Spectrum of paraneoplastic neurologic disorders in women with breast and gynecologic cancer. Medicine. 2003;82(3):216–23.

77. Ashour AA, Verschraegen CF, Kudelka AP, Kavanagh JJ. Paraneoplastic syndromes of gynecologic neoplasms. J Clin Oncol. 1997;15(3):1272–82.

78. Haggerty AF, Mantia-Smaldone G, Siegelman E, Livolsi V, Tanyi J. Surgical diagnosis of stage I fallopian tube cancer in

anti-Yo antibody paraneoplastic cerebellar degeneration. J Obstet Gynaecol: J Inst Obstet Gynaecol. 2015;35(1):100–1.

79. Peterson K, Rosenblum MK, Kotanides H, Posner JB. Paraneoplastic cerebellar degeneration. I. A clinical analysis of 55 anti-Yo antibody-positive patients. Neurology. 1992;42 (10):1931–7.

80. Shams'ili S, Grefkens J, de Leeuw B, van den Bent M, Hooijkaas H, van der Holt B, et al. Paraneoplastic cerebellar degeneration associated with antineuronal antibodies: analysis of 50 patients. Brain: J Neurol. 2003;126(Pt 6):1409–18.

81. Greenlee JE. Treatment of paraneoplastic cerebellar degeneration. Curr Treat Options Neurol. 2013;15(2):185–200.

82. Rodriguez M, Truh LI, O'Neill BP, Lennon VA. Autoimmune paraneoplastic cerebellar degeneration: ultrastructural localization of antibody-binding sites in Purkinje cells. Neurology. 1988;38 (9):1380–6.

83. Tanaka Y, Suzuki N, Takao M, Ichikawa A, Susumu N, Aoki D. Paraneoplastic cerebellar degeneration with fallopian tube adenocarcinoma. Gynecol Oncol. 2005;99(2):500–3.

84. Hetzel DJ, Stanhope CR, O'Neill BP, Lennon VA. Gynecologic cancer in patients with subacute cerebellar degeneration predicted by anti-Purkinje cell antibodies and limited in metastatic volume. Mayo Clin Proc. 1990;65(12):1558–63.

85. Rojas I, Graus F, Keime-Guibert F, Rene R, Delattre JY, Ramon JM, et al. Long-term clinical outcome of paraneoplastic cerebellar degeneration and anti-Yo antibodies. Neurology. 2000;55(5):713–5.

86. Hammack JE, Kimmel DW, O'Neill BP, Lennon VA. Paraneoplastic cerebellar degeneration: a clinical comparison of patients with and without Purkinje cell cytoplasmic antibodies. Mayo Clin Proc. 1990;65(11):1423–31.

87. Bradley WH, Dottino PR, Rahaman J. Paraneoplastic cerebellar degeneration in ovarian carcinoma: case report with review of immune modulation. Int J Gynecol Cancer. 2008;18 (6):1364–7.

88. Santillan A, Bristow RE. Paraneoplastic cerebellar degeneration in a woman with ovarian cancer. Nat Clin Pract Oncol. 2006;3 (2):108–12; quiz 1 p following 12.

89. Younes-Mhenni S, Janier MF, Cinotti L, Antoine JC, Tronc F, Cottin V, et al. FDG-PET improves tumour detection in patients with paraneoplastic neurological syndromes. Brain: J Neurol. 2004;127(Pt 10):2331–8.

90. Uchuya M, Graus F, Vega F, Rene R, Delattre JY. Intravenous immunoglobulin treatment in paraneoplastic neurological syndromes with antineuronal autoantibodies. J Neurol Neurosurg Psychiatry. 1996;60(4):388–92.

91. Keime-Guibert F, Graus F, Fleury A, Rene R, Honnorat J, Broet P, et al. Treatment of paraneoplastic neurological syndromes with antineuronal antibodies (Anti-Hu, anti-Yo) with a combination of immunoglobulins, cyclophosphamide, and methylprednisolone. J Neurol Neurosurg Psychiatry. 2000;68 (4):479–82.

92. Orange D, Frank M, Tian S, Dousmanis A, Marmur R, Buckley N, et al. Cellular immune suppression in paraneoplastic neurologic syndromes targeting intracellular antigens. Arch Neurol. 2012;69(9):1132–40.

93. Tuosto L, Cundari E, Gilardini Montani MS, Piccolella E. Analysis of susceptibility of mature human T lymphocytes to dexamethasone-induced apoptosis. Eur J Immunol. 1994;24 (5):1061–5.

94. Shams'ili S, de Beukelaar J, Gratama JW, Hooijkaas H, van den Bent M, van't Veer M, et al. An uncontrolled trial of rituximab for antibody associated paraneoplastic neurological syndromes. J Neurol. 2006;253(1):16–20.

95. Vernino S, O'Neill BP, Marks RS, O'Fallon JR, Kimmel DW. Immunomodulatory treatment trial for paraneoplastic neurological disorders. Neuro-Oncol. 2004;6(1):55–62.

96. Granerod J, Ambrose HE, Davies NW, Clewley JP, Walsh AL, Morgan D, et al. Causes of encephalitis and differences in their clinical presentations in England: a multicentre, population-based prospective study. Lancet Infect Dis. 2010;10(12):835–44.

97. Gable MS, Sheriff H, Dalmau J, Tilley DH, Glaser CA. The frequency of autoimmune N-methyl-D-aspartate receptor encephalitis surpasses that of individual viral etiologies in young individuals enrolled in the California Encephalitis Project. Clin Infect Dis. 2012;54(7):899–904.

98. Dalmau J, Lancaster E, Martinez-Hernandez E, Rosenfeld MR, Balice-Gordon R. Clinical experience and laboratory investigations in patients with anti-NMDAR encephalitis. Lancet Neurol. 2011;10(1):63–74.

99. Iizuka T, Sakai F, Ide T, Monzen T, Yoshii S, Iigaya M, et al. Anti-NMDA receptor encephalitis in Japan: long-term outcome without tumor removal. Neurology. 2008;70(7):504–11.

100. Sansing LH, Tuzun E, Ko MW, Baccon J, Lynch DR, Dalmau J. A patient with encephalitis associated with NMDA receptor antibodies. Nat Clin Pract Neurol. 2007;3(5):291–6.

101. Titulaer MJ, McCracken L, Gabilondo I, Armangue T, Glaser C, Iizuka T, et al. Treatment and prognostic factors for long-term outcome in patients with anti-NMDA receptor encephalitis: an observational cohort study. Lancet Neurol. 2013;12(2):157–65.

102. Tuzun E, Zhou L, Baehring JM, Bannykh S, Rosenfeld MR, Dalmau J. Evidence for antibody-mediated pathogenesis in anti-NMDAR encephalitis associated with ovarian teratoma. Acta Neuropathol. 2009;118(6):737–43.

103. Dabner M, McCluggage WG, Bundell C, Carr A, Leung Y, Sharma R, et al. Ovarian teratoma associated with anti-N-methyl D-aspartate receptor encephalitis: a report of 5 cases documenting prominent intratumoral lymphoid infiltrates. Int J Gynecol Pathol. 2012;31(5):429–37.

104. Gresa-Arribas N, Titulaer MJ, Torrents A, Aguilar E, McCracken L, Leypoldt F, et al. Antibody titres at diagnosis and during follow-up of anti-NMDA receptor encephalitis: a retrospective study. Lancet Neurol. 2014;13(2):167–77.

105. Dalmau J, Tuzun E, Wu HY, Masjuan J, Rossi JE, Voloschin A, et al. Paraneoplastic anti-N-methyl-D-aspartate receptor encephalitis associated with ovarian teratoma. Ann Neurol. 2007;61(1):25–36.

106. Dalmau J, Gleichman AJ, Hughes EG, Rossi JE, Peng X, Lai M, et al. Anti-NMDA-receptor encephalitis: case series and analysis of the effects of antibodies. Lancet Neurol. 2008;7(12):1091–8.

107. Muppidi S, Vernino S. Paraneoplastic neuropathies. Continuum. 2014;20(5 Peripheral Nervous System Disorders):1359–72.

108. Yamada M, Shintani S, Mitani K, Kametani H, Wada Y, Furukawa T, et al. Peripheral neuropathy with predominantly motor manifestations in a patient with carcinoma of the uterus. J Neurol. 1988;235(6):368–70.

109. Durmus H, Tuzun E, Icoz S, Akman-Demir G, Parman Y. Sensorimotor neuropathy associated with endometrioid endometrial carcinoma. Eur J Obstet Gynecol Reprod Biol. 2010;150(2):216–7.

110. Cavaletti G, Bogliun G, Marzorati L, Marzola M, Pittelli MR, Tredici G. The incidence and course of paraneoplastic neuropathy in women with epithelial ovarian cancer. J Neurol. 1991;238(7):371–4.

111. Antoine JC, Honnorat J, Camdessanche JP, Magistris M, Absi L, Mosnier JF, et al. Paraneoplastic anti-CV2 antibodies react with peripheral nerve and are associated with a mixed axonal and demyelinating peripheral neuropathy. Ann Neurol. 2001;49(2):214–21.

112. Rudnick E, Khakoo Y, Antunes NL, Seeger RC, Brodeur GM, Shimada H, et al. Opsoclonus-myoclonus-ataxia syndrome in neuroblastoma: clinical outcome and antineuronal antibodies-a report from the Children's Cancer Group Study. Med Pediatr Oncol. 2001;36(6):612–22.

113. Klaas JP, Ahlskog JE, Pittock SJ, Matsumoto JY, Aksamit AJ, Bartleson JD, et al. Adult-onset opsoclonus-myoclonus syndrome. Arch Neurol. 2012;69(12):1598–607.

114. Luque FA, Furneaux HM, Ferziger R, Rosenblum MK, Wray SH, Schold SC Jr, et al. Anti-Ri: an antibody associated with paraneoplastic opsoclonus and breast cancer. Ann Neurol. 1991;29(3):241–51.

115. Budde-Steffen C, Anderson NE, Rosenblum MK, Graus F, Ford D, Synek BJ, et al. An antineuronal autoantibody in paraneoplastic opsoclonus. Ann Neurol. 1988;23(5):528–31.

116. Lou E, Hensley ML, Lassman AB, Aghajanian C. Paraneoplastic opsoclonus-myoclonus syndrome secondary to immature ovarian teratoma. Gynecol Oncol. 2010;117(2):382–4.

117. Bataller L, Graus F, Saiz A, Vilchez JJ. Spanish Opsoclonus-Myoclonus Study G. Clinical outcome in adult onset idiopathic or paraneoplastic opsoclonus-myoclonus. Brain: J Neurol. 2001;124(Pt 2):437–43.

118. Hormigo A, Dalmau J, Rosenblum MK, River ME, Posner JB. Immunological and pathological study of anti-Ri-associated encephalopathy. Ann Neurol. 1994;36(6):896–902.

119. Bartos A. Effective high-dose clonazepam treatment in two patients with opsoclonus and myoclonus: GABAergic hypothesis. Eur Neurol. 2006;56(4):240–2.

120. Fernandes TD, Bazan R, Betting LE, da Rocha FC. Topiramate effect in opsoclonus-myoclonus-ataxia syndrome. Arch Neurol. 2012;69(1):133.

121. Falanga A, Donati MB. Pathogenesis of thrombosis in patients with malignancy. Int J Hematol. 2001;73(2):137–44.

122. Erturk NK, Erturk A, Basaran D, Ozgul N. Synchronous ovarian and endometrial endometrioid adenocarcinoma presenting with nonbacterial thrombotic endocarditis and pulmonary thromboembolism: adenocarcinoma with thrombotic events. Case Rep Obstet Gynecol. 2015;2015:825404.

123. Tadokoro Y, Sakaguchi M, Yagita Y, Furukado S, Okazaki S, Fujinaka T, et al. Ischemic stroke in patients with solid gynecologic tract tumors and coagulopathy. Eur Neurol. 2013;70(5–6):304–7.

124. Devulapalli S, Pinto N, Gandothra C, Jayam-Trouth A, Kurukumbi M. A rare case of occipital stroke as a consequence of nonbacterial thrombotic endocarditis in ovarian clear cell carcinoma: a case report. Case Rep Neurol. 2012;4(1):84–91.

125. Tanaka H, Ito M, Yoshida K, Asakura T, Taniguchi H. Nonbacterial thrombotic endocarditis complicated with stage Ia ovarian cancer. Int J Clin Oncol. 2009;14(4):369–71.

126. Chomette G, Auriol M, Baubion D, de Frejacques C. Non-bacterial thrombotic endocarditis. Autopsy study, clinico-pathological correlations (author's transl). Ann Med Interne (Paris). 1980;131(7):443–7.

127. Lee AY, Levine MN, Baker RI, Bowden C, Kakkar AK, Prins M, et al. Low-molecular-weight heparin versus a coumarin for the prevention of recurrent venous thromboembolism in patients with cancer. New Engl J Med. 2003;349(2):146–53.

128. Bohrer JC, Walters MD, Park A, Polston D, Barber MD. Pelvic nerve injury following gynecologic surgery: a prospective cohort study. Am J Obstet Gynecol. 2009;201(5):531 e1–7.

129. Hoffman MS, Roberts WS, Cavanagh D. Neuropathies associated with radical pelvic surgery for gynecologic cancer. Gynecol Oncol. 1988;31(3):462–6.

130. Cardosi RJ, Cox CS, Hoffman MS. Postoperative neuropathies after major pelvic surgery. Obstet Gynecol. 2002;100(2):240–4.

131. Irvin W, Andersen W, Taylor P, Rice L. Minimizing the risk of neurologic injury in gynecologic surgery. Obstet Gynecol. 2004;103(2):374–82.

132. Loos MJ, Scheltinga MR, Mulders LG, Roumen RM. The Pfannenstiel incision as a source of chronic pain. Obstet Gynecol. 2008;111(4):839–46.

133. Chan JK, Manetta A. Prevention of femoral nerve injuries in gynecologic surgery. Am J Obstet Gynecol. 2002;186(1):1–7.

134. Warner MA, Warner DO, Harper CM, Schroeder DR, Maxson PM. Lower extremity neuropathies associated with lithotomy positions. Anesthesiology. 2000;93(4):938–42.

135. Delanian S, Lefaix JL, Pradat PF. Radiation-induced neuropathy in cancer survivors. Radiotherapy Oncol: J Eur Soc Ther Radiol Oncol. 2012;105(3):273–82.

136. Georgiou A, Grigsby PW, Perez CA. Radiation induced lumbosacral plexopathy in gynecologic tumors: clinical findings and dosimetric analysis. Int J Radiat Oncol Biol Phys. 1993;26(3):479–82.

137. Aho K, Sainio K. Late irradiation-induced lesions of the lumbosacral plexus. Neurology. 1983;33(7):953–5.

138. Jaeckle KA. Neurologic manifestations of neoplastic and radiation-induced plexopathies. Semin Neurol. 2010;30(3):254–62.

139. Meyer LA, Bohlke K, Powell MA, Fader AN, Franklin GE, Lee LJ, et al. Postoperative radiation therapy for endometrial cancer: American Society of clinical oncology clinical practice guideline endorsement of the American Society for radiation oncology evidence-based guideline. J Clin Oncol. 2015;33(26):2908–13.

140. Han K, Milosevic M, Fyles A, Pintilie M, Viswanathan AN. Trends in the utilization of brachytherapy in cervical cancer in the United States. Int J Radiat Oncol Biol Phys. 2013;87(1):111–9.

141. Qayyum A, MacVicar AD, Padhani AR, Revell P, Husband JE. Symptomatic brachial plexopathy following treatment for breast cancer: utility of MR imaging with surface-coil techniques. Radiology. 2000;214(3):837–42.

142. Pritchard J, Anand P, Broome J, Davis C, Gothard L, Hall E, et al. Double-blind randomized phase II study of hyperbaric oxygen in patients with radiation-induced brachial plexopathy. Radiother Oncol: J Eur Soc Ther Radiol Oncol. 2001;58(3):279–86.

143. Bennett MH, Feldmeier J, Hampson N, Smee R, Milross C. Hyperbaric oxygen therapy for late radiation tissue injury. Cochrane Database Syst Rev. 2005;(3):CD005005.

144. Argyriou AA, Bruna J, Marmiroli P, Cavaletti G. Chemotherapy-induced peripheral neurotoxicity (CIPN): an update. Crit Rev Oncol Hematol. 2012;82(1):51–77.

145. von Schlippe M, Fowler CJ, Harland SJ. Cisplatin neurotoxicity in the treatment of metastatic germ cell tumour: time course and prognosis. Br J Cancer. 2001;85(6):823–6.

146. Argyriou AA, Polychronopoulos P, Iconomou G, Koutras A, Kalofonos HP, Chroni E. Paclitaxel plus carboplatin-induced peripheral neuropathy. A prospective clinical and electrophysiological study in patients suffering from solid malignancies. J Neurol. 2005;252(12):1459–64.

147. Krzakowski M, Ramlau R, Jassem J, Szczesna A, Zatloukal P, Von Pawel J, et al. Phase III trial comparing vinflunine with docetaxel in second-line advanced non-small-cell lung cancer previously treated with platinum-containing chemotherapy. J Clin Oncol. 2010;28(13):2167–73.

148. Grisold W, Cavaletti G, Windebank AJ. Peripheral neuropathies from chemotherapeutics and targeted agents: diagnosis, treatment, and prevention. Neuro-Oncol. 2012;14 Suppl 4:iv45–54.

149. Rybak LP, Mukherjea D, Jajoo S, Ramkumar V. Cisplatin ototoxicity and protection: clinical and experimental studies. Tohoku J Exp Med. 2009;219(3):177–86.

Megan L. Kruse and David M. Peereboom

Introduction

Sarcomas are malignant tumors that are derived from mesenchymal cells and can originate from a large variety of tissues including bone, muscle, fat, cartilage, and peripheral nerves. At least 50 different subtypes of soft tissue sarcoma have been described to date, which highlights the incredible heterogeneity existing within this tumor family [1]. Sarcomas are fairly rare tumors that account for approximately 1% all cancers overall. Although it is generally uncommon for sarcomas to occur within or metastasize to the CNS (approximately 3% of all brain metastases are sarcomas), there is concern that CNS involvement may become more common in the future due to better control of systemic disease through chemotherapy and radiation therapy without effective CNS treatment options [2]. Neurologic complications of sarcoma can also occur when the tumor is outside of the central nervous system specifically through extrinsic spinal cord compression, compression of peripheral nerves, or by paraneoplastic syndromes. This chapter will highlight common subtypes of sarcomas and the associated neurologic complications of the disease and its treatment.

Chondrosarcoma

Chondrosarcomas are malignant tumors that arise from a cartilaginous matrix. They can occur in any bone including those of the skull base where it is thought that they arise from embryonic cartilaginous remnants. As a group, chondrosarcomas account for 20–27% of primary malignancies

M.L. Kruse
Department of Hematology/Oncology, Cleveland Clinic,
9500 Euclid Ave, CA60, Cleveland, OH 44195, USA
e-mail: krusem@ccf.org

D.M. Peereboom (✉)
Burkhardt Brain Tumor and Neuro-Oncology Center, Cleveland
Clinic, 9500 Euclid Ave, CA51, Cleveland, OH 44195, USA
e-mail: peerebd@ccf.org

of bone [3]. Intracranial chondrosarcomas are rare, accounting for less than 0.2% of all intracranial tumors and approximately 6% of all skull base tumors [4]. They have been known to occur in the petrosal bone, occipital bone/clivus, sphenoid bone, frontal bone, and ethmoidal and parietal bones but can also arise from dural tissue [5]. Chondrosarcomas can also infrequently arise in the orbit and have potential for intracranial extension [6]. Metastasis from a systemic primary tumor may occur although this scenario is less commonly reported than primary skull base chondrosarcoma [7].

These tumors have no gender predominance and most commonly occur in the 3–4th decade of life although have been reported in both infants and the elderly [5]. Chondrosarcomas that occur outside of the head and neck are most commonly (90%) low-to-intermediate grade tumors that grow slowly and have low metastatic potential [8]. In contrast, intracranial chondrosarcomas have been reported to be more evenly distributed between lower grade tumors and the more aggressive mesenchymal subtype [5]. Chondrosarcomas can arise from preceding osteochrondromas or enchondromas, both of which are benign cartilaginous tumors. The congenital syndromes of Ollier disease and Maffucci syndrome are characterized by the presence of multiple enchondromas and a risk of chondrosarcoma of up to 50% [9–11].

Skull base chondrosarcomas commonly present with cranial nerve deficits. Oculomotor dysfunction was the most frequent cranial nerve deficit reported in a series of 192 patients with intracranial chondrosarcoma by Korten and colleagues [5]. The abducens nerve is particularly vulnerable to compression by these tumors due to proximity of the nerve to the skull base [12]. Other symptoms of intracranial chondrosarcomas include headache, hearing loss, sensory changes of the face/facial palsy, ataxia, hemiparesis, memory loss, and nausea/vomiting [5]. On imaging, these tumors may demonstrate bony destruction and calcification and can appear very similar to meningioma, making histologic examination crucial for diagnosis.

© Springer International Publishing AG 2018
D. Schiff et al. (eds.), *Cancer Neurology in Clinical Practice*,
DOI 10.1007/978-3-319-57901-6_27

The management of both intra- and extracranial chondrosarcomas relies heavily on surgical resection to obtain optimal outcomes. For extracranial chondrosarcomas, management with wide local excision is the preferred approach. Lower grade tumors may be amenable to intralesional curettage with subsequent local cryotherapy/chemical therapy (phenolization) although there is concern for higher rates of local recurrence and greater risk of metastasis [13–17]. Radiation therapy can be used in the event of incomplete resection to obtain the best local control and in situations where surgical resection is not possible or would be associated with unacceptable morbidity. These tumors, however, are generally considered relatively radioresistant [18, 19].

Treatment of intracranial chondrosarcoma is similar to that of extracranial lesions; however, complete resection is often not feasible due to the proximity of critical neurovascular structures. Use of conventional radiation therapy has also been limited because high doses of radiation, which can cause damage to cranial nerves and the brain stem, are often required to be effective for these slow-growing tumors. Newer approaches involve use of charged particle radiation therapy and stereotactic radiosurgery to overcome the issues with conventional surgery and radiation [20, 21].

Systemic chemotherapy has been used in the setting of recurrence and metastatic disease; however, its role is not clearly defined. In a 2003 review of 23 cases of intraspinal chondrosarcoma, 11 patients received chemotherapy with agents including ifosfamide, doxorubicin, cisplatin, etoposide, carboplatin, epirubicin, cyclophosphamide, and methotrexate [22]. Chondrosarcoma is known as a relatively chemoresistant tumor, and in the aforementioned review, improvement in CNS disease was seen in some patients although the number was too few to draw any definitive conclusions [22, 23].

A 2009 systematic review of 560 patients with intracranial chondrosarcoma reported a 5-year mortality rate of 12% with median survival of 24 months and an average survival time of 53 months [24]. In this review, mortality was significantly greater for patients with mesenchymal histology versus conventional histology (6% vs. 54%, respectively). Those patients treated with surgery alone had a 5-year mortality rate of 26%, while those who had postoperative radiation therapy had a 5-year mortality rate of 4%.

Malignant Fibrous Histiocytoma/Undifferentiated Pleomorphic Sarcoma

Malignant fibrous histiocytoma (MFH) is a soft tissue sarcoma pathologically consisting of fibrohistiocytic cells and spindle cells most commonly arranged in a storiform pattern [25]. In 2002, the World Health Organization (WHO) removed MFH as a formal diagnostic entity and renamed it "undifferentiated pleomorphic sarcoma" (UPS) in an attempt to reflect the uncertainty about the cell of origin for these tumors. UPS very rarely occurs in the central nervous system (<3% of cases) but has been described in the brain, dura, spine, peripheral nerves, and cranial bones [26, 27]. Intracranial UPS may represent a primary central nervous system tumor or a metastasis from a systemic primary tumor [27]. The most common intracranial sites are supratentorial and can mimic meningioma on imaging (Fig. 27.1a, b) [28, 29]. UPS has also been found in the cerebellum and at the cerebellar pontine angle [28]. While many of these tumors appear as mass lesions on imaging, one report describes a case of intracranial UPS that infiltrated the pons, cerebellum, and basal surface of the left temporal lobe without any visible mass [30]. On autopsy, these areas of the brain were found to contain anaplastic proliferation of spindle-shaped cells in a storiform pattern with immunophenotype studies consistent with UPS.

UPS is most commonly seen in middle-aged adults with no clear gender predominance [28]. The etiology of these tumors is also unclear although they may be associated with prior radiation or trauma to tumor site [31]. Neurologic symptoms related to an intracranial UPS vary depending on the location of the tumor with common symptoms being those of increased intracranial pressure such as headache. Neurologic complications can also arise from a UPS that arises outside the CNS in which case symptoms are related to compression of nearby peripheral nerves with resulting pain, altered sensation, or weakness. This is most often seen in the setting of retroperitoneal or lower extremity tumors. Paraneoplastic syndromes related to UPS can include opsoclonus-myoclonus syndrome and brain stem encephalitis [32, 33].

Surgical resection of UPS is the cornerstone of treatment [29]. The typical approach to treatment of these tumors when they occur outside the CNS consists of maximal safe resection followed by adjuvant chemotherapy and radiation. Consideration of doxorubicin-based combination chemotherapy has been previously proposed [34]; however, the effectiveness of chemotherapy for UPS is uncertain [29]. The approach to treatment of intracranial UPS also focuses on maximal safe resection often followed by radiation therapy. Utilization of chemotherapy is limited in this scenario as doxorubicin (the most well-studied chemotherapy used for systemic UPS) has poor blood-brain barrier penetration. Overall prognosis of UPS is generally poor due to frequent and rapid local recurrent following resection.

Solitary Fibrous Tumor/Hemangiopericytoma

Hemangiopericytoma (HPC) was originally described in 1942 as a soft tissue neoplasm thought to arise from pericytes, the cells that form the walls of capillaries and post-capillary

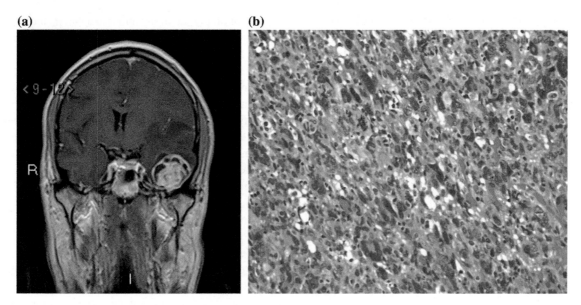

Fig. 27.1 A 34-year-old man presented with left-sided headaches, word finding difficulty, and short-term memory loss. Contrast-enhanced T1 coronal MRI (A) demonstrates a heterogeneously enhancing mass that appears to extend to the dura. CT scans of the chest, abdomen, and pelvis were negative. Resection of a mass that intraoperatively appeared to arise from the dura with left temporal mass May 2015 revealed a hypercellular lesion (B, H, and E) composed of pleomorphic cells with hyperchromatic, atypical nuclei. Immunostains and molecular tests for high-grade glioma (GFAP, OLIG2, S100, EGFR, IDHmt, and MGMT), carcinoma, melanoma, rhabdomyosarcoma, and leiomyosarcoma were all negative. The findings best supported a diagnosis of undifferentiated pleomorphic sarcoma

venules. Pathologically, HPC was defined by a distinctive "staghorn" branching pattern of vasculature [35]. While the term "hemangiopericytoma" is still used by neuropathologists, general consensus is that the tumors traditionally been called HPCs are actually quite heterogeneous. Previously, these tumors were classified separately as meningeal solitary fibrous tumors (SFTs) and hemangiopericytoma. The most recent WHO classification of central nervous system tumors, however, has grouped these tumors into a single entity named solitary fibrous tumor/hemangiopericytoma (SFT/HPC). [36]. Most of these tumors can be identified by STAT6 nuclear expression, which is detectable by immunohistochemistry [36]. In reviewing the literature on this topic, one may find the terms CNS HPC or intracranial HPC used to describe SFT/HPC of the CNS.

Solitary fibrous tumors have 3 typical primary locations: pleura, meninges, and extrathoracic soft tissue [37]. Most (80%) of pleural-based SFTs are benign. Pleural-based SFTs generally occur in the 5th–7th decade of life, occur equally in men and women, and have no clear risk factors. These tumors may cause symptoms characteristic of pleural irritation (pleuritic pain, cough, dyspnea) and have also been associated with paraneoplastic osteoarthropathy and paraneoplastic hypoglycemia [37–39]. Extrathoracic soft tissue SFTs also tend to occur in the 5th decade of life and occur equally in both genders. They generally present as painlessly enlarging soft tissue masses that may be asymptomatic until they cause compression of adjacent structures.

SFT/HPC represents 2–3% of all meningeal tumors and <1% of all intracranial tumors [40, 41]. These tumors generally occur in those aged 40–50 and have been suggested to have a gender distribution that is dependent on age. In a recent systematic review of over 500 patients with SFT/HPC, it was found that below age 45, the tumors were more common in men, while above age 45, they were more common in women [40]. The most common symptoms associated with intracranial HPC include headache and upper/lower limb weakness [42]. SFT/HPCs generally grow slowly although they can cause great morbidity due to their highly vascular and invasive nature. They often appear similar to a benign meningioma on radiographic studies, making preoperative diagnosis of HPC difficult.

Surgical resection is the most important component of management of all SFTs/HPCs. Multiple studies have demonstrated statistically significant improved overall survival in patients with SFT/HPC who had complete resection rather than incomplete resection [40]. The role of radiation therapy in management of intracranial HPC has been debated. Although the review by Ghose and colleagues showed a statistically improved survival when adjuvant radiation therapy was added to surgical resection [40], multiple other studies have been unable to show a survival benefit with addition of adjuvant radiation [43, 44]. Adjuvant radiation may play a role in decreasing local recurrence and improving time to local recurrence [41, 42, 45]. Adjuvant chemotherapy is not a standard component of management of localized soft tissue/pleural-based SFTs; however, response to chemotherapy (particularly doxorubicin) appears to be better in these tumors than in SFT/HPC [46]. There has been interest in using temozolomide and VEGF inhibitors in SFT/HPC with evidence showing response to this combination in small numbers of patients. However, a controlled, prospective trial is lacking [47].

SFT/HPCs tend to have high local recurrence rate but can also cause extracranial metastases. Although complete resection of the primary SFT/HPC improves overall survival, complete resection appears to have no impact on controlling rates of distant metastasis [40, 48]. The pattern of development of extracranial metastases requires long-term follow-up and awareness on the part of the provider as metastases can develop years after the primary tumor (typically 5–8 years but up to 20 years). Typical extracranial metastatic sites include bone, lung, and liver [37, 49, 50].

Rhabdomyosarcoma

Rhabdomyosarcoma (RMS) is a soft tissue sarcoma that is morphologically similar to other small round cell tumors but is specifically characterized by features of skeletal muscle including histological identification of cross-striations. This tumor is the most common soft tissue tumor of childhood but accounts for only 3–4% of pediatric cancers overall [51]. The majority of cases are diagnosed in children under the age of 6 with a slight male predominance and higher incidence in African Americans compared to Caucasians. Histologically, these tumors are classified as either embryonal or alveolar. Embryonal RMS is more commonly found in the head and neck or urinary tract, while alveolar-type RMS is more commonly found in the extremities [52]. No clear risk factors for RMS have been identified although there is an association with higher incidence with neurofibromatosis, Li–Fraumeni syndrome, Beckwith–Wiedemann syndrome, and Costello syndrome [53–56]. Despite the association with these syndromes, sporadic cases of RMS are most common. Rhabdomyosarcomas often present as areas of swelling either in the head and neck region or in the extremities with variable degrees of pain.

Primary intracranial RMS is very rare. Most CNS involvement with RMS occurs as a result of intracranial extension of tumors that occur in the head and neck (in areas such as the orbit, paranasal sinuses, middle ear, infratemporal fossa) rather than by lymphatic spread [57]. As in other sarcomas, brain metastases occur uncommonly with systemic RMS. The most common sites of metastases for RMS include bone marrow and lungs [57]. If brain metastases do occur, they generally develop with or after pulmonary metastases [58]. Neurologic symptoms associated with intracranial RMS, whether primary or metastatic, are largely dependent on the site of the tumor and can include headache, visual disturbance, papilledema, or proptosis with orbital tumors and nasal discharge due to sinus obstruction [52, 59]. Direct extension from these locations can result in leptomeningeal disease [60, 61].

Treatment of RMS generally involves use of combined modality therapy under guidelines developed by cooperative groups such as the Soft Tissue Sarcoma Committee of the Children's Oncology Group (formerly known as the Intergroup Rhabdomyosarcoma Study Group or IRSG). The use of multimodality therapy has been crucial in the improvement of survival rates in RMS in children [62]. Treatment decisions are based largely on a prognostic stratification system with the knowledge that prognosis of RMS is highly dependent on site of presentation. For example, a SEER database review of 558 cases of head and neck RMS reported from 1973 to 2007 showed 5-year survival rates of 49, 70, and 84% for parameningeal sites, non-parameningeal non-orbital sites, and orbital tumors, respectively [63]. Prognosis in adults is generally worse than in children, and studies have demonstrated that results of treatment are most favorable when adults are treated using pediatric clinical trial protocols (often enroll patients up to age 50) [64]. RMS tends to be quite radiosensitive, and radiation therapy has been a critical component of management of parameningeal primary tumors as well as metastatic intracranial disease [65]. Chemotherapy regimens for systemic RMS including vincristine, doxorubicin, and cyclophosphamide have limited utility for intracranial disease due to lack of blood-brain barrier penetration [64]. Once a patient develops cerebral metastases, survival is very short. In a series of over 400 pediatric patients with RMS, 2% of patients were found to have brain metastases and median survival was 2.7 months after diagnosis of brain metastases despite aggressive therapy [66].

Leiomyosarcoma

Leiomyosarcomas are soft tissue sarcomas that occur most commonly in the retroperitoneum, GI tract, uterus, and skin [67]. Primary CNS leiomyosarcoma is a very rare entity that has been reported more frequently in the HIV/AIDS era due to an association between development of leiomyosarcoma and EBV infection [68]. A similar rise in incidence has been seen in patients with solid organ transplant due to immunosuppression although the absolute incidence of primary CNS leiomyosarcoma remains very low [67]. Primary CNS leiomyosarcomas have been described from ages 4 to 72 years with no clear gender predominance [69–72]. Risk factors for development include immunosuppression as well as prior CNS radiation exposure [73]. As with other intracranial sarcomas, symptoms correlate with location of tumor and can include headache, motor deficits, and seizures. The prognosis of primary CNS leiomyosarcoma is poor with the longest reported overall survival of 32 months [69, 71, 74]. The approach to treatment of primary CNS leiomyosarcoma is not standardized due to the small number of cases; however, a multimodality approach utilizing surgical resection, radiation therapy, and chemotherapy is typically advocated [72]. Doxorubicin is the typical first-line chemotherapy for systemic leiomyosarcoma although dacarbazine, gemcitabine, and docetaxel are all reported to be active agents for leiomyosarcoma [23, 75]. It is unknown what the optimal chemotherapy regimen for CNS leiomyosarcoma is and outcome data are sparse.

Metastatic disease to the CNS from a systemic leiomyosarcoma is also very rare. To date, only 16 cases of CNS metastases from uterine leiomyosarcoma have been reported [67]. When CNS metastases do occur, they are generally found supratentorially with reports of involvement of the frontal and parietal lobes [76]. Treatment of brain metastases may include surgical resection, if feasible, though most commonly includes radiation, either whole-brain radiation therapy or stereotactic radiosurgery [77]. Prognosis once a patient develops CNS metastases from systemic leiomyosarcoma is also very poor and likely measured in months [67].

Malignant Peripheral Nerve Sheath Tumor

Malignant Peripheral Nerve Sheath Tumors (MPNSTs) are soft tissue sarcomas that arise from peripheral nerves. They can arise from any component of the nerve sheath including Schwann cells, fibroblasts, and perineural cells [78]. These tumors occur in approximately 0.001% of the general population but affect individuals with neurofibromatosis type 1 (NF1) at a higher rate with a 5–10% lifetime risk [79]. There is also a weak association with neurofibromatosis type 2 (NF2) [80]. Previous radiation exposure is an additional risk factor with approximately 10% of MPNSTs occurring in patients who have had prior radiation [81, 82]. MPNSTs occur in men and women with equal distribution and can occur at any age with a mean age of 40 years [83, 84]. The age of onset tends to be younger in patients with NF1. Intracranial MPNSTs are more common in men and are less likely to be associated with NF1 [83]. MPNSTs tend to occur most commonly in the extremities at sites of major nerve trunks like the sciatic nerve [78]. These tumors can also occur in the trunk or head and neck. Involvement of cranial nerves or intraosseous nerves is rare but can cause important neurologic symptoms including cranial nerve palsies and spinal cord compression [85, 86].

The presentation of MPNST commonly includes evidence of a painful enlarging mass. As these tumors originate from nerve sheaths, other common presenting symptoms are those of nerve compression including motor deficit or paresthesias in the innervated region of the particular nerve affected [78]. Intracranial involvement may occur with cranial nerves (primarily centered around the cerebellopontine angle but can also be intraventricular or intraparenchymal [87]. Presenting symptoms can be non-specific such as headache or dizziness. Other patients present with more specific signs of cranial nerve palsy. Karami and colleagues reported a case of MPNST of the vestibulocochlear nerve and brain stem in a young woman who presented with dizziness, headache, ataxia, and sudden unilateral hearing loss with hemifacial paralysis [85].

MPNSTs are generally aggressive tumors with high rates of local recurrent and metastasis via hematogenous spread. A review from 2014 reported a recurrence rate of MPNSTs as high as 40% with approximately two-thirds of patients experiencing metastatic spread (most commonly to lungs and bone) [78]. They also reported a poorer prognosis associated with larger tumors (variably defined as either greater than 5 cm or 7 cm depending on the series), those with higher histologic grade and those associated with NF1. Prognosis of intracranial MPNST also appears to be worse than extracranial disease with one review reporting 5-year overall survival of 14% [87].

Treatment of both extracranial and intracranial MPNSTs is focused on maximal safe surgical resection. These tumors have limited sensitivity to chemotherapy and radiation so the role of adjuvant therapy is unclear. Adjuvant radiation may improve local control rates although there is no clear survival benefit [88, 89]. A 2013 review of all reported cases ($n = 61$) of intracranial MPNST showed that nearly equal numbers of patients received partial resection and gross total resection. The majority of patients in this review received radiation after surgery, while very few (4 of 61) received chemotherapy [87]. Survival seems to be improved with adjuvant radiation therapy regardless of surgical results (partial or gross total resection) as the irradiated patients had a mean survival of 30 months with a 5-year survival of 30%, while unirradiated patients had a mean survival of 8.6 months with no survivors at 5 years. Notably, this study included 5 patients with history of NF1, and these patients were found to have survival from time of diagnosis of 3–5 months.

Osteosarcoma

Osteosarcoma is the most frequently occurring primary malignant tumor of bone [90] although it is rare overall and accounts for approximately 1% of all cancers in the USA annually [91]. It has a bimodal distribution in incidence with peaks occurring in adolescence and again at age over 65

[91]. In both adolescents and adults, males are more commonly affected than females. In children, African Americans are more commonly affected than whites; however, in adults, whites are more commonly affected than other races [91]. Predisposing factors include prior radiation and Paget's disease. Several genetic conditions also predispose to the development of osteosarcoma including hereditary retinoblastoma, Li-Fraumeni syndrome, and Rothmund–Thomson syndrome [92]. Typical sites of primary osteosarcoma include femur, tibia, humerus, and pelvis. Osteosarcomas usually present with bone pain. Osteosarcomas of the vertebral column and skull bones are rare. When the tumor involves the spine, presenting symptoms can include those of spinal cord compression. One case of primary osteosarcoma of the lamina of L2 presented with painless paraplegia in a young woman [93].

Osteosarcoma typically has a hematogenous route of spread with common metastatic sites including lung and other bones [94]. CNS metastasis of osteosarcoma is uncommon, occurring in only 2–6% of cases [95]. Pulmonary metastasis usually precedes CNS metastasis. A case report described an orbital metastasis of osteosarcoma in an eight-year-old girl, which presented as severe, progressive ptosis with associated visual disturbance after a minor orbital injury [96]. On evaluation, this patient was found to have a primary tumor of femur without pulmonary metastasis. A recent review of 55 cases of metastatic osteosarcoma involving the CNS showed that brain metastases have occurred throughout the cerebrum (with the frontal lobe being most common) and cerebellum in addition to the bones of the skull [90]. Treatment of these patients included a combination of surgical resection, whole-brain radiation therapy, or stereotactic radiosurgery. Chemotherapy may be used for osteosarcoma of the central nervous system; however, given the small number of cases reported in the literature, there is no consensus on optimal regimen to use. In a review of 19 cases of primary meningeal osteosarcoma, use of "standard osteosarcoma chemotherapy" was described [97]. Typical osteosarcoma regimens include doxorubicin with high-dose methotrexate and cisplatin [98]. Both methotrexate and cisplatin have known ability to penetrate the blood-brain barrier so are reasonable choices for treatment of CNS metastases [99]. Other agents used in osteosarcoma include ifosfamide and etoposide which also have been known to cross the blood-brain barrier [98, 99]. The overall mean survival for patients following diagnosis of brain metastases was 18.4 ± 30.4 months, highlighting the variability in clinical course [90].

Ewing's Sarcoma

Ewing's sarcoma accounts for approximately 6% of all childhood malignancies with peak incidence from age 10–15 years [100, 101]. Unlike osteosarcoma, Ewing's sarcoma rarely affects adults. Any bone can be affected; however, the femur, pelvis, and axial skeleton are most commonly involved [102]. The most common presenting symptom of Ewing's sarcoma is pain, which is typically progressive. The pain can often be exacerbated by activity and tends to be worse at night [103]. Up to 80% of patients have subclinical metastatic disease at the time of presentation [104]. Ewing's sarcoma has been known to metastasize to the CNS in 32–56% of cases with less than 2% of these cases comprising brain metastases [105]. More commonly, direct extension of tumor from location in bony elements of the spine causes CNS involvement. Symptoms of spine involvement can include back pain, radiculopathy, lower extremity weakness, or paresthesias. A recent review of 40 cases of Ewing's sarcoma brain metastases showed that the parietal lobe was most commonly affected followed by the frontal lobe, then the temporal/occipital lobes [90]. Management of primary Ewing's sarcoma is generally treated with multimodality therapy including chemotherapy, radiation, and surgical resection. In the review referenced above, management of Ewing's sarcoma brain metastases included surgical resection (25%), whole-brain radiation therapy (70%), stereotactic radiosurgery (18%), and conservative management (17%). The overall survival of these patients was 7.1 months (±7.7 months, range 0–24 months) after detection of metastatic disease to the brain [90].

Typical first-line chemotherapy regimens for Ewing's sarcoma include agents such as cyclophosphamide, doxorubicin, vincristine, etoposide, and ifosfamide [98]. Of these agents, etoposide and ifosfamide are known to be active in the CNS and this 5-drug regimen has been used previously in a case of primary intraspinal intradural extra-osseous Ewing's sarcoma [99, 106]. Other chemotherapy regimens used for systemic recurrence of Ewing's sarcoma including cyclophosphamide/topotecan, irinotecan/temozolomide, and gemcitabine have also been used in cases of CNS involvement by Ewing's sarcoma [107]. In a study of 18 children with CNS involvement by sarcoma (10 had Ewing's sarcoma), survival from time of CNS involvement until death, or last follow-up was similar between those receiving CNS-directed therapy (radiation/surgical resection) and chemotherapy, ranging from 2 to 6 months [107].

Gliosarcoma

Gliosarcoma is a rare primary brain tumor composed of a combination of malignant glial cells and mesenchymal elements. The mesenchymal elements of the tumor can show fibrosarcomatous, pleomorphic sarcomatous, leiomyosarcomatous, or osteosarcomatous patterns [108]. These tumors represent approximately 2% of glioblastomas (GBM) [109] and are molecularly identical to GBM with presumed sarcomatous metaplasia. They occur more commonly in men with typical age of onset in the 5th–6th decade of life [110, 111]. Gliosarcomas are most often found in the temporal lobe [111] and can present with symptoms such as headache and motor weakness [110]. These tumors have a similar clinical pattern of behavior as GBM overall although they have a unique propensity to metastasize extracranially. Involvement of the lungs, pancreas, bone marrow, and liver has all been reported with gliosarcoma [110, 112, 113]. Typical GBMs do not spread hematogenously but rather spread via the cerebrospinal fluid with resulting metastasis throughout the neuraxis [114–116]. Gliosarcomas also metastasize to other locations within the neuraxis as evidenced in the report of an intramedullary cervical spinal cord metastasis from a temporal lobe primary gliosarcoma by [117]. Prognosis for both glioblastoma and gliosarcoma is poor with overall survival on the order of months. In a 2009 review of all cases of glioblastoma and gliosarcoma reported in the SEER database of the US National Cancer Institute from 1988 to 2004, overall survival was slightly worse for gliosarcoma [118]. As this tumor is very rare, there is no standardized approach to treatment; however, surgical resection and radiation have been used [118]. Typically, these tumors are managed similarly to GBM and are generally included in GBM clinical trials.

Gastrointestinal Stromal Tumor

Gastrointestinal stromal tumors (GISTs) are mesenchymal tumors that arise from the interstitial cells of Cajal [119]. They commonly originate in the stomach and small intestine although they can occur throughout the GI tract or in extraintestinal sites such as the omentum or retroperitoneum [120–122]. GISTs account for up to 3% of all GI neoplasms and 5–7% of all sarcomas [123, 124]. Common presenting symptoms include abdominal pain, vomiting, anorexia, or bowel obstruction [122]. These tumors commonly metastasize, and up to one half of patients will have distant metastases at the time of diagnosis [125]. Common metastatic sites include the liver, peritoneum, and lung. CNS metastases are very rare although there have been reports of brain parenchymal lesions in both children and adults [122, 126]. Symptoms reported with intracranial space occupying

metastases include headache, weakness, and vomiting [122, 126]. There has also been a report of metastatic GIST involving the thoracic and lumbar spine which resulted in bilateral scapular tightness/pain and low back pain [125].

GISTs have traditionally been resistant to chemotherapy and radiation therapy [127]. Surgical resection is the treatment of choice for primary GIST [128]. Advances in treatment for relapsed or advanced disease occurred with the introduction of molecularly targeted therapy, specifically imatinib mesylate a small molecule kinase inhibitor. Lower concentrations of imatinib are achieved in the central nervous systems of both mice and humans [129, 130], which correlates with clinical observations of imatinib being ineffective in treatment of CNS metastases. Surgical resection has been utilized for management of intracranial or spinal metastases [119, 122, 125, 126].

Targeted Therapy for Sarcoma and Implications for CNS Involvement

Traditionally, sarcomas have been divided into groups based on site of origin and histopathologic features. More recently, effort has been directed to separating sarcomas into different categories based on their genetic characteristics. Some sarcomas are characterized by discrete genetic changes that may serve as the target for therapy, such as the 11:22 translocation seen in Ewing's sarcoma [1]. Other sarcomas are characterized by complex genetic changes that are not as easily targetable, such as leiomyosarcoma or undifferentiated pleomorphic sarcoma [1]. Identification of specific genetic targets or discovery of particular cellular pathways implicated in oncogenesis has opened the door for new drug development and testing of existing drugs in sarcoma with the hope of improving clinical outcomes.

Cellular pathways involved in angiogenesis have been an area of interest for drug development in sarcoma. Pazopanib is an angiogenesis inhibitor that targets VEGF receptors 1–3, PDGF receptor α/β, and c-kit that has recently been approved for use in patients with advanced soft tissue sarcomas who have received prior chemotherapy [1]. In the phase III PALETTE (pazopanib for metastatic soft tissue sarcoma) study, an improvement in progression-free survival was found for pazopanib compared to placebo (4.6 months vs. 1.6 months, respectively) with no difference in overall survival in the setting of advanced soft tissue sarcoma [131]. While no data exist for the use of pazopanib in sarcomas involving the CNS, there is a report of renal cell carcinoma brain metastases that were responsive to pazopanib [132]. This suggests that pazopanib may be helpful for intracranial disease. In this case report, the patient received whole-brain radiation therapy prior to pazopanib so it is unclear whether the drug has CNS activity on its own or whether the effect of radiation was necessary to allow CNS activity. In either case, pazopanib may have a role in treatment of sarcoma with CNS involvement. Although not FDA approved, agents including temozolomide/bevacizumab and sunitinib, which also have anti-angiogenic activity, have activity in small numbers of patients with hemangiopericytoma/solitary fibrous tumor extraskeletal myxoid chondrosarcoma and may be considered for off-label use with CNS involvement [47, 133, 134].

There has been interest in targeting the insulin-like growth factor 1 (IGF1) receptor in Ewing's sarcoma since it was discovered that the 11:22 translocation characteristic of Ewing's sarcoma produces a fusion protein (EWS-FLI1) that helps to upregulate IGF1 [135]. Two monoclonal antibody IGFR inhibitors, ganitumab and figitumumab, have been studied in Ewing's sarcoma. Although these agents have shown some activity in Ewing's sarcoma, the reported response rates are low and the duration of response is generally brief which has limited commercial development [1].

Mammalian target of rapamycin (mTOR) inhibition is another potential route of targeted therapy for sarcoma. mTOR inhibitors inhibit the PTEN pathway which has been implicated in the pathogenesis of different types of sarcomas [1, 136]. A phase II study of ridaforolimus in advanced bone and soft tissue sarcoma showed clinical benefit in 28% of patients with the majority experiencing stability of disease [137]. Results of this study prompted the phase III SUCCEED (Sarcoma Multi-Center Clinical Evaluation of the Efficacy of Ridaforolimus) study which investigated the role of ridaforolimus maintenance therapy in patients with metastatic soft tissue or bone sarcomas that have responded to chemotherapy. In this study of 711 patients with a variety of sarcoma types, there was a statistically significant improvement in progression-free survival with ridaforolimus maintenance versus placebo with no impact on overall survival [138]. As there was no overall survival benefit with ridaforolimus as maintenance therapy in metastatic sarcoma, the drug was not FDA approved for this indication; however, these results suggest that further evaluation of mTOR inhibitors in metastatic sarcoma (including those who have not responded to chemotherapy) may be warranted. There is also interest in combined use of mTOR inhibitors with IGFR inhibitors with phase I and II study data showing activity of this combination in bone and soft tissue sarcoma although further investigation is needed [139, 140].

While there are many promising targeted therapies for sarcoma, the appropriate patient population, clinical scenario, and sequence of therapies with regard to conventional chemotherapy, surgery, and radiation are yet to be determined. The potential for these agents to penetrate the blood-brain barrier will also need to be investigated prior to use in the CNS sarcoma population although they may currently have a role for disease outside the CNS causing neurologic symptoms by other means.

One strategy to select agents for patients with intracranial sarcomas is the use of next-generation sequencing (e.g., FoundationOne®, Cambridge, MA, USA) to determine genomic alterations in a patient's tumor that might be amenable to targeting with an agent that crosses the BBB.

Most importantly, patients with intracranial sarcoma should be included in clinical trials. This inclusion can occur in several venues. First, patients with intracranial sarcomas should be eligible for trials of systemic sarcoma. Such patients, who will likely constitute a small fraction of the patients accrued, might be included as an exploratory cohort that would not be included in determination of the primary endpoint(s). Any signal of activity would, however, be useful. Second, patients with intracranial sarcomas should be allowed to enter phase I clinical trials of new agents [141]. Third, these patients should be encouraged to enroll on biomarker-defined trials such as the Molecular Analysis for Therapy Choice (MATCH) Trial (NCT02465060) or the Signature array of clinical trials [142]. Although intracranial sarcomas are rare cancers, the determination of agents with potential activity should be pursued in the context of genomic sequencing and clinical trials.

Conclusion

Sarcomas are a diverse grouping of tumors that can create neurologic complications through direct CNS involvement or via proximity to peripheral nervous system structures. Outcomes for patients with sarcoma are generally poor when the CNS is involved and development of new treatment strategies is needed. There has been progress in the field of targeted therapy for systemic sarcomas; however, it is yet to be determined if these treatment approaches will be applicable to disease within the CNS.

References

1. Forscher C, Mita M, Figlin R. Targeted therapy for sarcoma. Biol: Targets Ther. 2014; 8:91–105.
2. Salvati M, D'Elia A, Frati A, et al. Sarcoma metastatic to the brain: a series of 35 cases and considerations from 27 years of experience. J Neurooncol. 2010;98(3):373–7.
3. Murphy MD, Walker WA, Wilson AJ, et al. From the archives of the AFIP: imaging of primary chondrosarcoma: radiologic-pathologic correlation. Radiographics. 2003;23:1245.
4. Cianfriglia F, Pompili A, Occhipinti E. Intracranial malignant cartilaginous tumours. Report of two cases and review of the literature. Acta Neurochirurgica (Wein). 1978;45:163–75.
5. Korten AG, Berg HJ, Spincemaille GH, et al. Intracranial chondrosarcoma: review of the literature and report of 15 cases. J Neurol Neurosurg Psychiatry. 1998;65:88–92.

6. Khouja N, Ben Amor S, Jemel H, et al. Mesenchymal extraskeletal chondrosarcoma of the orbit: report of a case and review of the literature. Surg Neurol. 1999;52:50–3.

7. Evans HL, Ayala AG, Romsdahl MM. Prognostic factors in chondrosarcoma of bone. A clinicopathologic analysis with emphasis on histologic grading. Cancer. 1977;40:818–31.

8. Angelini A, Guerra G, Mavrogenis AF, et al. Clinical outcome of central conventional chondrosarcoma. J Surg Oncol. 2012;106:929.

9. Silve C, Juppner H. Ollier disease. Orphanet J Rare Dis. 2006;1:37.

10. Liu J, Hudkins PG, Swee RG, et al. Bone sarcomas associated with Ollier's disease. Cancer. 1987;59:1376.

11. Albregts AE, Rapini RP. Malignancy in Maffucci's syndrome. Clin Dermatol. 1995;13:73.

12. Volpe NJ, Liebsch NJ, Munzenrider JE, et al. Neuro-ophthalmologic findings in chordoma and chondrosarcoma of the skull base. Am J Ophthalmol. 1993;115(1):97–104.

13. Leerapun T, Hugate RR, Inwards CY, et al. Surgical management of conventional grade I chondrosarcoma of long bones. Clin Orthop Relat Res. 2007;463:166.

14. van der Geest IC, de Valk MH, de Rooy JW, et al. Oncological and functional results of cryosurgical therapy of enchondromas and chondrosarcomas grade 1. J Surg Oncol. 2008;98:421.

15. Hickey M, Farrokhyar F, Deheshi B, et al. A systematic review and meta-analysis of intralesional versus wide resection for intramedullary grade I chondrosarcoma of the extremities. Ann Surg Oncol. 2011;18:1705.

16. Aarons C, Potter BK, Adams SC, et al. Extended intralesional treatment versus resection of low-grade chondrosarcomas. Clin Orthop Relat Res. 2009;467:2105.

17. Shearer D, Patt JC, Cizic A, et al. Curettage and cryotherapy for treatment of low grade chondrosarcoma. Proc Connect Tissue Surg Oncol Soc. 2006;12:760a.

18. Le A, Ball D, Pitman A, et al. Chondrosarcoma of bone complicating Ollier's disease: report of a favourable response to radiotherapy. Australas Radiol. 2003;47:322.

19. Normand AN, Ballo MT, Yasko AE, et al. Palliative radiation therapy for chondrosarcoma. Proc Connect Tissue Surgcal Oncol Soc. 2006;12:745a.

20. Uhl M, Mattke M, Welzel T, et al. High control rate in patients with chondrosarcoma of the skull base after carbon ion therapy: first report of long-term results. Cancer. 2014;120:1579.

21. Yasuda M, Bresson D, Chibbaro S, et al. Chordomas of the skull base and cervical spine: clinical outcomes associated with a multimodal surgical resection combined with proton-beam radiation in 40 patients. Neurosurg Rev. 2012;35(2):171–82.

22. Huang KF, Tzaan WC, Lin CY. Primary intraspinal mesenchymal chondrosarcoma. Chang Gung Med J. 2003;26:370–6.

23. Liebner DA. The indications and efficacy of conventional chemotherapy in primary and recurrent sarcoma. J Surg Oncol. 2015;111:622–31.

24. Bloch OG, Jian BJ, Yang I, et al. A systemic review of intracranial chondrosarcoma and survival. J Clin Neurosci. 2009;16(12):1547–51.

25. Fletcher CDM, Unni KK, Mertens F. World Health Organization classification of tumours: pathology and genetics of tumours of soft tissue and bone. 2002.

26. Hamalat A, And M, Caulet-Maugendre S, Guegan Y. Cerebellar malignant fibrous histiocytoma: case report and literature review. Neurosurgery. 2004;54:745–51.

27. Akimoto J, Takeda Y, Hasue M, et al. Primary meningeal malignant fibrous histiocytoma with cerebrospinal dissemination and pulmonary metastasis. Acta Neurochirurgica (Wein). 1998;140(11): 1191–96.

28. Harries AM, Mitchell R. Haemorrhagic cerebellar fibroud histiocytoma: case report and literature review. Br J Neurosurg. 2011;25(1):120–1.

29. Ozdemir M, Ozgural O, Bozkurt M, et al. Primary intracerebral malignant fibrous histiocytoma mimicking a meningioma. Turkish Neurosurg. 2012;22:475–7.

30. Sarrami AH, Setareh M, Afshar-Moghaddam N, et al. A case of intracranial malignant fibrous histiocytoma. J Res Med Sci. 2011;16(7):968–73.

31. Amendola BE, Amendola MA, McClatchey KD. Radiation-induced malignant fibrous histiocytoma: a report of five cases including two occurring post whole-brain irradiation. Cancer Invest. 1985;3(6):507–13.

32. Zamecnik J, Cerny R, Bartos A, et al. Paraneoplastic opsoclonus-myoclonus syndrome associated with malignant fibrous histiocytoma: neuropathological findings. Czecho-Slovak Pathol. 2004;40(2):63–7.

33. Corato M, Marinou-Aktipi K, Nano R, et al. Paraneoplastic brainstem encephalitis in a patient with malignant fibrous histiocytoma and atypical antineuronal antibodies. J Neurol. 2004;251(11):1415–7.

34. Camacho FM, Moreno JC, Murga M, et al. Malignant fibrous histiocytoma of the scalp: multidisciplinary treatment. J Eur Acad Dermatol Venereol. 1999;13:175–82.

35. Stout AP, Murray MR. Hemangiopericytoma: a vascular tumor featuring Zimmermann's pericytes. Ann Surg. 1942;116:26–33.

36. Louis D, Ohgaki H, Wiestler O, et al. Solitary fibrous tumor/hemangiopericytoma. World Health Organization classification of tumours of the central nervous system. 2016:249–254.

37. Penel N, Amela EY, Decanter G, et al. Solitary fibrous tumors and so-called hemangiopericytoma. Sarcoma. 2012;1–6.

38. England DM, Hochholzer L, McCarthy MJ. Localized benign and malignant fibrous tumors of the pleura: a clinicopathologic review of 223 cases. Am J Surg Pathol. 1989;13(8):640–58.

39. Kalebi AY, Hale MJ, Wong L, et al. Surgically cured hypoglycemia secondary to pleural solitary fibrous tumor: case report and update review on the doege-potter syndrome. J Cardiothorac Surg. 2009; 4(45).

40. Ghose A, Guha G, Kundu R, et al. CNS Hemangiopericytoma: a systemic review of 523 patients. Am J Clin Oncol. 2014:1–5.

41. Guthrie BL, Ebersold MJ, Scheithauer BW, et al. Meningeal hemangiopericytoma: histopathological features, treatment, and long-term follow-up of 44 cases. Neurosurgery. 1989;25:514–22.

42. Melone AG, D'Elia A, Santoro F, et al. Intracranial hemangiopericytoma-our experience in 30 years: a series of 43 cases and review of the literature. World Neurosurg. 2014; 81(3/4):556–62.

43. Ghia AJ, Allen PK, Mahajan A, et al. Intracranial hemangiopericytoma and the role of radiation therapy: a population based analysis. Neurosurg. 2013;72:203–9.

44. Rutkowski MJ, Sughrue ME, Kane AJ, et al. Predictors of mortality following treatment of intracranial hemangiopericytoma. J Neurosurg. 2010;113:333–9.

45. Schiariti M, Goetz P, El-Maghraby H, et al. Hemangiopericytoma: long-term outcome revisited. J Neurosurg. 2011;114:747–55.

46. Wong PP, Yagoda A. Chemotherapy of malignant hemangiopericytoma. Cancer. 1978;41:1256–60.

47. Park MS, Patel SR, Ludwig JA, et al. Activity of temozolomide and bevacizumab in the treatment of locally advanced, recurrent, and metastatic hemangiopericytoma and malignant solitary fibrous tumor. Cancer. 2011;117(21):4939–47.

48. Rutkowski MJ, Jian BJ, Bloch O, et al. Intracranial hemangiopericytoma: clinical experience and treatment consideration in a modern series of 40 adult patients. Cancer. 2012;118:1628–36.

49. Mena H, Ribas JL, Pezeshkpour GH, et al. Hemangiopericytoma of the central nervous system: a review of 94 cases. Hum Pathol. 1991;22(1):84–91.

50. Nonaka M, Kohmura E, Hirata M, et al. Metastatic meningeal hemangiopericytoma of thoracic spine. Clin Neurol Neurosurg. 1998;100(3):228–30.

51. Ries LAG, Harkins D, Krapcho M, et al. SEER Cancer Statistics Review, 1975–2003. Bethesda, MD: National Cancer Institute. http://seer.cancer.gov/csr/1975_2003.

52. Ahola DT, Provenzale JM, Longee DC. Metastatic rhabdomyosarcoma presenting as intracranial hemorrhage: imaging findings. Eur J Radiol. 1998;26:241–3.

53. Li FP, Fraumeni JF Jr. Soft-tissue sarcomas, breast cancer, and other neoplasms. A familial syndrome? Ann Intern Med. 1969;71:747.

54. Hartley AL, Birch JM, Marsden HB, et al. Neurofibromatosis in children with soft tissue sarcoma. J Pediatr Hematol Oncol. 1988;5:7.

55. DeBaun MR, Tucker MA. Risk of cancer during the first four years of life in children from the Beckwith-Wiedemann Syndrome Registry. J Pediatr. 1998;132:398.

56. Quezada E, Gripp KW. Costello syndrome and related disorders. Curr Opin Pediatr. 2007;19:636.

57. Hicks J, Flaitz C. Rhabdomyosarcoma of the head and neck in children. Oral Oncol. 2002;38:450–9.

58. Vannucci RC, Baten M. Cerebral metastatic disease in childhood. Neurology. 1974;24:981–5.

59. Chen SC, Bee YS, Lin MC, et al. Extensive alveolar-type paranasal sinus and orbit rhabdomyosarcoma with intracranial invasion treated successfully. J Chin Med Assoc. 2011;74:140–3.

60. Wharam MD Jr. Rhabdomyosarcoma of parameningeal sites. Semin Radiat Oncol. 1997;7(3):212–6.

61. Gerson JM, Jaffe N, Donaldson MH, et al. Meningeal seeding from rhabdomyosarcoma of the head and neck with base of the skull invasion: recognition of the clinical evolution and suggestions for management. Med Pediatr Oncol. 1978; 5(1):137–44.

62. Punyko JA, Mertens AC, Baker KS, et al. Long-term survival probabilities for childhood rhabdomyosarcoma. A population-based evaluation. Cancer. 2005;103(7):1475.

63. Turner JH, Richmon JD. Head and neck rhabdomyosarcoma: a critical analysis of population-based incidence and survival data. Otolaryngol-1 Head Neck Surg. 2011;145(6):967.

64. Ferrari A, Dileo P, Casanova M, et al. Rhabdomyosarcoma in adults: a retrospective analysis of 171 patientes treated at a single institution. Cancer. 2003;98:571–80.

65. Michalski JM, Meza J, Breneman JC, et al. Influence of radiation therapy parameters on outcome in children treated with radiation therapy for localized parameningeal rhabdomyosarcoma in intergroup rhabdomyosarcoma study group trials II through IV. Int J Radiat Oncol Biol Phys. 2004;59(4):1027.

66. Parasuraman S, Langston J, Rao BN, et al. Brain metastases in pediatric Ewing sarcoma and rhabdomyosarcoma: the St Jude Children's Research Hospital experience. J Pediatr Hematol Oncol. 1999;21(5):370–7.

67. Ritter AM, Amaker EH, Graham RS, et al. Central nervous system leiomyosarcoma in patients with acquired immunodeficiency syndrome. Report of two cases. J Neurosurg. 2000;92:688–92.

68. Eminger LA, Hall LD, Hesterman KS, et al. Epstein-Barr virus: dermatologic associations and implications. J Am Acad Dermatol. 2015;72(1):21–34.

69. Reddy Aeddula N, Pathireddy S, Samaha T, et al. Primary intracranial leiomyosarcoma in an immunocompetent adult. J Clin Oncol. 2011;29(14):e407–10.

70. Paulus W, Slowik F, Jellinger K. Primary intracranial sarcomas: Histopathological features of 19 cases. Histopathology. 1991;18:395–402.

71. Louis DN, Richardson EP Jr, Dickersin GR, et al. Primary intracranial leiomyosarcoma: case report. J Neurosurg. 1989;71:279–82.

72. Hussain S, Nanda A, Fowler M, et al. Primary intracranial leiomyosarcoma: report of a case and review of the literature. Sarcoma. 2006;52140

73. Toh CH, Wong HF, Jung SM, et al. Radiation-Induced skull base leiomyosarcoma presenting with intracranial hemorrhage. Br J Radiol. 2007;80:e212–5.

74. Espat NJ, Bilsky M, Lewis JJ, et al. Soft tissue sarcoma brain metastases: prevalence in a cohort of 3829 patients. Cancer. 2002;94:2706–11.

75. Reichardt P. Soft tissue sarcomas, a look into the future: different treatments for different subtypes. Future Oncol. 2014;10(8 Suppl.):19–27.

76. Melone GA, et al. Uterine leiomyosarcoma metastatic to the brain: case report. Tumori. 2008;94(6):856–60.

77. Yamada S, et al. A case of multiple brain metastases of uterine leiomyosarcoma with a literature review. J Surg Oncol. 2011;20 (4):e127–31.

78. Thway K, Fisher C. Malignant peripheral nerve sheath tumor: pathology and genetics. Ann Diagn Pathol. 2014;18:109–16.

79. Ferrari A, Bisogno G, Carli M. Management of childhood malignant peripheral nerve sheath tumor. Paediatr Drugs. 2007;9:239–48.

80. Gupta G, Maniker A. Malignant peripheral nerve sheath tumors. Neurosurg Focus. 2007:22(E21).

81. Ducatman BS, Scheithauer BW. Postirradiation neurofibrosarcoma. Cancer. 1983;51:1028–33.

82. Foley KM, Woodruff JM, Ellis FT, et al. Radiation-induced malignant and atypical peripheral nerve sheath tumors. Ann Neurol. 1980;7:311–8.

83. Ducatman BS, Scheithauer BW, Piepgras DG, et al. Malignant peripheral nerve sheath tumors. A clinicopathologic study of 120 cases. Cancer. 1986;57:2006–21.

84. Sandberg AA, Stone JF. Malignant peripheral nerve sheath tumors in the genetics and molecular biology of neural tumors. New Jersey: Humana; 2010.

85. Karami KJ, Kelkar PS, Verdon MP, et al. Malignant peripheral nerve sheath tumor of the vestibulocochlear nerve and brainstem: multimodality treatment with survival of 27 months. A case report and review of the literature. Neurosurgery. 2011;69(5): E1152–65.

86. Kumar VRR, Madhugiri VS, Sasidharan GM, et al. Multifocal spinal malignant peripheral nerve sheath tumor in an immunocompromised individual: case report and review of the literature. Eur Spine J. 2014;23(Supp 2):S236–41.

87. Voorhies J, Hattab EM, Cohen-Gadol AA. Malignant peripheral nerve sheath tumor of the abducens nerve and a review of the literature. World Neurosurgery. 2013;80:654e1–8.

88. Ferner RE, O'Doherty MJ. Neurofibroma and schwannoma. Curr Opin Neurol. 2002;15:679–84.

89. Carroll SL, Ratner N. How does the Schwann cell lineage form tumors in NF1? Glia. 2008;56:1590–605.

90. Shweikeh F, Bukavina L, Saeed K, et al. Brain metastasis in bone and soft tissues cancers: a review of incidence, interventions, and outcomes. Sarcoma. Vol. 2014, Article ID 475175, 19 p.

91. Mirabella L, Troisi RJ, Savage SA. Osteosarcoma incidence and survival rates from 1973 to 2004: data from the surveillance, epidemiology and end results program. Cancer. 2009;115:1531.

92. Hauben EI, Arends J, Vandenbroucke JP, et al. Multiple primary malignancies in osteosarcoma patients. Incidence and predictive

value of osteosarcoma subtype for cancer syndromes related with osteosarcoma. Eur J Hum Genet. 2003;11:611.

93. Korovessis P, Repanti M, Stamatakis M. Primary osteosarcoma of the L2 lamina presenting as "silent" paraplegia: case report and review of the literature. Eur Spine J. 1995;4(6):375–8.

94. Link MP, Gebhardt MC, Meyers PA. Osteosarcoma. Principles and practice of pediatric oncology. 5th ed. Philadelphia: Lippincott Williams & Wilkins; 2005:1075–113.

95. Kebudi R, Ayan I, Gorgun O, et al. Brain metastasis in pediatric extracranial solid tumors: survey and literature review. J Neurooncol. 2005;71(1):43–8.

96. Agrawal A. Osteosarcoma metastasis to the orbit presenting as severe proptosis following trivial trauma. J Clin Ophthalmol Res. 2014;2(3):155–7.

97. Dagcinar A, Bayrakli F, Yapicier O, et al. Primary meningeal osteosarcoma of the brain during childhood. J Neurosurg: Pediatr. 2008;1:325–9.

98. Meyers, PA. Systemic therapy for osteosarcoma and Ewing sarcoma. 2015 ASCO Educational Book. e644–47. Asco.org/edbook.

99. Muldoon LL, Soussain C, Jahnke K, et al. Chemotherapy delivery issues in central nervous system malignancy: a reality check. J Clin Oncol. 2007;25(16):2295–305.

100. Gurney JG, Swensen AR, Bulterys M. Malignant bone tumors in: cancer incidence and survival among children and adolescents. United States SEER program 1975–1995. National Cancer Institute; 1999.

101. Glass AG, Fraumeni JF Jr. Epideminology of bone cancer in children. J Natl Cancer Inst. 1970;44:187.

102. Nesbit ME Jr, Gehan EA, Burgert EO Jr, et al. Multimodaltherapy for the management of primary, non-metastatic Ewing's sarcoma of bone: a long-term follow-up of the First Intergroup study. J Clin Oncol. 1990;8(10):1664.

103. Grier H, Krailo M, Link M, et al. Improved outcome in non-metastatic Ewing's sarcoma (EWS) and PNET of bone with the addition of ifosfamide (I) and etoposide (E) to vincristine (V), Adriamycin (Ad), cyclophosphamide (C) and actinomycin (A): A Children's Cancer Group (CCG) and Pediatric Oncology Group (POG) report. (abstract). Proc Am Soc Clin Oncol. 1994;13:421.

104. Karosas AO. Ewing's sarcoma. Am J Healthsystem Pharm. 2010;67(19):1599–605.

105. Simpson RK Jr, Bruner JM, Leavens ME. Metastatic Ewing's sarcoma to the brain: case report. Surg Neurol. 1989;31(3):234–8.

106. Karikari IO, Mehta AI, Nimjee S, et al. Primary intradural extraosseous Ewing Sarcoma of the spine: case report and literature review. Neurosurgery. 2011;69(4):e995–9.

107. Postovsky S, Ash S, Ramu IN, et al. Central nervous system involvement in children with sarcoma. Oncology. 2003;65:118–24.

108. Charfi S, Ayadi L, Khabir A, et al. Gliosarcoma with osteosarcomatous features: a short illustrated review. Acta Neurochir. 2009;151:809–13.

109. Ohgaki H, Biernat W, Reis R, et al. "Gliosarcoma" World Health Organization classification of tumours. Pathol Genet: Tumours Nerv Syst. 2000:84–6.

110. Morantz RA, Feigin I, Ransohoff JD. Clinical and pathological study of 24 cases of gliosarcoma. J Neurosurg. 1976;45:398–408.

111. Galanis E. Clinical outcome of gliosarcoma compared with glioblastoma multiforme: North Central Cancer Treatment Group results. J Neurosurg. 1998;89:425–30.

112. Weaver D. Selective peripancreatic sarcoma metastases from primary gliosarcoma. J Neurosurg. 1984;61:599–601.

113. Pasquier B. Extraneural metastases of astrocytomas and glioblastomas: clinicopathological study of two cases and review of the literature. Cancer. 1980;45:112–25.

114. Nishio S. Ventricular and subarachnoid seeding of intracranial tumors of neuroectodermal origin- a study of 26 consecutive autopsy cases with ference to focal ependymal defect. Clin Neuropathol. 1982;1(2):83–91.

115. Onda K. Cerebral glioblastoma with cerebrospinal fluid dissemination: a clinicopathologic study of 14 cases examined by complete autopsy. Neurosurgery. 1989;25(4):533–40.

116. Onda K, Ryuichi T, Takeda N. Spinal metastases of cerebral glioblastoma: the value of commuted tomographic metrizamide myelography in the diagnosis. Surg Neurol. 1986;25:399–405.

117. Witwer BP, Salamat MS, Resnick DK. Gliosarcoma metastatic to the cervical spinal cord: case report and review of the literature. Surg Neurol. 2000;54:373–9.

118. Kozak KR, Mahadevan A, Moody JS. Adult gliosarcoma: epidemiology, natural history and factors associated with outcome. Neuro-Oncol. 2009;11:183–91.

119. Naoe H, Kaku E, Ido Y, et al. Brain metastasis from gastrointestinal stromal tumor: a case report and review of the literature. Case Rep Gastroenterol. 2011;5:583–9.

120. Kroep JR, Bovee JV, van der Molen AJ, et al. Extra-abdominal subcutaneous metastasis ofa gastrointestinal stromal tumor: report of a case and a review of the literature. J Cutan Pathol. 2009;36:565–9.

121. Corless CL, Fletcher JA, Heinrich MC. Biology of gastrointestinal stromal tumors. J Clin Oncol. 2004;22:3813–25.

122. Puri T, Gunabushanam G, Malik M, et al. Mesenteric gastrointestinal stromal tumour presenting as intracranial space occupying lesion. World J Surg Oncol. 2006;4:78.

123. Bor-Ren H, Hsien-Chih C, Tai-Ngar L, et al. Epidural metastases from a gastrointestinal stromal tumour. J Clin Neurosci. 2008;15:82–4.

124. Burkill GJ, Badran M, Al-Muderis O, et al. Malignant gastrointestinal stromal tumor: distribution, imaging features and pattern of metastatic spread. Radiology. 2003;226:527–32.

125. Slimack NP, Liu JC, Koski T, et al. Metastatic gastrointestinal stromal tumor to the thoracic and lumbar spine: first reported case and surgical treatment. Spine J. 2012;12:e7–12.

126. Jagannathan JP, Ramaiya NH, Shinagare AB. Intracranial metastasis from pediatric GI stromal tumor. J Clin Oncol. 2012;30(10):e122–5.

127. Rubin BP, Heinrich MC, Corless CL. Gastrointestinal stromal tumor. Lancet. 2007;369(9574):1731–41.

128. Demetri GD, Benjamin RS, Blanke CD, et al. NCCN task force report: management of patients with gastrointestinal stromal tumor (GIST)- update of the NCCN clinical practice guidelines. J Natl Compr Canc Netw. 2007;5(2 suppl):S1–29.

129. Wolff NC, Richardson JA, Egorin M, et al. The CNS is a sanctuary for leukemic cells in mice receiving imatinib mesylate for Bcr/Able induced leukemia. Blood. 2003;101:5010–3.

130. Petzer AL, Gunsilius E, Hayes M, et al. Low concentrations of ST1571 in the cerebrospinal fluid: a case report. Br J Haematol. 2002;117:623–5.

131. Van der Graaf WT, Blay JY, Chawla SP, et al. Pazopanib for metastatic soft tissue sarcoma (PALETTE): a randomized, double-blind, placebo-controlled phase 3 trial. Lancet. 2012;379(9829):1879–86.

132. Hingorani M, Dixit S, Maraveryas A. Pazopanib-induced regression of brain metastasis after whole brain palliative radiotherapy in metastatic renal cell cancer progressing on first-line sunitinib: a case report. World J Oncol. 2014;5(5–6):223–7.

133. Stacchiotti S, Negri T, Palassini E, et al. Sunitinib malate and figitumumab in solitary fibrous tumor: patterns and molecular bases of tumor response. Mol Cancer Ther. 2010;9(5):1286–97.

134. Dancey J, Krzyzanowska MK, Provencher DM, et al. NCIC CTG IND.206: a phase II umbrella trial of sunitinib or temsirolimus in advanced rare cancers. J Clin Oncol 2015;33(suppl; abstr 2594).

135. Pappo AS, Patel S, Crowley J, et al. Activity of R1507, a monoclonal antibody to the insulin-like growth factor-1 receptor (IGF1R) in patients with recurrent or refractory Ewing's sarcoma family of tumors. J Clin Oncol. 2010;28(suppl; abstr 10000).

136. Saito T, Oda Y, Kawaguchi K, et al. PTEN/MMAC1 gene mutation is a rare event in soft tissue sarcomas without specific balanced translocations. Int J Cancer. 2003;104(2):175–8.

137. Chawla SP, Tolcher AW, Staddon AP, et al. Updated results of a phase II trial of AP23573, a novel mTOR inhibitor in patients with advanced soft tissue or bone sarcomas. J Clin Oncol. 2006;24(suppl; abstr 9505).

138. Blay JY, Chawla SP, Ray-Coquard I, et al. Phase III, placebo-controlled trial (SUCCEED) evaluating ridaforolimus as maintenance therapy in advanced sarcoma patients following clinical benefit from prior standard cytotoxic chemotherapy: long-term (≥ 24 months) overall survival results. J Clin Oncol. 2012;30(suppl; abstr 10010).

139. Schwartz GK, Tap WD, Qin LX, et al. Cixutumumab and temsirolimus for patients with bone and soft-tissue sarcoma: a multicenter, open-label, phase 2 trial. Lancet Oncol. 2013;14(4):371–82.

140. Quek R, Wang Q, Morgan JA, et al. Combination mTOR and IGF-1R inhibition: phase 1 trial of everolimus and figitumumab in patients with advanced sarcomas and other solid tumors. Clin Cancer Res. 2011;17(4):871–9.

141. Wen PY, Schiff D, Cloughesy TF, et al. It is time to include patients with brain tumors in phase I trials in oncology. J Clin Oncol. 2011;29(24):3211–3.

142. Peguero JA, Knost JA, Bauer TM, et al. Successful implementation of a novel trial model: the signature program. J Clin Oncol. 2015;33(suppl; abstr 106).

Neurologic Complications of Head and Neck Cancer

Sepideh Mokhtari and Thomas J. Kaley

Background

Each year approximately 48,000 Americans are diagnosed with a head or neck cancer. Head and neck cancer accounts for approximately 3–5% of all newly diagnosed cases of cancer in the USA. The estimated number of diagnoses and deaths in 2014 were 59, 340, and 12,290, respectively [1]. Worldwide, more than 550,000 new cases with approximately 300,000 deaths are projected annually [2]. More than 90% of head and neck cancer is squamous cell carcinoma (HNSCC) in histology, and the majority of tumors are associated with smoking and alcohol use [1]. Most HNSCC are thought to arise from potentially malignant disorders (PMDs) such as leukoplakia, erythroplakia, oral lichen planus, oral submucous fibrosis, actinic cheilosis, and snuff patch [3]. The mucosa of the head and neck undergoes a change, perhaps due to carcinogen exposure, and becomes more susceptible to the development of many foci of malignant transformation (field cancerization theory) [4]. It is crucial to understand the biologic tumorigenesis of a second primary tumor to prevent relapse or multiple primary tumors after definitive therapy is delivered [5].

Over the last three decades, development of molecular biology has made major contributions to the basic understanding of tumorigenesis and identified multiple genes involved in the tumorigenesis process (i.e., p53 mutation/overexpression, erbB family, 9p21 deletion, 11q13 amplification, 17p loss, 3p loss, etc.) [6–11]. Over 50% of HNSCCs have TP53 gene mutation and over 50% demonstrate chromosomal loss of 17p, the site where the *TP53* gene resides [5]. The most targeted component of the Rb pathway is the p16INK4A tumor-suppressor gene, which inhibits the cyclin-dependent kinases 4 and 6. Loss of heterozygosity (LOH) at chromosomal region 9p21 (where p16INK4A resides) occurs in up to 80% of HNSCCs [6]. A Japanese series of 102 patients with larynx cancer treated surgically showed overexpression of cyclin D1, located at 11q13, in 57.8% of patients [9]. Chromosome 3p loss is seen in approximately 60% of HNSCC, which is one of the earliest events in the progression of HNSCC [11]. TP53 mutation often coincides with the loss of chromosome 3p, and the combination of these events is associated with a surprising decrease in survival time (1.9 years vs. >5 years for TP53 alone) [10].

Patients typically present with advanced local invasion, and symptoms vary with tumor location. Tumors of the oral cavity and oropharynx present with swelling or ulcer, odynophagia, dysphagia, otalgia, otitis, weight loss, and trismus. Laryngeal tumors present with hoarseness, stridor, dyspnea, or pain, which are also seen with common benign conditions [12, 13], thus leading to a delay in diagnosis. The findings of paresthesia and anesthesia, in the absence of a history of trauma, strongly suggest an invasive malignancy. Metastatic dissemination occurs through the submandibular, cervical, and jugular lymphatic pathways, and distant metastases most commonly target the lung [13].

Treatment

Surgical Treatment

Surgical treatment remains the mainstay of multi-modal treatment for oral cancers with the goal of adequate clearance of tumor tissue [14]. The treatment is determined based on stage and location of the head and neck cancer. For early-stage disease, surgery or brachytherapy is the treatment of choice, whereas for advanced-stage disease multi-disciplinary treatment including chemotherapy and

S. Mokhtari
Department of Neurology, H. Lee Moffitt Center, 12902 USF Magnolia Drive, Tampa, FL 33612, USA
e-mail: sepideh.mokhtari@moffitt.org

T.J. Kaley (✉)
Department of Neurology, Memorial Sloan Kettering Cancer Center, 1275 York Avenue, New York, NY 10065, USA
e-mail: kaleyt@mskcc.org

© Springer International Publishing AG 2018
D. Schiff et al. (eds.), *Cancer Neurology in Clinical Practice*,
DOI 10.1007/978-3-319-57901-6_28

radiation therapy is recommended. However, with surgery there is risk of disfigurement, trismus, speech impairment, and dysphagia [13]. After resection of large primary tumors, reconstructive surgery is required. Free tissue transfer is currently one of the most popular and reliable techniques for oral reconstruction [15].

The aim of surgical resection is adequate clearance of tumor tissue, since inadequate clearance can result in increased risks of local and regional recurrences, and decreased long-term survival rates [16]. Currently, three-dimensional 1-cm resection margins are considered acceptable. However, increasing the resection margins may result in increased functional morbidities [17–19]. For the past several decades, radical neck dissection (RND) is the gold standard for patients with positive cervical lymph nodes [14]. Interestingly, elective neck dissection is also considered when the risk of occult metastases is >20% [20].

RND involves complete removal of the lymphatic channels in the neck and many anatomical structures in the neck including the sternocleidomastoid muscle, spinal accessory nerve, and jugular vein, which are commonly injured. More recently, modified radical neck dissections (MRND) are being performed, which are less morbid and spare some of these structures [21]. MRND involves clearance of the cervical lymph nodes, with preservation of one or more of the following: the accessory nerve, internal jugular vein (IJV), and sternocleidomastoid muscle. Sentinel node biopsy has received considerable attention as a means of avoiding unnecessary lymph node dissection [22]. Postoperative radiotherapy or concurrent chemoradiotherapy is often recommended as adjuvant therapy for patients with multiple node metastases or extracapsular spread of tumors, since they often have recurrence after neck dissection [23–25].

Radiation Therapy

Radiation therapy (RT) plays an important role in the treatment of head and neck cancer, especially in cases of unresectable tumor or advanced tumors with cervical lymph node involvement and/or metastasis. RT could be used either as an effective alternative to surgery or a valuable adjunct to surgery and/or chemotherapy [13, 26]. In planning for advanced disease, it is important to consider the risk of recurrence, cosmetic and functional outcome, quality of life, speed of treatment, patient reliability, effectiveness of salvage therapy, and individualization of treatment options [27, 28].

Major high risk factors for recurrence are positive microscopic resection margins and extracapsular nodal extension. Other risk factors are ≥ 2 lymph node metastases with a diameter of 3 cm or more, perineural invasion, Level 4 (inferior internal jugular lymph node) or Level 5

(accessory nerve lymph node) lymph node metastasis in oropharyngeal cancer/oral cavity cancer and signs of vascular tumor embolism [28]. In the postoperative setting, the standard adjuvant therapy is concurrent chemotherapy and radiation to prevent recurrence in patients with high risk factors, with radiation alone for patients with intermediate risk and those at high risk for recurrence who are unsuitable for postoperative chemoradiotherapy [28].

Several studies have shown that concomitant chemoradiotherapy improves both locoregional control and survival compared with chemotherapy followed by RT [26, 29, 30]. Disease-free survival (DFS) was demonstrated in the Radiation Therapy Oncology Group (RTOG) 91-11 study to be significantly prolonged in patients who received chemoradiotherapy compared with RT alone [31]. In addition, elective RT can be beneficial in patients with clinically negative regional lymph nodes who have >20% increased risk of occult cervical nodal disease. The principal aim of either elective surgery or RT is to maximize the rate of control of the disease in the neck. Söderström and colleagues showed that RT fractionation in the head and neck resulted in significant risk reduction for regional recurrences of elective treatment [32].

Chemotherapy

Chemotherapy has been shown to be beneficial in recurrent disease or in the locally advanced previously untreated patients. Historically, the most common regimens for recurrent/metastatic HNSCC included cisplatin plus 5-FU, cisplatin plus a taxane, or single-agent methotrexate with unproven survival benefits [33–35]. Cisplatin has been a key agent and has shown to be effective [36, 37]. However, combination cytotoxic chemotherapy (cisplatin plus 5-fluorouracil, cisplatin plus paclitaxel, 5-fluorouracil plus hydroxyurea) has been a more standard treatment as a component of definitive chemoradiotherapy for locally advanced and unresectable disease.

A randomized phase II trial (RTOG 97-03) comparing outcomes with three doublet regimens in combination with RT in patients with advanced disease comparing cisplatin plus paclitaxel, cisplatin plus 5-fluorouracil, or hydroxyurea plus 5-fluorouracil showed cisplatin plus paclitaxel to have much better 2-year DFS, OS, and CR rates with less locoregional failure at 2 years [38]. Also, a combination of three chemotherapy agents has been used in recurrent or metastatic HNSCC. In a phase II study of paclitaxel, ifosfamide, and carboplatin (the TIC regimen) in patients with recurrent or metastatic head and neck squamous cell carcinoma, 59% experienced major response [39].

Understanding the molecular basis of HNSCC has led to the study of EGFR-targeting agents such as cetuximab and lapatinib [40]. The RTOG 90-03 trial demonstrated that high EGFR expression measured by immunohistochemistry was associated with a higher risk of both locoregional recurrence and death in comparison with tumors with EGFR expression below the median [41]. Based on the RTOG-0522 trial, there appears to be no benefit from adding cetuximab to cisplatin and RT in the curative setting.

The benefit of neoadjuvant chemotherapy is still controversial [42, 43]. For the most part, adjuvant chemotherapy is not indicated for postoperative HNSCC patients [28]. In a randomized trial comparing surgery and adjuvant RT versus concurrent chemoradiotherapy (CCRT) in patients with advanced, nonmetastatic HNSCC for patients with oral cavity cancer, survival was significantly better in those who underwent primary surgery compared with CCRT [44]. However, CCRT has been shown to have significant advantage over RT alone in the adjuvant setting for high-risk disease (defined as extracapsular extension and microscopic disease at the resection margin) [45].

The role of induction chemotherapy (ICT) has been reconsidered since the introduction of taxane–platinum-based(TPF) combinations that have proven to be superior to a platinum–fluorouracil (PF) schedule in locoregionally advanced disease. However, induction chemotherapy is not considered standard treatment in advanced disease [46]. Studies of induction chemotherapy, followed by chemoradiation, have failed to improve survival or decrease the risk of distant metastases [47, 48].

Neurologic Complications of Head and Neck Cancer

Neurologic complications of head and neck cancer are quite different from most other solid tumors. Brain metastases and leptomeningeal metastases are quite rare. However, due to the close proximity of the skull and brain, the brain is susceptible to both local spread of cancer as well as the toxicities of local therapies.

Direct Extension of Primary Tumor

The main routes of tumor extension include direct extension into the skull either through openings in the skull or through erosion of bone and creation of an opening, or via extension of long nerves [49]. Additionally, tumor may spread via lymphatics. The incidence rates of perineural spread range from 14 to 63.2%. Of head and neck tumors, the adenocystic carcinoma of the salivary gland, nasopharynx, oropharynx, or paranasal sinus is reported to have approximately 50% incidence rates of perineural growth [50].

Perineural spread of tumor is the most difficult to detect as patients typically present with rather nonspecific symptoms such as pain, numbness, or paresthesias. Careful neurologic examination can localize the lesion. Imaging is challenging as these tumors growing along nerves tend to do so linearly rather than creating a large bulky mass. MRI is the preferred imaging technique due to its superior soft tissue resolution. MRI can also examine the entire course of the nerve to detect skip lesions and plan for correct treatment (surgery vs. RT) targeting the entire extent of disease [49].

In a retrospective study of 89 patients who underwent radical surgery for oral tongue squamous cell carcinoma, perineural invasion was found in 27.0% of cases and the 5-year disease-specific survival (DSS) and overall survival rates for these patients were significantly lower than those without perineural invasion [51]. Perineural growth in HNSCC is often found in the fifth and seventh cranial nerves and their branches [52, 53]. This may be due to widespread innervation of the head and neck by these two nerves. In addition, these nerves meet at three different points and may provide routes for the cancer to spread from one nerve to the other [54]. See Fig. 28.1a, b.

When HNSCC has spread intracranially along peripheral nerves or cranial nerves, treatment may include surgery, intensity modulated radiation therapy (IMRT), or stereotactic radiosurgery (SRS). The surgical excision must always follow the path of the involved nerve until clear margins are obtained. The adjuvant therapy is mandatory; IMRT and SRS offer the advantage of reduced toxicity and, therefore, a better quality of life for these patients [55]. IMRT is preferred for large or diffuse intracranial spread. Even though SRS may provide effective local control with less morbidity for recurrent head and neck cutaneous squamous cell carcinoma, the rate of out-of-field failures remains unacceptably high [56].

Head and neck cancer can spread through thin bones of sinuses, cribriform plate, skull, orbit, and cavernous sinus and produce neurologic symptoms such as anosmia, cerebrospinal fluid leak, or frontal lobe syndromes. See Fig. 28.2a, b. In a study of 40 cases of head and neck cancers that sufficiently invaded adjacent skull, dura, or brain, the most common tumors were found to be sinonasal-origin tumors (n = 17) and cutaneous tumors (n = 10); others were olfactory neuroblastomas, middle ear-origin basal cell carcinoma, recurrent glomus jugulare, and orbital malignant hidradenoma [57]. The cavernous sinus invasion can be seen at the first presentation in advanced cases or in recurrent cases of nasopharyngeal carcinoma via the inferior orbital nerve. Patients may complain of diplopia, headache, proptosis, ptosis, or trigeminal paresthesias [58, 59]. The best imaging with highest specificity to detect bone erosion is multi-detector computed tomography (MDCT) with

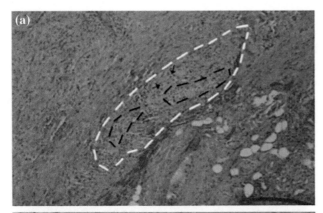

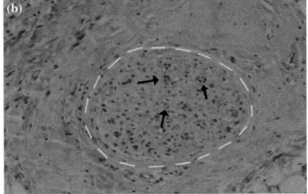

Fig. 28.1 Histological analysis of perineural invasion of HNSCC. Perineural (**a**) and intraneural invasions (**b**) by squamous cell carcinoma of the head and neck (H&E staining). *White dotted lines* indicate the nerve; *black dotted lines* indicate perineural invasion, and *black arrows* indicate intraneural invasion. (Used with permission of Elsevier from Roh et al. Perineural growth in head and neck squamous cell carcinoma: a review. Oral Oncol 2015; 51(1): 16–23.)

multi-planar reformations and bone and soft tissue algorithms [60].

Nasopharyngeal Carcinoma

Nasopharyngeal carcinoma (NPC) commonly presents with neurologic symptoms and complications. In a study of 381 patients with NPC, 113 (30%) were found to have neurologic complications. Sixteen percent presented with neurologic symptoms within one month to seven years. In two-thirds of patients, the neurologic picture began with either diplopia or sensory disturbance in the face. Neurologic examination revealed cranial nerve damage in almost all cases. The abducens nerve was involved in 68% of patients, the trigeminal in 47%, and the glossopharyngeal-vagus in 38%. Combinations of fifth and sixth cranial nerves were the most common [61]. NPC can also present with ptosis and a fourth nerve palsy. The frequency of diagnosed CN palsy in NPC ranges from 8.0 to 12.4%. NPC can invade upward and backward through the skull base to the cavernous sinus and

middle cranial fossa and invade CN II to VI (upper CN palsy). It may also involve the carotid space and invade CN XII as it exits through the hypoglossal canal, CN IX to XI as they emerge from the jugular foramen, and the cervical sympathetic nerves.

Invasion of brain parenchyma, dura, and leptomeninges is rare; however, a few cases have been documented [62, 63]. NPC may spread into the cavernous sinus from tumor surrounding the horizontal portion of the internal carotid artery, foramen ovale, orbital fissures, or directly through the skull base [64, 65]. MRI with contrast is the best study to detect CN, parenchymal, dural, or leptomeningeal involvement. It shows either enhancement of soft tissue tumor along the course of the nerve, or perineural spread, with enlargement or abnormal enhancement of the nerve, or neuroforaminal enlargement. Meningeal involvement appears as nodular enhancement, often along the floor of the middle cranial fossa or posterior to the clivus [65]. Clinicians need to maintain a high index of suspicion for dural metastasis in patients with radiographic signs (dural tale) of dural mass [62].

Orbital Tumor

Given the proximity of the nasal cavity and paranasal sinuses to the orbit, many tumors arising from these structures can cause orbital invasion via the inferior orbital fissure, optic canal, and superior orbital fissure [65, 66]. The incidence varies with the site of origin, histology, and aggressiveness of the particular tumor. Visual symptoms, including unilateral epiphora, proptosis, and diplopia, occur in 50% of patients with malignant sinonasal tumors and obviously relate to the site of disease with 62% of ethmoidal as opposed to 46% of nasal tumors producing orbital problems. Tumors may invade the orbit via preformed pathways, via neurovascular structures, or by direct extension through bone. Tumor extension into the orbit occurs particularly in ethmoid tumors, because of the thin lamina papyracea separating the two structures [67, 68].

Orbital invasion (bone erosion/invasion) occurs in 60–80% of maxillary sinus malignancies [69]. Orbital involvement is associated with a significant reduction in survival both in ethmoid and maxillary sinus tumors [68]. CT or MR with contrast is a good diagnostic tool for orbital metastasis [70]. Management consists of surgery in which the orbit is usually spared if there is no involvement of soft tissue, and orbital clearance when there is soft tissue involvement. Studies have not shown any significant difference in survival and recurrence rate in sparing the orbital content or including orbital clearance [69, 71]. Also, simultaneous combined conservative surgery, RT, and regional chemotherapy have been shown to have 5-year survival and local control to up to 60% [72, 73].

Fig. 28.2 Magnetic resonance images indicate perineural spread of head and neck cancer. MRI of carcinoma in a 67-year-old female in the **a** cavernous sinus which houses several cranial nerves, the foramen ovale where the V3 branch of the trigeminal nerve emerges from the brain, and **b** foramen rotundum where the V2 branch of the trigeminal nerve emerges from the brain. *White dotted lines* indicate perineural spread

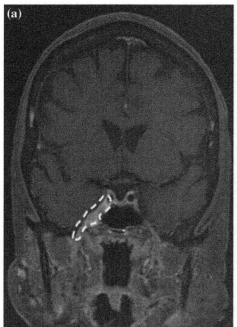
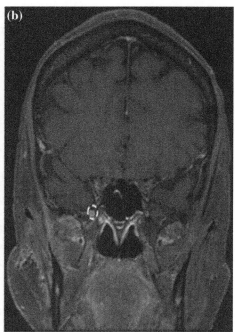

Skull Base Paragangliomas

Another tumor frequently manifesting neurologic symptoms is paraganglioma of the head and neck. These tumors are also known as chemodectomas or glomus tumors. The origin of these cells is from paraganglionic cells in the adventitial of the jugular bulb. The medial wall of the jugular bulb prevents tumor spread. However, once it is invaded, the tumor involves the lower cranial nerves and can also spread intracranially. Inferiorly, it spreads to the neck through the carotid foramen and the carotid sheath. These tumors are four to six times more common in women [74]. Approximately 30% of apparent familial head and neck paragangliomas are due to germ line mutations in one of the genes SDHB, SDHC, and SDHD. The risk of manifestation of the disease phenotype is only increased if the mutation is inherited through the paternal line [75].

These tumors are slow growing, but rarely can produce problems by local invasion. The four main locations of glomus tissue within the head and neck are as follows: (1) at the carotid bifurcation (carotid body tumor); (2) in the inferior ganglion region (ganglion nodosum) and cervical portion of the vagus nerve (glomus vagale); (3) in the jugular bulb region (glomus jugulare); and (4) in the middle ear cavity (glomus tympanicum, associated with the tympanic branch of the glossopharyngeal nerve). Glomus tympanicum is associated with the tympanic branch of the glossopharyngeal nerve and can produce pulsatile tinnitus and conductive hearing loss over a few years. Glomus vagale can grow rostrally and compress CN VII and VIII in the internal auditory canal causing loss hearing loss (in 60-80%) and pulsatile tinnitus and, in some cases, facial paralysis. Glomus jugulare can involve CN IX, X, and XI, causing hoarseness, dizziness, or dysphagia [74, 76, 77].

The best imaging modality to detect the extent of the lesion is high resolution CT (HRCT) and gadolinium-enhanced MRI. MRI is superior to CT scanning in providing exact delineation of glomus tumors and better differentiation of tumor from inflammatory tissue and areas of hemorrhages [76]. There is no consensus on the appropriate treatment for malignant paraganglioma. However, gross total surgical resection remains the mainstay of treatment. Postoperative irradiation has been shown to be beneficial in slowing the progression of residual disease and improving median overall survival by about 33 months [78, 79].

Metastatic Disease

Leptomeningeal Metastasis

The incidence of leptomeningeal disease in HNSCC is about 1–2% versus 5–10% in solid tumor SCC. Perineural invasion is the predominant route of spread to the meninges [80]. Leptomeningeal spread in head and neck cancer is rare and has a poor prognosis [81]. Unlike SCC of solid tumors, HNSCC rarely involves spinal cord and spinal nerve roots. Only one case of intramedullary spinal cord metastasis has been published [82]. The most sensitive imaging is currently MRI, which shows nodules or meningeal contrast enhancement [83]. Currently, treatment options include RT, intrathecal chemotherapy, or systemic therapy with CNS-penetrating agents. Epidermal growth factor receptor inhibitors and locally delivered chemotherapy may be effective in such cases [81].

Parenchymal Brain Metastases

Parenchymal brain metastases are very rare, and only a few case reports have been documented. The majority of these cases had long periods of time over which the patients had untreated primary disease [84, 85]. If brain metastasis appears in long-term survivors of HNSCC, there should also be high suspicion for a second primary malignancy. The origin of these brain metastases is either hematogenous (majority involving lung) or from CSF spread [86, 87]. In an autopsy of 2452 patients, 3% of all intracranial metastases were found in patients with HNSCC [87]. Over the past decade, there has been some rise in the incidence of brain metastasis from HNSCC. Some relate this rise to the increase in distant metastasis in patients with HNSCC who are HPV-positive [85]. In a study of 38 patients who underwent surgical excision of squamous cell carcinoma to the brain, 7 (18%) were from head and neck, and HPV-16 was detected in 4 (57%) of these HNSCC. In this study, invasive neurosurgical interventions, systemic chemotherapy, and RT were attempted to palliate symptoms in patients who presented with neurologic decline [85]. Hardee and colleagues recommend surveillance brain MRI for patients with long-standing untreated primary oral SCC [84].

Epidural Spinal Cord Compression

Epidural spinal cord compression is also very rare in HNSCC compared with other solid tumors. In a study of 759 patients with head and neck cancer, 5 developed epidural compression (1%) [88]. In two large studies from Memorial Sloan Kettering Cancer Center, one showed 6% of cases of epidural metastasis originated from HNSCC [89, 90]. Another study of 337 patients with epidural spinal cord compression at the Mayo Clinic found HNSCC accounted for 1.5% of all cases [91]. Rades and colleagues developed a scoring system based on eleven factors including age, gender, performance status, tumor site, time from cancer diagnosis until epidural spinal cord compression, affected vertebrae, walking ability, further osseous lesions, organ metastases, time developing motor deficits, and radiation regimen to estimate 6-month survival probabilities of these patients [92]. In general, aggressive treatment of spinal epidural compression (surgical resection and RT) is recommended to achieve long-term survival [88]. Due to the rarity of epidural spinal cord compression of HNSCC tumors, if they are seen in patients without evidence of disease for more than 2 years, clinicians should suspect a second primary malignancy.

Brachial Plexopathy

The brachial plexus is occasionally involved with advanced HNSCC. In a series of 75 patients at Memorial Sloan Kettering with brachial plexopathy due to neoplastic infiltration, only four patients had head and neck cancers [93]. These tumors will grow inferiorly, invading the superior plexus. The pattern of plexus involvement could be patchy due to irregular and random involvement of different areas of the plexus proximally and distally [94]. Contrary to radiation-induced plexopathy, neoplastic brachial plexopathy is painful and pain is the most common presenting symptom (75%) [93]. Prior neck dissection, concurrent chemotherapy, and maximum dose RT are significant risk factors for brachial plexopathy [95]. Treatment of metastatic plexopathy is palliative and includes RT to the tumor mass and chemotherapy [96].

Syncope and Glossopharyngeal Neuralgia

Glossopharyngeal neuralgia (GPN) is a rare complication of HNSCC [97, 98]. As in idiopathic cases, a brief severe stabbing pain felt in the ear, base of the tongue, tonsillar fossa, or beneath the angle of the jaw triggered by swallowing, talking, or coughing commonly exacerbates the pain. Syncope may accompany both idiopathic and tumor-related glossopharyngeal neuralgia in about 84% of cases [99]. In rare cases, GPN can present with syncope with no associated pain [100]. In nasopharyngeal carcinoma (NPC), syncope may be caused by parapharyngeal space extension, cervical lymph node involvement, and the invasion of the skull base causing lower cranial nerve palsies. This is mainly due to compression of the carotid sinus or glossopharyngeal nerve invasion [98]. During severe GPN pain, patients may experience pallor, followed by hypotension associated with bradycardia, which can lead to a loss of consciousness and associated tonic-clonic limb jerking movements [100]. Treatment for GPN includes anticonvulsant medications such as carbamazepine, gabapentin, phenytoin, oxcarbazepine, or pregabalin. For syncope, atropine should be used first, then RT with or without chemotherapy maybe effective [98, 100]. Rhizotomy and microvascular decompression of cranial nerves IX and X is the first surgical choice for pain relief [100].

Paraneoplastic Neurologic Syndrome

HNSCC rarely accounts for neurologic paraneoplastic syndromes (PNS). Among head and neck tumors, paraneoplastic SIADH is most commonly associated with squamous cell oral cavity cancer. Two retrospective studies reported an incidence of 2% in a series of 260 cases, and an incidence of 3% in 1436 patients [101, 102]. The resulting hyponatremia may produce encephalopathy and seizures. Hormonal hypercalcemia (HH) is the most common PNS in patients with HNSCC with an incidence of 2.6–7.2% and has a poor prognostic significance. Most of the reported cases of para-neoplastic HH with oral cancer were diagnosed after RT and/or chemotherapy. Patients may experience confusion or fatigue. Dermatologic PNS is less common, but when they occur, they may precede the diagnosis of the oral tumor. Acrokeratosis paraneoplastica is a dermatologic PNS associated with HNSCC. The treatment of the skin lesions is directly related to the eradication of the underlying neoplasm by surgery, chemotherapy, or RT [103].

Neurologic Complications of Treatment

Surgery

Resection of primary head and neck cancers often requires sacrifice of terminal branches of sensory nerves to the face, oral, and nasal cavity, the oropharynx and hypopharynx, or dermatomal branches of the upper cervical nerve roots. See Fig. 28.3. This typically causes severe side effects such as facial deformity, speech and swallowing difficulties, and chronic pain in the oral cavity, neck, face, or shoulder. The incidence of chronic pain approaches 40% at one year and 15% at five years. The accessory nerve and the nerves of the superficial cervical plexus are commonly injured and can cause typical and identifiable neuropathic pain syndromes [104]. Medications such as anticonvulsants (gabapentin, carbamazepine) are helpful in alleviating hyperalgesia and allodynia confined to a peripheral nerve in the acute

postoperative setting [105]. Postoperative physical therapy techniques prevent chronic shoulder pain syndromes [106].

The most characteristic postoperative neurologic complications seen in patients with head and neck cancer are those related to neck dissection. The standard radical neck dissection involves removal of the sternocleidomastoid, digastric, and stylohyoid muscles, the internal and external jugular veins, the submaxillary gland, and the spinal accessory nerve. Swift examined 24 patients who underwent a total of 33 radical neck dissections in the years from 1951 to 1967. All had shoulder weakness, droop (accessory nerve), and scapular winging (cervical plexus). He also found lesions of the mandibular branch of the facial nerve in 67%, hypoglossal nerve in 39%, sympathetic nerve fibers in 33%, the vagus nerve in 15%, and phrenic nerves in 10%. Patients with involvement of the carotid sheath were at greater postoperative risk of Horner's syndromes. Sensory loss was mostly limited to the ear, occiput, and supraclavicular regions [107]. However, recently there have been many attempts to spare the spinal accessory nerve, which has been shown to improve quality of life [108].

Carotid rupture is another significant neurologic complication from neck dissection or advanced HNSCC. Invasion of the carotid artery could also be seen by recurrent HNSCC. Many surgeons remove the affected carotid artery along with the tumor and do reconstruction of the vessel. Carotid artery rupture (carotid blowout) may occur either as a surgical complication in 3–5% of aggressive HNSCC resections, or in the setting of post-RT tumor resection [109, 110].

Fig. 28.3 Neural structures in the neck which might be injured by radical neck dissection. (Adapted with permission of Figure comes from [107])

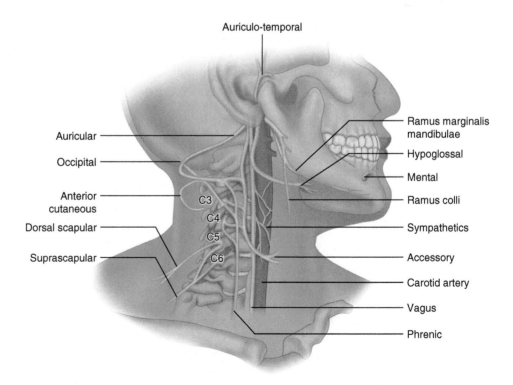

Auriculo-temporal

Auricular

Occipital

Anterior cutaneous

Dorsal scapular

Suprascapular

C3
C4
C5
C6

Ramus marginalis mandibulae

Hypoglossal

Mental

Ramus colli

Sympathetics

Accessory

Carotid artery

Vagus

Phrenic

Ligation of the common carotid or internal carotid artery was standard therapy; however, it led to major strokes. One study showed major neurologic complications with carotid ligation in an emergency setting of about 60% with mortality rates of 40% [110]. In a retrospective study of 28 patients with advanced head and neck malignancy who underwent carotid resection, 12 patients underwent immediate carotid artery resection and ligation, one patient died of severe neurologic deficits, two patients experienced neurologic deficits with good recovery, and one patient was moderately disabled [111]. This poor outcome has been significantly improved by endovascular techniques (e.g., coils, balloons, stents) [112].

Sacrifice of the internal jugular vein(IJV) can also produce major neurologic deficits such as increased intracranial pressure (ICP) [113]. This may be associated with headache, facial swelling, and cerebral edema resulting in seizures and obtundation. The symptoms may worsen in a supine patient due to the effects of impaired venous drainage upon ICP. Attempts have being made to spare the IJV; however, IJV preservation is associated with an increased risk of neck failure and a worse outcome mainly in patients with extra-capsular node involvement [114]. Benign intracranial hypertension has also been documented in either bilateral or unilateral RND due to resection of the dominant IJV in the presence of a hypoplastic or aplastic contralateral IJV or transverse sinus. In some cases, this can result in permanent visual loss. MRA is an effective technique to diagnose and follow these patients [115].

Radiotherapy

Radiotherapy for head and neck cancers typically involves the administration of 7000 cGy over six to seven weeks with a dose of 5600 cGy delivered to the areas of likely microscopic disease involvement, and 5000–5250 cGy delivered to areas at very low risk for presence of tumor [116]. Some patients with radiation injury to the cervical spinal cord experience Lhermitte's sign (LS) , which is an electric shock-like sensation, spreading along the spine in a cervico-caudal direction and also into both arms and legs upon forward flexion of the neck. Radiation can produce spinal cord toxicity in a transient form or reversible myelopathy characterized by LS, which appears soon after or within six months of RT with duration of weeks to six months [117]. The toxicity is due to demyelination of the ascending sensory axons. The incidence of LS developing in the context of transient radiation myelopathy was reported to be between 3.6 and 13% in large patient groups receiving RT for head and neck and thoracic malignancies [118]. At present, the maximum dose considered safe for spinal cord tolerance and the prevention of delayed radiation

myelopathy is 45–50 Gy delivered in 1.8–2 Gy daily fractions. When the spinal cord dose is kept below 50 Gy, the incidence of delayed radiation myelitis is very low [119]. In transient cases, MRI may be normal even if the patient has a severe neurologic deficit, as positive MRI findings appear only in delayed radiation myelitis [120]. In the absence of pain or other signs of myelopathy, close follow-up is all that is needed. However, occasionally patients with HNSCC develop serious late-delayed radiation myelopathy (incidence of 0.5–5%). The incidence increases with doses above 5500 cGy, high dose fractions, and longer length spinal cord in the radiation field [121]. Time of onset of symptoms following RT is variable and ranges from 12 months to eight years. Typical symptoms are those of a slowly progressive ascending sensorimotor disturbance. MRI has enabled both an early and specific diagnosis of radiation myelitis. Imaging reveals central cord swelling confined to the irradiated field and, in some cases, cord atrophy [122]. Clinical features of radiation myelopathy are discussed in Chap. 14. See Fig. 28.4a, b.

Patients with treated head and neck cancer may have focal neurologic symptoms and personality changes due to delayed cerebral radionecrosis. These lesions are usually in the frontal and temporal regions and on imaging may resemble high-grade gliomas or metastatic tumors. Histopathologic changes include fibrotic response of the meninges with pleomorphic and vacuolated fibroblasts, capillary hyperplasia, reactive astrocytes, and fibrosis of the blood vessels. Craniotomy is the recommended course of treatment [123] for symptoms unresponsive to corticosteroids or bevacizumab.

Cranial nerve palsy (CNP) is a rare complication of RT. In a study of 328 patients with nasopharyngeal carcinoma who received RT, 72 were found to have CNP after a mean follow-up of 11.2 years. The latency of palsy ranged from 0.6 to 16 years. Most patients develop CNP after two years. In those who received first course RT, CN IX and CNX were mostly affected (85%). In patients with reradiation, most had multiple upper cranial nerve injuries. Patients with facial–cervical field radiation had a significantly longer latency compared with patients who developed facial–cervical split fields [124]. In other studies, CNXII nerve has been shown to be most commonly affected [125].

Vasculopathy from RT for head and neck cancers may cause neurologic symptoms. The damage to small vessels and the endothelium can produce cerebral radionecrosis [123]. The injury to large vessels, such as the carotid artery, leads to stroke. The key mechanism of accelerated carotid atherosclerosis, endothelial damage, and fibrosis are due to tissue necrosis and inflammation caused by radiation. These mechanisms resemble morphologic features of spontaneous atherosclerosis [126]. Radiation-induced carotid disease is limited to the irradiated area and is less likely associated

(a)

(b)

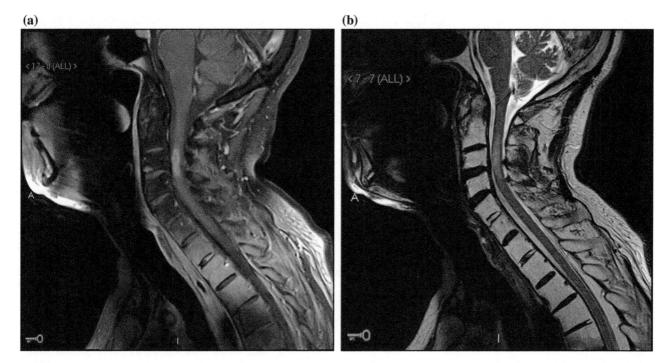

Fig. 28.4 Sagittal post-Gd and T2-weighted MR images of a 64-year-old man with six weeks of *right-sided* numbness from the neck down. He had received radiation (74 Gy) and concomitant chemotherapy three years earlier for squamous cell carcinoma of the hypopharynx. His cancer was in remission; body PET-CT and brain MRI were normal. He remained clinically stable without intervention, and follow-up MRI two years later showed resolution of contrast enhancement and the development of myelomalacia consistent with evolving radiation myelopathy

with atherogenic risk factors [127]. In a meta-analysis of 34 papers on radiation-induced carotid atherosclerosis, the authors found relative risk of stroke to be 5.6 in patients treated for head and neck cancer. The prevalence of carotid artery stenosis was increased by 16–55%, and carotid intima medial thickness was increased by 18–40% [128]. Carotid Doppler is recommended for long-term follow-up of these patients.

Chemotherapy

Cisplatin produces dose-related ototoxicity and peripheral neuropathy. It occasionally causes LS, which indicates the involvement of the centripetal branch of the sensory pathway within the spinal cord [129]. Chemotherapy protocols for head and neck cancers using cisplatin (commonly 100 mg/m^2 for every 3 weeks with concurrent radiation) rarely achieve the cumulative dose of cisplatin sufficient to produce a high incidence of peripheral neuropathy (cumulative dose $\geq$ 300 mg/m^2). Peripheral sensory neurotoxicities with platinum agents vary from paresthesias in fingers, loss of vibration, and ankle jerks to ataxic gait (loss of proprioception), which might be transient or irreversible. It damages peripheral nerves and dorsal root ganglia neurons, possibly because of progressive DNA-adduct accumulation

and inhibition of DNA repair pathways which mediate apoptosis [130]. However, severe neuropathy is seen in <1% of patients treated for head and neck cancer. Ototoxicity is another progressive and irreversible adverse effect of platinum chemotherapy with a high frequency of almost 88%; it usually presents bilaterally and may occur during or years after treatment [131]. Cisplatin accumulates in the cochlear tissue, forms DNA adducts, and causes inefficient and dysfunctional protein and enzyme synthesis leading to apoptosis of auditory sensory cells [132]. However, severe ototoxicity is seen in fewer than 5% of treated HNSCC patients. Cisplatin is almost always given in combination with other chemotherapy drugs and/or radiation, which could also be neurotoxic. However, the concurrent use of cisplatin/5-FU in moderate doses with radiation resulted in no instances of myelopathy or other CNS complications [133].

Other chemotherapeutic agents, including paclitaxel and docetaxel, are used in combination with cisplatin for treatment of head and neck cancer. This increases the risk of peripheral neuropathy. Paclitaxel-induced peripheral neuropathy is also associated with proximal muscle weakness [134]. The combination of paclitaxel, ifosfamide, and cisplatin (TIP regimen) is sometimes used for recurrent head and neck cancer, which can cause a higher incidence of peripheral neuropathy and fatigue. When cisplatin was replaced with carboplatin in the regimen (TIC), the side effects decreased significantly [39]. Other new chemotherapy agents, such as cetuximab, can cause peripheral neuropathy, fatigue, and weakness. However, there are not many cases reported in the literature.

Conclusion

Head and neck cancers, along with their treatments, can cause many neurologic complications. These are highlighted by the close proximity to the brain which proves challenging for treatment as well as offers the opportunity for cancers to extend directly into the cranium. Cranial neuropathies are quite common, mostly due to perineural spread of cancer. HNSCC rarely causes the more traditional CNS metastasis or leptomeningeal disease; however, when they occur, clinicians should suspect a second primary malignancy as a result of HNSCC treatment with chemotherapy and radiation. Surgical resection of head and neck cancer can cause significant neurologic complications such as cranial neuropathies, chronic pain syndrome, syncope, seizure, and stroke. Modified radical neck dissection and advanced endovascular techniques are some of the newer methods that have decreased the incidence of serious neurologic complications. Personality changes, myelopathy causing LS, and strokes are some of the serious adverse effects of RT and should be considered as a cause. Cisplatin is the most commonly used chemotherapy for HNSCC. Cisplatin in combination with other chemotherapy agents such as paclitaxel, ifosfamide, or docetaxel can increase the incidence of peripheral neuropathy.

References

1. Siegel RL, Miller KD, Jemal A. Cancer statistics, 2015. CA Cancer J Clin. 2015;65(1):5–29.
2. Jemal A, et al. Global cancer statistics. CA Cancer J Clin. 2011;61(2):69–90.
3. Warnakulasuriya S, Johnson NW, van der Waal I. Nomenclature and classification of potentially malignant disorders of the oral mucosa. J Oral Pathol Med. 2007;36(10):575–80.
4. Slaughter DP, Southwick HW, Smejkal W. Field cancerization in oral stratified squamous epithelium; clinical implications of multicentric origin. Cancer. 1953;6(5):963–8.
5. Sabharwal R, et al. Genetically altered fields in head and neck cancer and second field tumor. South Asian J Cancer. 2014;3(3):151–3.
6. Poeta ML, et al. TP53 mutations and survival in squamous-cell carcinoma of the head and neck. N Engl J Med. 2007;357(25):2552–61.
7. Gonzalez MV, et al. Loss of heterozygosity and mutation analysis of the p16 (9p21) and p53 (17p13) genes in squamous cell carcinoma of the head and neck. Clin Cancer Res. 1995;1(9):1043–9.
8. Kraft S, Granter SR. Molecular pathology of skin neoplasms of the head and neck. Arch Pathol Lab Med. 2014;138(6):759–87.
9. Dong Y, et al. Cyclin D1-CDK4 complex, a possible critical factor for cell proliferation and prognosis in laryngeal squamous cell carcinomas. Int J Cancer. 2001;95(4):209–15.
10. Gross AM, et al. Multi-tiered genomic analysis of head and neck cancer ties TP53 mutation to 3p loss. Nat Genet. 2014;46(9): 939–43.
11. Wu CL, et al. Deletion mapping on the short arm of chromosome 3 in squamous cell carcinoma of the oral cavity. Cancer Res. 1994;54(24):6484–8.
12. Vokes EE, et al. Head and neck cancer. N Engl J Med. 1993;328(3):184–94.
13. Huber MA, Tantiwongkosi B. Oral and oropharyngeal cancer. Med Clin North Am. 2014;98(6):1299–321.
14. Omura K. Current status of oral cancer treatment strategies: surgical treatments for oral squamous cell carcinoma. Int J Clin Oncol. 2014;19(3):423–30.
15. Sakuraba M, et al. Recent advances in reconstructive surgery: head and neck reconstruction. Int J Clin Oncol. 2013;18(4): 561–5.
16. Sutton DN, et al. The prognostic implications of the surgical margin in oral squamous cell carcinoma. Int J Oral Maxillofac Surg. 2003;32(1):30–4.
17. Wong LS, et al. Influence of close resection margins on local recurrence and disease-specific survival in oral and oropharyngeal carcinoma. Br J Oral Maxillofac Surg. 2012;50(2):102–8.
18. Mistry RC, Qureshi SS, Kumaran C. Post-resection mucosal margin shrinkage in oral cancer: quantification and significance. J Surg Oncol. 2005;91(2):131–3.
19. Meier JD, Oliver DA, Varvares MA. Surgical margin determination in head and neck oncology: current clinical practice. The results of an International American Head and Neck Society Member Survey. Head Neck. 2005;27(11):952–8.
20. Weiss MH, Harrison LB, Isaacs RS. Use of decision analysis in planning a management strategy for the stage N0 neck. Arch Otolaryngol Head Neck Surg. 1994;120(7):699–702.
21. Robbins KT, et al. Neck dissection classification update: revisions proposed by the American Head and Neck Society and the American Academy of otolaryngology-head and neck surgery. Arch Otolaryngol Head Neck Surg. 2002;128(7): 751–8.
22. Broglie MA, et al. Occult metastases detected by sentinel node biopsy in patients with early oral and oropharyngeal squamous cell carcinomas: impact on survival. Head Neck. 2013;35(5): 660–6.
23. Kowalski LP, et al. Prognostic significance of the distribution of neck node metastasis from oral carcinoma. Head Neck. 2000;22(3):207–14.
24. Shingaki S, et al. Impact of lymph node metastasis on the pattern of failure and survival in oral carcinomas. Am J Surg. 2003;185(3):278–84.
25. Bernier J, et al. Postoperative irradiation with or without concomitant chemotherapy for locally advanced head and neck cancer. N Engl J Med. 2004;350(19):1945–52.
26. Furness S et al. Interventions for the treatment of oral cavity and oropharyngeal cancer: chemotherapy. Cochrane Database Syst Rev 2011(4): Cd006386.
27. Peters J, et al. Evaluation of the dose for postoperative radiation therapy of head and neck cancer: first report of a prospective randomized trial. Int J Radiat Oncol Biol Phys. 1993;26(1):3–11.
28. Kiyota N, Tahara M, Fujii M. Adjuvant treatment for post-operative head and neck squamous cell carcinoma. Jpn J Clin Oncol. 2015;45(1):2–6.
29. Duvvuri U, Myers JN. Contemporary management of oropharyngeal cancer: anatomy and physiology of the oropharynx. Curr Probl Surg. 2009;46(2):119–84.

30. Haigentz MJr et al. Current trends in initial management of oropharyngeal cancer: the declining use of open surgery. Eur Arch Otorhinolaryngol. 2009;266(12):1845–55.

31. Forastiere AA, et al. Long-term results of RTOG 91-11: a comparison of three nonsurgical treatment strategies to preserve the larynx in patients with locally advanced larynx cancer. J Clin Oncol. 2013;31(7):845–52.

32. Soderstrom K, et al. Regional recurrence of oropharyngeal cancer after definitive radiotherapy: a case control study. Radiat Oncol. 2015;10(1):117.

33. Tannock IF. Chemotherapy for head and neck cancer. J Otolaryngol. 1984;13(2):99–104.

34. Al-Sarraf M. Chemotherapy strategies in squamous cell carcinoma of the head and neck. Crit Rev Oncol Hematol. 1984;1(4):323–55.

35. Glick JH, Zehngebot LM. Taylor SGt. Chemotherapy for squamous cell carcinoma of the head and neck: a progress report. Am J Otolaryngol. 1980;1(4):306–23.

36. Chan AT et al. Nasopharyngeal cancer: EHNS-ESMO-ESTRO clinical practice guidelines for diagnosis, treatment and follow-up. Ann Oncol 2012; 23 Suppl 7: vii83–5.

37. Chan AT, et al. Overall survival after concurrent cisplatin-radiotherapy compared with radiotherapy alone in locoregionally advanced nasopharyngeal carcinoma. J Natl Cancer Inst. 2005;97(7):536–9.

38. Brizel DM, et al. Hyperfractionated irradiation with or without concurrent chemotherapy for locally advanced head and neck cancer. N Engl J Med. 1998;338(25):1798–804.

39. Shin DM, et al. Phase II study of paclitaxel, ifosfamide, and carboplatin in patients with recurrent or metastatic head and neck squamous cell carcinoma. Cancer. 2001;91(7):1316–23.

40. Pancari P, Mehra R. Systemic therapy for squamous cell carcinoma of the head and neck. Surg Oncol Clin N Am. 2015;24(3):437–54.

41. Chung CH, et al. Integrating epidermal growth factor receptor assay with clinical parameters improves risk classification for relapse and survival in head-and-neck squamous cell carcinoma. Int J Radiat Oncol Biol Phys. 2011;81(2):331–8.

42. Hanna GJ, Haddad RI, Lorch JH. Induction chemotherapy for locoregionally advanced head and neck cancer: past, present, future? Oncologist. 2013;18(3):288–93.

43. Licitra L, et al. Primary chemotherapy in resectable oral cavity squamous cell cancer: a randomized controlled trial. J Clin Oncol. 2003;21(2):327–33.

44. Iyer NG, et al. Randomized trial comparing surgery and adjuvant radiotherapy versus concurrent chemoradiotherapy in patients with advanced, nonmetastatic squamous cell carcinoma of the head and neck: 10-year update and subset analysis. Cancer. 2015;121(10):1599–607.

45. Bernier J, et al. Defining risk levels in locally advanced head and neck cancers: a comparative analysis of concurrent postoperative radiation plus chemotherapy trials of the EORTC (#22931) and RTOG (# 9501). Head Neck. 2005;27(10):843–50.

46. Gregoire V, et al. Squamous cell carcinoma of the head and neck: EHNS-ESMO-ESTRO clinical practice guidelines for diagnosis, treatment and follow-up. Ann Oncol. 2010;21(Suppl 5):v184–6.

47. Cohen EE, et al. Phase III randomized trial of induction chemotherapy in patients with N2 or N3 locally advanced head and neck cancer. J Clin Oncol. 2014;32(25):2735–43.

48. Haddad R, et al. Induction chemotherapy followed by concurrent chemoradiotherapy (sequential chemoradiotherapy) versus concurrent chemoradiotherapy alone in locally advanced head and neck cancer (PARADIGM): a randomised phase 3 trial. Lancet Oncol. 2013;14(3):257–64.

49. Moonis G, et al. Patterns of perineural tumor spread in head and neck cancer. Magn Reson Imaging Clin N Am. 2012;20(3):435–46.

50. Barrett AW, Speight PM. Perineural invasion in adenoid cystic carcinoma of the salivary glands: a valid prognostic indicator? Oral Oncol. 2009;45(11):936–40.

51. Matsushita Y, et al. A clinicopathological study of perineural invasion and vascular invasion in oral tongue squamous cell carcinoma. Int J Oral Maxillofac Surg. 2015;44(5):543–8.

52. Panizza B, et al. Histopathological features of clinical perineural invasion of cutaneous squamous cell carcinoma of the head and neck and the potential implications for treatment. Head Neck. 2014;36(11):1611–8.

53. Catalano PJ, Sen C, Biller HF. Cranial neuropathy secondary to perineural spread of cutaneous malignancies. Am J Otol. 1995;16(6):772–7.

54. Roh J, et al. Perineural growth in head and neck squamous cell carcinoma: a review. Oral Oncol. 2015;51(1):16–23.

55. Frunza A, Slavescu D, Lascar I. Perineural invasion in head and neck cancers—a review. J Med Life. 2014;7(2):121–3.

56. Tang C, et al. Stereotactic radiosurgery for retreatment of gross perineural invasion in recurrent cutaneous squamous cell carcinoma of the head and neck. Am J Clin Oncol. 2013;36(3):293–8.

57. Serracino HS, Kleinschmidt-Demasters BK. Skull invaders: when surgical pathology and neuropathology worlds collide. J Neuropathol Exp Neurol. 2013;72(7):600–13.

58. Moona MS, Mehdi I. Nasopharyngeal carcinoma presented as cavernous sinus tumour. J Pak Med Assoc. 2011;61(12):1235–6.

59. de Bree R, et al. Intracranial metastases in patients with squamous cell carcinoma of the head and neck. Otolaryngol Head Neck Surg. 2001;124(2):217–21.

60. Arya S, Rane P, Deshmukh A. Oral cavity squamous cell carcinoma: role of pretreatment imaging and its influence on management. Clin Radiol. 2014;69(9):916–30.

61. Thomas JE, Waltz AJ. Neurological manifestations of nasopharyngeal malignant tumors. JAMA. 1965;192:95–8.

62. Kuo CL, Ho DM, Ho CY. Dural metastasis of nasopharyngeal carcinoma: rare, but worth considering. Singapore Med J. 2014;55(5):e82–4.

63. Rafee S, et al. A rare case of nasopharyngeal carcinoma with widespread CNS metastases. Ir Med J. 2014;107(6):180–1.

64. King AD, Bhatia KS. Magnetic resonance imaging staging of nasopharyngeal carcinoma in the head and neck. World J Radiol. 2010;2(5):159–65.

65. Razek AAKA, King A. MRI and CT of nasopharyngeal carcinoma. AJR Am J Roentgenol 2012; 198(1): 11–8.

66. Beckmann YY, et al. Third cranial nerve palsy as the presenting neuro-ophthalmic feature of nasopharyngeal carcinoma. J Neuroophthalmol. 2010;30(1):102–3.

67. Nunez F, et al. Sino-nasal adenocarcinoma: epidemiological and clinico-pathological study of 34 cases. J Otolaryngol. 1993;22(2):86–90.

68. Suarez C, et al. Management of the orbit in malignant sinonasal tumors. Head Neck. 2008;30(2):242–50.

69. Carrau RL, et al. Squamous cell carcinoma of the sinonasal tract invading the orbit. Laryngoscope. 1999;109(2 Pt 1):230–5.

70. Khan SN, Sepahdari AR. Orbital masses: CT and MRI of common vascular lesions, benign tumors, and malignancies. Saudi J Ophthalmol. 2012;26(4):373–83.

71. Imola MJ, Schramm VL Jr. Orbital preservation in surgical management of sinonasal malignancy. Laryngoscope. 2002;112(8 Pt 1):1357–65.

72. Nishino H, et al. Results of orbital preservation for advanced malignant maxillary sinus tumors. Laryngoscope. 2003;113(6):1064–9.

73. Jansen EP, et al. Does the combination of radiotherapy and debulking surgery favor survival in paranasal sinus carcinoma? Int J Radiat Oncol Biol Phys. 2000;48(1):27–35.

74. Jayashankar N, Sankhla S. Current perspectives in the management of glomus jugulare tumors. Neurol India. 2015;63(1):83–90.

75. Boedeker CC, et al. Clinical features of paraganglioma syndromes. Skull Base. 2009;19(1):17–25.

76. Mafee MF, et al. Glomus faciale, glomus jugulare, glomus tympanicum, glomus vagale, carotid body tumors, and simulating lesions. Role of MR imaging. Radiol Clin North Am. 2000; 38(5):1059–76.

77. Larson TC 3rd, et al. Glomus tympanicum chemodectomas: radiographic and clinical characteristics. Radiology. 1987; 163(3):801–6.

78. Chapman DB, et al. Clinical, histopathologic, and radiographic indicators of malignancy in head and neck paragangliomas. Otolaryngol Head Neck Surg. 2010;143(4):531–7.

79. Lee JH, et al. National cancer data base report on malignant paragangliomas of the head and neck. Cancer. 2002;94(3):730–7.

80. Redman BG, Tapazoglo E, Al-Sarraf M. Meningeal carcinomatosis in head and neck cancer. Report of six cases and review of the literature. Cancer. 1986;58(12):2656–61.

81. Pougnet I, et al. Carcinomatous myelitis and meningitis after a squamous cell carcinoma of the lip. Case Rep Oncol. 2014; 7(1):33–8.

82. Tornwall J, Snall J, Mesimaki K. A rare case of spinal cord metastases from oral SCC. Br J Oral Maxillofac Surg. 2008;46 (7):594–5.

83. Skripuletz T, et al. Meningeal carcinomatosis from penile squamous cell carcinoma. J Neurooncol. 2010;98(3):417–9.

84. Hardee PS, Hutchison LL. Intracranial metastases from oral squamous cell carcinoma. Br J Oral Maxillofac Surg. 2001; 39(4):282–5.

85. Ruzevick J, Olivi A, Westra WH. Metastatic squamous cell carcinoma to the brain: an unrecognized pattern of distant spread in patients with HPV-related head and neck cancer. J Neurooncol. 2013;112(3):449–54.

86. Ngan RK, et al. Central nervous system metastasis from nasopharyngeal carcinoma: a report of two patients and a review of the literature. Cancer. 2002;94(2):398–405.

87. Posner JB, Chernik NL. Intracranial metastases from systemic cancer. Adv Neurol. 1978;19:579–92.

88. Ampil FL, et al. Spinal epidural compression in head and neck cancer. Report of five cases. J Craniomaxillofac Surg. 1994; 22(1):49–52.

89. Gilbert RW, Kim JH, Posner JB. Epidural spinal cord compression from metastatic tumor: diagnosis and treatment. Ann Neurol. 1978;3(1):40–51.

90. Greenberg HS, Kim JH, Posner JB. Epidural spinal cord compression from metastatic tumor: results with a new treatment protocol. Ann Neurol. 1980;8(4):361–6.

91. Schiff D, et al. Neuroimaging and treatment implications of patients with multiple epidural spinal metastases. Cancer. 1998;83(8):1593–601.

92. Rades D, et al. Predicting survival of patients with metastatic epidural spinal cord compression from cancer of the head-and-neck. Anticancer Res. 2015;35(1):385–8.

93. Kori SH, Foley KM, Posner JB. Brachial plexus lesions in patients with cancer: 100 cases. Neurology. 1981;31(1):45–50.

94. Jaeckle KA. Neurologic manifestations of neoplastic and radiation-induced plexopathies. Semin Neurol. 2010;30(3): 254–62.

95. Chen AM, et al. Brachial plexus-associated neuropathy after high-dose radiation therapy for head-and-neck cancer. Int J Radiat Oncol Biol Phys. 2012;84(1):165–9.

96. Jaeckle KA. Nerve plexus metastases. Neurol Clin. 1991; 9(4):857–66.

97. Papay FA, et al. Evaluation of syncope from head and neck cancer. Laryngoscope. 1989;99(4):382–8.

98. Tang Y, Wang JM, Huang CH. Syncope in nasopharyngeal carcinoma: report of three cases and review of the literature. Changgeng Yi Xue Za Zhi. 1993;16(1):59–65.

99. Rushton JG, Stevens JC, Miller RH. Glossopharyngeal (vagoglossopharyngeal) neuralgia: a study of 217 cases. Arch Neurol. 1981;38(4):201–5.

100. Blumenfeld A, Nikolskaya G. Glossopharyngeal neuralgia. Curr Pain Headache Rep. 2013;17(7):343.

101. Talmi YP, Hoffman HT, McCabe BF. Syndrome of inappropriate secretion of arginine vasopressin in patients with cancer of the head and neck. Ann Otol Rhinol Laryngol. 1992;101(11):946–9.

102. Zohar Y, et al. Syndrome of inappropriate antidiuretic hormone secretion in cancer of the head and neck. Ann Otol Rhinol Laryngol. 1991;100(4 Pt 1):341–4.

103. Toro C, et al. Paraneoplastic syndromes in patients with oral cancer. Oral Oncol. 2010;46(1):14–8.

104. Burton AW, et al. Chronic pain in the cancer survivor: a new frontier. Pain Med. 2007;8(2):189–98.

105. Gilron I. Review article: the role of anticonvulsant drugs in postoperative pain management: a bench-to-bedside perspective. Can J Anaesth. 2006;53(6):562–71.

106. McNeely ML, et al. A pilot study of a randomized controlled trial to evaluate the effects of progressive resistance exercise training on shoulder dysfunction caused by spinal accessory neurapraxia/neurectomy in head and neck cancer survivors. Head Neck. 2004;26(6):518–30.

107. Swift TR. Involvement of peripheral nerves in radical neck dissection. Am J Surg. 1970;119(6):694–8.

108. Eickmeyer SM, et al. Quality of life, shoulder range of motion, and spinal accessory nerve status in 5-year survivors of head and neck cancer. PM R. 2014;6(12):1073–80.

109. Porto DP, Adams GL, Foster C. Emergency management of carotid artery rupture. Am J Otolaryngol. 1986;7(3):213–7.

110. Chaloupka JC, et al. Endovascular therapy for the carotid blowout syndrome in head and neck surgical patients: diagnostic and managerial considerations. AJNR Am J Neuroradiol. 1996;17(5):843–52.

111. Aslan I, et al. Management of carotid artery invasion in advanced malignancies of head and neck comparison of techniques. Ann Otol Rhinol Laryngol. 2002;111(9):772–7.

112. Zussman B, et al. Endovascular management of carotid blowout. World Neurosurg. 2012;78(1–2):109–14.

113. Sugarbaker ED, Wiley HM. Intracranial-pressure studies incident to resection of the internal jugular veins. Cancer. 1951;4(2): 242–50.

114. Gallo O, et al. Prognostic role of internal jugular vein preservation in neck dissection for head and neck cancer. J Surg Oncol. 2013;108(8):579–83.

115. Lam BL, et al. Pseudotumor cerebri from cranial venous obstruction. Ophthalmology. 1992;99(5):706–12.

116. Yom SS. Radiation treatment of head and neck cancer. Surg Oncol Clin N Am. 2015;24(3):423–36.

117. St Clair WH, et al. Spinal cord and peripheral nerve injury: current management and investigations. Semin Radiat Oncol. 2003;13(3):322–32.

118. Esik O, et al. A review on radiogenic Lhermitte's sign. Pathol Oncol Res. 2003;9(2):115–20.

119. Gemici C. Lhermitte's sign: review with special emphasis in oncology practice. Crit Rev Oncol Hematol. 2010;74(2):79–86.

120. Alfonso ER, et al. Radiation myelopathy in over-irradiated patients: MR imaging findings. Eur Radiol. 1997;7(3):400–4.

121. Abbatucci JS, et al. Radiation myelopathy of the cervical spinal cord: time, dose and volume factors. Int J Radiat Oncol Biol Phys. 1978;4(3–4):239–48.

122. Chan L, et al. Delayed radiation myelopathy after concurrent chemoradiation for hypopharyngeal-esophageal carcinoma. Acta Oncol. 2005;44(2):177–9.

123. Araoz C, Weems AM. Posttherapeutic cerebral radionecrosis: a complication of head and neck tumor therapy. South Med J. 1981;74(12):1485–8.

124. Rong X, et al. Radiation-induced cranial neuropathy in patients with nasopharyngeal carcinoma. A follow-up study. Strahlenther Onkol. 2012;188(3):282–6.

125. Berger PS, Bataini JP. Radiation-induced cranial nerve palsy. Cancer. 1977;40(1):152–5.

126. Cheng SW, Ting AC, Wu LL. Ultrasonic analysis of plaque characteristics and intimal-medial thickness in radiation-induced atherosclerotic carotid arteries. Eur J Vasc Endovasc Surg. 2002;24(6):499–504.

127. Halak M, et al. Neck irradiation: a risk factor for occlusive carotid artery disease. Eur J Vasc Endovasc Surg. 2002;23(4):299–302.

128. Gujral DM, et al. Radiation-induced carotid artery atherosclerosis. Radiother Oncol. 2014;110(1):31–8.

129. Cavaletti G, Alberti P, Marmiroli P. Chemotherapy-induced peripheral neurotoxicity in the era of pharmacogenomics. Lancet Oncol. 2011;12(12):1151–61.

130. Avan A, et al. Platinum-induced neurotoxicity and preventive strategies: past, present, and future. Oncologist. 2015;20(4):411–32.

131. Bertolini P, et al. Platinum compound-related ototoxicity in children: long-term follow-up reveals continuous worsening of hearing loss. J Pediatr Hematol Oncol. 2004;26(10):649–55.

132. Thomas JP, et al. High accumulation of platinum-DNA adducts in strial marginal cells of the cochlea is an early event in cisplatin but not carboplatin ototoxicity. Mol Pharmacol. 2006;70(1):23–9.

133. Denham JW, Abbott RL. Concurrent cisplatin, infusional fluorouracil, and conventionally fractionated radiation therapy in head and neck cancer: dose-limiting mucosal toxicity. J Clin Oncol. 1991;9(3):458–63.

134. Freilich RJ, et al. Motor neuropathy due to docetaxel and paclitaxel. Neurology. 1996;47(1):115–8.

Neurological Complications of Malignant Melanoma

29

Hamza Malek, Annise Wilson, and Jeffrey Raizer

Malignant Melanoma

Incidence and Age-Groups

Skin cancer is the most commonly diagnosed cancer in the USA. Melanoma comprises less than 2% of all skin cancer cases, but causes the majority of skin cancer deaths [1]. The highest incidence rates have been in Australia and New Zealand with approximately 60,000 cases per 100,000. Melanoma is the fifth most common cancer in men and the seventh most common cancer in women [1, 2].

According to the American Cancer Society, melanoma incidence rates have steadily risen over the past 30 years [3], though rates have begun to plateau in younger age-groups. Melanoma is the most common cancer among individuals 25–29 years of age. From 2007 to 2011, incidence rates have plateaued in individuals under 50, but increased by 2.6% per year in those over 50, especially in men [4]. The average age of diagnosis is 62. Pediatric melanoma is rare, accounting for 1–3% of all pediatric cancers and 1–4% of all melanoma cases [5]. The lifetime risk of melanoma is 2.4% in whites, 0.5% in Latinos, and 0.1% in African Americans. Between 2004 and 2007, the rates among whites were 25.4 per 100,000 men and 16.9 per 100,000 women [6, 7]. It is estimated that there will be 9940 deaths from melanoma in 2015. Overall, the mortality rates have remained stable since the 1980s despite increased incidence likely due to earlier detection at a curable stage [8].

In the 1990s, mortality rates in the USA declined among individuals aged 20–44 (39% in women, 29% in men), but increased in men over age 45 (70% among men aged 45–64 and 157% among men over age 65). It is theorized that the increased mortality in men over age 45 may be due to fewer self-examinations, a difference in biology in this patient population, or altered host defense mechanisms [9].

There has been an increase in the diagnosis of melanoma in young women over the past thirty years. According to SEER (Surveillance Epidemiology and End Results), there was an increase from 8.1 in 1975 to 17.4 in 2008 in women, while in men, the rate increased from 8.3 to 12.5 [10, 11]. The peak difference in gender incidence rates in young adults occurs between ages 20 and 24. It is important to note that this increased incidence was not observed in non-melanoma skin cancers, which suggests that other factors are involved such as hormones [12].

Risk Factors

Although anyone can develop melanoma, most patients with this cancer have fair skin. People with red or blond hair and green or blue eyes are at highest risk.

Ultraviolet radiation is well known to contribute to cases of melanoma via gene mutations, immunosuppression, cyclobutane pyrimidine dimers, and oxidative stress [13]. A history of sunburns or tanning also increases the risk of developing melanoma; indoor tanning increases the risk by 75%.

A family history of melanoma, especially in one or more first-degree relatives, also increases a person's chance of developing melanoma. Approximately 10% of individuals with melanoma have a family history. Familial melanoma occurs in 5–10% of patients and is consistent with an autosomal dominant, highly penetrant mutation [14]. Diagnosis typically occurs at an earlier age than sporadic cases with more than one primary melanoma visualized. This particular population is referenced as having Familial Melanoma Syndrome, Hereditary Dysplastic Nevus Syndrome,

H. Malek · A. Wilson · J. Raizer (✉)
Department of Neurology, Northwestern University,
710 North Lake Shore Drive, Abbott Hall, Rm 1123,
Chicago, IL 60611, USA
e-mail: jraizer@nm.org

H. Malek
e-mail: hamza.malek@northwestern.edu

A. Wilson
e-mail: annise.wilson@northwestern.edu

© Springer International Publishing AG 2018
D. Schiff et al. (eds.), *Cancer Neurology in Clinical Practice*,
DOI 10.1007/978-3-319-57901-6_29

or Familial Atypical Mole and Malignant Melanoma Syndrome [15, 16]. 30–40% of cases of familial melanoma are due to CDKN2A and CDK4 mutations [17]. Li-Fraumeni syndrome has also been linked to melanoma and may have an associated CDKN2A pathway [18, 19]. Numerous additional mutations can be found in melanoma [20–30].

There is a 5% chance that a person with a prior history of melanoma will develop melanoma again. A history of basal cell carcinoma or squamous cell carcinoma also increases risk of developing melanoma. Cutaneous melanomas have been associated with neurofibromas [31] and meningiomas [32].

Patients who have received solid organ transplants have a 2.4-fold increased incidence of melanoma as compared to the general population [33]. It is postulated that the immunocompromised state is the independent risk factor, though the immunosuppressant medication itself may also play a role [33]. Tumor necrosis factor (TNF)-α inhibitors have been noted to increase incidence of melanoma in a dose-dependent fashion [34].

There is a sevenfold increased relative risk of melanoma in individuals with Parkinson's disease. Conversely, those with melanoma have an increased risk of developing Parkinson's disease. It is unclear whether dopaminergic therapies (levodopa in particular) play a role [35–37].

Early Detection and Prevention

Melanoma begins in melanocytes which produce melanin, making the lesions black or brown, though they can also appear white, tan, or pink. Melanoma is more commonly found on the trunk and extremities in younger individuals and on the head or neck in older individuals. It is thought that melanomas located on the trunk are seen in the setting of multiple or atypical nevi, while head and neck melanomas are related to chronic actinic damage [8].

Staging and Treatment Overview

Clinical staging takes into account findings from a physical examination, biopsy or resection of the tumor, and imaging studies. Pathologic staging refers to the aforementioned clinical staging but also includes lymph node biopsy results [3].

The American Joint Commission on Cancer (AJCC) created a TNM system to stage melanoma, which can determine overall prognosis and help guide treatment [38]. The T stage stands for tumor classification and refers to the thickness of the melanoma. Depth of invasion is also referred to as the Breslow measurement, which involves using an ocular micrometer to measure from the granular layer of the epidermis to deepest point of invasion. The thickness is rated from 0 to 4 (measured in millimeters). Melanomas less than 1 mm thick are less likely to spread with increasing risk of spread overtime as thickness increases. An "a" or "b" may also be added and refers to mitotic rate and ulceration. A high mitotic rate is suggestive of a rapidly spreading melanoma, and ulceration refers to breakdown of the skin over the melanoma, both leading to a worse prognosis. Stage IA melanoma has a five-year survival rate of 97%.

The N stage refers to lymphatic spread and is rated 0–3 depending on whether there is lymph node or lymphatic channel involvement based on the sentinel lymph node biopsy. N2 and N3 can involve spread to surrounding skin (satellite tumors) or spread to surrounding lymph nodes areas (in-transit tumors). An "a, b, or c" may also be added; the "a" refers to microscopic spread only, "b" denotes that the melanoma involving the lymph nodes was either palpable or visible on imaging studies (macroscopic spread), and "c" refers to melanoma spread involving satellite tumors or spread to skin lymphatic channels surrounding the tumor.

The M stage stands for metastases and also includes LDH levels. It is rated 1 if there is any evidence of metastasis and a-c depending on whether serum LDH is elevated (c).

Patterns of Distant Metastases

The five- and ten-year survival rates for Stage IV melanoma are about 15–20% and 10–15%. The overall outcome is slightly improved if the serum LDH is normal or if the spread is only to distant lymph nodes or distant parts of the skin.

Melanomas metastasize via hematogenous or lymphatic spread. 25% of patients with metastatic melanoma have visceral metastases commonly located in the lung (18–36%), brain (12–20%), liver (14–20%), and bone (11–17%) [39, 40]. Other sites of metastases include the lymph nodes, soft tissue, and colon. Overall prognosis is poor with a median survival in untreated patients of 6–9 months, though this is dependent on LDH levels and location of the metastases [41].

CNS Metastases

Incidence

Melanoma is the third most common malignancy to metastasize to the brain, second only to lung and breast cancer [42, 43]. In one study, melanoma was the second most common type of brain metastasis, which may in part be due to improved therapies for breast cancer causing the incidence of brain metastases to plateau [44]. There is some evidence that melanoma, of all solid tumors, has the highest tendency to metastasize to the brain, occurring in up to 10% of patients with melanoma [42, 44, 45]. Half of the patients with stage IV melanoma have radiographic evidence of central nervous system (CNS) metastases, and autopsy series have found evidence of brain metastases in 70% of patients [14, 43, 46]. There does not appear to be an association with CNS metastases and involved lymph node characteristics, such as nodal region, size, number of involved nodes, or capsular spread [47].

Risk Factors for Developing CNS Metastases in Malignant Melanoma

There are multiple known risk factors for developing CNS metastases. Primary melanoma located in the head, neck, and the upper extremities is associated with an increased risk [14, 41, 48–50], perhaps due to proximity to the CNS. Uveal melanoma has a lower risk of CNS metastases than cutaneous melanoma [48].

The morphology of the primary melanoma is significantly related to the risk of cerebral metastases. Factors such as ulceration and/or superficial diameter of the skin lesions, and increased thickness as measured per Clark's Level or Breslow's Depth, increase brain metastases risk [1, 7, 9, 10].

Male gender may also increase risk of CNS metastases, perhaps because men develop melanoma of the head and neck more often [14, 48, 50–52]. Some studies suggest that patients over the age of 50 or 60 had an increased risk of CNS metastases [44, 53], while others showed no impact of age [50]. African Americans also seem to have a higher risk of CNS metastases compared to Caucasians [44].

Systemic findings can give insight to the risk of CNS metastases. The presence of visceral tumor metastases, especially in the liver or lung, is highly predictive and may precede the diagnosis of CNS metastases by only a few weeks [14, 48, 50]. In addition, metastatic melanoma of unknown origin has a higher risk of CNS metastases [48]. Elevation of serum LDH levels at the time of diagnosis of stage III or stage IV melanoma also increases the risk of CNS metastases [48, 50, 54, 55]. Melanoma that is BRAF- or NRAS-positive is also more likely than wild type to metastasize to the CNS [56].

Parenchymal Brain Metastases

The median time from diagnosing melanoma to developing CNS is two to four years [14, 42, 57]. Although CNS metastases tend to occur later on in the disease course, they

usually represent the first metastatic focus [58, 59]. Melanoma mainly spreads through the CNS via the vasculature rather than through local diffuse infiltration or well-demarcated growth [60]. In order to metastasize to the CNS, melanoma develops molecular characteristics that differentiate it from both the primary and extracranial tumors. These changes allow melanoma cells to penetrate the blood–brain barrier and may also give increased resistance to chemotherapy [61]. Both intracerebral and extracerebral metastases have identical ERK, p-ERK, and AKT immunohistochemistry staining patterns; however, intracerebral melanoma has been found to have hyperactivation of the AKT to p-AKT and loss of expression of PTEN. In addition, there was more activation of AKT to p-AKT in melanocytes cultured in an astrocyte medium than in a fibroblast medium. This suggests that the activation may be due to intracerebral factors. Furthermore, resistance to BRAF inhibitors (of melanoma brain metastases) seems to be related to the PI3K-AKT pathway and downstream signaling through MEK [62]. Additional traits that seem necessary for CNS metastases include expression of VEGF, STAT3, and heparinase activity [62–68].

The local CNS environment of a melanoma brain metastasis is unique and likely plays a role in promoting tumor survival and growth. One study evaluated 12 cytokines and chemokines of CSF samples of controls and CNS melanoma patients, finding a significant difference between the two. Chemokine CL22 and cytokines IL1α, CXCL10, CCL4, CCL17, and IL8 were all increased. There was also suggestion that the suppression of IL1α, IL4, IL5, and CCL22 with an elevation of CXCL10, CCL4, and CCL17 may be related to more aggressive CNS metastases [69]. These immunologic changes may help explain the activity of CTLA-4 and PD-1 inhibitors in brain metastases.

Clinical Presentation

The clinical manifestation of CNS melanoma metastases depends on their location and disease burden [14]. Patients often present with focal neurological symptoms, including cranial nerve dysfunction, motor weakness, or generalized symptoms such as cognitive impairment or seizures [50]. Around 40% of patients present with seizures at the time of their initial diagnosis [55]. An additional common initial presentation is headache with or without meningismus [14]. The CSF may have an increased opening pressure, elevated WBCs, and/or protein and may have decreased glucose [14]. There may also be abnormal EEG findings, with intermittent focal delta activity, localized higher frequency dysrhythmia, or sharp waves or spikes. EEG findings are sensitive but not very specific of CNS melanoma [14].

Radiographic Findings

The distribution of melanoma cerebral metastases is related to cerebral blood flow, with 85% of lesions in the cerebrum, 10–15% in the cerebellum, and 3–5% involving the brainstem. Lesions are usually within the gray-white matter junction [70–73]. Single metastases are present in one-fourth to one-third of patients on MRI [74]; however, compared with other primary tumors, melanoma is more likely to have multiple lesions [75–78].

As with other soft tissue cerebral lesions, MRI is more sensitive in diagnosing metastatic melanoma compared with CT, especially smaller lesions and infratentorial lesions [79–81]. Melanoma enhances with contrast and tends to be heterogenous in appearance (Fig. 29.1a–d). Lesions may have hemorrhage or necrosis within them. Because of the methemoglobin and melanin, melanoma commonly has increased intensity on T1-weighted imaging sequences before contrast. Due to the hemorrhagic nature, evidence of cerebral metastases can be found on gradient echo sequences. If leptomeningeal disease is present, enhancement may be seen in the cerebellar folio, leptomeninges, cranial nerves, or on the ependymal surface [82] (Fig. 29.2a, b).

Tumor Hemorrhage

Brain metastases from malignant melanoma have a hemmorhagic rate of 25–50% [73, 83–96]; even small lesions can lead to significant hemorrhage. Intratumoral hemorrhage presents with similar subacute progressive symptoms as non-hemorrhagic brain metastases [86]. They may also present with an abrupt onset of a headache with focal neurological deficits progressing into obtundation, while other will have worsening of their previous neurological deficits [86, 89, 97, 98]. Patients may be completely asymptomatic with BM found on screening MRI [84]. Hypertension and thrombocytopenia do not lead to the intratumoral hemorrhage [95].

Macroscopic bleeding is present in up to 80% of patients with cerebral melanoma metastases [86, 90]. Patients with multiple metastases tend to have bleeding into most of their lesions rather than an isolated hemorrhage [86]. In addition, up to 25% of patients who were previously thought not to have hemorrhage were found to have histological evidence of prior hemorrhage [90]. Hemorrhage may be intratumoral, adjacent to the tumor, or may present as a larger intracerebral hematoma surrounding scattered tumor fragments [89]. Intratumoral hemorrhage may be secondary to loss of vessel integrity associated with inter- and intratumoral necrosis and neovascularization [95]. The lesion size does not seem to affect the risk of developing a hemorrhage; lesions ranging from microscopic to 8 cm in diameter can bleed [89].

Intratumoral hemorrhage usually has non-contiguous enhancing lesions, with hemorrhage occurring outside of the basal ganglia region [86, 99], and enhancement adjacent to the blood clot [86, 97]. Neoplastic hemorrhage usually does not resolve on serial images and tends to have a heterogenous intensity pattern on spin-echo sequences [100].

One report showed that up to 50% of patients with cerebral melanoma may develop subdural hematomas [101]. Most subdural hematomas are asymptomatic, with only one-fourth of patients presenting with symptoms. Usually, patients will present with acute confusion or lethargy, and only 10% have focal neurological deficits [86]. It is thought that the etiology is secondary to neovascularization of tumor cells that spread to the leptomeninges [98, 102]. Thrombocytopenia is likely not related to the development of subdural hematomas [86].

Prognosis

Like other systemic metastases to the CNS, melanoma metastases carry a poor prognosis. CNS metastases are present in up to 75% of patients who die from the disease and are the cause of over half of all melanoma deaths [14, 42, 50, 103–105]. Patients with initial melanoma metastasis in the CNS may have a better prognosis than patients with initial metastasis elsewhere in the body [14, 46, 50]. Metastases to the lungs or liver have been found to worsen the prognosis [14, 50]. There is also a relationship with the prognosis and the location of the primary lesion, with head and neck lesions shortening the survival time [50]. In patients with >4-mm-thick melanomas, ulcerated primaries had a significantly worse five-year survival rate, even when controlling for thickness, mitotic rate, histotype, vascular involvement, and lymph node status [49]. Early hemorrhage also worsens the patient's prognosis [106]. Unsurprisingly, patients who respond to their initial management tend to have a better prognosis than those who fail their initial therapy [46].

The number and location of cerebral metastases discovered at diagnosis is another factor that worsens prognosis, with cerebellar and leptomeningeal metastases having a worse survival [46, 96]. The extent of extracranial metastases is associated with survival. The median survival in one study of patients with controlled extracranial disease activity was 12.7 months, which dropped to 3.9 months if the disease was active [96]. Hence, improving the prognosis for patients with CNS metastases necessitates also controlling systemic disease [96, 107].

The patient's clinical status is another prognostic factor. Patients who present with asymptomatic brain metastases or have a systemic response after their first treatment have an overall better prognosis [108]. Patients with Karnofsky

Fig. 29.1 Brain MRI reveals
hemorrhagic melanoma
metastasis in the left frontal, left
superior temporal, and right
posterior temporal lobes. **a, b**
Gradient echo sequence; **c, d** T1
post-contrast sequence

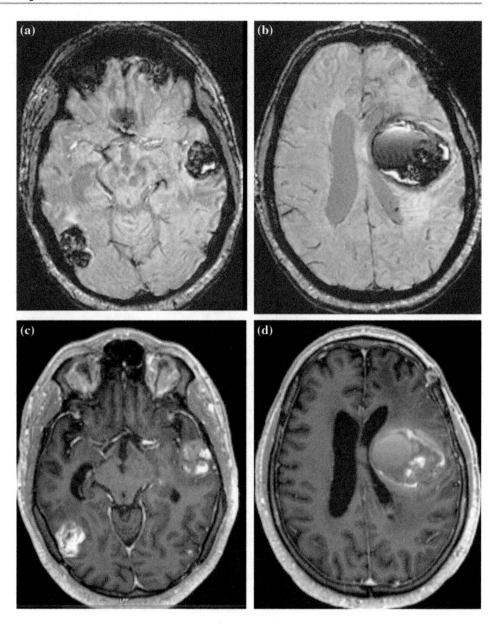

Performance Score (KPS) ≥ 90 do significantly better than
patients with a score ≤ 80 [96, 107]. In addition, patients
with a higher Recursive Partitioning Analysis (RPA) class
had a worsened survival. In one study comparing patients'
RPA classes, those who were class 1 had a median survival
of 12.7 months, class 2 had 4.9 months, and class 3 had
2.3 months [96].

When one study evaluated 17 patients surviving > three years from initial diagnosis of cerebral
metastases, some shared characteristics included the lack
of a primary lesion in the head and neck region, only a
single CNS lesion discovered at diagnosis, no visceral
metastases, and surgical resection performed as the initial
treatment [50].

Treatment Overview

Patients with untreated brain metastases have a median
survival between 3 and 8 weeks [52, 70, 109, 110]. Once a
patient develops CNS metastases, it is important that palliative care be a part of therapy discussions [57]. Although
current management can significantly prolong survival, in
particular for solitary brain metastases, the overall prognosis
remains poor [14]. This is largely due to melanoma being
characteristically radioresistant and chemoresistant. Moreover, in most cases, multiple metastases are found at presentation [45].

Some positive strides have been made in the past few
decades in the treatment of CNS melanoma. One study

Fig. 29.2 T1 post-contrast MRI revealing innumerable small enhancing brain lesions, all located along the surface of the brain, likely reflecting leptomeningeal carcinomatosis from melanoma

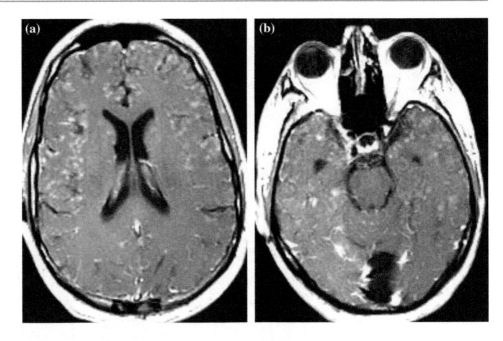

evaluating melanoma patients with cerebral metastases from 1986 to 2004 found that patients diagnosed before 1996 had an average survival of 4.14 months, while those diagnosed after 1996 had an average survival of 5.92 months. The increase may be due to a lead time bias since the use of MRIs has increased during this period of time; however, the number of patients who underwent SRS has also doubled likely improving the overall prognosis [46]. Current treatment options include surgical resection, stereotactic radiosurgery (SRS), whole-brain radiotherapy (WBRT), systemic therapy, and supportive care. An additional confounder of such retrospective can be selection bias, whereby therapies are often chosen based on a patient's burden of disease. Patients with less than three lesions and low tumor burden are usually treated with surgical resection or SRS. The patient with diffuse metastases and high tumor burden is usually treated with whole-brain radiotherapy, chemotherapy, or supportive care [46]. In general, WBRT has limited efficacy for the treatment of melanoma due to radioresistance. Radiosurgery is often more effective due to the ability to deliver a large fraction in a single dose, though this technique is often limited by the number and size of lesions.

Whole-Brain Radiation Therapy for Brain Metastases

Retrospective studies evaluating the effectiveness of WBRT and SRS have been challenging due to the selective bias of patients who undergo these treatments. WBRT is typically used in patients who have multiple cerebral metastases or leptomeningeal disease and therefore have an overall poorer prognosis [107]. However, evidence shows that patients with multiple intracerebral metastases receiving WBRT with SRS

as initial management increased the time before the patient developed further disease progression from two months to six months. In patients with single metastases, WBRT did not seem to affect disease progression in the same way. The impact on its effect of survival depends largely on whether intracranial disease or extracranial disease is the main driver of mortality in melanoma patients. If intracranial disease affects the mortality, then WBRT improves mortality by decreasing intracranial disease. The efficacy of salvage WBRT after SRS still remains in question [107]. Nevertheless, WBRT remains a viable option as initial treatment in patients where SRS is not indicated [96]. For limited burden of CNS disease, radiosurgery is preferred.

Surgery for Brain Metastases

Surgery remains as the initial standard of care for patients with brain melanoma metastases [45, 111]. The optimal surgical candidates are those with a good performance status (Karnofsky performance status of $\geq 90\%$), minimal comorbidity, and having up to three brain metastases [112]. The location of the cerebral metastases is also important. Patients with superficial metastases in relatively non-eloquent brain are better candidates for surgery [112]. Surgery should be considered in patients who have larger lesions (>3.5 cm) precluding the use of SRS, producing symptomatic edema, causing significant headaches, seizures, or mass effect threatening herniation. Surgery may also be performed to relieve mass effect or to evacuate hemorrhages produced by the tumors.

Technological advancements and improved surgical technique have helped to improve patient outcomes, with five-year survival rates increasing from 7 to 16% and median survival increasing from 7 to 12 months. Complete resection may produce control rates up to 85%, and incomplete resection can produce a palliative effect without improvement in overall survival. Post-resection, radiotherapy may be used to the surgical cavity or any additional lesions. If there are too many lesions for SRS, WBRT is preferred.

Radiosurgery for Brain Metastases

SRS tends to be the initial management in patients with 1–3 cerebral metastases [106], although data for more cerebral metastases exist and suggest that total volume of disease regardless of number of metastases is a strong predictor of benefit [113–115]. Most patients who undergo SRS only require one session [106]. The dose of radiation depends on the lesion size and volume, and it can range between 12 and 24 Gy [106]. The median survival after undergoing SRS ranges from 4.8 to 10.6 months [96, 106]. SRS may also be used for palliative management of symptoms later in the disease course, and there is evidence that patients with up to six metastases may benefit from SRS [96]. After patients fail their previous therapy, there seems to be no difference in survival if SRS is used as primary or salvage therapy [96]. In one study evaluating patients a median of 4.3 months after they had SRS, 6.1% had complete radiographic disappearance of their tumors, 32% had regression and 52.8% had no change, while 13.8% had progression [96]. The median time to appearance of new lesions after SRS was 4.2 months; increased lesion size and hemorrhagic metastases were predictors of SRS failure [96].

There is morbidity associated with SRS. Up to 10% of patients develop radiation necrosis on follow-up MRI, which can be visualized as increased contrast enhancement and signal changes. Only 7% of patients are symptomatic from this. In most of these cases, symptoms and radiographic changes completely resolve with a course of steroids. For the subset of patients refractory to steroids, a craniotomy or treatment with bevacizumab may be considered, although bevacizumab may increase the risk of hemorrhage [96, 116]. The patient's age, prior history of cranial irradiation, radiation dose, or tumor location does not seem to increase the risk of radiation effects. The only risk factor that has been correlated to developing these symptoms was radiation volume [96]. At a median of 4.3 months after SRS, 8.3% of patients had clinical improvement and 63.1% had stable disease, while 28.6% had clinically worsened. Among the patients who deteriorated, the most common cause was hemorrhage occurring in 45.8% of those patients. Adverse radiation effects and increased tumor burden, respectively, occurred in 27.1% of the patients. In addition, following radiosurgery, 13.1% of the patients required craniotomy, half for hemorrhage, 14% due to local progression, 11% due to new metastases, and 7% due to radiation injury [96].

Up to 22.3% of patients of all patients with melanoma brain metastasis may develop hemorrhage, with a majority of cases having undergone radiosurgery [96]. A history of hemorrhagic melanoma, increased tumor size, and radiosurgery volume were all risks of developing a hemorrhage [96]. The mean time from SRS to developing hemorrhage is 1.8 months. The potential role of SRS therapy in hemorrhage formation remains unclear but is thought to involve SRS-induced vascularized tumor necrosis.

Radiosurgery Versus Surgical Resection

SRS and surgical resection are both targeted methods for treating patients with few cerebral metastases to provide immediate relief. Both SRS and surgery seem to have similar tumor control rates with or without fractionated radiotherapy [117–123]. To date, there is no known randomized trial addressing the superiority of one over the other; however, there are some considerations which should be made before choosing a therapy. SRS is less expensive than surgery and may have an overall reduced morbidity [124]. Because SRS is associated with peritumoral edema or radiation necrosis oftentimes necessitating steroids, there is concern that the efficacy of immunotherapy will be hindered. Thus, in patients who are planning to receive immunotherapy, surgery may be preferred [125].

Systemic Therapy

Systemic therapy for melanoma CNS metastasis has many challenges. Extracranial melanoma is already very resistant to chemotherapy, and agents used must cross the blood–brain barrier [61]. In addition, because of the poor prognosis of patients with cerebral metastases, patients with CNS metastases tend to be excluded from clinical trials for systemic therapy, making the data on efficacy limited [126]. Until recently, even systemic melanoma responded poorly to the available systemic treatments, in part due to the intrinsic resistance of the disease.

Fotemustine, dacarbazine (DTIC), and temozolomide (TMZ) are chemotherapy agents used to treat extracranial melanoma metastases. All are alkylating agents with penetration into the CNS. Unfortunately, phase II trials showed that they were not as effective as hoped; TMZ and fotemustine had a response rate of 6 and 5.9%, respectively [57, 127]. Of note, the fotemustine study compared it to dacarbazine (DTIC), which at the time was the primary treatment for malignant melanoma. DTIC had a CNS response rate of 0%, and the study showed a trend toward fotemustine prolonging the time to brain metastases (22.7 vs. 7.2 months; $p = 0.059$) [126].

A multicenter, open-label, phase II trial with TMZ enrolled 151 patients with histologically confirmed melanoma metastases to the brain without prior radiotherapy or radiosurgery. Previously untreated patients were started on TMZ 200 mg/m^2/day for five days, and previously treated patients were started on TMZ 150 mg/m^2/day for five days every 28 days. Of the 117 patients who had no prior treatment, one patient had a complete response, seven had a partial response, and thirty-four had stable disease of the brain. Of the 34 patients who had previous therapy, one had a partial response and six had stable disease of the brain. Kaplan–Meier estimates of these groups showed progression-free survival of 1.2 and 1.0 months, and median survival or 3.5 and 2.2 months, for the previously untreated and treated groups, respectively. The improved response of the melanoma to TMZ in patients without prior treatment was speculated to be due to the melanoma cells being naïve to the chemotherapy. Disease progression occurred in 74% of patients and was the most common reason for discontinuation of the treatment. Of note, 6% of the patients had a response to temozolomide, comparable to the rates in the other visceral sites, suggesting it has similar efficacy for both. This also suggests that the reason other chemotherapy may have been failing at treating melanoma metastases was the difficulty in penetrating the blood–brain barrier [57]. One phase II pilot study substituting TMZ for DTIC reduced the incidence of CNS relapse, but it did not affect overall survival [128].

Thalidomide is an agent with both antiangiogenic and immunomodulatory effects. A phase II trial of 35 patients who had a WHO performance scale of ≤ 2 examined the effect of a thalidomide at doses starting at 100–400 mg/day over a span of four weeks. No patient had any response to brain metastases, although three had a partial response to their extracranial lesions. Four of the patients had stable CNS disease for over four months, suggesting some CNS activities. Twenty patients were placed on the maximum dose of 400 mg, with seven requiring dose reductions due to side effects that were reversible [129].

The potential to target molecular aberrations and mutations in melanoma brain metastasis has been the focus of recent research. Current studies are evaluating BRAF, NRAS, and KIT for melanoma metastases and BRAF for cerebral metastases [61]. The BRAF mutation is a particularly promising target with 50% of melanoma patients harboring the mutation [56]. There are two known mutation types: 71.9% have a substation of valine with glutamic acid at position 600, BRAF^{Val600E}, while 22.5% have a substitution with lysine, BRAF^{Val600K} [56]. There is currently no evidence of a relationship between KIT inhibitors and cerebral metastases [61].

BRAF works by phosphorylating and activating MEK proteins, which then activate MAP kinases. The MAP kinase pathway is responsible for regulating proliferation and survival of tumor cells [130]. BRAF inhibitors are currently the standard of care for patients who have BRAF^{V600E}-positive metastatic melanoma [54]. Dabrafenib acts as an ATP-competitive inhibitor against BRAF kinase and seems to work similarly on intracranial and extracranial metastases [131]. To what extent penetrates the blood–brain barrier remains unclear. A phase II trial investigated the effects of dabrafenib on patients harboring BRAF^{V600E} or BRAF^{V600K} mutations and at least one cerebral metastases between 5 and 40 mm. The patients were divided into two cohorts: cohort A contained 89 patients who had not received any previous treatments and cohort B contained 83 patients who had cerebral metastases with progression after receiving local treatment. The patients were started on dabrafenib 150 mg twice a day until disease progression, intolerable toxicity, or death. Using a modified version of the Response Evaluation Criteria in Solid Tumors (RECIST), for patients with BRAF^{V600E}, an intracranial response was found in 39.2% (29 of 74) in cohort A and 30.8% (20 of 65) in cohort B. Two of the patients in cohort A had a complete response to the therapy. The patients who were BRAF^{V600K}-positive had fewer overall responses, 1 of 15 in cohort A and 4 of 18 in cohort B. The global disease control rate was 80% in BRAF^{V600E}-positive and 50% in BRAF^{V600K}-positive patients. In these patients, serum LDH level made an impact on prognosis, with higher levels predicting slightly worsened response, and marginally shorter median progression-free survival and overall survival. The median survival was 33 weeks for cohort A and 31 weeks in cohort B [54].

Another inhibitor of BRAF kinase is vemurafenib. A phase III trial enrolled 371 patients with BRAF^{V600} and included patients with poor performance status, to provide vemurafenib to patients in medical need and to evaluate the tumor response. The patients were given oral vemurafenib 960 mg twice a day, and patients were followed up at a median of 2.8 months. The overall response rate was 54%, including 13 of 31 patients who had an ECOG PS of 2 or 3 and who normally would have been excluded from other studies for their poor prognosis. 20% of the patients had seizures; however, these were likely to be pre-existing and not related to therapy [132]. Of note, vemurafenib was only tested in patients with a positive 4800 BRAF^{V600} mutation, an allele-specific PCR test for BRAF^{V600E}. Therefore, unlike for dabrafenib which has been tested in BRAF^{V600E} and BRAF^{V600K}, its effectiveness against other mutation types is unknown [61]. There has been some evidence of patients with cerebral metastases on either dabrafenib or vemurafenib with a rare BRAF^{V600R} mutation responding to therapy [133].

Interleukin-2 (IL-2) has been used in patients with metastatic melanoma with some success; however, its use for cerebral metastases has been limited due to concerns of cerebral edema, intracerebral hemorrhage from thrombocytopenia, and neurotoxicity [61, 134].

Ipilimumab is a human IgG-1 monoclonal antibody that blocks cytotoxic T-lymphocyte-associated antigen 4 (CTLA-4), an inhibitor of T-cell activity. A phase 3 study was done to determine whether ipilimumab with DTIC improved overall survival. This study found significant improvement in survival; however, patients with cerebral metastases were excluded from the trial [135]. To further investigate this, a phase 2 study evaluated the treatment of ipilimumab in patients with evidence of cerebral metastasis. This study gave patients four days of ipilimumab 10 mg/kg/day every three weeks; patients stable at 24 weeks received additional doses every 12 weeks. The study enrolled 72 patients, dividing them into 51 patients without neurological symptoms (cohort A) and 21 patients who were symptomatic and receiving steroids (cohort B). After 12 weeks, 18% of the patients in cohort A and 5% in cohort B had disease control. The median survival in cohort A was 7 months, with two-year survival rate of 25%, while cohort B had a median survival of 3 months and a two-year survival of 10% (see Table 29.1 for further results from this study [136]).

To investigate whether chemotherapy-induced release of tumor antigens could amplify the effect of ipilimumab, a phase II study enrolled 86 patients with metastatic melanoma, 20 of which had asymptomatic brain metastases, for treatment with the combination of ipilimumab with fotemustine. Patients were given 10 mg/kg of ipilimumab every three weeks a total of four times in addition to fotemustine IV 100 mg/m² weekly for three weeks followed by once every three weeks from week 9 to week 24. Patients who had a clinical response were eligible for maintenance therapy every 12 weeks with ipilimumab from week 24 and every 3 weeks with fotemustine. By the end of the study, 46.5% of the patient achieved disease control, including 50% of those with brain metastases. The improved survival was theorized to be secondary to chemotherapy-induced release of tumor antigens amplifying the effect of ipilimumab [126].

The effect of radiotherapy on the tumorigenicity of ipilimumab via the potential release of tumor antigens has also been investigated. In this study, the median survival of patients who received ipilimumab in addition to radiotherapy was 18.3 months compared to 5.3 months (with radiotherapy alone). In addition, patients who underwent radiotherapy first had an overall survival of 18.4 months, while patients who received ipilimumab first had a survival of 8.1 months. Furthermore, four of the ten patients who received ipilimumab before radiotherapy had a partial response to the radiotherapy, while only 2 out of 22 who did not receive ipilimumab had a partial response to the radiotherapy [137].

Anti-programmed death 1 (PD-1) antibodies have also shown promise in treating BM. These antibodies block the interaction between PD-1 receptors on T-cells and the PDL-1 ligand expressed on tumor cells. Typically, when PD-1 attaches to its ligand, T-cells become inactivated and are unable to attack the tumor. Nivolumab and pembrolizumab both have shown promising results in some

Table 29.1 Summary of systemic therapy for cerebral melanoma metastases in patients who have not had previous therapy, unless otherwise specified

Study drug	# Of patients	OR	CR	PR	SD	PD	PFS	OS
DTIC	22	0	0	N/A	N/A	N/A	N/A	N/A
Fotemustine	22	5.90%	N/A	N/A	N/A	N/A	N/A	N/A
TMZ	117	6.84%	0.85%	5.98%	29.06%	46.15%	1.2 months	3.5 months
Thalidomide	35	0.00%	0.00%	0.00%	11.43%	100.00%	1.7 months	3.1 months
Debrafenib (BRAF Val600Glu)	74	39.19%	2.70%	36.49%	41.89%	12.16%	4 months	8.3 months
Debrafenib (BRAF Val600Lys)	15	6.67%	0.00%	6.67%	26.67%	40.00%	2 months	4 months
Vemurafenib with previous treatment	68	52.94%	0.00%	52.94%	27.94%	16.18%	N/A	N/A
Ipilimumab (asymptomatic, no steroids)	51	15.69%	0.00%	15.69%	7.84%	76.47%	1.4 months	7 months
Ipilimumab (symptomatic, steroids)	21	4.76%	4.76%	0.00%	4.76%	90.48%	1.2 months	3.7 months
Ipilimumab and fotemustine	20	50.00%	20.00%	30.00%	10.00%	50.00%	3 months	13.4 months
Ipilimumab before radiotherapy	10	40.00%	0.00%	40.00%	20.00%	40.00%	2.7 months	8.1 months
Ipilimumab after radiotherapy	12	16.67%	0.00%	16.67%	41.67%	41.67%	2.7 months	18.4 months

OR overall response (complete response + partial response), *CR* complete response, *PR* partial response, *SD* stable disease, *PD* progressive disease, *PFS* progression-free survival, *OS* overall survival. Data from Refs. [54, 57, 126, 127, 129, 132, 136, 137]

phase I studies [138], and pembrolizumab has shown activity in a phase II trial [139].

Overall, patients with metastatic melanoma should be considered for enrollment into a clinical trial. Multidisciplinary teams are critical to deciding the best overall approach to treatment. The patient's overall disease process, including performance status, rate of progression, presence of symptoms, and extracranial disease burden needs to be evaluated and taken into account prior to selecting a treatment strategy. Patients with one to three lesions should be evaluated as candidates for SRS or surgery with or without WBRT depending on the clinical status. If patients have multiple lesions, then WBRT might be initiated, and SRS or surgery may also be considered for symptomatic or adjuvant therapy. In patients with a BRAF^{V600} mutation, a BRAF inhibitor should be started as initial management, with local therapy for non-responsive or any progressive metastases. BRAF inhibitors should also be considered in patients who have failed local therapy. If patients are BRAF wild type, then local therapy would be the first-line management. Ipilimumab may also be co-administered with the local therapy; however, it is important to consider the possible negative impact steroids may have on the activity of ipilimumab. Table 29.1 has a summary of the current systemic treatment options available to patients with cerebral metastasis of melanoma. Finally, with all patients who have cerebral metastases, addressing goals of care should be a central part of discussions, attending to symptomatic treatment and palliative care [61].

Leptomeningeal Metastases

Breast cancer, lung cancer, and melanoma are the most common causes of leptomeningeal metastasis among solid tumors with melanoma comprising 17–25% of all cases [139]. The rate of spread of melanoma to the leptomeninges is 22–46% [14, 92, 140].

In melanoma, 19% of individuals with CNS metastases also had evidence of leptomeningeal involvement. This trend is also seen in other solid tumors [92]. Harstad and colleagues found that among 110 cases, the median interval from diagnosis of melanoma to leptomeningeal involvement was three years.

The overall prognosis for an individual with leptomeningeal metastasis is extremely poor, ranging from 8 to 16 weeks after diagnosis [18, 140]. The prognosis is slightly improved if leptomeningeal involvement is captured before the onset of neurological deficits [140].

LDH (lactate dehydrogenase) is a surrogate marker of systemic disease involvement in late-stage melanoma. Elevated serum LDH coupled with leptomeningeal disease is also associated with a poor prognosis [18].

Current treatment includes whole-brain radiation and intrathecal and systemic chemotherapy [139]. Intrathecal chemotherapy is preferred as the blood-CSF barrier is bypassed and systemic toxicity is reduced. Also, the half-life of cytotoxic agents is longer in the CSF as compared to plasma [140]. In cases of melanoma complicated by leptomeningeal metastases, methotrexate and cytarabine (ara-C) are most commonly used, followed by thiotepa. However, these agents are not particularly effective in melanoma. Ipilimumab, an anti-CTLA4 monoclonal antibody, and vemurafenib along with dabrafenib (therapies that target BRAF) have been shown to be effective in treating leptomeningeal metastases [141–143].

For a more complete review of leptomeningeal carcinomatosis please refer to Chap. 5.

Spinal Metastases

Most cases of bone metastases occur in the spine [144]. 5–17% of patients with stage IV melanoma have evidence of skeletal metastases which carries a poor prognosis with an estimated survival time of 4–6 months after diagnosis [145, 146]. The median time from diagnosis to discovery of bone metastases was 72 months [146]. Most spinal metastases are located extradurally (90%) with 5% intradural, and <1% intramedullary [147].

Patients have various presentations including pathologic fractures and cord compression. 5–10% of patients with known spinal metastases will go on to develop epidural compression [148, 149].

Melanoma comprises only 1–2% of all cases of metastatic epidural spinal cord compression [150]. Most cases of symptomatic compression occur in the thoracic spine (50–70%), followed by the lumbar spine (20–30%) and cervical spine (10–30%) [151].

Treatment options include resection, chemotherapy, radiation, intralesional debulking, spinal kyphoplasty, or stabilization and are aimed at local disease control and palliation. Coleman and colleagues [146] found that resection leads to increased overall survival as compared to other treatment options, with an estimated one-year survival rate of 24.8% but observed survival rate of 50% and a median overall survival of 11.8 months (mean 19 months). With resection, there is a risk of local recurrence which is managed with revision surgery, adjuvant radiotherapy, or a combination of the two [146]. Local recurrence is estimated to occur in 6–30% of resection cases [149]. Surgery is also useful for an unstable spine, pain relief in the setting of instability, or decompression [152].

As melanoma is known to be less radiosensitive than other cancers, overall response to radiation is fair at best, though when coupled with resection, improved outcomes have been reported [150]. Radiation options include conventional external beam radiotherapy (cEBRT) and spinal stereotactic radiosurgery (SSRS) [153]. Local recurrence after radiation appears to be dose-dependent [152].

For a complete review of spinal metastases please refer to Chap. 6.

Intramedullary Spinal Cord Metastases

Intramedullary tumors are extremely rare with an estimated 0.5 cases per 100,000 per year with melanoma being a less common cause (breast and lung cancers are the most common) [154]. Melanoma comprises 9% of intramedullary spinal cord metastases [155]. 8.5% of CNS metastases are secondary to intramedullary spinal cord metastases [156]. Melanoma that involves the spinal cord is usually intradural and extramedullary, while intramedullary melanoma is quite rare and is commonly found in the thoracic spine [157–159]. These metastases are thought to arise from melanocytes in the Virchow–Robin spaces.

For a complete review of intramedullary spinal metastases please refer to Chap. 6.

Plexus/Peripheral Nerve Metastases

In cases of metastatic melanoma, tumor spread can occur along the cervical plexus and cranial nerves [160–162]. Desmoplastic melanoma is a rare melanoma variant characterized by pleomorphic dermal spindle cells and most commonly occurs in the head and neck region followed by the extremities [163]. It is occasionally associated with lentigo maligna. There is typically neural invasion that histologically can resemble peripheral nerve sheath tumors. Staining is positive for S100 and collagen type IV with occasional positive staining with Melan-A, HMB-45, and tyrosinase [160].

Melanoma-Associated Retinopathy

Autoimmune retinopathy (AIR) encompasses cancer-associated retinopathy (CAR), melanoma-associated retinopathy (MAR), bilateral diffuse uveal melanocytic proliferation (BDUMP), and other AIRs. AIR refers to retinal degeneration from aberrant recognition of retinal antigens as autoantigens. It manifests as painless visual loss that progresses rapidly over weeks to months [164, 165]. An electroretinogram (ERG) reveals abnormal cone, rod, and even bipolar cell responses. Funduscopic examination can be variable; it can show retinal pigment epithelium (RPE) mottling or atrophic degenerative changes, optic disk pallor, attenuated retinal vessels indicative of retinal degeneration or be normal.

Cancer-associated retinopathy has been described as photoreceptor degeneration and is most commonly associated with small cell lung cancer, cervical cancer, and gynecological cancers. Melanoma accounts for 16% of CAR [166]. CAR usually presents at the onset of malignancy. Serum from patients with CAR reacts with recovering, which is a calcium-binding protein found in photoreceptors [164, 167]. CAR affects both cones and rods, with symptoms of rod dysfunction including nyctalopia, ring scotomas, extensive peripheral visual field deficits, and prolonged dark adaptation. Cone dysfunction presents with reduced visual acuity, decreased color perception, central scotomas, photoaversion, and prolonged glare after light exposure [166, 168]. CAR typically occurs over days to years [165]. The ERG may be abnormal, and the fundus usually appears normal early in the course. There is evidence of cone and rod photoreceptor degeneration on histological study [169]. CAR typically affects individuals over age 45 and is more prevalent in women (2:1) [164, 166]. Treatment of CAR is limited but consists of long-term immunosuppression, including corticosteroids [170]. Intravenous immunoglobulin (IVIG) is thought to only be effective when given before irreversible degeneration occurs [166]. Antioxidants may also be effective in controlling retinal degeneration [171].

MAR often presents after melanoma has metastasized, occurring on average 3.6 years after diagnosis [166, 172]. It is more common in men, typically occurs in patients in their 50s or older, and is seen in patients with uveal or metastatic cutaneous melanoma. Visual impairment can occur later in the course (progresses over months) and is characterized by photopsias (pulsating, flickering, or shimmering), nyctalopia, and painless vision loss in the midperiphery (central and paracentral scotomas) [164] all of which suggests rod dysfunction. The funduscopic examination can range from being completely normal to revealing vitreous cells, optic disk pallor, attenuated vessels, and retinal pigmented epithelium changes [172]. Bipolar cell function may be affected on ERG with normal photoreceptor cell function in some cases [172]. This is consistent with histopathological studies which show a reduced number of bipolar neurons with preserved photoreceptor cells [172]. Atrophy of trans-synaptic ganglion cells is also present [173]. MAR is associated with autoantibodies against bipolar cells, rhodopsin, transducing, alpha enolase, and arrestin, among others [164]. Laboratory testing includes evaluating for anti-retinal antibodies or immunohistochemical staining [174]. Treatment has not been shown to be particularly effective, but includes IV corticosteroids, plasmapheresis, IVIG, immunosuppression, radiation, and cytoreductive surgery [164, 172].

BDUMP can lead to bilateral vision loss and is characterized by rapid development of cataracts, exudative retinal detachments, multiple small red patches in the RPE, and multiple uveal melanocytic tumors with thickening of the uveal tract [175]. Visual changes precede the diagnosis of cancer. BDUMP is associated with melanoma, pancreatic and colorectal cancers, gynecological cancers, and lung cancer [164, 176]. BDUMP is quite rare with an average survival of 17 months [164]. Studies have suggested that plasmapheresis and radiation may be of use [177, 178].

Anti-Hu-Related Encephalomyelitis

Type 1 antineuronal nuclear autoantibodies (ANNA-1), also known as anti-Hu, are typically seen in small cell lung cancer, neuroblastoma, prostate, breast, Hodgkin, testicular cancers but can be associated with melanoma. Lucchinetti found that in 13% of cases of patients with ANNA-1, an unrelated primary malignancy was detected in addition to small cell lung cancer. Patients most commonly present with neuropathy (sensory more common than motor), cerebellar findings, limbic encephalitis, and cranial neuropathies [179].

Chronic Inflammatory Demyelinating Polyneuropathy

Several case reports have suggested a relationship between melanoma and CIDP. It must be noted that both Schwann cells and melanocytes are derived from neural crest cells. Gangliosides are an antigenic glycolipid component of melanocytes and are upregulated when malignant transformation of melanocytes occurs. CIDP, Guillain-Barre, and multifocal motor neuropathy with conduction block have been associated with an autoimmune response to gangliosides. Immunotherapy targeting the specific antigens has been shown to induce demyelinating polyneuropathies [180–183]. Demyelinating polyneuropathies have been reported in patients who received monoclonal anti-GM2 antibodies and in patients vaccinated with melanoma cell lysates [181].

Conclusion

CNS metastases in melanoma are diagnosed several years after the primary diagnosis and can present with focal neurological findings, seizures, and CSF abnormalities. The overall prognosis is poor, though the location of the lesion, degree of disease progression, response to treatment, and presence or absence of concurrent leptomeningeal disease all affects survival. Intratumoral hemorrhage is also very common and can present as macroscopic and microscopic on neuroimaging. Patients with metastatic melanoma should be enrolled in a clinical trial if they meet the criteria, though the high mortality

rate makes this difficult. Early treatment of melanoma is crucial and includes surgical resection, chemotherapy, and radiation. It has been shown that aggressive early management leads to improved outcomes. In patients with brain metastases or leptomeningeal disease and a high tumor burden, goals of care discussions should be a priority early in the course even if there are treatment options.

References

1. Nikolaou V, Stratigos AJ. Emerging trends in the epidemiology of melanoma. Br J Dermatol. 2014;170(1):11–9.
2. Society AC. Cancer facts and figures 2015. American Cancer Society (Internet); 2015. Available from: http://www.cancer.org/acs/groups/content/@editorial/documents/document/acspc-044552.pdf.
3. Melanoma Skin Cancer (Website). American Cancer Society; Updated 20 Mar 2015. Available from: http://www.cancer.org/cancer/skincancer-melanoma/.
4. Higgins HW, Lee KC, Galan A, Leffell DJ. Melanoma in situ: part I. Epidemiology, screening, and clinical features. J Am Acad Dermatol. 2015;73(2):181–90.
5. Downard CD, Rapkin LB, Gow KW. Melanoma in children and adolescents. Surg Oncol. 2007;16(3):215–20.
6. Kohler BA, Ward E, McCarthy BJ, Schymura MJ, Ries LA, Eheman C, et al. Annual report to the nation on the status of cancer, 1975–2007, featuring tumors of the brain and other nervous system. J Natl Cancer Inst. 2011;103(9):714–36.
7. Jemal A, Saraiya M, Patel P, Cherala SS, Barnholtz-Sloan J, Kim J, et al. Recent trends in cutaneous melanoma incidence and death rates in the United States, 1992–2006. J Am Acad Dermatol. 2011;65(5 Suppl 1):S17-25.e1-3.
8. Hoersch B, Leiter U, Garbe C. Is head and neck melanoma a distinct entity? A clinical registry-based comparative study in 5702 patients with melanoma. Br J Dermatol. 2006;155(4):771–7.
9. Ries Lag EM, Kosary CL et al. SEER cancer statistics review, 1975–2002: Bethesda, MD: National Cancer Institute; 2004. Available from: http://seer.cancer.gov/csr/1975_2002/.
10. Bradford PT, Anderson WF, Purdue MP, Goldstein AM, Tucker MA. Rising melanoma incidence rates of the trunk among younger women in the United States. Cancer Epidemiol Biomarkers Prev. 2010;19(9):2401–6 (a publication of the American Association for Cancer Research, cosponsored by the American Society of Preventive Oncology).
11. Purdue MP, Freeman LE, Anderson WF, Tucker MA. Recent trends in incidence of cutaneous melanoma among US Caucasian young adults. J Invest Dermatol. 2008;128(12):2905–8.
12. Liu F, Bessonova L, Taylor TH, Ziogas A, Meyskens FL Jr, Anton-Culver H. A unique gender difference in early onset melanoma implies that in addition to ultraviolet light exposure other causative factors are important. Pigment Cell Melanoma Res. 2013;26(1):128–35.
13. Kanavy HE, Gerstenblith MR. Ultraviolet radiation and melanoma. Semin Cutan Med Surg. 2011;30(4):222–8.
14. Amer MH, Al-Sarraf M, Baker LH, Vaitkevicius VK. Malignant melanoma and central nervous system metastases: incidence, diagnosis, treatment and survival. Cancer. 1978;42(2):660–8.
15. Kottschade LA, Grotz TE, Dronca RS, Salomao DR, Pulido JS, Wasif N, et al. Rare presentations of primary melanoma and

special populations: a systematic review. Am J Clin Oncol. 2014;37(6):635–41.

16. Leachman SA, Carucci J, Kohlmann W, Banks KC, Asgari MM, Bergman W, et al. Selection criteria for genetic assessment of patients with familial melanoma. J Am Acad Dermatol 2009;61 (4):677.e1-14.

17. Udayakumar D, Mahato B, Gabree M, Tsao H. Genetic determinants of cutaneous melanoma predisposition. Semin Cutan Med Surg. 2010;29(3):190–5.

18. Harstad L, Hess KR, Groves MD. Prognostic factors and outcomes in patients with leptomeningeal melanomatosis. Neuro Oncol. 2008;10(6):1010–8.

19. Hansen K, Gjerris F, Sorensen PS. Absence of hydrocephalus in spite of impaired cerebrospinal fluid absorption and severe intracranial hypertension. Acta Neurochir. 1987;86(3–4):93–7.

20. Valverde P, Healy E, Jackson I, Rees JL, Thody AJ. Variants of the melanocyte-stimulating hormone receptor gene are associated with red hair and fair skin in humans. Nat Genet. 1995;11 (3):328–30.

21. Williams PF, Olsen CM, Hayward NK, Whiteman DC. Melanocortin 1 receptor and risk of cutaneous melanoma: a meta-analysis and estimates of population burden. Int J Cancer J Int Du Cancer. 2011;129(7):1730–40.

22. Bishop DT, Demenais F, Iles MM, Harland M, Taylor JC, Corda E, et al. Genome-wide association study identifies three loci associated with melanoma risk. Nat Genet. 2009;41(8):920–5.

23. Barrett JH, Iles MM, Harland M, Taylor JC, Aitken JF, Andresen PA, et al. Genome-wide association study identifies three new melanoma susceptibility loci. Nat Genet. 2011;43 (11):1108–13.

24. Duffy DL, Iles MM, Glass D, Zhu G, Barrett JH, Hoiom V, et al. IRF4 variants have age-specific effects on nevus count and predispose to melanoma. Am J Hum Genet. 2010;87(1):6–16.

25. Bertolotto C, Lesueur F, Giuliano S, Strub T, de Lichy M, Bille K, et al. A SUMOylation-defective MITF germline mutation predisposes to melanoma and renal carcinoma. Nature. 2011;480(7375):94–8.

26. Yokoyama S, Woods SL, Boyle GM, Aoude LG, MacGregor S, Zismann V, et al. A novel recurrent mutation in MITF predisposes to familial and sporadic melanoma. Nature. 2011;480(7375):99–103.

27. Thomas NE, Edmiston SN, Alexander A, Millikan RC, Groben PA, Hao H, et al. Number of nevi and early-life ambient UV exposure are associated with BRAF-mutant melanoma. Cancer Epidemiol Biomarkers Prev. 2007;16(5):991–7 (a publication of the American Association for Cancer Research, cosponsored by the American Society of Preventive Oncology).

28. Besaratinia A, Pfeifer GP. Sunlight ultraviolet irradiation and BRAF V600 mutagenesis in human melanoma. Hum Mutat. 2008;29(8):983–91.

29. Handolias D, Salemi R, Murray W, Tan A, Liu W, Viros A, et al. Mutations in KIT occur at low frequency in melanomas arising from anatomical sites associated with chronic and intermittent sun exposure. Pigment Cell Melanoma Res. 2010;23(2):210–5.

30. Curtin JA, Busam K, Pinkel D, Bastian BC. Somatic activation of KIT in distinct subtypes of melanoma. J Clin Oncol. 2006;24 (26):4340–6.

31. Salvi PF, Lombardi A, Puzzovio A, Stagnitti F, Tisba M, Gaudinieri A, et al. Cutaneous melanoma with neurofibromatosis type 1: rare association? A case report and review of the literature. Ann Ital Chir. 2004;75(1):91–5.

32. Pal D, Bhargava D, Bucur SD, Shivane A, Chakrabarty A, Van Hille P. Metastatic malignant melanoma within meningioma with intratumoral infarct: report of an unusual case and literature review. Clin Neuropathol. 2010;29(2):105–8.

33. Dahlke E, Murray CA, Kitchen J, Chan AW. Systematic review of melanoma incidence and prognosis in solid organ transplant recipients. Transplant Res. 2014;3:10.

34. Long MD, Martin CF, Pipkin CA, Herfarth HH, Sandler RS, Kappelman MD. Risk of melanoma and nonmelanoma skin cancer among patients with inflammatory bowel disease. Gastroenterology. 2012;143(2):390-9.e1.

35. Zanetti R, Loria D, Rosso S. Melanoma, Parkinson's disease and levodopa: causal or spurious link? A review of the literature. Melanoma Res. 2006;16(3):201–6.

36. Bertoni JM, Arlette JP, Fernandez HH, Fitzer-Attas C, Frei K, Hassan MN, et al. Increased melanoma risk in Parkinson disease: a prospective clinicopathological study. Arch Neurol. 2010;67 (3):347–52.

37. Pan T, Li X, Jankovic J. The association between Parkinson's disease and melanoma. Int J Cancer J Int Du Cancer. 2011;128 (10):2251–60.

38. Gershenwald JE, Scolyer RA, Hess KR, et al. Melanoma of the Skin. In: American Joint Committee on Cancer. AJCC cancer staging manual, 8th ed. New York: Springer Nature; 2017.

39. Tas F. Metastatic behavior in melanoma: timing, pattern, survival, and influencing factors. J Oncol. 2012;2012:647684.

40. Kenchappa RS, Tran N, Rao NG, Smalley KS, Gibney GT, Sondak VK, et al. Novel treatments for melanoma brain metastases. Cancer Control. 2013;20(4):298–306.

41. Garbe C, Peris K, Hauschild A, Saiag P, Middleton M, Spatz A, et al. Diagnosis and treatment of melanoma. European consensus-based interdisciplinary guideline-update 2012. Eur J Cancer (Oxford, England: 1990). 2012;48(15):2375–90.

42. Qian M, Ma MW, Fleming NH, Lackaye DJ, Hernando E, Osman I, et al. Clinicopathological characteristics at primary melanoma diagnosis as risk factors for brain metastasis. Melanoma Res. 2013;23(6):461–7.

43. Gorantla V, Kirkwood JM, Tawbi HA. Melanoma brain metastases: an unmet challenge in the era of active therapy. Curr Oncol Rep. 2013;15(5):483–91.

44. Barnholtz-Sloan JS, Sloan AE, Davis FG, Vigneau FD, Lai P, Sawaya RE. Incidence proportions of brain metastases in patients diagnosed (1973 to 2001) in the Metropolitan Detroit Cancer Surveillance System. J Clin Oncol. 2004;22(14):2865–72.

45. Fonkem E, Uhlmann EJ, Floyd SR, Mahadevan A, Kasper E, Eton O, et al. Melanoma brain metastasis: overview of current management and emerging targeted therapies. Expert Rev. 2012;12(10):1207–15.

46. Davies MA, Liu P, McIntyre S, Kim KB, Papadopoulos N, Hwu WJ, et al. Prognostic factors for survival in melanoma patients with brain metastases. Cancer. 2011;117(8):1687–96.

47. Jackson JE, Burmeister BH, Burmeister EA, Foote MC, Thomas JM, Meakin JA, et al. Melanoma brain metastases: the impact of nodal disease. Clin Exp Metastasis. 2014;31(1):81–5.

48. Bedikian AY, Wei C, Detry M, Kim KB, Papadopoulos NE, Hwu WJ, et al. Predictive factors for the development of brain metastasis in advanced unresectable metastatic melanoma. Am J Clin Oncol. 2011;34(6):603–10.

49. Zettersten E, Sagebiel RW, Miller JR 3rd, Tallapureddy S, Leong SP, Kashani-Sabet M. Prognostic factors in patients with thick cutaneous melanoma (>4 mm). Cancer. 2002;94(4):1049–56.

50. Sampson JH, Carter JH Jr, Friedman AH, Seigler HF. Demographics, prognosis, and therapy in 702 patients with brain metastases from malignant melanoma. J Neurosurg. 1998;88 (1):11–20.

51. Hofmann MA, Coll SH, Kuchler I, Kiecker F, Wurm R, Sterry W, et al. Prognostic factors and impact of treatment in melanoma brain metastases: better prognosis for women? Dermatology. 2007;215(1):10–6.

52. Saha S, Meyer M, Krementz ET, Hoda S, Carter RD, Muchmore J, et al. Prognostic evaluation of intracranial metastasis in malignant melanoma. Ann Surg Oncol. 1994;1(1):38–44.

53. Azer MW, Menzies AM, Haydu LE, Kefford RF, Long GV. Patterns of response and progression in patients with BRAF-mutant melanoma metastatic to the brain who were treated with dabrafenib. Cancer. 2014;120(4):530–6.

54. Long GV, Trefzer U, Davies MA, Kefford RF, Ascierto PA, Chapman PB, et al. Dabrafenib in patients with Val600Glu or Val600Lys BRAF-mutant melanoma metastatic to the brain (BREAK-MB): a multicentre, open-label, phase 2 trial. Lancet Oncol. 2012;13(11):1087–95.

55. Lagerwaard FJ, Levendag PC, Nowak PJ, Eijkenboom WM, Hanssens PE, Schmitz PI. Identification of prognostic factors in patients with brain metastases: a review of 1292 patients. Int J Radiat Oncol Biol Phys. 1999;43(4):795–803.

56. Jakob JA, Bassett RL Jr, Ng CS, Curry JL, Joseph RW, Alvarado GC, et al. NRAS mutation status is an independent prognostic factor in metastatic melanoma. Cancer. 2012;118 (16):4014–23.

57. Agarwala SS, Kirkwood JM, Gore M, Dreno B, Thatcher N, Czarnetski B, et al. Temozolomide for the treatment of brain metastases associated with metastatic melanoma: a phase II study. J Clin Oncol. 2004;22(11):2101–7.

58. Hayward RD. Malignant melanoma and the central nervous system. A guide for classification based on the clinical findings. J Neurol Neurosurg Psychiatry. 1976;39(6):526–30.

59. Gottlieb JA, Frei E 3rd, Luce JK. An evaluation of the management of patients with cerebral metastases from malignant melanoma. Cancer. 1972;29(3):701–5.

60. Berghoff AS, Rajky O, Winkler F, Bartsch R, Furtner J, Hainfellner JA, et al. Invasion patterns in brain metastases of solid cancers. Neuro Oncol. 2013;15(12):1664–72.

61. Lyle M, Long GV. The role of systemic therapies in the management of melanoma brain metastases. Curr Opin Oncol. 2014;26(2):222–9.

62. Niessner H, Forschner A, Klumpp B, Honegger JB, Witte M, Bornemann A, et al. Targeting hyperactivation of the AKT survival pathway to overcome therapy resistance of melanoma brain metastases. Cancer Med. 2013;2(1):76–85.

63. Xie TX, Huang FJ, Aldape KD, Kang SH, Liu M, Gershenwald JE, et al. Activation of stat3 in human melanoma promotes brain metastasis. Can Res. 2006;66(6):3188–96.

64. Marchetti D, Li J, Shen R. Astrocytes contribute to the brain-metastatic specificity of melanoma cells by producing heparanase. Can Res. 2000;60(17):4767–70.

65. Murry BP, Blust BE, Singh A, Foster TP, Marchetti D. Heparanase mechanisms of melanoma metastasis to the brain: Development and use of a brain slice model. J Cell Biochem. 2006;97(2):217–25.

66. Davies MA, Stemke-Hale K, Lin E, Tellez C, Deng W, Gopal YN, et al. Integrated molecular and clinical analysis of AKT activation in metastatic melanoma. Clin Cancer Res. 2009;15(24):7538–46.

67. Kusters B, Leenders WP, Wesseling P, Smits D, Verrijp K, Ruiter DJ, et al. Vascular endothelial growth factor-A(165) induces progression of melanoma brain metastases without induction of sprouting angiogenesis. Can Res. 2002;62(2):341–5.

68. Yano S, Shinohara H, Herbst RS, Kuniyasu H, Bucana CD, Ellis LM, et al. Expression of vascular endothelial growth factor is necessary but not sufficient for production and growth of brain metastasis. Can Res. 2000;60(17):4959–67.

69. Lok E, Chung AS, Swanson KD, Wong ET. Melanoma brain metastasis globally reconfigures chemokine and cytokine profiles in patient cerebrospinal fluid. Melanoma Res. 2014;24(2):120–30.

70. Madajewicz S, Karakousis C, West CR, Caracandas J, Avellanosa AM. Malignant melanoma brain metastases. Review of Roswell Park Memorial Institute experience. Cancer. 1984;53 (11):2550–2.

71. Haar F, Patterson RH Jr. Surgical for metastatic intracranial neoplasm. Cancer. 1972;30(5):1241–5.

72. Delattre JY, Krol G, Thaler HT, Posner JB. Distribution of brain metastases. Arch Neurol. 1988;45(7):741–4.

73. Enzmann DR, Kramer R, Norman D, Pollock J. Malignant melanoma metastatic to the central nervous system. Radiology. 1978;127(1):177–80.

74. Yuh WT, Engelken JD, Muhonen MG, Mayr NA, Fisher DJ, Ehrhardt JC. Experience with high-dose gadolinium MR imaging in the evaluation of brain metastases. AJNR Am J Neuroradiol. 1992;13(1):335–45.

75. Beresford HR. Melanoma of the nervous system. Treatment with corticosteroids and radiation. Neurology. 1969;19(1):59–65.

76. Lang EF, Slater J. Metastatic brain tumors. Results of surgical and nonsurgical treatment. Surg Clin North Am. 1964;44:865–72.

77. Dasgupta T, Brasfield R. Metastatic melanoma: a clinicopathological study. Cancer. 1964;17:1323–39.

78. Stehlin JS, Jr., Hills WJ, Rufino C. Disseminated melanoma. Biologic behavior and treatment. Archives Surg (Chicago, Ill: 1960). 1967;94(4):495–501.

79. Kuhn MJ, Hammer GM, Swenson LC, Youssef HT, Gleason TJ. MRI evaluation of "solitary" brain metastases with triple-dose gadoteridol: comparison with contrast-enhanced CT and conventional-dose gadopentetate dimeglumine MRI studies in the same patients. Comput Med Imaging Graph Off J Comput Med Imaging Soc. 1994;18(5):391–9.

80. Nomoto Y, Miyamoto T, Yamaguchi Y. Brain metastasis of small cell lung carcinoma: comparison of Gd-DTPA enhanced magnetic resonance imaging and enhanced computerized tomography. Jpn J Clin Oncol. 1994;24(5):258–62.

81. Sze G, Milano E, Johnson C, Heier L. Detection of brain metastases: comparison of contrast-enhanced MR with unenhanced MR and enhanced CT. AJNR Am J Neuroradiol. 1990;11 (4):785–91.

82. Dewulf P, Demaerel P, Wilms G, Delanote G, Defloor E, Casselman J, et al. Cerebral metastatic malignant melanoma: CT and MR findings with pathological correlation. J Belge Radiol. 1993;76(5):318–9.

83. Scott M. Spontaneous intracerebral hematoma caused by cerebral neoplasms. Report of eight verified cases. J Neurosurg. 1975;42 (3):338–42.

84. Schold SC, Vurgrin D, Golbey RB, Posner JB. Central nervous system metastases from germ cell carcinoma of testis. Semin Oncol. 1979;6(1):102–8.

85. Dagi TF, Maccabe JJ. Metastatic trophoblastic disease presenting as a subarachnoid hemorrhage: report of two cases and review of the literature. Surg Neurol. 1980;14(3):175–84.

86. Graus F, Rogers LR, Posner JB. Cerebrovascular complications in patients with cancer. Medicine. 1985;64(1):16–35.

87. Madow L, Alpers BJ. Cerebral vascular complications of metastatic carcinoma. J Neuropathol Exp Neurol. 1952;11 (2):137–48.

88. Strang RR, Ljungdahl TI. Carcinoma of the lung with a cerebral metastasis presenting as subarachnoid haemorrhage. Med J Aust. 1962;49(1):90–1.

89. Mandybur TI. Intracranial hemorrhage caused by metastatic tumors. Neurology. 1977;27(7):650–5.

90. Wronski M, Arbit E. Surgical treatment of brain metastases from melanoma: a retrospective study of 91 patients. J Neurosurg. 2000;93(1):9–18.

91. Nussbaum ES, Djalilian HR, Cho KH, Hall WA. Brain metastases. Histology, multiplicity, surgery, and survival. Cancer. 1996;78(8):1781–8.

92. Byrne TN, Cascino TL, Posner JB. Brain metastasis from melanoma. J Neurooncol. 1983;1(4):313–7.

93. Retsas S, Gershuny AR. Central nervous system involvement in malignant melanoma. Cancer. 1988;61(9):1926–34.

94. Somaza S, Kondziolka D, Lunsford LD, Kirkwood JM, Flickinger JC. Stereotactic radiosurgery for cerebral metastatic melanoma. J Neurosurg. 1993;79(5):661–6.

95. Kondziolka D, Bernstein M, Resch L, Tator CH, Fleming JF, Vanderlinden RG, et al. Significance of hemorrhage into brain tumors: clinicopathological study. J Neurosurg. 1987;67(6):852–7.

96. Mathieu D, Kondziolka D, Cooper PB, Flickinger JC, Niranjan A, Agarwala S, et al. Gamma knife radiosurgery in the management of malignant melanoma brain metastases. Neurosurgery. 2007;60 (3):471–81 (discussion 81–2).

97. Little JR, Dial B, Belanger G, Carpenter S. Brain hemorrhage from intracranial tumor. Stroke J Cereb Circ. 1979;10(3):283–8.

98. Palmer FJ, Poulgrain AP. Metastatic melanoma simulating subdural hematoma. Case report. J Neurosurg. 1978;49(2):301–2.

99. Bitoh S, Hasegawa H, Ohtsuki H, Obashi J, Fujiwara M, Sakurai M. Cerebral neoplasms initially presenting with massive intracerebral hemorrhage. Surg Neurol. 1984;22(1):57–62.

100. Atlas SW, Grossman RI, Gomori JM, Hackney DB, Goldberg HI, Zimmerman RA, et al. Hemorrhagic intracranial malignant neoplasms: spin-echo MR imaging. Radiology. 1987;164 (1):71–7.

101. Madonick MJ, Savitsky N. Subarachnoid hemorrhage in melanoma of the brain. AMA Arch Neurol Psychiatry. 1951;65 (5):628–36.

102. Wolpert SM, Zimmer A, Schechter MM, Zingesser LH. The neuroradiology of melanomas of the central nervous system. Am J Roentgenol Radium Ther Nucl Med. 1967;101(1):178–87.

103. Budman DR, Camacho E, Wittes RE. The current causes of death in patients with malignant melanoma. Eur J Cancer (Oxford, England: 1990). 1978;14(4):327–30.

104. Einhorn LH, Burgess MA, Vallejos C, Bodey GP Sr, Gutterman J, Mavligit G, et al. Prognostic correlations and response to treatment in advanced metastatic malignant melanoma. Can Res. 1974;34(8):1995–2004.

105. Patel JK, Didolkar MS, Pickren JW, Moore RH. Metastatic pattern of malignant melanoma. A study of 216 autopsy cases. Am J Surg. 1978;135(6):807–10.

106. Neal MT, Chan MD, Lucas JT Jr, Loganathan A, Dillingham C, Pan E, et al. Predictors of survival, neurologic death, local failure, and distant failure after gamma knife radiosurgery for melanoma brain metastases. World Neurosurg. 2014;82(6):1250–5.

107. Dyer MA, Arvold ND, Chen YH, Pinnell NE, Mitin T, Lee EQ, et al. The role of whole brain radiation therapy in the management of melanoma brain metastases. Radiat. 2014;9:143.

108. Vecchio S, Spagnolo F, Merlo DF, Signori A, Acquati M, Pronzato P, et al. The treatment of melanoma brain metastases before the advent of targeted therapies: associations between therapeutic choice, clinical symptoms and outcome with survival. Melanoma Res. 2014;24(1):61–7.

109. Mendez IM, Del Maestro RF. Cerebral metastases from malignant melanoma. Can J Neurol Sci. 1988;15(2):119–23.

110. Mehta MP, Rozental JM, Levin AB, Mackie TR, Kubsad SS, Gehring MA, et al. Defining the role of radiosurgery in the management of brain metastases. Int J Radiat Oncol Biol Phys. 1992;24(4):619–25.

111. Sloan AE, Nock CJ, Einstein DB. Diagnosis and treatment of melanoma brain metastasis: a literature review. Cancer Control. 2009;16(3):248–55.

112. Paek SH, Audu PB, Sperling MR, Cho J, Andrews DW. Reevaluation of surgery for the treatment of brain metastases: review of 208 patients with single or multiple brain metastases treated at one institution with modern neurosurgical techniques. Neurosurgery. 2005;56(5):1021–34 (discussion-34).

113. Frakes JM, Figura ND, Ahmed KA, Juan TH, Patel N, Latifi K, et al. Potential role for LINAC-based stereotactic radiosurgery for the treatment of 5 or more radioresistant melanoma brain metastases. J Neurosurg. 2015:1–7.

114. Yamamoto M, Kawabe T, Sato Y, Higuchi Y, Nariai T, Watanabe S, et al. Stereotactic radiosurgery for patients with multiple brain metastases: a case-matched study comparing treatment results for patients with 2–9 versus 10 or more tumors. J Neurosurg. 2014;121(Suppl):16–25.

115. Baschnagel AM, Meyer KD, Chen PY, Krauss DJ, Olson RE, Pieper DR, et al. Tumor volume as a predictor of survival and local control in patients with brain metastases treated with gamma knife surgery. J Neurosurg. 2013;119(5):1139–44.

116. Levin VA, Bidaut L, Hou P, Kumar AJ, Wefel JS, Bekele BN, et al. Randomized double-blind placebo-controlled trial of bevacizumab therapy for radiation necrosis of the central nervous system. Int J Radiat Oncol Biol Phys. 2011;79(5):1487–95.

117. Mandell L, Hilaris B, Sullivan M, Sundaresan N, Nori D, Kim JH, et al. The treatment of single brain metastasis from non-oat cell lung carcinoma. Surgery and radiation versus radiation therapy alone. Cancer. 1986;58(3):641–9.

118. Flickinger JC, Kondziolka D, Lunsford LD, Coffey RJ, Goodman ML, Shaw EG, et al. A multi-institutional experience with stereotactic radiosurgery for solitary brain metastasis. Int J Radiat Oncol Biol Phys. 1994;28(4):797–802.

119. Patchell RA, Tibbs PA, Walsh JW, Dempsey RJ, Maruyama Y, Kryscio RJ, et al. A randomized trial of surgery in the treatment of single metastases to the brain. N Engl J Med. 1990;322 (8):494–500.

120. Auchter RM, Lamond JP, Alexander E, Buatti JM, Chappell R, Friedman WA, et al. A multiinstitutional outcome and prognostic factor analysis of radiosurgery for resectable single brain metastasis. Int J Radiat Oncol Biol Phys. 1996;35(1):27–35.

121. Mehta MP, Tsao MN, Whelan TJ, Morris DE, Hayman JA, Flickinger JC, et al. The American Society for therapeutic radiology and oncology (ASTRO) evidence-based review of the role of radiosurgery for brain metastases. Int J Radiat Oncol Biol Phys. 2005;63(1):37–46.

122. Smalley SR, Laws ER Jr, O'Fallon JR, Shaw EG, Schray MF. Resection for solitary brain metastasis. Role of adjuvant radiation and prognostic variables in 229 patients. J Neurosurg. 1992;77 (4):531–40.

123. O'Neill BP, Iturria NJ, Link MJ, Pollock BE, Ballman KV, O'Fallon JR. A comparison of surgical resection and stereotactic radiosurgery in the treatment of solitary brain metastases. Int J Radiat Oncol Biol Phys. 2003;55(5):1169–76.

124. Rutigliano MJ, Lunsford LD, Kondziolka D, Strauss MJ, Khanna V, Green M. The cost effectiveness of stereotactic radiosurgery versus surgical resection in the treatment of solitary metastatic brain tumors. Neurosurgery. 1995;37(3):445–53 (discussion 53–5).

125. Lonser RR, Song DK, Klapper J, Hagan M, Auh S, Kerr PB, et al. Surgical management of melanoma brain metastases in patients treated with immunotherapy. J Neurosurg. 2011;115 (1):30–6.

126. Di Giacomo AM, Ascierto PA, Pilla L, Santinami M, Ferrucci PF, Giannarelli D, et al. Ipilimumab and fotemustine in patients with advanced melanoma (NIBIT-M1): an open-label, single-arm phase 2 trial. Lancet Oncol. 2012;13(9):879–86.

127. Avril MF, Aamdal S, Grob JJ, Hauschild A, Mohr P, Bonerandi JJ, et al. Fotemustine compared with dacarbazine in patients with disseminated malignant melanoma: a phase III study. J Clin Oncol. 2004;22(6):1118–25.

128. Atkins MB, Gollob JA, Sosman JA, McDermott DF, Tutin L, Sorokin P, et al. A phase II pilot trial of concurrent biochemotherapy with cisplatin, vinblastine, temozolomide, interleukin 2, and IFN-alpha 2B in patients with metastatic melanoma. Clin Cancer Res. 2002;8(10):3075–81.

129. Vestermark LW, Larsen S, Lindelov B, Bastholt L. A phase II study of thalidomide in patients with brain metastases from malignant melanoma. Acta Oncol (Stockholm, Sweden). 2008;47 (8):1526–30.

130. Montagut C, Settleman J. Targeting the RAF-MEK-ERK pathway in cancer therapy. Cancer Lett. 2009;283(2):125–34.

131. Falchook G, Long G, Kurzrock R, Kim K, Arkenau H, Brown M, et al. RAF inhibitor dabrafenib (GSK2118436) is active in melanoma brain metastases, multiple BRAF genotypes and diverse cancers. Lancet. 2012;379(9829):1893–901.

132. Flaherty L, Hamid O, Linette G, Schuchter L, Hallmeyer S, Gonzalez R, et al. A single-arm, open-label, expanded access study of vemurafenib in patients with metastatic melanoma in the United States. Cancer J (Sudbury, Mass). 2014;20(1):18–24.

133. Klein O, Clements A, Menzies AM, O'Toole S, Kefford RF, Long GV. BRAF inhibitor activity in V600R metastatic melanoma–response. European Journal of Cancer. 2013;49(7):1797–8.

134. Guirguis LM, Yang JC, White DE, Steinberg SM, Liewehr DJ, Rosenberg SA, et al. Safety and efficacy of high-dose interleukin-2 therapy in patients with brain metastases. J Immunother (Hagerstown, Md: 1997). 2002;25(1):82–7.

135. Robert C, Thomas L, Bondarenko I, O'Day S, Weber J, Garbe C, et al. Ipilimumab plus dacarbazine for previously untreated metastatic melanoma. N Engl J Med. 2011;364(26):2517–26.

136. Margolin K, Ernstoff MS, Hamid O, Lawrence D, McDermott D, Puzanov I, et al. Ipilimumab in patients with melanoma and brain metastases: an open-label, phase 2 trial. Lancet Oncol. 2012;13 (5):459–65.

137. Silk AW, Bassetti MF, West BT, Tsien CI, Lao CD. Ipilimumab and radiation therapy for melanoma brain metastases. Cancer Med. 2013;2(6):899–906.

138. Weber JS, Kudchadkar RR, Yu B, Gallenstein D, Horak CE, Inzunza HD, et al. Safety, efficacy, and biomarkers of nivolumab with vaccine in ipilimumab-refractory or -naive melanoma. J Clin Oncol. 2013;31(34):4311–8.

139. Goldberg SB, Gettinger SN, Mahajan A, Chiang AC, Herbst RS, Sznol M, Tsiouris AJ, Cohen J, Vortmeyer A, Jilaveanu L, Yu J, Hegde U, Speaker S, Madura M, Ralabate A, Rivera A, Rowen E, Gerrish H, Yao X, Chiang V, Kluger HM. Pembrolizumab for patients with melanoma or non-small-cell lung cancer and untreated brain metastases: early analysis of a non-randomised, open-label, phase 2 trial. Lancet Oncol. 2016;17(7):976–83.

140. Le Rhun E, Taillibert S, Chamberlain MC. Carcinomatous meningitis: leptomeningeal metastases in solid tumors. Surg Neurol Int. 2013;4(Suppl 4):S265–88.

141. Bot I, Blank CU, Brandsma D. Clinical and radiological response of leptomeningeal melanoma after whole brain radiotherapy and ipilimumab. J Neurol. 2012;259(9):1976–8.

142. Simeone E, De Maio E, Sandomenico F, Fulciniti F, Lastoria S, Aprea P, et al. Neoplastic leptomeningitis presenting in a melanoma patient treated with dabrafenib (a V600EBRAF inhibitor): a case report. J Med Case Rep. 2012;6:131.

143. Lee JM, Mehta UN, Dsouza LH, Guadagnolo BA, Sanders DL, Kim KB. Long-term stabilization of leptomeningeal disease with whole-brain radiation therapy in a patient with metastatic melanoma treated with vemurafenib: a case report. Melanoma Res. 2013;23(2):175–8.

144. Bohm P, Huber J. The surgical treatment of bony metastases of the spine and limbs. J Bone Joint Surg Br. 2002;84(4):521–9.

145. Balch CM, Soong SJ, Murad TM, Smith JW, Maddox WA, Durant JR. A multifactorial analysis of melanoma. IV. Prognostic factors in 200 melanoma patients with distant metastases (stage III). J Clin Oncol. 1983;1(2):126–34.

146. Colman MW, Kirkwood JM, Schott T, Goodman MA, McGough RL 3rd. Does metastasectomy improve survival in skeletal melanoma? Melanoma Res. 2014;24(4):354–9.

147. Wong DA, Fornasier VL, MacNab I. Spinal metastases: the obvious, the occult, and the impostors. Spine. 1990;15(1):1–4.

148. Perrin RG, Livingston KE, Aarabi B. Intradural extramedullary spinal metastasis. A report of 10 cases. J Neurosurg. 1982;56 (6):835–7.

149. Lau D, Than KD, La Marca F, Park P. Independent predictors for local recurrence following surgery for spinal metastasis. Acta Neurochir. 2014;156(2):277–82.

150. Huttenlocher S, Sehmisch L, Rudat V, Rades D. Motor function and survival following radiotherapy alone for metastatic epidural spinal cord compression in melanoma patients. J Dermatol. 2014;41(12):1082–6.

151. Klimo P Jr, Schmidt MH. Surgical management of spinal metastases. Oncologist. 2004;9(2):188–96.

152. Joaquim AF, Ghizoni E, Tedeschi H, Pereira EB, Giacomini LA. Stereotactic radiosurgery for spinal metastases: a literature review. Einstein (Sao Paulo, Brazil). 2013;11(2):247–55.

153. Sellin JN, Gressot LV, Suki D, St Clair EG, Chern J, Rhines LD, et al. Prognostic factors influencing the outcome of 64 consecutive patients undergoing surgery for metastatic melanoma of the spine. Neurosurgery. 2015;77(3):386–93.

154. Adam Y, Benezech J, Blanquet A, Fuentes JM, Bousigue JY, Debono B, et al. Intramedullary tumors. Results of a national investigation in private neurosurgery. Neurochirurgie. 2010;56 (4):344–9.

155. Connolly ES, Jr., Winfree CJ, McCormick PC, Cruz M, Stein BM. Intramedullary spinal cord metastasis: report of three cases and review of the literature. Surg Neurol. 1996;46(4):329–37 (discussion 37–8).

156. Parikh S, Heron DE. Fractionated radiosurgical management of intramedullary spinal cord metastasis: a case report and review of the literature. Clin Neurol Neurosurg. 2009;111(10):858–61.

157. Salpietro FM, Alafaci C, Gervasio O, La Rosa G, Baio A, Francolini DC, et al. Primary cervical melanoma with brain metastases. Case report and review of the literature. J Neurosurg. 1998;89(4):659–66.

158. Caruso R, Marrocco L, Wierzbicki V, Salvati M. Intramedullary melanocytoma: case report and review of literature. Tumori. 2009;95(3):389–93.

159. Muthappan M, Muthu T, Hussain Z, Lamont D, Balakrishnan V. Cervical intramedullary melanocytoma: a case report and review of literature. J Clin Neurosci. 2012;19(10):1450–3.

160. Restrepo CE, Spinner RJ, Howe BM, Jentoft ME, Markovic SN, Lachance DH. Perineural spread of malignant melanoma from the mandible to the brachial plexus: case report. J Neurosurg. 2015;122(4):784–90.

161. Kwon SC, Rhim SC, Lee DH, Roh SW, Kang SK. Primary malignant melanoma of the cervical spinal nerve root. Yonsei Med J. 2004;45(2):345–8.

162. Chang PC, Fischbein NJ, McCalmont TH, Kashani-Sabet M, Zettersten EM, Liu AY, et al. Perineural spread of malignant melanoma of the head and neck: clinical and imaging features. AJNR Am J Neuroradiol. 2004;25(1):5–11.

163. Feng Z, Wu X, Chen V, Velie E, Zhang Z. Incidence and survival of desmoplastic melanoma in the United States, 1992–2007. J Cutan Pathol. 2011;38(8):616–24.

164. Grewal DS, Fishman GA, Jampol LM. Autoimmune retinopathy and antiretinal antibodies: a review. Retina (Philadelphia, Pa). 2014;34(5):827–45.

165. Weleber RG, Watzke RC, Shults WT, Trzupek KM, Heckenlively JR, Egan RA, et al. Clinical and electrophysiologic characterization of paraneoplastic and autoimmune retinopathies associated with antienolase antibodies. Am J Ophthalmol. 2005;139(5):780–94.

166. Adamus G. Autoantibody targets and their cancer relationship in the pathogenicity of paraneoplastic retinopathy. Autoimmun Rev. 2009;8(5):410–4.

167. Polans AS, Burton MD, Haley TL, Crabb JW, Palczewski K. Recoverin, but not visinin, is an autoantigen in the human retina identified with a cancer-associated retinopathy. Invest Ophthalmol Vis Sci. 1993;34(1):81–90.

168. Khan N, Huang JJ, Foster CS. Cancer associated retinopathy (CAR): an autoimmune-mediated paraneoplastic syndrome. Semin Ophthalmol. 2006;21(3):135–41.

169. Sawyer RA, Selhorst JB, Zimmerman LE, Hoyt WF. Blindness caused by photoreceptor degeneration as a remote effect of cancer. Am J Ophthalmol. 1976;81(5):606–13.

170. Ferreyra HA, Jayasundera T, Khan NW, He S, Lu Y, Heckenlively JR. Management of autoimmune retinopathies with immunosuppression. Arch Ophthalmol (Chicago, Ill: 1960). 2009;127(4):390–7.

171. Heckenlively JR, Ferreyra HA. Autoimmune retinopathy: a review and summary. Semin Immunopathol. 2008;30(2):127–34.

172. Keltner JL, Thirkill CE, Yip PT. Clinical and immunologic characteristics of melanoma-associated retinopathy syndrome: eleven new cases and a review of 51 previously published cases. J Neuro Ophthalmol Off J North Am Neuro Ophthalmol Soc. 2001;21(3):173–87.

173. Okel BB, Thirkill CE, Anderson K. An unusual case of melanoma-associated retinopathy. Ocular Immunol Inflamm. 1995;3(2):121–8.

174. Rahimy E, Sarraf D. Paraneoplastic and non-paraneoplastic retinopathy and optic neuropathy: evaluation and management. Surv Ophthalmol. 2013;58(5):430–58.

175. Gass JD, Gieser RG, Wilkinson CP, Beahm DE, Pautler SE. Bilateral diffuse uveal melanocytic proliferation in patients with occult carcinoma. Arch Ophthalmol (Chicago, Ill: 1960). 1990;108(4):527–33.

176. Mandelcorn E, McGuire K, Dixon W, Mandelcorn M. Ocular paraneoplastic syndrome: a case of bilateral diffuse uveal melanocytic proliferation. Retina (Philadelphia, Pa). 2009;29(9):1375–6.

177. Mets RB, Golchet P, Adamus G, Anitori R, Wilson D, Shaw J, et al. Bilateral diffuse uveal melanocytic proliferation with a positive ophthalmoscopic and visual response to plasmapheresis. Arch Ophthalmol (Chicago, Ill: 1960). 2011;129(9):1235–8.

178. Ritland JS, Eide N, Tausjo J. Bilateral diffuse uveal melanocytic proliferation and uterine cancer. A case report. Acta Ophthalmol Scand. 2000;78(3):366–8.

179. Lucchinetti CF, Kimmel DW, Lennon VA. Paraneoplastic and oncologic profiles of patients seropositive for type 1 antineuronal nuclear autoantibodies. Neurology. 1998;50(3):652–7.

180. Anthoney DA, Bone I, Evans TR. Inflammatory demyelinating polyneuropathy: a complication of immunotherapy in malignant melanoma. Ann Oncol. 2000;11(9):1197–200.

181. Palma JA, Martin-Algarra S. Chronic inflammatory demyelinating polyneuropathy associated with metastatic malignant melanoma of unknown primary origin. J Neurooncol. 2009;94(2):279–81.

182. Rousseau A, Salachas F, Baccard M, Delattre JY, Sanson M. Chronic inflammatory polyneuropathy revealing malignant melanoma. J Neurooncol. 2005;71(3):335–6.

183. Chau AM, Yu A, Keezer MR. Chronic inflammatory demyelinating polyneuropathy and metastatic melanoma. Can J Neurol Sci. 2013;40(5):750–2.

Joachim M. Baehring and Amy M. Chan

Introduction

Acute lymphoblastic leukemia (ALL) is the most common neoplasm in children, with 3000 newly diagnosed patients under age of 20 each year (SEER 2004–2008 data). Modern intensive systemic and intrathecal (IT) chemotherapy regimens have achieved 5-year event-free survival rates as high as 79–82% among children [1–3] and about 50% for adults [4]. Most cases are B-precursor cell ALL. About 10–15% of pediatric and 25% of adult cases represent the more aggressive T-cell ALL (T-ALL) subtype [5].

Acute myeloid leukemia (AML) is primarily a disease of aging, especially among those with previous cytotoxic therapy for solid tumor. It is most prevalent among adults over age 60 (15 per 100,000) [6]. Survival is poor. The most favorable cytogenetic subtypes, inv[7] or t[8, 9], achieve a 60% 3-year relapse-free survival (RFS) [10]. Survival in acute promyeloid leukemia has improved with all-trans retinoic acid. However, the 3-year RFS decreases to 20–30% if other poor prognostic factors are present. The "monosomal karyotype" has a median survival of only 6 months [8]. Pediatric disease has a somewhat different biology and can have up to 50% 5-year event-free survival [11].

Chronic lymphocytic leukemia (CLL) is a common (4.1 cases per 100,000 per year) [12] but diffuse group characterized by clonal proliferation of mature, typically CD5-positive B-cells [13]. It can be divided into two broad prognosis groups. The favorable "mutated" group (> 2% mutation in the VH gene from native clones) can survive for many years without therapy. The unfavorable "unmutated" group (CD38+ or ZAP-70+) has a rapidly fatal course [14].

In young adults, fludarabine-based regimens produce median progression-free survival (PFS) of 48 months [15]. Yet it carries significant infection risk among older patients as a result of profound leukopenia (56%) [15]. Alternative targeted therapies currently being investigated include monoclonal antibodies against B-cells (CD-20—rituximab, ofatumumab, obinutuzumab; CD-52—alemtuzumab) and small molecular inhibitors (fostamatinib, idelalisib, ibrutinib, dasatinib) [12].

Chronic myeloid leukemia (CML) is characterized by presence of the Philadelphia chromosome (t9;22; Ph+), and a reciprocal rearrangement and fusion of the *BCR* and *ABL* genes. It is predominantly a disease of adulthood (age 57–60) with annual incidence of 0.7–1.0 per 100,000 [16]. In the chronic phase, tyrosine kinase inhibitors (TKI) have dramatically improved overall 5-year survival to 89% [17]. However, resistance to TKI starts to emerge in the acceleration phase (15–19% blasts in blood; 30–49% blasts plus promyelocytes in marrow; platelets $<100 \times 10^9/L$; or clonal abnormality in Ph+ cells [7]). Despite four additional second-generation TKI (nilotinib, dasatinib, bosutinib and ponatinib) targeting various mutations [18, 19], acceleration phase patients still tend to evolve into a terminal acute leukemia-like blast phase (>20% blasts in blood).

Leukemic Infiltration or Compression of the Nervous System

Leptomeningeal Leukemia

The leptomeninges and spinal fluid (CSF) are sanctuary sites for leukemia. In autopsy series, CNS leukemic infiltrates were found in 81% of ALL cases, 46% of AML cases [20], 17% of CLL cases [21] and only in 1 out of 17 (6%) of CML cases [20]. Overall, myelogenous leukemia tends to have more prominent dural infiltration and less perivascular invasion [9, 22]. Mechanisms of leukemia entry into the

J.M. Baehring (✉)
Departments of Neurology and Neurosurgery, Yale School of Medicine, 15 York Street, New Haven, CT 06520, USA
e-mail: joachim.baehring@yale.edu

A.M. Chan
Department of Neurology, Yale School of Medicine, 15 York Street, New Haven, CT 06520, USA
e-mail: amy.chan@yale.edu

© Springer International Publishing AG 2018
D. Schiff et al. (eds.), *Cancer Neurology in Clinical Practice*,
DOI 10.1007/978-3-319-57901-6_30

CNS are thought to include translocation via the perforating vessels from the bone marrow, escape into the CSF via the choroid plexus, direct cerebral parenchymal invasion via brain capillaries, extravasation during hemorrhage, leptomeningeal infiltration via bony lesions, growth along nerve roots or iatrogenic via lumbar puncture [21, 23, 24]. Symptoms and signs of leptomeningeal leukemia include those related to meningeal irritation (headache, vomiting, lethargy), papilledema, visual disturbance from optic neuropathy, other cranial nerve dysfunctions (double vision, facial numbness, hearing loss), cerebellar symptoms, radiculopathies or cauda equina syndrome (Fig. 30.1a–f). Altered spinal fluid reabsorption may give rise to communicating hydrocephalus with a combination of cognitive decline, urgent micturition and gait apraxia. However, the most common patient (>70%) is asymptomatic [23, 25]. The most useful diagnostic tool is a lumbar puncture combined with modern molecular techniques. These include *BCR-ABL* fusion detection by fluorescence in situ hybridization (FISH) analysis for CML, flow cytometry and PCR amplification of the variable region of the immunoglobulin heavy chain (IgH) gene [26] for CLL. False negative rate of leptomeningeal enhancement by contrast enhanced MRI may be as high as 60–65% [27].

Treatment

As early as in the 1960s, "prophylactic" CNS irradiation (pCRT) plus intrathecal methotrexate (IT-MTX) reduced the cumulative risk for CNS dissemination of ALL in children from 60% [28] to around 4.5% [29]. However, this treatment regimen resulted in a substantial risk of delayed radiation-associated neurological toxicity and secondary

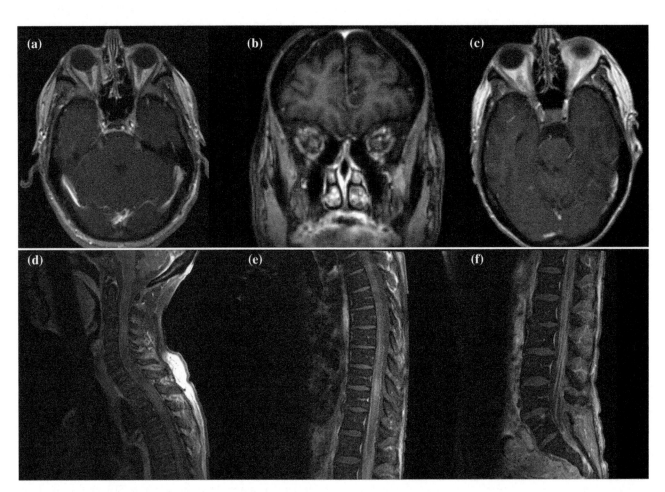

Fig. 30.1 a A 57-year-old man with acute lymphoblastic leukemia presented with right-sided Bell's palsy, a left-sided vocal cord paralysis and an abducens nerve palsy on the right. T1-weighted MRI brain with gadolinium showed thickening and enhancement of both trigeminal nerves diagnostic of meningeal dissemination of leukemia. **b–f** 63-year-old woman with relapsed pre-B-cell ALL. She described visual change in her right eye ("*a center black dot*") that progressed to complete blindness over two days. She also had a few weeks of back pain, perineal numbness, difficulty urinating and gait instability. T1-weighted MRI of brain and spine with gadolinium showed prominent enhancement of both optic nerves (**b**); abnormal linear leptomeningeal enhancement along the cerebellar folia (**c**); multifocal thickening and enhancement of the cervical and thoracic spinal cord as well as extensive enhancement of the cauda equina nerve roots. This is indicative of pial and cord infiltration by leukemia (**d–f**)

brain tumors. Currently, high-dose methotrexate and triple IT therapy (MTX, cytarabine (ARAC), prednisolone) have nearly eliminated pCRT in all except few high-risk patients (T-ALL; poor response to prednisone; t(4;11); t(9;22); t (1;19) with CNS involvement [30, 31]). These patients are either treated with a decreased pCRT dose (12 Gy; 6-year CNS relapse risk: 2.2%) [30, 32], or an intensified regimen including HD-MTX, asparaginase, dexamethasone and IT therapy (5-year CNS relapse rate of 2.6–2.7% [31, 33]).

For adults without overt CNS disease, multiple studies similarly showed that the combination of HD-MTX, IT-MTX and ARAC [34–36] reduces risk for CNS dissemination to 4–6%, comparable to previous pCRT protocols. For the 5–10% adults with overt CNS disease, treatments typically include IT chemotherapy, cranial radiation (CRT) followed by either allogeneic hematopoietic stem cell transplantation (HSCT) or chemotherapy intensification [36, 37]. This provides a 90% remission rate, comparable to patients without overt CNS disease. Nonetheless, CNS disease still carries an adverse prognosis, with 5-year overall survival rate at 29% compared to 38% without CNS disease ($p = 0.03$) [38].

In pediatric AML, there is no randomized study regarding the efficacy of pCRT. Contemporary protocols including systemic chemotherapy agents with good CNS penetration and intensified intrathecal therapy have demonstrated low rates of CNS relapse between 1.5 and 3% [39–41] in CNS-negative children and no adverse prognostic significance in children with low CNS disease burden [42, 43]. Many study groups now provide CRT only to children with cranial nerve infiltration or bulky disease impinging on important parameningeal structures who do not respond quickly to chemotherapy [11].

CNS involvement in adult AML patients is generally associated with a poorer prognosis [44, 45]. Adult patients with intermediate or unfavorable cytogenetic markers are recommended to receive standard allogeneic stem cell transplant (HSCT), investigational therapies or new approaches to HSCT [46]. One study using pre-HSCT routine diagnostic lumbar puncture identified up to 12% of patients with CNS disease involvement. The CNS+ patients treated with intrathecal chemotherapy had significantly poorer outcomes (RFS 6% at 5 years) than those who underwent additional irradiation (RFS-5 32%; $p = 0.004$) or those who were free of CNS disease (RFS-5 35%). This suggests a role of CNS irradiation boost in HSCT conditioning for CNS + AML patients [47].

Symptomatic CNS involvement by CLL is rare, with an estimated 1.5–3% incidence [48]. Neither risk factors nor optimal treatment have been well established. Case series showed that CNS involvement occurred across all Rai stages (Stage 0: 25%; I: 15%; II: 19%; III: 15%; IV: 24%) and CLL forms [49]. Treatment includes IT chemotherapy (MTX or

ARAC, twice weekly x 4; followed by weekly up to a total of 12 treatments), systematic fludarabine-based chemotherapy or radiation [49]. There is no randomized control study for efficacy. Case series showed no evidence of marked outcome differences between radiation alone (69%), IT therapy alone (76%) or both (86%) [49]. There is anecdotal evidence that IT therapy may be more efficacious in optic neuropathy [49–51]. Of note, there are reports of neurological symptom resolution [49] or long-term survival despite failure to clear the CSF of tumor cells [48]. Overall, this suggests that systemic disease control may be of most importance. CNS treatment should be aimed toward symptomatic relief only.

CNS involvement of CML is also rare. Risk factors are high tumor cell burden [52] or blast crisis [53]. Among high risk patients, incidence of meningeal dissemination may be as high as 46.7%, comparable to that in AML [54]. Risk factors combined with poor CNS penetration of imatinib [55] likely contribute to isolated CNS relapse months after achieving complete hematological and major cytogenetic response on imatinib [56]. Treatments for isolated CNS disease after imatinib failure include IT liposomal cytarabine [57], IT-MTX along with dexamethasone [58] or a TKI with increased CNS penetration, such as dasatinib [59]. Some investigators also consider allogeneic HSCT [56]. Orbital irradiation is provided for optic nerve infiltration. Otherwise roles for CNS irradiation and CNS prophylaxis have not been well established.

Spinal Cord Compression

Malignant spinal cord compression, estimated at a cumulative incidence of 2.5% among all cancer patients [60], is an uncommon but devastating complication. In about 0.3% [60] of acute leukemia patients, epidural deposits or vertebral destruction results in spinal cord compression. Early warning signs include localized pain from infiltration of the richly innervated periosteum, excruciating radicular pain from nerve root compression, motor paresis and spasticity ("leg heaviness," difficulty climbing stairs) followed by segmental sensory deficits and alarming symptoms of urinary retention and flaccid paresis. Emergency MRI studies of the entire spine should be pursued with care in excluding confounding etiologies such as epidural hemorrhage or abscess. Emergency treatment consists of dexamethasone and radiation therapy (40 Gy at 2 Gy/day in 20 fractions or biologically equivalent regimens).

Myeloid Sarcoma (Chloroma)

Myeloid sarcomas are immature myeloid mass lesions outside of the bone marrow. First described in 1811 [61],

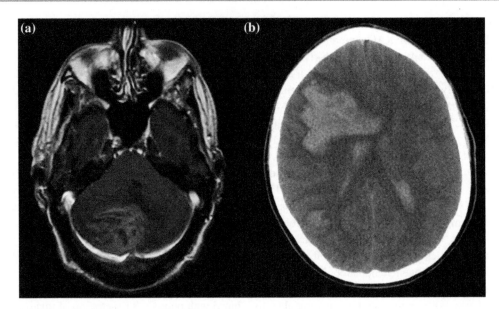

Fig. 30.2 **a** A 53-year-old man with history of AML presented with progressive headache and imbalance. T1-weighted MRI of the brain with gadolinium revealed an avidly enhancing mass in the posterior fossa. Biopsy confirmed chloroma. **b**. A 20-year-old man presented with a month of progressive lymphadenopathy and gum bleeding. Laboratory studies showed a marked leukocytosis (472,000/mcl), thrombocytopenia (16,000/mcl) as well as early signs of tumor lysis and disseminated intravascular coagulopathy. He suddenly complained of a headache, vomited and became unresponsive. Non-contrast computerized axial tomography of the head (**b**) showed a large right frontal hemorrhage with intra-ventricular extension, likely the result of cerebral leukostasis. He was emergently treated with leukapheresis followed by chemotherapy induction

these were later termed chloromas given a characteristic green color on cross sectioning from presence of myeloperoxidase. They can rarely involve the skull, orbits, periosteum, dura or meninges; invade the brain parenchyma; or cause spinal cord compression as described above (Fig. 30.2a). They are most common among AML patients with t(8;21) or inv(16) and certain morphological subtypes (FAB classification M2, M4, M5). In patients with known chronic myeloproliferative disorders, they often herald progression to AML. On non-contrast CT, chloromas most often are hyperdense masses with avid homogenous enhancement [62]. A biopsy and detailed immunohistochemistry for myeloid markers such as myeloperoxidase is required for accurate diagnosis. Treatment should be the same as for AML patients with CNS involvement [63] with the addition of external beam radiation as needed for bulky disease [64].

Richter Transformation

Richter transformation denotes the transformation of chronic lymphocytic leukemia into an aggressive lymphoma. CNS involvement is rare in this setting. Diffuse large B-cell lymphoma is the most common type [65].

Leukemic Infiltration of the Peripheral Nervous System

Asymmetric infiltration of peripheral nerves occurs in advanced stages of leukemia and may be confused with mononeuropathies of paraneoplastic, compressive or toxic origins. The incidence in autopsy series is much higher than in clinical studies [66]. Radiation is used for palliation and treatment of bulky disease.

Indirect Leukemia Effects

Cerebral Leukostasis Syndrome

Cerebral leukostasis occurs at blast counts exceeding 400,000/mcl and results in diffuse cerebral edema and increased intracranial pressure. Most commonly afflicted are patients with AML. Higher counts are usually required in lymphoblastic leukemia (ALL) since cells are smaller and less adherent than myeloid blasts [67]. Clustered cells within capillaries produce localized ischemic events at the same time as leukemic nodules appear in the white matter surrounding vessels. Patients complain of symptoms indicative of microcirculatory collapse such as transient hearing and vision loss. Treatment consists of leukapheresis, rapid initiation of chemotherapy and low-dose whole brain radiation therapy [68].

Intracranial Hemorrhage and Ischemic Stroke

Leukemia patients are at higher risk for cerebrovascular accidents from various mechanisms, including infective or non-bacterial thrombotic endocarditis, thrombocytopenia, dysfunctional platelets, coagulopathies and cerebral leukostasis [69, 70] (Fig. 30.2b). Chemotherapy regimens with L-asparaginase predispose to both venous and arterial thrombosis. Disseminated intravascular coagulopathy (DIC) is most common in acute promyelocytic (M3) or monocytic leukemia (M5) [71].

Paraneoplastic Neurological Syndromes

Paraneoplastic immune dysfunctions in the wider sense of the word are common among patients with CLL (10–25%) [72] and myelodysplastic syndrome (MDS) (10%) [73], in particular in MDS-derived chronic myelomonocytic leukemia (CMML). Presumably, leukemic cells [74, 75] can serve directly as immature antigen presenting cells or interfere with regulatory T-cell function [76]. The majority of cases are hematological disorders such as hemolytic anemia or thrombocytopenia. Anecdotally, paraneoplastic syndromes affecting the nervous system have been reported, including: acute demyelinating encephalomyelitis (ADEM) preceding pediatric ALL [77] and an aggressive case of CLL (Ki-67 > 30%) [78]; fulminant myopathy over 1 week with transient bone pain and fever [79] leading to diagnosis of ALL; limbic encephalitis associated with voltage-gated potassium channel antibody prior to relapsed AML [80]; and chronic inflammatory demyelinating polyneuropathy heralding transformation of MDS-chronic anemia to CMML and AML [75]. Almost all cases responded to leukemia treatment suggesting that indeed there was a pathogenetic link between the neurologic illness and leukemia. However, given the rarity of these disorders, coincidental occurrence cannot be excluded.

Complications of Leukemia Treatments

Complications of Chemotherapy

Neurologic toxicities to chemotherapeutic agents are rather common in the setting of leukemia. As treatment involves various modalities and chemotherapy combinations, the effect of any single agent is difficult to ascertain.

Methotrexate neurotoxicity is dependent upon mode of administration, dose and association with other neurotoxins, especially ionizing radiation. Within hours, IT methotrexate may cause chemical meningitis. Within hours to days of immediate-to-high IV doses or IT injection, patients can develop delayed leukoencephalopathy with stroke-like presentation manifesting as seizures, severe headache or transient focal neurological symptoms (sensory disturbance, aphasia, weakness) (Fig. 30.3a). Complete recovery is the rule. Re-exposure to methotrexate is possible without recurrence of the neurological syndrome. However, the dose is frequently reduced, or leucovorin rescue is intensified [81]. A chronic leukoencephalopathy with MRI evidence of demyelination is seen in recipients of IT or HD-MTX administered after cranial irradiation.

Cytarabine induces cerebellar and spinal cord toxicity [82]. The gait instability and incoordination, within weeks of therapy, is more pronounced in recipients of high-dose cytarabine, elderly patients and those with impaired renal function. Therapy should be ceased.

L-asparaginase has been linked to thrombotic and hemorrhagic cerebrovascular complications in 1–2% of patients. Patients are at risk for arterial and venous thrombosis [83]. These complications are likely due to depletion of plasma proteins involved in coagulation and fibrinolysis. Fresh frozen plasma is provided as an emergency treatment but also as prophylaxis in patients who suffered a complication during a previous cycle. Dural sinus thrombosis (Fig. 30.3b) is treated with anticoagulation, often combined with fresh frozen plasma or antithrombin III concentrate.

Vincristine produces a cumulative dose-related disorder of sensory nerves in the face or extremities giving rise to tingling or burning paresthesia or jaw pain. Autonomic involvement leads to gastrointestinal dysmotility and abdominal cramping. Some improvement is noted with cessation of treatment and with neuropathic pain medications such as gabapentin or amitriptyline. Once weakness (e.g., foot drop) ensues, the drug has to be discontinued.

Fludarabine affects the peripheral and central nervous system at high doses. A highly morbid acute toxic leukoencephalopathy with cognitive dysfunction, decreased levels of consciousness and vision changes has been described [84, 85]. Risk factors include older age, decreased renal function, previous fludarabine-based transplant [85] and polymorphisms leading to high activity of the pro-drug-converting enzyme deoxycytidine (CdR) kinase in the brain [86].

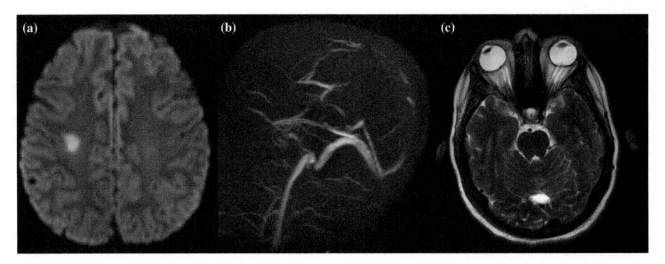

Fig. 30.3 **a** A 14-year-old boy with pre-B-cell ALL awoke with left face and arm numbness and weakness five days after intrathecal methotrexate administration. Diffusion weighted images showed restriction of water diffusion in the right centrum semiovale. He recovered within two days receiving supportive care only. **b.** A 17-year-old boy undergoing induction therapy for pre-T-cell ALL which included L-asparaginase awoken one morning with a headache as well as right arm and leg weakness. He then had a focal motor seizure involving his right side. Magnetic resonance venogram with contrast (**b**) showed extensive filling defects in the superior sagittal sinus confirming cerebral venous thrombosis. **c** A 20-year-old woman with acute promyelocytic leukemia (APML) had an insidious onset of a holocephalic headache, double vision and transient visual obscurations with Valsalva maneuver while undergoing therapy with all-trans retinoic acid. T2-weighted MRI showed a partially empty sella turcica, mild tortuosity of the optic nerves and widening of the optic nerve sheaths. Lumbar puncture showed an increased opening pressure indicative of pseudotumor cerebri

All-trans retinoic acid treatment can be complicated by pseudotumor cerebri (Fig. 30.3c).

Complications of Ionizing Radiation

Increasing emphasis has been placed on substitution of "safe" chemotherapeutic agents for whole brain radiation for CNS prophylaxis and treatment of CNS disease in leukemia patients. Depending on total and single fraction dose, WBRT alone or combined with intrathecal or systemic methotrexate is associated with irreversible white matter changes and cognitive dysfunction [87, 88]. This dysfunction likely reflects the underlying calcific microangiopathy affecting the white matter [89, 90]. WBRT is also associated with aresorptive hydrocephalus poorly responsive to ventriculoperitoneal shunting.

Neuroendocrine difficulties are dependent on dose and age at the time of exposure. The growth hormone (GH) axis is most sensitive and can be the only axis affected following irradiation of less than 30 Gy [91]. Even at 18 Gy, a subtle insufficiency of the GH axis during the puberty growth spurt is observed [92]. Treatment is available with early hormone replacement therapy.

A seven-fold excess of all cancers and a 22-fold increase in the risk of central nervous system tumors have been observed among leukemia patients [93]. Radiation-induced tumors occur at a median latency of 6 years (range 0.9–15 years) [32]. High-grade glioma (median latency 9 years) and meningioma (median latency 19 years) arise with equal frequency (Fig. 30.4). The risk is dose dependent [94].

Opportunistic Infection (OI)

In general, B-lymphocyte dysfunction predisposes the host to encapsulated bacterial infections (e.g., Streptococcus, Hemophilus, Klebsiella). Rituximab, a CD-20 specific monoclonal antibody that is effective in treating CLL, is also known to reactivate viral infections such as hepatitis B, cytomegalovirus, herpes simplex virus, varicella zoster virus, West Nile virus and JC virus (Fig. 30.5a) [95]. Allogeneic stem cell transplantation requiring immunosuppressive therapy results in T-lymphocyte dysfunction, which predisposes to infections with fungi (Fig. 30.5b), viruses (e.g., human herpesvirus 6, JC virus), parasites (toxoplasmosis) or fastidious organisms (listeria, mycobacteria) [96]. Routine screening and prophylactic administration of acyclovir or ganciclovir for high-risk patients have essentially eliminated cytomegalovirus encephalitis [97]. Diagnosis of OI can be challenging, as clinical and radiographic presentations may be atypical. An example is cerebral toxoplasmosis, which may lack characteristic features such as rim-enhancement and vasogenic edema on MRI (Fig. 30.5c).

Among patients with AML, invasive fungal infection is a leading cause of mortality [98, 99]. Systemically, the most

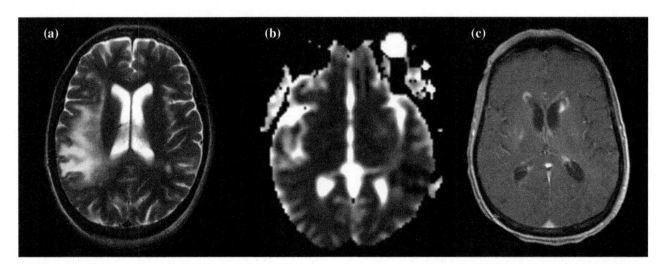

Fig. 30.4 A 38-year-old man who had received prophylaxis cranial radiation (pCRT) as part of childhood ALL treatment presented with a sudden onset of headache and mild right hemiparesis. Workup revealed a left parietal hematoma (not shown). After resolution of the hematoma, T1-weighted MRI brain with gadolinium showed a heterogeneously enhancing mass lesion. Stereotactic biopsy demonstrated glioblastoma

common organisms are mold (64% of cases; 90% aspergillus, <5% zygomycetes) followed by yeast (35% of cases; 90% candida, <5% cryptococcus) [99]. CNS aspergillosis or zygomycosis can present as abscesses or hemorrhagic strokes from angioinvasive fungal hyphae causing mycotic aneurysm, vasculitis and venous occlusion [100]. Candida and cryptococcus have a predilection for the meninges and present as meningitis or diffuse cerebral micro-abscesses [101]. For candida meningitis, the IDSA Practice guidelines [102] recommend intravenous amphotericin B plus flucytosine. However, treatment success with liposomal amphotericin for aspergillus [103] and zygomycetes [104] has been limited. Voriconazole is now considered first-line therapy for CNS aspergillosis [105]. Posaconazole has shown some promise against zygomycetes [106, 107].

Of special note, alemtuzumab, a monoclonal antibody directed against CD52, suppresses B-lymphocyte and natural killer cells for up to 6 months and CD4+ and CD8 + T-lymphocyte for years. In one report, almost 9% of patients who received alemtuzumab conditioning developed Guillain–Barre syndrome or myelitis associated with varicella zoster virus (VZV) or human herpesvirus-7 [108]. Post-transplant acute limbic encephalitis (PALE; amnesia, hyponatremia, abnormal EEG) has also been associated with human herpesvirus-6, particularly after receiving alemtuzumab [109, 110].

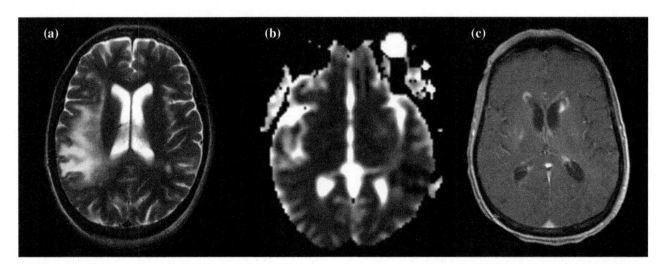

Fig. 30.5 **a** A 68-year-old woman was admitted with progressive confusion one year after completion of fludarabine therapy for CLL. On examination, there was left hemineglect, anosagnosia, somatagnosia and a mild left hemiparesis. T2-weighted MRI brain showed confluent T2 hyperintensities in the right frontoparietal region extending through the splenium of the corpus callosum into the deep white matter of the left hemisphere. Cerebrospinal fluid analysis revealed amplifiable JC virus DNA confirming the diagnosis of progressive multifocal leukoencephalopathy. **b** Aspergillus abscess in the left temporal lobe in a 48-year-old woman after allogeneic stem cell transplantation (apparent diffusion coefficient (ADC) map). **c** A 64-year-old gentleman status post allogeneic stem cell transplant for peripheral T-cell lymphoma/leukemia presented with progressive delirium. T1-weighted MRI brain with contrast revealed multiple small irregularly enhancing lesions. Brain biopsy revealed toxoplasma tachyzoites

Non-infectious Complications of Bone Marrow and Stem Cell Transplantation

Reversible posterior encephalopathy syndrome (PRES) is a clinical syndrome comprised of headache, seizures and vision loss observed in patients on chronic immunosuppression with cyclosporine or tacrolimus and various chemotherapeutic agents. It is named after its MRI correlate [111]. Blood pressure management and modification of immunosuppressive therapy usually lead to complete recovery.

Graft versus host disease (GVH) involving the CNS is rare, and a pathogenetic link to cerebral vasculitis-like syndrome is difficult to establish. However, a few cases of primary CNS angiitis have been described in recipients of allogeneic bone marrow or peripheral blood stem cell transplants [112, 113]. There may be some benefits from cyclophosphamide or corticosteroid treatment.

Immune reconstitution inflammatory syndrome (IRIS), a dramatic and often dysfunctional inflammatory response to systemic or CNS infections after a rapid rise in CD4+ count, occurs during engraftment after stem cell transplantation or after discontinuation of immunosuppression. It has been reported after treatment for cryptococcal meningitis, tuberculosis meningitis, toxoplasmosis and VZV meningoencephalitis [114, 115]. IRIS affecting the eye has been reported after CMV retinitis [116]. Corticosteroid treatment is aimed at edema suppression.

Post-Transplant Lymphoproliferative Disorder (PTLD) after allogeneic stem cell transplantation often reflects EBV reactivation or recent infection. Isolated CNS manifestations are rare. If identified at an early stage of transformation, the process may be reversed by administration of corticosteroids, reduction of the dose of immunosuppression or provision of radiation therapy. Whether antiviral therapy is of additional benefit is unproven. For later stage disease or disease unresponsive to these manipulations, treatment with rituximab may be successful [117], although its poor penetration into the CNS may hamper its efficacy in primary CNS PTLD.

References

1. Moricke A, Reiter A, Zimmermann M, Gadner H, Stanulla M, et al. Risk-adjusted therapy of acute lymphoblastic leukemia can decrease treatment burden and improve survival: treatment results of 2169 unselected pediatric and adolescent patients enrolled in the trial ALL-BFM 95. Blood. 2008;111:4477–89.
2. Moghrabi A, Levy DE, Asselin B, Barr R, Clavell L, et al. Results of the Dana-Farber Cancer Institute ALL Consortium Protocol 95-01 for children with acute lymphoblastic leukemia. Blood. 2007;109:896–904.
3. Pui CH, Sandlund JT, Pei D, Campana D, Rivera GK, et al. Improved outcome for children with acute lymphoblastic leukemia: results of total therapy study XIIIB at St Jude Children's Research Hospital. Blood. 2004;104:2690–6.
4. DeAngelo DJ, Pui C-H. Acute lymphoblastic leukemia and lymphoblastic lymphoma. American Society of Hematology Self-Assessment Program; 2013:491–507.
5. Ferrando AA, Neuberg DS, Staunton J, Loh ML, Huard C, et al. Gene expression signatures define novel oncogenic pathways in T cell acute lymphoblastic leukemia. Cancer Cell. 2002;1:75–87.
6. Dores GM, Devesa SS, Curtis RE, Linet MS, Morton LM. Acute leukemia incidence and patient survival among children and adults in the United States, 2001–2007. Blood. 2012;119:34–43.
7. Swerdllow SH, Campo E, Harris NL. WHO classification of tumours of haematopoietic and lymphoid tissues. France: IARC Press; 2008. p. 32–7.
8. Breems DA, Van Putten WL, De Greef GE, Van Zelderen-Bhola SL, Gerssen-Schoorl KB, et al. Monosomal karyotype in acute myeloid leukemia: a better indicator of poor prognosis than a complex karyotype. J Clin Oncol Off J Am Soc Clin Oncol. 2008;26:4791–7.
9. Moore EW, Thomas LB, Shaw RK, Freireich EJ. The central nervous system in acute leukemia: a postmortem study of 117 consecutive cases, with particular reference to hemorrhages, leukemic infiltrations, and the syndrome of meningeal leukemia. Arch Intern Med. 1960;105:451–68.
10. de Lima M, Strom SS, Keating M, Kantarjian H, Pierce S, et al. Implications of potential cure in acute myelogenous leukemia: development of subsequent cancer and return to work. Blood. 1997;90:4719–24.
11. Pui CH, Howard SC. Current management and challenges of malignant disease in the CNS in paediatric leukaemia. Lancet Oncol. 2008;9:257–68.
12. Hallek M. Chronic lymphocytic leukemia: 2015 update on diagnosis, risk stratification, and treatment. Am J Hematol. 2015;90:446–60.
13. Rozman C, Montserrat E. Chronic lymphocytic leukemia. N Engl J Med. 1995;333:1052–7.
14. Chiorazzi N, Rai KR, Ferrarini M. Chronic lymphocytic leukemia. N Engl J Med. 2005;352:804–15.
15. Eichhorst BF, Busch R, Hopfinger G, Pasold R, Hensel M, et al. Fludarabine plus cyclophosphamide versus fludarabine alone in first-line therapy of younger patients with chronic lymphocytic leukemia. Blood. 2006;107:885–91.
16. Hoglund M, Sandin F, Simonsson B. Epidemiology of chronic myeloid leukaemia: an update. Ann Hematol. 2015;94(Suppl 2): S241–7.
17. Druker BJ, Guilhot F, O'Brien SG, Gathmann I, Kantarjian H, et al. Five-year follow-up of patients receiving imatinib for chronic myeloid leukemia. N Engl J Med. 2006;355:2408–17.
18. Baccarani M, Deininger MW, Rosti G, Hochhaus A, Soverini S, et al. European Leukemia Net recommendations for the management of chronic myeloid leukemia. Blood. 2013;122:872–84.
19. National Comprehensive Cancer N. Clinical practice guidelines in oncology. Chronic myelogenous leukemia v. 2. Fort Washington, PA: nccn; 2010.
20. Bojsen-Moller M, Nielsen JL. CNS involvement in leukaemia. An autopsy study of 100 consecutive patients. Acta pathologica, microbiologica, et immunologica Scandinavica. Section A, Pathology 1983;91:209–16.
21. Cramer SC, Glaspy JA, Efird JT, Louis DN. Chronic lymphocytic leukemia and the central nervous system: a clinical and pathological study. Neurology. 1996;46:19–25.
22. Hoogerbrugge PM, Hagenbeek A. Leptomeningeal infiltration in rat models for human acute myelocytic and lymphocytic leukemia. Leuk Res. 1985;9:1397–404.

23. Reske-Nielsen E, Petersen JH, Sogaard H, Jensen KB. Letter: Leukaemia of the central nervous system. Lancet (London, England) 1974;1:211–2.

24. Azzarelli V, Roessmann U. Pathogenesis of central nervous system infiltration in acute leukemia. Arch Pathol Lab Med. 1977;101:203–5.

25. Gassas A, Krueger J, Alvi S, Sung L, Hitzler J, Lieberman L. Diagnosis of central nervous system relapse of pediatric acute lymphoblastic leukemia: Impact of routine cytological CSF analysis at the time of intrathecal chemotherapy. Pediatr Blood Cancer. 2014;61:2215–7.

26. Garicochea B, Cliquet MG, Melo N, del Giglio A, Dorlhiac-Llacer PE, Chamone DA. Leptomeningeal involvement in chronic lymphocytic leukemia identified by polymerase chain reaction in stored slides: a case report. Mod Pathol. 1997;10: 500–3.

27. Chamberlain MC, Sandy AD, Press GA. Leptomeningeal metastasis: a comparison of gadolinium-enhanced MR and contrast-enhanced CT of the brain. Neurology. 1990;40:435–8.

28. Weinstein HJTN. Leukemias and Lymphomas of Childhood. In: Lawrence TS, DeVita VT, Rosenberg SA, editors. Cancer. Principles and practice of oncology. Philadelphia: Lippincott-Raven; 1997: 2145–65.

29. Aur RJ, Hustu HO, Verzosa MS, Wood A, Simone JV. Comparison of two methods of preventing central nervous system leukemia. Blood. 1973;42:349–57.

30. Moricke A, Zimmermann M, Reiter A, Henze G, Schrauder A, et al. Long-term results of five consecutive trials in childhood acute lymphoblastic leukemia performed by the ALL-BFM study group from 1981 to 2000. Leukemia. 2010;24:265–84.

31. Pui CH, Campana D, Pei D, Bowman WP, Sandlund JT, et al. Treating childhood acute lymphoblastic leukemia without cranial irradiation. N Engl J Med. 2009;360:2730–41.

32. Loning L, Zimmermann M, Reiter A, Kaatsch P, Henze G, et al. Secondary neoplasms subsequent to Berlin-Frankfurt-Munster therapy of acute lymphoblastic leukemia in childhood: significantly lower risk without cranial radiotherapy. Blood. 2000;95:2770–5.

33. Veerman AJ, Kamps WA, van den Berg H, van den Berg E, Bokkerink JP, et al. Dexamethasone-based therapy for childhood acute lymphoblastic leukaemia: results of the prospective Dutch Childhood Oncology Group (DCOG) protocol ALL-9 (1997–2004). Lancet Oncol. 2009;10:957–66.

34. Stock W, Johnson JL, Stone RM, Kolitz JE, Powell BL, et al. Dose intensification of daunorubicin and cytarabine during treatment of adult acute lymphoblastic leukemia: results of Cancer and Leukemia Group B Study 19802. Cancer. 2013;119:90–8.

35. Kantarjian HM, O'Brien S, Smith TL, Cortes J, Giles FJ, et al. Results of treatment with hyper-CVAD, a dose-intensive regimen, in adult acute lymphocytic leukemia. J Clin Oncol Off J Am Soc Clin Oncol. 2000;18:547–61.

36. Sancho JM, Ribera JM, Oriol A, Hernandez-Rivas JM, Rivas C, et al. Central nervous system recurrence in adult patients with acute lymphoblastic leukemia: frequency and prognosis in 467 patients without cranial irradiation for prophylaxis. Cancer. 2006;106:2540–6.

37. Reman O, Pigneux A, Huguet F, Vey N, Delannoy A, et al. Central nervous system involvement in adult acute lymphoblastic leukemia at diagnosis and/or at first relapse: results from the GET-LALA group. Leuk Res. 2008;32:1741–50.

38. Lazarus HM, Richards SM, Chopra R, Litzow MR, Burnett AK, et al. Central nervous system involvement in adult acute lymphoblastic leukemia at diagnosis: results from the international ALL trial MRC UKALL XII/ECOG E2993. Blood. 2006;108:465–72.

39. Tomizawa D, Tabuchi K, Kinoshita A, Hanada R, Kigasawa H, et al. Repetitive cycles of high-dose cytarabine are effective for childhood acute myeloid leukemia: long-term outcome of the children with AML treated on two consecutive trials of Tokyo Children's Cancer Study Group. Pediatr Blood Cancer. 2007;49:127–32.

40. Liang DC, Chan TT, Lin KH, Lin DT, Lu MY, et al. Improved treatment results for childhood acute myeloid leukemia in Taiwan. Leukemia. 2006;20:136–41.

41. Gibson BE, Wheatley K, Hann IM, Stevens RF, Webb D, et al. Treatment strategy and long-term results in paediatric patients treated in consecutive UK AML trials. Leukemia. 2005;19:2130–8.

42. Woods WG, Kobrinsky N, Buckley J, Neudorf S, Sanders J, et al. Intensively timed induction therapy followed by autologous or allogeneic bone marrow transplantation for children with acute myeloid leukemia or myelodysplastic syndrome: a Childrens Cancer Group pilot study. J Clin Oncol. 1993;11:1448–57.

43. Abbott BL, Rubnitz JE, Tong X, Srivastava DK, Pui CH, et al. Clinical significance of central nervous system involvement at diagnosis of pediatric acute myeloid leukemia: a single institution's experience. Leukemia. 2003;17:2090–6.

44. Castagnola C, Nozza A, Corso A, Bernasconi C. The value of combination therapy in adult acute myeloid leukemia with central nervous system involvement. Haematologica. 1997;82:577–80.

45. Sanders KE, Ha CS, Cortes-Franco JE, Koller CA, Kantarjian HM, Cox JD. The role of craniospinal irradiation in adults with a central nervous system recurrence of leukemia. Cancer. 2004;100:2176–80.

46. Estey EH. Acute myeloid leukemia: 2012 update on diagnosis, risk stratification, and management. Am J Hematol. 2012;87:89–99.

47. Mayadev JS, Douglas JG, Storer BE, Appelbaum FR, Storb R. Impact of cranial irradiation added to intrathecal conditioning in hematopoietic cell transplantation in adult acute myeloid leukemia with central nervous system involvement. Int J Radiat Oncol Biol Phys. 2011;80:193–8.

48. Hanse MC, Van't Veer MB, van Lom K, van den Bent MJ. Incidence of central nervous system involvement in chronic lymphocytic leukemia and outcome to treatment. J Neurol 2008;255:828–30.

49. Moazzam AA, Drappatz J, Kim RY, Kesari S. Chronic lymphocytic leukemia with central nervous system involvement: report of two cases with a comprehensive literature review. J Neurooncol. 2012 Jan 1;106(1):185–200.

50. Mowatt L, Matthews T, Anderson I. Sustained visual recovery after treatment with intrathecal methotrexate in a case of optic neuropathy caused by chronic lymphocytic leukemia. J Neuro Ophthalmol. 2005;25:113–5.

51. Cash J, Fehir KM, Pollack MS. Meningeal involvement in early stage chronic lymphocytic leukemia. Cancer. 1987;59:798–800.

52. Altintas A, Cil T, Kilinc I, Kaplan MA, Ayyildiz O. Central nervous system blastic crisis in chronic myeloid leukemia on imatinib mesylate therapy: a case report. J Neurooncol. 2007;84:103–5.

53. Kim HJ, Jung CW, Kim K, Ahn JS, Kim WS, et al. Isolated blast crisis in CNS in a patient with chronic myelogenous leukemia maintaining major cytogenetic response after imatinib. J Clin Oncol. 2006;24:4028–9.

54. Saikia TK, Dhabhar B, Iyer RS, Nanjangud G, Gopal R, et al. High incidence of meningeal leukemia in lymphoid blast crisis of chronic myelogenous leukemia. Am J Hematol. 1993;43:10–3.

55. Wolff NC, Richardson JA, Egorin M, Ilaria RL Jr. The CNS is a sanctuary for leukemic cells in mice receiving imatinib mesylate for Bcr/Abl-induced leukemia. Blood. 2003;101:5010–3.

56. Lindhorst SM, Lopez RD, Sanders RD. An unusual presentation of chronic myelogenous leukemia: a review of isolated central nervous system relapse. J Natl Compr Cancer Netw JNCCN 2013;11:745–9 (quiz 50).

57. Aichberger KJ, Herndlhofer S, Agis H, Sperr WR, Esterbauer H, et al. Liposomal cytarabine for treatment of myeloid central nervous system relapse in chronic myeloid leukaemia occurring during imatinib therapy. Eur J Clin Invest. 2007;37:808–13.

58. Isobe Y, Sugimoto K, Masuda A, Hamano Y, Oshimi K. Central nervous system is a sanctuary site for chronic myelogenous leukaemia treated with imatinib mesylate. Intern Med J. 2009;39:408–11.

59. Inverardi D, Lazzarino M, Morra E, Bernasconi P, Merante S, et al. Extramedullary disease in Ph'-positive chronic myelogenous leukemia: frequency, clinical features and prognostic significance. Haematologica. 1990;75:146–8.

60. DA Loblow NL, WJ Mackillop. A population—based study of malignant spinal cord compression in Ontario. Clin Oncol. 2003;15:211–7.

61. Burns A. Head and neck. In: Observations of surgical anatomy. London; 1811: 364 pp.

62. Cervantes GC, Zuzan. Intracranial CNS manifestations of myeloid sarcoma in patients with acute myeloid leukemia: review of the literature and three case reports from the author's institution. J Clin Med. 2015;4:1102–12.

63. Baikaidi MCS, Tallman MS, Damon L, Walker A, Marcucci G, Sholi A, Morris GJ. 75-year-old Woman with thoracic spinal cord compression and chloroma (granulocytic sarcoma). Semin Oncol. 2012;39:37–46.

64. Binder CTM, Haase D, Humpe A, Kneba M. Isolated meningeal chloroma (granulocytic sarcoma)—a case report and review of literature. Ann Hematol. 2000;79:459–62.

65. O'Neill BPHT, Banks P, O'Fallon JR, Earle JD. Primary central nervous system lymphoma as a variant of Richter's syndrome in two patients with chronic lymphocytic leukemia. Cancer. 1989;64(6):1296–300.

66. Jellinger KRT. Involvement of the central nervous system in malignant lymphomas. Pathol Anat Histol. 1976;370:345–62.

67. Choo-Kang LRJD, Fehr JJ, Eskenazi AE, Toretsky JA. Cerebral edema and priapism in an adolescent with acute lymphoblastic leukemia. Pediatr Emerg Care. 1999;15:110–2.

68. Pineda AAVE. Applications of therapeutic apheresis in patients with malignant disease. Oncologist. 1997;2:94–103.

69. Noguchi T, Ikeda K, Yamamoto K, Ashiba A, Yoshida I, et al. Severe bleeding tendency caused by leukemic infiltration and destruction of vascular walls in chronic neutrophilic leukemia. Int J Hematol. 2001;74:437–41.

70. Quinn JADL. Neurologic emergencies in the cancer patient. Semin Oncol. 2000;27:311–21.

71. Graus FRL, Posner JB. Cerebrovascular complications in patients with cancer. Medicine (Baltimore). 1985;64:16–35.

72. Tj H. Autoimmune complications of chronic lymphocytic leukemia. Semin Oncol. 2006;33:230–9.

73. Enright HJH, Vercellotti G, et al. Paraneoplastic autoimmune phenomena in patients with myelodysplastic syndromes: response to immunosuppressive therapy. Br J Haematol. 1995;91:403–8.

74. Maverakis E, Goodarzi H, Wehrli LN, Ono Y, Garcia MS. The etiology of paraneoplastic autoimmunity. Clin Rev Allergy Immunol. 2012;42:135–44.

75. Isoda A, Sakurai A, Ogawa Y, Miyazawa Y, Saito A, et al. Chronic inflammatory demyelinating polyneuropathy accompanied by chronic myelomonocytic leukemia: possible pathogenesis

76. Hamblin TJ. Autoimmune complications of chronic lymphocytic leukemia. Semin Neurol. 2006;33:230–9.

77. Kaur S, Dhingra B, Singh V, Chandra J, Narula MK. Neurological paraneoplastic syndrome as presentation of leukemia. J Pediatr Hematol Oncol. 2013;35:e214–6.

78. DeVito N, Mui K, Jassam Y, Taylor L, Pilichowska M, Cossor F. Small lymphocytic lymphoma presenting as a paraneoplastic syndrome with acute central nervous system demyelination. Clin Lymphoma Myeloma Leuk. 2014;14:e131–5.

79. Kameda G, Vieker S, Duck C, Blaes F, Langler A. Paraneoplastic myopathy as a very rare manifestation of acute lymphoblastic leukemia. Klin Padiatr. 2010;222:386–7.

80. Alcantara M, Bennani O, Verdure P, Leprêtre S, Tilly H, Jardin F. Voltage-gated potassium channel antibody paraneoplastic limbic encephalitis associated with acute myeloid leukemia. Case Reports Oncol. 2013;6:289–92.

81. Mahoney DHJ, Shuster JJ, Nitschke R, Lauer SJ, Steuber CP, Winick N, et al. Acute neurotoxicity in children with B-precursor acute lymphoid leukemia: an association with intermediate-dose intravenous methotrexate and intrathecal triple therapy-a Pediatric Oncology Group study. J Clin Oncol. 1998;16:1712–22.

82. LE Damon MR, Linker CA. The association between high-dose cytarabine neurotoxicity and renal insufficiency. J Clin Oncol. 1989;7:1563–8.

83. Feinberg WMSM. Cerebrovascular complications of L-asparaginase therapy. Neurology. 1988;38:127–33.

84. Annaloro C, Costa A, Fracchiolla NS, Mometto G, Artuso S, et al. Severe fludarabine neurotoxicity after reduced intensity conditioning regimen to allogeneic hematopoietic stem cell transplantation: a case report. Clin Case Rep. 2015;3:650–5.

85. Beitinjaneh A, McKinney AM, Cao Q, Weisdorf DJ. Toxic leukoencephalopathy following fludarabine-associated hematopoietic cell transplantation. Biology Blood Marrow Trans J Am Soc Blood Marrow Trans. 2011;17:300–8.

86. Spriggs DR, Stopa E, Mayer RJ, Schoene W, Kufe DW. Fludarabine phosphate (NSC 312878) infusions for the treatment of acute leukemia: phase I and neuropathological study. Cancer Res. 1986;46:5953–8.

87. Butler RWHJ, Steinherz PG, Meyers PA, Finlay JL. Neuropsychologic effects of cranial irradiation, intrathecal methotrexate, and systemic methotrexate in childhood cancer. J Clin Oncol. 1994;12:2621–9.

88. Mulhern RKFD, Ochs J. A prospective comparison of neuropsychologic performance of children surviving leukemia who received 18-Gy, 24-Gy, or no cranial irradiation. J Clin Oncol. 1991;9:1348–56.

89. Lovblad KKP, Ozdoba C, Ramelli G, Remonda L, Schroth G. Pure methotrexate encephalopathy presenting with seizures: CT and MRI features. Pediatr Radiol. 1998;28:86–91.

90. TL Phillips. Early and late effect of radiation of normal tissues. In: Gutin PH, Leibel SA, Sheline GE, editors. Radiation injury to the nervous system. New York: Raven; 1991:37–55.

91. Darzy KHSA. Hypopituitarism following radiotherapy. Pituitary. 2009;12:40–50.

92. Crowne EC, Moore C, Wallace WH, Ogllvy-Stuart AL, Addison GM, Morris-Jones PH, Shalet SM. A novel variant of growth hormone (GH) insufficiency following low dose cranial irradiation. Clin Endocrinol 1992;36:59–68.

93. Neglia JPMA, Robison LL, Kim TH, Newton WA, Ruymann FB, et al. Second neoplasms after acute lymphoblastic leukemia in childhood. N Engl J Med. 1991;325:1330–6.

94. Walter AWHM, Pui CH, Hudson MM, Ochs JS, Rivera GK, et al. Secondary brain tumors in children treated for acute

of autoimmunity in myelodysplastic syndrome. Int J Hematol. 2009;90:239–42.

lymphoblastic leukemia at St Jude Children's Research Hospital. J Clin Oncol. 1998;16:3761–7.

95. Aksoy S, Harputluoglu H, Kilickap S, Dede DS, Dizdar O, et al. Rituximab-related viral infections in lymphoma patients. Leuk Lymphoma. 2007;48:1307–12.

96. Pruitt AA. Central nervous system infections in cancer patients. Semin Neurol. 2010;30:296–310.

97. DU Maschke M, Prumbaum M, Kastrup O, Turowski B, Schaefer UW, et al. Opportunistic CNS infection after bone marrow transplantation. Bone Marrow Transpl. 1999;23:1167–76.

98. Auberger J, Lass-Florl C, Ulmer H, Nogler-Semenitz E, Clausen J, et al. Significant alterations in the epidemiology and treatment outcome of invasive fungal infections in patients with hematological malignancies. Int J Hematol. 2008;88:508–15.

99. Pagano L, Fau Caira M, Candoni A, Offidani M, Fianchi L, Martino B, et al. The epidemiology of fungal infections in patients with hematologic malignancies: the SEIFEM-2004 study. Haematologica. 2006;91(8):1068–75.

100. Sasaki T, Mineta M Fau, Kobayashi K, Masakatsu A, Obata M. Zygomycotic invasion of the central nervous system. Jpn J Radiol. 2010;28(5):376–380.

101. Mattiuzzi G, Giles FJ. Management of intracranial fungal infections in patients with haematological malignancies. Br J Haematol. 2005;131(3):287–300.

102. Pappas PG, Rex JH, Sobel JD, Filler SG, Dismukes WE, et al. Guidelines for treatment of candidiasis. Clin Infect Dis. 2004;38:161–89.

103. Pagano LRP, Montillo M, Cenacchi A, Nosari A, Tonso A, et al. Localization of aspergillosis to the central nervous system among patients with acute leukemia: report of 14 cases. Gruppo Italiano Malattie Ematologiche dell'Adulto Infection Program. Clin Infect Dis. 1996;23:628–30.

104. Khoury HAD, Miller G, Goodnough L, Brown R, DiPersio J. Resolution of invasive central nervous system aspergillosis in a transplant recipient. Bone Marrow Transpl. 1997;20:179–80.

105. Al-Abdely HM, Alothman AF, Salman JA, Al-Musawi T, Almaslamani M, et al. Clinical practice guidelines for the treatment of invasive Aspergillus infections in adults in the middle east region: expert panel recommendations. J Infec Pub Health. 2014;7:20–31.

106. Caggiano G, Cantisani P, Rolli M, Gianfreda CD, Pizzolante M, Montagna MT. The importance of a proper aetiological diagnosis in the management of patients with invasive mycoses: a case report of a brain abscess by Scedosporium apiospermum. Mycopathologia. 2011;172:317–22.

107. Greenberg RNMK, van Burik JA, Raad I, Abzug MJ, Anstead G, et al. Posaconazole as salvage therapy for zygomycosis. Antimicrob Agents Chemother. 2006;50:126–33.

108. Avivi ICS, Kottaridis P, et al. Neurological complications following alemtuzumab-based reduced-inten- sity allogeneic transplantation. Bone Marrow Transpl. 2004;34:137–42.

109. Seeley WWMF, Holmes TM, et al. Post-transplant acute limbic encephalitis: clinical features and relationship to HHV6. Neurology. 2007;69:156–65.

110. Pruitt AA. CNS infections in patients with cancer. Continuum (Minneapolis, Minn.) 2012;18:384–405.

111. Hinchey JCC, Appignani B, Breen J, Pao L, Wang A, et al. A reversible posterior leukoencephalopathy syndrome. N Engl J Med. 1996;334:494–500.

112. Ma MBG, Pulliam J, Jezek D, Baumann RJ, Berger JR. CNS angiitis in graft vs host disease. Neurology. 2002;59:1994–7.

113. Padovan CS, Bise K, Hahn J, Sostak P, Holler E, et al. Angiitis of the central nervous system after allogeneic bone marrow transplantation? Stroke. 1999;30:1651–6.

114. Airas LPM, Roytta M, et al. Central nervous system immune reconstitution inflammatory syndrome (IRIS) after hematopoietic SCT. Bone Marrow Transpl. 2010;45:593–6.

115. Ingram PRHR, Leahy MF, Dyer JR. Cryptococcal immune reconstitution inflammatory syndrome following alemtuzumab therapy. Clin Infect Dis. 2007;44:e115–7.

116. Cesaro SBM, Pillon M, et al. Immune reconstitution complicated by CMV retinitis in a pediatric patient 1200 who underwent haploidentical CD34 selected hematopoietic stem cell transplant for acute lymphoblastic leukemia. Int J Hematol. 2008;88:145–8.

117. Milpied NVB, Parquet N, Garnier JL, Antoine C, Quartier P, et al. Humanized anti-CD20 monoclonal antibody (Rituximab) in post transplant B-lymphoproliferative disorder: a retrospective analysis on 32 patients. Ann Oncol. 2000;11:113–6.

Lakshmi Nayak and Christian Grommes

Introduction

Systemic lymphoma can affect any level of the nervous system, including the central (brain, spinal cord, meninges) or the peripheral (nerve root, plexus, peripheral nerve, neuromuscular junction, muscle) nervous system. Neurologic complications may result from direct invasion or compression of these structures, or indirect involvement via paraneoplastic syndromes. Vascular and infectious complications are additional examples of non-invasive involvement of the nervous system by lymphoma. Therapy-related complications as a result of chemotherapy, biologics, radiation, and stem cell transplant are covered in separate chapters (Chaps. 14–20) in this book.

This chapter will cover complications of non-Hodgkin's and Hodgkin's lymphoma (HL) and briefly discuss paraneoplastic syndromes associated with lymphoma as this topic is covered in detail in Chap. 13.

Complications Associated with Non-Hodgkin's Lymphoma (NHL)

Direct Complications of NHL

Epidemiology and Risk Factors

Systemic NHL can lead to involvement of the nervous system at the time of initial diagnosis, but more frequently at relapse. The central nervous system (CNS) is affected and the sole site of involvement in the majority of cases. The median time to development of CNS disease is less than a year, though for many can be within 6 months or less of initial treatment, which may be related to subclinical CNS disease at the time of initial diagnosis [1]. CNS relapse may occur as an isolated event or in conjunction with systemic relapse.

The risk of secondary CNS lymphoma varies depending on several factors with an overall incidence of 2–7% [1–5]. Risk factors associated for CNS involvement include the histologic subtype, site of disease, advanced disease, and rituximab use during initial treatment:

- Histologic subtypes: Patients with aggressive subtypes of NHL are at a higher risk of development of CNS involvement [2]. The incidence is up to 30–50% in Burkitt and lymphoblastic lymphoma, 5% in diffuse large B cell lymphoma (DLBCL), 2–4% in peripheral T cell lymphoma, and <5% in indolent lymphomas including mantle cell lymphoma [6–9]. Mycosis fungoides with large cell transformation has an increased risk of CNS relapse [10].
- Primary Site: An increased risk of CNS relapse is seen with lymphomatous involvement of the testes, orbit, and paranasal sinuses [4, 7, 11]. Intravascular lymphoma is also seen frequently in association with CNS disease in up to 40% of patients [12, 13]. Other sites with an increased risk of CNS involvement include kidneys, adrenal glands, breast, bone marrow (large cell involvement), and epidural disease [6].
- Other risk factors: These include age >60, performance status >1, advanced stage disease (stage III/IV), involvement of >1 extranodal site, high International Prognostic Index (IPI), or elevated serum lactate dehydrogenase level [2, 3].

Double-hit lymphomas (DHL) characterized by the presence of cytogenetic *MYC* and *BCL2* and/or *BCL6* rearrangements are associated with 4–7% risk of CNS involvement at diagnosis with a 3-year cumulative risk of CNS

L. Nayak (✉)
Department of Neuro-Oncology, Dana-Farber Cancer Institute, 450 Brookline Avenue, DA2120, Boston, MA 02215, USA
e-mail: lakshmi_nayak@dfci.harvard.edu

C. Grommes
Department of Neurology, Memorial Sloan Kettering Cancer Center, 1275 York Avenue, New York, NY 10065, USA
e-mail: grommesc@mskcc.org

© Springer International Publishing AG 2018
D. Schiff et al. (eds.), *Cancer Neurology in Clinical Practice*,
DOI 10.1007/978-3-319-57901-6_31

relapse at 13% [14–16]. DLBCL co-expressing *MYC/BCL2*, or those that are CD5 positive have a propensity for developing CNS relapse [16, 17].

The impact of rituximab on CNS relapse is unclear. Several studies have shown that addition of rituximab to first-line chemotherapy treatment of NHL reduces the incidence of CNS relapses [18–21]. Other studies indicate no difference in relapse rates with rituximab [22–24].

Central Nervous System Involvement

CNS involvement from systemic NHL can involve the brain, spinal cord, leptomeninges, or dura in isolation or in combination. Signs and symptoms are based on the site of NHL in the CNS. Patients typically present with acute or subacute development of symptoms. Brain and spine MRI help to identify lesions and extent of disease in the CNS. This is followed by lumbar puncture for CSF and/or brain biopsy to confirm diagnosis. It is important to evaluate the presence of co-existing systemic disease by body CT and/or PET in addition to bone marrow biopsy if needed. Treatment options include systemic and/or intrathecal chemotherapy, high-dose chemotherapy, and autologous stem cell transplant and radiation. The overall prognosis is poor.

Leptomeningeal Metastases

Incidence and Clinical Features

Leptomeningeal metastases or lymphomatous meningitis is the most common CNS complication of NHL occurring in 6–8% of NHL patients [25]. Conversely, the primary cancer in 11–24% of patients with leptomeningeal metastases is lymphoma [26, 27] Patients often present with cranial nerve palsies, seen in up to 80% of patients [28]. One or multiple cranial nerves may be involved. There is a predilection for cranial nerves II, III, V, VI, and VII, although virtually any cranial nerve may be affected. Other symptoms such as radiculopathies, pain, focal motor or sensory symptoms, gait imbalance, mental status changes, or seizures may occur [25, 29]. Leptomeningeal disease may lead to hydrocephalus and raised intracranial pressure with the resulting symptoms of headaches, nausea, vomiting, visual obscurations and depressed level of consciousness. About one-fourth of patients with leptomeningeal disease may have concurrent brain metastases [30].

Diagnosis

Brain and spine MRI with and without gadolinium is recommended to all patients suspected with CNS involvement of NHL, although the sensitivity of imaging in hematologic malignancies is only about 50% [31]. Subarachnoid nodular enhancement involving the cauda equina and lumbosacral nerve roots, enhancement of the cerebellar folia, basal

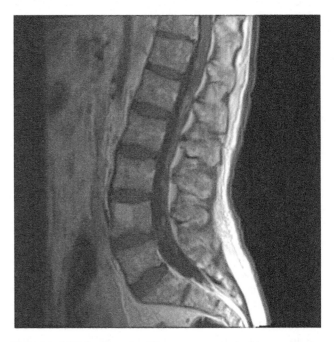

Fig. 31.1 MRI lumbar spine T1 post-contrast sagittal image showing leptomeningeal enhancement of the cauda equina and lumbosacral nerve roots in a 74-year-old man with a transformed follicular lymphoma, presenting with headaches, tinnitus, diplopia, and radicular pain in the right leg. CSF studies confirmed involvement by lymphoma

cisterns, or cranial nerves may be seen (Fig. 31.1). Hydrocephalus may also be noted. CT and PET scans are not ideal imaging modalities to diagnosis leptomeningeal metastases. It is important to obtain MRI before lumbar puncture for CSF studies as the procedure may lead to intracranial hypotension and associated pachymeningeal enhancement, which may mimic leptomeningeal enhancement particularly in the spine [32]. CSF studies suggestive of leptomeningeal metastases include elevated protein and white cells, and low glucose. CSF beta-2 microglobulin and lactate dehydrogenase may also be elevated. CSF cytology for identification of malignant cells is the definitive diagnostic test, although the sensitivity may be as low as 50% on the first lumbar puncture increasing to 90% on the 3rd lumbar puncture [33–35]. Other CSF studies helpful in making the diagnosis include flow cytometry and polymerase chain reaction (PCR) amplification of IgH gene or T-cell receptor [36].

Treatment

Intrathecal chemotherapy is often used to treat leptomeningeal metastases from hematologic malignancies as it is relatively well tolerated, particularly in those with normal intracranial pressure with no evidence of bulky disease or CSF outflow obstruction. Oncologists prefer to use intrathecal chemotherapy when patients have concurrent systemic disease as it can be easily combined with the systemic chemotherapy. An ommaya reservoir may be placed surgically for easier drug administration. Methotrexate and cytarabine separately or in combination with hydrocortisone may be used intrathecally. Liposomal cytarabine allows for a longer interval between treatments (every 2 weeks) and possibly a better response [37]. Intrathecal rituximab with or without liposomal cytarabine has also been tried [38]. Toxicity associated with intrathecal chemotherapy may include chemical meningitis, acute or subacute encephalopathy, and hydrocephalus.

Systemic chemotherapy with high-dose methotrexate and cytarabine is considered for bulky disease [39, 40]. Other agents such as nitrosoureas and thiotepa have been used. Often, systemic chemotherapy is used in combination with intrathecal chemotherapy.

While patients may respond to the above treatment, the risk of recurrence is very high and high-dose chemotherapy followed by autologous stem cell rescue should be considered for young patients with chemosensitive disease [41–44].

Whole brain radiation has been used before or after chemotherapy in the treatment of leptomeningeal metastases. There is a significant risk of neurotoxicity from the combination of chemotherapy and radiation [45], and so it is usually reserved for palliation and/or refractory disease. Cauda and lower nerve root or base of skull involvement can be treated with focal radiation particularly in patients not responding to chemotherapy or for palliation of symptoms.

Brain Metastases

Incidence and Clinical Features

Prior studies have shown that parenchymal or brain metastases are less common than leptomeningeal metastases from NHL, accounting for 16% of CNS involvement. However, more recent studies have demonstrated that 50–75% of the patients with CNS involvement develop brain relapse only [18–20, 46]. Signs and symptoms may be focal or generalized depending on the site and number of lesions. Patients may develop progressive focal motor or sensory symptoms, gait abnormalities, mental status changes, or symptoms and signs of raised intracranial pressure. Cranial nerve deficits are often seen. Seizures and headaches are less common, but can occur. Involvement of the brain by intravascular lymphoma can lead to strokes.

Diagnosis

Gadolinium-enhanced MRI of the brain is the optimal imaging for the CNS. Brain metastases can occur anywhere within the brain and appear as single or multiple, homogenously enhancing lesions on T1 post-contrast sequences of MRI. See Fig. 31.2a, b. There is associated surrounding edema as evidenced by T2 hyperintensity. The appearance is radiographically similar to primary CNS lymphoma (PCNSL) with a common site being deep gray matter. The differential includes primary brain malignancy such as glioma or other neurologic disorders, such as infectious, vascular, inflammatory, demyelinating, or autoimmune conditions. Diagnosis is made by evaluation of CSF or by brain biopsy for pathologic confirmation.

Treatment

Systemic chemotherapy with high-dose methotrexate (HD-MTX) is the standard treatment for lymphoma in the brain parenchyma [47–49]. This is associated with high response rates that are typically not durable. Addition of high-dose

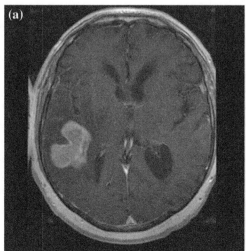 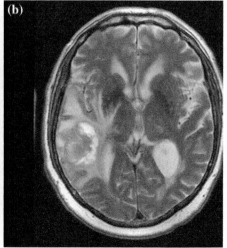

Fig. 31.2 MRI brain T1 post-contrast (**a**) and T2 axial (**b**) images showing contrast-enhancing right parietal lesion with surrounding T2 changes and mass effect in a 78-year-old man with testicular lymphoma treated with chemotherapy and CNS prophylaxis with intrathecal methotrexate, presenting 3 years later with cognitive impairment and Left leg weakness. Brain biopsy confirmed diagnosis of lymphoma

cytarabine and rituximab, which are used in treatment of PCNSL, may be considered [50, 51]. Some studies have combined HD-MTX with ifosfamide or procarbazine. More recently, studies with high-dose chemotherapy followed by autologous stem cell rescue have shown improved survival in patients with CNS involvement by NHL [41–44]. Intrathecal chemotherapy may be considered in combination with systemic chemotherapy especially in patients with CSF involvement, but by itself it is not recommended due to inadequate brain penetration. Radiation is typically used for palliative treatment in secondary CNS lymphoma, particularly in those who do not respond to or are not candidates for systemic chemotherapy. Whole brain radiation may be considered for brain involvement. Involved field radiation is typically not recommended in CNS lymphoma due to its invasiveness and extent of disease, but may be considered for palliation and symptom management. While craniospinal radiation would treat the full extent of disease particularly in leptomeningeal metastases or disease with brain and spinal cord involvement, it is associated with significant morbidity including neurologic side effects, fatigue, and bone marrow toxicity.

Corticosteroids can help with symptom management by reducing tumor burden and associated edema. They also have direct lymphocytolytic effects, and so should be held prior to obtaining pathologic diagnosis.

Spinal Cord Metastases

Incidence and Clinical Features
Intramedullary spinal cord metastases from NHL are rare [52]. Often, spinal cord involvement is a result of epidural disease or in conjunction with leptomeningeal metastases. Patients may present with signs and symptoms of a myelopathy such as weakness, sensory level, spasticity, and bladder/bowel dysfunction. Spinal cord lesions may be present at multiple levels.

Diagnosis
Total spine MRI with and without gadolinium contrast is optimal for evaluation of spinal cord metastases, which typically show intramedullary contrast-enhancing lesions with associated cord edema. There may be involvement of the cauda equina associated with intradural lesions or leptomeningeal enhancement along the cord and nerve roots. Spinal cord biopsies are typically not performed due to the risk of permanent neurologic deficits and reserved for cases in which CSF is negative and the clinical and radiographic picture are not suggestive of lymphoma.

Treatment
For acute onset and progressive myelopathy, corticosteroids are helpful with symptom management, followed by focal radiation. Chemotherapy is considered when neurologic symptoms are mild.

Dural and Epidural Metastases

Incidence and Clinical Features
Dural and epidural metastases typically occur in the spine as a result of vertebral body, intervertebral foramina or paraspinal muscle involvement of NHL [52]. Patients typically present with signs and symptoms of cord compression or cauda equina syndrome depending on the location in the spine. Patients may present with back pain or weakness. Back pain in a patient with systemic NHL particularly with known bony involvement should raise the suspicion for epidural spinal cord compression.

Dural metastases in the brain are less common and cause symptoms from compression of the brain and mass effect. Patients may present with headache, seizures, or focal deficits based on the location and size of the lesion.

Diagnosis
Spine and brain MRI are useful for diagnosis. Occasionally, leptomeningeal metastases may also be present. Biopsy may be considered in patients without a known diagnosis of NHL.

Treatment
Cord compression is a neurosurgical emergency, and surgery and decompression may be necessary in unstable cases. High-dose corticosteroids, such as dexamethasone, are used for acute management. NHL is radiosensitive and in patients with a known diagnosis emergent radiation is preferred. Chemotherapy is typically not preferred in patients with cord compression as neurologic and radiographic response is slower than with radiation.

Peripheral Nervous System Involvement

Plexopathy

Clinical Features
Direct compression or infiltration by NHL can lead to plexopathies. Symptoms include severe pain in addition to weakness and sensory loss in the distribution of the involved levels of the plexus. The differential includes radiation induced plexopathy and paraneoplastic plexopathy, both which may be seen as indirect complications of NHL. The distinguishing feature is pain, which typically indicates lymphomatous plexopathy.

Diagnosis
Imaging with MRI demonstrates enhancement of the involved plexus (Fig. 31.3). Rarely, biopsy is employed for diagnosis.

Fig. 31.3 MRI brachial plexus T1 post-contrast coronal image showing contrast enhancement of the right brachial plexus in a 26-year-old man with an aggressive double-hit lymphoma presenting with right arm pain and weakness associated with atrophy

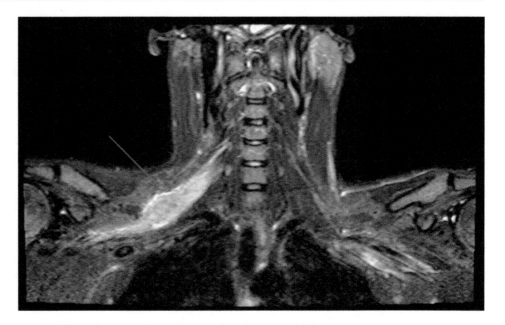

Treatment

Focal radiation or chemotherapy is used for treatment of lymphomatous plexopathy. Radiation also helps with quicker pain relief.

Peripheral Neuropathy

Clinical Features

Neurolymphomatosis or lymphomatous involvement of nerve roots and peripheral nerves is a rare complication of NHL [53, 54]. Patients typically present with a painful peripheral neuropathy or radiculopathy. Mononeuropathies of the sciatic, median or radial nerves may be seen. Occasional cranial nerves are also involved. Motor or sensory nerves can be involved. This may also be seen in association with plexopathies. Pain is absent in 25–50% of the cases.

Diagnosis

PET imaging is helpful in diagnosis of neurolymphomatosis. The involved areas show increased uptake. MRI is also useful when the involved segment of nerve is imaged.

Treatment

Chemotherapy and focal radiation are the modalities of treatment.

Chemotherapy-induced and paraneoplastic peripheral neuropathy are described in detail in other chapters.

Myopathy

Lymphomatous involvement of the muscle is rare. The most common form of muscle involvement in NHL is related to corticosteroid induced proximal myopathy, which is discussed in Chap. 19. The muscle (dermatomyositis and polymyositis) and neuromuscular junction may be involved in paraneoplastic syndromes from NHL (later in this chapter and reviewed in Chap. 13 in detail).

Central Nervous System Prophylaxis

The issue of CNS prophylaxis in NHL is controversial. There is minimal consensus with regards to which patients should be treated, the optimal treatment, and the timing of treatment due to lack of adequate evidence to date [6, 55]. In general, patients with aggressive histologic subtypes, such as Burkitt's and lymphoblastic lymphoma and intravascular lymphoma, should certainly undergo frontline therapies with CNS-directed treatment. Others associated with risk factors as outlined earlier in this chapter should undergo baseline evaluation for evidence of CNS disease at initial diagnosis and be considered for CNS prophylaxis. Systemic high-dose methotrexate and high-dose cytarabine with or without intrathecal methotrexate are utilized to reduce the risk of CNS relapse in high-risk patients [56, 57].

Indirect Complications of NHL

Paraneoplastic Syndromes

Classic paraneoplastic neurologic syndromes are rare in lymphomas and different from those seen in association with solid tumors. The incidence of paraneoplastic syndromes is higher in HL, and the type and frequency differ between NHL and HL [58]. Onconeural antibodies are often absent except with paraneoplastic cerebellar degeneration (more common in HL). Dermatomyositis, polymyositis, and sensorimotor neuropathies are seen in association with NHL. Brainstem and limbic encephalitis, neuromyotonia, and motor neuron disease have also been reported [58, 59]. A detailed description of paraneoplastic neurologic syndrome is available in Chap. 13.

Vascular Complications: Intravascular Lymphoma

Clinical Features

Intravascular lymphoma, previously known as angiotropic lymphoma, is a rare and aggressive extranodal DLBCL characterized by lymphoma cells within the vascular lumen, particularly capillaries. It can involve any organ; the skin and the CNS being the most common sites [12]. CNS involvement occurs in up to 40% of the cases. Clinical presentation includes fever, cutaneous lesions, neurologic symptoms, pain, and fatigue. In the nervous system, signs and symptoms are related to ischemic events from occlusion of small arteries by malignant cells. Neurologic presentation can be varied, in the form of acute focal neurologic deficits, subacute encephalopathy, myelopathy, polyneuropathy, mononeuritis multiplex, or myopathy. CNS and skin involvement is uncommon in the hemophagocytosis variant of intravascular lymphoma reported in Japanese patients.

Diagnosis

Brain MRI demonstrates T2 hyperintense lesions with restricted diffusion. The lesions may or may not on enhance on administration of gadolinium contrast. Cerebral angiography may show occlusions of medium or small vessels. Skin biopsy or occasionally bone marrow biopsy may be diagnostic. Occasionally, brain biopsy may be necessary.

Treatment

The overall prognosis is poor, and prompt diagnosis followed by rapid institution of treatment is of importance to prevent widespread progressive disease. Treatment involves addition of high-dose methotrexate and rituximab to systemic anthracycline-based regimens. High-dose chemotherapy followed by autologous stem cell rescue should be considered in younger patients for improved relapse-free rates.

Treatment-Related Complications

Neurologic complications can result from the various treatment modalities for NHL including chemotherapy, radiation, autologous stem cell transplant, and allogeneic transplant. Please refer to Chaps. 14–20 for specific treatment-related complications.

Complications Associated with Hodgkin's Lymphoma

Direct Involvement of the Central Nervous System

Brain Metastases

Incidence and Clinical Features

Parenchymal metastases are less common in HL than in other lymphomas with an incidence rate of only 0.2–0.5% [60–62]. Women and men are equally affected [63]. No specific risk factors have been identified for intracranial HL disease [64], but a role of Epstein Barr virus infections has been suggested [65, 66]. Hematogenous dissemination is the most common route for spread to the brain. HL brain metastases are almost exclusively found in patients with advanced and/or refractory disease but may also be present at diagnosis. Very rarely, the brain can be the sole site of disease (primary CNS HL) [65]. Clinical signs and symptoms depend on the location of the parenchymal metastases and include cranial neuropathies (55%), headache (36%), weakness (35%), papilledema (19%), nausea and vomiting (17%), memory problems (17%), seizures (14%), and gait difficulties (5%) [67]. B symptoms, including weight loss, night sweat, and fevers, are uncommon in patients with CNS involvement and only present with concomitant systemic disease.

Diagnosis

Usually, HL presents as solitary brain metastatic lesions within the subcortical and periventricular white matter, with well circumscribed contrast-enhanced lesions on MRI and multiple lesions are uncommon. Metastases are found mainly in the brain parenchyma (67%), dura (19%) and pituitary gland (3%) [67]. Dural lesions may have the radiological appearance of a meningioma [68] and should raise suspicion in a patient with HL. Brain biopsy or evaluation of CSF may be performed for confirmation of diagnosis.

Treatment

Due to its rarity and the lack of prospective clinical trials, treatment options are not well established. Surgery, radiation (whole brain radiation or stereotactic focal radiation), and several different chemotherapeutic regimens (MVPP:

mustine, vinblastine, vincristine, bleomycin, etoposide, prednisone; Stanford V: mechlorethamine, doxorubicin, vinblastine, vincristine, bleomycin, etoposide, prednisone; ABVD: doxorubicin, bleomycin, vinblastine, dacarbazine; IVAC: if osphamide, etoposide, and high-dose cytarabine [63]) have been used. There seems to be an improved response rate and survival in early diagnosed and aggressively treated patients who received combination radiochemotherapy [61, 63]. CNS prophylaxis is not routinely recommended in HL [61].

Spinal Metastases

Incidence and Clinical Features

The spine can be affected by HL through intramedullary metastases or epidural involvement. Intramedullary involvement is extremely rare and arises from hematogenous spread or by centripetal tumor growth along spinal nerve roots with secondary invasion of the spinal cord [69, 70]. Epidural HL is more common and estimated to be found in 0.2–5% of cases [69]. As with brain metastases, epidural disease is mainly seen in patients with advanced disease. The mixed cellularity histology seems to have a higher predilection for development of epidural compression [71] and the thoracic spinal cord is most commonly affected site of the spinal cord. Epidural HL is typically diagnosed in the setting of preexisting extranodal disease [72]. Clinical signs of spinal involvement and cord compression are not unique to HL and include back pain, weakness, sensory level, autonomic dysfunction (painless urinary retention, fecal incontinence, and impotence), and ataxia.

Diagnosis

Radiographic evaluation by spine MRI with and without gadolinium is optimal, followed by CSF or tissue analysis, although spinal cord biopsy is rarely performed.

Treatment

Spinal HL responds well to radiation and/or chemotherapy. Surgery is reserved for patients with spinal instability and progressive neurologic deficits [73]. The degree of motor deficits remains the single most important prognostic factor for outcome and recovery of function after treatment.

Leptomeningeal Disease

Incidence and Clinical Features

Although lymphomatous involvement of the leptomeninges is very rare in HL, it can develop at any time during the course of disease [74, 75]. Leptomeningeal disease usually affects the base of the skull and conus medullaris, resulting in the development of global cerebral dysfunction and multiple cranial neuropathies.

Diagnosis

Cerebrospinal fluid (CSF) studies generally reveal elevated protein and lymphocytic pleocytosis. The identification of Reed-Sternberg cells in the CSF cytology is a definitive indicator of HL-related leptomeningeal metastases [76]. Additionally, if eosinophilic pleocytosis is identified, one should consider HL-related leptomeningeal metastases [74].

Treatment

No standard treatment exists for HL-related leptomeningeal disease, but intrathecal chemotherapy may play a role in these patients. If untreated, patients die from their disease within weeks to months.

Indirect Effects on the Central Nervous System

Many of the indirect effects of HL are similar for both HL and NHL. The indirect effects preferentially found in HL are described in the following section.

Vascular Complications: Primary Angiitis of the CNS

Clinical Features

HL has been associated with a rare non-infectious granulomatous angiitis affecting exclusively the small vessels of the brain and spinal cord [77–79]. Primary angiitis of the CNS was first described by Cravioto and Feigin in 1959 [80] and its pathogenesis has not been well established but associations with hypersensitivity, autoimmune reactions, and viral infections have been suggested [77, 81]. Neurologic signs and symptoms are the main clinical findings as the lack of changes in extracranial vessels leads to a paucity of systemic symptoms. Depending of the site of CNS involvement, the patients can develop headaches, encephalopathy, seizures, confusion, focal stroke-like deficits, and multifocal infarcts [82]. The rarely occurring spinal lesions can manifest as cord compression or transverse myelitis.

Diagnosis

The diagnosis of primary angiitis of the CNS and HL is often made simultaneously or closely correlated in time [77]. The diagnosis is challenging because there exist no specific findings on MRI, CSF analysis, or cerebral angiography; in fact, these results can appear normal [83]. One should be suspicious of this entity if the cerebral angiography identifies multifocal and segmental narrowing of blood vessels, or microaneurysm formation. Ultimately, the diagnosis requires a biopsy of the leptomeninges or brain parenchyma demonstrating focal and segmental non-necrotizing granulomatous inflammation of small vessels. Other conditions associated with primary angiitis of the CNS include herpes zoster, HIV, and Sjögren syndrome.

Treatment

No evidence-based treatment strategies are available for the treatment of primary angiitis of the CNS associated with HL, but the combination of corticosteroids and immunosuppression with specific treatment of HL should be initiated. Unfortunately, results are usually disappointing.

Infectious Complications

Patients with HL are at a higher risk for opportunistic infections of the CNS. HL associated alteration of cell-mediated immunity through functional and quantitative deficits of CD4+ T-cells weaken the patient's ability to withstand microorganisms. Additionally, suppressed immunity in the setting of staging splenectomy in combination with chemotherapy or radiotherapy further increases the risk of infection. Therefore, both the incidence and severity of infections are increased in HL patients and can lead to life threatening illnesses of the CNS. These infections range from fungal and protozoan pathogens, including Cryptococcus neoformans and toxoplasma gondii, to common bacterial (Listeria meningitis; brain abscess with Nocardia asteroides) and viral agents, particularly the herpes and papova groups of viruses [84, 85]. Zoster can occur at any time during the course of HL and account for 25% of infection in HL patients [84]. Disease can be disseminated in up to 20% of cases. The most common neurologic complications include encephalitis/meningitis, shingles (thoracic > lumbar > cervical dermatome), and post-herpetic neuralgia [86].

One of the most severe CNS infections observed in HL patients is progressive multifocal leukoencephalopathy (PML) caused by the papovavirus John Cunningham virus (JC virus). This virus is widely distributed in humans by late childhood but rarely cause CNS pathology in normal hosts. In immunocompromised HL patients, the JC virus can have devastating effects. Patients affected by PML develop variable clinical presentation which can include progressive weakness, encephalopathy, headaches, visual changes, dysarthria, and ataxia [87]. On imaging, multiple confluent perivascular white matter changes that are hyperintense on T2/FLAIR sequences can be observed [88]. The ultimate diagnosis can be achieved by the identification of JC virus through viral PCR in the CSF or biopsy material. Before 1990, most PML cases occurred among persons with Hodgkin disease, whereas in recent years, with the development of purine analogs, hematopoietic stem cell transplantation procedures, and rituximab, most PML cases occur among non–HIV-infected persons with NHL or chronic lymphocytic leukemia [89].

Paraneoplastic Syndromes

Paraneoplastic syndromes occur in 1–5% of patients with HL [90]. HL is mainly associated with subacute cerebellar degeneration (Anti-Yo, Anti-Tr), limbic encephalitis (Anti-Hu), subacute necrotic neuropathy and chronic motor neuropathy [91–93]. The CSF in these patients can be abnormal in early stages, displaying a mild pleocytosis and an increase in the total protein value [94]. Paraneoplastic syndromes and clinical signs can develop prior to a cancer diagnosis and should trigger a thorough work-up for malignancy. For a more detailed overview and description of paraneoplastic syndromes, see Chap. 13.

Conclusion

Lymphoma can affect the nervous system at any level both directly and indirectly. Direct invasion or compression of brain, spinal cord, or meninges can result in numerous nervous system complications. Indirectly lymphoma can result in several paraneoplastic syndromes and affect the CNS by increasing risk of infectious and vascular complications. A thorough understanding of how lymphoma affects the nervous system can aid in the identification of complications and implementation of therapy when appropriate.

References

1. Bernstein SH, Unger JM, Leblanc M, Friedberg J, Miller TP, Fisher RI. Natural history of CNS relapse in patients with aggressive non-Hodgkin's lymphoma: a 20-year follow-up analysis of SWOG 8516—the Southwest Oncology Group. J Clin Oncol. 2009;27(1):114–9.
2. Hollender A, Kvaloy S, Nome O, Skovlund E, Lote K, Holte H. Central nervous system involvement following diagnosis of non-Hodgkin's lymphoma: a risk model. Ann Oncol. 2002;13(7):1099–107.
3. van Besien K, Ha CS, Murphy S, et al. Risk factors, treatment, and outcome of central nervous system recurrence in adults with intermediate-grade and immunoblastic lymphoma. Blood. 1998;91(4):1178–84.
4. Boehme V, Zeynalova S, Kloess M, et al. Incidence and risk factors of central nervous system recurrence in aggressive lymphoma–a survey of 1693 patients treated in protocols of the German High-Grade Non-Hodgkin's Lymphoma Study Group (DSHNHL). Ann Oncol. 2007;18(1):149–57.
5. Tomita N, Yokoyama M, Yamamoto W, et al. Central nervous system event in patients with diffuse large B-cell lymphoma in the rituximab era. Cancer Sci. 2012;103(2):245–51.

6. Cheah CY, Seymour JF. Central nervous system prophylaxis in non-Hodgkin lymphoma: who, what, and when? Curr Oncol Rep. 2015;17(6):25.

7. Hill QA, Owen RG. CNS prophylaxis in lymphoma: who to target and what therapy to use. Blood Rev. 2006;20(6):319–32.

8. Pro B, Perini G. Central nervous system prophylaxis in peripheral T-cell lymphoma. Blood. 2010;115(26):5427.

9. Oinonen R, Franssila K, Elonen E. Central nervous system involvement in patients with mantle cell lymphoma. Ann Hematol. 1999;78(3):145–9.

10. Vu BA, Duvic M. Central nervous system involvement in patients with mycosis fungoides and cutaneous large-cell transformation. J Am Acad Dermatol. 2008;59(2 Suppl 1):S16–22.

11. Zucca E, Conconi A, Mughal TI, et al. Patterns of outcome and prognostic factors in primary large-cell lymphoma of the test is in a survey by the international Extranodal Lymphoma study group. J Clin Oncol. 2003;21(1):20–7.

12. Ferreri AJ, Campo E, Seymour JF, et al. Intravascular lymphoma: clinical presentation, natural history, management and prognostic factors in a series of 38 cases, with special emphasis on the 'cutaneous variant'. Br J Haematol. 2004;127(2):173–83.

13. Shimada K, Murase T, Matsue K, et al. Central nervous system involvement in intravascular large B-cell lymphoma: a retrospective analysis of 109 patients. Cancer Sci. 2010;101(6):1480–6.

14. Oki Y, Noorani M, Lin P, et al. Double hit lymphoma: the MD Anderson cancer center clinical experience. Br J Haematol. 2014;166(6):891–901.

15. Petrich AM, Gandhi M, Jovanovic B, et al. Impact of induction regimen and stem cell transplantation on outcomes in double-hit lymphoma: a multicenter retrospective analysis. Blood. 2014;124(15):2354–61.

16. Cheah CY, Oki Y, Westin JR, Turturro F. A clinician's guide to double hit lymphomas. Br J Haematol. 2015;168(6):784–95.

17. Miyazaki K, Yamaguchi M, Suzuki R, et al. CD5-positive diffuse large B-cell lymphoma: a retrospective study in 337 patients treated by chemotherapy with or without rituximab. Ann Oncol. 2011;22(7):1601–7.

18. Boehme V, Schmitz N, Zeynalova S, Loeffler M, Pfreundschuh M. CNS events in elderly patients with aggressive lymphoma treated with modern chemotherapy (CHOP-14) with or without rituximab: an analysis of patients treated in the RICOVER-60 trial of the German High-Grade Non-Hodgkin Lymphoma Study Group (DSHNHL). Blood. 2009;113(17):3896–902.

19. Shimazu Y, Notohara K, Ueda Y. Diffuse large B-cell lymphoma with central nervous system relapse: prognosis and risk factors according to retrospective analysis from a single-center experience. Int J Hematol. 2009;89(5):577–83.

20. Villa D, Connors JM, Shenkier TN, Gascoyne RD, Sehn LH, Savage KJ. Incidence and risk factors for central nervous system relapse in patients with diffuse large B-cell lymphoma: the impact of the addition of rituximab to CHOP chemotherapy. Ann Oncol. 2010;21(5):1046–52.

21. Mitrovic Z, Bast M, Bierman PJ, et al. The addition of rituximab reduces the incidence of secondary central nervous system involvement in patients with diffuse large B-cell lymphoma. Br J Haematol. 2012;157(3):401–3.

22. Feugier P, Virion JM, Tilly H, et al. Incidence and risk factors for central nervous system occurrence in elderly patients with diffuse large-B-cell lymphoma: influence of rituximab. Ann Oncol. 2004;15(1):129–33.

23. Yamamoto W, Tomita N, Watanabe R, et al. Central nervous system involvement in diffuse large B-cell lymphoma. Eur J Haematol. 2010;85(1):6–10.

24. Tai WM, Chung J, Tang PL, et al. Central nervous system (CNS) relapse in diffuse large B cell lymphoma (DLBCL): pre- and post-rituximab. Ann Hematol. 2011;90(7):809–18.

25. Mead GM, Kennedy P, Smith JL, et al. Involvement of the central nervous system by non-Hodgkin's lymphoma in adults. A review of 36 cases. Q J Med. 1986;60(231):699–714.

26. Clarke JL, Perez HR, Jacks LM, Panageas KS, Deangelis LM. Leptomeningeal metastases in the MRI era. Neurology. 2010;74(18):1449–54.

27. Kaplan JG, DeSouza TG, Farkash A, et al. Leptomeningeal metastases: comparison of clinical features and laboratory data of solid tumors, lymphomas and leukemias. J Neurooncol. 1990;9(3):225–9.

28. Hoerni-Simon G, Suchaud JP, Eghbali H, Coindre JM, Hoerni B. Secondary involvement of the central nervous system in malignant non-Hodgkin's lymphoma. A study of 30 cases in a series of 498 patients. Oncology. 1987;44(2):98–101.

29. Yoshida S, Morii K, Watanabe M, Saito T. Characteristic features of malignant lymphoma with central nervous system involvement. Surg Neurol. 2000;53(2):163–7.

30. Ferreri AJ, Assanelli A, Crocchiolo R, Ciceri F. Central nervous system dissemination in immunocompetent patients with aggressive lymphomas: incidence, risk factors and therapeutic options. Hematol Oncol. 2009;27(2):61–70.

31. Freilich RJ, Krol G, DeAngelis LM. Neuroimaging and cerebrospinal fluid cytology in the diagnosis of leptomeningeal metastasis. Ann Neurol. 1995;38(1):51–7.

32. Chamberlain MC, Glantz M, Groves MD, Wilson WH. Diagnostic tools for neoplastic meningitis: detecting disease, identifying patient risk, and determining benefit of treatment. Semin Oncol. 2009;36(4 Suppl 2):S35–45.

33. Glantz MJ, Cole BF, Glantz LK, et al. Cerebrospinal fluid cytology in patients with cancer: minimizing false-negative results. Cancer. 1998;82(4):733–9.

34. Glass JP, Melamed M, Chernik NL, Posner JB. Malignant cells in cerebrospinal fluid (CSF): the meaning of a positive CSF cytology. Neurology. 1979;29(10):1369–75.

35. Wasserstrom WR, Glass JP, Posner JB. Diagnosis and treatment of leptomeningeal metastases from solid tumors: experience with 90 patients. Cancer. 1982;49(4):759–72.

36. Bromberg JE, Breems DA, Kraan J, et al. CSF flow cytometry greatly improves diagnostic accuracy in CNS hematologic malignancies. Neurology. 2007;68(20):1674–9.

37. Glantz MJ, LaFollette S, Jaeckle KA, et al. Randomized trial of a slow-release versus a standard formulation of cytarabine for the intrathecal treatment of lymphomatous meningitis. J Clin Oncol. 1999;17(10):3110–6.

38. Rubenstein JL, Li J, Chen L, et al. Multicenter phase 1 trial of intraventricular immunochemotherapy in recurrent CNS lymphoma. Blood. 2013;121(5):745–51.

39. Bokstein F, Lossos A, Lossos IS, Siegal T. Central nervous system relapse of systemic non-Hodgkin's lymphoma: results of treatment based on high-dose methotrexate combination chemotherapy. Leuk Lymphoma. 2002;43(3):587–93.

40. Fischer L, Korfel A, Kiewe P, Neumann M, Jahnke K, Thiel E. Systemic high-dose methotrexate plus ifosfamide is highly effective for central nervous system (CNS) involvement of lymphoma. Ann Hematol. 2009;88(2):133–9.

41. Bromberg JE, Doorduijn JK, Illerhaus G, et al. Central nervous system recurrence of systemic lymphoma in the era of stem cell transplantation–an international primary central nervous system lymphoma study group project. Haematologica. 2013;98(5):808–13.

42. Kasamon YL, Jones RJ, Piantadosi S, et al. High-dose therapy and blood or marrow transplantation for non-Hodgkin lymphoma with central nervous system involvement. Biol Blood Marrow Transplant J Am Soc Blood Marrow Transplant. 2005;11(2):93–100.

43. Korfel A, Elter T, Thiel E, et al. Phase II study of central nervous system (CNS)-directed chemotherapy including high-dose

chemotherapy with autologous stem cell transplantation for CNS relapse of aggressive lymphomas. Haematologica. 2013;98 (3):364–70.

44. Maziarz RT, Wang Z, Zhang MJ, et al. Autologous haematopoietic cell transplantation for non-Hodgkin lymphoma with secondary CNS involvement. Br J Haematol. 2013;162(5):648–56.

45. Correa DD, Shi W, Abrey LE, et al. Cognitive functions in primary CNS lymphoma after single or combined modality regimens. Neuro-oncology. 2012;14(1):101–8.

46. Kumar A, Vanderplas A, LaCasce AS, et al. Lack of benefit of central nervous system prophylaxis for diffuse large B-cell lymphoma in the rituximab era: findings from a large national database. Cancer. 2012;118(11):2944–51.

47. Doolittle ND, Abrey LE, Shenkier TN, et al. Brain parenchyma involvement as isolated central nervous system relapse of systemic non-Hodgkin lymphoma: an international primary CNS lymphoma collaborative group report. Blood. 2008;111(3):1085–93.

48. Patrij K, Reiser M, Watzel L, et al. Isolated central nervous system relapse of systemic lymphoma (SCNSL): clinical features and outcome of a retrospective analysis. German medical science: GMS e-journal 2011; 9: Doc11.

49. van Besien K, Gisselbrecht C, Pfreundschuh M, Zucca E. Secondary lymphomas of the central nervous system: risk, prophylaxis and treatment. Leuk Lymphoma. 2008;49(Suppl 1):52–8.

50. Shah GD, Yahalom J, Correa DD, et al. Combined immunochemotherapy with reduced whole-brain radiotherapy for newly diagnosed primary CNS lymphoma. J Clin Oncol. 2007;25 (30):4730–5.

51. Rubenstein JL, Hsi ED, Johnson JL, et al. Intensive chemotherapy and immunotherapy in patients with newly diagnosed primary CNS lymphoma: CALGB 50202 (Alliance 50202). J Clin Oncol. 2013;31(25):3061–8.

52. DeAngelis LM, Posner JB. Neurologic complications of cancer. New York: Oxford University Press; 2009.

53. Grisariu S, Avni B, Batchelor TT, et al. Neurolymphomatosis: an international primary CNS lymphoma collaborative group report. Blood. 2010;115(24):5005–11.

54. Tomita M, Koike H, Kawagashira Y, et al. Clinicopathological features of neuropathy associated with lymphoma. Brain J Neurol. 2013;136(Pt 8):2563–78.

55. McMillan A, Ardeshna KM, Cwynarski K, et al. Guideline on the prevention of secondary central nervous system lymphoma: British Committee for Standards in Haematology. Br J Haematol. 2013;163(2):168–81.

56. Abramson JS, Hellmann M, Barnes JA, et al. Intravenous methotrexate as central nervous system (CNS) prophylaxis is associated with a low risk of CNS recurrence in high-risk patients with diffuse large B-cell lymphoma. Cancer. 2010;116(18):4283–90.

57. Arkenau HT, Chong G, Cunningham D, et al. The role of intrathecal chemotherapy prophylaxis in patients with diffuse large B-cell lymphoma. Ann Oncol. 2007;18(3):541–5.

58. Graus F, Arino H, Dalmau J. Paraneoplastic neurological syndromes in Hodgkin and non-Hodgkin lymphomas. Blood. 2014;123(21):3230–8.

59. Briani C, Vitaliani R, Grisold W, et al. Spectrum of paraneoplastic disease associated with lymphoma. Neurology. 2011;76(8):705–10.

60. Wood NL, Coltman CA. Localized primary extranodal Hodgkin's disease. Ann Intern Med. 1973;78(1):113–8.

61. Sapozink MD, Kaplan HS. Intracranial Hodgkin's disease. A report of 12 cases and review of the literature. Cancer. 1983;52(7):1301–7.

62. Todd ID. Intracranial lesions in Hodgkin's disease. Proc Roy Soc Med. 1967;60(8):734–6.

63. Gerstner ER, Abrey LE, Schiff D, et al. CNS Hodgkin lymphoma. Blood. 2008;112(5):1658–61.

64. Sheehan T, Cuthbert RJ, Parker AC. Central nervous system involvement in haematological malignancies. Clin Lab Haematol. 1989;11(4):331–8.

65. Biagi J, MacKenzie RG, Lim MS, Sapp M, Berinstein N. Primary Hodgkin's disease of the CNS in an immunocompetent patient: a case study and review of the literature. Neuro-oncology. 2000;2 (4):239–43.

66. Alexander FE, Jarrett RF, Lawrence D, et al. Risk factors for Hodgkin's disease by Epstein-Barr virus (EBV) status: prior infection by EBV and other agents. Br J Cancer. 2000;82 (5):1117–21.

67. Hirmiz K, Foyle A, Wilke D, et al. Intracranial presentation of systemic Hodgkin's disease. Leuk Lymphoma. 2004;45(8):1667–71.

68. Johnson MD, Kinney MC, Scheithauer BW, et al. Primary intracerebral Hodgkin's disease mimicking meningioma: case report. Neurosurgery 2000; 47(2): 454–6; discussion 6–7.

69. Higgins SA, Peschel RE. Hodgkin's disease with spinal cord compression. A case report and a review of the literature. Cancer. 1995;75(1):94–8.

70. Citow JS, Rini B, Wollmann R, Macdonald RL. Isolated, primary extranodal Hodgkin's disease of the spine: case report. Neurosurgery 2001; 49(2): 453–6; discussion 6–7.

71. Cuttner J, Meyer R, Huang YP. Intracerebral involvement in Hodgkin's disease: a report of 6 cases and review of the literature. Cancer. 1979;43(4):1497–506.

72. Friedman M, Kim TH, Panahon AM. Spinal cord compression in malignant lymphoma. Treatment and results. Cancer. 1976;37 (3):1485–91.

73. Grimm S, Chamberlain M. Hodgkin's Lymphoma: a review of neurologic complications. Adv Hematol. 2011;2011:624578.

74. Patchell R, Perry MC. Eosinophilic meningitis in Hodgkin disease. Neurology. 1981;31(7):887–8.

75. Cervantes F, Montserrat E, Rozman C. Eosinophilic meningitis in Hodgkin's disease. Ann Intern Med. 1979;91(6):930.

76. Sachdeva MU, Suri V, Malhotra P, Srinivasan R. Cerebrospinal fluid infiltration in Hodgkin lymphoma: a case report. Acta Cytol. 2008;52(5):623–6.

77. Rosen CL, DePalma L, Morita A. Primary angiitis of the central nervous system as a first presentation in Hodgkin's disease: a case report and review of the literature. Neurosurgery 2000; 46(6): 1504–8; discussion 8–10.

78. Delobel P, Brassat D, Danjoux M, et al. Granulomatous angiitis of the central nervous system revealing Hodgkin's disease. J Neurol. 2004;251(5):611–2.

79. Fuehrer NE, Hammack JE, Morris JM, Kaufmann TJ, Giannini C. Teaching NeuroImages: granulomatous angiitis of the CNS associated with Hodgkin lymphoma. Neurology. 2011;77(19):e110–1.

80. Cravioto H, Feigin I. Noninfectious granulomatous angiitis with a predilection for the nervous system. Neurology. 1959;9:599–609.

81. Slivnick DJ, Ellis TM, Nawrocki JF, Fisher RI. The impact of Hodgkin's disease on the immune system. Semin Oncol. 1990;17 (6):673–82.

82. Birnbaum J, Hellmann DB. Primary angiitis of the central nervous system. Arch Neurol. 2009;66(6):704–9.

83. Younger DS, Hays AP, Brust JC, Rowland LP. Granulomatous angiitis of the brain. An inflammatory reaction of diverse etiology. Arch Neurol. 1988;45(5):514–8.

84. Mazur MH, Dolin R. Herpes zoster at the NIH: a 20 year experience. Am J Med. 1978;65(5):738–44.

85. Abate G, Corazzelli G, Ciarmiello A, Monfardini S. Neurologic complications of Hodgkin's disease: a case history. Ann Oncol. 1997;8(6):593–600.

86. Correale J, Monteverde DA, Bueri JA, Reich EG. Peripheral nervous system and spinal cord involvement in lymphoma. Acta Neurol Scand. 1991;83(1):45–51.

87. Tan CS, Koralnik IJ. Progressive multifocal leukoencephalopathy and other disorders caused by JC virus: clinical features and pathogenesis. Lancet Neurol. 2010;9(4):425–37.

88. Sahraian MA, Radue EW, Eshaghi A, Besliu S, Minagar A. Progressive multifocal leukoencephalopathy: a review of the neuroimaging features and differential diagnosis. Eur J Neurol. 2012;19(8):1060–9.

89. Garcia-Suarez J, de Miguel D, Krsnik I, Banas H, Arribas I, Burgaleta C. Changes in the natural history of progressive multifocal leukoencephalopathy in HIV-negative lymphoproliferative disorders: impact of novel therapies. Am J Hematol. 2005;80 (4):271–81.

90. Vickers SM, Niederhuber JE. Hodgkin's disease associated with neurologic paraneoplastic syndrome. South Med J. 1997;90 (8):839–44.

91. Hammack J, Kotanides H, Rosenblum MK, Posner JB. Paraneoplastic cerebellar degeneration. II. Clinical and immunologic findings in 21 patients with Hodgkin's disease. Neurology. 1992;42(10):1938–43.

92. Graus F, Dalmau J, Valldeoriola F, et al. Immunological characterization of a neuronal antibody (anti-Tr) associated with paraneoplastic cerebellar degeneration and Hodgkin's disease. J Neuroimmunol. 1997;74(1–2):55–61.

93. Cehreli C, Payzin B, Undar B, Yilmaz U, Alakavuklar MN. Paraneoplastic cerebellar degeneration in association with Hodgkin's disease: a report of two cases. Acta Haematol. 1995;94 (4):210–3.

94. Darnell RB, Posner JB. Paraneoplastic syndromes involving the nervous system. N Engl J Med. 2003;349(16):1543–54.

Neurologic Complications of Plasma Cell Dyscrasias

32

Elie Naddaf and Michelle L. Mauermann

Abbreviations	
AL	Primary systemic amyloidosis
CBC	Complete blood count
CIDP	Chronic inflammatory demyelinating polyradiculoneuropathy
CNS	Central nervous system
CSF	Cerebrospinal fluid
DADS-M	Distal acquired demyelinating symmetric neuropathy with M protein
EMG	Electromyography
FLC	Kappa-lambda free light chains
INCAT	Inflammatory neuropathy cause and treatment
M protein	Monoclonal protein
MGUS	Monoclonal gammopathy of undetermined significance
MM	Multiple myeloma
PNS	Peripheral nervous system
SCT	Stem cell transplant
SPEP	Serum protein electrophoresis
TTR	Transthyretin
WM	Waldenström macroglobulinemia

Introduction

Plasma cell dyscrasias are a group of disorders resulting from monoclonal proliferation of a B cell clone and are accompanied by the secretion of monoclonal immunoglobulins. They are often associated with neurologic involvement most frequently affecting the peripheral nervous system. Neurologic complications can be caused by direct effect of the plasma cells themselves or indirect effect through their secreted proteins including immunoglobulins. However, in many situations, the underlying pathogenic process is yet to be discovered. In patients with a peripheral neuropathy and a monoclonal gammopathy, the type of the monoclonal protein, the neuropathy phenotype, and laboratory findings can help establish the diagnosis (Table 32.1).

Monoclonal Gammopathy of Undetermined Significance

Immunoglobulins are made of two heavy chains and two light chains. Heavy chains can be of IgG, IgA, IgM, IgD or IgE subtype. Light chains are either kappa (κ) or lambda (λ) subtype. A monoclonal population of B lymphocytes or plasma cells may produce one type of immunoglobulin, creating a monoclonal gammopathy. Monoclonal

E. Naddaf · M.L. Mauermann (✉)
Department of Neurology, Mayo Clinic, 200 First St. SW, Rochester, MN 55905, USA
e-mail: mauermann.michelle@mayo.edu

E. Naddaf
e-mail: naddaf.elie@mayo.edu

© Springer International Publishing AG 2018
D. Schiff et al. (eds.), *Cancer Neurology in Clinical Practice*,
DOI 10.1007/978-3-319-57901-6_32

Table 32.1 Plasma cell dyscrasias

Hematologic disorder	Most common monoclonal protein type	Neuropathy phenotype	Autonomic involvement	Helpful laboratory markers
Monoclonal gammopathy of undetermined significance	IgM kappa	Length-dependent, sensory predominant, demyelinating with prolonged distal latencies	–	Anti-MAG antibodies
Waldenström macroglobulinemia	IgM kappa[b]	Length-dependent, sensory predominant, axonal or demyelinating with prolonged distal latencies	–	Hemoglobin, platelet count (thrombocytopenia), IgM levels, β2-microglobulin
Immunoglobulin light chain amyloidosis	Lambda more than kappa	Length-dependent, sensory and motor, axonal	+++	24-h urine total protein, complete blood count, creatinine, alkaline phosphatase, troponin, brain natriuretic peptide, or N-terminal pro-brain natriuretic peptide levels
Multiple myeloma[a]	IgG more often than IgA	Length-dependent, sensory and motor, axonal	±	Hemoglobin, calcium, creatinine, 24-h urine total protein
POEMS syndrome	IgG or IgA, lambda	Polyradiculoneuropathy, sensory and motor, demyelinating	+	Platelet count (thrombocytosis), VEGF, endocrine studies, CSF protein

[a]Multiple myeloma-associated neuropathy, without amyloid
[b]Waldenstrom macroglobulinemia by definition is IgM kappa

gammopathies can be associated with an underlying malignant plasma cell dyscrasia such as multiple myeloma or Waldenström macroglobulinemia. They can also cause primary amyloidosis with multi-organ involvement including the peripheral nervous system. When monoclonal gammopathies are found in isolation without evidence of an associated hematological malignancy, they are called a monoclonal gammopathy of undetermined significance or MGUS. To be called MGUS, the plasma cell content of the bone marrow has to be less than 10%, the monoclonal protein spike less or equal to 3 g/dL and there should be no evidence of end-organ damage (hypercalcemia, renal insufficiency, anemia or bone lesions) [1].

MGUS is found in approximately 3.2 percent among persons 50 years of age or older, 5.3 percent among persons 70 years of age or older and 7.5 percent among those 85 years of age or older [2]. The risk of progression from MGUS to a malignant plasma cell dyscrasia is about 1 percent per year [3]. Risk factors for malignant transformation include monoclonal protein of 1.5 g/dL or greater, non-IgG subtype, and abnormal kappa-lambda-free light chains (FLC) ratio (<0.26 or >1.65) [3, 4].

Laboratory Evaluation

Serum protein electrophoresis and immunofixation should be performed when looking for a monoclonal gammopathy. Immunofixation is more sensitive for detection of monoclonal proteins when compared to electrophoresis [5].

Serum-free light chain (FLC) ratio can also be done to further increase the sensitivity [6]. When detected, the amount of the monoclonal protein (M protein) needs to be quantified in both serum and urine (via 24-h urine collection). A complete blood count (CBC), serum electrolytes including calcium, renal function assessment, and skeletal survey should be done to assess for end-organ damage. Bone marrow aspirate and biopsy may be performed for individuals with high-risk features [7].

Given the risk of progression detailed above, routine follow-up testing should be performed. There is no consensus on the frequency of testing; nonetheless, it should be tailored to the size of the monoclonal protein and risk factor profile [7]. Usually, we monitor with SPEP and serum FLC ratio at 6 months then yearly thereafter. Urine protein electrophoresis is performed if an M spike was initially found in urine.

MGUS Neuropathy

In the general population, the prevalence of length-dependent peripheral neuropathy is about 1.66% [8]. MGUS is found in up to 10% of patients with peripheral neuropathy seen at a tertiary referral center [9]. Due to the common occurrence of both peripheral neuropathy and MGUS, which increases with age, it is important to determine whether their presence is purely a chance association or whether the neuropathy is secondary to the process causing the monoclonal gammopathy. In the general population, IgG

Fig. 32.1 Overrepresentation of IgM monoclonal protein in patients with peripheral neuropathy

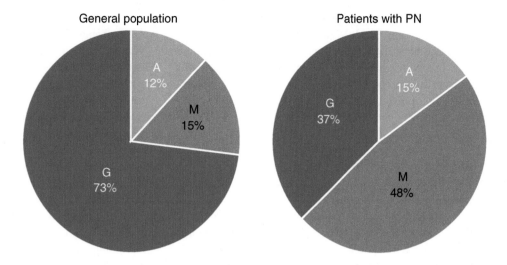

is the most common monoclonal gammopathy, while IgM is the most frequent monoclonal gammopathy found in patients with peripheral neuropathy (Fig. 32.1) [10, 11]. Laboratory work up, electrodiagnostic testing, and the neuropathy phenotype may help resolving this dilemma.

The classic phenotype of MGUS neuropathy is called DADS-M or distal acquired demyelinating symmetric neuropathy with M protein [12]. It affects men more than women usually between the fourth and ninth decade. Initially, the symptoms are predominantly sensory; however, mild distal lower limb weakness is not uncommon and patients might present with, or evolve into a disabling polyradiculoneuropathy with proximal and distal weakness. MGUS neuropathy is most commonly associated with IgM kappa monoclonal gammopathy. On electrodiagnostic testing, patients typically have demyelinating features with slowing of motor conduction velocities and marked prolongation of distal latencies implying terminal nerve involvement. Sensory potentials are typically reduced or absent.

Antibodies against myelin-associated glycoprotein (MAG) are found in nearly half of DADS-M patients. In patients with MAG positivity, the IgM binds to the peripheral nerve MAG causing widening of the myelin lamellae that can be seen on electron microscopy [13–16]. However, the clinical presentation and course of DADS-M is the same in the presence or absence of MAG antibodies [11, 17] and MAG positivity may be seen in amyloid neuropathy patients and in IgM MGUS without neuropathy [18]. Therefore, subdividing patients with MGUS neuropathy into two categories, based on the presence of anti-MAG antibodies, is of uncertain clinical significance.

DADS-M is often considered a subtype of chronic inflammatory demyelinating polyradiculoneuropathy (CIDP) [12, 19]. DADS-M was distinguished from CIDP as patients with CIDP and IgM MGUS were found to respond poorly to conventional CIDP treatment [11, 12, 20]. On the other

hand, there was no difference in response between CIDP patients with and without IgA or IgG MGUS. Therefore, the presence of IgA and IgG in CIDP patients might be just an incidental finding. Furthermore, the evidence of an association of IgA or IgG MGUS with peripheral neuropathy in general remains unclear.

In summary, there is no definitive way to determine with confidence whether a MGUS and peripheral neuropathy have a causal relationship in a specific patient. Therefore, the clinician should gather as much evidence as possible before assuming the patient has a paraproteinemic neuropathy guided by the clinical phenotype, electrodiagnostic findings, the type of the monoclonal protein (IgM vs. non-IgM) and the presence of anti-MAG antibodies.

MGUS Neuropathy Management

Multiple case reports and case series using different immunomodulating agents have been published with varying results. Some clinical trials only included patients with IgM anti-MAG neuropathies, while others treated all patients with IgM neuropathy regardless of anti-MAG status. A 2012 Cochrane Review did not find enough evidence to support the use of intravenous immunoglobulin, interferon alfa-2a, cyclophosphamide and steroids, and plasma exchange in IgM anti-MAG neuropathies [21]. Earlier small studies suggested possible benefit with rituximab [22, 23]. Subsequently, a double-blinded, placebo-controlled trial of rituximab in IgM anti-MAG neuropathy was performed [24]. The study did not meet the primary outcome of an absolute improvement on the inflammatory neuropathy cause and treatment (INCAT) sensory score at 12 months. However, there was evidence of some improvement in secondary outcomes including the INCAT disability scale in 20% of patients and self-evaluation scale.

Currently, there is no reliable evidence to support the use of immunotherapy in IgM neuropathy. Thus, treatment decision has to be made on a case by case basis. Treatment is usually offered for very young patients or older patients with significant disability. Patients with proximal weakness resembling a polyradiculoneuropathy tend to respond better to treatment [25].

Waldenström Macroglobulinemia

Waldenström macroglobulinemia (WM) is a lymphoplasmacytic lymphoma associated with IgM monoclonal gammopathy. Diagnosis is usually made via a bone marrow biopsy demonstrating a lymphoplasmacytic infiltration with a predominantly intertrabecular pattern, supported by appropriate immunophenotypic studies, and regardless of the IgM protein concentration [26]. WM affects men more than women (2:1) [27]. Patients most commonly present in their seventh decade with fatigue related to the underlying anemia. Clinical manifestations include peripheral neuropathy, hepatomegaly, splenomegaly, lymphadenopathy, and hyperviscosity syndrome.

Most commonly, WM is a chronic disease with a 5-year relative survival rate of about 78% [28, 29]. Prognostic factors associated with poor outcome include: age > 65 years, Hemoglobin $\leq$ 11.5 g/dL, platelet count $\leq$ 100,000/µL, β2-microglobulin > 3, and monoclonal IgM concentration > 7 g/dL [27].

CNS Complications of Waldenström Macroglobulinemia

Hyperviscosity syndrome is characterized by skin and mucosal bleeding, retinopathy with retinal hemorrhages mimicking central vein occlusion, and central nervous system (CNS) involvement (intracerebral hemorrhage, seizures, vertigo and altered level of consciousness including coma) [30]. In addition to hyperviscosity syndrome, CNS involvement can result from direct infiltration by lymphoplasmacytic cells known as Bing-Neel syndrome. MRI of the brain and cerebrospinal fluid (CSF) studies help establish the diagnosis. Furthermore, patients may also develop Bing-Neel syndrome without evidence of CNS infiltration. The underlying mechanism remains unclear but could be related to intraparenchymal IgM deposition [31]. When the CNS is involved, large cell transformation needs to be ruled out.

Waldenström Macroglobulinemia Neuropathy

The peripheral neuropathy associated with WM is clinically indistinguishable from IgM-MGUS neuropathy. It is a predominantly sensory neuropathy with the most common symptom being foot numbness resulting in sensory ataxia.

Nerve conduction studies and EMG demonstrate that WM neuropathy is more commonly axonal with only 27% of patients having demyelinating features compared to 62% of patients with IgM-MGUS neuropathy [32]. The degree of axonal loss on nerve conduction studies/EMG and on teased nerve fibers is similar to that seen in IgM-MGUS, which likely accounts for the similar type and severity of impairments. Patients with WM have much higher IgM levels (median 3100 mg/dL) and much greater presence of anemia (median hemoglobin of 11.8 g/dL) when compared to patients with IgM MGUS (median IgM level of 650 mg/dL and median hemoglobin of 14.4 g/dL) [32]. While none of these findings in isolation can rule in or rule out WM, they should nonetheless serve as helpful clues to prompt further evaluation and hematology consultation.

CT scan of the chest, abdomen, and pelvis identifying hepatosplenomegaly or lymphadenopathy and bone marrow biopsy with lymphoplasmacytic infiltrate can establish the diagnosis of WM.

Waldenström Macroglobulinemia Management

Given the relatively good long-term survival of patients with WM, potential toxicity of therapy should be taken in consideration and treatment should be tailored depending on disease severity [27]. Observation is recommended for asymptomatic patients. Patients with hemoglobin < 11 g/dL or platelet < 120,000/µL and patients with early disease including patients with WM neuropathy, hemolytic anemia or glomerulonephritis may be treated with one cycle of rituximab as a single agent. Patients with advanced disease including patients with bulky disease, profound cytopenias (hemoglobin $\leq$ 10 g/dL or platelets < 100,000/µL), or hyperviscosity symptoms should be treated with rituximab, cyclophosphamide, and dexamethasone [33]. Ibrutinib, an inhibitor of the Bruton's tyrosine kinase, has been recently reported to be effective in WM-pretreated patients [34]. Plasmapheresis should be offered for patients with hyperviscosity symptoms. Autologous stem cell transplantation may be considered in relapsing/refractory cases [33].

Primary Amyloidosis

Amyloidosis includes a group of disorders resulting from the deposition of insoluble amyloid fibrils in various tissues including peripheral nerves. Amyloidosis is classified by the subunit of protein compromising the amyloid fibril [35]. Amyloidosis associated with peripheral neuropathy includes primary systemic amyloidosis (AL) and familial amyloidosis. Familial amyloidosis is most commonly due to mutations in the transthyretin (TTR) and less often, apolipoprotein A-1 or gelsolin [36]. On biopsy specimen, amyloid consists of a homogenous amorphous material that stains pink with hematoxylin and eosin and metachromatically with methyl violet or crystal violet. Positive reactivity is seen on Congo red staining with apple-green birefringence when seen under polarized light (Fig. 32.2a–c).

Amyloidosis is not always systemic. It can be localized to a specific site such as the skin, urinary tract or peripheral nerves.

Immunoglobulin Light-Chain Amyloidosis

AL amyloidosis results from the deposit of monoclonal light chains, kappa or lambda, in various tissues including the heart, kidneys, gastrointestinal tract, and peripheral nerves. Changes in the secondary and tertiary structure of the light chains result in the formation of insoluble beta-pleated sheets that disrupt organ function. Rarely, primary amyloidosis can be associated with a heavy-chain fragment [37].

AL amyloid has an incidence of 8 per 1 million people per year and median age of onset of 62 years [38]. It is uncommon in patients under the age of 40 [39]. It affects men more than women (ratio of 2:1) [40]. The most common symptoms are fatigue and weight loss in nearly half of the patients [40]. Cardinal clinical findings, including macroglossia, facial purpura, hepatosplenomegaly, and submandibular salivary gland enlargement, are present in a minority of cases. At time of diagnosis, nephrotic syndrome, with or without renal failure, is found in 28% of patients, carpal tunnel syndrome in 21%, peripheral neuropathy in 17%, congestive heart failure in 17%, and orthostatic hypotension in 11% [39]. Survival depends on the extent of cardiac involvement. Typically, patients develop a cardiomyopathy that results in congestive heart failure and/or cardiac arrhythmias that can result in sudden death [41]. With the use of high-dose chemotherapy, the availability of new chemotherapeutic agents, the decrease in post-stem cell transplant (SCT) mortality, and the better selection of SCT eligible patients, there is evidence of improvement in overall survival rate [42]. Currently, the median survival is about 2–4 years [43]. Nonetheless, the survival rate can vary from less than 6 months for patients with overt cardiac failure, to a 10-year survival of 43% after autologous stem cell transplantation (SCT) [44].

AL Amyloidosis Neuropathy

Peripheral neuropathy affects 15–20% of patients with AL amyloidosis [39]. The most common pattern of amyloidosis

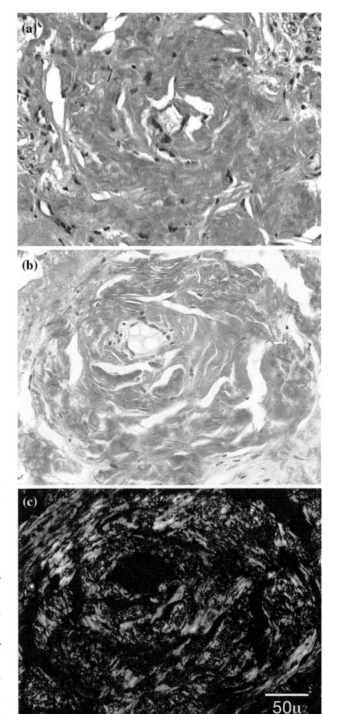

Fig. 32.2 A representative case of amyloidosis in nerve **a** Hematoxylin and eosin demonstrates amyloid deposition around endoneurial vessels, which is **b** congophilic and shows **c** *apple-green* birefringence under polarized light. (Used with permission of Oxford University Press from Mauermann ML, Tracy JA, Singer W. Autonomic Neuropathies. In: Bennarroch E, ed: Autonomic Neurology. Oxford: Oxford University Press; 2014.)

neuropathy (including both AL and familial forms) is seen in about two-thirds of patients and consists of generalized autonomic failure with a painful, length-dependent, sensorimotor peripheral neuropathy [45]. In some patients, the generalized autonomic failure may be associated with a painless, length-dependent, sensorimotor peripheral neuropathy or can happen in isolation. Less likely, patients can have a length-dependent, sensorimotor peripheral neuropathy without generalized autonomic failure or can have generalized autonomic failure associated with a small-fiber neuropathy [45].

The length-dependent peripheral neuropathy starts distally in the feet and spreads more proximally with time. It usually affects the hands when it reaches the knee level. Patients often report numbness, tingling, burning, stabbing pains, and weakness. On physical examination, patients commonly have pan-modality sensory loss including both large-fiber (light touch, vibration and proprioception) and small-fiber (pain, temperature) modalities. However, as mentioned above, patients may only have a small-fiber neuropathy with selective loss of pain and temperature sensation.

Autonomic involvement can affect the cardiovascular, gastrointestinal, and genitourinary systems. The most frequent symptom is orthostatic intolerance, followed by gastrointestinal symptoms including postprandial diarrhea or vomiting, severe constipation, and gastroparesis [46]. Genitourinary involvement manifests with erectile dysfunction early on and dysuria and urinary retention later with disease progression [36]. Patients also commonly have sweating abnormalities. Light-near dissociation of pupillary reactions (Argyll-Robertson pupil) may be observed.

Localized deposit of amyloid, termed amyloidoma, can cause a focal neuropathy by compression or amyloid deposition within the nerve [47, 48]. Rarely, the whole IgM molecule forms deposits within the nerve without amyloid-associated proteins [49, 50]. Morphologically, the deposition of the whole IgM molecule mimics amyloid, but does not stain with Congo red.

Laboratory Evaluation

Nerve conduction studies/EMG typically shows a length-dependent axonal, sensorimotor peripheral neuropathy. However, in a pure small-fiber neuropathy, NCS/EMG will be normal. If clinically indicated, quantitative sudomotor axon reflex testing, thermoregulatory sweat test, and/or skin biopsy to determine epidermal nerve fiber density may be used to evaluate for small-fiber involvement. Autonomic reflex screening usually shows generalized adrenergic, cardiovagal, and sudomotor dysfunction.

Screening for suspected AL amyloidosis should include serum and urine immunofixation as well as an immunoglobulin free light-chain assay [51]. When amyloidosis is suspected, tissue confirmation is required. Biopsy of the iliac crest bone marrow combined with abdominal subcutaneous fat aspiration will identify amyloid deposits in 85% of patients with amyloidosis [51]. If these are unrevealing, a biopsy of an affected tissue should be considered. Thereafter, amyloid protein composition should be determined by mass spectrometry [52, 53]. Screening for other organ involvement should include an echocardiography, 24-h urine total protein measurement, measurement of complete blood count, creatinine level, alkaline phosphatase level, troponin and N-terminal pro-brain natriuretic peptide levels [51].

AL Amyloidosis Management

It is crucial to make the diagnosis of AL amyloidosis early on as it has major treatment implications, and delay in diagnosis may affect eligibility for stem cell transplant. SCT is the treatment of choice for AL amyloidosis with survival rates of 53% for patients with a complete response and 43% for all treated patients [44, 54]. Unfortunately, only 20–25% of patients are eligible for SCT at diagnosis. Eligibility requirements include NT-proBNP <5000 ng/mL, troponin T < 0.06 ng/mL, age < 70 years, <3 organs involved, and serum creatinine ≤ 1.7 mg/dL [51]. SCT-ineligible patients should be given a chemotherapeutic regimen such as melphalan–dexamethasone or cyclophosphamide–bortezomib–dexamethasone. In patients with a peripheral neuropathy, some therapies, including bortezomib and thalidomide, should be used with caution due to the high risk of a length-dependent, sensory-predominant, axonal neuropathy as will be detailed in multiple myeloma section [55].

Multiple Myeloma

Multiple myeloma (MM) is a malignant plasma cell disorder. It is more common in men with an average age of onset of 66 years and annual incidence of 4.3 cases per 100,000 people [56]. Patients usually present with fatigue, weight loss, bone pain, and recurrent infections. A majority of patients have an associated monoclonal protein (>90%) with IgG kappa being the most common (34%) [57]. The main features of MM that reflect end-organ damage include hypercalcemia, renal insufficiency, anemia, and bone involvement [58].

MM neurologic complications can involve both the central (CNS) and peripheral (PNS) nervous systems. They can be caused by different mechanisms:

1. Direct tissue damage via infiltration by neoplastic cells or compression
2. Indirect effect via autoimmune processes (e.g., paraneoplastic), amyloid deposition, or toxic metabolic derangements caused by end-organ damage
3. Iatrogenic effect related to chemotherapeutic drugs.

Laboratory Evaluation

Laboratory evaluation should include serum and urine monoclonal protein screen as detailed in the monoclonal gammopathy section. Investigation should also evaluate for end-organ damage and bone involvement via skeletal survey or low-dose CT scan without contrast. The diagnosis of MM requires the presence of a monoclonal protein (except in non-secretory MM), plasma cell count greater than or equal to 10% on bone marrow evaluation by bone marrow aspirate or biopsy, and presence of end-organ damage [59]. In the absence of end-organ damage, MM can be diagnosed if bone marrow plasma cell count is ≥ 60% [60].

CNS Complications

Spinal Cord Compression

MM has predilection for bone and bone marrow. Bone health relies on a balance between bone resorption mediated mainly by osteoclasts and bone formation by osteoblasts. In MM patients, the balance is disrupted favoring osteoclast activity, resulting in bone friability and the development of lytic lesions. Consequently, spinal cord compression can result from a vertebral fracture or from an expanding myelomatous lesion in the marrow cavity of the vertebrae. Less often, spinal cord compression is due to an extramedullary plasmacytoma [61].

Patients with thoracic spinal cord compression usually present with acute severe back pain, weakness and/or numbness in lower limbs with or without bowel and bladder symptoms. Spasticity may not be present upon presentation. Furthermore, patients may present with slowly progressive symptoms and dull pain. Less often, the compression is at the level of the cervical spinal cord with symptoms involving the upper limbs as well.

Spinal cord compression requires immediate attention. Urgent imaging of the spinal cord helps establish the diagnosis. Immediate treatment with high-dose corticosteroids is recommended, helping to alleviate the pain and improve neurologic deficits. Decompression surgery or radiotherapy will generally follow.

CNS Myelomatosis

Direct CNS infiltration by myelomatous cells is rare. MM can involve the leptomeninges or the brain parenchyma. Patients may present with a wide range of symptoms such as symptoms related to intracranial hypertension, cranial nerve involvement, nerve root involvement, pituitary malfunction, diffuse cerebral dysfunction, and focal deficits depending on the site of infiltration [62]. Intracranial plasmacytomas are rare and most commonly resulting from direct extension of a skull lesion [63]. Brain MRI with contrast and CSF studies helps establish the diagnosis.

Hyperviscosity

Hyperviscosity syndrome is seen in multiple myeloma and Waldenström macroglobulinemia. It is due to the increased protein content of the blood and the large molecular size, abnormal polymerization, and abnormal shape of immunoglobulin molecules. Symptoms of hyperviscosity usually appear when the normal serum viscosity of 1.4–1.8 cp reaches 4–5 cp [64]. Patients with hyperviscosity syndrome usually present with focal neurologic symptoms, visual disturbances, and bleeding as detailed previously in the Waldenström macroglobulinemia section.

Toxic-Metabolic Encephalopathy

Encephalopathy in a patient with multiple myeloma warrants a thorough investigation to assess for metabolic derangements or electrolyte abnormalities due to end-organ damage or medication side effects. Renal involvement can result in uremia, metabolic acidosis, and electrolyte abnormalities especially hyperkalemia. Hypercalcemia can present with altered mental status, tetany, seizures, or focal neurologic deficits. Interestingly, patients with MM can have hyperammonemia in the absence of liver involvement [65]. Moreover, patients may develop hypoperfusion encephalopathy in the setting of low cardiac output. Cardiotoxicity can be seen in autologous stem cell transplant patients treated with cyclophosphamide and/or melphalan [66, 67], and in patients treated with proteasome inhibitors (bortezomib and carfilzomib) [68–70]. Nonetheless, hyperviscosity syndrome and CNS involvement need to be considered in encephalopathic patients.

PNS Complications

Compression and Infiltration

Cranial nerves and nerve roots can be involved secondary to leptomeningeal infiltration, adjacent bony lesions, or plasmacytomas. A notable syndrome is the numb-chin syndrome caused by lytic lesions of the mandible and involvement of the mental or inferior alveolar nerve [71]. About 10% of MM patients have mandibular bony lesions [72].

Multiple Myeloma-Associated Peripheral Neuropathy

Clinically, 5–20% of multiple myeloma patients have evidence of peripheral neuropathy. Including patients with subclinical peripheral neuropathy detected solely on electrodiagnostic testing, the incidence of peripheral neuropathy in untreated MM is about 39% [73].

Most commonly, the peripheral neuropathy associated with MM is progressive, length-dependent, and sensorimotor. On examination, there is evidence of pan-modality sensory loss, mild distal weakness, and reduced or absent ankle reflexes. Nerve conduction studies show low to absent compound muscle and sensory action potentials, with mild slowing of motor conduction velocities [74]. Rarely, multiple myeloma patients can present with a pure sensory neuropathy or ganglionopathy, or a motor polyradiculoneuropathy [74].

Patients with multiple myeloma-associated peripheral neuropathy do not usually have marked pain or autonomic involvement. Therefore, a painful neuropathy or marked autonomic involvement should prompt considering neuropathy secondary to amyloidosis or treatment-emergent peripheral neuropathy as alternative diagnoses (Table 32.2).

Treatment-Emergent Peripheral Neuropathy

With the advent of new therapeutic agents, especially bortezomib and thalidomide, in improving multiple myeloma outcomes, treatment-emergent peripheral neuropathy has become the leading cause of peripheral neuropathy in multiple myeloma patients. Chemotherapeutic drug neurotoxicity has major impact on management, as it often requires dose reduction or even premature discontinuation of an otherwise successful drug. Furthermore, it makes the choice of an alternative treatment agent difficult, as many of the available drugs are associated with peripheral neuropathy. As peripheral neuropathy can be seen in up to 39% of patients with untreated multiple myeloma, it may be challenging to determine whether the peripheral neuropathy is related to the treatment or the disease itself. Hence, it is crucial to screen the patients for symptoms and signs of a preexisting peripheral neuropathy, and consider baseline nerve conduction studies prior to starting chemotherapy.

Proteasome Inhibitors

Bortezomib is a reversible proteasome inhibitor preventing the proteasomal elimination of ubiquinated proteins. Based on in vitro experiments using rat dorsal root ganglia neurons, bortezomib alters microtubule polymerization and axonal transport [75]. The incidence of bortezomib-associated neuropathy increases with cumulative doses and is often dose limiting. With the conventional regimen using intravenous bortezomib twice a week, about a half to two-thirds of multiple myeloma patients develop treatment-emergent peripheral neuropathy [76, 77]. Replacing with subcutaneous bortezomib or weekly doses of IV bortezomib has shown a reduction in the incidence of peripheral neuropathy to approximately 40% [78, 79]. Patients with pre-existing peripheral neuropathy are more prone to develop a severe treatment-emergent peripheral neuropathy interfering with activity of daily living [80]. Bortezomib-associated neuropathy is typically a painful, distal, and sensory-predominant polyneuropathy. All sensory modalities are usually affected. Nerve conduction studies usually demonstrate low sensory nerve action potentials. Less commonly, patients may develop a severe, motor-predominant, polyradiculoneuropathy with demyelinating features on nerve conduction studies and elevated CSF protein [81, 82]. Recognizing bortezomib-associated neuropathy is important as it may be reversible in majority of patients with dose reduction or discontinuation [76, 80.] Newer proteasome inhibitors, such as carfilzomib, have a lower incidence of treatment-emergent peripheral neuropathy [83].

Thalidomide

Thalidomide is an immunomodulatory drug with multiple mechanisms of action. It is thought to cause dorsal root ganglia degeneration [84]. The development of thalidomide-associated neuropathy is dependent on the cumulative dose and more so, the treatment duration. 38% of patients develop

Table 32.2 Multiple myeloma neuropathies

Neuropathy subtype	Painful	Sensory versus motor	Autonomic involvement	Treatment
MM-associated without amyloid	±	Sensory more than motor	±	Treating the underlying disorder
MM-associated with amyloid	++	Sensory and motor	+++	SCT for eligible patients
Treatment-emergent (Bortezomib, thalidomide)	++	Sensory	+	Dose reduction or discontinuation of the offending agent

MM multiple myeloma, *SCT* stem cell transplant

it at 6 months and 73% at 12 months [85]. Similar to bortezomib-associated neuropathy, thalidomide-associated neuropathy is usually painful, predominantly sensory and length-dependent. Nerve conduction studies demonstrate low amplitude sensory nerve action potentials and sometimes low amplitude compound muscle action potentials as well. The symptoms can present after treatment has stopped and may progress for several months after discontinuation of thalidomide. Peripheral nerve damage may be irreversible. Treatment-emergent peripheral neuropathy is less commonly seen with lenalidomide and pomalidomide [83].

Management

Treating the underlying plasma cell dyscrasia is the mainstay of multiple myeloma-associated peripheral neuropathy treatment. Current treatment options include autologous stem cell transplant as well as varied chemotherapeutic regimens. Risk stratification via cytogenetic markers help guiding treatment decisions [60, 86]. For treatment-emergent peripheral neuropathy, reducing the dose of the offending agent is recommended; however, total discontinuation may become necessary.

POEMS Syndrome

POEMS syndrome is a rare paraneoplastic disorder due to an underlying plasma cell neoplasm. Other names for POEMS syndrome include Takatsuki syndrome, Crow-Fukase syndrome or osteosclerotic myeloma. The POEMS acronym refers to several common clinical features—peripheral neuropathy, organomegaly, monoclonal plasma cell disorder and skin changes [87]. These are some but not all of the clinical features of this syndrome. Criteria for diagnosis have been established for POEMS syndrome (Table 32.3). Patients must have a monoclonal plasma cell disorder and peripheral neuropathy. There must also be one of the three other major criteria, which include Castleman disease, sclerotic bones lesions and elevated vascular endothelial growth factor, and one of the six minor criteria (detailed in Table 32.3). Due to the high prevalence of diabetes mellitus and thyroid abnormalities, this diagnosis alone cannot meet the minor criteria. The monoclonal plasma cell disorder is almost always lambda (>95%) [88].

Neuropathy in POEMS Syndrome

Peripheral neuropathy is required for the diagnosis of POEMS syndrome and is typically the dominant, but not always the presenting, feature of the illness. The neuropathy presents initially in the feet and progresses symmetrically in a length-dependent manner [89, 90]. Patients present with sensory symptoms (numbness, paresthesias and pain) followed by motor involvement. At the time of evaluation, the neuropathy can either be a distal symmetric sensorimotor peripheral neuropathy or a sensorimotor polyradiculoneuropathy with significant proximal involvement and hypo- or areflexia. The weakness is often severe such that 45% of patients are in a wheelchair at the time of evaluation and some are even bedbound [90]. Nerve conduction studies and electromyography demonstrate both axonal loss and demyelination [88]. The lower limb motor and sensory responses are severely reduced or absent. Upper limb studies demonstrate reduced motor and sensory amplitudes, slowed conduction velocities and prolonged distal latencies. Conduction block and temporal dispersion may be seen. F-wave latencies are prolonged. Due to the proximal involvement, areflexia and EMG characteristics, these patients are often mistaken for chronic inflammatory demyelinating polyneuropathy. However, differentiating characteristics include more frequent positive neuropathic symptoms and pain, more severe distal lower limb weakness, and nerve conduction studies demonstrating greater axonal loss in the lower limbs with uniform slowing and greater involvement of intermediate nerve segments [88, 91].

Laboratory Evaluation

In cases of suspected POEMS syndrome or a CIDP-like illness, it is imperative to search thoroughly for a monoclonal protein in both the serum and the urine. Finding an IgG or IgA lambda monoclonal gammopathy acts as a red flag for considering the diagnosis and pursuing further evaluation. The evaluation should include a skeletal survey as osteosclerotic lesions occur in approximately 95% of patients. Lesions can be densely sclerotic, lytic with a sclerotic rim or have a mixed soap-bubble appearance [92]. Bone marrow biopsy should be performed to evaluate for a monoclonal plasma cell disorder that is found in two-thirds of patients (91% lambda) but often comprises less than 5% of the bone marrow. There is also megakaryocyte hyperplasia and megakaryocyte clustering [93].

Laboratory studies should include CBC for thrombocytosis [94], studies of endocrine function and alternative causes of peripheral neuropathy. Computed tomography of the chest, abdomen and pelvis can assess for organomegaly and lymphadenopathy as well as signs of extravascular volume overload. The cytokine VEGF (vascular endothelial growth factor) correlates best with disease activity and is markedly increased in POEMS. A plasma level greater than 200 pg/mL has a specificity of 95% and sensitivity of 68% in support of a diagnosis of POEMS syndrome [95]. CSF

Table 32.3 Criteria for the diagnosis of polyneuropathy, organomegaly, endocrinopathy, monoclonal plasma cell disorder, and skin changes (POEMS) syndrome[a,b]

►**Mandatory major criteria**
Polyneuropathy (typically demyelinating)
Monoclonal plasma cell proliferative disorder (almost always lambda)
►**Other major criteria (one required for diagnosis)**
Castleman disease[c]
Sclerotic bone lesions
Elevated vascular endothelial growth factor
►**Minor criteria (one required for diagnosis)**
Organomegaly (e.g., splenomegaly, hepatomegaly, or lymphadenopathy)
Extravascular volume overload (e.g., edema, pleural effusion, or ascites)
Endocrinopathy (e.g., adrenal, thyroid,[d] pituitary, gonadal, parathyroid, pancreatic[d])
Skin changes (e.g., hyperpigmentation, hypertrichosis, glomeruloid hemangiomata, plethora, acrocyanosis, flushing, white nails)
Papilledema
Thrombocytosis/polycythemia[e]
►**Other signs and symptoms**
Clubbing
Weight loss
Hyperhidrosis
Pulmonary hypertension/restricted lung disease
Thrombotic diatheses
Diarrhea
Low vitamin B_{12} level

[a]Used with permission of John Wiley and Sons from Dispenzieri A. POEMS syndrome: update on diagnosis, risk-stratification, and management. Am J Hematol 2012 Aug [cited 2015 Jun 16];87(8):804–14

[b]The diagnosis of POEMS syndrome is confirmed when both of the mandatory major criteria, one of the three other major criteria, and one of the six minor criteria are present

[c]There is a Castleman disease variant of POEMS syndrome that occurs without evidence of a clonal plasma cell disorder that is not accounted for in this table. This entity should be considered separately

[d]Because of the high prevalence of diabetes mellitus and thyroid abnormalities, this diagnosis alone is not sufficient to meet this minor criterion

[e]Approximately 50% of patients will have bone marrow changes that distinguish it from a typical monoclonal gammopathy of undetermined significance or myeloma bone marrow. Anemia and/or thrombocytopenia are distinctively unusual in this syndrome unless Castleman disease is present

evaluation typically demonstrates albuminocytologic dissociation (the presence of an elevated CSF protein in the absence of an elevated cell count) [88].

POEMS Management

Treatment for POEMS syndrome is aimed at the underlying monoclonal plasma cell disorder. The method of treatment depends on the number of bone lesions as well as the presence of plasma cell involvement in the bone marrow. If there are one to three bone lesions without bone marrow involvement, patients are typically referred for curative doses of radiation to the affected sites. Patients who are candidates for radiation therapy have a better overall survival [35]. A 4-year overall survival of 97% and event-free survival of 52% has been reported [96]. Patients with more than 2 or 3 lesions or bone marrow evidence of a clonal population of plasma cells are referred for systemic treatment. This includes systemic chemotherapy or autologous stem cell transplantation (SCT). An alkylator-based regimen is most commonly used with lenalidomide, thalidomide and bortezomib as promising alternatives. High-dose chemotherapy with SCT is effective with one study demonstrating a progression-free survival of 98% and 75% at 1 and 5 years, respectively [97]. The peripheral neuropathy also improves following SCT with marked improvement in neuropathy impairment scores, modified Rankin Scale and nerve conduction study parameters over 5 years [90].

Conclusion

Monoclonal gammopathies and peripheral neuropathy both commonly occur. A true association can be difficult to determine and plasma cell dyscrasias can be challenging to diagnose. Collaboration between an experienced hematologist and neurologist is crucial to deliver the best possible care to the patient. This requires a comprehensive knowledge of the evaluation of monoclonal gammopathies as well as a thorough understanding of the neuropathy phenotypes and their associations with certain gammopathy subtypes. An organized approach to establish the correct diagnosis is fundamental in caring for these patients.

References

1. Group IMW. Criteria for the classification of monoclonal gammopathies, multiple myeloma and related disorders: a report of the International Myeloma Working Group. Br J Haematol. 2003;121(5):749–57.
2. Kyle RA, Therneau TM, Rajkumar SV, Larson DR, Plevak MF, Offord JR, et al. Prevalence of monoclonal gammopathy of undetermined significance. N Engl J Med. 2006;354(13):1362–9.
3. Kyle RA, Therneau TM, Rajkumar SV, Offord JR, Larson DR, Plevak MF, et al. A long-term study of prognosis in monoclonal gammopathy of undetermined significance. N Engl J Med. 2002;346(8):564–9.
4. Rajkumar SV, Kyle RA, Therneau TM, Melton LJ, Bradwell AR, Clark RJ, et al. Serum free light chain ratio is an independent risk factor for progression in monoclonal gammopathy of undetermined significance. Blood. 2005;106(3):812–7.
5. Vrethem M, Larsson B, von Schenck H, Ernerudh J. Immunofixation superior to plasma agarose electrophoresis in detecting small M-components in patients with polyneuropathy. J Neurol Sci. 1993;120(1):93–8.
6. Katzmann JA, Abraham RS, Dispenzieri A, Lust JA, Kyle RA. Diagnostic performance of quantitative kappa and lambda free light chain assays in clinical practice. Clin Chem. 2005;51(5):878–81.
7. Berenson JR, Anderson KC, Audell RA, Boccia RV, Coleman M, Dimopoulos MA, et al. Monoclonal gammopathy of undetermined significance: a consensus statement. Br J Haematol. 2010;150(1): 28–38.
8. Hoffman EM, Staff NP, Robb JM, St Sauver JL, Dyck PJ, Klein CJ. Impairments and comorbidities of polyneuropathy revealed by population-based analyses. Neurology 2015 Apr 1;84(16):1644–51.
9. Kelly JJ, Kyle RA, O'Brien PC, Dyck PJ. Prevalence of monoclonal protein in peripheral neuropathy. Neurology. 1981;31(11):1480–3.
10. Ramchandren S, Lewis RA. An update on monoclonal gammopathy and neuropathy. Curr Neurol Neurosci Rep. 2012;12(1):102–10.
11. Gosselin S, Kyle RA, Dyck PJ. Neuropathy associated with monoclonal gammopathies of undetermined significance. Ann Neurol. 1991;30(1):54–61.
12. Katz JS, Saperstein DS, Gronseth G, Amato AA, Barohn RJ. Distal acquired demyelinating symmetric neuropathy. Neurology. 2000;54(3):615–20.
13. Lombardi R, Erne B, Lauria G, Pareyson D, Borgna M, Morbin M, et al. IgM deposits on skin nerves in anti-myelin-associated glycoprotein neuropathy. Ann Neurol. 2005;57(2):180–7.
14. Ellie E, Vital A, Steck A, Boiron JM, Vital C, Julien J. Neuropathy associated with "benign" anti-myelin-associated glycoprotein IgM gammopathy: clinical, immunological, neurophysiological pathological findings and response to treatment in 33 cases. J Neurol. 1996;243(1):34–43.
15. Latov N, Hays AP, Sherman WH. Peripheral neuropathy and anti-MAG antibodies. Crit Rev Neurobiol. 1988;3(4):301–32.
16. Vallat JM, Jauberteau MO, Bordessoule D, Yardin C, Preux PM, Couratier P. Link between peripheral neuropathy and monoclonal dysglobulinemia: a study of 66 cases. J Neurol Sci. 1996;137(2): 124–30.
17. Suarez GA, Kelly JJ. Polyneuropathy associated with monoclonal gammopathy of undetermined significance: further evidence that IgM-MGUS neuropathies are different than IgG-MGUS. Neurology. 1993;43(7):1304–8.
18. Garces-Sanchez M, Dyck PJ, Kyle RA, Zeldenrust S, Wu Y, Ladha SS, et al. Antibodies to myelin-associated glycoprotein (anti-Mag) in IgM amyloidosis may influence expression of neuropathy in rare patients. Muscle Nerve. 2008;37(4):490–5.
19. Simmons Z, Albers JW, Bromberg MB, Feldman EL. Presentation and initial clinical course in patients with chronic inflammatory demyelinating polyradiculoneuropathy: comparison of patients without and with monoclonal gammopathy. Neurology. 1993; 43(11):2202–9.
20. Dyck PJ, Low PA, Windebank AJ, Jaradeh SS, Gosselin S, Bourque P, et al. Plasma exchange in polyneuropathy associated with monoclonal gammopathy of undetermined significance. N Engl J Med. 1991;325(21):1482–6.
21. Lunn MPT, Nobile-Orazio E. Immunotherapy for IgM anti-myelin-associated glycoprotein paraprotein-associated peripheral neuropathies. Cochrane Database Syst Rev 2012 Jan;5: CD002827.
22. Dalakas MC, Rakocevic G, Salajegheh M, Dambrosia JM, Hahn AF, Raju R, et al. Placebo-controlled trial of rituximab in IgM anti-myelin-associated glycoprotein antibody demyelinating neuropathy. Ann Neurol. 2009;65(3):286–93.
23. Benedetti L, Briani C, Grandis M, Vigo T, Gobbi M, Ghiglione E, et al. Predictors of response to rituximab in patients with neuropathy and anti-myelin associated glycoprotein immunoglobulin M. J Peripher Nerv Syst. 2007;12(2):102–7.
24. Léger J-M, Viala K, Nicolas G, Créange A, Vallat J-M, Pouget J, et al. Placebo-controlled trial of rituximab in IgM anti-myelin-associated glycoprotein neuropathy. Neurology. 2013;80(24):2217–25.
25. Gorson KC, Ropper AH, Weinberg DH, Weinstein R. Treatment experience in patients with anti-myelin-associated glycoprotein neuropathy. Muscle Nerve. 2001;24(6):778–86.
26. Owen RG, Treon SP, Al-Katib A, Fonseca R, Greipp PR, McMaster ML, et al. Clinicopathological definition of Waldenstrom's macroglobulinemia: consensus panel recommendations from the Second International Workshop on Waldenstrom's Macroglobulinemia. Semin Oncol. 2003;30(2):110–5.
27. Gertz MA. Waldenström macroglobulinemia: 2015 update on diagnosis, risk stratification, and management. Am J Hematol. 2015;90(4):346–54.
28. Kristinsson SY, Eloranta S, Dickman PW, Andersson TM-L, Turesson I, Landgren O, et al. Patterns of survival in lymphoplasmacytic lymphoma/Waldenström macroglobulinemia: a population-based study of 1,555 patients diagnosed in Sweden from 1980 to 2005. Am J Hematol. 2013;88(1):60–5.
29. Castillo JJ, Olszewski AJ, Cronin AM, Hunter ZR, Treon SP. Survival trends in Waldenström macroglobulinemia: an analysis of the surveillance, epidemiology end results database. Blood. 2014; 123(25):3999–4000.
30. Gertz MA. Waldenstrom's Macroglobulinemia. Oncologist AlphaMed Press; 2000 Feb 1;5(1):63–7.

31. Fintelmann F, Forghani R, Schaefer PW, Hochberg EP, Hochberg FH. Bing-Neel syndrome revisited. Clin Lymphoma Myeloma. 2009;9(1):104–6.

32. Klein CJ, Moon J-S, Mauermann ML, Zeldenrust SR, Wu Y, Dispenzieri A, et al. The neuropathies of Waldenström's macroglobulinemia (WM) and IgM-MGUS. Can J Neurol Sci. 2011;38(2):289–95.

33. Ansell SM, Kyle RA, Reeder CB, Fonseca R, Mikhael JR, Morice WG, et al. Diagnosis and management of Waldenström macroglobulinemia: Mayo stratification of macroglobulinemia and risk-adapted therapy (mSMART) guidelines. Mayo Clin Proc. 2010;85(9):824–33.

34. Treon SP, Tripsas CK, Meid K, Warren D, Varma G, Green R, et al. Ibrutinib in previously treated Waldenström's macroglobulinemia. N Engl J Med. 2015;372(15):1430–40.

35. Dispenzieri A, Kyle RA, Lacy MQ, Rajkumar SV, Therneau TM, Larson DR, et al. POEMS syndrome: definitions and long-term outcome. Blood. 2003;101(7):2496–506.

36. Planté-Bordeneuve V, Said G. Familial amyloid polyneuropathy. Lancet Neurol. 2011;10(12):1086–97.

37. Solomon A, Weiss DT, Murphy C. Primary amyloidosis associated with a novel heavy-chain fragment (AH amyloidosis). Am J Hematol. 1994;45(2):171–6.

38. Gertz MA, Rajkumar SV. Primary systemic amyloidosis. Curr Treat Options Oncol. 2002;3(3):261–71.

39. Kyle RA, Gertz MA. Primary systemic amyloidosis: clinical and laboratory features in 474 cases. Semin Hematol. 1995;32(1): 45–59.

40. Kyle RA, Greipp PR. Amyloidosis (AL). Clinical and laboratory features in 229 cases. Mayo Clin Proc. 1983;58(10):665–83.

41. Cueto-Garcia L, Tajik AJ, Kyle RA, Edwards WD, Greipp PR, Callahan JA, et al. Serial echocardiographic observations in patients with primary systemic amyloidosis: an introduction to the concept of early (asymptomatic) amyloid infiltration of the heart. Mayo Clin Proc. 1984;59(9):589–97.

42. Kumar SK, Gertz MA, Lacy MQ, Dingli D, Hayman SR, Buadi FK, et al. Recent improvements in survival in primary systemic amyloidosis and the importance of an early mortality risk score. Mayo Clin Proc. 2011;86(1):12–8.

43. Merlini G, Stone MJ. Dangerous small B-cell clones. Blood. 2006;108(8):2520–30.

44. Cordes S, Dispenzieri A, Lacy MQ, Hayman SR, Buadi FK, Dingli D, et al. Ten-year survival after autologous stem cell transplantation for immunoglobulin light chain amyloidosis. Cancer. 2012;118(24):6105–9.

45. Wang AK, Fealey RD, Gehrking TL, Low PA. Patterns of neuropathy and autonomic failure in patients with amyloidosis. Mayo Clin Proc. 2008;83(11):1226–30.

46. Kelly JJ, Kyle RA, O'Brien PC, Dyck PJ. The natural history of peripheral neuropathy in primary systemic amyloidosis. Ann Neurol. 1979;6(1):1–7.

47. Sadek I, Mauermann ML, Hayman SR, Spinner RJ, Gertz MA. Primary systemic amyloidosis presenting with asymmetric multiple mononeuropathies. J Clin Oncol. 2010;28(25):e429–32.

48. Ladha SS, Dyck PJB, Spinner RJ, Perez DG, Zeldenrust SR, Amrami KK, et al. Isolated amyloidosis presenting with lumbosacral radiculoplexopathy: description of two cases and pathogenic review. J Peripher Nerv Syst. 2006;11(4):346–52.

49. Figueroa JJ, Bosch EP, Dyck PJB, Singer W, Vrana JA, Theis JD, et al. Amyloid-like IgM deposition neuropathy: a distinct clinico-pathologic and proteomic profiled disorder. J Peripher Nerv Syst. 2012;17(2):182–90.

50. Vallat J-M, Magy L, Richard L, Piaser M, Sindou P, Calvo J, et al. Intranervous immunoglobulin deposits: an underestimated mechanism of neuropathy. Muscle Nerve. 2008;38(1):904–11.

51. Gertz MA. Immunoglobulin light chain amyloidosis: 2014 update on diagnosis, prognosis, and treatment. Am J Hematol. 2014; 89(12):1132–40.

52. Klein CJ, Vrana JA, Theis JD, Dyck PJ, Dyck PJB, Spinner RJ, et al. Mass spectrometric-based proteomic analysis of amyloid neuropathy type in nerve tissue. Arch Neurol. 2011;68(2):195–9.

53. Vrana JA, Gamez JD, Madden BJ, Theis JD, Bergen HR, Dogan A. Classification of amyloidosis by laser microdissection and mass spectrometry-based proteomic analysis in clinical biopsy specimens. Blood. 2009;114(24):4957–9.

54. Sanchorawala V, Skinner M, Quillen K, Finn KT, Doros G, Seldin DC. Long-term outcome of patients with AL amyloidosis treated with high-dose melphalan and stem-cell transplantation. Blood. 2007;110(10):3561–3.

55. Staff NP, Windebank AJ. Peripheral neuropathy due to vitamin deficiency, toxins, and medications. Continuum (Minneap Minn) 2014 Oct;20(5 Peripheral Nervous System Disorders):1293–306.

56. Kyle RA, Therneau TM, Rajkumar SV, Larson DR, Plevak MF, Melton LJ. Incidence of multiple myeloma in Olmsted County, Minnesota: Trend over 6 decades. Cancer. 2004;101(11):2667–74.

57. Kyle RA, Gertz MA, Witzig TE, Lust JA, Lacy MQ, Dispenzieri A, et al. Review of 1027 patients with newly diagnosed multiple myeloma. Mayo Clin Proc. 2003;78(1):21–33.

58. Mikhael JR, Dingli D, Roy V, Reeder CB, Buadi FK, Hayman SR, et al. Management of newly diagnosed symptomatic multiple myeloma: updated Mayo stratification of Myeloma and risk-adapted therapy (mSMART) consensus guidelines 2013. Mayo Clin Proc. 2013;88(4):360–76.

59. Kyle RA, Rajkumar SV. Criteria for diagnosis, staging, risk stratification and response assessment of multiple myeloma. Leukemia. 2009;23(1):3–9.

60. Vincent Rajkumar S. Multiple myeloma: 2014 Update on diagnosis, risk-stratification, and management. Am J Hematol 2014 Oct;89(10):999–1009.

61. Zhang J, Zhong Y. Clinical analysis of 36 multiple myeloma patients with extramedullary plasmacytoma invasion of the spinal canal. Hematol Oncol. 2015;33(2):75–9.

62. Schluterman KO, Fassas AB-T, Van Hemert RL, Harik SI. Multiple myeloma invasion of the central nervous system. Arch Neurol 2004 Sep;61(9):1423–9.

63. Joukhadar R, Chiu K. Sellar plasmacytomas: a concise review. Pituitary. 2012;15(2):146–9.

64. Mehta J, Singhal S. Hyperviscosity syndrome in plasma cell dyscrasias. Semin Thromb Hemost. 2003;29(5):467–71.

65. Talamo G, Cavallo F, Zangari M, Barlogie B, Lee C-K, Pineda-Roman M, et al. Hyperammonemia and encephalopathy in patients with multiple myeloma. Am J Hematol. 2007;82(5):414–5.

66. Zver S, Zadnik V, Cernelc P, Kozelj M. Cardiac toxicity of high-dose cyclophosphamide and melphalan in patients with multiple myeloma treated with tandem autologous hematopoietic stem cell transplantation. Int J Hematol. 2008;88(2):227–36.

67. Kozelj M, Zver S, Zadnik V. Long term follow-up report of cardiac toxicity in patients with multiple myeloma treated with tandem autologous hematopoietic stem cell transplantation. Radiol Oncol. 2013;47(2):161–5.

68. Gupta A, Pandey A, Sethi S. Bortezomib-induced congestive cardiac failure in a patient with multiple myeloma. Cardiovasc Toxicol. 2012;12(2):184–7.

69. Aota Y, Gotoh A, Hanyu N, Honma T, Morisaki M, Yokoyama T, et al. Bortezomib-associated acute congestive heart failure in a patient with multiple myeloma. Rinsho Ketsueki. 2015;56(1):44–7.

70. Grandin EW, Ky B, Cornell RF, Carver J, Lenihan DJ. Patterns of cardiac toxicity associated with irreversible proteasome inhibition in the treatment of multiple myeloma. J Card Fail. 2015;21(2): 138–44.

71. Tejani N, Cooper A, Rezo A, Pranavan G, Yip D. Numb chin syndrome: a case series of a clinical syndrome associated with malignancy. J Med Imaging Radiat Oncol. 2014;58(6):700–5.
72. Scutellari PN, Orzincolo C. Mandibular lesions in multiple myeloma. Radiol Med. 1992;83(3):219–23.
73. Walsh JC. The neuropathy of multiple myeloma. An electrophysiological and histological study. Arch Neurol. 1971;25(5):404–14.
74. Kelly JJ, Kyle RA, Miles JM, O'Brien PC, Dyck PJ. The spectrum of peripheral neuropathy in myeloma. Neurology. 1981;31(1):24–31.
75. Staff NP, Podratz JL, Grassner L, Bader M, Paz J, Knight AM, et al. Bortezomib alters microtubule polymerization and axonal transport in rat dorsal root ganglion neurons. Neurotoxicology. 2013;39:124–31.
76. Richardson PG, Xie W, Mitsiades C, Chanan-Khan AA, Lonial S, Hassoun H, et al. Single-agent bortezomib in previously untreated multiple myeloma: efficacy, characterization of peripheral neuropathy, and molecular correlations with response and neuropathy. J Clin Oncol. 2009;27(21):3518–25.
77. San Miguel JF, Schlag R, Khuageva NK, Dimopoulos MA, Shpilberg O, Kropff M, et al. Bortezomib plus melphalan and prednisone for initial treatment of multiple myeloma. N Engl J Med. 2008;359(9):906–17.
78. Moreau P, Pylypenko H, Grosicki S, Karamanesht I, Leleu X, Grishunina M, et al. Subcutaneous versus intravenous administration of bortezomib in patients with relapsed multiple myeloma: a randomised, phase 3, non-inferiority study. Lancet Oncol. 2011;12(5):431–40.
79. Bringhen S, Larocca A, Rossi D, Cavalli M, Genuardi M, Ria R, et al. Efficacy and safety of once-weekly bortezomib in multiple myeloma patients. Blood. 2010;116(23):4745–53.
80. Richardson PG, Briemberg H, Jagannath S, Wen PY, Barlogie B, Berenson J, et al. Frequency, characteristics, and reversibility of peripheral neuropathy during treatment of advanced multiple myeloma with bortezomib. J Clin Oncol. 2006;24(19):3113–20.
81. Ravaglia S, Corso A, Piccolo G, Lozza A, Alfonsi E, Mangiacavalli S, et al. Immune-mediated neuropathies in myeloma patients treated with bortezomib. Clin Neurophysiol. 2008;119(11):2507–12.
82. Mauermann ML, Blumenreich MS, Dispenzieri A, Staff NP. A case of peripheral nerve microvasculitis associated with multiple myeloma and bortezomib treatment. Muscle Nerve. 2012;46(6):970–7.
83. Richardson PG, Delforge M, Beksac M, Wen P, Jongen JL, Sezer O, et al. Management of treatment-emergent peripheral neuropathy in multiple myeloma. Leukemia. 2012;26(4):595–608.
84. Giannini F, Volpi N, Rossi S, Passero S, Fimiani M, Cerase A. Thalidomide-induced neuropathy: a ganglionopathy? Neurology. 2003;60(5):877–8.
85. Mileshkin L, Stark R, Day B, Seymour JF, Zeldis JB, Prince HM. Development of neuropathy in patients with myeloma treated with thalidomide: patterns of occurrence and the role of electrophysiologic monitoring. J Clin Oncol. 2006;24(27):4507–14.
86. Fonseca R, Bergsagel PL, Drach J, Shaughnessy J, Gutierrez N, Stewart AK, et al. International Myeloma Working Group molecular classification of multiple myeloma: spotlight review. Leukemia. 2009;23(12):2210–21.
87. Bardwick PA, Zvaifler NJ, Gill GN, Newman D, Greenway GD, Resnick DL. Plasma cell dyscrasia with polyneuropathy, organomegaly, endocrinopathy, M protein, and skin changes: the POEMS syndrome. Report on two cases and a review of the literature. Med (Baltimore). 1980;59(4):311–22.
88. Mauermann ML, Sorenson EJ, Dispenzieri A, Mandrekar J, Suarez GA, Dyck PJ, et al. Uniform demyelination and more severe axonal loss distinguish POEMS syndrome from CIDP. J Neurol Neurosurg Psychiatry. 2012;83(5):480–6.
89. Kelly JJ, Kyle RA, Miles JM, Dyck PJ. Osteosclerotic myeloma and peripheral neuropathy. Neurology. 1983;33(2):202–10.
90. Karam C, Klein CJ, Dispenzieri A, Dyck PJB, Mandrekar J, D'Souza A, et al. Polyneuropathy improvement following autologous stem cell transplantation for POEMS syndrome. Neurology. 2015;84(19):1981–7.
91. Nasu S, Misawa S, Sekiguchi Y, Shibuya K, Kanai K, Fujimaki Y, et al. Different neurological and physiological profiles in POEMS syndrome and chronic inflammatory demyelinating polyneuropathy. J Neurol Neurosurg Psychiatry. 2012;83(5):476–9.
92. Dispenzieri A. POEMS syndrome: 2014 update on diagnosis, risk-stratification, and management. Am J Hematol. 2014;89(2):214–23.
93. Dao LN, Hanson CA, Dispenzieri A, Morice WG, Kurtin PJ, Hoyer JD. Bone marrow histopathology in POEMS syndrome: a distinctive combination of plasma cell, lymphoid, and myeloid findings in 87 patients. Blood. 2011;117(24):6438–44.
94. Naddaf E, Dispenzieri A, Mandrekar J, Mauermann ML. Thrombocytosis distinguishes POEMS syndrome from chronic inflammatory demyelinating polyneuropathy. Muscle Nerve. 2015;52(4):658–9.
95. D'Souza A, Hayman SR, Buadi F, Mauermann M, Lacy MQ, Gertz MA, et al. The utility of plasma vascular endothelial growth factor levels in the diagnosis and follow-up of patients with POEMS syndrome. Blood. 2011;118(17):4663–5.
96. Humeniuk MS, Gertz MA, Lacy MQ, Kyle RA, Witzig TE, Kumar SK, et al. Outcomes of patients with POEMS syndrome treated initially with radiation. Blood. 2013;122(1):68–73.
97. D'Souza A, Lacy M, Gertz M, Kumar S, Buadi F, Hayman S, et al. Long-term outcomes after autologous stem cell transplantation for patients with POEMS syndrome (osteosclerotic myeloma): a single-center experience. Blood. 2012;120(1):56–62.

Neurologic Complications of Pediatric Systemic Cancer

Elizabeth S. Duke, Scott L. Pomeroy, and Nicole J. Ullrich

Introduction

Cancer is the most common disease-related cause of death for children under the age of 20 years and remains the fourth most common cause of all deaths, after accidents, suicide and homicide [1]. The most frequently arising cancers in children include leukemia and central nervous system tumors, which comprise nearly half of new cases [2]. Brain tumors are the second most common malignancy of childhood and the most common solid tumors, representing approximately 25% of childhood cancers (Fig. 33.1).

Despite an increasing incidence in pediatric cancers (13 per 100,000 in 1975 compared to 17.7 per 100,000 in 2012), there has been an overall decline in cancer mortality of approximately 50% over the same time period [3]. However, despite an equal increase in incidence of brain tumors, the decrease in mortality was only 20% between 1975 and 2012. The apparent increase in pediatric cancers may be, in part, related to earlier identification, increased access to care, and wider availability of advanced imaging and other diagnostic techniques. Nearly two-thirds of children diagnosed with cancer in the mid-1980s are now 20-year survivors of their disease [4], and these numbers are expected to increase as advancements continue in detection and treatment options. As survival continues to improve, the detrimental consequences of treatment on the nervous system, in particular the developing nervous system, are now better appreciated. Precise frequencies and attribution of these effects to the underlying tumor or its treatment are often quite difficult to determine.

As with adults, the incidence of neurologic complications from systemic cancer in children has been increasing. This may be partly due to the better overall recognition of these types of issues, but is also likely a reflection of improved overall survival, particularly in the pediatric population. In the adult population, neurologic effects have been well documented; it is estimated that as many as two-thirds of patients with cancer develop some type of neurological problem during the course of their illness and therapy [5–7]. Neurologic complications of childhood solid malignant tumors have been increasingly described over the past decade, with exact incidence difficult to determine, although the rate may be as high as one-third of patients [8–10]. In general, the focus of prior studies has been on metastatic disease in children [11–13].

As is well appreciated, children are not "mini-adults." Cancer presentation, manifestations, response to therapies and late effects often differ in children compared to the adult population. Rather than focusing on a particular tumor subtype in children, as has been done for the adult malignancies, this chapter will focus on the unique aspects of pediatric cancer in general. In children as with adults, these complications can be divided into direct tumor-related effects including metastases and paraneoplastic disorders, as well as indirect treatment-related effects from chemotherapy, surgery, cranial irradiation and stem cell transplant (Table 33.1).

Direct Neurologic Effects

Brain Metastases

Metastases of systemic cancers to the brain are the most common intracranial tumor in adults, with 15–40% of patients with advanced cancer developing CNS involvement

E.S. Duke · S.L. Pomeroy
Department of Neurology, Boston Children's Hospital,
300 Longwood Avenue, Fegan 11, Boston, MA 02215, USA
e-mail: elizabeth.duke@childrens.harvard.edu

S.L. Pomeroy
e-mail: scott.pomeroy@childrens.harvard.edu

N.J. Ullrich (✉)
Department of Neurology, Boston Children's Hospital,
333 Longwood Avenue, Boston, MA 02215, USA
e-mail: nicole.ullrich@childrens.harvard.edu

© Springer International Publishing AG 2018
D. Schiff et al. (eds.), *Cancer Neurology in Clinical Practice*,
DOI 10.1007/978-3-319-57901-6_33

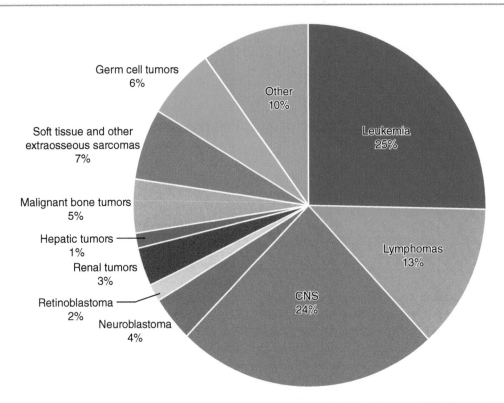

Fig. 33.1 Incidence of pediatric cancers. Age-adjusted and age-specific SEER cancer incidence rates, 2008–2012, all races, male and female, ages 0–19. (Created from data in Howlader N, Noone AM, Krapcho M, Garshell J, Miller D, Altekruse SF et al. Childhood Cancer by the ICCC, Table 29.1: Incidence Rates by Age at Diagnosis: Age-Adjusted and Age-Specific SEER Cancer Incidence Rates, 2008–2012. By International Classification of Childhood Cancer (ICCC) Group and Subgroup and Age at Diagnosis (including myelodysplastic syndromes and Group III benign brain/CNS tumors. All Races, Males and Females. In: SEER Cancer Statistics Review, 1975–2012. National Cancer Institute, Bethesda, MD. 2015. https://seer.cancer.gov/archive/csr/1975_2012/browse_csr.php?sectionSEL=29&pageSEL=sect_29_table.01.html)

Table 33.1 Neurologic complications of cancer in children

Direct, cancer-related toxicities	Treatment-related/iatrogenic
Local compression	Headache
Metastatic disease	Seizure
Leptomeningeal carcinomatosis	Neuropathy
Paraneoplastic syndromes	Toxic/metabolic encephalopathy
Indirect, non-metastatic neurologic effects	Cerebral infarction
Seizure	Drug-specific effects
Headache/migraine	Radiation complications
Tic disorder, movement disorder	Central nervous system infections
Static encephalopathy	Effects of stem cell transplantation

[14–17]. By contrast, central nervous system metastases are much less common in most extracranial pediatric solid tumors, with an estimated 1.5–2.5% incidence in clinical series and 6–13% in autopsy series [12, 18–22]. In adults, the most common primary cancers that metastasize to the brain are lung, breast, melanoma, renal and colorectal. In children, CNS seeding is common in leukemia, but rarer in solid extracranial primary tumors, with the most common being adrenal/renal tumors and sarcomas (Table 33.2) [12, 13, 19, 21, 23]. Similar to cancer incidence in general, the incidence of metastases in pediatric populations seems to be increasing, perhaps due to more effective treatments of the primary cancer, prolonged survival of patients and improvement in neuroimaging techniques. However, most studies are small and there remains debate as to whether routine surveillance for brain metastases is warranted in all patients [24].

Because of the relative rarity of brain metastases in children, information regarding presenting symptoms, pattern of spread, management and further prognosis is quite

Table 33.2 Solid tumors that lead to brain metastases in children

Primary tumor type	Frequency (range) (%)
Osteosarcoma	5–13
Ewing sarcoma	0–17
Soft tissue sarcoma	2–14
Wilms tumor	1–13
Germ cell tumor	0–50
Neuroblastoma	0–8
Other	2–19

Other = retinoblastoma, hepatoblastoma, melanoma, malignant schwannoma, lung cancer
Data from Refs. [12, 13, 19, 21, 173]

limited. Children are thought to have more rapid onset of neurologic manifestations compared with adults, perhaps because of a higher proliferative rate of pediatric malignancies [21]. Symptoms are dependent on location of disease and can result from increased intracranial pressure, local compression or disturbance of the tumor microenvironment. The most commonly reported symptoms include headache, nausea, vomiting, hemiparesis, cranial nerve palsies, mental status changes and seizures, the latter with an incidence ranging from 8 to 60% [8, 19, 21].

Patterns of metastatic spread differ by primary tumor site. Pediatric patients who have solid tumors with pulmonary metastases are more likely to have brain metastases, suggesting a hematogenous spread of tumor emboli from the pulmonary metastases [19, 20]. In neuroblastoma, by contrast, metastases are thought to arise from adjacent bone metastases, and in these cases, local invasion of the skull or brain parenchyma and spinal metastases are seen, rather than isolated parenchymal lesions [21, 24]. Additionally, patients with acute myeloid leukemia (AML) can get chloromas (granulocytic sarcomas), which are a subset of parenchymal metastases defined as an extramedullary manifestation of AML in any organ including the brain [25].

Pediatric brain metastases are most often solitary and supratentorial, and by the time CNS involvement is discovered, prognosis tends to be poor despite aggressive therapy. In most cases, surgical extirpation is not attempted, but over time potential treatments have expanded to include stereotactic radiosurgery, whole brain radiation therapy, chemotherapy and targeted agents [22, 26]. In one recent study, patients with Wilms tumor had the longest survival after the diagnosis of CNS metastasis, yet the 1-year survival rates remain approximately 50%. Independent of underlying pathology or treatment, studies report a median survival of 1–12 months after diagnosis of CNS metastases; even with control of brain disease, the majority of patients die of other systemic disease [8, 12, 18–21, 23, 24].

Leptomeningeal and Spinal Metastatic Disease

Leptomeningeal metastases are found most frequently in children with leukemia or primary CNS malignancy [27–29]. Prior to the use of prophylactic CNS therapy, nearly 50% of children with leukemia had CNS disease, which was the major cause of treatment failure, even after bone marrow transplantation [28, 30]. Now, fewer than 10% of patients have CNS leukemia; it is these patients at highest risk who are treated with a combination of intrathecal methotrexate, with or without cytarabine and dexamethasone, and craniospinal irradiation [28]. Leptomeningeal lymphoma is more common in those patients with concurrent disease of the bone marrow [29, 31–33]. Solid tumors can have a leptomeningeal component, either at presentation, as an isolated event, or associated with local disease progression. This is seen most frequently with retinoblastoma [34], neuroblastoma [35–37], rhabdomyosarcoma [38], melanoma [39, 40], and Ewing's sarcoma [41, 42], and most commonly with advanced systemic disease.

Diagnosis of leptomeningeal disease is confirmed with sampling of cerebrospinal fluid and imaging studies. A negative cytology does not preclude the diagnosis; in adults, initial CSF was positive in 55–70%, but the yield increases to 80–92% with repeated CSF sampling [31, 43]. The diagnosis of CSF leukemia requires definable blasts in the CSF, with a stratification based on number of leukocytes and blasts detected. For germ cell tumors, elevated tumor markers such as alpha fetoprotein and human chorionic gonadotropin may support the diagnosis of leptomeningeal metastases, along with simultaneous serum marker studies. Other potential clues include elevated opening pressure, decreased glucose and increased protein. Imaging studies may be helpful to show bulky disease and to assess CSF flow dynamics.

Leptomeningeal disease and spinal cord compression are both thought to be more treatable and have a better prognosis in children than in adults. Leptomeningeal disease can be bulky, nodular and more focal in nature or have more widespread and diffuse involvement. The most frequent mode of metastases is to the epidural or subarachnoid space or by metastatic spread to the cord parenchyma. Presenting features, therefore, reflect the pattern of involvement and may include both non-specific and focal neurologic symptoms; these symptoms can be the presentation of underlying malignancy in children, either with or without concurrent symptoms of the underlying neoplasm [8, 44]. Patients may also be asymptomatic clinically, with the diagnosis made by surveillance of CSF cytology and/or neuroimaging studies [27]. The most common presentation of leptomeningeal disease is from symptoms of increased intracranial pressure, including headache, nausea and vomiting. There may also be involvement of the cranial nerves or spinal cord involvement with weakness, sensory loss, pain, ataxia or paraparesis. The most common non-traumatic cause of paraparesis in children is neoplastic spinal cord compression [45]. Symptoms of spinal cord compression often include back pain, lower extremity weakness, paresthesias and urinary retention [8, 18, 27, 46]. Occasionally, leptomeningeal disease can mimic a mass lesion in the cerebellum by infiltrating cerebellar pathways [47]. For leukemia, the most common neurologic symptoms overall include weakness and back pain, even without leptomeningeal infiltration [44]. Lymphoma, by contrast, is more likely to show direct meningeal infiltration with spinal cord compression and/or cranial neuropathy [48]. Neuroblastoma may present with spinal cord compression due to epidural spinal metastases.

Treatment for spinal cord compression can include a combination of decompressive laminectomy and/or high-dose steroids followed by therapeutic irradiation and intrathecal and/or systemic chemotherapy. In children, laminectomy is avoided as much as possible, particularly in young patients, because of concerns for development of anterior subluxation, kyphosis or scoliosis; surgery is reserved for cases with rapid neurologic deterioration [49]. Children with neuroblastoma producing spinal cord compression from local disease are often treated with chemotherapy alone (Fig. 33.2).

Paraneoplastic Disorders

Paraneoplastic neurological syndromes, which are thought to be autoimmune phenomena associated with specific cancers and marked by specific autoantibodies, are rare complications of malignancy that are seen much more frequently in the adult population. These syndromes affect <1% of all patients with cancer and often occur while the primary tumor is small and otherwise asymptomatic [50–52].

Paraneoplastic syndromes can be broken down into four categories based on the mechanism of action of the

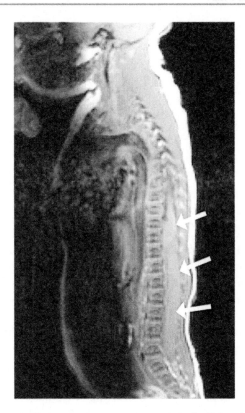

Fig. 33.2 Sagittal magnetic resonance imaging of a 3-day-old infant, who presented with paraparesis and found to have spinal neuroblastoma and spinal cord compression. He was treated with chemotherapy alone. At 15 months, he now is crawling and standing with stander device

autoantibodies [53]. First are the neuromuscular paraneoplastic disorders including myasthenia gravis, Lambert-Eaton myasthenic syndrome, autoimmune autonomic neuropathy, Isaacs syndrome (acquired neuromyotonia) and inflammatory myopathies (polymyositis, dermatomyositis). In these cases, autoantibodies to the NMJ or peripheral nerve membrane have direct physiologic effects and generally respond to immunosuppressive treatment (steroids, IVIG, plasmapheresis). Second are the classical paraneoplastic disorders with antibodies that mark a cell-mediated immune response, but which do not directly cause disease and thus have a poor response to immunotherapy; these include the anti-Hu, anti-Ma/Ta and anti-Yo syndromes that can lead to encephalomyelitis, limbic encephalitis or cerebellar degeneration, respectively. Third are autoantibodies to intracellular synaptic and neuronal surface proteins, such as anti-GAD65, which may be directly pathogenic or mark a T-cell response, as there is often a mixed response to immunotherapy. And finally, there are autoantibodies to extracellular surface epitopes of CNS synaptic and other neuronal membrane proteins that do have direct effects, such as anti-NMDA receptor syndrome and many others that are actively being identified.

Although paraneoplastic disorders are less common in children, as identification of antigenic neuronal membrane proteins continues to progress, the incidence will likely increase. The classic example in pediatric cancer is opsoclonus-myoclonus syndrome (OMS), which is commonly associated with neuroblastoma. OMS is defined by the classical acute onset of rapid and chaotic eye movements, myoclonic jerks and appendicular and axial ataxia. It can also be associated with behavioral changes and emotional lability. OMS is associated with underlying neuroblastoma in more than one half of cases and occurs in 2–3% of all children with neuroblastoma [54, 55]. A thorough search for neuroblastoma is necessary in all patients with OMS. Despite continued research, there does not appear to be a universal autoantibody detectable, although an autoimmune pathogenesis has been suspected, particularly with the favorable response to steroids and intravenous immunoglobulin [56]. Children with OMS are more likely to have serum antineuronal antibodies than other children with neuroblastoma, but the anti-Ri antibodies detected in adult cases of this syndrome are less frequently identified in children [57].

In at least half of these cases, OMS is the first presenting symptom of the neuroblastoma; the presence of OMS is often thought to portend a more favorable prognosis, with almost all being small, stage I–II, non-*MYCN* amplified tumors. Despite a better oncologic prognosis, there can be acute as well as chronic neurologic effects [54, 55, 58–60]. Personality changes, developmental regression with loss of speech and language, and motor deficits may remain significant, and many children will continue to experience severe learning and language deficits [61]. Surgical removal of the tumor in addition to prompt and strong immunosuppression remains the mainstay of therapy; however, very few children actually receive early therapy [62]. There was a recently completed Children's Oncology Group randomized phase III trial for patients with OMS and neuroblastoma to determine the efficacy of immunosuppressive therapy with cyclophosphamide, prednisone and IVIG in treating OMS, with final results still pending (NCT00033293) [63].

A second paraneoplastic neurologic syndrome, paraneoplastic limbic encephalitis (PLE), has been better defined over the past decade. PLE is thought to be not a single entity, but rather a subset of autoimmune disorders with antineuronal antibodies that primarily affect the limbic system [64]. There is an ever-increasing number of antineuronal antibodies identified, the most common in pediatrics being the anti-NMDA receptor syndrome, seen most frequently in young women with ovarian teratomas. The illness often begins with a viral prodrome, followed by behavioral or cognitive changes, then variably with seizures, movement disorders, eye movement abnormalities and/or autonomic dysfunction. Without treatment, the illness often culminates in coma, but is often improved with immunomodulators [65]. Additionally, antibodies to the metabotropic glutamate receptor 5 (mGluR5) have been described in patients with

Hodgkin lymphoma who experience the "Ophelia syndrome," a constellation of altered mental status, insomnia, short-term memory loss, depression and cognitive impairment [66, 67].

Paraneoplastic neurologic syndromes are clinically heterogeneous and can be quite difficult both to recognize and to diagnose; more research is needed to further understand their pathophysiology and efficacy of treatments with immunotherapy, which appears to depend on the underlying mechanism of action of the specific autoantibody.

Indirect and Treatment-Related Neurologic Complications

Treatment of pediatric cancer is generally tailored to the underlying tumor type and location, as in adults. While these treatments are critical, from surgery to chemotherapy to radiation to stem cell transplant, they often have neurologic side effects that can be long lasting. These complications include headaches, seizures, altered mental status, cerebral infarctions, peripheral neuropathies, sleep disturbances, cognitive effects and secondary tumors. Chemotherapy-related effects in children are in many cases similar to those experienced and reported in adults. The incidence of neurotoxicity from acute lymphoblastic leukemia (ALL) therapy is thought to range from 5% to 18% [68–70]. In addition to toxicities of chemotherapy, radiation and stem cell transplant have their own unique concerns. This section will review some general complications of cancer treatment in children and will discuss several chemotherapeutic agents and their more common neurotoxic effects (Table 33.3).

Headaches

Headaches in children are a common neurologic complaint and the most common cause for neurologic consultation in children with cancer; the difficulty lies in determining the underlying etiology (Table 33.4) [71]. Typical causes of headache can be seen, such as migraine or tension-type headaches. Of 147 childhood ALL survivors in at least 1-year of remission and 5 years from diagnosis, more than 40% had new-onset headaches; of those, approximately 1/3 were migraine, 1/3 were tension-type headache and 1/3 were mixed [72].

Treatment-specific causes of headache can occur, such as adverse drug reactions, post-LP headaches and posterior reversible encephalopathy syndrome (PRES). Common drug effects include fever, anemia or pseudotumor cerebri. Low pressure headaches after lumbar puncture, with or without intrathecal chemotherapy, are frequent with an incidence that ranges from 8% overall [73] to as much as 50% in the

Table 33.3 Commonly used chemotherapeutic drugs, frequency and type of neurologic side effects

Drug	Common, >10%	Uncommon, <10%	Rare, <1%
Methotrexate	Leukoencephalopathy, esp. with radiotherapy	Myelitis, arachnoiditis	Seizure
Cytarabine		Ataxia, arachnoiditis	
Vincristine	Peripheral/autonomic neuropathy		Seizures
Asparaginase	Mental status Δ		Sinus thrombosis
Corticosteroids	Myopathy, tremor, behavioral Δ		Psychosis, seizures, neuropathy
Cisplatin/carboplatin	Hearing loss		Peripheral neuropathy, seizure
Cyclosporine	Tremor	Seizure, Leukoencephalopathy	
Thalidomide		Neuropathy	

Table 33.4 Most common reasons for neurologic assessment in children with systemic cancer

Reason for neurologic evaluation	% complaints
Headache	34.9
Back/neck pain	25
Limb pain/sensory change	12
Extremity weakness	7.1
Seizure	7
Altered mental status	8.4
Visual complaints/diplopia	6.5

Used with permission of Elsevier from Antunes et al. [75]

adolescent population [74]. PRES is seen particularly in the setting of hypertension, induction chemotherapy or treatment with immunosuppressive agents (e.g., cyclosporine, tacrolimus and corticosteroids).

Complications of the disease itself can cause headaches, from metastases to infection to vascular injury (arterial occlusion, venous sinus thrombosis, hemorrhage). For systemic cancers, brain metastases are the most common structural cause of headache, followed by infections such as abscess and meningitis, and less frequently by intracranial hemorrhage [71]. The significant immunosuppression induced by many cancer treatments makes patients susceptible to many microorganisms, with life-threatening infections mainly caused by viruses (herpesvirus, VZV, CMV) or fungi. Structural disease should be excluded even in the absence of localizing signs, as 25% of children with systemic cancer and headache have an underlying structural lesion [75].

Seizures

The second most frequent reason for neurologic consultation is seizures, which occur in children with both solid tumors and hematologic malignancies, as well as children undergoing bone marrow transplantation. Seizures in children are more frequent than in adults and can result from either tumor- or treatment-related toxicity. Seizure risk may be increased in those patients who are known to have central nervous system involvement. All types of seizures may be observed in children who are treated with chemotherapy. Seizures without evidence for mass lesion are reported in 8–10% of children with leukemia and lymphoma [76, 77], though it is estimated that as many as 50% of children with solid tumors who experience a seizure have an underlying structural abnormality [71]. A thorough evaluation must be performed to search for intracranial lesions, infection, encephalopathy and stroke as potential etiologies.

Primary CNS causes of seizure include primary brain tumor, parenchymal or leptomeningeal metastases, ischemic or hemorrhagic stroke, PRES, leukoencephalopathy or intracranial infection (meningitis, cerebritis, abscess). At least 15% of brain tumor patients will have seizures, which may result from disruption of peritumoral environment, tumoral edema, adjacent scar, local hypoxia, acidosis or metabolic changes that affect neuronal excitability and epileptogenesis in tumor cells [78]. In brain tumor patients, several factors affect the incidence of seizures, including age, location, histology and grade of the tumor. Low-grade and slow-growing tumors tend to be more epileptogenic. Cortical lesions in the temporal, frontal and parietal lobes are more often correlated with seizures than tumors in the occipital lobe or posterior fossa [79].

Treatment-related causes of seizures include toxic-metabolic effects of chemotherapy (cyclosporine, asparaginase, imipenem), medication toxicity or withdrawal, radiation injury, renal or liver failure, latent non-CNS infection, and electrolyte abnormalities (SIADH, hypoglycemia, hypomagnesemia, hypo- or hypercalcemia) [80]. The strongest association with seizures and chemotherapy has been reported with methotrexate, which is used to treat many pediatric cancers, including ALL, lymphoma and sarcomas. Estimates of seizure frequency suggest that 7–20% of children with ALL experience seizures at some point during the course of therapy [76, 81, 82]. One study of survivors of ALL showed that 13% of children had experienced a seizure at some point during their treatment, and all reported patients except one experienced seizure after intrathecal methotrexate or subcutaneous asparaginase [77]. Other agents known to lower seizure threshold include cisplatin and vincristine, as both of these agents can pass through the blood-brain barrier and can secondarily induce seizures secondary to electrolyte disturbances from hypocalcemia, hypomagnesemia or hyponatremia.

Seizure prophylaxis must be carefully considered to determine whether medications are needed and, if so, the specific choice. The choice of anticonvulsant may be challenging, particularly as many of the more traditional anticonvulsants, such as phenytoin, carbamazepine and phenobarbital, can affect metabolism of chemotherapeutic drugs by inducing increased activity of the cytochrome p450 system [83, 84]. This may result in decreased tumor therapy efficacy, decreased seizure control and/or unexpected toxicity. Newer AEDs, especially those without significant drug–drug interactions, are becoming accepted as first-line seizure treatment in children who require ongoing seizure prophylaxis [85, 86].

Change in Mental Status

Alteration of mental status is a relatively common occurrence in children undergoing chemotherapy and has been reported in as many as 11% of children during the course of treatment [87]. Similar to headache and seizure, altered mental status can have multiple etiologies in patients with cancer, both disease- and treatment-related. As in the adult population, the underlying cause of mental status changes in children is toxic-metabolic encephalopathy in two-thirds of the cases and structural causes in the other one-third [71]. Many different agents are known to cause changes in level of alertness and/or somnolence in children, including

asparaginase, cisplatin, ifosfamide, methotrexate (including intrathecal), cytarabine, cyclosporine, etoposide and vincristine. Independent of chemotherapy, opioids, benzodiazepines, H2-blockers, antihistamines and antibiotics may cause delirium as well. Although medications may ultimately be the culprit, it is important to eliminate other potential causes, such as seizure, cerebrovascular event, infection, hemorrhage or metabolic derangement, so as to address potentially treatable sources.

Cerebral Infarction

Stroke is becoming an increasingly recognized complication in pediatric cancer patients. As in adults, cerebral infarction in childhood cancer patients may be ischemic or hemorrhagic. Etiologies range from disease-related complications of hypercoagulability, disseminated intravascular coagulation, thrombocytopenia or hemorrhagic metastases, to treatment-related complications of chemotherapy (venous sinus thrombosis, meningitis) or radiation (small and large vessel vasculopathy) [88, 89]. Stroke manifestations may be age-related. In the younger child, presentation may be more insidious with irritability, altered level of alertness and seizures while older children often report headaches, focal deficits such as visual change, speech impairment, weakness and seizures [90, 91].

Ischemic stroke is seen secondary to direct thrombosis, septic emboli, non-septic embolic disease, venous sinus thrombosis or disseminated intravascular coagulation. One large study of children with leukemia reported a 0.47% prevalence of ischemic stroke, all of which were sinovenous thrombosis (Fig. 33.3) [92]. Despite a relatively high frequency of elevated white blood cell counts and decreased platelets in children with cancer, the overall rate of strokes is thought to be quite low as a result of these risk factors. Strokes from chemotherapy itself have been more commonly associated with asparaginase and methotrexate [87, 93, 94]. In the pediatric population, neurologic outcome after sinovenous thrombosis was related to underlying clinical features such as seizures, impaired level of consciousness, coincident intracranial hemorrhage, deep venous location, lack of antithrombotic therapy and young age, less than six years [95–98].

Hemorrhagic stroke is a serious risk in acute leukemia patients, typically due coagulation abnormalities and most often occurring during induction therapy. Intracranial hemorrhage is reported to be the second leading cause of mortality in AML patients, accounting for up to 70% in some series [99]. Treatment with L-asparaginase is an additional risk factor. Superficial siderosis is a less common complication in CNS tumor patients, with deposition of

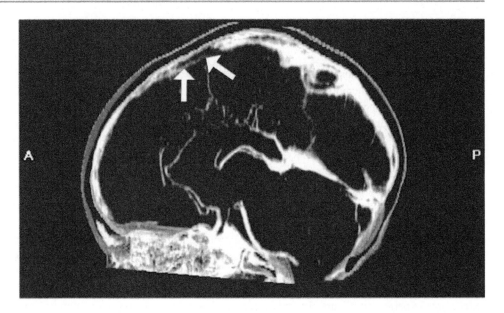

hemosiderin in the subarachnoid space leading to sensorineural deafness, cerebellar ataxia and myelopathy due to recurrent hemorrhage [100].

Radiation therapy is a primary risk factor for cerebral infarction [101]. Patients with hematologic malignancies and primary brain tumors who receive radiation therapy are at high risk, generally in a dose-dependent manner [102]. Location of radiation is another risk factor for cerebral infarction, with mantle radiation in Hodgkin's disease (thought to trigger cardiac valvular dysfunction and carotid artery disease) and radiation to the Circle of Willis in suprasellar tumors both increasing risk [103]. Radiation contributes to weakening of the microvasculature within the blood-brain barrier and increasing capillary permeability, leading to increased inflammation and thrombosis of small vessels [104]. Inflammation also leads to premature atherosclerosis, intimal fibrosis and macrophage activation that can lead to stenosis or thrombus [105]. Damaged vasculature can lead to abnormal dilation and tortuosity, causing vascular malformation, aneurysm or moyamoya syndrome, and this risk is higher in children with neurofibromatosis type 1 [106, 107]. These changes can result in seizures, headaches and potentially life-threatening hemorrhage. Hemorrhagic strokes presenting as delayed hemorrhagic radiation vasculopathy, separate from tumor recurrence or secondary tumor and unrelated to treatment dose, have been reported after radiation alone or radiation in combination with systemic chemotherapy in children [108].

Motor Deficits/Neuropathy

Pediatric oncology patients experience motor deficits for a variety of reasons, with localization potentially anywhere along the neural axis. Motor deficits can occur due to primary tumor or metastatic compression of fibers along the motor strip, supplementary motor areas or corticospinal tract. In the brainstem, cranial nerve deficits may also be observed, particularly in patients who already have some cranial nerve dysfunction.

In the spinal cord, acute cord compression is a neurologic emergency in children as in adults and must be investigated emergently for potentially reversible causes. Spinal cord compression occurs in 3–5% of children with cancer, most commonly if the tumor involves epidural or subarachnoid space [109]. Childhood tumors implicated include neuroblastoma, sarcomas, non-Hodgkin lymphoma and germ cell tumors. Symptoms include motor or sensory deficits, sphincter abnormalities or back pain. Steroids should be given immediately, followed by MRI to confirm diagnosis, then more definitive treatment with surgical decompression, radiation and/or chemotherapy. Some patients have persistent neurologic deficits, with severity of deficits at time of diagnosis most predictive of long-term symptoms.

The most well-studied nerve injury in cancer patients is chemotherapy-induced peripheral neuropathy (CIPN), which is known to damage axon, cell body or myelin depending on the mechanism of action. CIPN can be difficult to assess in children due to limited verbal expression and vocabulary to express specific symptoms. Nerve damage is generally length-dependent, with longest axons displaying abnormalities first. Risk factors include higher dose of chemotherapy with specific agents, intensity of treatment schedule, multimodal treatment, preexisting neuropathy and genetic predisposition (e.g., decreased expression of CYP3A5) [110]. Some of the more common agents used in pediatrics include vincristine, a mitotic inhibitor that inhibits tubulin polymerization and can cause sensory, motor and autonomic neuropathies as well as platinum-based agents that bind with DNA strands and induce apoptotic cell death [111]. Platinum drugs more commonly lead to high frequency sensorineural hearing loss; ototoxic effects are related to total dose and often synergistic in patients who have also received cranial irradiation. The underlying mechanism is thought to be related to permanent damage to the mitochondria of the hair cells. Taxanes and epothilones, microtubule-stabilizing agents, can contribute to peripheral neuropathy by inhibition of axonal transport [110]. Finally, the newer antibody and enzyme inhibitor therapies are less well studied, but agents such as bortezomib appear to affect dorsal root ganglion cells, leading to moderate to severe neuropathic pain [112].

Damage to the neuromuscular junction and muscle itself can also occur, due to treatment toxicity or paraneoplastic syndromes. Residual deficits are present in many long-term cancer survivors, with one study documenting sensation, vibration and reflex deficits in adult survivors of childhood ALL treated with vincristine >20 years after completion of treatment [113]. Studies are being conducted to analyze agents with potential neuroprotective factors in children receiving these treatments. In addition to physical and occupational rehabilitation, treatment of neuropathic pain with gabapentin, pregabalin and various antidepressants are being studied in children.

Sleep Disorders

Sleep problems are common in the general population, and even more so in children and adolescents with chronic medical conditions, including cancer. Like many of the other comorbidities described in this chapter, sleep dysfunction can be due to specific cancer-related factors (direct brain injury, chemotherapy, cranial radiation, pain, seizures, endocrinopathies, medications) or other genetic and environmental factors including familial predisposition, stress and other mental health problems [114].

The specific sleep disturbances seen are varied and include symptoms from cancer-related fatigue and excessive daytime sleepiness (EDS) to insomnia, parasomnias and restless leg syndrome [115]. There are limited studies of the prevalence of sleep problems in children with cancer, but the Childhood Cancer Survivorship Study (CCSS) found that 19% of adult survivors were in the most fatigued range, 16.7% reported disrupted sleep and 14% reported EDS [116].

Sleep disorders are particularly common in patients with CNS tumors and metastases; one study showed 46% of children with a neoplasm of the hypothalamus, thalamus or brainstem had sleep-disordered breathing (obstructive sleep apnea, central sleep apnea) and 80% had EDS [117]. In children with leukemia, insomnia was the most common sleep problem identified (39%), especially in patients receiving high-dose steroid treatment. Sleep irregularities are not solely a result of obstructive sleep apnea; for example, in craniopharyngiomas, direct injury to the hypothalamus can result in disruption of circadian rhythms [118].

Sleep dysfunction is associated with reduced quality of life in pediatric cancer patients and should be addressed regularly, and if indicated, objectively measured with a validated sleep scale, actigraphy, multiple sleep latency test and/or nocturnal polysomnography [119, 120]. For treatment, lifestyle modifications should be trialed including weight loss, exercise, avoiding daytime naps and treatment of thyroid hormone or cortisol deficiency. Pharmacotherapy options include melatonin at bedtime or stimulants in cases of EDS related to delayed sleep phase syndrome [121].

Cognitive Effects

Neurocognitive late effects are a multidimensional, globally impacting and potentially modifiable problem in survivors of childhood cancer. The nature and severity of deficits depend on the patient's neurodevelopmental stage at the time of diagnosis and treatment. One study estimated that 40–50% of acute lymphoblastic leukemia survivors and 70–80% of brain tumor survivors would require special education services during their school years [122]. The cognitive domains most typically affected include memory, attention, processing speed and executive functioning, in addition to motor skills and psychosocial functioning [123]. Risk factors include young age at time of treatment, female gender and dose intensity of treatment.

In a study of nearly 3000 adolescent and young adult survivors of cancer (ages 11–21 years at diagnosis) compared with siblings, the patients had significantly increased rates of depression and anxiety and more problems with task efficiency, emotional regulation and memory [124]. Brain tumor survivors are especially vulnerable to neurocognitive dysfunction given the aggressive CNS-directed therapies required for treatment of their tumors. Deficits can be due to direct brain injury from the tumor (type, size, location), its treatment (surgery, radiation or systemic effects of chemotherapy), or disease-related complications; all of which are further modified by the surrounding environment and psychosocial factors of the child [125].

Craniospinal radiation is particularly injurious, with destruction of white matter tracts and/or failure to develop white matter at a rate consistent with the developmental stage of the child implicated as the mechanism by which cognitive deficits occur [126]. A unique deficit described in children treated for posterior fossa tumors is cerebellar mutism, a typically transient syndrome of paucity of speech often accompanied by emotional and behavioral dysregulation that evolves after cerebellar injury and occurs in approximately 25% of children following posterior fossa tumor surgery [127].

Strategies for prevention of these neurocognitive deficits include more directed therapies specific to tumor subtype, focused surgical resections with improved imaging and mapping of eloquent cortex, and research in molecularly targeted therapies that may spare use of whole brain radiation [128].

Secondary Tumors

Pediatric cancer survivors are at risk of developing secondary tumors up to decades after their initial diagnosis. This is likely due to various treatments including radiation and chemotherapy, in addition to underlying genetic predispositions [129].

The Childhood Cancer Survivor Study (CCSS) has a population of nearly 15,000 five-year survivors of childhood cancer who were treated from 1970 to 1986, and in a study to assess the cumulative incidence of subsequent neoplasms at 30 years after diagnosis, they found that nearly 10% of survivors developed a second neoplasm [130]. Patients surviving Hodgkin lymphoma and Ewing sarcoma were at greatest risk, compared to patients with kidney cancer who had a decreased risk of subsequent neoplasms. Other risk factors include female sex and radiation therapy exposure. A recent study found a relationship between less telomere content and treatment-related thyroid cancer, suggesting that shorter telomeres may contribute to certain subsequent neoplasms in childhood cancer survivors [131].

In the CCSS cohort, the secondary cancers that occurred most commonly included non-melanoma skin cancer, bone cancer, thyroid cancer, head and neck cancer, breast cancer, CNS malignancies (particularly meningiomas) and soft tissue sarcoma [132]. Age at primary diagnosis affected type of secondary neoplasm: younger age at diagnosis (<10 years) increased risk for meningioma, malignant CNS tumor, sarcoma and thyroid cancer. Older age at diagnosis increased risk for breast, non-melanoma skin and other solid organ cancers. The median time to first occurrence of a subsequent malignant neoplasm was just under 18 years, with shorter period for leukemia and longer period for GI cancers [130]. Diet and lifestyle factors have not been well studied to understand their impact on these associations.

The overall mortality rate due to recurrence or progression of a primary malignancy is 0.44%/year [133]. This rate decreases as time from diagnosis increases (9.9 deaths/1000 person-years at 5–9 years from diagnosis vs. 0.5 deaths/1000 person-years at >30 years from diagnosis), whereas the mortality rate due to subsequent neoplasm

increases (1.3 at 5–9 years vs. 4.6 at >30 years). The standardized mortality ratio (SMR) from subsequent neoplasms is 15.2, which is higher than other causes including pulmonary death (SMR 8.8), cardiac death (SMR 7.0), external causes such as accidents/homicides/suicides (SMR 0.9) and all other causes (SMR 2.6) [133]. More studies are needed to further assess risk related to specific primary diagnoses, determine appropriate screening protocols and continue to balance maximizing cure rates while minimizing long-term effects of cancer treatments.

Drug-Specific Effects

Several chemotherapeutic agents, which are used with much higher frequency in children based on underlying disease prevalence, are known to have quite specific neurologic effects. These offending agents include methotrexate, cytarabine, vincristine, asparaginase and corticosteroids. However, because standard therapy often relies on combinations of chemotherapy, it is sometimes difficult to isolate the offending agent.

Methotrexate is often implicated as a major cause of acute neurologic issues. All of the major risk factors for methotrexate-induced neurotoxicity, including use in higher doses [134], intrathecal administration [135], young age at time of treatment [136, 137], and concurrent use of cranial irradiation [137], are applicable in the pediatric age group. The characteristic radiographic finding in patients with associated neurotoxicity is thought to be reversible leukoencephalopathy, radiographically signified by hyperintense regions on T2-weighted MRI that are typically located in the periventricular white matter [137, 138]. These white matter changes often recover spontaneously, but some patients have irreversible lesions [139]. Chemical arachnoiditis/aseptic meningitis occurs in 10–60% of patients receiving intrathecal therapy with acute onset headache, meningismus, nausea, vomiting and altered mental status [140]. CSF analysis typically shows pleocytosis but cultures are negative. Transverse myelopathy is an uncommon complication of intrathecal methotrexate, more common with exposure to radiation, repeated injections or leukemic CNS infiltration [99]. Recovery is variable; pathology demonstrates a vacuolar necrotizing demyelination of the spinal cord and brainstem [140].

One of the mainstays of therapy for children with acute lymphoblastic leukemia is asparaginase, which functions by depletion of downstream stores of l-asparagine and aspartic acid. Secondary toxicities from asparaginase include alteration of coagulation and hypersensitivity reactions. Reported central nervous system complications include cerebral hemorrhage and cerebral thrombosis [141]. Defects in coagulation are thought to result from an imbalance of the

607 Neurologic Complications of Pediatric Systemic Cancer

pro- and anticoagulating systems, leading to decreased antithrombin III, protein S and protein C. Common presenting symptoms of sinus venous thrombosis, associated with secondary parenchymal hemorrhage, include headache, seizure and increased intracranial pressure. These symptoms were all evident in this 5-year-old boy with ALL, who experienced a sagittal sinus thrombosis, for which additional therapy with asparaginase had to be discontinued and fractionated low-molecular weight heparin was initiated (Fig. 33.3).

Vincristine is one of the basic components of therapy for leukemia as well as many central nervous system tumors, including low-grade glioma. Vincristine is thought to impair motor function by causing a peripheral neuropathy, which manifests as decreased deep tendon reflex responses, decreased peripheral motor abilities, motor clumsiness and decreased distal sensation [142, 143]. Although considered reversible, these effects can last months to years after completion of therapy, and signs of motor problems have been reported up to five years after therapy for ALL when patients are followed with careful electromyographic studies [144]. Other agents such as thalidomide can produce a peripheral neuropathy, which may continue to progress even after cessation of treatment [145].

Newer biologically targeted agents are being studied that may be able to deliver specific anticancer effects while limiting damage to healthy tissue. Data are still limited in children, and more neurotoxicity may occur in the pediatric population because some agents target pathways that control tumorigenesis or neural maturation [146]. Further investigation is needed into long-term neurologic effects.

Neurologic Effects of Radiation in Children

Radiation therapy remains an important component of cancer treatment. Like many other therapies, radiation has non-specific cytotoxic effects on the adjacent nervous system when used to treat malignancies located in close proximity to the brain and spinal cord. Although tissue thresholds have been established, individual persons may have individual radiation tolerances. Moreover, patients may experience different complications related to age, disease status, concomitant therapies, length of survival and radiation features such as dose, size of the field and fractionation schema [147]. Radiation, used alone or in combination with chemotherapy, is associated with significant adverse neurologic effects, including headache, neuropathy, neurocognitive deficits, endocrine abnormalities, sleep dysfunction, secondary neoplasms and cerebrovascular disease. Radiation injury can affect each level of the nervous system and can be acute (at the time of therapy), subacute (within six months of treatment) or delayed (6 months to years after completion of

therapy). Acute and subacute symptoms tend to be reversible, whereas delayed injury often is not.

Acute radiation encephalopathy is rare and more frequently occurs in patients with already increased intracranial pressure and vasogenic edema surrounding the tumor; symptoms typically improve with steroids [140]. Subacute radiation encephalopathy can be seen from one to six months after treatment, with headache, nausea, worsening or reappearance of original neurologic symptoms, and occasionally "somnolence syndrome," a profound lethargy described in children receiving cranial irradiation for a primary brain tumor or CNS prophylaxis for acute leukemia [148].

Delayed complications from radiation include focal-enhancing lesions of radiation necrosis, leukoencephalopathy, myelopathy or neuropathy, vasculopathy, endocrinopathy and secondary tumor formation (atypical meningiomas, gliomas, nerve sheath tumors) [149]. There are ongoing studies of drug-based approaches for neuroprotection, including statins, antioxidants, anti-inflammatory agents and antiangiogenic drugs [140]. A unique post-radiation syndrome is SMART (stroke-like migraine after radiation therapy) characterized by prolonged and usually reversible episodes of headache and focal deficits including seizures [150]. MRI shows ribbon-like cortical and leptomeningeal enhancement along with gyral thickening (Fig. 33.4) with focal slowing on EEG and hypermetabolism on PET. Treatment includes symptomatic headache control, AEDs as needed and avoidance of vasoconstrictive agents [151].

The two most common forms of neurologic sequelae after radiation in children are related to cognitive and neuroendocrine damage. The frequency, degree of and etiology of neurocognitive dysfunction is less than completely elucidated, and the exact relationship between radiotherapy and the volume and dose of radiotherapy and degree of cognitive damage is unclear. Cognitive deficits are progressive in nature, and younger children are more likely to suffer the most severe damage; but no patient of any age is free of risk of damage [152, 153]. In addition to core deficits in attention and concentration [154], declines of intelligence and impairment of working memory and information processing are also seen after cranial irradiation [155, 156]. Due to growing concerns that larger doses of radiation contributed to worse cognitive declines in children with ALL, a reduction in dose from 2400 to 1800 cGy was attempted, but significant declines in IQ persisted, perhaps confounded by the fact that as radiation doses were reduced, doses of methotrexate were increased [157, 158].

There continues to be renewed interest in reduction of total radiation dose, both for solid tumors and primary brain tumors. For example, while it is thought that preventive therapy to the central nervous system with intrathecal chemotherapy and/or irradiation reduces the probability of relapse in patients with ALL, currently cranial irradiation is

Fig. 33.4 Magnetic resonance imaging of diffuse leptomeningeal enhancement with gyral thickening in the left parietal and occipital thought to represent sequela of radiation therapy (SMART syndrome)

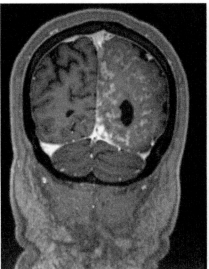 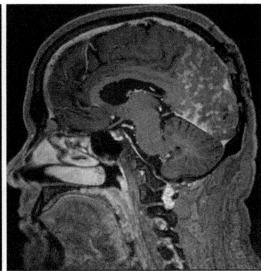

reserved for patients with central nervous system relapse or high-risk disease. Other potential interventions include using cognitive remediation as an educational strategy to improve preparedness and on task performance [159]. In addition, stimulant medications are sometimes used to help improve cognitive performance [160].

Thyroid hormone and growth hormone impairment are the most common forms of neuroendocrine dysfunction after cranial irradiation in children [161, 162]. Radiation to the brain can lead to dysregulation of the hypothalamic-pituitary axis, especially affecting regulators of growth. Higher doses of radiation can lead to more widespread effects. Early puberty is now recognized and is often treated with gonadotrophin-releasing hormone analogs in order to maximize final height. Radiation to the spine and adjuvant chemotherapy can both lead to long-term consequences including decreased fertility and premature ovarian failure [163].

Current Children's Oncology Group recommendations for survivors of childhood cancers who received radiation are stratified based on dose [164]. Those who received >40 Gy to the neck region should have annual neurologic examinations and assessment for diminished carotid pulses/presence of carotid bruits, and diagnostic imaging of carotid arteries as clinically indicated and in most cases 10 years after radiation therapy. Those who received >18 Gy cranial irradiation should have annual neurologic examinations and brain MRI/MRA as clinically indicated. Referrals to endocrinology should be made if radiation dose >30 Gy or for signs of poor growth, precocious puberty, thyroid dysfunction or other abnormalities of the HPA axis.

Neurologic Effects of Stem Cell Transplantation in Children

Hematopoietic stem cell transplantation (HSCT) is now used as the main treatment for a large number of heritable and acquired diseases, including leukemia, lymphoma, histiocytosis and myelodysplastic syndrome as well as refractory anemias. HSCT is an effective, yet intensive, therapy used in the treatment of several pediatric malignancies, and neurologic complications are an important cause of transplant-related morbidity, affecting 10–25% of pediatric patients undergoing transplant [165].

Neurotoxicity can be seen pre-transplant (secondary to drugs used for marrow ablation during conditioning) or post-transplant (secondary to ongoing pancytopenia, metabolic disturbances, graft vs. host vs. tumor effects) [166–168]. Drug-related effects including encephalopathy, seizures and PRES are common, especially with calcineurin inhibitors and busulfan [165]. Infections are also common, with opportunistic organisms and fungi being difficult to diagnose in many cases. Cerebrovascular dysfunction varies from intracranial hemorrhage secondary to thrombocytopenia or infection, to vasculitis to cardiac emboli to global cerebral ischemia [169].

Graft versus host disease (GVHD) can affect both the central and peripheral nervous systems [170]. Manifestations in the PNS include polymyositis, myasthenia gravis and chronic inflammatory demyelinating polyneuropathy (CIDP), often developing late in the course of transplantation at a time of reduction in immunosuppressive therapy. In the CNS, GVHD is rare but has been described with variable

Table 33.5 Risk factors for neurologic complications after stem cell transplantation

Risk factors for transplant-related neurologic complications
Total body irradiation
Allogeneic donor (particularly if unrelated donor)
Acute graft versus host disease grade >2
Drug-related neurotoxicity

Data from Refs. [166, 167]

presentations: meningitis, vasculitis with focal parenchymal hemorrhage, focal lymphocytic encephalitis or acute demyelinating encephalomyelitis.

In a large series of 272 consecutive children undergoing allogeneic or autologous hematopoietic stem cell transplant for both hematologic and non-hematologic diseases, 13.6% developed severe neurologic events [167]. These events typically occurred within the first year, with a median of 90 days after transplant. The most frequent complications were related to neurotoxicity from cyclosporine A. This was followed by what was thought to be irreversible late effects from irradiation and reversible and irreversible effects from chemotherapy. In another large series, which included children and adults, neurologic complications were present at an even higher frequency of more than 50%; moreover, overall survival was significantly worse in patients with major neurologic issues [166]. Of the group with severe neurologic sequelae, mortality ranged from 6 to 30% [167, 168].

Risk factors for neurologic complications after transplant include more immunosuppressive drugs, mismatched transplantation, AML, grade II or higher GVHD, allogeneic transplants (compared to autologous) and the use of total body irradiation [167] (Table 33.5). Underlying disease type was not an independent risk factor in the development of post-transplant complications. Neurologic complications continue to cause significant mortality for patients undergoing HSCT, with diverse causes and clinical features. Even after reduced-intensity stem cell transplantation (RIST), CNS complications remain a significant problem, particularly after umbilical cord blood transplantation, which has the potential for a rare, unique side effect of limbic encephalopathy [171].

Conclusions

Outcomes for children with cancer have improved significantly over the past several decades, with greater than 80% of patients today becoming 5-year survivors [172]. As therapies improve, we continue to learn more about the long-term side effects of cancer treatment. As is now better appreciated, therapy for cancer can lead to long-lasting neurologic toxicity, particularly in the setting of the developing nervous system. Many of the complications of the disease itself and the therapies for

cancer in children are often not appreciated until many years after the completion of therapy. The precise mechanisms by which neurotoxicity in childhood or young adulthood translates to later functioning are not yet fully elucidated, but long-term follow-up into adulthood for survivors of childhood cancer is critical. Future cooperative group studies should include systematic neurologic assessment of childhood cancer patients to better determine the incidence of neurologic sequelae and therefore provide a means to prevent and/or ameliorate these late effects.

References

1. Osterman MJ, Kochanek KD, MacDorman MF, Strobino DM, Guyer B. Annual summary of vital statistics: 2012–2013. Pediatrics. 2015;135(6):1115–25.
2. Howlader N, Noone AM, Krapcho M, Garshell J, Miller D, Altekruse SF, et al. Childhood cancer by the ICCC, Table 29.1: incidence rates by age at diagnosis. In: SEER cancer statistics review, 1975–2012. National Cancer Institute, Bethesda, MD. 2015. http://seer.cancer.gov/csr/1975_2012/. Based on November 2014 SEER data submission, posted to the SEER web site 23 April 2015.
3. Howlader N, Noone AM, Krapcho M, Garshell J, Miller D, Altekruse SF, et al. Childhood cancer, Table 28.2: annual incidence rates by site. In: SEER cancer statistics review, 1975–2012. National Cancer Institute, Bethesda, MD. 2015. http://seer.cancer.gov/csr/1975_2012/. Based on November 2014 SEER data submission, posted to the SEER web site 23 April 2015. Accessed 18 Aug 2015.
4. Howlader N, Noone AM, Krapcho M, Garshell J, Miller D, Altekruse SF, et al. Childhood cancer, Table 28.11: relative survival by year of diagnosis, ages 0–19, both sexes. In: SEER cancer statistics review, 1975–2012. National Cancer Institute, Bethesda, MD. 2015. http://seer.cancer.gov/csr/1975_2012/. Based on November 2014 SEER data submission, posted to the SEER web site 23 April 2015. Accessed 18 Aug 2015.
5. Clouston PD, DeAngelis LM, Posner JB. The spectrum of neurological disease in patients with systemic cancer. Ann Neurol. 1992;31(3):268–73.
6. Gilbert MR, Grossman SA. Incidence and nature of neurologic problems in patients with solid tumors. Am J Med. 1986;81(6):951–4.
7. Patchell RA, Posner JB. Neurologic complications of systemic cancer. Neurol Clin. 1985;3(4):729–50.
8. Weyl-Ben Arush M, Stein M, Perez-Nachum M, Dale J, Babilsky H, Zelnik N, et al. Neurologic complications in pediatric solid tumors. Oncology. 1995;52(2):89–92.

9. Tasdemiroglu E, Patchell RA, Kryscio R. Neurological complications of childhood malignancies. Acta Neurochir (Wien). 1999;141(12):1313–21.

10. Goldsby RE, Liu Q, Nathan PC, Bowers DC, Yeaton-Massey A, Raber SH, et al. Late-occurring neurologic sequelae in adult survivors of childhood acute lymphoblastic leukemia: a report from the childhood cancer survivor study. J Clin Oncol. 2010;28(2):324–31.

11. Baram TZ, van Tassel P, Jaffe NA. Brain metastases in osteosarcoma: incidence, clinical and neuroradiological findings and management options. J Neurooncol. 1988;6(1):47–52.

12. Graus F, Walker RW, Allen JC. Brain metastases in children. J Pediatr. 1983;103(4):558–61.

13. Vannucci RC, Baten M. Cerebral metastatic disease in childhood. Neurology. 1974;24(10):981–5.

14. Boring CC, Squires TS, Tong T, Montgomery S. Cancer statistics, 1994. CA Cancer J Clin. 1994;44(1):7–26.

15. Subramanian A, Harris A, Piggott K, Shieff C, Bradford R. Metastasis to and from the central nervous system—the 'relatively protected site'. Lancet Oncol. 2002;3(8):498–507.

16. Soffietti R, Ruda R, Mutani R. Management of brain metastases. J Neurol. 2002;249(10):1357–69.

17. Puhalla S, Elmquist W, Freyer D, Kleinberg L, Adkins C, Lockman P, et al. Unsanctifying the sanctuary: challenges and opportunities with brain metastases. Neuro-oncology. 2015;17(5):639–51.

18. Bouffet E, Marec-Berard P, Thiesse P, Carrie C, Risk T, Jouvet A, et al. Spinal cord compression by secondary epi- and intradural metastases in childhood. Childs Nerv Syst. 1997;13(7):383–7.

19. Bouffet E, Doumi N, Thiesse P, Mottolese C, Jouvet A, Lacroze M, et al. Brain metastases in children with solid tumors. Cancer. 1997;79(2):403–10.

20. Deutsch M, Orlando S, Wollman M. Radiotherapy for metastases to the brain in children. Med Pediatr Oncol. 2002;39(1):60–2.

21. Kebudi R, Ayan I, Gorgun O, Agaoglu FY, Vural S, Darendeliler E. Brain metastasis in pediatric extracranial solid tumors: survey and literature review. J Neurooncol. 2005;71(1):43–8.

22. Wiens AL, Hattab EM. The pathological spectrum of solid CNS metastases in the pediatric population. J Neurosurg Pediatr. 2014;14(2):129–35.

23. Tasdemiroglu E, Patchell RA. Cerebral metastases in childhood malignancies. Acta Neurochir (Wien). 1997;139(3):182–7.

24. Suki D, Khoury Abdulla R, Ding M, Khatua S, Sawaya R. Brain metastases in patients diagnosed with a solid primary cancer during childhood: experience from a single referral cancer center. J Neurosurg Pediatr. 2014;14(4):372–85.

25. Cervantes GM, Cayci Z. Intracranial CNS manifestations of myeloid sarcoma in patients with acute myeloid leukemia: review of the literature and three case reports from the author's institution. J Clin Med. 2015;4(5):1102–12.

26. Brastianos PK, Curry WT, Oh KS. Clinical discussion and review of the management of brain metastases. J Natl Compr Cancer Netw JNCCN. 2013;11(9):1153–64.

27. Neville KA, Blaney SM. Leptomeningeal cancer in the pediatric patient. Cancer Treat Res. 2005;125:87–106.

28. Bleyer WA, Byrne TN. Leptomeningeal cancer in leukemia and solid tumors. Curr Probl Cancer. 1988;12(4):181–238.

29. Chamberlain MC, Nolan C, Abrey LE. Leukemic and lymphomatous meningitis: incidence, prognosis and treatment. J Neurooncol. 2005;75(1):71–83.

30. Evans AE, Gilbert ES, Zandstra R. The increasing incidence of central nervous system leukemia in children. (Children's Cancer Study Group A). Cancer. 1970;26(2):404–9.

31. Kaplan JG, DeSouza TG, Farkash A, Shafran B, Pack D, Rehman F, et al. Leptomeningeal metastases: comparison of clinical features and laboratory data of solid tumors, lymphomas and leukemias. J Neurooncol. 1990;9(3):225–9.

32. Giglio P, Gilbert MR. Neurologic complications of non-Hodgkin's lymphoma. Curr Oncol Rep. 2005;7(1):61–5.

33. Glass J. Neurologic complications of lymphoma and leukemia. Semin Oncol. 2006;33(3):342–7.

34. Meli FJ, Boccaleri CA, Manzitti J, Lylyk P. Meningeal dissemination of retinoblastoma: CT findings in eight patients. AJNR Am J Neuroradiol. 1990;11(5):983–6.

35. Blatt J, Fitz C, Mirro J Jr. Recognition of central nervous system metastases in children with metastatic primary extracranial neuroblastoma. Pediatr Hematol Oncol. 1997;14(3):233–41.

36. Kellie SJ, Hayes FA, Bowman L, Kovnar EH, Langston J, Jenkins JJ 3rd, et al. Primary extracranial neuroblastoma with central nervous system metastases characterization by clinicopathologic findings and neuroimaging. Cancer. 1991;68(9):1999–2006.

37. Shaw PJ, Eden T. Neuroblastoma with intracranial involvement: an ENSG Study. Med Pediatr Oncol. 1992;20(2):149–55.

38. Parasuraman S, Langston J, Rao BN, Poquette CA, Jenkins JJ, Merchant T, et al. Brain metastases in pediatric Ewing sarcoma and rhabdomyosarcoma: the St. Jude Children's Research Hospital experience. J Pediatr Hematol Oncol. 1999;21(5):370–7.

39. Rodriguez-Galindo C, Pappo AS, Kaste SC, Rao BN, Cain A, Jenkins JJ, et al. Brain metastases in children with melanoma. Cancer. 1997;79(12):2440–5.

40. Allcutt D, Michowiz S, Weitzman S, Becker L, Blaser S, Hoffman HJ, et al. Primary leptomeningeal melanoma: an unusually aggressive tumor in childhood. Neurosurgery. 1993;32(5):721–9 (discussion 9).

41. Yu L, Craver R, Baliga M, Ducos R, Warrier R, Ward K, et al. Isolated CNS involvement in Ewing's sarcoma. Med Pediatr Oncol. 1990;18(5):354–8.

42. Trigg ME, Makuch R, Glaubiger D. Actuarial risk of isolated CNS involvement in Ewing's sarcoma following prophylactic cranial irradiation and intrathecal methotrexate. Int J Radiat Oncol Biol Phys. 1985;11(4):699–702.

43. Wasserstrom WR, Glass JP, Posner JB. Diagnosis and treatment of leptomeningeal metastases from solid tumors: experience with 90 patients. Cancer. 1982;49(4):759–72.

44. Aysun S, Topcu M, Gunay M, Topaloglu H. Neurologic features as initial presentations of childhood malignancies. Pediatr Neurol. 1994;10(1):40–3.

45. Raffel C. Spinal cord compression by epidural tumors in childhood. Neurosurg Clin N Am. 1992;3(4):925–30.

46. Huang LT, Hsiao CC, Weng HH, Lui CC. Neurologic complications of pediatric systemic malignancies. J Formos Med Assoc. 1996;95(3):209–12.

47. Armstrong T, Gilbert MR. Central nervous system toxicity from cancer treatment. Curr Oncol Rep. 2004;6(1):11–9.

48. Tomita N, Kodama F, Sakai R, Koharasawa H, Hattori M, Taguchi J, et al. Predictive factors for central nervous system involvement in non-Hodgkin's lymphoma: significance of very high serum LDH concentrations. Leuk Lymphoma. 2000;38(3–4):335–43.

49. Raffel C, Neave VC, Lavine S, McComb JG. Treatment of spinal cord compression by epidural malignancy in childhood. Neurosurgery. 1991;28(3):349–52.

50. Darnell RB, Posner JB. Paraneoplastic syndromes involving the nervous system. N Engl J Med. 2003;349(16):1543–54.

51. Braik T, Evans AT, Telfer M, McDunn S. Paraneoplastic neurological syndromes: unusual presentations of cancer. A practical review. Am J Med Sci. 2010;340(4):301–8.

52. Zaborowski MP, Spaczynski M, Nowak-Markwitz E, Michalak S. Paraneoplastic neurological syndromes associated with ovarian tumors. J Cancer Res Clin Oncol. 2015;141(1):99–108.

53. Lancaster E. Paraneoplastic disorders. Continuum. 2015;21(2 Neuro-oncology):452–75.
54. Pranzatelli MR. The neurobiology of the opsoclonus-myoclonus syndrome. Clin Neuropharmacol. 1992;15(3):186–228.
55. Rudnick E, Khakoo Y, Antunes NL, Seeger RC, Brodeur GM, Shimada H, et al. Opsoclonus-myoclonus-ataxia syndrome in neuroblastoma: clinical outcome and antineuronal antibodies-a report from the Children's Cancer Group Study. Med Pediatr Oncol. 2001;36(6):612–22.
56. Pranzatelli MR. The immunopharmacology of the opsoclonus-myoclonus syndrome. Clin Neuropharmacol. 1996;19(1):1–47.
57. Posner JB. Paraneoplastic opsoclonus/myoclonus: B cells, T cells, both, or neither? Neurology. 2004;62(9):1466–7.
58. Russo C, Cohn SL, Petruzzi MJ, de Alarcon PA. Long-term neurologic outcome in children with opsoclonus-myoclonus associated with neuroblastoma: a report from the Pediatric Oncology Group. Med Pediatr Oncol. 1997;28(4):284–8.
59. Altman AJ, Baehner RL. Favorable prognosis for survival in children with coincident opso-myoclonus and neuroblastoma. Cancer. 1976;37(2):846–52.
60. Rothenberg AB, Berdon WE, D'Angio GJ, Yamashiro DJ, Cowles RA. The association between neuroblastoma and opsoclonus-myoclonus syndrome: a historical review. Pediatr Radiol. 2009;39(7):723–6.
61. Mitchell WG, Davalos-Gonzalez Y, Brumm VL, Aller SK, Burger E, Turkel SB, et al. Opsoclonus-ataxia caused by childhood neuroblastoma: developmental and neurologic sequelae. Pediatrics. 2002;109(1):86–98.
62. Tate ED, Allison TJ, Pranzatelli MR, Verhulst SJ. Neuroepidemiologic trends in 105 US cases of pediatric opsoclonus-myoclonus syndrome. J Pediatr Oncol Nurs. 2005;22(1):8–19.
63. Children's Oncology Group. Cyclophosphamide and prednisone with or without immunoglobulin in treating abnormal muscle movement in children with neuroblastoma (NCT00033293). 2002–2015. https://clinicaltrials.gov/ct2/show/NCT00033293. Accessed 25 May 2017.
64. Didelot A, Honnorat J. Update on paraneoplastic neurological syndromes. Curr Opin Oncol. 2009;21(6):566–72.
65. Titulaer MJ, McCracken L, Gabilondo I, Armangue T, Glaser C, Iizuka T, et al. Treatment and prognostic factors for long-term outcome in patients with anti-NMDA receptor encephalitis: an observational cohort study. Lancet Neurol. 2013;12(2):157–65.
66. Lancaster E, Martinez-Hernandez E, Titulaer MJ, Boulos M, Weaver S, Antoine JC, et al. Antibodies to metabotropic glutamate receptor 5 in the Ophelia syndrome. Neurology. 2011;77(18):1698–701.
67. Mat A, Adler H, Merwick A, Chadwick G, Gullo G, Dalmau JO, et al. Ophelia syndrome with metabotropic glutamate receptor 5 antibodies in CSF. Neurology. 2013;80(14):1349–50.
68. Shuper A, Stark B, Kornreich L, Cohen IJ, Aviner S, Steinmetz A, et al. Methotrexate treatment protocols and the central nervous system: significant cure with significant neurotoxicity. J Child Neurol. 2000;15(9):573–80.
69. Mahoney DH Jr, Shuster JJ, Nitschke R, Lauer SJ, Steuber CP, Winick N, et al. Acute neurotoxicity in children with B-precursor acute lymphoid leukemia: an association with intermediate-dose intravenous methotrexate and intrathecal triple therapy—a Pediatric Oncology Group study. J Clin Oncol. 1998;16(5):1712–22.
70. Kuskonmaz B, Unal S, Gumruk F, Cetin M, Tuncer AM, Gurgey A. The neurologic complications in pediatric acute lymphoblastic leukemia patients excluding leukemic infiltration. Leuk Res. 2006;30(5):537–41.
71. Antunes NL. Acute neurologic complications in children with systemic cancer. J Child Neurol. 2000;15(11):705–16.
72. Sadighi ZS, Ness KK, Hudson MM, Morris EB, Ledet DS, Pui CH, et al. Headache types, related morbidity, and quality of life in survivors of childhood acute lymphoblastic leukemia: a prospective cross sectional study. Eur J Paediatr Neurol: EJPN: Off J Eur Paediatr Neurol Soc. 2014;18(6):722–9.
73. Ramamoorthy C, Geiduschek JM, Bratton SL, Miser AW, Miser JS. Postdural puncture headache in pediatric oncology patients. Clin Pediatr (Phila). 1998;37(4):247–51.
74. Wee LH, Lam F, Cranston AJ. The incidence of post dural puncture headache in children. Anaesthesia. 1996;51(12):1164–6.
75. Antunes NL, De Angelis LM. Neurologic consultations in children with systemic cancer. Pediatr Neurol. 1999;20(2):121–4.
76. Ochs JJ, Bowman WP, Pui CH, Abromowitch M, Mason C, Simone JV. Seizures in childhood lymphoblastic leukaemia patients. Lancet. 1984;2(8417–18):1422–4.
77. Maytal J, Grossman R, Yusuf FH, Shende AC, Karayalcin G, Lanzkowsky P, et al. Prognosis and treatment of seizures in children with acute lymphoblastic leukemia. Epilepsia. 1995;36(8):831–6.
78. Gertsch EA, Ullrich NJ. Seizures in children treated for a primary brain tumor: risk factors, evaluation and management. Future Neurol. 2014;9(6):626–37.
79. van Breemen MS, Wilms EB, Vecht CJ. Epilepsy in patients with brain tumours: epidemiology, mechanisms, and management. Lancet Neurol. 2007;6(5):421–30.
80. Avila EK, Graber J. Seizures and epilepsy in cancer patients. Curr Neurol Neurosci Rep. 2010;10(1):60–7.
81. Mahoney DH Jr, Shuster JJ, Nitschke R, Lauer S, Steuber CP, Camitta B. Intensification with intermediate-dose intravenous methotrexate is effective therapy for children with lower-risk B-precursor acute lymphoblastic leukemia: A Pediatric Oncology Group study. J Clin Oncol. 2000;18(6):1285–94.
82. Winick NJ, Bowman WP, Kamen BA, Roach ES, Rollins N, Jacaruso D, et al. Unexpected acute neurologic toxicity in the treatment of children with acute lymphoblastic leukemia. J Natl Cancer Inst. 1992;84(4):252–6.
83. Zamboni WC, Gajjar AJ, Heideman RL, Beijnen JH, Rosing H, Houghton PJ, et al. Phenytoin alters the disposition of topotecan and N-desmethyl topotecan in a patient with medulloblastoma. Clin Cancer Res. 1998;4(3):783–9.
84. Villikka K, Kivisto KT, Maenpaa H, Joensuu H, Neuvonen PJ. Cytochrome P450-inducing antiepileptics increase the clearance of vincristine in patients with brain tumors. Clin Pharmacol Ther. 1999;66(6):589–93.
85. Tibussek D, Distelmaier F, Schonberger S, Gobel U, Mayatepek E. Antiepileptic treatment in paediatric oncology—an interdisciplinary challenge. Klin Padiatr. 2006;218(6):340–9.
86. Wells EM, Gaillard WD, Packer RJ. Pediatric brain tumors and epilepsy. Semin Pediatr Neurol. 2012;19(1):3–8.
87. DiMario FJ Jr, Packer RJ. Acute mental status changes in children with systemic cancer. Pediatrics. 1990;85(3):353–60.
88. Reddingius RE, Patte C, Couanet D, Kalifa C, Lemerle J. Dural sinus thrombosis in children with cancer. Med Pediatr Oncol. 1997;29(4):296–302.
89. Packer RJ, Rorke LB, Lange BJ, Siegel KR, Evans AE. Cerebrovascular accidents in children with cancer. Pediatrics. 1985;76(2):194–201.
90. Lynch JK, Hirtz DG, DeVeber G, Nelson KB. Report of the National Institute of Neurological Disorders and Stroke workshop on perinatal and childhood stroke. Pediatrics. 2002;109(1):116–23.
91. deVeber G, Andrew M, Adams C, Bjornson B, Booth F, Buckley DJ, et al. Cerebral sinovenous thrombosis in children. N Engl J Med. 2001;345(6):417–23.

92. Santoro N, Giordano P, Del Vecchio GC, Guido G, Rizzari C, Varotto S, et al. Ischemic stroke in children treated for acute lymphoblastic leukemia: a retrospective study. J Pediatr Hematol Oncol. 2005;27(3):153–7.

93. Fleischhack G, Solymosi L, Reiter A, Bender-Gotze C, Eberl W, Bode U. Imaging methods in diagnosis of cerebrovascular complications with L-asparaginase therapy. Klin Padiatr. 1994;206(4):334–41.

94. Ott N, Ramsay NK, Priest JR, Lipton M, Pui CH, Steinherz P, et al. Sequelae of thrombotic or hemorrhagic complications following L-asparaginase therapy for childhood lymphoblastic leukemia. Am J Pediatr Hematol Oncol. 1988;10(3):191–5.

95. von Mering M, Stiefel M, Brockmann K, Nau R. Deep cerebral venous sinus thrombosis often presents with neuropsychologic symptoms. J Clin Neurosci. 2003;10(3):310–2.

96. Buccino G, Scoditti U, Patteri I, Bertolino C, Mancia D. Neurological and cognitive long-term outcome in patients with cerebral venous sinus thrombosis. Acta Neurol Scand. 2003;107 (5):330–5.

97. de Bruijn SF, de Haan RJ, Stam J. Clinical features and prognostic factors of cerebral venous sinus thrombosis in a prospective series of 59 patients. For The Cerebral Venous Sinus Thrombosis Study Group. J Neurol Neurosurg Psychiatry. 2001;70(1):105–8.

98. Lanthier S, Carmant L, David M, Larbrisseau A, de Veber G. Stroke in children: the coexistence of multiple risk factors predicts poor outcome. Neurology. 2000;54(2):371–8.

99. Vagace JM, de la Maya MD, Caceres-Marzal C, Gonzalez de Murillo S, Gervasini G. Central nervous system chemotoxicity during treatment of pediatric acute lymphoblastic leukemia/lymphoma. Crit Rev Oncol/Hematol. 2012;84(2):274–86.

100. Kumar N. Superficial siderosis: associations and therapeutic implications. Arch Neurol. 2007;64(4):491–6.

101. Partap S. Stroke and cerebrovascular complications in childhood cancer survivors. Semin Pediatr Neurol. 2012;19(1):18–24.

102. Bowers DC, Liu Y, Leisenring W, McNeil E, Stovall M, Gurney JG, et al. Late-occurring stroke among long-term survivors of childhood leukemia and brain tumors: a report from the Childhood Cancer Survivor Study. J Clin Oncol. 2006;24 (33):5277–82.

103. Campen CJ, Kranick SM, Kasner SE, Kessler SK, Zimmerman RA, Lustig R, et al. Cranial irradiation increases risk of stroke in pediatric brain tumor survivors. Stroke; J Cereb Circ. 2012;43(11):3035–40.

104. Yuan H, Gaber MW, Boyd K, Wilson CM, Kiani MF, Merchant TE. Effects of fractionated radiation on the brain vasculature in a murine model: blood-brain barrier permeability, astrocyte proliferation, and ultrastructural changes. Int J Radiat Oncol Biol Phys. 2006;66(3):860–6.

105. Stewart FA, Hoving S, Russell NS. Vascular damage as an underlying mechanism of cardiac and cerebral toxicity in irradiated cancer patients. Radiat Res. 2010;174(6):865–9.

106. Fajardo LF. The pathology of ionizing radiation as defined by morphologic patterns. Acta Oncol. 2005;44(1):13–22.

107. Ullrich NJ, Robertson R, Kinnamon DD, Scott RM, Kieran MW, Turner CD, et al. Moyamoya following cranial irradiation for primary brain tumors in children. Neurology. 2007;68(12):932–8.

108. Poussaint TY, Siffert J, Barnes PD, Pomeroy SL, Goumnerova LC, Anthony DC, et al. Hemorrhagic vasculopathy after treatment of central nervous system neoplasia in childhood: diagnosis and follow-up. AJNR Am J Neuroradiol. 1995;16 (4):693–9.

109. Henry M, Sung L. Supportive care in pediatric oncology: oncologic emergencies and management of fever and neutropenia. Pediatr Clin North Am. 2015;62(1):27–46.

110. Gilchrist L. Chemotherapy-induced peripheral neuropathy in pediatric cancer patients. Semin Pediatr Neurol. 2012;19(1):9–17.

111. Lavoie Smith EM, Li L, Chiang C, Thomas K, Hutchinson RJ, Wells EM, et al. Patterns and severity of vincristine-induced peripheral neuropathy in children with acute lymphoblastic leukemia. J Peripher Nerv Syst: JPNS. 2015;20(1):37–46.

112. Cata JP, Weng HR, Burton AW, Villareal H, Giralt S, Dougherty PM. Quantitative sensory findings in patients with bortezomib-induced pain. J Pain. 2007;8(4):296–306.

113. Ness KK, Hudson MM, Pui CH, Green DM, Krull KR, Huang TT, et al. Neuromuscular impairments in adult survivors of childhood acute lymphoblastic leukemia: associations with physical performance and chemotherapy doses. Cancer. 2012;118 (3):828–38.

114. Rosen GM, Shor AC, Geller TJ. Sleep in children with cancer. Curr Opin Pediatr. 2008;20(6):676–81.

115. Kaleyias J, Manley P, Kothare SV. Sleep disorders in children with cancer. Semin Pediatr Neurol. 2012;19(1):25–34.

116. Mulrooney DA, Ness KK, Neglia JP, Whitton JA, Green DM, Zeltzer LK, et al. Fatigue and sleep disturbance in adult survivors of childhood cancer: a report from the childhood cancer survivor study (CCSS). Sleep. 2008;31(2):271–81.

117. Rosen G, Brand SR. Sleep in children with cancer: case review of 70 children evaluated in a comprehensive pediatric sleep center. Supportive Care Cancer: Off J Multinatl Assoc Supportive Care Cancer. 2011;19(7):985–94.

118. Lipton J, Megerian JT, Kothare SV, Cho YJ, Shanahan T, Chart H, et al. Melatonin deficiency and disrupted circadian rhythms in pediatric survivors of craniopharyngioma. Neurology. 2009;73(4):323–5.

119. van Litsenburg RR, Huisman J, Hoogerbrugge PM, Egeler RM, Kaspers GJ, Gemke RJ. Impaired sleep affects quality of life in children during maintenance treatment for acute lymphoblastic leukemia: an exploratory study. Health Qual Life Outcomes. 2011;9:25.

120. Erickson JM, Beck SL, Christian BR, Dudley W, Hollen PJ, Albritton KA, et al. Fatigue, sleep-wake disturbances, and quality of life in adolescents receiving chemotherapy. J Pediatr Hematol Oncol. 2011;33(1):e17–25.

121. Morgenthaler TI, Kapur VK, Brown T, Swick TJ, Alessi C, Aurora RN, et al. Practice parameters for the treatment of narcolepsy and other hypersomnias of central origin. Sleep. 2007;30(12):1705–11.

122. Nathan PC, Patel SK, Dilley K, Goldsby R, Harvey J, Jacobsen C, et al. Guidelines for identification of, advocacy for, and intervention in neurocognitive problems in survivors of childhood cancer: a report from the Children's Oncology Group. Arch Pediatr Adolesc Med. 2007;161(8):798–806.

123. Robinson KE, Kuttesch JF, Champion JE, Andreotti CF, Hipp DW, Bettis A, et al. A quantitative meta-analysis of neurocognitive sequelae in survivors of pediatric brain tumors. Pediatr Blood Cancer. 2010;55(3):525–31.

124. Prasad PK, Hardy KK, Zhang N, Edelstein K, Srivastava D, Zeltzer L, et al. Psychosocial and neurocognitive outcomes in adult survivors of adolescent and early young adult cancer: a report from the childhood cancer survivor study. J Clin Oncol. 2015;33(23):2545–52.

125. Ullrich NJ, Embry L. Neurocognitive dysfunction in survivors of childhood brain tumors. Semin Pediatr Neurol. 2012;19(1):35–42.

126. Mulhern RK, Merchant TE, Gajjar A, Reddick WE, Kun LE. Late neurocognitive sequelae in survivors of brain tumours in childhood. Lancet Oncol. 2004;5(7):399–408.

127. Küper M, Timmann D. Cerebellar mutism. Brain Lang. 2013;127 (3):327–33.

128. Castellino SM, Ullrich NJ, Whelen MJ, Lange BJ. Developing interventions for cancer-related cognitive dysfunction in childhood cancer survivors. J Natl Cancer Inst. 2014;106(8).

129. Marks AM, Packer RJ. A review of secondary central nervous system tumors after treatment of a primary pediatric malignancy. Semin Pediatr Neurol. 2012;19(1):43–8.

130. Friedman DL, Whitton J, Leisenring W, Mertens AC, Hammond S, Stovall M, et al. Subsequent neoplasms in 5-year survivors of childhood cancer: the Childhood Cancer Survivor Study. J Natl Cancer Inst. 2010;102(14):1083–95.

131. Gramatges MM, Liu Q, Yasui Y, Okcu MF, Neglia JP, Strong LC, et al. Telomere content and risk of second malignant neoplasm in survivors of childhood cancer: a report from the Childhood Cancer Survivor Study. Clin Cancer Res. 2014;20 (4):904–11.

132. Meadows AT, Friedman DL, Neglia JP, Mertens AC, Donaldson SS, Stovall M, et al. Second neoplasms in survivors of childhood cancer: findings from the Childhood Cancer Survivor Study cohort. J Clin Oncol. 2009;27(14):2356–62.

133. Armstrong GT, Liu Q, Yasui Y, Neglia JP, Leisenring W, Robison LL, et al. Late mortality among 5-year survivors of childhood cancer: a summary from the Childhood Cancer Survivor Study. J Clin Oncol. 2009;27(14):2328–38.

134. Jaffe N, Takaue Y, Anzai T, Robertson R. Transient neurologic disturbances induced by high-dose methotrexate treatment. Cancer. 1985;56(6):1356–60.

135. Gowan GM, Herrington JD, Simonetta AB. Methotrexate-induced toxic leukoencephalopathy. Pharmacotherapy. 2002;22(9):1183–7.

136. Chessells JM, Cox TC, Kendall B, Cavanagh NP, Jannoun L, Richards S. Neurotoxicity in lymphoblastic leukaemia: comparison of oral and intramuscular methotrexate and two doses of radiation. Arch Dis Child. 1990;65(4):416–22.

137. Matsumoto K, Takahashi S, Sato A, Imaizumi M, Higano S, Sakamoto K, et al. Leukoencephalopathy in childhood hematopoietic neoplasm caused by moderate-dose methotrexate and prophylactic cranial radiotherapy—an MR analysis. Int J Radiat Oncol Biol Phys. 1995;32(4):913–8.

138. Asato R, Akiyama Y, Ito M, Kubota M, Okumura R, Miki Y, et al. Nuclear magnetic resonance abnormalities of the cerebral white matter in children with acute lymphoblastic leukemia and malignant lymphoma during and after central nervous system prophylactic treatment with intrathecal methotrexate. Cancer. 1992;70(7):1997–2004.

139. Antunes NL, Small TN, George D, Boulad F, Lis E. Posterior leukoencephalopathy syndrome may not be reversible. Pediatr Neurol. 1999;20(3):241–3.

140. Nolan CP, DeAngelis LM. Neurologic complications of chemotherapy and radiation therapy. Continuum. 2015;21(2 Neuro-oncology):429–51.

141. Kieslich M, Porto L, Lanfermann H, Jacobi G, Schwabe D, Bohles H. Cerebrovascular complications of L-asparaginase in the therapy of acute lymphoblastic leukemia. J Pediatr Hematol Oncol. 2003;25(6):484–7.

142. Casey EB, Jellife AM, Le Quesne PM, Millett YL. Vincristine neuropathy. Clinical and electrophysiological observations. Brain. 1973;96(1):69–86.

143. Harila-Saari AH, Huuskonen UE, Tolonen U, Vainionpaa LK, Lanning BM. Motor nervous pathway function is impaired after treatment of childhood acute lymphoblastic leukemia: a study

with motor evoked potentials. Med Pediatr Oncol. 2001;36 (3):345–51.

144. Lehtinen SS, Huuskonen UE, Harila-Saari AH, Tolonen U, Vainionpaa LK, Lanning BM. Motor nervous system impairment persists in long-term survivors of childhood acute lymphoblastic leukemia. Cancer. 2002;94(9):2466–73.

145. Fleming FJ, Vytopil M, Chaitow J, Jones HR Jr, Darras BT, Ryan MM. Thalidomide neuropathy in childhood. Neuromuscul Disord. 2005;15(2):172–6.

146. Wells EM. Nageswara Rao AA, Scafidi J, Packer RJ. Neurotoxicity of biologically targeted agents in pediatric cancer trials. Pediatr Neurol. 2012;46(4):212–21.

147. Cross NE, Glantz MJ. Neurologic complications of radiation therapy. Neurol Clin. 2003;21(1):249–77.

148. Kelsey CR, Marks LB. Somnolence syndrome after focal radiation therapy to the pineal region: case report and review of the literature. J Neurooncol. 2006;78(2):153–6.

149. Greene-Schloesser D, Robbins ME, Peiffer AM, Shaw EG, Wheeler KT, Chan MD. Radiation-induced brain injury: a review. Front Oncol. 2012;2:73.

150. Partap S, Walker M, Longstreth WT Jr, Spence AM. Prolonged but reversible migraine-like episodes long after cranial irradiation. Neurology. 2006;66(7):1105–7.

151. Armstrong AE, Gillan E, DiMario FJ Jr. SMART syndrome (stroke-like migraine attacks after radiation therapy) in adult and pediatric patients. J Child Neurol. 2014;29(3):336–41.

152. Butler RW, Haser JK. Neurocognitive effects of treatment for childhood cancer. Ment Retard Dev Disabil Res Rev. 2006;12 (3):184–91.

153. Mulhern RK, Butler RW. Neurocognitive sequelae of childhood cancers and their treatment. Pediatr Rehabil. 2004;7(1):1–14 (discussion 5–6).

154. Rodgers J, Horrocks J, Britton PG, Kernahan J. Attentional ability among survivors of leukaemia. Arch Dis Child. 1999;80 (4):318–23.

155. Fletcher JM, Copeland DR. Neurobehavioral effects of central nervous system prophylactic treatment of cancer in children. J Clin Exp Neuropsychol. 1988;10(4):495–537.

156. Schatz J, Kramer JH, Ablin A, Matthay KK. Processing speed, working memory, and IQ: a developmental model of cognitive deficits following cranial radiation therapy. Neuropsychology. 2000;14(2):189–200.

157. Mulhern RK, Fairclough D, Ochs J. A prospective comparison of neuropsychologic performance of children surviving leukemia who received 18-Gy, 24-Gy, or no cranial irradiation. J Clin Oncol. 1991;9(8):1348–56.

158. Duffner PK. Risk factors for cognitive decline in children treated for brain tumors. Eur J Paediatr Neurol: EJPN: Off J Eur Paediatr Neurol Soc. 2010;14(2):106–15.

159. Butler RW. Attentional processes and their remediation in childhood cancer. Med Pediatr Oncol. 1998;Suppl 1:75–8.

160. Mulhern RK, Khan RB, Kaplan S, Helton S, Christensen R, Bonner M, et al. Short-term efficacy of methylphenidate: a randomized, double-blind, placebo-controlled trial among survivors of childhood cancer. J Clin Oncol. 2004;22(23):4795–803.

161. Gleeson HK, Shalet SM. The impact of cancer therapy on the endocrine system in survivors of childhood brain tumours. Endocr Relat Cancer. 2004;11(4):589–602.

162. Cohen LE. Endocrine late effects of cancer treatment. Endocrinol Metab Clin North Am. 2005;34(3):769–89, xi.

163. Brougham MF, Wallace WH. Subfertility in children and young people treated for solid and haematological malignancies. Br J Haematol. 2005;131(2):143–55.

164. Children's Oncology Group. Long-term follow-up guidelines for survivors of childhood, adolescent, and young adult cancers,

Version 4.0. Children's Oncology Group, Monrovia, CA. 2014. http://www.survivorshipguidelines.org/. Accessed 24 Aug 2015.

165. Azik F, Yazal Erdem A, Tavil B, Bayram C, Tunc B, Uckan D. Neurological complications after allogeneic hematopoietic stem cell transplantation in children, a single center experience. Pediatric transplantation. 2014;18(4):405–11.

166. Antonini G, Ceschin V, Morino S, Fiorelli M, Gragnani F, Mengarelli A, et al. Early neurologic complications following allogeneic bone marrow transplant for leukemia: a prospective study. Neurology. 1998;50(5):1441–5.

167. Faraci M, Lanino E, Dini G, Fondelli MP, Morreale G, Dallorso S, et al. Severe neurologic complications after hematopoietic stem cell transplantation in children. Neurology. 2002;59(12):1895–904.

168. Denier C, Bourhis JH, Lacroix C, Koscielny S, Bosq J, Sigal R, et al. Spectrum and prognosis of neurologic complications after hematopoietic transplantation. Neurology. 2006;67(11):1990–7.

169. Coplin WM, Cochran MS, Levine SR, Crawford SW. Stroke after bone marrow transplantation: frequency, aetiology and outcome. Brain: J Neurol. 2001;124(Pt 5):1043–51.

170. Pruitt AA, Graus F, Rosenfeld MR. Neurological complications of transplantation: part I: hematopoietic cell transplantation. Neurohospitalist. 2013;3(1):24–38.

171. Kishi Y, Miyakoshi S, Kami M, Ikeda M, Katayama Y, Murashige N, et al. Early central nervous system complications after reduced-intensity stem cell transplantation. Biol Blood Marrow Transplant. 2004;10(8):561–8.

172. Adamson PC. Improving the outcome for children with cancer: Development of targeted new agents. CA Cancer J Clin. 2015;65 (3):212–20.

173. Paulino AC, Nguyen TX, Barker JL Jr. Brain metastasis in children with sarcoma, neuroblastoma, and Wilms' tumor. Int J Radiat Oncol Biol Phys. 2003;57(1):177–83.

Neurological Complications of Cancer and Cancer Therapies in Long-Term Survivors

Isabel Arrillaga

Introduction

The advent of improved cancer therapies has increased patient survivorship and with it the need to better understand the long-term sequelae of cancer and cancer therapies. With earlier detection methods and improved treatments, the number of cancer survivors by the year 2020 is estimated to reach approximately 20 million [1]. As this number increases, so does our awareness of the long-term neurological complications of cancer treatments. Among several cancer treatment-related side effects, neurotoxicity can be particularly severe and impact quality of life and overall functioning [2–4]. Given the inherent susceptibility of the developing nervous system to toxicity and an estimated high survival rates of up to 80% [5, 6], survivors of childhood cancers are affected disproportionately. Much of what we know about the long-term neurological complications of cancer and cancer therapies has been learned from research on survivors of childhood cancers.

This chapter will focus on several common long-term neurological side effects of cancer and cancer treatments, with some emphasis on CNS toxicity in long-term survivors of pediatric cancers. Some of the most common CNS complications to be discussed below include impaired cognition, seizures, cerebrovascular events, and peripheral neuropathy. A discussion of these complications in acute and subacute treatment settings can be found in earlier chapters of this text.

Cognitive Impairment

Cognitive impairment is a potentially long-lasting and late side effect of cancer and cancer treatments that can greatly impact quality of life and overall functioning [7]. Pediatric

I. Arrillaga (✉)
Department of Neurology/Neuro-Oncology,
Massachusetts General Hospital, 55 Fruit Street,
Yawkey 9E, Boston, MA 02114, USA
e-mail: iarrillaga@mgh.harvard.edu

© Springer International Publishing AG 2018
D. Schiff et al. (eds.), *Cancer Neurology in Clinical Practice*,
DOI 10.1007/978-3-319-57901-6_34

oncology patients are particularly vulnerable to the damaging effects of radiation and chemotherapy on the developing brain, and cognitive dysfunction has been reported in up to 40% of childhood cancer survivors. Neurocognitive difficulties have also been reported in adult cancer survivors [8–16]. Various cognitive domains can be impacted including attention, memory, and processing speed [17, 18].

Cognition in Survivors of Pediatric CNS Tumors

About 20% of pediatric tumors arise in the CNS. The 5-year overall survival of pediatric primary brain tumor patients has been estimated at more than 75% [5], with many survivors at risk of pervasive neurocognitive impairment decades after diagnosis and treatment [19–27]. Pediatric brain tumor patients experience up to a 20-fold increased frequency of severe impairment compared to the general population 20 years after diagnosis [28], and cognitive declines of 20–40 IQ points are not uncommon [20, 23, 29]. Importantly, subjective cognitive complaints do not mirror objective declines in cognition, despite significant functional implications. In one study, fewer than 10% of survivors reported severe cognitive impairment despite 50% being severely impaired in performance-based measures [28], highlighting the need for clinical assessment in addition to patient-reported outcomes when assessing cognition in this population. Despite subjective awareness of deficits, the functional implications of severe cognitive decline are tremendous, with observed reduced attainment of expected adult developmental milestones including education, employment, independent living [28], and possibly a lower socioeconomic attainment [20].

Cranial and craniospinal irradiation have been a well-known risk factor for impairment in cognition in children and adult survivors of pediatric brain tumors [5, 24, 30–33], particularly in areas of memory and executive functioning [34–37]. There is a correlation between radiation dose and IQ [38, 39]. Moreover, it is estimated that, when irradiated at age less than 7 years, nearly 100% of children require special education; after 7 years of age approximately 50% of children require special education [33]. The temporal lobe is particularly vulnerable to effects of radiation; higher dose levels to this region are associated with higher risk for memory impairment [21]. Newer treatment techniques have been aimed at minimizing dose and target volume, though the long-term benefit of these techniques has yet to be established.

While the precise mechanisms underlying radiation-induced cognitive dysfunction remain elusive, damage to hippocampal neurogenesis may be involved. Studies in animal models have demonstrated that therapeutic doses of cranial irradiation virtually ablate neurogenesis and that this inhibition of neurogenesis correlates with impaired performance on hippocampal-dependent memory tests [33, 40, 41]. Surprisingly, irradiation does not simply deplete the stem cell population, but rather disrupts the microenvironment that normally supports hippocampal neurogenesis [40, 42]. This microenvironmental perturbation is due largely to irradiation-induced microglial inflammation and anti-inflammatory therapy with the non-steroidal anti-inflammatory agent indomethacin partially restores hippocampal neurogenesis and function in rodents [42]. Additional possible mechanisms underlying radiation-induced cognitive dysfunction include white matter dysfunction, altered regional blood flow due to microvascular disease and acute and chronic oxidative stress and inflammatory responses [43–45].

Cognition in pediatric brain tumor survivors is also affected by factors other than radiation. In survivors with no exposure to radiation, there exists a 17-fold increase in the prevalence of impaired cognitive flexibility, and a fivefold increase in the prevalence of impairments in short- and long-term memory. Additionally, up to 37% of these survivors are severely impaired on at least one measure of processing speed [28].

Treatment of pediatric brain tumors may include cranial irradiation and/or cytotoxic chemotherapy; both have been implicated in the pathophysiology of cancer treatment-induced cognitive decline. Additional factors that have been associated with neurocognitive outcome include tumor site [46], age at diagnosis [47], history of seizures and hydrocephalus with shunt placement [20, 28]. After adjustment for exposure to cranial irradiation, Brinkman and colleagues found that seizures conferred a 50% increase in the risk of cognitive impairment [28]. This may be related to the use of anticonvulsant medications or the cumulative neurobiological and physiologic consequences of recurrent

seizures. Likewise, the same group reported that a history of hydrocephalus with shunt placement conferred 40% increased risk of memory impairment [28], possibly related to hippocampal vulnerability to hydrocephalus [48].

Cognition in Survivors of Non-CNS Pediatric Cancers

Pediatric survivors of non-CNS cancers are also at risk of developing clinically significant impairment in neurocognitive functioning [6]. The incidence of impairment in at least one cognitive domain has been reported as high as 21% [49]. Most of these data have been derived from studies on survivors of childhood leukemias [50–56] and lymphomas. These studies suggest that cranial irradiation, chemotherapy (in particular high dose systemic and intrathecal) [57], stem cell transplant [58], and other treatments such as corticosteroids [55, 58] may be involved in the etiology of cognitive dysfunction in these patients. Additional factors associated with neurocognitive outcome in this patient population include age at diagnosis and female sex [49, 57, 59–62].

Acute lymphoblastic leukemia (ALL) represents the largest diagnostic group of survivors of childhood cancers, and the best studied. Neurocognitive impairment in this population is pervasive and long lasting, being reported up to 26 years after diagnosis, well into adulthood [53, 63]. Deficits in attention, memory, intelligence, processing speed, and executive functioning have been reported [53, 59, 64–66]. Until recently, these impairments had been largely attributed to prophylactic cranial irradiation [50, 53].

Cranial irradiation affects cognition in a dose-dependent manner [53], and, in this population, dose thresholds remain debatable. Recent reports suggest that a dose of less than 18 Gy may reduce risk [31, 67]. Withholding radiation and treating with chemotherapy alone may further reduce risk [31, 67] and has been an impetus for the omission of radiation therapy for most patients with childhood ALL. Instead, systemic and intrathecal chemotherapy is used to establish CNS prophylaxis.

Chemotherapy also has a significant impact on cognition in this population [6, 18, 60, 68–72]. Krull et al. [53] recently demonstrated that significant cognitive impairments were common among survivors of childhood ALL treated with chemotherapy only. Likewise, a recent meta-analysis assessing long-term neurocognitive functioning after chemotherapy-only regimens among survivors of childhood ALL revealed significant moderate impairment across multiple neurocognitive domains, with intelligence most affected [56]. Additional information is needed on the functional implications of these impairments though certainly patient and families should be provided with appropriate educational planning and surveillance.

Imaging correlates to neurocognitive outcomes in ALL survivors have been discovered, providing an understanding of some of the mechanistic underpinnings of late cognitive deficits and suggesting a role of white matter changes in neurocognitive changes secondary to cancer treatments. Specifically, smaller brain white matter volumes have been associated with larger deficits in attention, memory, intelligence, and academic achievement [73–75]. Additionally, fractional anisotropy (a measure related to degree of myelination) has been associated with IQ in childhood survivors of ALL.

Though limited, additional data exist to suggest that cognition is affected in childhood survivors of other non-CNS cancers. Intriguingly, some of these reports suggest that cognition can be affected by indirect mechanisms of treatment and not by direct CNS toxicity. Krull et al. [76] reported that adult long-term survivors of pediatric Hodgkin disease (HD) were at significant risk for neurocognitive decline. Importantly, this finding was associated with cardiopulmonary dysfunction attributable to standard care treatment with thoracic radiation and anthracyclines or bleomycin. Cardiopulmonary morbidity was further linked with cerebrovascular pathology as evidenced by multifocal leukoencephalopathy and hemosiderin deposits in the brain. This notable CNS finding was sixfold higher in HD survivors than in comparable cohorts and suggests a mechanism whereby pulmonary and cardiac dysfunction may lead to cognitive decline in this population. Primary prevention strategies have been sought and include reduction or omission of mantle field radiation, though these patients likely remain at risk given known cardiopulmonary side effects of anthracyclines and bleomycin.

Cognitive outcomes in long-term survivors of childhood osteosarcoma have also been evaluated [77]. Pediatric osteosarcoma has a 70% survival rate, largely due to advances in treatment including adjuvant chemotherapy with intravenous methotrexate. In addition, historical treatment regimens have incorporated anthracyclines, bleomycin, and alkylating agents, all chemotherapies known to affect cardiopulmonary function. The prevalence of cognitive decline in this population was found to be high, and this was not completely related to treatment with methotrexate. Maximum plasma concentrations, median clearance, and median/cumulative exposure to systemic methotrexate were not associated with cognitive impairment. Instead, any grade 3 or 4 adverse chronic conditions such as cardiac, pulmonary, or endocrine dysfunction were associated with poorer memory and slower processing speed. These results suggest that chronic health conditions related to cancer and cancer treatment can have a significant impact on cognition, in some cases more so that direct toxicity from treatment itself.

Cognition in Survivors of Adult Cancers

The incidence of post-treatment cognitive impairment in survivors of adult cancers ranges from 15 to 61% [78] and may be among the most frequently reported post-treatment symptoms of cancer survivors [79]. Effects can be worse immediately after treatment with some improvement over time [78] or with little recovery, leading to long-lasting impairment [10, 16, 80, 81]. Alternatively, patients may develop symptoms months to years following treatment [14]. Deficits in memory, executive function, processing speed, and attention appear most frequently [82]. Age [83, 84] and baseline cognitive reserve [83] have been identified as risk factors to neurotoxic effects of chemotherapy.

The mechanisms underlying effects of chemotherapy on the brain remain elusive, but may involve direct neurotoxic injury of hippocampal progenitor cells [85–87]. Such effects on hippocampal neurogenesis may help explain the delayed impact of treatment on cognition. Chemotherapy-induced increases in oxidative stress [88], white matter damage [86, 89], and reduced brain vascularization [78] may also be involved. Imaging studies have provided additional information about the structural and functional pathology associated with chemotherapy exposure. Reductions in hippocampal and frontal white and gray matter have been documented in cancer patients treated with chemotherapy [90, 91]. Advanced imaging studies using functional MRI, PET, and diffusion tensor MRI have provided additional albeit limited understanding of the pathophysiology of cognitive changes associated with chemotherapy [78].

Cerebrovascular Events

Numerous studies have shown that cancer survivors are at increased risk for stroke. The potential consequences of a stroke can be devastating leading to overt physical and cognitive disabilities, but can also be subtle and worsen cognitive impairment related to other factors. Cranial irradiation, in a dose-dependent fashion, is a particularly strong predictor of stroke risk [92–97]. The cumulative stroke risk in survivors treated with 50+ Gy has been estimated at 12% between 10 and 30 years of post-diagnosis [96]. Importantly, the elevated stroke risk conferred by cranial irradiation in childhood persists into early adulthood and continues to increase decades after treatment [96, 98, 99].

Radiation increases risk of arteriopathies such as moyamoya. Arteriopathies can lead to small and large vessel necrosis and has been identified as the most common risk factor for recurrent stroke in cancer survivors [100]. They typically occur shortly after completion of radiation, with one report estimating a median of 55 months from the time of radiation to discovery [101]. Since stroke risk persists decades after treatment, a second mechanism for delayed arteriopathy may exist.

Atherosclerosis is a more common cause of stroke in all comers and has also been linked with radiation [102–105]. The cumulative risk of stroke in survivors of childhood cancer treated with cranial irradiation increases fourfold for patients with additional atherosclerotic risk factors such as hypertension, diabetes, or black race [96], but is not solely dependent on these additional factors. A better understanding of the role of arteriopathy and atherosclerosis in the mechanism of stroke in cancer survivors would have significant implication for primary prevention, in particular in childhood cancer survivors. As it stands, the increased risk of stroke in cancer survivors suggests that frequent screening for modifiable stroke risk factors needs to be considered.

Seizures

Seizures are a common occurrence in both adults and children with brain tumors with an incidence near 30% [2]. The incidence of ongoing seizures in long-term survivors of pediatric brain tumors is as high as 14–25% [19, 106]. Seizures in this population are recognized as one of the most significant neurological complications of childhood brain tumors as they can occur frequently and at any time from diagnosis to years later. Moreover, they negatively impact quality of life [107]. Tumor pathology, extent of tumor resection and tumor recurrence are all risk factors [106]. In addition, treatment such as surgery, radiation, and chemotherapy can increase risk for seizures. In an analysis of a large cohort of survivors through the Childhood Cancer Survivor Study, patients with a history of radiation dose greater than 30 Gy to a cortical region of the brain had twofold risk of developing seizure as a late effect of treatment [19]. In this population, concurrent use of medications such as antidepressants and antibiotics, as well secondary medical complications such as infection or bleeding, can also lower seizure thresholds and increase risk [106].

Survivors of pediatric non-CNS cancers are likewise at increased risk for seizure as reported in a study assessing neurological morbidity in survivors of childhood ALL, which reported seizures in 11% of study participants [4]. History of CNS involvement of disease was associated with seizures, but additional factors such as cranial irradiation and chemotherapy likely also played a role [4].

Seizures themselves can be quite burdensome to cancer survivors, limiting functionality and quality of life in many cases, and affecting brain function in some. Moreover, additional side effects from the treatment of seizures with antiepileptic drugs (AEDs) can be equally as disturbing. Many of these agents have been associated with fatigue, and cognitive impairment, in addition to many non-neurological side effects. Thus, even infrequent seizures can impact overall medical health and quality of life.

Peripheral Neuropathy

Chemotherapy-Induced Peripheral Neuropathy

In comparison with the central nervous system, the peripheral nervous system (PNS) has better regeneration capacity. Notwithstanding, peripheral nerve toxicity, typically related to chemotherapy (chemotherapy-induced peripheral neuropathy, CIPN), can be debilitating, long lasting, and sometimes permanent [108, 109]. Until recently, this type of toxicity had remained an underestimated and under-recognized clinical problem in cancer survivors [110], perhaps because the accepted paradigm was that of a reversible condition. The evidence of long-term persistence of symptoms is now clear, in part due to the availability of large cancer registries such as Patient-Reported-Outcomes Following Initial Treatment of Long Term Evaluation of Survivorship (PROFILES) [110]. This has led to increased attention to this topic, so much so that the National Comprehensive Cancer Network recently expanded its guidelines for survivorship to address CIPN [111]. The hope is that with the increased attention, research in this field will continue to expand.

Most of the evidence supporting long-term CIPN in cancer survivors comes from studies of patient with breast, colorectal, and ovarian cancers who are typically exposed to neurotoxic agents. In one study of patients treated with oxaliplatin, 79% reported ongoing peripheral neuropathy after a median of 29 months from treatment [112]. Another study reported that over 25% of patients treated with oxaliplatin had NCI-CTC grade 3 symptoms 2 years after treatment. More compelling have been results from analysis of PROFILES data that revealed the persistence of CIPN up to 11 years post-treatment [113]. Cumulative dose was associated with worse outcomes [114].

Additional reports have revealed that CIPN can result in functional impairment. In a recent study, 89% of cancer survivors treated with oxaliplatin reported at least one symptom of neuropathy at 7 years from completion of therapy [115]. Importantly, due to their peripheral nerve symptoms, up to 24% of these survivors had difficulties driving, and 60% reported difficulties with exercise [115].

Functional consequences are further evidenced by reports that reveal an increased propensity to falls, with some series reporting up to 20% of patients with cancer and CIPN reporting falls [116, 117]. Motor neuropathy associated with taxanes use in breast cancer has been most strongly associated with increased propensity for falls [117]. Importantly, while clearly prevalent in cancer survivors, CIPN remains underreported by patients [118], suggesting that practitioners must be vigilant for symptoms and be educated to recognize early signs of the condition.

CIPN is also prevalent in adult survivors of pediatric cancers. In patients treated with either vinca alkaloids or platinum agents, the prevalence at a median of 25 years from diagnosis can be as high as 20 and 17.5% for long-term motor and sensory impairments, respectively [119]. In platinum-treated testicular cancer survivors, 22% had detectable peripheral neuropathy 23–33 years after therapy, and 6% had disabling neuropathy up to 22 and 15 years out from treatment, respectively [120, 121]. Clinical evidence for peripheral neuropathy as measured by EMG/NCS has also been reported in nearly 30% of survivors of childhood ALL at a mean of 7.4 years post-treatment [122]. CIPN in this population likely increases the risk for functional performance limitations, as evidenced by objective decreases in mobility and poor performance on a walk test and a timed "up and go" test [119].

Unfortunately, there are no proven preventive therapies for CIPN. There are data to support the role of duloxetine in the treatment of neuropathic pain related to CIPN, though relief is typically incomplete. No convincing data exist to support the use of other agents such as tricyclic antidepressants, gabapentine, or topical lidocaine, despite data supporting their utility in other neuropathic nerve conditions. Practitioners will often try these agents regardless of their success in these other conditions. Additional research with these agents is needed. Although no protective or curative agents exist, early detection of symptoms is important, in particular for children, as rehabilitative services and equipment may improve symptoms and provide strengthening and joint protection which in the long run could minimize functional limitations. For a compete discussion of CIPN including pathogenesis, clinical features, and evidence for treatment, please refer to Chap. 15 of this text.

Radiation-Induced Peripheral Neuropathy (RIPN)

Radiation-induced peripheral neuropathy (RIPN) is a less well-recognized, studied phenomenon, largely because it is more rare than its counterpart CIPN. The functional implications, however, can be equally severe [123]. RIPN has long been considered irreversible [124] and is associated with fibrotic changes to the nerves. The pathogenesis may be related to progressive fibrosis driven by reactive oxidative species and inflammatory mediators, ultimately resulting in demyelination, direct axonal injury, and nerve ischemia [125, 126].

A classic example of this type of neuropathy is a brachial plexopathy that can occur when radiation is directed at the chest, axillary region, thoracic outlet, or neck [127]. The incidence has decreased over the past six decades due impart to better radiation techniques and decreased doses. In the 1950s, the incidence was close to 65%, while now the incidence is only 1–2% [125], with 40–75% of cases resulting from radiation for breast cancer [128, 129]. Timing of symptom presentation varies widely, ranging anywhere from one year to decades after completion of treatment [130]. Presentation also varies ranging from mild sensory symptoms to debilitating pain and motor dysfunction. For a complete discussion of RIPN including pathogenesis, clinical features, and evidence for treatment, please refer to Chap. 14 of this text.

Summary

Neurological complications of cancer and cancer therapies are common in survivors of both adult and childhood cancers. Common complications often include cognitive deficits, strokes, seizures, and peripheral neuropathy. Importantly, these side effects are often associated with limitations in normal functioning, and impairment in quality of life. Much remains to be learned about the pathophysiology underlying many of these complications. This knowledge will ideally aid in the discovery of preventive and curative strategies, where currently there are none. Early recognition of these complications and risk for complications is crucial to provide both functional and psychological support to survivors and their families.

References

1. Jemal A, et al. Cancer statistics, 2009. CA: A Cancer J Clin. 2009;59(4):225–49.
2. Liigant A, et al. Seizure disorders in patients with brain tumors. Eur Neurol. 2001;45(1):46–51.
3. Luyken C, et al. The spectrum of long-term epilepsy-associated tumors: long-term seizure and tumor outcome and neurosurgical aspects. Epilepsia. 2003;44(6):822–30.
4. Khan RB, et al. Neurologic morbidity and quality of life in survivors of childhood acute lymphoblastic leukemia: a prospective cross-sectional study. J Cancer Surviv. 2014;8(4):688–96.
5. Howlander N, Krapcho M, et al. SEER Cancer statistics review, 1975–2011. Bethesda, MD: National Cancer Institute; 2011.
6. Anderson FS, Kunin-Batson AS. Neurocognitive late effects of chemotherapy in children: the past 10 years of research on brain structure and function. Pediatr Blood Cancer. 2009;52(2):159–64.

7. Mitby PA, et al. Utilization of special education services and educational attainment among long-term survivors of childhood cancer: a report from the childhood cancer survivor study. Cancer. 2003;97(4):1115–26.

8. van Dam FS, et al. Impairment of cognitive function in women receiving adjuvant treatment for high-risk breast cancer: high-dose versus standard-dose chemotherapy. J Natl Cancer Inst. 1998;90(3):210–8.

9. Schagen SB, et al. Cognitive deficits after postoperative adjuvant chemotherapy for breast carcinoma. Cancer. 1999;85(3):640–50.

10. Brezden CB, et al. Cognitive function in breast cancer patients receiving adjuvant chemotherapy. J Clin Oncol. 2000;18 (14):2695–701.

11. Hurria A, et al. Cognitive function of older patients receiving adjuvant chemotherapy for breast cancer: a pilot prospective longitudinal study. J Am Geriatr Soc. 2006;54(6):925–31.

12. Ahles TA, Saykin A. Cognitive effects of standard-dose chemotherapy in patients with cancer. Cancer Investig. 2001;19 (8):812–20.

13. Schagen SB, et al. Late effects of adjuvant chemotherapy on cognitive function: a follow-up study in breast cancer patients. Ann Oncol. 2002;13(9):1387–97.

14. Wefel JS, et al. The cognitive sequelae of standard-dose adjuvant chemotherapy in women with breast carcinoma: results of a prospective, randomized, longitudinal trial. Cancer. 2004;100 (11):2292–9.

15. Schagen SB, et al. Change in cognitive function after chemotherapy: a prospective longitudinal study in breast cancer patients. J Natl Cancer Inst. 2006;98(23):1742–5.

16. Weis J, Poppelreuter M, Bartsch HH. Cognitive deficits as long-term side-effects of adjuvant therapy in breast cancer patients: 'subjective' complaints and 'objective' neuropsychological test results. Psycho-oncology. 2009;18(7):775–82.

17. Campbell LK, et al. A meta-analysis of the neurocognitive sequelae of treatment for childhood acute lymphocytic leukemia. Pediatr Blood Cancer. 2007;49(1):65–73.

18. Moleski M. Neuropsychological, neuroanatomical, and neurophysiological consequences of CNS chemotherapy for acute lymphoblastic leukemia. Arch Clin Neuropsychol. 2000;15 (7):603–30.

19. Packer RJ, et al. Long-term neurologic and neurosensory sequelae in adult survivors of a childhood brain tumor: childhood cancer survivor study. J Clin Oncol. 2003;21(17):3255–61.

20. Ellenberg L, et al. Neurocognitive status in long-term survivors of childhood CNS malignancies: a report from the childhood cancer survivor study. Neuropsychology. 2009;23(6):705–17.

21. Armstrong GT, et al. Region-specific radiotherapy and neuropsychological outcomes in adult survivors of childhood CNS malignancies. Neuro Oncol. 2010;12(11):1173–86.

22. Anderson NE. Late complications in childhood central nervous system tumour survivors. Curr Opin Neurol. 2003;16(6):677–83.

23. Mulhern RK, et al. Late neurocognitive sequelae in survivors of brain tumours in childhood. Lancet Oncol. 2004;5(7):399–408.

24. Mulhern RK, et al. Neurocognitive consequences of risk-adapted therapy for childhood medulloblastoma. J Clin Oncol. 2005;23 (24):5511–9.

25. Mabbott DJ, et al. Core neurocognitive functions in children treated for posterior fossa tumors. Neuropsychology. 2008;22 (2):159–68.

26. Nagel BJ, et al. Early patterns of verbal memory impairment in children treated for medulloblastoma. Neuropsychology. 2006;20 (1):105–12.

27. Ris MD, et al. Intellectual outcome after reduced-dose radiation therapy plus adjuvant chemotherapy for medulloblastoma: a Children's Cancer Group study. J Clin Oncol. 2001;19(15):3470–6.

28. Brinkman TM, et al. Long-term neurocognitive functioning and social attainment in adult survivors of pediatric CNS tumors: results from the St Jude lifetime cohort study. J Clin Oncol. 2016;34(12):1358–67.

29. Ellenberg L, et al. Factors affecting intellectual outcome in pediatric brain tumor patients. Neurosurgery. 1987;21(5):638–44.

30. Smibert E, et al. Risk factors for intellectual and educational sequelae of cranial irradiation in childhood acute lymphoblastic leukaemia. Br J Cancer. 1996;73(6):825–30.

31. Spiegler BJ, et al. Change in neurocognitive functioning after treatment with cranial radiation in childhood. J Clin Oncol. 2004;22(4):706–13.

32. Palmer SL, et al. Predicting intellectual outcome among children treated with 35–40 Gy craniospinal irradiation for medulloblastoma. Neuropsychology. 2003;17(4):548–55.

33. Monje M. Cranial radiation therapy and damage to hippocampal neurogenesis. Dev Disabil Res Rev. 2008;14(3):238–42.

34. Jain N, et al. Neuropsychological outcome following intensity-modulated radiation therapy for pediatric medulloblastoma. Pediatr Blood Cancer. 2008;51(2):275–9.

35. Palmer SL, Reddick WE, Gajjar A. Understanding the cognitive impact on children who are treated for medulloblastoma. J Pediatr Psychol. 2007;32(9):1040–9.

36. Dennis M, et al. Neuropsychological sequelae of the treatment of children with medulloblastoma. J Neurooncol. 1996;29(1):91–101.

37. Aarsen FK, et al. Cognitive deficits and predictors 3 years after diagnosis of a pilocytic astrocytoma in childhood. J Clin Oncol. 2009;27(21):3526–32.

38. Grill J, et al. Long-term intellectual outcome in children with posterior fossa tumors according to radiation doses and volumes. Int J Radiat Oncol Biol Phys. 1999;45(1):137–45.

39. Kieffer-Renaux V, et al. Patterns of neuropsychological deficits in children with medulloblastoma according to craniospatial irradiation doses. Dev Med Child Neurol. 2000;42(11):741–5.

40. Monje ML, et al. Irradiation induces neural precursor-cell dysfunction. Nat Med. 2002;8(9):955–62.

41. Raber J, et al. Radiation-induced cognitive impairments are associated with changes in indicators of hippocampal neurogenesis. Radiat Res. 2004;162(1):39–47.

42. Monje ML, Toda H, Palmer TD. Inflammatory blockade restores adult hippocampal neurogenesis. Science. 2003;302(5651):1760–5.

43. Zhao W, Diz DI, Robbins ME. Oxidative damage pathways in relation to normal tissue injury. Br J Radiol. 2007;80(1):S23–31.

44. Lee WH, et al. Irradiation induces regionally specific alterations in pro-inflammatory environments in rat brain. Int J Radiat Biol. 2010;86(2):132–44.

45. Soussain C, et al. CNS complications of radiotherapy and chemotherapy. Lancet. 2009;374(9701):1639–51.

46. Mulhern RK, et al. Neuropsychological status of children treated for brain tumors: a critical review and integrative analysis. Med Pediatr Oncol. 1992;20(3):181–91.

47. Sands SA, et al. Long-term quality of life and neuropsychologic functioning for patients with CNS germ-cell tumors: from the first international CNS germ-cell tumor study. Neuro Oncol. 2001;3 (3):174–83.

48. Savolainen S, et al. MR imaging of the hippocampus in normal pressure hydrocephalus: correlations with cortical Alzheimer's disease confirmed by pathologic analysis. AJNR Am J Neuroradiol. 2000;21(2):409–14.

49. Kadan-Lottick NS, et al. Neurocognitive functioning in adult survivors of childhood non-central nervous system cancers. J Natl Cancer Inst. 2010;102(12):881–93.

50. Ochs J, et al. Comparison of neuropsychologic functioning and clinical indicators of neurotoxicity in long-term survivors of childhood leukemia given cranial radiation or parenteral methotrexate: a prospective study. J Clin Oncol. 1991;9 (1):145–51.

51. Mahoney DH Jr, et al. Acute neurotoxicity in children with B-precursor acute lymphoid leukemia: an association with intermediate-dose intravenous methotrexate and intrathecal triple therapy—a Pediatric Oncology Group study. J Clin Oncol. 1998;16(5):1712–22.

52. Cousens P, et al. Cognitive effects of cranial irradiation in leukaemia: a survey and meta-analysis. J Child Psychol Psychiatry. 1988;29(6):839–52.

53. Krull KR, et al. Neurocognitive outcomes decades after treatment for childhood acute lymphoblastic leukemia: a report from the St Jude lifetime cohort study. J Clin Oncol. 2013;31(35):4407–15.

54. Mulhern RK, et al. Memory function in disease-free survivors of childhood acute lymphocytic leukemia given CNS prophylaxis with or without 1,800 cGy cranial irradiation. J Clin Oncol. 1988;6(2):315–20.

55. Waber DP, et al. Cognitive sequelae in children treated for acute lymphoblastic leukemia with dexamethasone or prednisone. J Pediatr Hematol Oncol. 2000;22(3):206–13.

56. Iyer NS, et al. Chemotherapy-only treatment effects on long-term neurocognitive functioning in childhood ALL survivors: a review and meta-analysis. Blood. 2015;126(3):346–53.

57. Langer T, et al. CNS late-effects after ALL therapy in childhood. Part III: neuropsychological performance in long-term survivors of childhood ALL: impairments of concentration, attention, and memory. Med Pediatr Oncol. 2002;38(5):320–8.

58. Wefel JS, Witgert ME, Meyers CA. Neuropsychological sequelae of non-central nervous system cancer and cancer therapy. Neuropsychol Rev. 2008;18(2):121–31.

59. Copeland DR, et al. Neuropsychological sequelae of childhood cancer in long-term survivors. Pediatrics. 1985;75(4):745–53.

60. Brown RT, et al. Cognitive and academic late effects among children previously treated for acute lymphocytic leukemia receiving chemotherapy as CNS prophylaxis. J Pediatr Psychol. 1998;23(5):333–40.

61. Waber DP, et al. Late effects of central nervous system treatment of acute lymphoblastic leukemia in childhood are sex-dependent. Dev Med Child Neurol. 1990;32(3):238–48.

62. von der Weid N, et al. Intellectual outcome in children and adolescents with acute lymphoblastic leukaemia treated with chemotherapy alone: age- and sex-related differences. Eur J Cancer. 2003;39(3):359–65.

63. Krull KR, et al. Reliability and validity of the childhood cancer survivor study neurocognitive questionnaire. Cancer. 2008;113 (8):2188–97.

64. Giralt J, et al. Long-term neuropsychologic sequelae of childhood leukemia: comparison of two CNS prophylactic regimens. Int J Radiat Oncol Biol Phys. 1992;24(1):49–53.

65. Kingma A, et al. Academic career after treatment for acute lymphoblastic leukaemia. Arch Dis Child. 2000;82(5):353–7.

66. Meadows AT, et al. Declines in IQ scores and cognitive dysfunctions in children with acute lymphocytic leukaemia treated with cranial irradiation. Lancet. 1981;2(8254):1015–8.

67. Kadan-Lottick NS, et al. Comparison of neurocognitive functioning in children previously randomly assigned to intrathecal methotrexate compared with triple intrathecal therapy for the treatment of childhood acute lymphoblastic leukemia. J Clin Oncol. 2009;27(35):5986–92.

68. Mahone EM, et al. Motor and perceptual timing deficits among survivors of childhood leukemia. J Pediatr Psychol. 2007;32 (8):918–25.

69. Espy KA, et al. Chemotherapeutic CNS prophylaxis and neuropsychologic change in children with acute lymphoblastic leukemia: a prospective study. J Pediatr Psychol. 2001;26(1):1–9.

70. Hill DE, et al. Visual and verbal short-term memory deficits in childhood leukemia survivors after intrathecal chemotherapy. J Pediatr Psychol. 1997;22(6):861–70.

71. Copeland DR, et al. Neuropsychologic effects of chemotherapy on children with cancer: a longitudinal study. J Clin Oncol. 1996;14(10):2826–35.

72. Kingma A, et al. No major cognitive impairment in young children with acute lymphoblastic leukemia using chemotherapy only: a prospective longitudinal study. J Pediatr Hematol Oncol. 2002;24(2):106–14.

73. Reddick WE, et al. Smaller white-matter volumes are associated with larger deficits in attention and learning among long-term survivors of acute lymphoblastic leukemia. Cancer. 2006;106 (4):941–9.

74. Carey ME, et al. Reduced frontal white matter volume in long-term childhood leukemia survivors: a voxel-based morphometry study. AJNR Am J Neuroradiol. 2008;29(4):792–7.

75. Lesnik PG, et al. Evidence for cerebellar-frontal subsystem changes in children treated with intrathecal chemotherapy for leukemia: enhanced data analysis using an effect size model. Arch Neurol. 1998;55(12):1561–8.

76. Krull KR, et al. Neurocognitive function and CNS integrity in adult survivors of childhood hodgkin lymphoma. J Clin Oncol. 2012;30(29):3618–24.

77. Edelmann MN, et al. Neurocognitive and patient-reported outcomes in adult survivors of childhood osteosarcoma. JAMA Oncol. 2016;2(2):201–8.

78. Ahles TA, Root JC, Ryan EL. Cancer- and cancer treatment-associated cognitive change: an update on the state of the science. J Clin Oncol. 2012;30(30):3675–86.

79. Boykoff N, Moieni M, Subramanian SK. Confronting chemobrain: an in-depth look at survivors' reports of impact on work, social networks, and health care response. J Cancer Surviv Res Pract. 2009;3(4):223–32.

80. Ahles TA, et al. Neuropsychologic impact of standard-dose systemic chemotherapy in long-term survivors of breast cancer and lymphoma. J Clin Oncol. 2002;20(2):485–93.

81. Schagen SB, et al. Neurophysiological evaluation of late effects of adjuvant high-dose chemotherapy on cognitive function. J Neurooncol. 2001;51(2):159–65.

82. Janelsins MC, et al. An update on cancer- and chemotherapy-related cognitive dysfunction: current status. Semin Oncol. 2011;38(3):431–8.

83. Ahles TA, Fau-Saykin AJ, et al. Longitudinal assessment of cognitive changes associated with adjuvant treatment for breast cancer: impact of age and cognitive reserve. J Clin Oncol. 2010;28(29):4434–40.

84. Kesler SR, Kent JS, O'Hara R. Prefrontal cortex and executive function impairments in primary breast cancer. Arch Neurol. 2011;68(11):1447–53.

85. Dietrich J, et al. CNS progenitor cells and oligodendrocytes are targets of chemotherapeutic agents in vitro and in vivo. J Biol. 2006;5(7):22.

86. Han R, et al. Systemic 5-fluorouracil treatment causes a syndrome of delayed myelin destruction in the central nervous system. J Biol. 2008;7(4):12.

87. Hyrien O, Dietrich J, Noble M. Mathematical and experimental approaches to identify and predict the effects of chemotherapy on neuroglial precursors. Can Res. 2010;70(24):10051–9.

88. Konat GW, et al. Cognitive dysfunction induced by chronic administration of common cancer chemotherapeutics in rats. Metab Brain Dis. 2008;23(3):325–33.

89. Ahles TA, Saykin AJ. Candidate mechanisms for chemotherapy-induced cognitive changes. Nat Rev Cancer. 2007;7(3):192–201.

90. McDonald BC, et al. Gray matter reduction associated with systemic chemotherapy for breast cancer: a prospective MRI study. Breast Cancer Res Treat. 2010;123(3):819–28.

91. Deprez S, et al. Longitudinal assessment of chemotherapy-induced structural changes in cerebral white matter and its correlation with impaired cognitive functioning. J Clin Oncol. 2012;30(3):274–81.

92. Haddy N, et al. Relationship between the brain radiation dose for the treatment of childhood cancer and the risk of long-term cerebrovascular mortality. Brain. 2011;134(Pt 5):1362–72.

93. Bowers DC, et al. Stroke as a late treatment effect of Hodgkin's disease: a report from the Childhood Cancer Survivor Study. J Clin Oncol. 2005;23(27):6508–15.

94. Harrington CB, et al. It's not over when it's over: long-term symptoms in cancer survivors—a systematic review. Int J Psychiatry Med. 2010;40(2):163–81.

95. van den Beuken-van Everdingen MH, et al. Prevalence of pain in patients with cancer: a systematic review of the past 40 years. Ann Oncol. 2007;18(9):1437–49.

96. Mueller S, et al. Radiation, atherosclerotic risk factors, and stroke risk in survivors of pediatric cancer: a report from the childhood cancer survivor study. Int J Radiat Oncol Biol Phys. 2013;86 (4):649–55.

97. Amir Z, Neary D, Luker K. Cancer survivors' views of work 3 years post diagnosis: a UK perspective. Eur J Oncol Nurs. 2008;12(3):190–7.

98. Bowers DC, et al. Late-occurring stroke among long-term survivors of childhood leukemia and brain tumors: a report from the childhood cancer survivor study. J Clin Oncol. 2006;24 (33):5277–82.

99. Mueller S, et al. Risk of first and recurrent stroke in childhood cancer survivors treated with cranial and cervical radiation therapy. Int J Radiat Oncol Biol Phys. 2013;86(4):643–8.

100. Fullerton HJ, et al. Recurrent stroke in childhood cancer survivors. Neurology. 2015;85(12):1056–64.

101. Ullrich NJ, et al. Moyamoya following cranial irradiation for primary brain tumors in children. Neurology. 2007;68(12):932–8.

102. Plummer C, et al. Ischemic stroke and transient ischemic attack after head and neck radiotherapy: a review. Stroke. 2011;42 (9):2410–8.

103. Dorresteijn LD, et al. Increased carotid wall thickening after radiotherapy on the neck. Eur J Cancer. 2005;41(7):1026–30.

104. Meeske KA, et al. Premature carotid artery disease in pediatric cancer survivors treated with neck irradiation. Pediatr Blood Cancer. 2009;53(4):615–21.

105. Cavaletti G, Marmiroli P. Chemotherapy-induced peripheral neurotoxicity. Nat Rev Neurol. 2010;6(12):657–66.

106. Ullrich NJ, et al. Incidence, risk factors, and longitudinal outcome of seizures in long-term survivors of pediatric brain tumors. Epilepsia. 2015;56(10):1599–604.

107. Sato I, et al. Impact of late effects on health-related quality of life in survivors of pediatric brain tumors: motility disturbance of limb(s), seizure, ocular/visual impairment, endocrine abnormality, and higher brain dysfunction. Cancer Nurs. 2014;37(6):E1–14.

108. Mols F, et al. Chemotherapy-induced neuropathy and its association with quality of life among 2- to 11-year colorectal cancer survivors: results from the population-based PROFILES registry. J Clin Oncol. 2013;31(21):2699–707.

109. Beijers A, et al. Chemotherapy-induced peripheral neuropathy and impact on quality of life 6 months after treatment with chemotherapy. J Community Support Oncol. 2014;12(11):401–6.

110. Cavaletti G, Alberti P, Marmiroli P. Chemotherapy-induced peripheral neurotoxicity in cancer survivors: an underdiagnosed clinical entity? Am Soc Clin Oncol Educ Book. 2015;35:e553–60.

111. Kvale E, Urba SG. NCCN guidelines for survivorship expanded to address two common conditions. J Natl Compr Canc Netw. 2014;12(5 Suppl):825–7.

112. Park SB, et al. Long-term neuropathy after oxaliplatin treatment: challenging the dictum of reversibility. Oncologist. 2011;16 (5):708–16.

113. Mols F, et al. Chemotherapy-induced peripheral neuropathy and its association with quality of life: a systematic review. Support Care Cancer. 2014;22(8):2261–9.

114. Beijers AJ, et al. Peripheral neuropathy in colorectal cancer survivors: the influence of oxaliplatin administration. Results from the population-based PROFILES registry. Acta Oncol. 2015;54(4):463–9.

115. Tofthagen C, et al. Oxaliplatin-induced peripheral neuropathy's effects on health-related quality of life of colorectal cancer survivors. Support Care Cancer. 2013;21(12):3307–13.

116. Tofthagen C, Visovsky C, Berry DL. Strength and balance training for adults with peripheral neuropathy and high risk of fall: current evidence and implications for future research. Oncol Nurs Forum. 2012;39(5):E416–24.

117. Gewandter JS, et al. Falls and functional impairments in cancer survivors with chemotherapy-induced peripheral neuropathy (CIPN): a University of Rochester CCOP study. Support Care Cancer. 2013;21(7):2059–66.

118. Armes J, et al. Patients' supportive care needs beyond the end of cancer treatment: a prospective, longitudinal survey. J Clin Oncol. 2009;27(36):6172–9.

119. Ness KK, et al. Chemotherapy-related neuropathic symptoms and functional impairment in adult survivors of extracranial solid tumors of childhood: results from the St. Jude lifetime cohort study. Arch Phys Med Rehabil. 2013;94(8):1451–7.

120. Glendenning JL, et al. Long-term neurologic and peripheral vascular toxicity after chemotherapy treatment of testicular cancer. Cancer. 2010;116(10):2322–31.

121. Strumberg D, et al. Evaluation of long-term toxicity in patients after cisplatin-based chemotherapy for non-seminomatous testicular cancer. Ann Oncol. 2002;13(2):229–36.

122. Ramchandren S, et al. Peripheral neuropathy in survivors of childhood acute lymphoblastic leukemia. J Peripher Nerv Syst. 2009;14(3):184–9.

123. Pradat PF, Delanian S. Late radiation injury to peripheral nerves. Handb Clin Neurol. 2013;115:743–58.

124. Gillette EL, et al. Late radiation injury to muscle and peripheral nerves. Int J Radiat Oncol Biol Phys. 1995;31(5):1309–18.

125. Delanian S, Lefaix JL, Pradat PF. Radiation-induced neuropathy in cancer survivors. Radiother Oncol. 2012;105(3):273–82.

126. Brown MR, Ramirez JD, Farquhar-Smith P. Pain in cancer survivors. Br J Pain. 2014;8(4):139–53.

127. Chen AM, et al. Brachial plexus-associated neuropathy after high-dose radiation therapy for head-and-neck cancer. Int J Radiat Oncol Biol Phys. 2012;84(1):165–9.

128. Kori SH, Foley KM, Posner JB. Brachial plexus lesions in patients with cancer: 100 cases. Neurology. 1981;31(1):45–50.

129. Fathers E, et al. Radiation-induced brachial plexopathy in women treated for carcinoma of the breast. Clin Rehabil. 2002;16 (2):160–5.

130. Johansson S. Radiation induced brachial plexopathies. Acta Oncol. 2006;45(3):253–7.

Index

Printed by Printforce, the Netherlands